Drug-Induced Ocular Side Effects

Drug-Induced Ocular Side Effects

EIGHTH EDITION

FREDERICK "FRITZ" T. FRAUNFELDER, MD
Professor
Department of Ophthalmology
Oregon Health and Science University
Casey Eye Institute
Portland, OR, USA

FREDERICK "RICK" W. FRAUNFELDER, MD, MBA
Associate Dean of Faculty Affairs
Chair of Department of Ophthalmology
Roy E. Mason and Elizabeth Patee Mason Distinguished Professor of Ophthalmology
University of Missouri – Columbia School of Medicine
Mason Eye Institute
Columbia, MO, USA

Associate Editor:

BREE JENSVOLD-VETSCH, BS
National Registry of Drug-Induced Ocular Side Effects
Department of Ophthalmology
Oregon Health and Science University
Casey Eye Institute
Portland, OR, USA

For additional online content visit ExpertConsult.com

ELSEVIER

London   New York   Oxford   Philadelphia   St Louis   Sydney   2021

First edition 1976
Second edition 1982
Third edition 1989
Fourth edition 1996
Fifth edition 2000
Sixth edition 2008
Seventh edition 2015
Eighth edition 2020

Notices

Practitioners and researchers must always rely on their own experience and knowledge in evaluating and
using any information, methods, compounds or experiments described herein. Because of rapid advances
in the medical sciences, in particular, independent verification of diagnoses and drug dosages should be
made. To the fullest extent of the law, no responsibility is assumed by Elsevier, authors, editors or contribu-
tors for any injury and/or damage to persons or property as a matter of products liability, negligence or
otherwise, or from any use or operation of any methods, products, instructions, or ideas contained in the
material herein.

ISBN: 978-0-323-65375-6
e-Book ISBN: 978-0-323-67401-0
INK ISBN: 978-0-323-67402-7

Content Strategist: Kayla Wolfe
Content Development Specialist: Nani Clansey
Project Manager: Joanna Souch
Design: Patrick Ferguson
Illustration Manager: Theresa McBryan
Marketing Manager: Claire McKenzie

Printed in the the United States of America

Last digit is the print number: 9   8   7   6   5   4   3   2

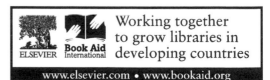

Working together
to grow libraries in
developing countries

www.elsevier.com • www.bookaid.org

Table of Contents

Preface

This is the eighth edition of *Drug-Induced Ocular Side Effects*. This book is intended as a *guide* to help the busy clinician decide whether a visual problem is related to a medication. The clinician's past experience, the known natural course of the disease, the adverse effects of similarly structured compounds, and previous reports all help physicians make their decisions. Unfortunately, there have been only limited attempts to apply rigorous science to the clinical ocular toxicology of marketed products. There are many variables, and there is a paucity of research dollars available to assess cause-and-effect relationships between drugs and visual adverse events. The clinician needs to keep in mind the marked variability of how each human metabolizes or reacts to the drug or its metabolites. A change in the expected course of a disease after starting a drug should heighten the physician's suspicion of a drug-related event. Peer-review journals have difficulty in accepting papers on potential visual side effects of drugs because causation, once the drug is marketed, is usually difficult to prove by scientific parameters. Clinical ocular toxicology primarily relies on case reports, case series, and spontaneous reporting systems. Although we have attempted to classify a suspected adverse event with our impression as to causality (i.e. *certain, probable, possible, unlikely, conditional/ unclassified*), one needs to remember that this is based on less powerful scientific evidence. We continue to review spontaneous reports from the US Food and Drug Administration (Bethesda, Maryland), World Health Organization (Uppsala, Sweden), and the National Registry of Drug-Induced Ocular Side Effects (Casey Eye Institute, Oregon Health & Science University, Portland, Oregon). The classification system categories are meant to be "signals," and any intended causality may be unsubstantiated. Our rationale is there may be a pattern in a subset of the user population that we feel the clinician should consider in possible patient adverse drug reactions. This is only a guide for the busy clinician and will always be a work in progress. We welcome your input.

F.T. Fraunfelder, MD
F.W. Fraunfelder, MD, MBA

List of Contributors

Wiley A. Chambers, MD
Clinical Professor of Ophthalmology
Adjunct Assistant Professor of Computer Medicine
George Washington University School of Medicine
Washington, DC, USA

Michael F. Marmor, MD
Professor of Ophthalmology, Emeritus
Byers Eye Institute at Stanford
Stanford University School of Medicine
Palo Alto, CA, USA

Instructions to Users

The basic format used in each section of ocular side effects is:

Class: The general category of the primary action of the drug, chemical, or herb is given.

Generic Name: The recommended International Nonproprietary Name (rINN) for each drug is listed, which is designated by the World Health Organization. In parentheses is the United States National Formulary name or other commonly accepted names.

Proprietary Name: The United States trade names are given, but this is not an all-inclusive listing. In a group of drugs, the number before a generic name for both the systemic and ophthalmic forms corresponds to the number preceding the proprietary drug. International trade names and multi-ingredient preparations are not listed unless indicated.

Primary Use: The class of medicine and its current use in the management of various conditions are listed.

OCULAR SIDE EFFECTS:

Systemic Administration: Ocular side effects are reported from articular, auricular, cutaneous, epidural, implant, infiltration, intradermal, inhalation, intra-arterial, intracarotid, intramuscular, intrapleural, intraspinal, intrathecal, intratympanic, intrauterine, intravenous, nasal, oral, percutaneous, perineural, rectal, subcutaneous, sublingual, topical, transdermal, urethral, or vaginal administration or environmental exposure.

Local Ophthalmic Use or Exposure: Ocular side effects are reported from topical ocular application or eyelid, intracameral, intralesional, intraocular, intravitreal, parabulbar, periocular, retrobulbar, subconjunctival, or subtenon injection.

Inadvertent Ocular Exposure: Ocular side effects are reported due to accidental ocular exposure.

Inadvertent Systemic Exposure: Ocular side effects are reported due to accidental systemic exposure from topical ophthalmic medications.

The ocular side effects are listed as *certain, probable, possible, unlikely,* and *conditional/unclassified.* This classification is based, in part, on the system established by the World Health Organization. There are debatable scientific bases for our opinions. They are only intended

as guides for the clinician and are the results of "educated" conjectures from the authors, F. T. Fraunfelder and F. W. Fraunfelder. The name of the preparation in the parentheses adjacent to an adverse reaction indicates that this is the only drug in the group reported to have caused this side effect.

SYSTEMIC SIDE EFFECTS:

Systemic Administration: Systemic side effects are reported from ophthalmic medications administered by an intramuscular, intravenous, or oral route.

Local Ophthalmic Use or Exposure: Systemic side effects are reported from topical ocular application or intracameral, intraocular, periocular, retrobulbar, or subconjunctival injection.

The listing as to certainty of causality is the same as that used by systemic medications.

WHO CLASSIFICATION SYSTEM

Where data are available (i.e. published or submitted for publication), we have classified medication adverse reactions, in part, according to the following World Health Organization Causality Assessment of Suspected Adverse Reactions Guide.

Certain: A clinical event, including laboratory test abnormality, occurring in a plausible time relationship to drug administration and that cannot be explained by concurrent disease or other drugs or chemicals. The response to withdrawal of the drug (dechallenge) should be clinically plausible. The event must be definitive pharmacologically or phenomenologically, using a satisfactory rechallenge procedure if necessary.

Probable/Likely: A clinical event, including laboratory test abnormality, with a reasonable time sequence to administration of the drug, unlikely to be attributed to concurrent disease or other drugs or chemicals, and that follows a clinically reasonable response on withdrawal (dechallenge). Rechallenge information is not required to fulfill this definition.

Possible: A clinical event, including laboratory test abnormality, with a reasonable time sequence to administration of the drug, but that could also be explained by concurrent disease or other drugs or chemicals. Information on drug withdrawal may be lacking or unclear.

Unlikely: A clinical event, including laboratory test abnormality, with a temporal relationship to drug administration that makes a causal relationship improbable and in which other drugs, chemicals, or underlying disease provide plausible explanations.

Conditional/Unclassified: A clinical event, including laboratory test abnormality, reported as an adverse reaction about which more data are essential for a proper assessment, or the additional data are under examination.

Clinical Significance: A concise overview of the general importance of the ocular side effects produced is given. Not all side effects listed are reported for each drug and are only a guide for ocular side effects for the class of drugs.

References: References have been limited to the most informative articles, the most current, or those with the most complete bibliography.

Further Reading: Other publications that are useful.

Recommendations: For specific medications, we make recommendations on following patients for probable related effects on the visual system. This was often done in consultation with other coworkers interested in the specific drug; however, this is only intended as a possible guide.

Index of Side Effects: The lists of adverse ocular side effects due to preparations are intended in part to be indexes in themselves. The adverse ocular reactions are not separated in this index as to route of administration.

CHAPTER 1

National Registry of Drug-Induced Ocular Side Effects

FREDERICK W. FRAUNFELDER, MD • FREDERICK T. FRAUNFELDER, MD

RATIONALE

In a specialized area such as ophthalmology, it is not common for a practitioner to see the patient volume necessary to make a correlation between possible cause and effect of medication-related ocular disease. Post-marketing observational studies from multiple sources permit the evaluation of drug safety in a real-world setting where off-label use and various practice patterns occur. There is no question that this has limited ability to determine causation, but it can detect signals that alert the clinician as to adverse drug events. In subspecialty areas of medicine with comparatively limited markets, sometimes this is all that we have. A national registry specifically interested in a specialized area of medicine has filled a need, as shown by the more than three decades of the National Registry of Drug-Induced Ocular Side Effects (NRDIOSE).

The NRDIOSE, which is based at the Casey Eye Institute in Portland, Oregon, USA (www.eyedrugregistry.com), is a clearinghouse of spontaneous reports collected mostly from ophthalmologists from around the world. It is the only database that collects only eye-related adverse drug reactions (ADRs). The MedWatch program run by the US Food and Drug Administration (FDA) (https://www.fda.gov/safety/medwatch-fda-safety-information-and-adverse-event-reporting-program) collects ADRs on all organ systems in the United States and is another source for reporting data and requesting data. The Uppsala Monitoring Center, a branch of the World Health Organization (WHO) in Uppsala, Sweden (www.who-umc.org), collects spontaneous reports on all organ systems from around the world and has more than 70 national centers that report to them, including the FDA. Finally, clinicians and patients frequently report an ADR directly to the drug company, who in turn periodically submits these spontaneous reports to the FDA.

Regardless of where an ADR is submitted, the various organizations mentioned here can be contacted with questions about an ADR or how many types of reports exist for specific drug–ADR combinations. The NRDIOSE provides this information free of charge to ophthalmologists, and the FDA is required to provide this information to the public through the Freedom of Information Act. The WHO may charge a fee, depending on the type of information requested. The information from pharmaceutical companies should eventually end up in the FDAs MedWatch database.

Spontaneous reporting databases have adopted statistical analyses methods of interpreting ADRs. At the Uppsala Monitoring Center, for instance, a quantitative method for data mining the WHO database is part of the signal detection strategy. Their method is called the Bayesian Confidence Propagation Neural Network (BCPNN). An Information Component (IC) number is calculated based on a statistical dependency between a drug and an ADR calculated on the frequency of reporting. The IC value does not give evidence of causality between a drug and an ADR; it is only an indication or signal that it may be necessary to study the individual case reports in the WHO database. The IC value calculation is a tool that can guide the WHO to create a hypothesis of association between drugs and ADRs among the over 3 million case reports in the WHO database.

This method of analysis is also being adopted within the pharmaceutical industry and at the FDA. The NRDIOSE is also able to use the IC values because its staff are consultants to the WHO. If a clinician suspects an ADR, especially if it may be a new drug-induced ocular side effect, he or she is encouraged to report this to the NRDIOSE. Access to the website is free.

OBJECTIVES OF THE NATIONAL REGISTRY OF DRUG-INDUCED OCULAR SIDE EFFECTS
The Registry

- To establish a national center where possible drug-, chemical-, or herbal-induced ocular side effects can be accumulated.

- To review possible drug-induced ocular side-effects data collected through the FDA, WHO Monitoring Center, and our registry.
- To compile data in the world literature on reports of possible drug-, chemical-, or herbal-induced ocular side effects.
- To make available these data to physicians who feel they have a possible drug-induced ocular side effect.

HOW TO REPORT A SUSPECTED REACTION

The cases of primary interest are those adverse ocular reactions not previously recognized or those that are rare, severe, serious, or unusual. To be of value, data should be complete and follow the basic format shown here:

Age:

Gender:

Suspected drug:

Suspected reaction date of onset:

Route, dose, and when drug started:

Improvement after suspected drug stopped. If restarted, did adverse reaction recur?:

Other drug(s) taken at time of suspected adverse reaction:

Other disease(s) or diagnosis(es) present:

Comments   optional (your opinion if drug induced, probably related, possibly related, or unrelated):

Your name and address (optional):

Send to:

Frederick T. Fraunfelder, Co-Director

National Registry of Drug-Induced Ocular Side Effects, Casey Eye Institute, Oregon Health Sciences University, 515 SW Campus Drive, Portland, Oregon 97239-4197

http://www.eyedrugregistry.com

E-mail: eyedrug@ohsu.edu

FURTHER READING

Bate A, Lindquist M, Edwards IR, et al. A Bayesian neural network method for adverse drug reaction signal generation. *Eur J Clin Pharmacol.* 1998;54:315–321.

Bate A, Lindquist M, Edwards IR, et al. A data mining approach for signal detection and analysis. *Drug Saf.* 2002;25:393–397.

Bate A, Lindquist M, Orre R, et al. Data mining analyses of pharmacovigilance signals in relation to relevant comparison drugs. *Eur J Clin Pharmacol.* 2002;58:483–490.

Bate A, Orre R, Lindquist M, et al. Explanation of data mining methods. *BMJ.* http://www.bmj.com/cgi/content/full/322/7296/1207/DC1.html.

Coulter DM, Bate A, Meyboom RH, et al. Antipsychotic drugs and heart muscle disorder in international pharmacovigilance: a data mining study. *BMJ.* 2001;322:1207–1209.

Lindquist M, Stahl M, Bate A, et al. A retrospective evaluation of a data mining approach to aid finding new adverse drug reaction signals in the WHO international database. *Drug Saf.* 2000;23:533–542.

Orre R, Lansener A, Bate A, et al. Bayesian neural networks with confidence estimations applied to data mining. *Comput Stat Data Anal.* 2000;34:473–493.

Spigset O, Hagg S, Bate A. Hepatic injury and pancreatitis during treatment with serotonin reuptake inhibitors: data from the World Health Organization (WHO) database of adverse drug reactions. *Int Clin Psychopharmacol.* 2003;18:157–161.

Van Puijenbroek EM, Bate A, Leufkens HG, et al. A comparison of measures of disproportionality for signal detection in spontaneous reporting systems for adverse drug reaction. *Pharmacoepidemiol Drug Saf.* 2002;11:3–10.

CHAPTER 2

Ocular Drug Delivery and Toxicology

FREDERICK T. FRAUNFELDER, MD

Drug delivery to the eye is a complex process. The eye is unique in the body in many ways that affect its pharmacology and toxicology. It includes several different cell types and functions basically as a self-contained system. The rate and efficacy of drug delivery differ in healthy and diseased eyes. Variables affecting delivery include age, genetic ancestry, and route of administration. The complexities of delivery, toxicology, or both are greatly influenced by patient compliance, especially in the management of glaucoma, which requires multiple topical ocular medications to be given at one sitting each day, often multiple times daily. Each time and method of drug delivery modify the therapeutic and toxicologic response.

Ocular toxicology is dependent on the concentration of the drug, frequency of application, speed of removal, and whether the drug reaches sensitive cells such as the corneal endothelium, lens epithelium, or macula in toxic concentrations. Of equal importance is the vehicle for delivery and the pH, buffering systems, and preservatives necessary for optimum drug delivery. Each adds its own potentially toxic effect to this complex picture. Originally, much of ocular pharmacology and toxicology was conducted by trial and error, often with local corner pharmacies compounding medications. Today, the ocular pharmaceutical industry is acutely aware of potential problems and is continuously researching and producing medications, usually with fewer side effects and delivered by better medications.

TOPICAL OCULAR ADMINISTRATION

This is by far the most commonly used method of drug delivery to the eye. Topically administered medications are convenient, easy to reapply, and relatively inexpensive. This method concentrates the pharmacologic activity of the drug on/in the eye while limiting systemic reactions. Local toxic responses are increased, however, especially with lifelong use, as with glaucoma medications. Unlike medication given orally, topical ocular medications reach systemic circulation while avoiding the first-order pass effect through the liver. A drug absorbed through the nasal mucosa or conjunctiva "drains" to the right atrium and ventricle. The blood containing the drug is then pumped to the head before returning to the left atrium and ventricle. The second passage is through the liver, where the primary detoxification occurs before going to the right atrium. When medications are orally administered, the first pass includes absorption from the gut through the liver, where, depending on the drug, up to 90% of the agent is detoxified before going to the right atrium. Thus oral medications are metabolized during the first pass, whereas ocularly or nasally administered drugs are not metabolized until the second pass. This is the reason why therapeutic blood levels, and accompanying systemic side effects, may occur from topical ocular medications. Other factors include racial differences in metabolism, as with timolol. One percent of people with Japanese or Chinese genetic ancestry, 2.4% of African Americans, and 8% of those with European ancestry do not have the p450 enzyme CYP2D6 that is necessary to metabolize this drug. The lack of this enzyme significantly enhances systemic blood levels of timolol.[1]

BASIC PHARMACOLOGY AND TOXICOLOGY OF TOPICAL MEDICATIONS

Ocular toxicology is based on pharmacokinetics – how the drug is absorbed, including its distribution, metabolism, and elimination – as well as pharmacodynamics, the action of the drug on the body. This bioavailability is influenced by age, body weight, sex, and eye pigmentation. It is also affected by the disease process, interactions with other drugs, and mode of delivery. Only a small percentage of any topically applied drug enters the eye. At best, 1–10% of topical ocular solutions are absorbed by ocular tissues.[2] This absorption is governed by ocular contact time, drug concentration, tissue permeability, and characteristics of the cornea and pericorneal tissue. Nearly all solutions will leave the conjunctival sac, or cul-de-sac, within 15–30 seconds of application.[3] The average volume of the cul-de-sac is 7 μL, with 1 additional μL in the precorneal tear film.[4] The cul-de-sac may hold 25–30 μL of an eye drop; however, blinking will decrease this volume markedly and rapidly, so that, at most, only 10 μL remain for longer than a few seconds. The drop size of commercial drugs varies from 25 μL to more than 56 μL.[4] In a healthy eye, one not affected by disease, lid manipulation to instill the drug will double or triple the normal basal tear flow exchange rate of 16% per minute, thereby decreasing ocular contact time via dilution.[4]

The cornea is the primary site of intraocular drug absorption from topical drug application. This is a complex process that favors small, moderately lipophilic drugs that are partially nonionized under physiologic conditions. Although the cornea is a five-layer structure, it has significant barriers to absorption into the eye. It can be visualized as three layers, like a sandwich, with a hydrophilic stroma flanked by lipophilic epithelium and endothelial layers.[4]

Topically administered drugs are also absorbed via the conjunctiva, sclera, and lacrimal system. The total surface area of the conjunctiva is 17 times the corneal surface area.[4] The conjunctiva allows absorption of lipophilic agents to a lesser degree than the cornea, but it is relatively permeable to hydrophilic drugs. The sclera is porous via nerve and blood vessel tracts, but otherwise fairly resistant to penetration. Hydrophilic agents may pass through it 80 times faster than through the cornea; however, the lacrimal system can remove the drug 100 times faster than the cornea and conjunctiva can absorb it.[4,5]

Clearly, overflow from every administration of eye drops occurs not only over the eyelid but also in the lacrimal outflow system. Lynch et al showed that 2.5% phenylephrine topically applied to the eyes of newborn babies in 8-μL or 30-μL aliquots produced no difference in pupillary response.[6] However, neonates who received the 30-μL dosage had double the plasma concentrations of phenylephrine of those who received 8 μL, increasing the potential for systemic complications.

INTRAOCULAR DISTRIBUTION

Once a drug reaches the inside of the eye, anatomic barriers play a major role in where it ends up. Drugs that enter primarily through the cornea seldom penetrate behind the lens. The pattern of aqueous humor flow and the physical barriers of the iris and ciliary body help keep the drug anterior. It is not uncommon for a drug to be more concentrated in the ciliary body than in the aqueous humor due to scleral absorption directly into the ciliary body, with less fluid exchange than in the aqueous humor. In addition, pigmented tissue reacts differently to different drugs. For example, lipid-soluble mydriatics that are more slowly absorbed by pigmented cells will dilate dark pupils more slowly, resulting in longer duration but a decrease in maximum dilation.[7]

Drug distribution is markedly affected by eye inflammation. Tissue permeability is increased, allowing greater drug availability. However, as Mikkelson et al have demonstrated, protein binding may decrease drug availability 75–100% in inflamed eyes.[8] The protein–drug complex decreases bioavailability. Increases in aqueous or tear protein, such as mucus, are also factors in bioavailability, as is the increased tearing that may wash away a drug before it can be absorbed.[8]

PRESERVATIVES

Preservatives are important parts of topical ocular medications, not only to prolong shelf life but also to disrupt the corneal and conjunctival epithelium to allow greater drug penetration.

Preservatives such as benzalkonium have been shown to have antibacterial properties almost as great as those of topical ocular antibiotics. Even in exceedingly low concentrations, benzalkonium causes significant cell damage by emulsification of the cell-wall lipids. De Saint Jean et al report cell-growth arrest and death at concentrations as low as 0.0001%.[9] Short-term use seldom causes clinically significant damage to healthy corneas and conjunctiva other than superficial epithelial changes. However, with long-term use, e.g. in patients with glaucoma and dry eye, preservatives in topical eye medication may cause adverse effects. Hong et al have shown induction of squamous metaplasia by chronic application of glaucoma medications containing preservatives.[10] This may progress to more severe side effects, as shown in Table 2.1.

VEHICLES FOR TOPICAL OCULAR MEDICATION DELIVERY

Aqueous solutions: With aqueous solutions, ingredients are fully dissolved within a solution. Benefits include easy application and few visual side effects. The main drawback is a short ocular contact time, which leads to poor absorption and limited bioavailability. Nevertheless, this is still the most commonly used means of delivering topical ocular medications. Solutions may congregate in the lacrimal sac (Fig. 2.1).

TABLE 2.1
Preservative Ocular Side Effects

Eyelids and Conjunctiva	Cornea
Allergic reactions	Punctate keratitis
Hyperemia	Edema
Erythema	Pseudomembrane formation
Blepharitis	Decreased epithelial microvilli
Conjunctiva, papillary	Vascularization
Edema	Scarring
Pemphigoid lesion with	Delayed wound-healing symblepharon
Squamous metaplasia	Increased transcorneal permeability
Contact allergies	Decreased stability of tear film Squamous metaplasia

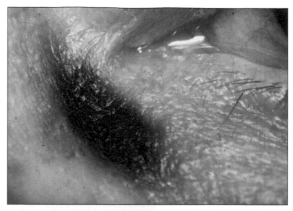

FIG. 2.1 Chronic use of silver nitrate solutions causes staining of the lacrimal sac and surrounding tissue[18].

Suspensions: With this vehicle, the active ingredient is in a fine particulate form suspended in a saturated solution of the same medication. This method allows for longer contact time with greater bioavailability. Its drawbacks include the necessity of vigorously shaking the container before application and a possible increase in foreign-body sensation after application because of the deposition of particles in the corneal tear film.

Ointments: These consist of semisolid lipoid preparations containing lipid-soluble drugs. They are designed to melt at body temperature and are dispersed by the shearing action of blinking. Ointments are frequently entrapped in lashes, fornices, and canthal areas, which are capable of acting as reservoirs. They can also become entrapped in corneal defects (Fig. 2.2); e.g. ointment at the base of the lashes comes in contact with the skin. Because ointment will melt when it comes in contact with the skin, the ointment at the base of the lashes reaches the eye in a continuous process of becoming entrapped in the lashes and remelting into the eye. Ointments have high bioavailability and require less frequent dosing than other methods but suffer by being difficult to administer. Other problems include variable dosing (it is difficult to control the amount applied) and possible unacceptability to patients due to blurred vision and cosmetic disfigurement.

Pledgets: Pledgets (small absorbent pads saturated with medication) may be used to deliver high concentrations of drugs directly to the ocular surface for relatively prolonged periods. This method of drug delivery to the eye is not approved by the US Food and Drug Administration. Pledgets of vasoconstrictors to limit bleeding in keratorefractive surgery have been shown to cause significant systemic reactions, including hypertension, cardiac arrest, subarachnoid hemorrhage, convulsions, and death.[11]

Injections: Subconjunctival injections allow medication to be concentrated locally, with high bioavailability and limited systemic side effects. Wine et al suggested that the mechanism of drug delivery may be in part simple leakage of the drug through the needle-puncture site with subsequent absorption through the cornea.[12] McCartney et al showed that subconjunctival injections of hydrocortisone did penetrate the overlying sclera and that the injection site should be located directly over the area of pathology.[13]

Intracameral injections are administered directly to the anterior chamber of the eye and are most frequently used to place viscoelastics. Although small amounts of antibiotics may also be administered, some of these drugs pose risks to the corneal endothelium, and cataracts, corneal opacities, anterior uveitis, and neovascularization are possible.

Intravitreal injections have become increasingly popular due to their efficacy against macular degeneration, bacterial and fungal endophthalmitis, and viral retinitis. Each drug has its own toxicity profile; however, these injections are so commonly done that the volumes, concentrations, and vehicles are well tested, and complications are within an acceptable risk–benefit ratio.

Other delivery devices: Ocuserts (small plastic membranes impregnated with medication); collagen corneal shields (biodegradable contact-lens–shaped clear

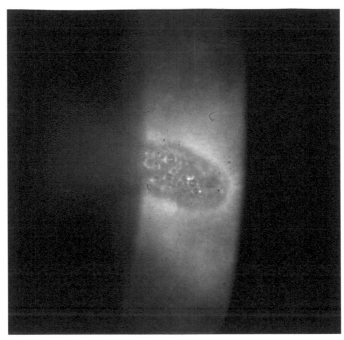

FIG. 2.2 Corneal defects may entrap ointment on the surface, creating ointment globules[18].

films made to dissolve within 12–72 hours); contact lenses; and various other delivery systems, including nanoparticles, liposomes, emulsions, and gels, have either made it to market with limited success or are still in the research pipeline.

TOXICITY RESPONSES

Anterior segment: Toxicity produces an inflammatory response without prior exposure to the host, whereas hypersensitivity responses require prior exposure. In general, allergic reactions involve repeated exposure to the antigen and sufficiently elapsed time to allow the immune system to react. Depending on the potency of the sensitizing agent or the strength of the immune system, this may vary from a few days to years.[14] The clinical diagnosis of a toxic response is usually presumptive, whereas in allergic reactions conjunctival scraping may reveal eosinophils or basophils. One of the most common signs of ocular toxicity from topical medication is hyperemia. This reaction includes burning and irritation, usually without itching, occurring after starting an offending agent, with classic symptoms of intracanthal eyelid edema and erythema (Fig. 2.3). There are no definitive confirmatory tests. In more severe cases, a papillary hyperemia with a watery mucoid type of

discharge is evident. If the cornea is involved, this may present as a superficial punctate keratitis, usually more severe inferiorly or inferior nasally. Occasionally, intraepithelial microcysts may be seen, although these are more commonly seen with chemical toxicity. If the reaction is severe enough or goes unrecognized, it may become full blown with corneal ulceration, limbal neovascularization, anterior uveitis, cataracts, and damage to the lacrimal outflow system. The diagnosis is confirmed if clearing occurs after stopping the offending drug and the eye and adnexa improve markedly.

Drugs can induce a condition such as ocular pemphigoid, a syndrome of nonprogressive toxic reactions, which are self-limiting once the drug is discontinued. This condition is clinically and histologically identical to idiopathic ocular pemphigoid and includes a conjunctival cicatricial process with scarring of the fornix and tarsal conjunctiva, corneal and conjunctival keratinization, corneal vascularization, and lacrimal outflow scarring with occlusion.

Almost any type of pathology can be seen as a result of a toxic response in the anterior segment. Systemic medications affect the anterior segment and occur via secretion of the drug into the tears with secondary changes due to the drug or its metabolites on ocular structures (Fig. 2.4). If the drug is secreted in the tears

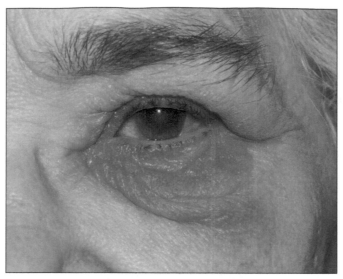

FIG. 2.3 Allergic reaction[18].

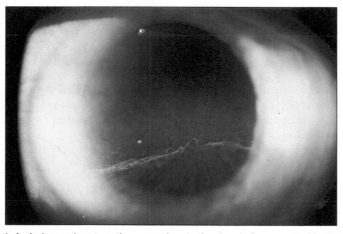

FIG. 2.4 Amiodarone keratopathy secondary to the drug being secreted in the tears[18].

and deposited in the conjunctiva or cornea, it may produce changes in color vision or visual changes. The key to recognizing a toxic response is a high degree of suspicion that the pattern of symptoms and signs is not characteristic for the clinician's differential diagnosis. A toxic effect is due to a pharmacologic effect from a drug that damages a structure or disturbs its function. An irritation is an inflammatory effect unrelated to sensitization or cellular immunity.

Ciliary body: Ciliary body ultrasound has shown bilateral choroidal effusions caused by various systemic drugs that may cause bilateral narrow-angle glaucoma.

Lens: It is difficult to identify which drugs are weak cataractogenic agents because these studies often require large numbers of patients. Findings are also difficult to confirm because instrumentation or classification systems are often cumbersome and costly. Some drugs used in the past, such as MER-29 (triparanol), caused acute lens changes, but cataractogenic drugs in current use are slow to cause lens changes, which may take many years to develop. In general, a drug-induced lens change is fairly specific for that drug. For example, both topical and systemic corticosteroid medications produce posterior subcapsular

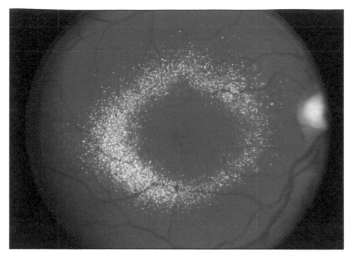

FIG. 2.5 Canthaxanthine perimacular deposition[18].

opacities. Early recognition may in some cases reverse these changes, but this is rare for almost all drug-induced cataracts.

Posterior segment: As newer classes of drugs are introduced, we are seeing more adverse retinal and optic nerve abnormalities. Whereas in the past visual acuity, color vision testing, and ophthalmoscopy were our primary tools for investigating retinal and optic nerve changes, electrophysiology testing is now being used with improved instrumentation and better standardization of methodology. Drugs can cause blood vessels to narrow, dilate, leak, swell, and hemorrhage. They can also cause pigmentary changes, photoreceptor damage, or inflammation. There can be deposition of the drug or its metabolites into the retina, as well as lipidosis. A drug can cause edema of the choroid, exudative detachment, or retinal detachment (Fig. 2.5).

Elevation of intraocular pressure: Adverse ocular effects may cause acute glaucoma by dilation of the pupil or ciliary body effusions, by vasodilatation, by affecting the mucopolysaccharides in the trabecula (secondary to uveitis), or by means of a substance that interferes with aqueous outflow. Drugs or preservatives may, on chronic exposure, deposit in the ocular outflow system causing ocular pressure elevation.

Neurologic disorders: Multiple drugs can affect the extraocular muscles, causing weakness or paralysis, which in turn leads to ptosis, nystagmus, oculogyric crisis, or lid retraction. Direct neurotoxicity to the retina or optic nerve can occur, as can secondary optic nerve edema from benign intracranial hypertension.

Miscellaneous: Eyelash, eyebrow, and orbital disturbance reactions such as poliosis, madarosis, and exophthalmos or enophthalmos can also occur.

Newer methods of delivery and new drugs have brought on side effects and toxicities not seen or recognized previously. The various metabolic pathways of patients and multiple variables such as drug, food, or disease interactions make recognition more difficult. Also, the basic incidence is often small, which makes an association difficult to prove.

HOW TO APPLY TOPICAL OCULAR MEDICATION
Applying Medication to Someone Else[15]
1. Tilt the person's head back so he or she is looking up toward the ceiling. Grasp the lower eyelid below the lashes and gently pull it away from the eye (Fig. 2.6A).
2. Apply one drop of solution or a match-head–sized amount of ointment into the pocket between the lid and the eye (Fig. 2.6B). The external eye holds only about one quarter to one half of a drop, so don't waste medicine by applying two drops.
3. As the person looks down, gently lift the lower eyelid to make contact with the upper lid (Fig. 2.6C). The person should keep their eyelid closed for 3 minutes.

Applying Your Own Medication[15]
1. Tilt your head back. Rest your hand on your cheek and grasp your lower eyelid below the lashes. Gently lift the lid away from your eye. Next, hold the

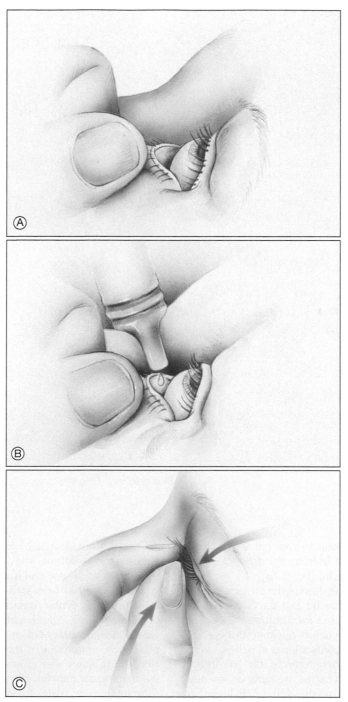

FIG. 2.6 (A–C)[15]

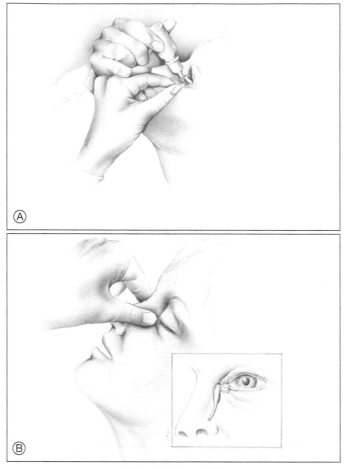

FIG. 2.7 **(A** and **B)**[15]

dropper over and as near to your eye as you feel is safe, resting the hand holding the dropper on the hand holding your eyelid (Fig. 2.7A).

2. Look up and apply one drop of the medication into the pocket between the lid and the eye. Close the eyelid and keep it closed for 3 minutes. Blot away any excess medication before opening your eye.

When applying eye medications, it is best to ask someone else to apply them for you. It is very important to wash your hands before applying eye medication. The person receiving medication should keep their eyes closed for 3 minutes after application. Blot excess fluid from the inner corner of the lids before opening the eyes. This is especially important with glaucoma medication. Wait 5–10 minutes between drug applications when applying more than one eye medication.

All medications should be kept at room temperature because cool solutions stimulate tearing. This causes the drug to be diluted and may cause epiphora.

Lid closure has been well documented as dramatically increasing ocular contact time and decreasing lacrimal drainage.[16] Zimmerman et al demonstrated that merely closing the eyelids for 3 minutes can decrease plasma concentrations of timolol by 65% when measured 60 minutes after topical application.[17] Likewise, the therapeutic benefits of nasolacrimal occlusion are substantial, particularly for drugs absorbed from nonconjunctival routes. Pressure over the lacrimal sac can allow for a decrease in both the frequency and dose of topical ocular agents (Fig. 2.7B). It may be difficult for patients to perform nasolacrimal occlusion routinely, so this technique is not used as frequently as it should be.

REFERENCES

1. Edeki T, He H, Wood AJ. Pharmacogenetic explanation for excessive beta-blockage following timolol eye drops. Potential for oral ophthalmic drug interaction. *JAMA.* 1995;274:1611–1613.

2. Schoenwald RD. The control of drug bioavailability from ophthalmic dosage forms. In: Smolen VF, Ball VA, eds. *Controlled Drug Bioavailability. Bioavailability Control by Drug Delivery System Design.* Vol 3. New York: John Wiley; 1985:257–306.

3. Shell JW. Pharmacokinetics of topically applied ophthalmic drugs. *Surv Ophthalmol.* 1982;26:207–218.

4. Mishima S, Gasset A, Klyce Jr SD, et al. Determination of tear volume and tear flow. *Invest Ophthalmol.* 1966;5:264–276.

5. Van Ootegham MM. Factors influencing the retention of ophthalmic solutions on the eye surface. In: Saettone MF, Bucci M, Speiser P, eds. *Ophthalmic Drug Delivery. Fidia Research Series.* Vol. 11. Berlin: Springer Verlag; 1987:7–18.

6. Lynch MG, Brown RH, Goode SM, et al. Reduction of phenylephrine drop size in infants achieves equal dilation with decreased systemic absorption. *Arch Ophthalmol.* 1987;105:1364–1365.

7. Harris LS, Galin MA. Effect of ocular pigmentation on hypotensive response to pilocarpine. *Am J Ophthalmol.* 1971;72:923–925.

8. Mikkelson TJ, Charai S, Robinson JR. Altered bioavailability of drugs in the system due to drug protein interaction. *J Pharmacol Sci.* 1973;62:1648–1653.

9. De Saint Jean M, Brignole F, Bringuier AF, et al. Effects of benzalkonium chloride on growth and survival of Chang conjunctival cells. *Invest Ophthalmol Vis Sci.* 1999;40:619–630.

10. Hong S, Lee CS, Seo KY, et al. Effects of topical antiglaucoma application on conjunctival impression cytology specimens. *Am J Ophthalmol.* 2006;142:185–186.

11. Fraunfelder FW, Fraunfelder FT, Jensvold B. Adverse systemic effects from pledgets of topical ocular phenylephrine 10%. *Am J Ophthalmol.* 2002;134:624–625.

12. Wine NA, Gornall AG, Basu PK. The ocular uptake of subconjunctively injected C14 hydrocortisone. Part 1. Time and major route of penetration in a normal eye. *Am J Ophthalmol.* 1964;58:362–366.

13. McCartney HJ, Drysdale IO, Gornall AG, et al. An autoradiographic study of the penetration of subconjunctively injected hydrocortisone into the normal and inflamed rabbit eye. *Invest Ophthalmol.* 1965;4:297–302.

14. Abelson MB, Torkildsen G, Shapiro A. Thinking outside the eye dropper. *Rev Ophthalmol.* 2005;12:78–80.

15. Fraunfelder FT. Ways to diminish systemic side effects. In: Vaughan D, Asbury T, eds. *General Ophthalmology.* 15th ed. Norwalk, CT: Appleton and Lange; 1999:68–73.

16. Fraunfelder FT. Extraocular fluid dynamics: how best to apply topical ocular medication. *Tran Am Ophthalmol Soc.* 1976;74:457–487.

17. Zimmerman TJ, Sharir M, Nardin GF, et al. Therapeutic index of epinephrine and dipivefrin with nasolacrimal occlusion. *Am J Ophthalmol.* 1992;114:8–13.

18. Fraunfelder FT. *Chronic use of silver nitrate solutions causes staining of the lacrimal sac and surrounding tissue; Corneal defects may entrap ointment on the surface, creating ointment globules; Allergic reaction; Amiodarone keratopathy, secondary to the drug being secreted in the tears; Canthaxanthine perimacular deposition [photographs].* Portland (OR): Casey Eye Institute, Oregon Health & Science University; ©1990. 5 photographs: color.

CHAPTER 3

Methods for Evaluating Drug-Induced Visual Side Effects

WILEY A. CHAMBERS, MD

This chapter reflects the views of the author and should not be construed to represent the US Food and Drug Administration's (FDA's) views or policies.

RISK

All drug products have some risk. If there is pharmacologic activity due to the drug product, there is also a risk of adverse events from the pharmacologic activity. Risk is generally best assessed in controlled clinical studies. Unfortunately, in the case of low-incident events, this is not always possible. A risk may not be identified until after the drug product has been commercially marketed. At that time, it is often difficult to determine the number of people who have been exposed to the drug product. If the number of people exposed cannot be accurately determined, the exact frequency or likelihood of a side effect cannot be accurately determined.

The assessment of risk generally improves as more individuals receive the drug product. Although it would be extremely helpful to know the full risk profile of every drug product before release into commercial marketing, usually the full risk profile is not completely known until after the drug product has been marketed, and sometimes not until years later.

SELECTING DIAGNOSTIC TESTS

A wide variety of diagnostic testing modalities may be used to detect and evaluate a suspected ocular toxicity. Although it is theoretically possible to perform each of these tests on any individual who is suspected to have an abnormality, the time, expense, resources, and ability of the patient to cooperate must be taken into consideration. In broad terms, these tests may be divided into two main categories. The first covers methods capable of detecting objective anatomic changes, and the second covers methods capable of detecting functional changes. The former category of tests is not necessarily better than the latter; they simply measure different things.

The number of tests needed to characterize an abnormality (or deviation) will vary with the abnormality being evaluated and the extent to which it needs to be characterized. Screening tests may be used to superficially scan for irregularities without fully quantitating the extent of the anomaly, but there should be a justified reason for the selection of each test. Each test should be appropriate for the type of potential event in question.

As noted earlier, it may be theoretically possible to perform many tests, but consideration of the following questions can help narrow the choice:
1. What are the findings from any nonclinical toxicology studies in nonhuman animals?
2. What abnormalities are expected based on the known pharmacologic action of the drug?
3. What is the route of administration of the drug?
4. How widely is the drug distributed throughout the human body?
5. How serious is the potential abnormality?
6. How likely is the test to detect an abnormality?
7. How invasive is the test?

When possible, it is recommended that nonclinical toxicology studies be conducted before conducting human toxicology studies. Ideally, nonclinical studies should be conducted using higher multiples ($2\times$, $10\times$, $100\times$) of the doses proposed for humans (based on concentration and/or frequency of administration). The duration of dosing should be at least as long as planned in humans (up to 9 months). It is helpful to compare multiple different dose levels in these studies. The findings of the nonclinical toxicology studies should then be used to help guide the initial tests to be conducted in humans. Although the events observed in nonhuman studies may not be duplicated in human studies, there is frequently some overlap. It is therefore important to assess the potential for these events.

For example, an important characteristic that may be determined in nonclinical studies is whether or not a drug product binds to melanin. Melanin is found widely in the eye, and products that bind to it may cause ocular toxicities. If a drug product has been found to bind to melanin, it would be important to know whether the nonclinical studies demonstrated abnormalities in electroretinograms (ERGs). If a drug product is found to bind to melanin and demonstrates ERG abnormalities in animals, it would be prudent to monitor best corrected distance visual acuity, color vision, automated threshold static visual fields, ocular coherence tomography (OCT), and dilated fundus photographs of subjects in clinical studies.

Histopathology in the nonclinical studies can be important. If in nonclinical studies, a retinal lesion or retinal drug deposit is observed in animals, best corrected distance visual acuity, color vision, threshold static visual field, OCT, and fundus photographs should be monitored in clinical studies of humans. Drug products that cause retinal lesions and ERG changes in nonhuman animals often cause toxicity in humans as well.

If in nonclinical studies, lens opacity is observed in animals, then best corrected distance visual acuity and lens photography or the use of a standardized lens grading system should be included in clinical studies of humans.

The structure of the drug, nonclinical pharmacology studies, and clinical pharmacology studies may be helpful in identifying the expected pharmacologic actions of the drug. To the extent that the pharmacologic action potentiates or interferes with ocular functions, ocular tests may be planned to quantitate the enhancement or interference of the function. For example, drug products that affect the sympathomimetic system are likely to affect intraocular pressure (IOP) and pupil size. It is therefore important to perform tonometry and pupil size measurements to quantitate the expected changes. Drug products that affect the cholinergic system are likely to affect IOP, pupil size, tear production, and the corneal surface. Tests such as tonometry, pupil size measures, Schirmer tear tests, and rose bengal or lissamine green corneal staining may be useful.

The seriousness of a potential adverse event should influence the effort spent on characterizing the likelihood of the event to occur and any factors that may mitigate or enhance its occurrence. It is most helpful to be able to predict events that can cause irreversible changes and in particular events that can lead to irreversible blindness. To the extent that these events are associated with warning signs or symptoms, some of these events may be preventable.

FREQUENCY

The frequency of a potential adverse event occurring will influence the methods used to characterize the event. For the reasons discussed later, the likelihood of detecting rare events (such as those that occur in fewer than 1 per 10,000 subjects) in controlled clinical studies is rare. Other methods must be used to study the events. In cases where the frequency of events is dose dependent and increases with increasing dose, it may be possible to study in a clinical trial the potential for the event in patients by administering artificially high doses in study subjects.

The frequency of a potential event occurring in the general population, and more importantly, in the population of patients likely to take a particular drug product, may make recognizing an association with that particular drug product difficult. Ocular events, such as nonarteritic ischemic optic neuropathy (NAION), occur very rarely. NAION events occur most frequently in patients with known risk factors for them, such as crowded optic discs, coronary artery disease, diabetes, hyperlipidemia, hypertension, older age, and smoking. If patients who have any of these conditions take a drug product and then have a NAION event, it is extremely difficult to determine whether the drug product, the other risk factors, or both contributed to the event.

It should also be recognized that some serious events may occur too infrequently to be able to be adequately studied. Taken at the extreme, if an event is so rare that it is expected to occur in 1 in 7 billion patients, even if it results in total blindness, the frequency is so low that no one would expect to ever see another case.

TOPICAL ADMINISTRATION

The route of administration will affect the particular areas of the eye that are exposed to the drug product. Direct application of a drug product to the eye increases the likelihood that significant concentrations of the drug reach the eye. As a general rule, the following tests are recommended for all subjects of all drug products administered topically to the eye:

1. Best corrected distance visual acuity
2. Dilated slit lamp of anterior segment
3. Dilated indirect fundoscopy or photography
4. Pupil diameter
5. Applanation tonometry
6. Assessment of symptoms in the first minute after topical application

Additionally, a subset of patients receiving a drug product topically administered to the eye should have corneal endothelial cell counts.

ORDER OF TESTING

The order of conducting the tests is important. A number of tests are capable of producing temporary ocular abnormalities or temporarily masking ocular abnormalities. If the order of the tests is not chosen carefully, some of the temporary ocular abnormalities caused by earlier tests will be detected by later tests and incorrectly attributed to the drug product. For example, applanation tonometry requires the use of an anesthetic agent. The anesthetic's effect may last up to 30 minutes and may mask ocular discomfort produced by the test product.

TIMING OF TESTING

Whenever possible, the inclusion of a baseline test before exposure to a drug product is extremely helpful in the interpretation of any suspected abnormalities. It is also helpful to have a post drug-exposure test to determine whether any abnormality is reversible or permanent. Besides these two time points, additional testing is dependent on the drug and the particular test.

FUNCTIONAL TESTS
Visual Acuity

Visual acuity is the most commonly used and universally understood measure of visual function. It is important to measure visual acuity because it provides a simultaneous measurement of central corneal clarity, central lens clarity, central macular function, and optic nerve conduction. If it is normal, it provides a quick assessment of this central ocular pathway. If it is abnormal, however, it does not distinguish between the many causes of an abnormality.

Visual acuity should be measured as best corrected distance visual acuity. A recent refraction is required to obtain the best corrected visual acuity. Although the traditional distance used to measure visual acuity was 20 feet or 6 meters, distance vision can be measured at any distance from 3 feet or greater. The closer the subject is to the target, the more important it is to limit potential movement of the head and prevent the subject from moving closer to the test object, artificially increasing the visual angle. The use of a 4-meter distance for refractions has the advantage of being one quarter of a diopter in lens power from a theoretical infinite distance. Each eye should be tested separately. The test should be conducted using a high-contrast chart with an equal number of letters per line and equal spacing between lines. The stroke width of the letters should be smaller on each succeeding line so that the visual angle needed to identify the letters is reduced by two-thirds per line.

The result of a visual acuity test should be reported as a log-MAR value (log of the minimum angle of resolution). Normal visual acuity for most adults is approximately −0.1 on this scale, which is equivalent to 20/16 on a Snellen visual acuity chart. A two-line or greater change from one visit to the next in a single patient should suggest additional investigation. A three-line or greater change in a single individual is usually considered clinically significant. In the evaluation of a group of subjects, changes in the mean logMAR score and in shift tables created by categorizing subjects by gains and losses in zero, one, two, three, or more lines of visual acuity are often helpful in recognizing changes in visual acuity.

Additional measures of visual acuity, such as best corrected near visual acuity, uncorrected distance visual acuity, and uncorrected near visual acuity, are rarely necessary unless it is not possible to perform a best corrected distance visual acuity. Although abnormalities may occur that alter near visual acuity without affecting best corrected distance visual acuity, these abnormalities are better characterized by measuring the accommodative amplitude together with any observed changes in refractive power in association with the best corrected distance visual acuity. Refractive power can be measured by either a manifest refraction or a cycloplegic refraction. When evaluating the effect of a drug product on refractive power, it is usually best not to perform a cycloplegic refraction, as the pharmacologic action of the cycloplegic agent may alter the results.

Color Vision

Color vision is a test of macular function because there are relatively few cones outside the macular area. There is a large variety of color vision tests with different degrees of sensitivity and specificity. The different color tests are most commonly distinguished by their ability to screen for color vision defects versus quantitating color defects, as well as their ability to detect common congenital defects in color vision (red-green confusion) versus typical acquired defects in color vision (blue-yellow confusion). Each eye should be tested separately. The gold-standard test of color vision is the Farnsworth Munsell (FM) 100 hue color test. The FM 100 hue color test can be used to detect both red-green and blue-yellow confusion, and to some degree it can quantitate the extent of the confusion. The FM 100 hue color test consists of four trays of color caps that are arranged in sequential hue. The test is scored on the basis of caps that are placed out of order and, when plotted, can provide both the magnitude and type of deviation. However, the FM 100 hue color test has a learning curve associated with improvements in scores during the first few test administrations.

Subsets of the FM 100 hue color test can also be used to screen for color vision abnormalities. These subsets include 40 and 28 hue tests. The sensitivity of these tests progressively decreases as fewer caps are tested. These tests are also known as the *Lanthony 40 hue, Lanthony 28 hue, Roth 28 hue,* or *FM 28 hue desaturated tests.*

Another subset of the FM 100, the 15 hue test, including the desaturated versions of the 15 hue (Farnsworth D15 and Lanthony D15), is not always sensitive enough to detect mild losses in color vision. This test, the Hardy Rand and Rittler (HRR) color vision test, and the SPP2 color vision test are useful as screening tests for color vision defects.

The following tests are generally not useful in testing acquired color vision defects because they do not evaluate blue-yellow confusion: Ishihara test, SPP1, and Dvorine color vision tests. These tests predominantly provide an evaluation of red-green confusion.

Visual Fields

Visual field tests can be broadly divided into several categories. These categories include manual versus automated perimetry tests, static versus kinetic perimetry tests, threshold versus suprathreshold perimetry tests, white light target versus colored targets, and central field versus peripheral field perimetry tests. When automated, threshold perimetry tests are generally the preferred methods for evaluating drug-induced visual field defects; the use of static versus kinetic, central versus peripheral, and white versus color filtered light is dependent on the particular abnormality being investigated. For most drug-induced visual field defects, automated threshold, static, central 24-degree, white object perimetry testing is adequate to detect potential defects. Perimetry programs that meet these criteria include the Humphrey 30-1, 30-2, 24-1, 24-2, SITA Fast and SITA Standard Visual Field Tests, and the Octopus 30-1 and 30-2 Visual Field Tests.

Reporting of visual fields should always include the actual thresholds determined for each field point and the number of false positives, false negatives, and fixation losses. A significant learning curve is demonstrated by most subjects who take a visual field test. This learning curve should be expected to take place over at least the first three tests completed in each eye. The learning curve most commonly results in a significant increase in mean threshold values for normal individuals.

In cases where there is an expectation that rods will be affected more than cones, an automated peripheral white object perimeter testing program is preferred, e.g. the Humphrey P-60 and FF-120 visual field tests. In cases where there is an expectation that the cones will be affected more than the rods, an automated color filtered, central visual field test is preferred.

The most widely used kinetic test can be performed with a Goldmann perimeter. It is important that the same technician performs the testing with a Goldmann perimeter from visit to visit to reduce the chances of variability in the field due to operator differences.

The Amsler grid test may help identify central macular changes. It is occasionally useful as a screening test in assessing drug toxicity when there are drug deposits in the macular area.

Contrast Sensitivity Testing

Contrast sensitivity testing has often not been included in toxicity testing because it was assumed that the measurements would overlap with other tests already included. When performed using standardized methodologies, contrast sensitivity testing is capable of measuring aspects of visual function that may not otherwise typically be measured by visual acuity, color vision, or visual field tests. When testing for toxicity purposes, multiple different levels of contrast should be included.

Electroretinography

International standards of electroretinography testing are set by the International Society for Clinical Electrophysiology of Vision (ISCEV). These standards provide complete details on the conduct of the testing parameters, including the light stimuli. If ISCEV standards are not followed, an explanation for why they were not followed should be included. For interpretation purposes, it is important to report full numerical results and graphs when reporting electroretinography findings.

Testing is expected to measure both rod and cone functions in a variety of stimuli. From a toxicology standpoint, amplitudes and/or latent times must usually change by at least 40% to be considered clinically significant. Electroretinography testing is often the most informative method available for assessing retinal function in nonhuman animals. It is a mainstay in testing drug products that bind to melanin and/or produce retinal lesions (seen by ophthalmoscopy, OCT, or histology). Development of a particular drug product is often stopped if it is shown to cause both retinal lesions and decreased amplitudes on electroretinography testing. Electroretinography abnormalities in nonhuman animal studies alone are not necessarily predictive of human injury.

Photostress Tests

Retinal damage may sometimes be manifested in delays in recovery time. Photostress tests may be helpful in identifying this type of injury if the effect is widespread throughout the retina. There is considerable subject-to-subject variability in photostress test evaluations, and therefore it is usually difficult to detect an abnormality unless the injury is great or the number of subjects tested is very large.

Double Vision and Ocular Motility

Complaints of double vision must first be assessed to determine if the double vision is uniocular or binocular. The Worth 4 DOT test can be used to assess this. If the double vision is binocular, assessments of ocular motility in nine fields of gaze should be conducted and cover/uncover tests should be conducted to assess phorias and tropias. This is one of the few times when both eyes should be tested simultaneously.

Pupil Measurements

Pupillary measurements provide an opportunity to test responses to ocular stimuli. It is important that pupillary diameters be measured under reproducible controlled settings of light and accommodation. Pupillary responses to light stimuli and to accommodation should be measured separately. Pupillary responses in one eye due to a light stimulus in the other eye should also be measured separately from the pupillary response to a light stimulus in the same eye. Pupillary measurements may be made in a variety of ways. It is rarely necessary to measure pupil responses to a sensitivity of more than a tenth of a millimeter.

Corneal Sensitivity

There are relatively few methods to quantitatively measure corneal sensitivity. The most commonly used instrument is the Cochet-Bonnet esthesiometer. This instrument can discriminate between fairly large changes in corneal sensitivity.

Corneal Thickness

The corneal endothelial cells provide an effective pump system that, when functioning properly, keeps the cornea thin. Corneal thickness, therefore, although an anatomic measurement, can be a surrogate for corneal endothelial cell function. There are two common corneal pachymetry methods – optical and ultrasonic. For the purposes of assessing corneal endothelial cell function, either can be useful as long as the same instrument is used consistently in a subject.

OBJECTIVE ANATOMIC METHODS

For most ocular tissues, electronic digital images provide the best method for recording anatomic findings. These electronic photographs generally provide opportunities for more complete analysis and characterization. A large number of different areas of the eye can be well imaged. These areas include all five layers of the corneal surface, corneal surface topography, corneal thickness, corneal clarity, anterior chamber depth, anterior chamber inflammation, lens thickness, lens clarity, nerve fiber thickness, vitreous inflammation, vitreous traction, retinal surface irregularities, retinal vasculature, optic nerve size, and optic cup size and contour.

Cornea and Conjunctiva

As external, relatively clear structures, the cornea and conjunctiva can be evaluated by direct observation. Direct observation can be aided by the magnification provided by a slit lamp or a confocal microscope. The application of different stains such as fluorescein, lissamine green, or rose bengal can help by differentially staining various cells or tissues. Fluorescein stain is incorporated when epithelial cells are dead or missing; lissamine green and rose bengal stains are incorporated when epithelial cells are injured and have lost some of their functionality. These stains are useful in assessing corneal or conjunctival epithelial damage.

Corneal endothelial cells, if exposed to a toxic substance, are among the most sensitive in the eye to ocular damage, and because they are not regenerated in humans, they provide a permanent marker of damage. Endothelial cell counts measure damage to the corneal endothelium.

The best method for recording corneal or conjunctival changes is with electronic images by digitalized photography. This method is generally most useful for future analysis and characterization. When this is not possible, predefined scales may be used to capture a description of any findings.

Tear Film

The production of tears may be affected by different pharmacologic agents in terms of both the quantity and quality of the tears produced. The effects on tear quantity may be evaluated by Schirmer tear test (anesthetized and nonanesthetized conditions). The effects on tear quality may be evaluated by tear breakup time.

Lens

Any evaluation of a lens change should include the type of lens change, as well as the size and the location of the change. Digital photography remains the gold standard for evaluating lens clarity, although a single photograph is rarely capable of capturing all aspects of the lens. Multiple photographs taken on and off the central axis, and including but not limited to retroillumination, are useful in assessing lens clarity and therefore cataract development. If this is not available, a predefined scale system with reference photographs for each point on the scale is useful. It is extremely useful to grade posterior subcapsular changes, cortical changes, and nuclear changes separately because often they may be independent of one another.

Lens opacities tend to occur slowly. Whereas direct trauma to the lens can cause opacities to develop within minutes, hours, or days, most milder injuries take weeks to months or years to develop. Corticosteroid drug products, which are well known to cause cataracts even when administered intraocularly, may take up to 2 years to cause clinically recognizable lens changes. It is recommended that when a drug product is to be administered for a period of 6 weeks or more, lens changes be monitored at 6-month intervals for at least 2 years.

At least as important as the size of an opacity in the lens is the location of that opacity in the lens. Although all opacities in a lens are important and may spread to other areas of the lens, the initial location may have more impact on the immediate clinical consequences and help characterize a particular toxicity. Opacities that occur in the posterior portion of the lens generally cause more interference with sight than opacities that occur in the anterior portion of the lens. Opacities that occur in the center of the visual axis cause the most interference with sight. Drug-induced toxicities tend to first occur more commonly in the posterior portion of the lens.

It is not always possible to directly appreciate the impact of a lens change on an individual patient's visual acuity. In some of these cases, visual acuity will change before any lens opacity becomes noticeable. Visual acuity should therefore always be measured when evaluating patients for lens changes.

Anterior Chamber

The position of the lens and consequently the size and shape of the anterior chamber can be affected by pharmacologic agents. This is best assessed by slit lamp examinations and diagnostic ultrasound measurements. Pharmacologically induced angle closure may be first identified by cases of elevated IOP in association with refractive changes.

Retina

Both color digital photography and OCT are the current gold standards for evaluating the retinal surface. Fluorescein angiography (FA) and indocyanine green (ICG) angiography provide separate and additional information on the retinal vasculature. Direct fundoscopy and indirect fundoscopy, although capable of detecting retinal abnormalities, often provide more limited views with less magnification. Direct fundoscopy may include the use of a direct ophthalmoscope or the use of a slit lamp with an additional 78D or 90D lens. The ability to follow fundus photographs and OCT images over time makes these methods superior to direct or indirect fundoscopy.

Intraocular Pressure

The measurement of IOP for the purposes of toxicology assessments can be adequately made by applanation tonometry. The invasiveness of more accurate measures is usually not warranted. In the rare cases where a more exact estimate of aqueous production is needed, tonography can be performed.

NUMBER OF PATIENTS TO TEST

Common events are easier to identify and characterize than more unusual ones. It is customary to attempt to identify events that occur at a frequency of 1% or higher before the commercial distribution of a drug product. Mathematical principles of probability dictate that when the true event incidence is 1% or higher, to have a 95% chance of observing at least one event, 300 subjects must be monitored. This is often referred to as the rule of three.[1]

The rule of three states that to detect events that would occur at X% or more, you need Y patients, where 3 / Y = X. Applying this rule suggests that if a true incidence rate of 10% is to be identified, at least 30 patients need to be studied. If an incidence rate of 5% is to be detected, 60 patients must be studied. If an incidence rate of 0.1% is to be detected, 3000 patients must be studied.

SUMMARY

Many potential ocular toxicities can occur as the result of administering a pharmacologic agent. Ocular toxicity tests should be used to investigate potential adverse events that might be either frequent or serious. There should be a justified reason for the selection of each test, and each test should be appropriate for the event in question.

REFERENCE

1. Hanley JA, Lippman-Hand A. If nothing goes wrong, is everything all right? Interpreting zero numerators. *JAMA.* 1983;249:1743–1745.

CHAPTER 4

Anti-Infectives

CLASS: AMEBICIDES

Generic Names:
1. Broxyquinoline; 2. diiodohydroxyquinoline (iodoquinol).

Proprietary Names:
1. Starogyn; 2. Sebaquin, Yodoxin.

Primary Use
These amebicidal drugs are effective against *Entamoeba histolytica*.

Ocular Side Effects
Systemic administration – oral
Certain
1. Decreased vision
2. Optic atrophy
3. Optic neuritis – subacute myelo-optic neuropathy (SMON)
4. Nystagmus
5. Toxic amblyopia
6. Macular edema
7. Macular degeneration
8. Diplopia
9. Absence of foveal reflex
10. Color vision defect – purple spots on white background

Clinical Significance
Major toxic ocular effects may occur with long-term oral administration of these amebicidal drugs, especially in children. Since they are given orally for *E. histolytica*, most reports come from the Far East. Data suggest that these amebicides may cause SMON. This neurologic disease has a 19% incidence of decreased vision and a 2.5% incidence of toxic amblyopia. It has been suggested that in patients being treated for acrodermatitis enteropathica, which is a disease of inherited zinc deficiency, optic atrophy may be secondary to zinc deficiency instead of diiodohydroxyquinoline. Because long-term quinolone exposure has been shown to result in accumulation of the drug in pigmented tissues, retinal degenerative changes may be observed. The best overall review of this subject is in Grant et al.[1]

Generic Name:
Emetine hydrochloride.

Proprietary Name:
Multi-ingredient preparations only.

Primary Use
This alkaloid is effective in the treatment of acute amebic dysentery, amebic hepatitis, and amebic abscesses.

Ocular Side Effects
Systemic administration – subcutaneous or intramuscular injection near toxic levels
Certain
1. Irritation
   a. Lacrimation
   b. Hyperemia
   c. Photophobia
   d. Foreign body sensation
2. Eyelids or conjunctiva
   a. Hyperemia
   b. Edema
   c. Urticaria
   d. Purpura
   e. Eczema
3. Cornea
   a. Superficial punctate keratitis
   b. Erosions
4. Pupils
   a. Mydriasis
   b. Absence of reaction to light
5. Decreased accommodation
6. Decreased vision
7. Visual fields
   a. Scotomas – central
   b. Constriction
8. Retinal and optic nerve
   a. Ischemia
   b. Hyperemia optic nerve

Inadvertent ocular exposure
Certain
1. Irritation
   a. Lacrimation

b. Hyperemia
c. Photophobia
2. Eyelids or conjunctiva
   a. Allergic reactions
   b. Conjunctivitis – nonspecific
   c. Blepharospasm
3. Cornea
   a. Keratitis
   b. Ulceration

Conditional/unclassified
1. Iritis
2. Secondary glaucoma

Clinical Significance

Although this is a limited-use drug and most of the data are from the older literature, the basic ingredient in ipecac is emetine hydrochloride, which is used off-label to induce vomiting in patients with anorexia nervosa. Emetine hydrochloride is somewhat unique in that somewhere between 4 and 10 hours after exposure in humans, the drug is probably secreted in the tears to give significant bilateral foreign body sensation, epiphora, photophobia, lid edema, blepharospasm, and conjunctival hyperemia. Because the drug is seldom used for longer than 5 days, these signs and symptoms quickly resolve once the drug is discontinued.[1] At normal dosages, these are probably the only ocular side effects, but at higher doses Jacovides described optic nerve and retinal ischemic changes with pupillary, accommodation, vision, and visual field abnormalities.[2] These are all transitory with complete recovery.

Emetine hydrochloride is highly toxic when inadvertent direct ocular exposure occurs. This rarely causes significant scarring with permanent corneal opacities, with or without iritis and secondary glaucoma.

CLASS: ANTHELMINTICS

Generic Name:
Diethylcarbamazine citrate.

Proprietary Name:
Hetrazan.

Primary Use
This antifilarial drug is particularly effective against *Wuchereria bancrofti*, *Wuchereria malayi*, *Onchocerca volvulus*, and *Loa*.

Ocular Side Effects
Systemic administration – secondary to the drug-induced death of the organism
Certain
1. Eyelids or conjunctiva
   a. Allergic reactions
   b. Conjunctivitis – nonspecific
   c. Edema
   d. Urticaria
   e. Nodules
2. Uveitis
3. Cornea – probably drug related
   a. Fluffy punctate opacities
   b. Punctate keratitis
4. Chorioretinitis
5. Visual field defects
6. Chorioretinal pigmentary changes
7. Loss of eyelashes or eyebrows
8. Toxic amblyopia

Local ophthalmic use or exposure – topical ocular application
Certain
1. Eyelids or conjunctiva
   a. Allergic reactions
   b. Erythema
   c. Edema
2. Irritation
   a. Lacrimation
   b. Hyperemia
   c. Photophobia
   d. Pain
3. Cornea – probably drug related
   a. Fluffy punctate opacities
   b. Punctate keratitis
   c. Corneal opacities

Clinical Significance

Adverse ocular reactions to diethylcarbamazine are rare; however, severe reactions depend in large part on which organism is being treated. Drug-induced death of the filaria can result in a severe allergic reaction due to the release of foreign protein. Nodules may form in the area of the dead worm from a secondary inflammatory reaction. This reaction in the eye may be so marked that toxic amblyopia follows. Newer drugs that kill the organism more slowly are being used, with fewer ocular side effects. The use of diethylcarbamazine eye drops for treatment of ocular onchocerciasis produces dose-related inflammatory reactions similar to those seen with systemic use of the drug. Local ocular effects may include globular limbal infiltrates, severe vasculitis, pruritus, and erythema.

Generic Name:
Mepacrine hydrochloride.

Proprietary Name:
Atabrine.

Primary Use
This methoxyacridine drug is effective in the treatment of tapeworm infestations and in the prophylaxis and treatment of malaria.

Ocular Side Effects
Systemic administration – oral
Certain
1. Decreased vision
2. Yellow, white, clear, brown, blue, or gray punctate deposits
   a. Conjunctiva
   b. Cornea
   c. Nasolacrimal system
   d. Sclera
3. Cornea
   a. Corneal edema
   b. Superficial punctate keratitis
4. Color vision defect
   a. Objects have yellow, green, blue, or violet tinge
   b. Colored haloes around lights – mainly blue
5. Eyelids or conjunctiva
   a. Blue-black hyperpigmentation
   b. Yellow discoloration
   c. Urticaria
6. Photophobia
7. Visual hallucinations

Probable
1. Posterior subcapsular cataracts

Possible
1. Macula – bull's-eye appearance with thinning and clumping of the pigment epithelium
2. Eyelids or conjunctiva
   a. Exfoliative dermatitis
   b. Eczema

Inadvertent direct ocular exposure
Certain
1. Irritation
   a. Lacrimation
   b. Pain
2. Eyelids, conjunctiva, or cornea
   a. Edema
   b. Yellow or yellow-green discoloration
3. Blue haloes around lights

Clinical Significance
Adverse ocular reactions due to mepacrine are common, but most are reversible and fairly asymptomatic. Systemic mepacrine can stain eyelids, conjunctiva, cornea, and sclera yellow and the basal layers of the conjunctival epithelium blue-gray. This is probably due to the drug being present in the tears. The pigmentary deposition and/or corneal edema may cause complaints of decreased vision, as well as yellow, blue, green, or violet vision. These changes are reversible once the drug is discontinued. This may or may not be associated with a superficial keratitis. Drug-induced corneal edema may be precipitated in sensitive individuals, especially those with hepatic dysfunction. This can occur with dosages as low as 0.10 g per day and may take several weeks of therapy to occur. If the drug is discontinued, this will resolve; but if the drug is restarted, the edema will occur again in a few days. Cumming et al, in the Blue Mountain Eye Study, found an association between mepacrine and posterior subcapsular cataracts.[1] Reports of optic neuritis, scotoma, and enlarged blind spots are usually single case reports over 50 years ago and are not substantiated as a cause-and-effect relationship. Direct ocular exposure to mepacrine occurs either from exposure to the dust during its manufacture or self-infection.[2,3] This drug can stain the eyelids, cornea, and conjunctiva. Significant corneal changes, including severe edema and folds in Descemet's membrane, may occur. Color vision changes can also occur. These changes are reversible.

Generic Name:
Piperazine.

Proprietary Name:
Piperazine.

Primary Use
This anthelmintic drug is used in the treatment of ascariasis and enterobiasis.

Ocular Side Effects
Systemic administration – oral
Probable
1. Decreased vision
2. Color vision defect

3. Decreased accommodation
4. Miosis
5. Nystagmus
6. Visual hallucinations
7. Paresis of extraocular muscles
8. Visual sensations
   a. Flashing lights
   b. Entopic light flashes
9. Eyelids or conjunctiva
   a. Allergic reactions
   b. Edema
   c. Photosensitivity
   d. Urticaria
   e. Purpura
10. Lacrimation

Possible
1. Eyelids or conjunctiva – eczema

Conditional/unclassified
1. Cataract

Clinical Significance
Although a number of ocular side effects have been attributed to piperazine, they are rare, reversible, and usually of little clinical importance. Adverse ocular reactions generally occur only in instances of overdose or in cases of impaired renal function or in systemic neurotoxic states. A few cases of well-documented extraocular muscle paresis have been reported. There are suggestions that this is a cataractogenic drug, but this is unproven.

Generic Name:
Thiabendazole.

Proprietary Name:
Mintezol.

Primary Use
This benzimidazole drug is used in the treatment of enterobiasis, strongyloidiasis, ascariasis, uncinariasis, trichuriasis, and cutaneous larva migrans. It has been advocated as an antimycotic in corneal ulcers.

Ocular Side Effects
Systemic administration – oral
Probable
1. Decreased vision
2. Color vision defect – objects have yellow tinge
3. Abnormal visual sensations
4. Eyelids or conjunctiva

a. Allergic reactions
b. Hyperemia
c. Edema
d. Urticaria
5. Visual hallucinations

Possible
1. May aggravate or cause ocular sicca
2. Eyelids or conjunctiva
   a. Erythema multiforme
   b. Exfoliative dermatitis
   c. Lyell syndrome

Clinical Significance
Although thiabendazole is a potent therapeutic drug, it has surprisingly few reported ocular or systemic toxic side effects. Ocular side effects that occur are transitory, reversible, and seldom of clinical importance. However, a mother and daughter, after only a few doses, developed ocular sicca, xerostomia, cholangiostatic hepatitis, and pancreatic dysfunction.[1] Rex et al and Davidson et al reported cases similar to this.[2,3] Some feel these reactions may represent allergic responses to the dead parasites rather than direct drug effects. This drug may induce ocular pemphigoid-like syndrome.

CLASS: ANTIBIOTICS

Generic Name:
Amikacin sulfate.

Proprietary Name:
Amikin.

Primary Use
This intraocularly and systemically administered aminoglycoside is primarily used for Gram-negative infections.

Ocular Side Effects
Systemic administration – intravenous or oral
Certain
1. Decreased vision
2. Eyelids or conjunctiva
   a. Urticaria
   b. Purpura

Local ophthalmic use or exposure – intravitreal injection
Certain
1. Macular infarcts

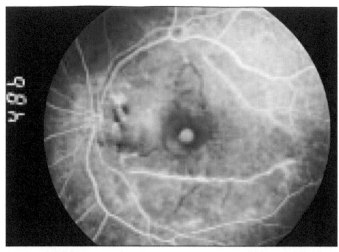

FIG. 4.1 Amikacin retinal toxicity: diffuse arteriolar occlusion as seen on fluorescein angiography.[5]

2. Retina
   a. Toxicity (Fig. 4.1)
   b. Degeneration

Clinical Significance

This aminoglycoside rarely causes ocular side effects when given orally. Ophthalmologists' interest in this antibiotic is primarily for intravitreal injections, usually in combination with a cephalosporin for management of endophthalmitis. Gentamicin has been the aminoglycoside of choice for intravitreal injections until reports of macular infarcts occurred. Amikacin was shown to be less toxic to the retina than gentamicin, so many surgeons started using it intravitreally. However, now cases of retinal infarcts have been reported with this drug, with perifoveal capillaries becoming occluded, as per fluorescein angiography. D'Amico et al found lysosomal inclusions in the retinal pigment epithelium secondary to amikacin.[1] Campochiaro pointed out the role of the dependent position of the macula at the time of intravitreal injection, with the resultant potential increased concentration of this drug over the macula.[2-4] Aminoglycosides have a known toxic effect on ganglion and other neural cells of the retina. Doft et al, from the Endophthalmitis Vitreous Study Group, felt that the data were not compelling enough to suggest a different antibiotic, and they continue to recommend amikacin as the empirical standard to date.[5,6] There are more than 30 spontaneous reports of macular infarct associated with amikacin use. However, based on risk–benefit ratios, along with the available clinical data, Doft's recommendation seems reasonable. This is, however, an area of controversy among retinal specialists shown by Galloway et al.[7,8]

Generic Names:

1. Amoxicillin; 2. ampicillin; 3. nafcillin sodium; 4. piperacillin; 5. ticarcillin monosodium.

Proprietary Names:

1. Amoxil, Augmentin, DisperMox, Moxatag, Moxilin, Sumox, Trimox; 2. Principen, Unasyn; 3. Nafcil; 4. Pipracil, Zosyn; 5. Timentin.

Primary Use

Semisynthetic penicillins are primarily effective against staphylococci, streptococci, pneumococci, and various other Gram-positive and Gram-negative bacteria.

Ocular Side Effects
Systemic administration – oral
Certain

1. Eyelids or conjunctiva
   a. Allergic reactions
   b. Blepharoconjunctivitis
   c. Edema
   d. Photosensitivity
   e. Urticaria

Probable

1. Myasthenia gravis – aggravated
   a. Diplopia
   b. Ptosis
   c. Paresis of extraocular muscles

Possible
1. Eyelids or conjunctiva
   a. Erythema multiforme
   b. Exfoliative dermatitis
   c. Lyell syndrome

Local ophthalmic use or exposure – topical ocular application or subconjunctival injection
Certain
1. Irritation – primarily with subconjunctival injection
   a. Hyperemia
   b. Pain
   c. Edema
2. Eyelids or conjunctiva
   a. Allergic reactions
   b. Edema
3. Conjunctival necrosis (nafcillin) – subconjunctival injection

Clinical Significance
Surprisingly few ocular side effects other than dermatologic- or hematologic-related conditions have been reported with the semisynthetic penicillins. The incidence of allergic skin reactions due to ampicillin, however, may be high. Periorbital or eyelid edema may be the most common adverse ocular effect. Ampicillin and other semisynthetic penicillins may unmask or aggravate ocular signs of myasthenia gravis. Perez-Roca et al reported a case of an 11-year-old child with acute diplopia and near vision due to transient convergence palsy possibly related to amoxicillin use.[1] Nafcillin has been reported to cause conjunctival necrosis with subconjunctival injections. Many, and maybe all, of these drugs can be found in the tears in therapeutic levels and can cause local reactions if the patients are sensitive to the drug.

Generic Names:
1. Azithromycin; 2. clarithromycin; 3. clindamycin; 4. erythromycin.

Proprietary Names:
1. Azasite, Zithromax, Zithromax Tri-Pak, Zithromax Z-Pak, Zmax; 2. Biaxin, Biaxin XL; 3. Cleocin, Cleocin Ovules, Cleocin Pediatric, Cleocin T, CLIN, Clinda-Derm, Clindacin ETZ, Clindacin PAC, Clindacin-P, Clindagel, ClindaMax, ClindaReach, Clindesse, Clindets, Evoclin, PledgaClin; 4. Akne-Mycin, ATS, Delmycin, E-Base, E-Mycin, EES, Emcin Clear, EMGEL, Emgal, Eramycin, Ery-Ped, Ery-Tab, ERYC, Erycette, Eryderm, Erygel, Erymax, EryPed, Erythra Derm, Erythrocin, Erythrocin Lactobionate, Erythrocin Stearate, Ilosone, Ilotycin, PCE, PCE Dispertab, Robimycin Robitabs, Romycin, Staticin, T-Stat.

Primary Use
Azithromycin, clarithromycin, and erythromycin are macrolides, and clindamycin is an antibiotic with similar properties. These bactericidal antibiotics are effective against Gram-positive or Gram-negative organisms.

Ocular Side Effects
Systemic administration – intramuscular, intravenous, or oral
Certain
1. Color vision defect – blue-yellow defect (erythromycin)
2. Eyelids or conjunctiva
   a. Allergic reactions
   b. Hyperemia
   c. Photosensitivity
   d. Edema
   e. Urticaria
3. Visual hallucinations (clarithromycin)

Probable
1. Myasthenia gravis – aggravated (azithromycin, clarithromycin, erythromycin)
   a. Diplopia
   b. Ptosis
   c. Paresis of extraocular muscles

Possible
1. Cornea – subepithelial deposits (clarithromycin)
2. Eyelids or conjunctiva
   a. Exfoliative dermatitis
   b. Lyell syndrome (erythromycin)
   c. Myasthenic crisis (intravenous azithromycin)
4. Uveitis

Local ophthalmic use or exposure – topical ocular application or subconjunctival injection
Certain
1. Irritation
   a. Hyperemia
   b. Pain
   c. Edema
2. Eyelids or conjunctiva
   a. Allergic reactions
   b. Edema

Possible
1. Mydriasis (erythromycin)
2. Cornea – subepithelial deposits (clarithromycin)

3. Unmask myasthenia gravis (traumatized ocular surface)
4. Elevate prothrombin times (traumatized ocular surface)

Local ophthalmic use or exposure – intracameral injection
Certain
1. Uveitis (erythromycin)
2. Corneal edema (erythromycin)
3. Lens damage (erythromycin)

Local ophthalmic use or exposure – retrobulbar or subtenon injection
Possible
1. Irritation (clindamycin)
2. Optic neuritis (clindamycin)
3. Optic atrophy (clindamycin)
4. Diplopia (clindamycin)

Clinical Significance

Few significant adverse ocular reactions due to either systemic or topical ocular use of these antibiotics are seen. Clinicians may overlook in the elderly patient the effect of these drugs causing lid edema and blame it on age. Nearly all ocular side effects are transitory and reversible after the drug is discontinued. Pradhan et al reported myasthenia crisis after intravenous (IV) azithromycin.[1] Dramatic improvement after IV calcium in these patients suggests azithromycin probably caused presynaptic suppression of acetylcholine release. In severe infections or ocular trauma, where absorption may be enhanced, topical ocular antibiotics may cause myasthenia gravis signs and symptoms. Most adverse ocular reactions are secondary to dermatologic or hematologic conditions. A well-documented, rechallenged, idiosyncratic response to topical ocular application of erythromycin causing mydriasis has been reported in a spontaneous case report. Also, an interaction of erythromycin with carbamazepine causing mydriasis and gaze-evoked nystagmus has been reported. Parker et al reported erythromycin ointment causing increased prothrombin times with rechallenge data.[2] There are spontaneous reports of Stevens-Johnson syndrome after topical ophthalmic erythromycin ointment application. Clarithromycin, with both oral and topical ocular exposure, has been associated with subepithelial infiltrate when treating mycobacterium avium complex. When the drug was stopped, the deposits were absorbed. Visual hallucinations due to clarithromycin have only been seen when the drug was used in peritoneal dialysis.

Recommendations

1. This group of antibiotics can cause significant eyelid edema that recovers off the medication. Plastic surgery should be delayed until off the medication. Surgery may not be necessary.
2. Topical ocular or systemic medications may unmask myasthenia gravis.

Generic Name:

Bacitracin.

Proprietary Names:

Ak-Tracin, Baci-IM, Ocu-Tracin.

Primary Use

This polypeptide bactericidal drug is primarily effective against Gram-positive cocci, *Neisseria*, and organisms causing gas gangrene.

Ocular Side Effects

Systemic administration – oral
Certain
1. Decreased vision
2. Eyelids or conjunctiva
   a. Allergic reactions
   b. Edema
   c. Urticaria

Probable
1. Myasthenia gravis – aggravated
   a. Diplopia
   b. Ptosis
   c. Paresis of extraocular muscles

Local ophthalmic use or exposure – topical ocular application or subconjunctival injection
Certain
1. Irritation
2. Eyelids or conjunctiva
   a. Allergic reactions
   b. Blepharoconjunctivitis
   c. Edema
   d. Urticaria
3. Keratitis
4. Delayed corneal wound healing

Local ophthalmic use or exposure – intracameral injection
Certain
1. Uveitis
2. Corneal edema
3. Lens damage

Inadvertent orbital injection (ointment)
Possible
1. Orbital compartment syndrome (Fig. 4.2)

Clinical Significance

Ocular side effects from either systemic or ocular administration of bacitracin are rare. Myasthenia gravis is more commonly seen if systemic bacitracin is used in combination with neomycin, kanamycin, polymyxin, or colistin. With increasing use of "fortified" bacitracin solution (10,000 units per mL), marked conjunctival irritation and keratitis may occur, especially if the solutions are used frequently. The potential of decreased wound healing with prolonged use of any topical antibiotic, especially fortified solution, may occur. Severe ocular or periocular allergic reactions, although rare, have been seen due to topical ophthalmic bacitracin application. An anaphylactic reaction was reported after the use of bacitracin ointment.[1] Caraballo et al reported an anaphylactic reaction that occurred during the application of scleral buckle placement for retinal detachment surgery, which was soaked in 150 units per mL bacitracin solution.[2] Using a stepwise approach, bacitracin was identified as the causative drug. Orbital compartment syndrome, acute proptosis, chemosis, increased intraocular pressure, decreased vision, and ophthalmoplegia were reported by Castro et al immediately after endoscopic sinus surgery secondary to inadvertent exposure to bacitracin ointment.[3]

Generic Name:

Benzathine benzylpenicillin (benzathine G penicillin).

Proprietary Names:

Bicillin L-A, Permapen.

Primary Use

This bactericidal penicillin is effective against streptococci, *Staphylococcus aureus*, gonococci, meningococci, pneumococci, *Treponema pallidum*, *Clostridium*, *Bacillus anthracis*, *Corynebacterium diphtheriae*, and several species of *Actinomyces*.

Ocular Side Effects

Systemic administration – intramuscular
Certain
1. Mydriasis
2. Decreased accommodation
3. Diplopia
4. Papilledema secondary to pseudotumor cerebri
5. Decreased vision

6. Visual hallucinations
7. Visual agnosia
8. Eyelids or conjunctiva
   a. Allergic reactions
   b. Erythema
   c. Blepharoconjunctivitis
   d. Edema
   e. Urticaria

Possible
1. Eyelids or conjunctiva
   a. Lupoid syndrome
   b. Lyell syndrome
2. Cystoid macular edema

Local ophthalmic use or exposure – topical ocular application or subconjunctival injection
Certain
1. Irritation
2. Eyelids or conjunctiva – allergic reactions

Local ophthalmic use or exposure – intracameral injection
Certain
1. Uveitis
2. Corneal edema
3. Lens damage

Clinical Significance

Systemic administration of penicillin rarely causes ocular side effects. The most serious adverse reaction is papilledema secondary to elevated intracranial pressure. The incidence of allergic reactions is greater in patients with Sjögren syndrome or rheumatoid arthritis than in other individuals. Saleh et al reported cystoid macular edema worsening after IV penicillin, probably due to an inflammatory reaction to treponemal antigens released after antibiotic treatment for syphilis.[1] Most ocular side effects due to penicillin are transient and reversible. Kawasaki et al showed electroretinogram (ERG) changes with intravitreal injections of penicillin.[2] Topical ocular administration results in a high incidence of sensitivity reactions.

Generic Names:

1. Cefaclor; 2. cefadroxil; 3. cefalexin (cephalexin); 4. cefazolin sodium; 5. cefditoren pivoxil; 6. cefoperazone sodium; 7. cefotaxime; 8. cefotetan disodium; 9. cefoxitin sodium; 10. cefradine; 11. ceftazidime; 12. ceftizoxime sodium; 13. ceftriaxone sodium; 14. cefuroxime; 15. cefuroxime axetil.

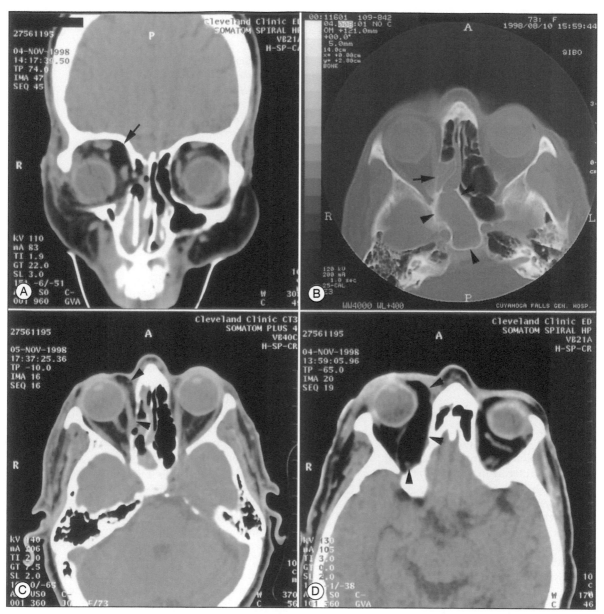

FIG. 4.2 **(A)** Preoperative axial computed tomography (CT) scan of the orbit showing orbital compartment syndrome caused by bacitracin ointment. This is shown by opacification of the right posterior ethmoid air cells and the right sphenoid sinus. The long arrow identifies the location of the ethmoidal opacification, and the short bullets outline the opacified right sphenoid sinus. **(B)** Axial CT scan obtained immediately after surgery showing the abnormal hypointense area along the medial orbital wall *(bullets)*. The superior ophthalmic vein is temporal to the radiolucent area. **(C)** Coronal CT scan immediately after surgery showing a relatively hypodense area within the right superior nasal orbit *(arrow)*. The right globe is displaced inferiorly and laterally. The Hounsfield units in this area were −147H, compatible with bacitracin ointment (−140 H to −160H). **(D)** The CT scan was repeated 1 day after surgery. The new CT shows a significant decrease in the orbital volume of the bacitracin ointment. Bullets outline the anterior and posterior extent of the medial orbital foreign material.[3]

Proprietary Names:

1. Ceclor, Ceclor CD; 2. Duricef; 3. Biocef, Cefanex, Daxbia, Keflex, Keftab; 4. Ancef, Kefzol, Zolicef; 5. Spectracef; 6. Cefobid; 7. Claforan; 8. Cefotan; 9. Mefoxin; 10. Velosef; 11. Ceptaz, Fortaz, Tazicef, Tazidime; 12. Cefizox; 13. Rocephin; 14. Alti-Cefuroxime, Ceftin, Kefurox, Zinacef; 15. Alti-Cefuroxime, Ceftin, Kefurox, Zinacef.

Primary Use

Cephalosporins are effective against streptococci, staphylococci, pneumococci, and strains of *Escherichia coli, Pneumococci mirabilis,* and *Klebsiella.*

Ocular Side Effects

Systemic administration – intramuscular, intravenous, or oral
Probable

1. Eyelids or conjunctiva
   a. Allergic reactions
   b. Erythema
   c. Conjunctivitis – nonspecific
   d. Edema
   e. Urticaria
2. Visual hallucinations

Possible

1. Periorbital edema
2. Nystagmus

Conditional/unclassified

1. Corneal edema – peripheral (cefaclor)
2. Acute macular neuroretinopathy

Local ophthalmic use or exposure – intracameral injection (cefuroxime)
Certain

1. Macula
   a. Edema
   b. Cystoid changes
   c. Infarct (overdose)
2. Retina
   a. Edema
   b. Serous retinal detachment
   c. Vasculitis (overdose)
   d. Atrophy
   e. Hemorrhagic infarction
3. Uveitis (overdose)
4. Abnormal electroretinogram (ERG) (overdose)
5. Visual field changes (overdose)
6. Optic nerve atrophy (overdose)

Conditional/unclassified

1. Corneal edema (overdose)

Local ophthalmic use or exposure – topical ocular application or subconjunctival cefuroxime injection
Certain

1. Irritation
   a. Hyperemia
   b. Pain
   c. Edema
2. Eyelids or conjunctiva
   a. Allergic reactions
   b. Edema
   c. Urticaria

Clinical Significance

These cephalosporins differ minimally in terms of ocular side effects. Although most are given only orally, a few are given intramuscularly, intravenously, or intracamerally. Oral cephalosporins seldom cause ocular side effects, and if they do, they are reversible. In less than 1% a nonspecific conjunctivitis may occur with cefaclor.[1] For each of these drugs there are spontaneous case reports of eyelid edema; periorbital edema was the most commonly reported event. Akam et al described acute uveitis 5 days after oral cefuroxime axetil.[2] This was associated with a systemic hypersensitivity reaction. Kraushar et al reported an anaphylactic reaction to intravitreal cefazolin.[3] There is significant cross-sensitivity within this group, as well as with penicillin. Platt described a generalized allergic event of type III hypersensitivity with reversible limbal hyperemia, mild conjunctivitis, and peripheral corneal edema in a patient taking cefaclor.[4]

With the marked increase in use of intracameral cefuroxime injections for prophylaxis post–cataract endophthalmitis, adverse effects at accepted dosage levels may be seen. The most common are macular edema and retinal edema of various degrees. D'Amico Ricci et al, Gimenez-de-la-Linde et al, Kontos et al, Xiao et al, Faure et al, and multiple spontaneous case reports have described various macular changes.[5-9] It is most often cystoid edema involving the outer nuclear layer (ONL) with an overlying serous retinal detachment. This usually only involves the posterior pole, but cases involving the peripheral retina have also been reported. This occurs within the first 24 hours, with visual loss of 20/60 to 20/400. All reported cases cleared with almost full recovery within 6–7 days. In a prospective, randomized, double-masked, clinical study of intracameral injections at the end of cataract surgery (34 patients in the cefuroxime group and 28 in the balanced salt solution group), Gupta et al showed no change in macular thickness between the 2 groups.[10] Hann et al questioned some parts of the study; regardless, this shows that at the current used dosage, these changes are an uncommon event.[11]

The other group of problems comes from overdosage or inadvertent intracameral injection. Ciftci et al, Le Du et al, Delyfer et al, Qureshi et al, and Wong et al have published reports that mirror, to a degree, side effects at a normal dosage (1 mg/0.1 mL).[12-16] The dosage may vary as high as 70+ times this concentration. What differs at this dosage is the degree of anterior chamber reaction, corneal edema and/or uveitis, abnormal retinal leakage, the greater extent of macular edema, and serous retinal detachment. There is only 1 case report of the cornea edema and/or uveitis, and it cleared after 2 weeks. Of greater concern seems to be an associated hemorrhagic infarct, which may affect the macular and/or optic nerve. This may cause irreversible retinal, macular, and optic nerve changes. In general, serous retinal detachments, retinal edema, and macular edema improve in 5–7 days with various degrees of recovery. Cataract extraction procedures with associated vitreous loss or posterior capsule tears may be risk factors for poorer outcomes. Delyfer et al described 6 patients with the classic syndrome, including vasculitis, but without hemorrhagic infarcts.[14] These all resolved with satisfactory outcomes. All patients received 40–50 times the normal dosage. No case has postoperative surgical intervention. They suggest, however, long-term retinal function studies should be assessed with repeated ERGs.

Generic Name:
Chloramphenicol.

Proprietary Names:
Ak-Chlor, Chloromycetin, Chloroptic.

Primary Use
This bacteriostatic dichloroacetic acid derivative is particularly effective against *Salmonella typhi*, *Haemophilus influenzae* meningitis, rickettsia, and the lymphogranuloma-psittacosis group and is useful in the management of cystic fibrosis.

Ocular Side Effects
Systemic administration – intramuscular, intravenous, or oral
Certain
1. Decreased vision
2. Retrobulbar or optic neuritis
3. Visual fields
   a. Scotomas – central and paracentral
   b. Constriction
4. Optic atrophy
5. Toxic amblyopia
6. Color vision defect – objects have yellow tinge
7. Eyelids or conjunctiva
   a. Allergic reactions
   b. Conjunctivitis – nonspecific
   c. Edema
   d. Urticaria
8. Decreased accommodation
9. Pupils
   a. Mydriasis
   b. Absence of reaction to light
10. Blindness

Local ophthalmic use or exposure – topical ocular application or subconjunctival injection
Certain
1. Irritation
2. Eyelids or conjunctiva
   a. Allergic reactions
   b. Conjunctivitis – nonspecific
   c. Depigmentation
3. Keratitis

Possible
1. Eyelids or conjunctiva – anaphylactic reaction

Local ophthalmic use or exposure – intracameral injection
Certain
1. Uveitis
2. Corneal edema
3. Lens damage

Systemic Side Effects
Local ophthalmic use or exposure – topical ocular application
Possible
1. Aplastic anemia
2. Various blood dyscrasias

Clinical Significance

Ocular side effects from systemic chloramphenicol administration are uncommon in adults but may occur more frequently in children, especially if the total dose exceeds 100 g or if therapy lasts more than 6 weeks. Optic neuritis with secondary optic atrophy is the most serious side effect. These are most often of acute onset and bilateral, and optic neuritis is much more frequent than retrobulbar neuritis. The first sign may be sudden visual loss with cecocentral scotoma.

Topical ophthalmic application causes infrequent ocular side effects. Although chloramphenicol has fewer allergic reactions than neomycin, those due to chloramphenicol are often more severe. Like other antibiotics, this drug may cause latent hypersensitivity, which may last for many years. Topical ocular chloramphenicol probably has fewer toxic effects on the corneal epithelium than other antibiotics. Berry et al pointed out, however, that after 14 days this is no longer true, and it is second only to gentamicin in toxicity tested in in-vitro studies on human corneal epithelium.[1]

Almost 70 cases of blood dyscrasia or aplastic anemia after topical ocular chloramphenicol have been reported in the literature or to spontaneous reporting systems, with 19 fatalities. It is unknown if there is a direct cause-and-effect relationship.[2] The risk of developing pancytopenia or aplastic anemia after oral chloramphenicol treatment is 13 times greater than the risk of idiopathic aplastic anemia in the general population. Two forms of hemopoietic abnormalities, idiosyncratic and dose related, may occur after systemic chloramphenicol. Although the latter response is unlikely from topical ophthalmic use of the drug, the incidence of the idiosyncratic response is unknown and indeed is a highly controversial topic. The topical eye drop form of chloramphenicol became available in 1948, and the first fatality from eye drops was reported in 1955. In 1982, Fraunfelder et al reported another fatality associated with this medication.[3] A subsequent research letter in 1993 reviewed all known case reports of this adverse drug reaction, with 23 blood dyscrasias leading to 12 deaths.[4] In 2007, chloramphenicol eye drops related to aplastic anemia and blood dyscrasias were classified as "probable" according to World Health Organization criteria based upon the known published case reports and spontaneous reports.[5] Within 2 years of the 1982 case report of death associated with topical ocular chloramphenicol, sales in the United States declined by 90%, and the *Physicians' Desk Reference* (PDR) placed a black box warning that read "…ocular chloramphenicol should not be used unless there is no alternative."[6] However, most countries continued to use the eye drop form of chloramphenicol. In 2002, England made it the first-line drug of choice for conjunctivitis, and it was made available over the counter without the need for a prescription. The epidemiologic studies include publications from around the world, including Canada, Spain, Bahrain, Israel, Germany, Bulgaria, Sweden, and the United Kingdom. The most specific study in regard to the incidence of aplastic anemia was by Laporte et al.[7] The investigators performed a case-control surveillance of aplastic anemia in a community of 4.2 million inhabitants (Barcelona, Spain) from 1980 to 1995 (67.2 million person-years). A case population risk estimate was made based on sales figures of ocular chloramphenicol during the study period. Three cases and 5 controls had been exposed to ocular chloramphenicol during the study period, and the adjusted odds ratio was 3.77 (95% confidence interval). Two cases had been exposed to other drugs associated with aplastic anemia. The incidence of aplastic anemia among users of ocular chloramphenicol was 0.36 cases per million weeks of treatment. The incidence among nonusers was 0.04. Extrapolation from these data led to the estimate of a less than 1-per-million treatment courses. Other population studies stated the number of case reports in their country and compared it with the number of exposures. A multicenter study, including patients from Sweden, the United States, Thailand, and Israel, found no cases of aplastic anemia or blood dyscrasia in subjects representing 185 million person-years that had received chloramphenicol eye drops. In all of these population studies, the authors concluded that the data do not implicate chloramphenicol eye drops as causing this adverse reaction, as the incidence of idiopathic or other drug-related instances of blood dyscrasias could account for all of the known case reports.

From literature reviews, case reports, and book chapters on this subject we have come to some conclusions. First, topical ocular chloramphenicol "possibly" can cause blood dyscrasias and aplastic anemia, and the latter is frequently fatal. Second, it is not possible to quantify the risk, although it appears to be very rare. Quoted incidence is 1 in 1 million; however, these data are based on a very small number of case reports. Third, it is likely that there are genetically susceptible individuals to this idiosyncratic reaction and that it is not possible to identify who these subjects are.

Recommendations

Recommendations for topical ocular chloramphenicol are as follows:

1. Topical ocular chloramphenicol probably should not be used on any patient with a family history of a blood dyscrasia without informed consent.

2. Its use is preferably limited to 7–14 days.
3. Only 1 drop should be used at a time. Consider limiting systemic absorption by closing the lids for 3 minutes after drop application and removing excess drug at the inner canthus with a tissue before opening the eyelids.
4. Physicians must make their own judgments as to the risk–benefit ratio in using this drug topically. Informed consent may be prudent in some cases.

Generic Names:
1. Ciprofloxacin; 2. sparfloxacin; 3. tosufloxacin.

Proprietary Names:
1. Cetraxal, Ciloxan, Cipro, Cipro IV, Cipro XR, Otiprio, Proquin; 2. Zagam, Zagam Respipac; 3. Ozex.

Primary Use
These fluoroquinolone antibacterial drugs are used primarily against most Gram-negative aerobic bacteria and many Gram-positive aerobic bacteria.

Ocular Side Effects
Systemic administration – intravenous and oral (primarily ciprofloxacin)
Certain
1. Visual sensations
   a. Glare phenomenon
   b. Lacrimation
   c. Flashing lights
2. Photosensitivity
3. Abnormal visually evoked response (VER)

Probable
1. Eyelids
   a. Pruritus
   b. Edema
   c. Urticaria
   d. Hyperpigmentation
2. Visual hallucinations
3. Myasthenia gravis – aggravated
   a. Diplopia
   b. Ptosis
   c. Paresis or extraocular muscles

Possible
1. Nystagmus
2. Retinal detachment (ciprofloxacin)
   a. Photopsias
   b. Vitreous floaters
   c. Vitreous hemorrhage

3. Eyelids or conjunctiva
   a. Erythema multiforme
   b. Erythema nodosum
   c. Exfoliative dermatitis
   d. Lyell syndrome

Conditional/unclassified
1. Optic neuropathy (reversible)
2. Uveitis
3. Acute visual loss
4. Papilledema secondary to pseudotumor cerebri

Local ophthalmic use or exposure – topical ocular application
Certain
1. Irritation
   a. Pain
   b. Burning sensation
   c. Lacrimation
   d. Foreign body sensation
2. Eyelids
   a. Crusting – crystalline
   b. Edema
   c. Allergic reactions
   d. Pruritus
3. Cornea
   a. Precipitates – white (Fig. 4.3)
   b. Keratitis
   c. Infiltrates
   d. Superficial punctate keratitis
4. Conjunctiva
   a. Hyperemia
   b. Chemosis
5. Decreased vision
6. Photophobia

Systemic Side Effects
Local ophthalmic use or exposure – topical ocular application
Certain
1. Metallic taste
2. Dermatitis
3. Nausea

Conditional/unclassified
1. Psychosis
2. Seizures
3. Pediatric warning: arthropathy (theoretically under age 12)

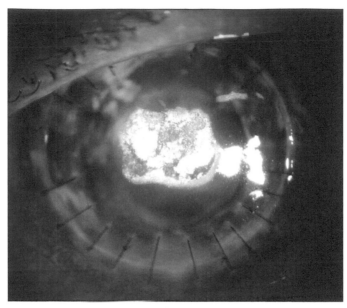

FIG. 4.3 White corneal deposits from topical ocular ciprofloxacin application in corneal transplant.[18]

Clinical Significance

Ciprofloxacin causes relatively few and minor ocular side effects from systemic use. Of all drug-induced side effects seen with this drug, 12% involve the skin. Exacerbations of myasthenia symptoms involving the eye are well documented, but rare. Visual sensations, such as increased glare and increased brightness of color or lights, occur occasionally. From spontaneous reporting systems there are only a few cases of possible optic neuropathy and pseudotumor cerebri with papilledema. Vrabec et al described a case of acute bilateral "count fingers" visual loss associated with ciprofloxacin, which slowly improved after discontinuing the drug.[1] Ciprofloxacin may cause diplopia from possible extraocular muscle tendinitis.[2] From the 171 case reports submitted to spontaneous reporting systems, and although the data were incomplete, this ocular side effect seemed to have resolved with discontinuation of the drug and was transient.

More recently, retinal detachments have been associated with ciprofloxacin therapy. Etminan et al reported a 4 in 10,000 person-years risk of a retinal detachment associated with ciprofloxacin therapy.[3] Han et al postulated that ciprofloxacin may interfere with the vitreous collagen, and Albini postulated a direct cytotoxic affect to the retina.[4,5] Raguideau et al, in a large database study, supported oral fluoroquinolone use and the occurrence of retinal detachments.[6]

VanderBeek wrote an editorial on this study and pointed out possible problems in interpreting the data.[7] In a population-based study, it was found that there was no association of rhegmatogenous retinal detachments or symptomatic retinal breaks with oral fluoroquinolones.[8] Fife et al, in 2 large database case-control studies, also found no association with retinal pathology.[9] To date, it is still unclear if retinal pathology occurs with oral fluoroquinolones. Sandhu et al, in a retrospective cohort study, found no association with oral fluoroquinolones and uveitis, but found these drugs were more often used in systemic diseases that cause uveitis.[10]

Ciprofloxacin ophthalmic solutions are generally well tolerated. Transient ocular burning and discomfort, however, occur in approximately 10% of patients. Seldom does this necessitate discontinuation of the drug. The main side effect is the deposition of the drug as a white crystalline deposit, especially on abraded corneal epithelium or stroma. This may occur in approximately 15–20% of patients using either solution or ointment. Leibowitz as well as Wilhelmus et al showed this is pure ciprofloxacin deposit with continued antibacterial properties.[11,12] Patients under 40 years old and those above 70 years old have a 4 times increased deposition rate compared with those 40–70 years of age. pH affects the precipitation of the antibiotic, as well as sicca and more alkaline surface in the elderly. Precipitates may start as early as 24 hours after starting therapy, may resolve while on full therapy, and can be irrigated off. These deposits may last a few weeks after the drug is discontinued. Other than a foreign body sensation, these deposits are usually well tolerated. The precipitates may not alter the rate of infection, but they may impede epithelialization. Patwardhan et al reported delay from recovery from viral ocular surface infections secondary to topical ocular ciprofloxacin.[13] Sparfloxacin and tosufloxacin are infrequently used compared with ciprofloxacin, so their ocular side effects profile is not as complete. It is clear, however, when given as topical ocular medication that their corneal profile is the same as ciprofloxacin.[14,15] Other ocular side effects secondary to topical ocular application occur in less than 1% of patients.

Systemic reactions may occur from topical ocular ciprofloxacin. The primary ones are a metallic or foul taste occurring in 5% of patients and nausea in 1%. There is a warning based on animal work to not use this drug in patients 12 years and younger for fear of causing degenerative articular changes in weight-bearing joints. There are no human data to support this. Tripathi et al reported an acute psychosis following topical ocular ciprofloxacin with supporting data that oral ciprofloxacin can cause the same.[16] Malladi et al reported topical ocular ciprofloxacin may have caused a reduction in a patient's serum phenytoin levels, allowing breakthrough seizures to occur.[17]

Generic Names:

1. Demeclocycline hydrochloride; 2. doxycycline; 3. minocycline hydrochloride; 4. oxytetracycline; 5. tetracycline hydrochloride.

Proprietary Names:

1. Declomycin; 2. Acticlate, Adoxa, Adoxa Pak, Alodox, Atridox, Avidoxy, Doryx, Doxal, Doxy 100, Doxy 200, Monodoxyne NL, Monodox, Morgidox 1x, Morgidox 2x, NutriDox, Ocudox, Oracea, Oraxyl, PerioStat, Targadox, Vibra-Tabs, Vibramycin; 3. Arestin, Dynacin, Minocin, Minocid PAC, Solodyn, Ximino; 4. Terramycin; 5. Achromycin V, Actisite, Emtet-500, Panmycin, Sumycin.

Primary Use

These bacteriostatic derivatives of polycyclic naphthacene carboxamide are effective against a wide range of Gram-negative and Gram-positive organisms, mycoplasmas, and members of the lymphogranuloma-psittacosis group.

Ocular Side Effects
Systemic administration – intravenous or oral
Certain
1. Myopia
2. Photophobia
3. Decreased vision
4. Eyelids or conjunctiva
   a. Erythema
   b. Edema
   c. Yellow or green discoloration or deposits (doxycycline, tetracycline, minocycline)
   d. Urticaria
5. Sclera – blue-gray, dark blue, or brownish scleral pigmentation (minocycline) (Fig. 4.4)
6. Retinal pigmentation (minocycline)
7. Visual hallucinations
8. May aggravate or cause ocular sicca
9. Decreased contact lens tolerance

Probable
1. Pseudotumor cerebri
2. Myasthenia gravis – aggravated
   a. Diplopia
   b. Ptosis
   c. Paresis of extraocular muscles

Possible
1. Eyelids or conjunctiva
   a. Lupoid syndrome
   b. Erythema multiforme
   c. Lyell syndrome

Local ophthalmic use or exposure – topical application or subconjunctival injection
Certain
1. Irritation
2. Eyelids or conjunctiva
   a. Allergic reactions
   b. Conjunctivitis – nonspecific
3. Keratitis
4. Yellow-brown corneal discoloration (with drug-soaked hydrophilic lenses)

Local ophthalmic use or exposure – intracameral injection
Certain
1. Uveitis
2. Corneal edema
3. Lens damage

Ocular teratogenic effects
Probable
1. Corneal pigmentation – permanent

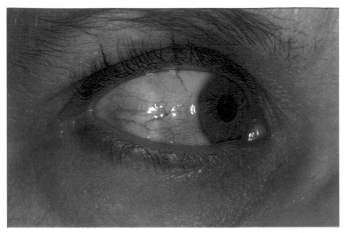

FIG. 4.4 Minocycline blue pigmentation of the sclera.[3]

Clinical Significance

Systemic or ocular use of the tetracyclines rarely causes significant ocular side effects. Although a large variety of drug-induced ocular side effects have been attributed to tetracyclines, most are reversible. This group of drugs can cause pseudotumor cerebri. This is most commonly reported with tetracycline and minocycline. Minocycline possibly possesses greater lipid solubility as it passes into cerebrospinal fluid; therefore it may cause this side effect more readily. Increased intracranial pressure is not dose related and may occur as early as 4 hours after first taking the drug or may occur after many years of drug usage. Although the papilledema may resolve once the drug is discontinued, the visual loss may be permanent.[1] Paresis or paralysis of extraocular muscles may occur secondary to pseudotumor cerebri. This can occur in any age group. Gardner et al felt that this side effect may have been related to an underlying genetic susceptibility.[2] Many patients are obese, which is a risk factor for pseudotumor cerebri and clouds the picture of the role of causation of this drug in this disease. However, most who work in this area feel that tetracycline can cause pseudotumor cerebri. The tetracyclines have been implicated in aggravating or unmasking myasthenia gravis with its own associated ocular findings. Tetracycline has caused hyperpigmentation in light-exposed skin and yellow-brown pigmentation of light-exposed conjunctiva after long-term therapy. This occurs in about 3% of patients taking 400–1600 g. Oral minocycline can cause scleral pigmentation. The pigmentation is most prominent in sun-exposed areas. However, minocycline can cause hyperpigmentation in non–sun-exposed areas, i.e. the roof of the mouth.[3] The pigmentation may resolve over a number of years if the drug is discontinued, or the stain may be permanent. This side effect may be an indication to stop the drug for cosmetic reasons.[3] Yellow-brown discoloration of the cornea can occur if hydrophilic contact lenses are presoaked in tetracycline before ocular application. Bradfield et al described retinal pigmentation after oral minocycline in 1 case.[4] There are reports in the literature and spontaneous reports of dark gray-blue or black deposits in the central macular area in patients on minocycline.[5,6] Spectral-domain optic coherence tomographic scan places these nodular deposits at the level of the pigment epithelium.[6] These patients are often on these medications for a few decades. To date, the only reports of retinal pigmentation have been in patients on minocycline. All tetracycline drugs are photosensitizers, and they may enhance any or all light-induced ocular changes. Doxycycline may be the greatest photosensitizer in this group, with minocycline being the least. However, even with minocycline, in susceptible patients, significant ocular and periocular photosensitivity reactions may occur. Shah et al described 3 cases of ocular and periocular photosensitivity, 1 occurring after only 1 exposure and another after 2 weeks of therapy.[7] The latter was the most severe and had the clinical appearance of an arc-welding injury. This includes intense bilateral photophobia, blepharospasm, lid edema, marked papillary conjunctivitis, and superficial punctate keratitis. This cleared within 2 days after stopping the drug. These

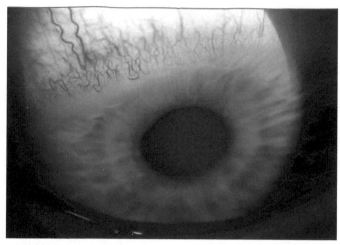

FIG. 4.5 Marginal peripheral ulcerative keratitis (nonstaining) from systemic filgrastim treatment.[2]

drugs are secreted in a crystalline form in the tear film, often in therapeutic concentration. Therefore oral intake may cause or increase ocular irritation in patients with sicca or contact lenses. Long-term therapy may allow the drug or its metabolites to mix with calcium concretions, which may take on characteristics of the drug, such as yellow color and fluorescence. Permanent discoloration of the cornea has been seen in infants whose mothers received high doses of tetracycline during pregnancy.

Generic Name:
Filgrastim.

Proprietary Names:
Neupogen, Zarxio.

Primary Use
A 175 amino acid protein used to prevent infection in neutropenic patients who are receiving myelosuppressive therapy for nonmyeloid malignancies.

Ocular Side Effects
Systemic administration – intravenous
Possible
1. Irritation
   a. Hyperemia
   b. Pain
   c. Foreign body sensation
2. Cornea
   a. Peripheral marginal subepithelial infiltrates
   b. Marginal peripheral ulcerative keratitis (nonstaining) (Fig. 4.5)
3. Photophobia

Conditional/unclassified
1. Anterior uveitis – mild
2. Cataract (high dosage) (infant)

Clinical Significance
There are 2 reports in which bilateral marginal ulcerative keratitis occurred 2–4 days after receiving IV filgrastim.[1,2] There were subepithelial infiltrates similar to those connected to connective tissue disorders such as Wegener granulomatosis. This is associated with ocular hyperemia, foreign body sensation, and significant ocular irritation. There are only 2 such reports for the many thousands of patients who have been exposed to this drug, so this is a rare event or may not even be drug related. One case resolved with the only treatment being artificial tears after the drug was discontinued. In the other case, the patient continued the drug and the eyes were treated with topical ocular steroids, and the infiltrate cleared within 24 hours. There are a few similar cases in the spontaneous reporting systems.

Aljaouni et al reported a single case of a 7-month-old male requiring extensive filgrastim therapy who developed bilateral cataracts after 4 months.[3] The authors felt that this was a rare dose-related, filgrastim-induced lens change requiring cataract extraction.

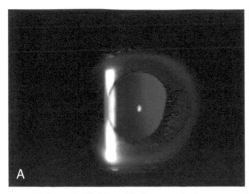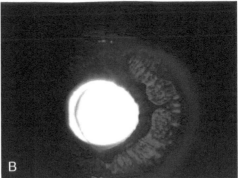

FIG. 4.6 Right and left eye anterior segment photograph. Positive iris transillumination.[13]

Generic Names:
1. Gatifloxacin; 2. levofloxacin; 3. moxifloxacin hydrochloride; 4. norfloxacin; 5. ofloxacin.

Proprietary Names:
1. Tequin, Zymar, Zymaxid; 2. Iquix, Levaquin, Levaquin Leva-Pak, Quixin; 3. Avelox, Avelox ABC Pack, Avelox IV, Moxeza, Vigamox; 4. Noroxin; 5. Floxin, Ocuflox.

Primary Use
These quinolone antibacterial drugs are used primarily against most Gram-negative aerobic bacteria and many Gram-positive aerobic bacteria.

Ocular Side Effects
Systemic administration – intravenous or oral
Probable
1. Eyelids
   a. Hyperpigmentation
   b. Edema
   c. Urticaria
2. Conjunctiva
   a. Hyperemia
   b. Hypersensitivity
3. Visual sensations
   a. Decreased vision
   b. Glare phenomenon (norfloxacin)
   c. Lacrimation
4. Photosensitivity (ofloxacin)
5. Pain

Possible
1. Bilateral acute iris transillumination (BAIT)
   a. Anterior pigment dispersion
   b. Iris

   i. Transillumination defects (Fig. 4.6)
   ii. Atrophy
   iii. Change in color
   iv. Posterior synechiae
   c. Glaucoma
   d. Dyscoria
2. Anterior uveitis
3. Diplopia
4. Pseudotumor cerebri
5. Eyelids or conjunctiva
   a. Erythema multiforme
   b. Erythema nodosum
   c. Exfoliative dermatitis
   d. Lyell syndrome

Conditional/unclassified
1. Visual hallucinations (ofloxacin)
2. Nystagmus (ofloxacin)
3. Toxic optic neuropathy (moxifloxacin)
4. Myasthenia gravis – aggravated

Local ophthalmic use or exposure – topical ocular application
Certain
1. Irritation
   a. Pain
   b. Burning sensation
   c. Lacrimation
   d. Foreign body sensation
2. Eyelids
   a. Edema
   b. Allergic reactions
   c. Pruritus
3. Cornea (Fig. 4.7)
   a. Precipitates – white (rare)
   b. Keratitis

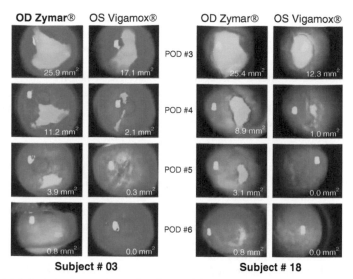

FIG. 4.7 Epithelial defect size on postoperative days 3–6 in two study participants. Slit-lamp photographs were taken with cobalt blue filter after instillation of topical fluorescein drops (original magnification ×16). The photographs on the left represent a patient whose moxifloxacin-treated eye healed on day 6 and whose gatifloxacin-treated eye healed on day 7. This subject also has a peripheral corneal infiltrate on postoperative day 4. The photographs on the right represent a patient whose moxifloxacin-treated eye healed on postoperative day 5 and whose gatifloxacin-treated eye healed on day 7. Calculated surface area of epithelial defects is shown at bottom right of each photograph.[21]

   c. Infiltrates
   d. Superficial punctate keratitis
4. Conjunctiva
   a. Hyperemia
   b. Chemosis
   c. Papillary conjunctivitis
5. Decreased vision
6. Photophobia
7. Miosis (moxifloxacin)

Systemic Side Effects
Local ophthalmic use or exposure – topical ocular application
Certain
1. Dermatitis
2. Nausea

Possible
1. Pediatric warning: arthropathy (theoretically under age 12)

Clinical Significance
Other than some recently suggested possible side effects, systemic administration of this class of drugs is seldom of major clinical significance. These drugs are probably secreted in the tears, which can cause irritation and decreased vision. There are surprisingly few and seldom severe adverse systemic effects from these quinolones. Although hypersensitivity reactions occur, they are uncommon. Photosensitivity may occur rarely, but it appears to be seen most frequently with ofloxacin. Visual sensations are more common with ciprofloxacin and occasionally with norfloxacin. Topical ocular quinolones are generally well tolerated. Ocular pain, erythema, pruritus photophobia, and epiphora occur in a small percentage of patients. Seldom is corneal precipitation of these drugs seen as with ciprofloxacin; however, there are reports with ofloxacin and norfloxacin.[1-3] Awwad et al reported corneal intrastromal gatifloxacin crystal deposits after penetrating keratoplasty, with follow-up discussion by Wittpenn and Cavanaugh.[4-6] Donnenfeld et al reported that topical ocular moxifloxacin can cause papillary miosis, possibly due to prostaglandin release into the anterior chamber.[7] Because moxifloxacin does not contain the preservative benzalkonium chloride, topical ocular toxicity may be less overall.

Over the past decade a confusing, undetermined possible association of this class of drugs with a "pseudo-uveitis" with iritis or iritis alone has been reported. Cases are rare, but a pattern is apparent. This possible drug-induced side effect has been called BAIT syndrome.[8-15] It has primarily been seen with moxifloxacin. Onset may be a few days after starting the drug, but more often after a few weeks to months. It consists of bilateral, irreversible iris transillumination defects and pigment dispersion in the anterior chamber, often with secondary pigment dispersion glaucoma. The pattern varies with severity and is largely dependent on time of discovery. The first sign of onset is often photophobia. Late stages include severe glaucoma, posterior synechiae, dyscoria, changes in iris color, cataracts, and dense iris atrophy. Occasionally this may be unilateral or discovered before the second eye is involved. BAIT syndrome has only been seen in phakic eyes, most likely because posteroanterior clearance of the drug may be impaired.[12] Occasionally there is an associated significant uveitis.[9]

Hinkle et al have shown uveitis associated in rare instances with all fluoroquinolones.[16] However, only a "possible" association could be made. Eadie et al, using a case-control study, found that moxifloxacin and ciprofloxacin appear to increase the risk of uveitis, with levofloxacin posing less of a risk.[17]

There are well over 200+ possible cases in the literature and spontaneous reports of diplopia associated with this class of drugs.[18] This may even be a "probable" to "certain" association based on a number of positive dechallenge and rechallenge cases. Onset may be with a few days to many months after starting the drug. Causation is unknown, but these drugs can cause a tendinitis and tendon rupture in 0.4% of cases.[19] This diplopia is completely reversible when the drug is discontinued. Sodhi et al pointed out that this diplopia may also signal pseudotumor cerebri, which this class of drugs has also been implicated with.[20]

Generic Name:
Gentamicin sulfate.

Proprietary Names:
Garamycin, Genoptic, Genoptic SOP, Gentacidin, Gentafair, Gentak, Gentasol, Ocu-Mycin.

Primary Use
This aminoglycoside is effective against *Pseudomonas aeruginosa*, *Aerobacter*, *E. coli*, *K. pneumoniae*, and *Proteus*.

Ocular Side Effects
Systemic administration – intramuscular, intravenous, or topical
Probable
1. Decreased vision
2. Papilledema secondary to pseudotumor cerebri
3. Loss of eyelashes or eyebrows
4. Eyelids
   a. Photosensitivity
   b. Urticaria
5. Myasthenia gravis – aggravated
   a. Diplopia
   b. Ptosis
   c. Paresis of extraocular muscles
6. Visual hallucinations
7. Oscillopsia

Systemic administration – intratympanic injection
Local ophthalmic use or exposure – topical application or subconjunctival injection
Certain
1. Conjunctiva
   a. Hyperemia
   b. Mucopurulent discharge
   c. Chemosis
   d. Ulceration – necrosis
   e. Mild papillary hypertrophy
   f. Delayed healing
   g. Localized pallor
   h. Pseudomembranous conjunctivitis
2. Eyelids
   a. Allergic reactions
   b. Blepharoconjunctivitis
   c. Depigmentation
3. Cornea
   a. Superficial punctate keratitis
   b. Ulceration
   c. Delayed healing
4. Periocular ulcerative dermatitis (newborn)

Probable – subconjunctival injection
1. Scleral-retinal toxicity and necrosis
2. Extraocular and periocular muscle myopathy
3. Mydriasis

Possible – subconjunctival injection
1. Toxic anterior segment syndrome

Certain
1. Skew extraocular muscle deviation

2. Diplopia
3. Nystagmus

***Local ophthalmic use or exposure –
intravitreal or intraocular injection***
Certain
1. Retina
   a. Infarcts
   b. Retinal edema
   c. Hemorrhages
   d. Opacities
   e. Pigmentary changes
   f. Degeneration
2. Vitreous opacities
3. Optic nerve changes, including atrophy
   a. Retinal edema
   b. Occlusion
   c. Hemorrhages
   d. Ischemia

Clinical Significance

Surprisingly few drug-induced ocular side effects from systemic administration of gentamicin have been reported. Pseudotumor cerebri with secondary papill-edema and visual loss after systemic use of gentamicin are the most clinically significant side effects. Other adverse ocular effects are reversible and transitory after discontinued use of the drug. Marra et al described 2 cases of self-limiting oscillopsia, probably secondary to gentamicin-induced ototoxicity.[1]

Topical ocular gentamicin may cause significant local side effects, the most common being a superficial punctate keratitis. Chronic use can also cause keratinization of the lid margin and blepharitis. Skin depigmentation in blacks, primarily when topical ocular gentamicin was associated with eye-pad use, has been reported. Conjunctival necrosis, especially with fortified solutions, may occur. This is found most often in the inferior nasal conjunctiva and starts as a localized area of hyperemia or pallor that usually stains with fluorescein. The lesions start after 5–7 days on either gentamicin solution or ointment and resolve within 2 weeks after discontinuing the drug. Bullard et al reported 4 cases of pseudomembranous conjunctivitis after topical ocular gentamicin.[2] These also occurred inferiorly and started with intense focal bulbar conjunctival hyperemia, mucopurulent discharge, and palpebral conjunctival papillae. The membranes appeared 4–7 days after starting therapy and resolved 4–5 days after the drug was stopped. A worldwide shortage of erythromycin or tetracycline ophthalmic ointment resulted in the use of gentamicin ophthalmic ointment for the prophylaxis of ophthalmic neonatorum. Numerous reports, including Nathawad et al, Merlob et al, and Binenbaum et al, reported characteristic periocular ulcerative dermatitis that occurred within 1–2 days after exposure and resolved within 2–3 weeks.[3-5] Conjunctiva was uninvolved. This contact dermatitis was felt to occur due to a vaso-occlusive effect of the gentamicin or an irritative effect of the antibiotic or its preservative, paraben. Libert et al and D'Amico et al described lamellated cytoplasmic storage inclusion containing lipid material in the conjunctiva secondary to gentamicin injections.[6,7] Awan described paresthesia of the eyes from topical ocular gentamicin and pupillary dilation from subconjunctival injections.[8] Chapman et al showed that subconjunctival injections of gentamicin could cause muscle fiber degeneration with myopathy causing ocular motility impairment.[9]

Intraocular gentamicin has caused severe retinal ischemia, rubeosis, iritis, neovascular glaucoma, optic atrophy, and blindness. A number of cases of inadvertent intraocular injections have been reported in the literature and to spontaneous reporting systems. The degree of ocular damage is primarily dependent on trauma of the injection, volume of the injection, location of the injection, and concentration of the drug. Injections into the anterior chamber are rarely devastating, in part due to early recognition, small volume, and immediate irrigation. Koban et al reported toxic anterior segment syndrome after inadvertent overdose of gentamicin in the anterior chamber.[10] Inadvertent posterior injection may result in elevated intraocular pressure with secondary vascular occlusions. In addition, trauma of the injection itself may cause intraocular bleeding and retinal detachment.

Although there are earlier publications outlining posterior gentamicin toxicity from intravitreal injections, Campochiaro et al, along with the follow-up letter to the editor by Grizzard, gives the most complete picture.[11,12] In essence, even 0.1 mg of gentamicin may cause significant changes because gravity allows the drug to concentrate in a dependent area for an indefinite period. If this dependent area is in the fovea, permanent visual changes have occurred. Fluorescein angiograms show discrete geographic involvement, with the nonperfusion not corresponding to the vascular pattern. Campochiaro et al and Grizzard et al pointed out that the topography and the abrupt "cookie cutter" margins suggest an event mediated by the drug in contact with the retinal surface.[12,13] These findings show that a localized infarct is the end result of the gentamicin toxicity. Visual acuity loss has included cases of blindness. Additional findings have included retinal opacities, retinal hemorrhages and edema, neovascular glaucoma, retinal pigmentary degeneration, and optic atrophy.

Heath Jeffery et al reported macular hole formation possibly caused by subconjunctival gentamicin injection seeping through an unsutured 25-gauge sclerotomy.[14]

Gentamicin is given by intratympanic injection for the management of Meniere's disease. Leon Ruiz et al and Dresner et al reported total or near-full skew deviation and head tilt after a number of months of gentamicin treatment.[15,16] Complex cyclotorsion, gaze stability, vestibulo-ocular reflex, and diplopia may occur.

Generic Name:
Kanamycin sulfate.

Proprietary Name:
Kantrex.

Primary Use
This aminoglycoside is effective against Gram-negative organisms and in drug-resistant *Staphylococcus*.

Ocular Side Effects
Systemic administration – intramuscular or intravenous
Certain
1. Decreased vision
2. Eyelids or conjunctiva – allergic reactions

Probable
1. Myasthenia gravis – aggravated
   a. Diplopia
   b. Ptosis
   c. Paresis of extraocular muscles

Conditional/unclassified
1. Optic neuritis

Local ophthalmic use or exposure – subconjunctival injection
Certain
1. Irritation
2. Eyelids or conjunctiva – allergic reactions

Clinical Significance
Systemic and ocular side effects due to kanamycin are quite rare. Myasthenia gravis occurs more frequently if kanamycin is given in combination with other antibiotics, such as neomycin, gentamicin, polymyxin B, colistin, or streptomycin. Allergic reactions with cross-sensitivity have been reported for gentamycin, but not for neomycin.[1] Adverse ocular reactions to this drug are reversible, transitory, and seldom have residual complications. Although optic neuritis has been reported to be associated with this drug, it has not been proven.

Generic Name:
Linezolid.

Proprietary Name:
Zyvox.

Primary Use
A synthetic antibiotic (oxazolidinone) for use in drug-resistant bacterial infections.

Ocular Side Effects
Systemic administration – intravenous or oral
Certain
1. Decreased vision
2. Color vision defect
3. Optic neuropathy (Fig. 4.8)
   a. Peripapillary nerve fiber layer edema – initially inferior to the disc
   b. Microhemorrhages
   c. Hyperemia – initially inferior to the disc
   d. Temporal pallor
   e. Atrophy
4. Visual field defects
   a. Centrocecal scotomas
   b. Arcuate scotomas
5. Blindness

Possible
1. Cataracts (newborn)

Clinical Significance
The use of this antibiotic is primarily in patients who have a drug-resistant organism, often in a life-threatening circumstance. Ocular symptoms, although rare, are seldom seen in the first 28 days of therapy other than decreased vision. Azamfirei et al reported a possible case of severe neuropathy after 16 days.[1]

The initial complete review of linezolid neuropathy is by Javaheri et al.[2] Their seminal case is a 6-year-old male taking linezolid for 1 year who developed bilateral optic neuropathy with 20/400 vision OU, disc edema, hyperemia, and peripapillary retinal nerve fiber layer swelling confirmed by optic coherence tomography.

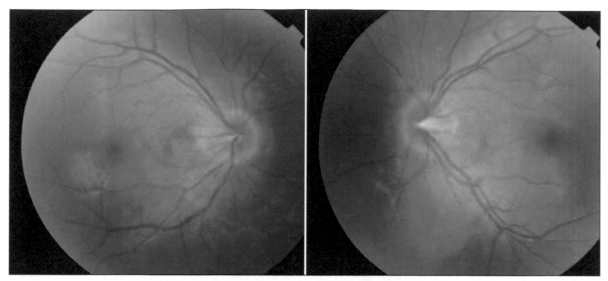

FIG. 4.8 Bilateral temporal disc pallor from systemic linezolid treatment.[11]

After linezolid was discontinued, in 3 months vision was 20/20 OU, with the only disc abnormality a bilateral mild temporal pallor. This classic presentation of toxic linezolid neuropathy has been confirmed.[3] If the drug is stopped at these early findings, full recovery usually occurs at 3 months. Even at late stages of recognition, some recovery is expected. Otherwise, irreversible visual loss may occur. Lee et al described a case of severe bilateral optic neuropathy with bilateral central scotoma after 2 months of treatment with linezolid.[4] The drug was continued for 6 more months, and the patient's visual acuity decreased to 20/200- and 20/300. Three months after stopping the drug, visual acuity was 20/50 and 20/25; however, there was no effect on the peripheral neuropathy. Javaheri et al and Wang et al have reported linezolid-related mitochondrial optic neuropathies.[2,5] The clinical features include slow, progressive, bilateral loss of central vision; dyschromatopsia; central or cecocentral scotoma; and loss of high spatial frequency contrast sensitivity.[5] Patients often describe the visual loss as a central haze or dark cloud. Pain is not a feature. The optic disc may initially show inferior hyperemia or edema. Over time, temporal pallor of the disc may occur. Over 200 cases have been reported in the literature and spontaneous reports.

There are cases of optic neuropathy due to this drug in children.[2,6] Linam et al have suggested monthly ophthalmic examinations after ≥3 months of therapy. If long-term therapy is needed, a baseline examination may be indicated.[7]

Ishii et al, based on 1 case, suggested that microcystic spaces occur in the inner retina and resolve when the drug is discontinued.[8]

There is a report of cataracts and thrombocytopenia in a newborn after linezolid exposure. In this case, vacuoles were located in the peripheral lens and near the posterior lens capsule.[9] These cleared shortly after stopping the drug.

Patients on linezolid are often very ill and bedridden; therefore ophthalmic testing may need to be done at the bedside. Polypharmacy is universal, and various drug side effects caused by other drugs cloud the diagnosis.[10]

Recommendations[10]

1. Perform an ophthalmic evaluation at 3–4 months after starting the drug, and if the patient remains on the drug without visual symptoms, perform further evaluations every 2–3 months. Baseline examination after 1 month of therapy, although ideal, may not be cost-effective.

2. If the patient is on linezolid more than 28 days and bedridden, ocular examination should include near visual acuity (with presbyopic correction), color testing (HRR or Cambridge Colour Test), red Amsler grid, and observation of optic discs. If the patient is moveable, then visual fields (24-2) and optic coherence tomography (OCT) of the nerve fiber layer at the disc margin should be considered.

3. If any visual changes occur, i.e. decreased vision, color vision abnormalities, or any visual field change, the patient should see an ophthalmologist.
4. If diagnosis of optic neuropathy is suspected, a risk–benefit ratio is needed to determine if it is appropriate to continue the medication. Permanent visual loss, including legal blindness, has occurred if the drug is continued; therefore informed consent is essential.

Generic Name:
Nalidixic acid.

Proprietary Name:
Generic only.

Primary Use
This bactericidal naphthyridine derivative is effective against *E. coli*, *Aerobacter*, and *Klebsiella*. Its primary clinical use is against *Proteus*.

Ocular Side Effects
Systemic administration – oral
Certain
1. Visual sensations
   a. Glare phenomenon
   b. Flashing lights – white or colored
   c. Scintillating scotomas – may be colored
2. Color vision defect – objects have green, yellow, blue, or violet tinge
3. Papilledema secondary to pseudotumor cerebri
4. Decreased vision
5. Eyelids or conjunctiva
   a. Photosensitivity
   b. Edema
   c. Urticaria

Probable
1. Photophobia
2. Paresis of extraocular muscles
3. Decreased accommodation
4. Nystagmus
5. Visual hallucinations

Possible
1. Eyelids or conjunctiva – lupoid syndrome

Clinical Significance
Numerous ocular side effects due to nalidixic acid have been reported. The most common adverse ocular reaction is a curious visual disturbance, which includes brightly colored appearances of objects as the main feature. This often appears soon after the drug is taken. Temporary visual loss has also occurred and lasted from half an hour to 72 hours. Probably the most serious ocular reaction is papilledema secondary to elevated intracranial pressure. Most of the reports concerning pseudotumor cerebri deal with children and adolescents, the oldest being 20 years of age. A large series of pseudotumor cerebri occurred in infants below 6 months of age given 100–150 mg/kg/day for acute bacillary dysentery.[1] Use of nalidixic acid during pregnancy carries the possible prenatal risk of increased intracranial pressure. Most adverse ocular reactions due to nalidixic acid are transitory and reversible if the dosage is decreased or the drug is discontinued.

Generic Name:
Neomycin sulfate.

Proprietary Names:
Mycifradin, Neo-fradin, Neo-tab.

Primary Use
These bactericidal aminoglycosidic drugs are effective against *P. aeruginosa*, *Aerobacter*, *K. pneumoniae*, *Proteus vulgaris*, *E. coli*, *Salmonella*, *Shigella*, and most strains of *S. aureus*.

Ocular Side Effects
Systemic administration – neomycin powder to mucous membranes
Probable
1. Myasthenia gravis – aggravated
   a. Diplopia
   b. Ptosis
   c. Paresis of extraocular muscles
2. Decreased or absent pupillary reaction to light

Local ophthalmic use or exposure – topical application or subconjunctival injection
Certain
1. Irritation
   a. Hyperemia
   b. Pain
   c. Edema
   d. Burning sensation
2. Eyelids or conjunctiva
   a. Allergic reactions
   b. Erythema
   c. Blepharoconjunctivitis – follicular
   d. Urticaria
3. Punctate keratitis

Conditional/unclassified
1. Nystagmus (in DMSO ointment)

Local ophthalmic use or exposure –
intracameral injection
Certain
1. Uveitis
2. Corneal edema
3. Lens damage

Clinical Significance

These drugs are not used parenterally because of nephrotoxicity and ototoxicity. There are well-documented reports of decreased or absent pupillary reactions due to application of neomycin to the pleural or peritoneal cavities during a thoracic or abdominal operation.

Topical ocular application of neomycin has been reported to cause allergic conjunctival or lid reactions in 4% of patients using this drug. If neomycin is used topically for longer than 7–10 days on inflammatory dermatosis, the incidence of allergic reaction is increased 13-fold over matched controls. Neomycin preparations for minor infections should rarely be used more than 7–10 days. Also, if the patient has been previously exposed to neomycin, there is a significantly higher chance of an allergic response. In one study, neomycin was found to be 1 of the 3 most common drugs causing periocular allergic contact dermatitis. Rarely will neomycin be given alone in topical ocular medication. Often a steroid is added, which may mask the incidence of hypersensitivity reactions. Additional antibiotics are frequently added to increase the antimicrobial spectrum. Some feel that of the more commonly used topical ocular antibiotics, neomycin has the greatest toxicity to the corneal epithelium. It probably produces plasma membrane injury and cell death, primarily of the superficial cell layers, with chronic topical exposure. Dohlman described tiny snowflakes on the corneal epithelial surface, along with superficial punctate keratitis persisting for weeks after topical ocular neomycin use.[1] After long-term ocular exposure to neomycin, fungi superinfections have been reported. Nystagmus has been reported in a 9-year-old child after topical treatment of the skin with 1% neomycin in 11% dimethyl sulfoxide ointment (DMSO).

Generic Name:
Nitrofurantoin.

Proprietary Names:
Furadantin, Macrodantin, Macrobid.

Primary Use
This bactericidal furan derivative is effective against specific organisms that cause urinary tract infections, especially *E. coli*, enterococci, and *S. aureus*.

Ocular Side Effects
Systemic administration – oral
Certain
1. Irritation
   a. Lacrimation
   b. Burning sensation
   c. Epiphora
2. Decreased vision
3. Eyelids or conjunctiva
   a. Allergic reactions
   b. Photosensitivity
   c. Edema
   d. Urticaria
   e. Loss of eyelashes or eyebrows
4. Color vision defect – objects have yellow tinge

Probable
1. Optic neuritis
2. Papilledema secondary to pseudotumor cerebri
3. Myasthenia gravis – aggravated
   a. Diplopia
   b. Ptosis – unilateral or bilateral
   c. Paresis of extraocular muscle

Possible
1. Retinal – crystalline retinopathy (long-term therapy)
2. Eyelids or conjunctiva
   a. Lupoid syndrome
   b. Erythema multiforme
   c. Lyell syndrome

Conditional/unclassified
1. Constricted visual field
2. Achromatopsia

Ocular Teratogenic Effects
Systemic administration - oral
Possible
1. Anophthalmia
2. Microphthalmos

Clinical Significance
A unique ocular side effect secondary to nitrofurantoin is a severe ocular pruritus, burning, and tearing reaction, which may persist long after discontinuing the drug. Aggravating or causing ocular myasthenia has been well documented with nitrofurantoin. This is probably due to interference in the transmission

of the neurologic impulse pharmacologically to the resting muscle.[1] In addition, various degrees of polyneuropathies with demyelination and degeneration of sensory and motor nerves have occurred with long-term use of nitrofurantoin, probably on a toxic basis. Pseudotumor cerebri associated with nitrofurantoin therapy has been reported.[2] Khwaja et al reported an acute case of bilateral decreased vision, achromatopsia, and visual field constriction with complete recovery 2 weeks after discontinuing nitrofurantoin.[3] Ibanez et al reported an intraretinal crystalline deposit in both eyes of a 69-year-old male who for 19 years received nitrofurantoin daily for a chronic urinary tract infection.[4]

Crider et al reported congenital ocular defects secondary to nitrofurantoins from data from the National Birth Defects Prevention Study.[5]

Generic Name:
Polymyxin B sulfate.

Proprietary Name:
Generic and multi-ingredient preparations only.

Primary Use
This bactericidal polypeptide is effective against Gram-negative bacilli, especially *P. aeruginosa*.

Ocular Side Effects
Systemic administration – intramuscular, intrathecal, intravenous, or topical
Probable
1. Myasthenia gravis – aggravated
   a. Diplopia
   b. Ptosis
   c. Paresis of extraocular muscles
2. Decreased vision
3. Diplopia
4. Nystagmus
5. Mydriasis

Local ophthalmic use or exposure – topical application or subconjunctival injection
Certain
1. Irritation – pain
2. Eyelids or conjunctiva – allergic reactions
   a. Pruritus
   b. Edema
   c. Erythema

Probable
1. Myasthenia gravis – aggravated
   a. Diplopia
   b. Ptosis
   c. Paresis of extraocular muscles
2. Anaphylactic reaction

Local ophthalmic use or exposure – intracameral injection
Certain
1. Uveitis
2. Corneal edema
3. Lens damage

Possible
1. Anaphylactic reaction

Clinical Significance
Although ocular side effects due to polymyxin B sulfate are well documented, they are quite rare and seldom of major clinical importance. The drug is rarely used by itself as a topical ocular medication, so the true incidence of side effects is difficult to determine. Myasthenia gravis is transitory and does occur from topical ocular administration. To date, we are unaware of systemic polymyxin B sulfate toxicity from topical ocular medication other than transitory neuromuscular transmission defects, such as myasthenia gravis–type clinical syndrome. Some systemic absorption may occur, e.g. if the drug is given every hour for corneal ulcers. There are reports of anaphylactic reactions from topical polymyxin B–bacitracin applications. The clinically important side effects are secondary to intracameral injections, where permanent changes to the cornea and lens have been reported. Although extremely rare, anaphylaxis secondary to polymyxin B–trimethoprim eye drops in a 2-year-old child has been reported.[1]

Generic Names:
1. Sulfacetamide sodium; 2. sulfadiazine; 3. sulfafurazole (sulfisoxazole); 4. sulfamethizole; 5. sulfamethoxazole; 6. sulfanilamide; 7. sulfasalazine; 8. sulfathiazole.

Proprietary Names:
1. Ak-Sulf, Bleph-10, Carmol, Cetamide, Isopto Cetamide, Klaron, Mexar, Ocu-Sul, Ocusulf-10, Ovace, Ovace Plus, RE-10, Rosula NS, Seb-Prev, Sodium Sulamyd, Sulf-10, Sulfac, Vanocin; 2. Multi-ingredient preparation only; 3. Gantrisin; 4. Multi-ingredient preparation only; 5. Multi-ingredient preparation only; 6. AVC; 7. Azulfidine, Azulfidine En-Tabs, Sulfazine, Sulfazine EC; 8. Multi-ingredient preparation only.

Primary Use
The sulfonamides are bacteriostatic drugs effective against most Gram-positive and some Gram-negative organisms.

Ocular Side Effects
Systemic administration – oral
Certain
1. Decreased vision
2. Myopia – transitory
3. Irritation
   a. Lacrimation
   b. Photosensitivity
4. Keratitis
5. Color vision defect – objects have yellow or red tinge
6. Periorbital edema
7. Visual hallucinations
8. Decreased anterior chamber depth – may precipitate acute glaucoma
9. Eyelids or conjunctiva
   a. Allergic reactions
   b. Conjunctivitis – nonspecific
   c. Urticaria
   d. Purpura
   e. Pemphigoid lesion with or without symblepharon
   f. Loss of eyelashes or eyebrows
10. Contact lenses stained yellow
11. Uveitis

Possible
1. Optic neuritis
2. Myasthenia gravis – aggravated
   a. Diplopia
   b. Ptosis
   c. Paresis of extraocular muscles
3. Papilledema secondary to pseudotumor cerebri
4. Vivid, light lavender–colored retinal vascular tree
5. Eyelids or conjunctiva
   a. Lupoid syndrome
   b. Erythema multiforme
   c. Exfoliative dermatitis
   d. Lyell syndrome

Local ophthalmic use or exposure – topical ocular application
Certain
1. Irritation
2. Eyelids or conjunctiva
   a. Allergic reactions
   b. Conjunctivitis – follicular
   c. Deposits
   d. Photosensitivity
   e. Hyperemia
3. Delayed corneal wound healing

Possible
1. Eyelids or conjunctiva
   a. Lupoid syndrome
   b. Erythema multiforme

Conditional/unclassified
1. Cornea – peripheral immune ring

Clinical Significance
Although there are numerous reported ocular side effects from systemic sulfa medication, most are rare and reversible. Probably the most common ocular side effect seen in patients on systemic therapy is myopia. This is transient, with or without induced astigmatism, usually bilateral, and may exceed several diopters. This is most likely due to an increased anteroposterior lens diameter secondary to ciliary body edema. In rare instances, this may decrease the depth of the anterior chamber or possibly cause a choroidal effusion, inducing angle-closure glaucoma.[1] Tilden et al reported 12 cases of uveitis attributed to systemic use of sulfonamide derivatives.[2] Most of the cases were bilateral, occurring within 24 hours to as long as 8 days after first exposure to the sulfonamide. Three patients had a positive rechallenge with a recurrence of bilateral uveitis within 24 hours. Some of the patients had systemic findings of Stevens-Johnson syndrome, erythema multiforme, diffuse macular-vesicular rashes, stomatitis, glossitis, and granulomatous hepatitis. Optic neuritis has been reported even in low oral dosages and is usually reversible with full recovery of vision.[3]

The ophthalmologist should be aware that anaphylactic reactions, Stevens-Johnson syndrome, and exfoliative dermatitis have all been reported, although rarely from topical ocular administration of sulfa preparations. Fine et al reported a single case of toxic epidermal necrolysis within 2 hours after ocular application of sulfonamide.[4] In a letter to the editor, Waller et al discussed the phrase "supports a causal relationship."[5] Ocular irritation from crystalline sulfa in the tears may occur. Gutt et al reported immune rings in the peripheral cornea associated with topical ocular sulfamethoxazole.[6]

Generic Name:
Telithromycin.

Proprietary Name:
Ketek.

Primary Use
A fairly new class of antibacterial drugs, ketolides are used in the management of community-acquired

pneumonia, acute exacerbation of chronic bronchitis, or acute bacterial sinusitis.

Ocular Side Effects
Systemic administration – oral
Certain
1. Decreased vision
2. Difficulty focusing
3. Delayed accommodation

Probable
1. Visual field disturbance (various scotomas)
2. Myasthenia gravis – aggravated
   a. Diplopia
   b. Ptosis
   c. Paresis or extraocular muscles

Clinical Significance
Telithromycin causes a reversible, bilateral, central decreased vision and a delay in accommodation, most frequently described as a delay in focusing when adjusting from near to far vision. This occurs in approximately 0.8% of patients and is twice as frequent in women than men. Typically, it first occurs within 1–3 days after starting therapy and at the time of peak blood levels of the drug. The effect occurs within 1–2 hours after dosing and lasts a mean of 2 hours. In some patients this may happen after each dose, but in others the visual side effects no longer occur after 1–3 days. The visual side effects may or may not occur if the patient retakes the drug at a later date. Visual field changes and diplopia are very rare events. Most patients with visual symptoms maintain normal visual acuities, but some patients should modify their activities, such as driving and operating machinery. The *Physicians' Desk Reference* (PDR) states an incidence of severe visual impairment, moderate decreased vision, or mild diplopia occurring from 0–2%.[1] Telithromycin has the potential to exacerbate myasthenia gravis in patients who have a preexisting myasthenia. Taking the drug at bedtime may eliminate some of the ocular side effects. These side effects are said to occur in part due to the drug's anticholinergic effect.

Generic Name:
Tobramycin.

Proprietary Names:
TOBI, Tobradex, Zylet.

Primary Use
This aminoglycoside is effective against many Gram-negative organisms, including *P. aeruginosa, E. coli, K.* *pneumoniae, Proteus, Enterobacter,* and some Gram-positive organisms, including staphylococci and streptococci.

Ocular Side Effects
Systemic administration – intramuscular or intravenous
Certain
1. Decreased vision
2. Nystagmus

Probable
1. Myasthenia gravis – aggravated
   a. Diplopia
   b. Ptosis
   c. Paresis of extraocular muscles

Conditional/unclassified
1. Color vision defect
2. Visual hallucinations

Local ophthalmic use or exposure – topical ocular application
Certain
1. Eyelids and conjunctiva
   a. Hyperemia
   b. Edema
   c. Burning sensation – pain
   d. Pruritus
   e. Allergic reactions
   f. Conjunctival necrosis (fortified solutions) (Fig. 4.9)
2. Epiphora
3. Superficial punctate keratitis
4. Photosensitivity

Probable
1. Myasthenia gravis – aggravated
   a. Diplopia
   b. Ptosis
   c. Paresis of extraocular muscles

Tobramycin-soaked collagen shield
Certain
1. Cornea
   a. Keratitis
   b. Edema
   c. Endothelial damage

Inadvertent ocular exposure – intraocular injection
Certain
1. Optic atrophy

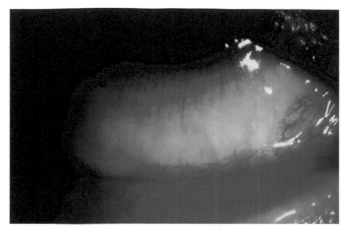

FIG. 4.9 Bulbar conjunctival ischemia and necrosis from topical tobramycin. [8]

2. Retinal degeneration

Inadvertent ocular exposure – subconjunctival injection
Probable
1. Macular infarction

Inadvertent ocular exposure – ointment in anterior chamber
Probable
1. Uveitis
2. Glaucoma

Clinical Significance

Few drug-induced ocular side effects from systemic administration of tobramycin have been reported. Decreased vision is rare and transitory. Nystagmus occurs secondary to tobramycin-induced vestibular toxicity. This drug can induce or aggravate myasthenia gravis by interfering with neuromuscular transmission.[1] Other findings are so rare it is difficult to prove they are drug related.

Topical ocular toxicity of tobramycin is totally dependent on concentration, frequency, and the integrity of the corneal epithelium and stoma. In nonfortified solutions, the incidences of hypersensitivity reactions occur in about 3–4% of patients. Superficial punctate keratitis is rare, seen primarily with frequent dosing or with fortified solutions. By stopping the drug, ocular tissues return to normal in a few days, but occasionally it may require over a month. Systemic absorption from topical ocular application is minimal with normal anterior segments; however, with ulcerated corneas or with fortified solutions, absorption can occur. There is a case report by Khella et al of exacerbation of myasthenia gravis by topical ocular tobramycin, betaxolol, and dexamethasone.[2] There are a few spontaneous case reports of topical ocular tobramycin, alone or in a steroid combination, causing or enhancing myasthenia gravis. These patients had chronic renal disease with probable increased serum blood levels of the drug. One of these cases resulted in a lawsuit. There is also a spontaneous case report of anaphylaxis after a topical ocular combination of tobramycin, a steroid, and Naphcon-A.

Systemic absorption and local toxicity significantly increase in collagen-soaked tobramycin shields. Garzozi et al reported a case of inadvertent tobramycin ophthalmic ointment entering the anterior chamber through a microperforation after radial keratectomy.[3] This was followed by 3 episodes of uveitis and glaucoma. The endothelial cell count was reduced by one-third, and the iris texture was slightly atrophic compared with the fellow eye. Animal studies confirm the toxicity of tobramycin to the corneal endothelial cell. Retinal degeneration and optic atrophy have followed inadvertent intraocular injection of tobramycin.[4] Intraocular complications have probably occurred from subconjunctival injection, with the drug entering the eye through the cataract wound, or after glaucoma surgery.[5,6] Campochiaro et al reported 3 cases of macular infarctions after subconjunctival injections or tobramycin.[7]

Generic Name:
Trimethoprim.

Proprietary Name:
Primsol.

Primary Use

Used systemically in the management of urinary traction infections. Also used in combination with polymyxin B as a topical ocular antibiotic.

Ocular Side Effects

Systemic administration – oral
Possible
1. Uveitis
2. Photophobia
3. May aggravate or cause ocular sicca
4. Periorbital edema
5. Photosensitivity

Local ophthalmic use or exposure with polymyxin B
Certain
1. Irritation
   a. Hyperemia
   b. Pain
2. Eyelids or conjunctiva
   a. Allergic reactions
   b. Edema

Clinical Significance

All ocular side effects appear to be reversible with no lasting sequelae. Uveitis is not proven, with 3 case reports in the literature, although there are an additional 14 cases in the spontaneous reporting systems.[1-3] If uveitis occurs when starting or on this antibiotic, consider stopping the drug because to date there is no evidence that the uveitis will resolve without doing so. Sulfonamides are often given with trimethoprim, and sulfonamide is a known cause of uveitis, so some of these cases may not be due to trimethoprim.[4,5] The drug is well known to cause xerostomia, so possibly it could also aggravate or cause ocular sicca. Trimethoprim is a photosensitizing drug, so it may cause some ocular photophobia or eyelid changes. Topical ocular trimethoprim at commercial dosages seldom causes ocular side effects.

CLASS: ANTIFUNGAL DRUGS

Generic Name:
Amphotericin B.

Proprietary Names:
Abelcet, AmBisome, Amphocin, Amphotec, Fungizone.

Primary Use

This polyene fungistatic drug is effective against *Blastomyces, Histoplasma, Cryptococcus, Coccidioides, Candida,* and *Aspergillus.*

Ocular Side Effects

Systemic administration – intrathecal or intravenous
Probable
1. Decreased vision – transitory

Possible
1. Uveitis
2. Paresis of extraocular muscles

Conditional/unclassified
1. Retinal exudates
2. Diplopia
3. Blindness (intravenous)

Local ophthalmic use or exposure – topical ocular application or subconjunctival injection
Certain
1. Irritation
   a. Pain
   b. Burning sensation
2. Punctate keratitis
3. Eyelids or conjunctiva
   a. Allergic reactions
   b. Ulceration
   c. Conjunctivitis – follicular
   d. Necrosis (subconjunctival injection)
   e. Nodules (subconjunctival injection)
   f. Yellow discoloration (subconjunctival injection)
4. Uveitis
5. Hyphema
6. Delayed wound healing

Local ophthalmic use or exposure – intracameral injection
Certain
1. Uveitis
2. Corneal edema

Probable
1. Lens damage

Clinical Significance

Seldom are significant ocular side effects seen from systemic administration of amphotericin B, except with intrathecal or intravenous injections. In general, transitory decreased vision is the most common ocular side effect. Allergic reactions are so rare that initially it was felt they did not even occur. Li et al reported that after intravenous amphotericin B, a patient with previously bilateral normal vision went to irreversible light perception within 10 hours and optic atrophy within 10 weeks.[1] Intravenous amphotericin B rarely causes uveitis.[2] There are occasional spontaneous case reports of this side effect.

Topical ocular administration of amphotericin B can produce significant conjunctival and corneal irritative responses. This drug can affect cell membranes and allow increased penetration of other drugs through the cornea. There have been rare reports of marked iridocyclitis with small hyphema occurring after each exposure of topical ocular amphotericin B. The formation of salmon-colored, raised nodules can occur secondary to subconjunctival injection, especially if the dosage exceeds 5 mg.[3] These regress somewhat with time. The injection of this drug subconjunctivally or subcutaneously can cause permanent yellowing. Some clinicians feel that amphotericin B is too toxic to the tissue to be given subconjunctivally. However, in extreme circumstances, even intracorneal injections have been done.[4]

Intravitreal administration of amphotericin B is used for endophthalmitis and corneal ulcers. Sharma et al injected intracameral amphotericin B in the dose of 5–10 μg in 1 mL of 5% dextrose. Overall, 81% had no complications, 11% developed anterior uveitis, and 3.6% developed endothelial toxicity or lens changes.[5] Payne et al described 3 cases of inadvertent, higher-than-normal concentrations of this drug with resultant cataracts, intraocular inflammation, and rhegmatogenous retinal detachment.[6]

Generic Name:
Griseofulvin.

Proprietary Names:
Fulvicin P/G, Fulvicin U/F, Grifulvin V, Gris-PEG, Grisactin.

Primary Use
This oral antifungal drug is effective against tinea infections of the nails, skin, and hair.

Ocular Side Effects
Systemic administration – oral
Certain
1. Decreased vision
2. Visual hallucinations
3. Eyelids or conjunctiva

 a. Allergic reactions
 b. Hyperemia
 c. Edema
 d. Photosensitivity
 e. Urticaria

Probable
1. Papilledema secondary to pseudotumor cerebri

Possible
1. Eyelids or conjunctiva
 a. Lupoid syndrome
 b. Exfoliative dermatitis
 c. Erythema multiforme

Conditional/unclassified
1. Macular edema (transient)
2. Systemic lupus erythematosus (SLE)
3. Superficial corneal opacities
4. Color vision defect

Clinical Significance
Systemic griseofulvin rarely causes ocular side effects, but severe allergic reactions with secondary ocular involvement may occur. Decreased vision rarely occurs and seldom requires stopping the drug except in cases of pseudotumor cerebri. Delman et al reported a single case of unilateral, greenish vision with transient macular edema possibly secondary to this drug.[1] There is a case of bilateral superficial corneal deposits resembling Meesman's corneal dystrophy with ocular injection and superficial punctate keratitis, which was reported to the spontaneous reporting systems, that resolved within 1 week after discontinuation of the drug. This drug is photosensitizing, and increased light exposure increases the prevalence of eyelid and conjunctival reactions.

Generic Name:
Voriconazole.

Proprietary Name:
VFEND.

Primary Use
This triazole antifungal drug's greatest use is in aspergillosis infections.

Ocular Side Effects
Systemic administration – intravenous or oral
Certain
1. Decreased vision

2. Altered or enhanced visual perception
3. Photosensitivity
4. Color vision defect
5. Visual hallucinations
6. Abnormal electroretinogram (ERG)

Possible
1. Eyelids or conjunctiva – erythema multiforme
2. Cutaneous rash and photosensitivity (when used with retinol)

Conditional/unclassified
1. Visual field changes
   a. Cecocentral scotomas
   b. Arcuate scotoma
2. Optic neuropathy

Clinical Significance
The adverse ocular side effects of voriconazole are complicated by the underlying disease that it is used to treat. The "adverse reaction" data in the *Physicians' Desk Reference* (PDR) mirror this, with many reactions that are possibly not due to the drug.[1] To date, all ocular drug reactions appear to be reversible.

Voriconazole has unique ocular side effects. The most common visual complaints are altered or enhanced visual perception, "enhanced perception of light," "brighter lights and objects," decreased or "hazy" vision, and photophobia ("dazzle" or "glare").[2] The onset of these symptoms occurs within 15–30 minutes after exposure (more rapid with IV than oral), with a mean duration of 30–60 minutes (IV more prolonged than oral). In rare instances, these visual phenomena may last 1–2 weeks. With repeat exposure, the incidence and severity of the visual reaction decrease in most patients. The altered visual perceptions are reversible and seldom cause a patient to discontinue using the drug. This reaction occurs in up to 38% of patients, most frequently in the very young and the elderly, and is more pronounced when given intravenously. Humphrey visual field testing showed overall a slight drop in mean sensitivity, resolving in a few days after the drug was discontinued. Patients are most often unaware of decreased color vision and/or any changes in their visual field. Visual hallucinations occurred in 4.7% of patients exposed to voriconazole.[3-5]

The certainty of these visual effects due to voriconazole is a combination of positive rechallenges, high incidences, typical pattern of onset and course, and data to show peak onset associated with peak serum levels. The mechanism of voriconazole on the visual system possibly is a retinal effect. Possibly, voriconazole may keep the retinal receptors in an artificially "light-adapted" state, acting on the mechanism of the photo transductor cascade and/or horizontal cell coupling. The importance of these studies to the ophthalmologist is that most findings to date are reversible and nearly always of short duration. Kadikoy et al reported a single case of persistent photopsia.[6] Laties et al reported a long-term, multicenter, open-label comparative center study trial that showed no evidence of an effect of voriconazole on long-term visual function.[7] There have been scattered spontaneous reports of optic neuropathy and retinal vascular disturbances, but most patients who receive this drug have systemic fungal diseases and are on multiple medications. To date there are no data to prove that these findings are due to voriconazole. Six pediatric cystic fibrosis patients also on retinol experienced a dermatologic photosensitivity reaction probably due to increased serum retinol or its metabolites due to inhibition of hepatic enzymes, which break down retinol, by voriconazole.[8]

Recommendations[1]
If voriconazole is used beyond 28 days, the manufacturer suggests that visual acuity, visual fields, and color perception be monitored. Extra caution should be used in children.

CLASS: ANTILEPROSY DRUGS

Generic Name:
Clofazimine.

Proprietary Name:
Lamprene.

Primary Use
This phenazine derivative is used in the treatment of leprosy and also as an anti-inflammatory in psoriasis, discoid lupus, and pyoderma gangrenosum.

Ocular Side Effects
Systemic administration – oral
Certain
1. Irritation
2. Decreased vision
3. Eyelids or conjunctiva
   a. Pigmentation (red-brown)
   b. Discoloration of lashes
   c. Perilimbal crystalline deposits
4. Tears
   a. Discoloration
   b. Crystalline drug in tears

c. May aggravate or cause ocular sicca
5. Cornea verticillata – polychromatic crystalline deposits
6. Photosensitivity
7. Crystalline deposits – brownish/reddish
   a. Iris
   b. Conjunctiva
   c. Sclera

Probable
1. Retina
   a. Variable macular pigmentary changes
   b. Bull's-eye maculopathy
   c. Abnormal electroretinogram (ERG)

Possible
1. Lens – bluish discoloration

Clinical Significance
This phenazine derivative can cause dose-related ocular changes mimicking those of chloroquine. Reversible reddish pigmentation of the skin, conjunctiva, and cornea can be seen. Polychromatic crystals have been found in the tear film, giving it a reddish appearance. Findings include fine, reddish-brown subepithelial corneal lines and perilimbal crystalline deposits seen on biomicroscopy. These crystals have been seen on the iris and possibly the lens. This rarely interferes with vision, and the crystalline deposits can disappear within a few months to many years after clofazimine has been discontinued. It is unclear if this drug can cause ocular sicca. It is more likely that the crystals act as an aggravation in patients with clinical or subclinical ocular sicca. These crystals may give a foreign body sensation and symptomatology consistent with a sicca-like syndrome. In one series, up to 50% of patients had some form of conjunctival pigmentation, 12% had variable changes in their vision, 25% had ocular irritation, and 32% had crystals in their tears.[1] Craythorn et al, Cunningham et al, Forester et al, and Agarwal reported that this drug can produce bull's-eye maculopathy.[2-5] Kasturi et al reported maculopathy in a vitiliginous patient.[6] Visual loss can be permanent, even if the drug is discontinued.

Generic Name:
Dapsone.

Proprietary Name:
Aczone.

Primary Use
This sulfone is used in the treatment of leprosy and ocular pemphigoid.

Ocular Side Effects
Systemic administration – oral
Certain
1. Decreased vision
2. Eyelids or conjunctiva
   a. Edema
   b. Hyperpigmentation
   c. Urticaria
   d. Purpura
   e. Hypersensitivity reaction
3. Retina
   a. Necrosis
   b. Macular exudates
   c. Intraretinal hemorrhages
   d. Peripheral powdery deposits
4. Optic nerve
   a. Optic neuritis
   b. Optic atrophy – toxic states
5. Photosensitivity
6. Visual hallucinations

Possible
1. Eyelids or conjunctiva
   a. Erythema multiforme
   b. Exfoliative dermatitis
   c. Lyell syndrome
2. Ischemic optic neuropathy

Clinical Significance
Dapsone has few ocular side effects except in massive doses or in the presence of a glucose-6-phosphate dehydrogenase deficiency. Daneshmend et al, Kenner et al, and Alexander et al described retinal and optic nerve findings in overdosed patients.[1-3] These included massive retinal necrosis, yellow-white lesions in the macula, intraretinal hemorrhages, and varying degrees of optic nerve damage. Alexander et al described 2 cases, 1 with long-term therapy of dapsone and another case of overdose in an attempted suicide.[3] There was massive deposition of grayish-white material in the macula with a relatively clear fovea. Scattered powdery deposits were seen in the peripheral retina. They felt that the drug or its metabolites were in the inner layers of the retina. This cleared over time. Permanent blindness has occurred in some cases. At lower doses, these findings may be seen in patients with glucose 6-phosphatedehydrogenase deficiency.[4] Darkening of skin color may be due to iatrogenic cyanosis, as a slate gray discoloration characteristic of drug-induced methemoglobinemia. Some patients under treatment with dapsone for leprosy have been known to develop lagophthalmos and posterior synechiae, but these effects are probably due to the disease rather than to the drug.[5]

Chaliulias et al described a single case where possible hemolysis secondary to dapsone in conjunction with insulin-dependent diabetes mellitus was likely responsible for delayed blood flow and decreased oxygenation of the optic nerve head.[6] This possibly caused a nonarteritic anterior ischemic optic neuropathy.

Hanuschk et al described a case of dapsone-induced methemoglobinemia and hemolytic anemia that caused severe ischemic retinal injury.[7]

The *Physicians' Desk Reference* (PDR) states a 10% incidence of iritis in patients on this drug.[8] However, this is due to the diseases the drug is used for and is not a drug side effect.

CLASS: ANTIMALARIAL DRUGS

Generic Names:
1. Chloroquine phosphate; 2. hydroxychloroquine sulfate.

Proprietary Names:
1. Aralen; 2. Plaquenil, Quineprox.

Primary Use
These aminoquinolines are used in the treatment of malaria, extraintestinal amebiasis, rheumatoid arthritis, and lupus erythematosus.

Ocular Side Effects
Systemic administration – oral
Certain
1. Decreased vision
2. Cornea
   a. Punctate – yellowish to white opacities
   b. Lineal – whorl-like pattern, primarily in palpebral aperture
   c. Enhanced Hudson-Stähli line
   d. Transient edema
   e. Decreased sensitivity
3. Retina and/or macula
   a. Perifoveal granularity of retinal pigment epithelium (early)
   b. Bull's-eye appearance of the macula, with thinning and clumping of pigment epithelium
   c. Attenuation of vascular tree
   d. Peripheral fine granular pigmentary changes
   e. Prominent choroidal pattern
   f. Angiography changes
      i Parafoveal retinal pigment epithelium window defects (early)
      ii. Window defects in annular pattern
      iii Choroidal filling defects (late)
   g. Decreased or absent foveal reflex

4. Abnormal sensory testing
   a. Critical flicker fusion
   b. Macular recovery times
   c. Decreased dark adaptation
   d. Electrooculogram (EOG) and electroretinogram (ERG) changes
5. Tear film
   a. Drugs found in tear film
   b. May aggravate or cause ocular sicca
   c. Decreased contact lens tolerance
6. Decreased accommodation
7. Visual fields
   a. Scotoma – annular, central, paracentral
   b. Constriction
   c. Hemianopsia
8. Eyelids and conjunctiva
   a. Pigmentary changes – hyper or hypo effects
   b. Yellow, bluish, or blackish deposits
   c. Photosensitivity reactions
   d. Blepharospasm or clonus
   e. Poliosis
9. Optic atrophy (late)
10. Color vision defect
   a. Blue-yellow defects (early)
   b. Red-green defects (late)
   c. Objects have yellow, green, or blue tinge
   d. Colored haloes around lights
11. Choroidal thinning – especially choriocapillaris

Probable
1. Posterior subcapsular cataract (chloroquine)
2. Night blindness (late) (chloroquine)
3. Myasthenia gravis – aggravated
   a. Diplopia
   b. Ptosis
   c. Paresis of extraocular muscle
4. Oculogyric crisis

Possible
1. Pigment epithelium detachment (hydroxychloroquine)

Clinical Significance
Although hydroxychloroquine is widely used in Britain, North America, and Australia, chloroquine may be more common in Europe, South America, and Asia. Hydroxychloroquine use has markedly increased because it has become a first-line drug for some forms of arthritis and lupus erythematosus, cancer chemotherapy, and diabetes. Probably all side effects seen with chloroquine can also be seen with hydroxychloroquine.

Corneal deposits due to chloroquine have no direct relationship to posterior segment disease and may be seen as early as 3 weeks after starting the medication. Corneal changes may first appear as a Hudson-Stähli line or an increase in a preexisting Hudson-Stähli line. Probably more common is a whorl-like pattern known as *cornea verticillata*. It is known that a number of drugs and diseases can cause this pattern, in which morphologic, histologic, and electron microscopic findings are identical. "Amphophilic" drugs, such as chloroquine, amiodarone, and chlorpromazine, form complexes with cellular phospholipids, which cannot be metabolized by lysosomal phospholipases; therefore these intracellular deposits occur and are visible in the superficial portion of the cornea.

Corneal deposits due to hydroxychloroquine may be of more clinical importance as an indication to hunt more aggressively for retinal toxicity. These deposits suggest drug retention and the need for regular screening. These are best seen with a dilated pupil and retroillumination. These deposits are finer and less extensive than with chloroquine. Easterbrook has found these corneal deposits to be possible indicators of hydroxychloroquine macular toxicity.[1] Corneal deposits occasionally cause haloes around lights. All corneal deposits are reversible. Hydroxychloroquine crystals have been found in the tear film, which may aggravate some sicca patients and contact lens wearers.[2]

Toxic maculopathy is usually reversible only in its earliest phases. At the 2018 Association of Research in Ophthalmology meeting, Marmor reported that once a patient has retinal pigment epithelial damage from hydroxychloroquine toxicity, the disease will never stop progressing.[3] If these drugs have caused skin, eyelid, corneal (hydroxychloroquine), or hair changes, this may be an indicator of possible drug-induced retinopathy. Asian patients may develop hydroxychloroquine toxicity more in a pericentral pattern rather than the typical parafoveal (bull's-eye) pattern.[4] Progression on the drug differs as well.[5] Ahn et al pointed out the need to do wide-field optic coherence tomography (OCT) scans to screen Asian patients taking hydroxychloroquine.[6] Night blindness has been reported late with chloroquine toxicity.[7-9] Although there are no citations for night blindness associated with hydroxychloroquine, there are 13 unsubstantiated cases in the spontaneous reports. The bull's-eye macula is not diagnostic for chloroquine-induced disease because a number of other entities can cause this same clinical picture. Although retinal toxicity occurs in patients taking hydroxychloroquine, the incidence is much lower than with chloroquine. To date, Osadchy et al have shown no ocular toxicity in children exposed to in utero antimalarial drugs.[10]

Chloroquine and hydroxychloroquine belong to the quinolone family of drugs, which can affect the nervous system, including cranial nerves. This may be the reason that, in rare instances, extraocular muscles are involved. This may also explain accommodation problems. In addition, these drugs can aggravate or unmask myasthenia gravis.[11]

Before pigment epithelium of the retina is involved, progression rarely lasts beyond a year. If, however, the fovea is threatened and the pigment epithelium is involved, the progression may continue for years, even leading to legal blindness.

Subcapsular cataracts have been attributed to chloroquine usage, but not hydroxychloroquine to date.[12] In more severe diseases such as rheumatoid arthritis, patients are taking or have been taking other medications, such as steroids, which also cause posterior subcapsular lens changes.

Annual examinations for drug-induced toxicity is not recommended in part due to cost–benefit ratio data. Some patients without major risk factors may require it based in part on their personality in a litigious society. With high dosages used in cancer therapy, hydroxychloroquine can cause retinal toxicity within 1–2 years. Leung et al reported retinal toxicity at 15 months after starting high-dose hydroxychloroquine.[13]

Management of Antimalarials to Minimize Retinopathy

MICHAEL F. MARMOR, MD

The antimalarials chloroquine and hydroxychloroquine are valuable drugs in the treatment of SLE and rheumatoid disease, both for effectiveness and for a lack of systemic side effects. However, they can become retinotoxic with excessive dosage or many years of use. The ophthalmologist needs to be aware of proper management to advise rheumatologists and patients and to screen effectively for early toxicity before it threatens vision.[14]

EPIDEMIOLOGY

The best estimates of dose, duration, and retinal toxicity come from a study of 2,361 patients using hydroxychloroquine for more than 5 years.[15] These data showed that calculating dose by real rather than ideal weight gives the most accurate estimation of risk, especially for smaller women, who are a high percentage of the SLE population. Fig. 4.10 shows Kaplan-Meier curves of risk at different dosages. Patients with daily dose <5 mg/kg real weight of hydroxychloroquine have <1% risk of toxicity up to 5 years of usage, and <2% up to 10 years. The risk rises quickly after that, but it is still modest for patients being followed and screened. If a patient is clinically normal on examination (Fig. 4.11), the risk of developing toxicity in the next year using <5 mg/kg real weight is still only 4% after 20 years of use. Because doses and environmental factors vary among individuals, there is no single number (such as cumulative dose/kg) that signifies risk of toxicity; one must look at the curves. Beyond dose and duration, the two major risk factors are renal insufficiency (because the kidneys are the major excretion route) and tamoxifen usage (a retinal toxin in its own right).

DOSE MANAGEMENT

The key to minimizing retinopathy is proper daily dosage, along with screening, and prescribing rheumatologists should be informed. There are no good conversion

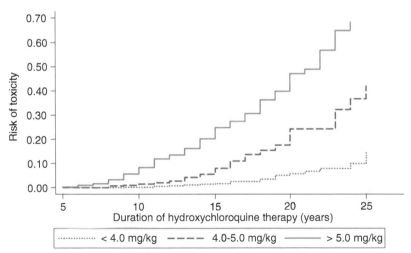

FIG. 4.10 Kaplan-Meier curves showing the cumulative risk of retinopathy over time. When usage is 4.0–5.0 mg/kg, the risk is very low within the first 5–10 years, but it rises markedly thereafter.[15]

data between the toxicity of hydroxychloroquine and chloroquine, but older literature on the incidence of bull's-eye retinopathy suggested that staying <2.3 mg/kg of chloroquine would be roughly equivalent to <5 mg/kg of hydroxychloroquine. Unfortunately, hydroxychloroquine comes only in 200-mg tablets, and chloroquine in 250 mg tablets, which raises the question of how intermediate doses can be prescribed. In fact, it is simple, because these drugs distribute and stabilize very slowly in the body. Thus one can calculate the proper weekly dose, and use two, one, or zero tablets on different days of the week to achieve the desired weekly total.

SIGNS OF RETINAL DAMAGE

The textbook description of chloroquine or hydroxychloroquine retinopathy is a bull's eye of parafoveal depigmentation, but this is advanced disease with a high likelihood of central visual loss. With modern technology, one can (and should) recognize damage at a much earlier stage before any fundus changes are visible (Fig. 4.12). Automated visual fields are very sensitive to early functional damage, especially if a SITA protocol is used so that statistical pattern deviations can be assessed (grayscale field diagrams are noisy). Spectral density optical coherence tomography (SD-OCT) is less sensitive but more specific and objective.

SD-OCT will show early breakup in the ellipsoid zone (EZ) line and thinning of the ONL before there is any abnormality in the RPE (see Fig. 4.12). These changes usually begin inferiorly (or inferonasally or inferotemporally) rather than superiorly. This pattern of early damage is typically parafoveal for people of European or Caucasian descent, but individuals of Asian heritage will more often show the initial damage eccentrically, near the vascular arcades (Fig. 4.13).[4–6]

SCREENING RECOMMENDATIONS

There are usually no symptoms of chloroquine or hydroxychloroquine retinopathy until late severe stages. Thus prospective screening is critical.[14] By the first year of usage, a good fundus examination should be performed (and other tests as indicated) to rule out underlying retinal disease that might contraindicate use of a retinal toxin or might obscure the reading of screening tests. These include retinal dystrophies, diseases with marked field loss, and macular degeneration that affects retinal thickness and vision. A few drusen are not a contraindication. If there is no underlying disease or special risk factor, annual screening can be deferred for 5 years. After 5 years, annual screening is advised, ideally with both an automated visual field and SD-OCT, and this should continue indefinitely. For

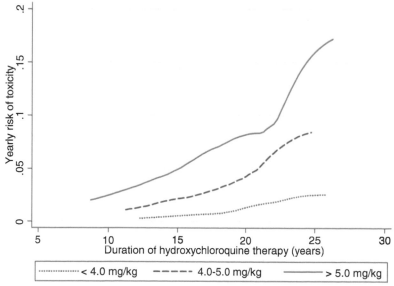

FIG. 4.11 Incremental annual risk of toxicity for a patient who is free of retinopathy at a given point in time. The annual risk is low within the first 10 years of use, but it rises with longer durations of therapy.[15]

Fundus photograph   Spectral-domain OCT   10-2 Pattern deviation and threshold

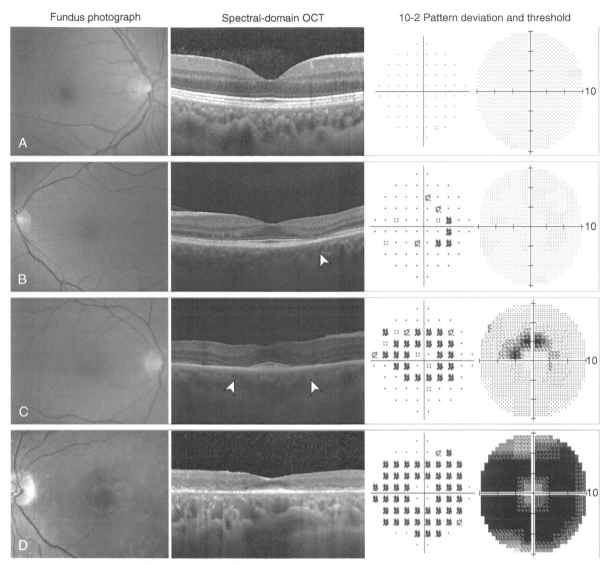

FIG. 4.12 Progressive changes in hydroxychloroquine retinopathy for Caucasian patients. From left to right: fundus appearance, SD-OCT, 10-2 field pattern deviation and grayscale. From top to bottom: **(A)** normal eye; **(B)** early damage with temporal SD-OCT thinning and mild field loss; **(C)** moderate damage with no fundus changes or RPE loss, but more severe SD-OCT and field changes; **(D)** severe retinopathy with a prominent bull's-eye macular lesion, RPE damage on SD-OCT, and a dense ring scotoma.[15]

Caucasians, 10-2 visual fields are required; for Asians both 10-2 and either 24-2 or 30-2 are advised (using a SITA Fast program to minimize time). Fundus examination is insensitive and should not be used as a screening test.

IMPLICATIONS OF RETINOPATHY

If fields or SD-OCT show possible but borderline findings, other tests such as multifocal electroretinogram (ERG) or fundus autofluorescence can be added to rule pathology in or out. Or the patient can be retested in a

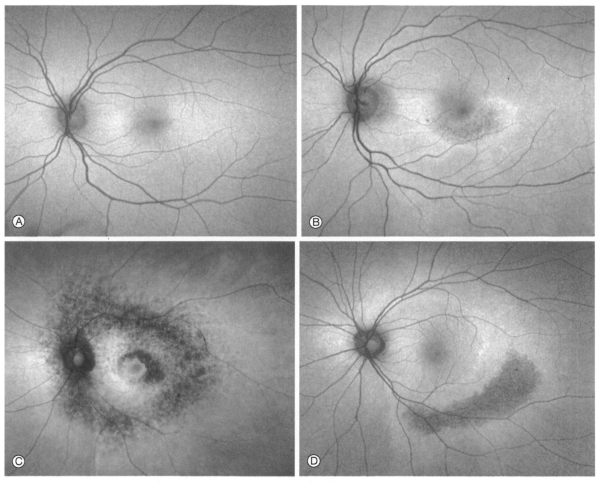

FIG. 4.13 Widefield fundus autofluorescence images showing severe hydroxychloroquine retinopathy (RPE loss) with different patterns of damage. Note the inferior predilection. **(A)** Normal. **(B)** Parafoveal pattern. **(C)** Mixed pattern (advanced damage). **(D)** Pericentral and arcade pattern (Asian eyes).[4]

few months (because toxicity does not progress very fast) to evaluate consistency or progression of abnormalities. In general, it is best to have two confirmatory tests before stopping an excellent drug that keeps patients off of steroids and immune-suppressive medication. Fortunately, retinopathy detected early, before any RPE damage (on SD-OCT or in the fundus), will stabilize when hydroxychloroquine is stopped. At these early stages there may be some partial ring scotoma, but this is rarely symptomatic and central vision is unaffected. Once the RPE is involved, however, the damage can continue to progress for decades, as if the retinopathy had turned into a dystrophy.[16] Central vision is at risk over these ensuing years, and there is no specific therapy. These drugs

should be stopped, if medically feasible, once there is unmistakable evidence of early toxic damage.

CONCLUSIONS

Concern over retinal toxicity of the antimalarials is valid, but fear of it should not prevent their use. These drugs can often be maintained for decades, with little risk of retinal damage or visual loss, if they are prescribed at a proper dose and patients are followed with proper screening.

Generic Name:
Mefloquine hydrochloride.

Proprietary Name:
Lariam.

Primary Use
This drug is primarily used in the treatment of malaria.

Ocular Side Effects
Systemic administration – oral
Certain
1. Decreased vision
2. Eyelids or conjunctiva
   a. Urticaria
   b. Rash
   c. Pruritus
3. Visual hallucinations

Probable
1. Diplopia

Possible
1. Eyelids of conjunctiva
   a. Erythema multiforme
   b. Exfoliative dermatitis

Conditional/unclassified
1. Maculopathy
2. Optic neuritis

Clinical Significance
This drug was developed for resistant malaria, but has become a favorite for malaria prevention. It does not cause deposits in the cornea or retina, which are seen with other commonly used antimalarial drugs. Palmer et al pointed out that at least 20% of patients taking this drug complain of diplopia.[1] This figure is much higher than reported by others. In fact, the *Physicians' Desk Reference* (PDR) does not list diplopia as a side effect due to mefloquine.[2] Around 1% of patients taking prophylactic dosages have had visual hallucinations lasting a few seconds or up to 1 hour. This occurs after each dosage. There does not appear to be a relationship between total dosage of mefloquine and the onset of neuropsychiatric side effects.

Walker et al reported a single case of maculopathy related to mefloquine use; however, the case was complicated by prior vascular occlusion.[3] Jain et al reported a single case of diplopia and central serous chorioretinopathy in a patient on multiple antimalarial medications.[4] The authors felt mefloquine was involved. There are 8 cases of central serous maculopathy in the spontaneous reports. The side effect is unproven, and with the volume and length of time the drug has been available, it's probably an "unlikely" association.

De Mendonca Melo et al and Fujii et al described cases of optic neuritis, enlarged blind spots, and visual field defects.[5,6] There are no other cases in the literature or spontaneous reporting systems.

In 2 manufacturer-sponsored clinical studies, no evidence was found that this drug increases the risk of eye disorders.[7,8] In their series, there were some minimal changes in visual acuity, rare neuro-ophthalmic events, and 9 cases of maculopathy. Most cases reported as due to the drug could be explained via other pathology. However, the authors warned that any ocular changes in patients on this drug should be seen by an ophthalmologist.

Generic Name:
Quinine sulfate.

Proprietary Name:
Qualaquin.

Primary Use
This alkaloid is effective in the management of nocturnal leg cramps, myotonia congenita, and resistant *Plasmodium falciparum*. It is also used in attempted abortions. Ophthalmologically it is useful in the treatment of eyelid myokymia.

Ocular Side Effects
Systemic administration – oral
Certain
1. Decreased vision – all gradations of visual loss, from transient blindness to permanent visual loss
2. Iris
   a. Depigmentation
   b. Diffuse atrophy
3. Pupils
   a. Mydriasis
   b. Decreased or absent reaction to light
   c. Irregular – oval
   d. Vermiform motions
4. Retinal or macular
   a. Edema
   b. Degeneration – atrophy
   c. Pigmentary changes (Fig. 4.14)
   d. Exudates
   e. Vasodilatation followed by vasoconstriction
   f. Absence of foveal reflex
   g. Cherry red spot – macula
   h. Abnormal electroretinogram (ERG), electrooculogram (EOG), visual evoked potential (VEP), or critical flicker fusion

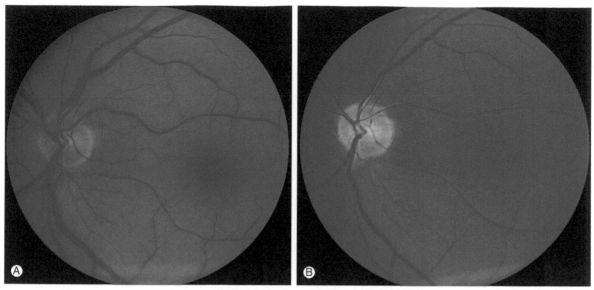

FIG. 4.14 **(A)** Quinine retinopathy with palish opalescent retina and **(B)** quinine retinopathy with fibrotic sheathing, pale disc, and arterial attenuation.[15]

5. Visual sensations
   a. Distortion due to flashing lights
   b. Distortion of images secondary to sensations of waves
6. Optic nerve
   a. Papilledema
   b. Pallor
   c. Atrophy
7. Color vision defect
   a. Red-green or blue-yellow defect
   b. Objects have red or green tinge
8. Visual fields
   a. Scotomas
   b. Constriction
9. Eyelids or conjunctiva
   a. Allergic reactions
   b. Edema
   c. Photosensitivity
   d. Purpura
   e. Urticaria
   f. May aggravate or cause ocular sicca
10. Night blindness
11. Visual hallucinations

Probable
1. Myasthenia gravis – aggravated
   a. Diplopia
   b. Ptosis
   c. Paresis of extraocular muscle

Possible
1. Eyelids or conjunctiva – erythema multiforme

Conditional/unclassified
1. Myopia – transitory
2. Granulomatous uveitis
3. Acute glaucoma
4. Vertical nystagmus

Ocular teratogenic effects
Conditional/unclassified
1. Optic nerve hypoplasia

Clinical Significance
Quinine has been used for centuries, and serious ocular side effects occur mainly in deliberate, self-harm situations. It is also used as a diluent for many "street drugs" and as a method of terminating a pregnancy. An excellent overview of almost 300 articles on this subject can be found in Grant's *Toxicology of the Eye.*[1] Quinine seldom causes significant ocular side effects at normal dosage, although Waddell reported 2 cases.[2] In rare instances, hypersensitivity reactions or long-term low dosages can cause significant ocular effects. In cases of massive exposure, visual loss may be sudden or progressive over a number of hours or days. In large overdose situations, retinal arteriolar constriction, venous congestion, pronounced retinal and papillary edema, and permanent loss of the peripheral vision field may

occur. Complete, irreversible loss of vision may occur, but most patients have some return of vision. Boland et al gave an excellent overview of 165 patients who were hospitalized with quinine poisoning, of whom 42% had significant visual side effects.[3] Mild cases may show only minimal macular changes by Amsler grid, decreased vision, or some constriction of the visual field. Zahn et al showed that early ERG may be normal; however, in late ERG, scotopic b-waves and a-waves are altered.[4] Su et al described distinctive ERG abnormalities secondary to inner retinal atrophy.[5] Hustead reported that in individuals hypersensitive to quinine, a granulomatous uveitis may occur.[6] Segal et al reported shallowing of the anterior chamber precipitating narrow-angle glaucoma.[7] Schuman reported a case of acute bilateral transitory myopia.[8] The pupil is commonly affected, probably on a vasotoxic basis. The usual effect is mydriasis and decreased reaction to light all the way to severe atrophy of the iris.[9-11] Smidt et al suggested that quinine can cause or aggravate ocular sicca.[12] Worden et al and others have noted that chronic overuse of tonic water (which contains quinine) can cause toxic quinine effects in the eye.[13]

According to the evidence presently available, the etiology of the toxic effect of quinine seems to involve not only an early effect on the outer layers of the retina and pigment epithelium but also probably a direct effect on retinal ganglion cells and optic nerve fibers, as well as vasculotoxic effects.

Quinine can cause optic nerve hypoplasia and decreased vision, including blindness, in the offspring secondary to prenatal maternal ingestion.

Recommendations[14]
This drug should not be used in patients with optic neuritis or tinnitus; it may exacerbate these conditions.

CLASS: ANTIPROTOZOAL DRUGS

Generic Name:
Metronidazole.

Proprietary Names:
First-Metronidazole 100, First-Metronidazole 50, Flagyl, Flagyl ER, Flagyl IV, Flagyl RTU, MetroCream, Metro IV, MetroGel, MetroGel Vaginal, MetroGel-Vaginal, MetroLotion, Noritate, Nuvessa, Nydamaz, Rosadan, Vandazole, Vitazol.

Primary Use
This nitroimidazole derivative is an antibacterial and antiprotozoal drug effective in the treatment of trichomoniasis, amebiasis, giardiasis, and anaerobic bacterial infections.

Ocular Side Effects
Systemic administration – intravenous, oral, or topical
Certain
1. Decreased vision
2. Photosensitivity
3. Retrobulbar or optic neuritis
   a. Visual field changes
      i. Scotoma
      ii. Enlarged blind spot
   b. Color vision defect
4. Eyelids or conjunctiva
   a. Erythema
   b. Conjunctivitis – nonspecific
   c. Eyelid edema
   d. Periorbital edema
   e. Urticaria
5. Diplopia
6. Myopia – reversible

Probable
1. Oculogyric crisis
2. Visual hallucinations

Possible
1. Uveitis (worsens)

Local ophthalmic use or exposure – topical ocular application
Certain
1. Irritation
2. Burning
3. Erythema
4. Epiphora

Ocular teratogenic effects
Conditional/unclassified
1. Telecanthus

Clinical Significance
Ocular side effects due to the systemic use of metronidazole are unusual and are mostly reversible on discontinuation of the drug. One of the most common ocular side effects in the spontaneous reporting systems is periocular and eyelid edema (443 cases). The most serious ocular side effects affect the nervous system. These appear to be most common on long-term therapy. Retrobulbar and optic neuritis are the most common.[1-5] This is associated with color vision defects, decreased

vision, and various scotomas. This may be unilateral initially, but with time most are bilateral. Stopping the drug, in general, causes complete recovery. The drug may cause vestibulopathy with secondary extraocular muscle abnormalities, cerebellopathy with downbeat nystagmus, and abduction defects.[6,7] Grinbaum et al reported a case with rechallenge data showing this drug can cause a reversible myopia.[8] Oculogyric crisis has been reported in 17 patients in the spontaneous reporting systems.[9]

Turnbull et al reported worsening of uveitis after starting this drug, which was probably secondary to dying parasites with the release of antigens.[10]

Topical periocular application is said to be of value in acne rosacea. Use on the eyelid with inadvertent ocular exposure may cause ocular irritation, but to date, no permanent ocular side effects have been reported.

A midline facial defect, including telecanthus, has been reported after maternal use of this drug during the first trimester.[11] There is little to support the concern that this drug used orally has any teratogenic effects.

Generic Name:
Suramin sodium.

Proprietary Name:
Generic only.

Primary Use
This nonmetallic polyanion is effective in the treatment of trypanosomiasis and is used as adjunctive therapy in onchocerciasis and AIDS. Recently this drug has been used in anticancer therapy.

Ocular Side Effects
Systemic administration – intravenous
Certain
1. Decreased vision
2. Intraepithelial inclusions
   a. Cornea
   b. Conjunctiva
   c. Anterior lens epithelium
3. Cornea
   a. Keratitis
   b. Superficial punctate keratitis
   c. Erosions
   d. Vortex keratopathy
4. Hypermetropia
5. Irritation
   a. Lacrimation
   b. Photophobia
   c. Conjunctivitis
   d. Foreign body sensation

6. Eyelids or conjunctiva
   a. Edema
   b. Urticaria

Clinical Significance
When suramin sodium is used in the management of parasitic disease, it is difficult to differentiate an adverse drug effect from the adverse reaction of the death of the intraocular organism. However, Hemady et al, in a study of 114 patients, reported that suramin sodium for metastatic cancer of the prostate had an incidence of 16.6% of ocular signs and symptoms.[1] These include bilateral, whorl-like corneal deposits, often with foreign body sensation and lacrimation. This was also associated with decreased vision and a hyperopic shift in a range of +0.75 to +2.00 diopters. This refractive change was persistent throughout the course of treatment. No patients showed a decrease in baseline best-corrected vision, and the drug was not considered dose limiting due to ocular toxicity. In patients with AIDS on high-dose suramin sodium, Teich et al reported not only vortex keratopathy but also fine, cream-colored, deep epithelial or subepithelial deposits.[2] Holland et al described these as light golden-brown deposits starting on the lower portion of the cornea and progressing into a whorl keratopathy that involved the whole cornea.[3] One patient had these deposits on the anterior lens epithelium. These deposits histologically are identified as membranous lamellar inclusion bodies, the same as with other drug-induced lipid storage diseases produced by lysosomal enzyme inhibition.

Generic Name:
Tryparsamide.

Proprietary Name:
Generic only.

Primary Use
This organic arsenical is used in the treatment of trypanosomiasis as a backup to safer drugs.

Ocular Side Effects
Systemic administration – intravenous
Certain
1. Constriction of visual fields
2. Decreased vision
3. Visual sensations
   a. Smokeless fog
   b. Shimmering effect
4. Optic neuritis
5. Optic atrophy
6. Toxic amblyopia

Clinical Significance

The most serious and common adverse drug reactions due to tryparsamide involve the eye. Incidence of ocular side effects varies from 3–20% of cases, with constriction of visual fields followed by decreased vision as the characteristic sequence. Almost 10% of individuals taking tryparsamide experience visual changes consisting of "shimmering" or "dazzling," which may persist for days or even weeks. If the medication is not immediately discontinued following these visual changes, the pathologic condition of the optic nerve may become irreversible and progress to blindness. Due to the severity of side effects of this drug on the optic nerve, it has generally been replaced by melarsoprol.

CLASS: ANTITUBERCULAR DRUGS

Generic Name:
Cycloserine.

Proprietary Name:
Seromycin.

Primary Use
This isoxazolidone is effective against certain Gram-negative and Gram-positive bacteria and *Mycobacterium tuberculosis*.

Ocular Side Effects
Systemic administration – intravenous
Certain
1. Decreased vision
2. Eyelids or conjunctiva
   a. Allergic reactions
   b. Conjunctivitis – nonspecific
   c. Photosensitivity
3. Trichomegaly

Probable
1. Visual hallucinations
2. Flickering vision

Conditional/unclassified
1. Optic nerve
   a. Neuritis
   b. Atrophy

Clinical Significance
Even though ocular complications due to cycloserine are quite rare, this drug is primarily used in combination with other drugs; therefore pinpointing cause and effect for an ocular side effect is very difficult. An increased number of eyelashes (hypertrichosis) has been reported and may prompt the clinical suspicion of an immune system abnormality.[1] Optic nerve damage, including optic neuritis and atrophy, has been reported, but these data are not conclusive.

Generic Name:
Ethambutol hydrochloride.

Proprietary Name:
Myambutol.

Primary Use
Ethambutol is a tuberculostatic drug that is effective against *M. tuberculosis*.

Ocular Side Effects
Systemic administration – oral
Certain
1. Color vision defect – red-green or blue-yellow defect
2. Decreased vision
3. Contrast sensitivity – decreased
4. Visual evoked potential – decreased
5. Electroretinogram (ERG) changes
6. Visual fields
   a. Scotomas – annular, central, or centrocecal
   b. Constriction
   c. Hemianopsia
   d. Enlarged blind spot
7. Optic nerve
   a. Retrobulbar or optic neuritis
   b. Papilledema
   c. Peripapillary atrophy
   d. Atrophy (Fig. 4.15)

Probable
1. Optic nerve
   a. Microhemorrhages
   b. Hyperemia
2. Photophobia
3. Retinal or macular
   a. Retinitis
   b. Vascular disorder
   c. Edema
   d. Pigmentary changes

Possible
1. Hemorrhages
2. Paresis of extraocular muscles

Unconditional/unclassified
1. Mydriasis

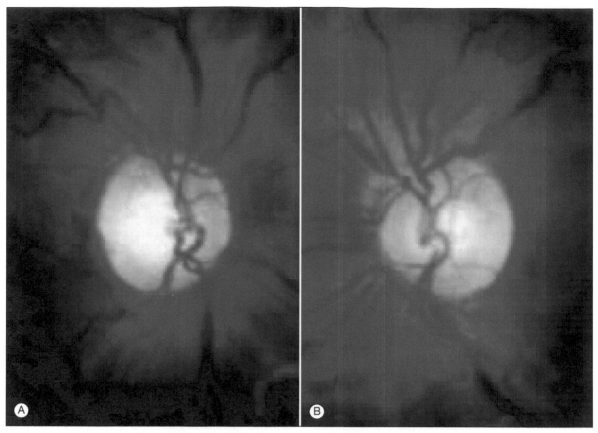

FIG. 4.15 **(A)** Right and **(B)** left optic nerve atrophy secondary to ethambutol.[7]

2. Spasms
3. Visual hallucinations

Clinical Significance

Ethambutol is still a first-line drug used in the multi-drug treatment of tuberculosis. Its use is on the increase because more resistant forms of tuberculosis are occurring. The most significant adverse effect of ethambutol is optic or retrobulbar neuritis, which is usually bilateral but can be asymmetric. Ethambutol toxicity may affect only the small-caliber papillomacular bundle axons, and optic atrophy will not develop until months after the fibers are lost. This means objective findings on the fundus examination are frequently absent. Optic neuropathy may occur, on average, at 2–5 months after starting therapy. The earliest ophthalmologic findings in toxic optic neuropathy from ethambutol may be loss of visual acuity, color vision loss, or central scotomas. Ethambutol also has an affinity for the optic chiasm, with bitemporal visual field defects manifesting toxicity.

Some authors have proposed electrophysiologic tests to screen for toxicity due to ethambutol.

A multifocal ERG may be of value to diagnose and monitor patients taking ethambutol, and full-field ERGs and electrooculograms (EOGs), also have demonstrated abnormalities. Contrast sensitivity measurement may also be useful in detecting subclinical ethambutol toxic optic neuropathy. OCT shows promise as a screening tool to detect subclinical optic neuropathy. Kim et al felt that pattern visual evoked potential (VEP) and retinal nerve fiber layer OCT (RNFL OCT) are suitable tests for early detection of subclinical ethambutol-induced ocular toxicity.[1]

Isoniazid is frequently prescribed concomitantly with ethambutol for tuberculosis due to multiple cases of drug resistance to single-drug therapy. Isoniazid has also been associated with optic neuropathy, and differentiating toxicity due to ethambutol versus isoniazid can be challenging. In general, the toxicity from isoniazid is less frequent, less severe, and usually reversible. When in doubt, a dechallenge with isoniazid and/or ethambutol may need to be undertaken after consultation with the primary care physician.

Once a defect is found and the ethambutol is discontinued, occasionally the abnormality may continue to progress for 1–2 months. The vast majority will improve over weeks to many months to complete recovery. However, there are over 200 well-documented cases of permanent visual loss, including blindness. Some authors feel that patients with initial severe central visual loss before the drug is stopped have the poorest prognosis for full recovery. Although direct toxic effects to the retina are supported by abnormal visual evoked cortical potentials and patterned ERGs, the clinical retinal findings are rare but may include macular edema and pigmentary disturbances.[2] Conventional ERG findings remain controversial as to clinical usefulness. Dotti et al described a case of ethambutol-induced optic neuropathy aggravating a genetic predisposition for optic nerve pathology.[3]

Bouffard et al reported a case of ethambutol-induced optic neuritis with full recovery after discontinuing the drug.[4] Ten years later the drug was started again without any optic nerve side effects.

Recommendations

1. Obtain informed consent before assuming care for patients taking ethambutol, explaining that optic neuropathy can occur at any dose, despite regular ophthalmic examinations and that the vision loss can be severe and irreversible.
2. Obtain a baseline examination to include a visual field test, color vision test, dilated fundus and optic-nerve examination, and visual acuity.
3. If any visual symptoms occur, discontinue the medication and see an ophthalmologist.
4. Frequency of examination is monthly for doses greater than 15 mg/kg/day[4]; however, monthly examinations at lower doses may be necessary for patients at increased risk for toxicity:
   a. Diabetes mellitus
   b. Chronic renal failure
   c. Alcoholism
   d. Elderly
   e. Children
   f. Other ocular defects
   g. Ethambutol-induced peripheral neuropathy
5. Consider discontinuation of ethambutol after any signs of loss of visual acuity, color vision, or a visual field defect.
6. Consider OCT or contrast sensitivity testing, as these tests could pick up early ethambutol toxicity not detected with the baseline examination.

7. Some suggest that if no improvement occurs in visual signs after 4 months of being off the drug, hydroxocobalamin therapy should be considered, but this is not proven.[5] If the vision does not improve 10–15 weeks after ethambutol discontinuation, parenteral administration of 40 mg of hydroxocobalamin daily over a 10- to 28-week period has been suggested as a possible treatment. Also consider glutamate antagonists in limiting the ocular side effects of ethambutol during drug therapy.[6] There are also data to suggest that cases of optic nerve toxicity should be treated with 100–250 mg of oral zinc sulfate 3 times daily. The bottom line is that the best way to treat this entity is unknown.

Generic Name:
Ethionamide.

Proprietary Name:
Trecator-Sc.

Primary Use
This isonicotinic acid derivative is effective against *M. tuberculosis* and *M. leprae*. It is indicated in the treatment of patients when resistance to primary tuberculostatic drugs has developed.

Ocular Side Effects
Systemic administration – oral
Probable
1. Decreased vision
2. Diplopia
3. Eyelids or conjunctiva
   a. Allergic reactions
   b. Erythema
   c. Pellegra-like syndrome
   d. Urticaria
4. Photophobia
5. Color vision defect – heightened color perception
6. Visual hallucinations

Possible
1. Eyelids of conjunctiva – exfoliative dermatitis

Conditional/unclassified
1. Optic neuropathy

Clinical Significance
The incidence of adverse ocular effects due to ethionamide is quite small and seldom of clinical significance. Although certain adverse effects occur at

low dosage levels, they usually do not continue even if the dosage is increased. Optic neuritis has been reported but in so few cases that it is difficult to pinpoint a cause-and-effect relationship. The *Physicians' Desk Reference* (PDR) lists incidences of diplopia and/or optic neuritis at 0–0.1%.[1] In the spontaneous reporting systems, there is only 1 case of optic neuropathy and 4 cases of diplopia.

Generic Name:
Isoniazid.

Proprietary Names:
Laniazid, Nydrazid.

Primary Use
This hydrazide of isonicotinic acid is effective against *M. tuberculosis*.

Ocular Side Effects
Systemic administration – intramuscular, intravenous, or oral (often in combination with other anti-infective drugs)
Certain
1. Decreased vision
2. Optic nerve
   a. Retrobulbar or optic neuritis
   b. Papilledema
   c. Optic atrophy
3. Visual fields
   a. Scotomas
   b. Constriction
   c. Hemianopsia
4. Eyelids or conjunctiva
   a. Allergic reactions
   b. Edema
   c. Urticaria
5. Color vision defect – red-green defect
6. Decreased accommodation
7. Photophobia
8. Visual hallucinations

Probable
1. Eyelids of conjunctiva
   a. Lupoid syndrome
   b. Erythema multiforme
   c. Exfoliative dermatitis
   d. Lyell syndrome
2. Uveitis

Possible
1. Ciliochoroidal effusion

Conditional/unclassified
1. Cornea
   a. Keratitis
   b. Brownish infiltrates
2. Extraocular muscles
   a. Paresis
   b. Nystagmus
3. Retinal nerve fiber layer – decrease

Clinical Significance
Clear associations between isoniazid and its side effects are often difficult because it is mostly used in combination therapy. Some of these ocular side effects are a Jarisch-Herxheimer reaction (endotoxin-like production secondary to the death of microorganisms).[1] Isoniazid can induce a peripheral neuritis in 5–20% of patients. The drug interferes with pyridoxine metabolism. This is probably the cause of optic neuritis. A large number of published cases include a combination of isoniazid and ethambutol, which also causes optic nerve disease, likely by a different mechanism. Kim et al showed progressive decrease in the retinal nerve fiber layer in patients taking multiple antitubercular drugs.[2] None were taking isoniazid alone. There are a number of cases with a full return of vision without sequelae by giving pyridoxine. The association seems "certain." There are cases, however, of optic atrophy and permanent blindness, especially if the side effect goes unrecognized. Rarely, extraocular muscles may be involved, possibly by the same mechanism.[3]

Honegger et al found that about one-third of patients on isoniazid had some impairment of accommodation.[4] This was transient and reversible. Neff described a single case with positive rechallenge in which isoniazid caused brownish corneal infiltrates and anterior uveitis.[5]

Gan et al described a case of bilateral decreased vision, conjunctival injection, 2+ flare and cells, and shallow 360-degree serous choroidal effusion after 1 week of taking isoniazid for tuberculosis prophylaxis.[6] This cleared within 3 days of stopping the drug with no recurrence.

Generic Name:
Rifabutin.

Proprietary Name:
Mycobutin.

Primary Use
This drug is used in the treatment of *Mycobacterium avium*, leprosy tuberculosis, staphylococcal infections,

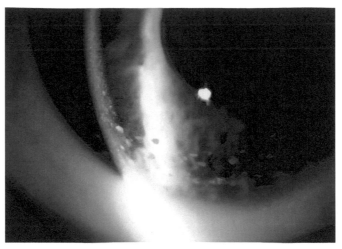

FIG. 4.16 Keratic deposits on the posterior surface of the cornea from systemic rifabutin.[9]

brucellosis, HIV patients, atypical mycobacteria, and Legionnaires' disease. It is also used in the prophylaxis of *Haemophilus*, meningococcal meningitis, and *Mycobacterium avium*.

Ocular Side Effects
Systemic administration – oral
Certain
1. Uveitis
   a. Anterior (from fine stellate keratic precipitates to large hypopyon)
   b. Posterior
   c. Panuveitis
   d. Hypopyon
2. Decreased vision
3. Photophobia
4. Pain
5. Conjunctiva
   a. Hyperemia
   b. Microhemorrhages
6. Vitreous body
   a. Vitritis
   b. Yellow-white opacities
7. Contact lens staining
8. Retina
   a. Microhemorrhages
   b. Vasculitis
9. Eyelids
   a. Contact dermatitis
   b. Rashes
   c. Orange-tan discoloration
10. Cornea
    a. Deep stromal fine or large stellate deposits (Fig. 4.16)
11. Lacrimation – rose color

Probable
1. Staining intraocular lens (IOL) – rose color
2. Macular edema
3. Deposits on anterior surface of the lens
4. Full-field electroretinogram (ERG) – reduction

Conditional/unclassified
1. Cornea
   a. Opacities
   b. Ulcers

Clinical Significance
Uveitis associated with rifabutin is the predominant ocular side effect with this drug. Fraunfelder et al reported 113 cases of rifabutin-associated uveitis from spontaneous reporting systems.[1] Shafran et al performed a prospective randomized study of 119 patients, 59 of whom received rifabutin in combination with clarithromycin and ethambutol.[2] About 40% of those who received rifabutin developed uveitis, about two-thirds bilateral, with an onset mean of 65 days. The uveitis may occur within 2 weeks to 7 months after starting the drug. The inflammatory-like response may involve only the anterior segment or, rarely, the whole uvea. It may be mild, with only fine peripheral endothelial deposits without uveitis, to a fulminating panuveitis with significant

posterior corneal and vitreal deposits. It may or may not be associated with hypopyon; significant vitritis, including vitreal opacities; or, in rare instances, a retinal vasculitis.[3] Although it is most commonly associated with HIV-infected patients who are often on other antibiotics concomitantly, this entity is now being reported in immune-suppressed patients, patients without AIDS on rifabutin alone, and in immune-competent persons. The uveitis is more common in patients on rifabutin along with clarithromycin or fluconazole. These drugs may elevate rifabutin serum levels by inhibition of the hepatic microsomal cytochrome P 450 system, which metabolizes rifabutin. The uveitis is unique, in part because topical ocular steroids, even in fulminating cases, often clear the intraocular inflammation quite rapidly.[4] This ocular inflammatory response clears on topical ocular steroids and stopping the drug. There are a few cases where the drug was not discontinued and the uveitis cleared on its own. The etiology of this uveitis is unknown, and some postulate the possibility of interaction of multiple drugs, an altered immune system, underlying infections, or drug-related factors contributing to the development of this uveitis syndrome. Smith et al described bilateral, peripheral, endothelial, stellate-shaped deposits in children with HIV disease on rifabutin.[5] Confocal studies place these deposits in the deep stroma rather than on the endothelium.[6] Williams et al described these as endothelial.[7] Rifabutin can stain multiple body fluids, including tears and aqueous humor. It has a potential to stain silicone, i.e. contact lenses or IOLs.[8] High doses of rifabutin have also been associated with an orange-tan discoloration of the skin, as well as the sclera and oral mucosa. There are several reports in the spontaneous reporting systems of corneal ulceration and opacities, but these data are unconfirmed.

Generic Name:
Rifampin.

Proprietary Names:
Rifadin, Rimactane.

Primary Use
Systemic
This bactericidal as well as bacteriostatic drug is effective against *Mycobacteria*, many Gram-positive cocci, and some Gram-negative, including *Neisseria* species and *H. influenzae*.

Ophthalmic
This drug is used for treatment of ocular *Chlamydia* infections.

Ocular Side Effects
Systemic administration – intravenous or oral
Certain
1. Decreased vision
2. Eyelids or conjunctiva
    a. Hyperemia
    b. Erythema
    c. Blepharoconjunctivitis
    d. Edema
    e. Yellow or red discoloration
    f. Urticaria
    g. Purpura
    h. Pemphigoid lesion
    i. Hypersensitivity reactions
3. Lacrimation
4. Color vision defect – red-green defect
5. Tears and/or contact lenses stained orange
    a. Periorbital edema

Possible
1. Eyelids of conjunctiva
    a. Lupoid syndrome
    b. Exfoliative dermatitis

Local ophthalmic use or exposure – ointment
Certain
1. Irritation
    a. Lacrimation
    b. Hyperemia
    c. Pain
    d. Edema

Clinical Significance
Ocular side effects from systemic rifampin are quite variable. Reactions may include conjunctival hyperemia, mild blepharoconjunctivitis, or painful severe exudative conjunctivitis. The latter includes markedly congested palpebral and bulbar conjunctiva with thick white exudates.[1] Although not all patients seem to secrete this drug or a by-product in their tears, Lyons, as well as Fraunfelder, reported orange-red staining of contact lenses and the inability to wear lenses while taking this drug.[2,3] Systemic rifampin may stain other body fluids as well, but this discoloration disappears once the drug is discontinued. Ocular side effects seen with this drug appear to occur more frequently during intermittent treatment than during daily treatment and are reversible when the drug has been discontinued. In animals, this drug accumulates in ocular pigment, but there are no data for this in humans. Topical ocular use of 1% rifampin ointment has been reported to cause approximately a 10% incidence of adverse

ocular effects, which are primarily due to irritation and include discomfort, tearing, lid edema, and conjunctival hyperemia. The irritation, discomfort, and tearing usually last only 10–50 minutes after the application of the ointment.

Generic Name:

Thioacetazone (amithiozone).

Proprietary Names:

Conteben, Tibione.

Primary Use

This tuberculostatic drug is effective against *M. tuberculosis* and *M. leprae*. This drug is also used for lupus vulgaris.

Ocular Side Effects

Systemic administration – oral
Certain

1. Decreased vision
2. Irritation
   a. Photosensitivity
   b. Pain
   c. Burning sensation
3. Eyelids or conjunctiva
   a. Allergic reactions
   b. Hyperemia
   c. Blepharoconjunctivitis
   d. Hypertrichosis

Possible

1. Eyelids or conjunctiva
   a. Erythema multiforme
   b. Exfoliative dermatitis
   c. Lyell syndrome

Conditional/unclassified

1. Retinal edema
2. Color vision defect
3. Scotoma

Clinical Significance

Numerous adverse ocular reactions due to thioacetazone have been seen. Skin manifestations have been the most frequent. Nearly all ocular side effects are reversible and are of minor clinical significance. One instance of irreversible toxic amblyopia with a central scotoma and decreased color vision has been reported; however, the patient was also receiving aminosalicylic acid.

REFERENCES

Drugs: Broxyquinoline and diiodohydroxyquinoline

1. Grant WM, Schuman JS. *Toxicology of the Eye.* 4th ed. Springfield, IL: Charles C Thomas; 1993:282–283, 842–843.

Drug: Emetine hydrochloride

1. Fontana G. The effect of emetine on the cornea. *Arch Ottalmol Ocu (Italian).* 1948;52:115–132.
2. Jacovides O. Troubles visuels a la suite d'injections fortes d'emetine. *Arch Ophtalmol (Paris).* 1923;40:657.

Drug: Mepacrine hydrochloride

1. Cumming RG, Mitchell P. Medications and cataract – The Blue Mountains Eye Study. *Ophthalmology.* 1998;105(9):1751–1757.
2. Mann I. "Blue haloes" in Atebrin workers. *Br J Ophthalmol.* 1947;31:40–46.
3. Somerville-Large LB. Mepicrine and the eye. *Br J Ophthalmol.* 1947;31:191–192.

Drug: Thiabendazole

1. Fink AI, MacKay CJ, Cutler SS. Sicca complex and cholangiostatic jaundice in two members of a family probably cause by thiabendazole. *Ophthalmology.* 1979;86(10):1892–1896.
2. Rex D, Lumeng L, Eble J, et al. Intrahepatic cholestasis and sicca complex after thiabendazole. *Gastroenterology.* 1983;85:718–721.
3. Davidson RN, Weir WRC, Kaye GL, et al. Intrahepatic cholestasis after thiabendazole. *Trans R Soc Trop Med Hyg.* 1988;82:620.

Drug: Amikacin sulfate

1. D'Amico DJ, Caspers-Velu L, Libert J, et al. Comparative toxicity of intravitreal aminoglycoside Antibiotics. *Am J Ophthalmol.* 1985;100:264–275.
2. Campochiaro PA, Conway BP. Aminoglycoside toxicity – A survey of retinal specialists: implications for ocular use. *Arch Ophthalmol.* 1991;109:946–950.
3. Campochiaro PA, Green WR. Toxicity of intravitreous ceftazidime in primate retina. *Arch Ophthalmol.* 1992;110:1625–1629.
4. Campochiaro PA, Lim JI. The Aminoglycoside Toxicity Study Group. Aminoglycoside toxicity in the treatment of endophthalmitis. *Arch Ophthalmol.* 1994;112:48–53.
5. Doft BH, Barza M. Ceftazidime or amikacin: choice of intravitreal antimicrobials in the treatment of postoperative endophthalmitis. *Arch Ophthalmol.* 1994;112:17–18.
6. Doft BH, Barza M. Macular infarction after intravitreal amikacin. *Br J Ophthalmol.* 2004;88:850.
7. Galloway G, Ramsay A, Jordan K. Macular infarction after intravitreal amikacin: mounting evidence against amikacin. *Br J Ophthalmol.* 2002;86:359–360.
8. Galloway G, Ramsay A, Jordan K, et al. Macular infarction after intravitreal amikacin: authors' reply. *Br J Ophthalmol.* 2004;88:1228.

Drugs: Amoxicillin, ampicillin, nafcillin sodium, piperacillin, ticarcillin monosodium

1. Perez-Roca F, Alfaro Juarez A, Sanchez Merino C, et al. Convergence palsy secondary to amoxicillin. *Arch Soc Esp Oftalmol.* 2016;91(12):589–591.

Drugs: Azithromycin, clarithromycin, clindamycin, erythromycin

1. Pradhan S, Pardasani V, Ramteke K. Azithromycin-induced myasthenic crisis: reversibility with calcium gluconate. *Neurol India.* 2009;57(3):352–353.
2. Parker DL, Hoffmann TK, Tucker MA, et al. Elevated international normalized ration associated with concurrent use of ophthalmic erythromycin and warfarin. *Am J Health Syst Pharm.* 2010;67:38–41.

Drug: Bacitracin

1. Fisher AA, Adams RM. Anaphylaxis following the use of bacitracin ointment. *Am Acad Dermatol.* 1987;16:1057.
2. Caraballo J, Binkley E, Han I, et al. Intraoperative anaphylaxis to bacitracin during scleral buckle surgery. *Ann Allergy Asthma Immunol.* 2017;119(6):559–560.
3. Castro E, Seeley M, Kosmorsky G, et al. Orbital compartment syndrome caused by intraorbital bacitracin ointment after endoscopic sinus surgery. *Am J Ophthalmol.* 2000;130:376–378.

Drug: Benzathine benzylpenicillin (benzathine G penicillin)

1. Saleh MG, Campbell JP, Yang P, et al. Ultra-wide-field fundus autofluorescence and spectral-domain optic coherence tomography findings in syphilitic outer retinitis. *Ophthalmic Surg Lasers Imaging Retina.* 2017;48(3):208–215.
2. Kawasaki K, Ohnogi J. Nontoxic concentration of antibiotics for intravitreal use – evaluated by human in vitro ERG. *Doc Ophthalmol.* 1989;70:301–308.

Drugs: Cefaclor, cefadroxil, cefalexin (cephalexin), cefazolin sodium, cefditoren pivoxil, cefoperazone sodium, cefotaxime, cefotetan disodium, cefoxitin sodium, cefradine, ceftazidime, ceftizoxime sodium, ceftriaxone sodium, cefuroxime, cefuroxime axetil

1. Cefaclor. 2018 Retrieved from http://www.pdr.net.
2. Akman C, Duran A, Kalafat UM, et al. Uveitis attack and drug reaction due to cefuroxime axetil. *Cutan Ocul Toxicol.* 2016;35(3):254–256.
3. Kraushar MF, Nussbaum P, Kisch AL. Anaphylactic reaction to intravitreal cefazolin (letter). *Retina.* 1994;14(2):187–188.
4. Platt LW. Bilateral peripheral corneal edema after cefaclor therapy. *Arch Ophthalmol.* 1990;108:175.
5. D'Amico Ricci G, Airaghi G, Boscia F, et al. Spectral-domain optical coherence tomography and fluorescein angiography features of cystoid macular edema with serous

retinal detachment secondary to intracameral cefuroxime administration. *JCRS Online Case Rep.* 2016;4(4):84–89.
6. Gimenez-de-la-Linde M, Gimenez-Alcantara B, Barañano-Alcaide R, et al. Macular oedema after uncomplicated cataract surgery. Possible relationship with the volume of intracameral cefuroxime. *Arch Soc Esp Oftalmol.* 2017;92(1):49–50.
7. Kontos A, Mitry D, Althauser S, et al. Acute serous macular detachment and cystoid macular edema after uncomplicated phacoemulsification using standard dose subconjunctival cefuroxime. *Cutan Ocul Toxicol.* 2014;33(3):233–234.
8. Xiao H, Liu X, Guo X. Macular edema with serous retinal detachment post-phacoemulsification followed by spectral domain optical coherence tomography: a report of two cases. *BMC Res Notes.* 2015;8:647.
9. Faure C, Perreira D, Audo I. Retinal toxicity after intracameral use of a standard dose of cefuroxime during cataract surgery. *Doc Ophthalmol.* 2015;130(1):57–63.
10. Gupta MS, McKee HDR, Saldaña M, et al. Macular thickness after cataract surgery with intracameral cefuroxime. *J Cataract Refract Surg.* 2005;31(6):1163–1166.
11. Hann JV, Lee LR. Macular thickness after cataract surgery with intracameral cefuroxime. *J Cataract Refract Surg.* 2006;32(4):545:author reply 545.
12. Ciftci S, Ciftci L, Dag U. Hemorrhagic retinal infarction due to inadvertent overdose of cefuroxime in cases of complicated cataract surgery: retrospective case series. *Am J Ophthalmol.* 2014;157(2):421–425.
13. Le Du B, Pierre-Kahn V. Early macular edema after phacoemulsification and suspected overdose of cefuroxime: report of six cases. *J Fr Ophtalmol.* 2014;37(3):202–210.
14. Delyfer MN, Rougier MB, Leoni S, et al. Ocular toxicity after intracameral injection of very high doses of cefuroxime during cataract surgery. *J Cataract Refract Surg.* 2011;37(2):271–278.
15. Qureshi F, Clark D. Macular infarction after inadvertent intracameral cefuroxime. *J Cataract Refract Surg.* 2011;37(6):1168–1169.
16. Wong DC, Waxman MD, Herrinton LJ, et al. Transient macular edema after intracameral injection of a moderately elevated dose of cefuroxime during phacoemulsification surgery. *JAMA Ophthalmol.* 2015;133(10):1194–1197.

Drug: Chloramphenicol

1. Berry M, Gurung A, Easty DL. Toxicity of antibiotics and antifungal on cultured human corneal cells: effect of mixing, exposure and concentration. *Eye.* 1995;9(Pt 1):110–115.
2. Fraunfelder FW, Fraunfelder FT. Restricting topical ocular chloramphenicol eye drop use in the United States. Did we overreact? *Am J Ophthalmol.* 2013;156(3):420–422.
3. Fraunfelder FT, Bagby Jr GC, Kelly DJ. Fatal aplastic anemia following topical administration of ophthalmic chloramphenicol. *Am J Ophthalmol.* 1982;93:356–360.

4. Fraunfelder FT, Morgan RL, Yunis AA. Blood dyscrasias and topical ophthalmic chloramphenicol. *Am J Ophthalmol.* 1993;115(6):812–813.

5. Fraunfelder FW, Fraunfelder FT. Scientific challenges in postmarketing surveillance of ocular adverse drug reactions. *Am J Ophthalmol.* 2007;143:145–149.

6. *Physicians' Desk Reference.* 42nd ed. Oradell, NJ: Medical Economics Co; 1988.

7. Laporte JR, Vidal X, Ballarin E, et al. Possible association between ocular chloramphenicol and aplastic anaemia – the absolute risk is very low. *Br J Clin Pharm.* 1998;46(2):181–184.

Drugs: Ciprofloxacin, sparfloxacin, tosufloxacin

1. Vrabec TR, Sergott RC, Jaeger EA, et al. Reversible visual loss in a patient receiving high-dose ciprofloxacin hydrochloride. *Ophthalmology.* 1990;97(6):707–710.

2. Fraunfelder FW, Fraunfelder FT. Diplopia and fluoroquinolones. *Ophthalmology.* 2009;116:1814–1817.

3. Etminan M, Forooghian F, Brophy JM, et al. Oral fluoroquinolones and the risk of retinal detachment. *JAMA.* 2012;307(13):1414–1419.

4. Han DP, Szabo A. Flashes, floaters, and oral fluoroquinolones. *JAMA Ophthalmol.* 2013;131(1):91–93.

5. Albini TA, Karakousis PC, Abbey AM, et al. Association between oral fluoroquinolones and retinal detachment. *Am J Ophthalmol.* 2012;154(6):919–921.

6. Raguideau F, Lemaitre M, Dray-Spira R, et al. Association between oral fluoroquinolone use and retinal detachment: a case-only design study of 27,540 retinal detachments. *JAMA Ophthalmol.* 2016;134(4):415–421.

7. VanderBeek BL. Oral fluoroquinolones, retinal detachments and claims database studies. *JAMA Ophthalmol.* 2016;134(4):422–423.

8. Kapoor KG, Hodge DO, Sauver JL, et al. Oral fluoroquinolones and the incidence of rhegmatogenous retinal detachment and symptomatic retinal breaks. *Ophthalmology.* 2014;121(6):1269–1273.

9. Fife D, Zhu V, Voss E, et al. Exposure to oral fluoroquinolones and the risk of retinal detachment: retrospective analyses of two large healthcare databases. *Drug Saf.* 2014;37(3):171–182.

10. Sandhu HS, Brucker AJ, Ma L, et al. Oral fluoroquinolones and the risk of uveitis. *JAMA Ophthalmol.* 2016;134(1):38–43.

11. Leibowitz HW. Clinical evaluation of ciprofloxacin 0.3% ophthalmic solution for treatment of bacterial keratitis. *Am J Ophthalmol.* 1991;112:34S–47S.

12. Wilhelmus KR, Abshire RL. Corneal ciprofloxacin precipitation during bacterial keratitis. *Am J Ophthalmol.* 2003;136:1032–1037.

13. Patwardhan A, Khan M. Topical ciprofloxacin can delay recovery from viral ocular surface infection. *J Roy Soc Med.* 2005;98:274–275.

14. Agarwal AK, Ram J, Singh R. Sparfloxacin-associated corneal epithelial toxicity. *BMJ Case Rep Sept.* 2014;19.

15. Kim YD, Kim MK, Wee WR, et al. Tosufloxacin deposits in compromised corneas. *Optom Vis Sci.* 2014;91(9):e241–e244.

16. Tripathi A, Chen SI. Acute psychosis following the use of topical ciprofloxacin. *Arch Ophthalmol.* 2002;120:665–666.

17. Malladi SS, Liew EK, Ng XT, et al. Ciprofloxacin eye drops-induced subtherapeutic serum phenytoin levels resulting in breakthrough seizures. *Singapore Med J.* 2014;55(7):e114–e115.

18. Krachmer JH, Palay DA. *Cornea Atlas.* 2nd ed. London: Mosby Elsevier; 2006.

Drugs: Demeclocycline hydrochloride, doxycycline, minocycline hydrochloride, oxytetracycline, tetracycline hydrochloride

1. Chiu AM, Cheunkongkaew WL, Cornblath WT, et al. Minocycline treatment and pseudotumor cerebri syndrome. *Am J Ophthalmol.* 1998;126(1):116–121.

2. Gardner K, Cox T, Digre KB. Idiopathic intracranial hypertension associated with tetracycline use in fraternal twins: case reports and review. *Neurology.* 1995;45:6–10.

3. Fraunfelder FT, Randall JA. Minocycline-induced scleral pigmentation. *Ophthalmology.* 1997;104(6):936–938.

4. Bradfield YS, Robertson DM, Salomao DR, et al. Minocycline-induced ocular pigmentation. *Arch Ophthalmol.* 2003;121:114–145.

5. Jung JJ, Chen MH, Sorenson AL, et al. Swept-source optical coherence tomography and OCT angiography of minocycline-induced retinal and systemic hyperpigmentation. *Ophthalmic Surg Lasers Imaging Retina.* 2016;47(4):356–361.

6. Wilson ME, Sridhar J, Garg SJ, et al. Spectral-domain optical coherence tomographic imaging of pigmented retinal pigment epithelial deposits in a patient with prolonged minocycline use. *JAMA Ophthalmol.* 2015;133(11):1360–1362.

7. Shah W, De Cock R. Actinic keratoconjunctivitis and minocycline (letter). *Eye.* 1999;13(Pt 1):119–120.

Drug: Filgrastim

1. Esmaeli B, Ahmadi MA, Kim S, et al. Marginal keratitis associated with administration of filgrastim and sargramostim in a healthy peripheral blood progenitor cell donor. *Cornea.* 2002;21:621–622.

2. Fraunfelder FW, Harrison D. Peripheral ulcerative keratitis associated with filgrastim. *Cornea.* 2007;26:368–369.

3. Aljaouni SK, Aljedani HM. Cataract associated with high-dose hematopoietic colony stimulating factor, case report and literature review. *Saudi Pharm J.* 2010;18(2):107–110.

Drugs: Gatifloxacin, levofloxacin, moxifloxacin hydrochloride, norfloxacin, ofloxacin

1. Desai C, Desai KJ, Shah UH. Ofloxacin induced hypersensitivity reaction. *J Assoc Physicians India.* 1999;47:349.

2. Claerhout I, Kestelyn PH, Meire F, et al. Corneal deposits after the topical use of ofloxacin in two children with vernal keratoconjunctivitis. *Br J Ophthalmol.* 2003;87:646.

3. Castillo A, Benitez del Castillo JM, Toledano N, et al. Deposits of topical norfloxacin in the treatment of bacterial keratitis. *Cornea*. 1997;16:420–423.

4. Awwad ST, Haddad W, Wang MX, et al. Corneal intrastromal gatifloxacin crystal deposits after penetrating keratoplasty. *Eye Contact Lens*. 2004;30:169–172.

5. Wittpenn JR. Crystallization of gatifloxacin after penetrating keratoplasty. *Eye Contact Lens*. 2005;31:93.

6. Cavanagh HD. Response: crystallization of gatifloxacin after penetrating keratoplasty. *Eye Contact Lens*. 2005;31:93.

7. Donnenfeld EP, Chruscicki DA, Bitterman A, et al. A comparison of fourth generation fluoroquinolones gatifloxacin 0.3% and moxifloxacin 0.5% in terms of ocular tolerability. *Curr Med Res Opin*. 2004;20:1753–1758.

8. Bringas-Calva R, Iglesias-Cortinas D. Acute and bilateral uveitis secondary to moxifloxacin. *Arch Soc Esp Oftalmol (Spain)*. 2004;79:357–359.

9. Duncombe A, Gueudry J, Massy N, et al. Severe pseudouveitis associated with moxifloxacin therapy. *J Fr Ophtalmol*. 2013;36(2):146–150.

10. Cano-Parra J, Diaz-Llopis M. Drug induced uveitis. *Arch Soc Esp Oftalmol*. 2005;80:137–149.

11. Morshedi RG, Bettis DI, Moshirfar M, et al. Bilateral acute iris transillumination following systemic moxifloxacin for respiratory illness: report of two cases and review of the literature. *Ocul Immunol Inflamm*. 2012;20(4):266–272.

12. Knape RM, Sayyad FE, Davis JL. Moxifloxacin and bilateral acute transillumination. *J Ophthalmic Inflamm Infect*. 2013;3(1):10.

13. Nascimento HM, Sousa JM, Campos MS, et al. Acute iris depigmentation following systemic moxifloxacin. *Clinics (Sao Paulo)*. 2013;68(7):899–900.

14. Broens A, Collignon N. Moxifloxacin and iris transillumination. *Revue Medicale de Liege*. 2016;71(7-8):321–323.

15. Den Beste KA, Okeke C. Trabeculotomy ab interno with trabectome as surgical management for systemic fluoroquinolone-induced pigmentary glaucoma: a case report. *Medicine (Baltimore)*. 2017;96(43):e7936.

16. Hinkle DM, Dacey MS, Mandelcorn E, et al. Bilateral uveitis associated with fluoroquinolone therapy. *Cutan Ocul Toxicol*. 2012;31(2):111–116.

17. Eadie B, Etminan M, Mikelberg FS. Risk for uveitis with oral moxifloxacin: a comparative safety study. *JAMA Ophthalmol*. 2015;133(1):81–84.

18. Fraunfelder FW, Fraunfelder FT. Diplopia and fluoroquinolones. *Ophthalmology*. 2009;116(9):1814–1817.

19. Muzi F, Gravanta G, Tati E, et al. Fluoroquinolones-induced tendinitis and tendon rupture in kidney transplant recipients: 2 cases and a review of the literature. *Transplant Proc*. 2007;39:1673–1675.

20. Sodhi M, Sheldon CA, Carleton B, et al. Oral fluoroquinolones and risk of secondary pseudotumor cerebri syndrome: nested case-control study. *Neurology*. 89(8):792–795.

21. Burka JM, Bower KS, Vanroekel C, et al. The effect of fourth-generation fluoroquinolones gatifloxacin and moxifloxacin on epithelial healing following photorefractive keratectomy. *Am J Ophthalmol*. 2005;140:83–87.

Drug: Gentamicin sulfate

1. Marra TR, Reynolds Jr NC, Stoddard JJ. Subjective oscillopsia ("jiggling vision") presumably due to aminoglycoside ototoxicity. *J Clin Neuroophthalmol*. 1988;8:35–38.

2. Bullard SR, O' Day DM. Pseudomembranous conjunctivitis following topical gentamicin therapy. *Arch Ophthalmol*. 1997;115:1591–1592.

3. Nathawad R, Mendez H, Ahmad A, et al. Severe ocular reactions after neonatal ocular prophylaxis with gentamicin ophthalmic ointment. *Pediatr Infect Dis J*. 2011;30(2):175–176.

4. Merlob P, Metzker A. Neonatal orbital irritant contact dermatitis caused by gentamicin ointment. *Cutis*. 1996;57:429–430.

5. Binenbaum G, Bruno CJ, Forbes BJ, et al. Periocular ulcerative dermatitis associated with gentamicin ointment prophylaxis in newborns. *J Pediatr*. 2010;156:320–321.

6. Libert J, Ketelbant-Balasse PE, Van Hoof F, et al. Cellular toxicity of gentamicin. *Am J Ophthalmol*. 1979;87:405–411.

7. D'Amico DJ, Kenyon KP. Drug-induced lipidoses of the cornea and conjunctiva. *Int Ophthalmol*. 1981;4:67–76.

8. Awan KJ. Mydriasis and conjunctival paresthesia from local gentamicin. *Am J Ophthalmol*. 1985;99:723–724.

9. Chapman JM, Abdelatif OMA, Cheeks L, et al. Subconjunctival gentamicin induction of extraocular toxic muscle myopathy. *Ophthalmic Res*. 1992;24:189–196.

10. Koban Y, Genc S, Bilgin G, et al. Toxic anterior segment syndrome following phacoemulsification secondary to overdose of intracameral gentamicin. *Case Rep Med*. 2014;2014:143564.

11. Campochiaro PA, Lim JI. Aminoglycoside toxicity in the treatment of endophthalmitis. *Arch Ophthalmol*. 1994;112:48–53.

12. Grizzard WS. Aminoglycoside toxicity in the treatment of endophthalmitis (letter). *Arch Ophthalmol*. 1995;113:262–263.

13. Campochiaro PA. Aminoglycoside toxicity in the treatment of endophthalmitis (letter). *Arch Ophthalmol*. 1995;113:262–263.

14. Heath Jeffery RC, Bowden FJ, Essex RW. Subconjunctival gentamicin-induced macular toxicity following suture less 25-gauge vitrectomy. *Clin Exp Ophthalmol*. 2017;45(3):301–304.

15. Leon Ruiz M, Izquierdo Esteban L, Parra Santiago A, et al. Binocular vertical diplopia following chemical labyrinthectomy with gentamicin: a case report and review of the literature. *Neurologia*. 2016;31(7):503–505.

16. Dresner SM, Kung NH, Palko JR, et al. Skew deviation and partial ocular tilt reaction due to intratympanic gentamicin injection, with review of the literature. *Neuroophthalmology*. 2017;41(5):268–270.

Drug: Kanamycin sulfate

1. Sanchez-Perez J, Lopez MP, De Vega Haro JM, et al. Allergic contact dermatitis from gentamicin in eyedrops, with cross-reactivity to kanamycin but not neomycin. *Contact Dermatitis*. 2001;44(1):54.

Drug: Linezolid

1. Azamfirei L, Copotoiu S-M, Branzaniuc K, et al. Complete blindness after optic neuropathy induced by short-term linezolid treatment in a patient suffering from muscle dystrophy. *Pharmacoepidem Dr S.* 2007;16:402–404.
2. Javaheri M, Khurana RN, O'Hearn TM, et al. Linezolid-induced optic neuropathy: a mitochondrial disorder? *Br J Ophthalmol.* 2007;91(1):111–115.
3. Brown J, Aitken SL, van Manen RP, et al. Potential for linezolid-related blindness: a review of spontaneous adverse event reports. *Pharmacotherapy.* 2011;31(6):585–590.
4. Lee S, Kang BH, Ryu WY, et al. Is severe and long-lasting linezolid-induced optic neuropathy reversible? *Intern Med.* 2018;57(24):3611–3613.
5. Wang MY, Sadun AA. Drug-related mitochondrial optic neuropathies. *J Neuroophthalmol.* 2013;33(2):172–178.
6. Nambia S, Rellosa N, Wassel RT, et al. Linezolid-associated peripheral and optic neuropathy in children. *Pediatrics.* 2011;127(6):e1528–e1532.
7. Linam WM, Wesselkamper K, Gerber MA. Peripheral neuropathy in an adolescent treated with linezolid. *Pediatr Infect Dis J.* 2009;28(2):149–151.
8. Ishii N, Kinouchi R, Inoue M, et al. Linezolid-induced optic neuropathy with a rare pathological change in the inner retina. *Int Ophthalmol.* 2016;36(6):761–766.
9. Ilarslan E, Aydin B, Kabatas EU, et al. Cataract in a preterm newborn: a possible side effect of linezolid therapy. *J Coll Physicians Surg Pak.* 2014;24(suppl 3):S281–S283.
10. Sotgiu G, Centis R, D'Ambrosio L, et al. Efficacy, safety and tolerability of linezolid containing regimens in treating MDR-TB and XDR-TB: systematic review and meta-analysis. *Eur Respir J.* 2012;40:1430–1442.
11. Sadun AA. Metabolic optic neuropathies. *Semin Ophthalmol.* 2002;17(1):29–32.

Drug: Nalidixic acid

1. Van Dyk HJL, Swan KC. Drug-induced pseudotumor cerebri. In: Leopold IH, ed. *Symposium on Ocular Therapy.* 4th ed. St Louis: Mosby; 1969:71–77.

Drug: Neomycin sulfate

1. Dohlman CH. Reply to query). *Arch Ophthalmol.* 1966;76:902.

Drug: Nitrofurantoin

1. Wittbrodt ET. Drugs and myasthenia gravis: an update. *Arch Intern Med.* 1997;157(4):399–408.
2. Mushet GR. Pseudotumor and nitrofurantoin therapy. *Arch Neurol.* 1977;34:257.
3. Khwaja GA, Duggal A, Kulkarni A, et al. Nitrofurantoin-induced reversible achromatopsia and visual field constriction defect. *JIACM.* 2015;16(1):90–92.
4. Ibanez HE, Williams DF, Boniuk I. Crystalline retinopathy associated with long-term nitrofurantoin therapy: case report. *Arch Ophthalmol.* 1994;112:304–305.
5. Crider KS, Cleves MA, Reefhuis J, et al. Antibacterial medication use during pregnancy and risk of birth defects: National Birth Defects Prevention Study. *Arch Pediat Adol Med.* 2009;163(11):978–985.

Drug: Polymyxin B sulfate

1. Henao MP, Ghaffari G. Anaphylaxis to polymyxin B-trimethoprim eye drops. *Ann Allergy Asthma Immunol.* 2016;116(4):372.

Drugs: Sulfacetamide sodium, sulfadiazine, sulfafurazole (sulfisoxazole), sulfamethizole, sulfamethoxazole, sulfanilamide, sulfasalazine, sulfathiazole

1. Waheep S, Feldman F, Velos P, et al. Ultrasound biomicroscopic analysis of drug-induced bilateral angle-closure glaucoma associated with supraciliary choroidal effusion. *Can J Ophthalmol.* 2003;38:299–302.
2. Tilden ME, Rosenbaum JT, Fraunfelder FT. Systemic sulfonamides as a cause of bilateral, anterior uveitis. *Arch Ophthalmol.* 1991;109:67–69.
3. Lane RJ, Routledge PA. Drug-induced neurological disorders. *Drugs.* 1983;26:124–147.
4. Fine HF, Kim E, Eichenbaum KD, et al. Toxic epidermal necrolysis induced by sulfonamide eyedrops. *Cornea.* 2008;27(9):1068–1069.
5. Waller SG. Skepticism and science (letter to the editor). *Cornea.* 2010;29(2):244.
6. Gutt L, Feder JM, Feder RS, et al. Corneal ring formation after exposure to sulfamethoxazole. *Arch Ophthalmol.* 1988;106:726–727.

Drug: Telithromycin

1. Telithromycin. 2018 Retrieved from http://www.pdr.net.

Drug: Tobramycin

1. Kaeser HE. Drug-induced myasthenic syndromes. *Acta Neurol Scand.* 1984;70(suppl 100):39–47.
2. Khella SL, Kozart D. Unmasking and exacerbation of myasthenia gravis by ophthalmic solutions: betaxolol, tobramycin, and dexamethasone. A case report (letter). *Muscle Nerve.* 1997;20(5):631.
3. Garzozi HJ, Muallem MS, Harris A. Recurrent anterior uveitis and glaucoma associated with inadvertent entry of ointment into the anterior chamber after radial keratotomy. *J Cataract Refract Surg.* 1999;25:1685–1687.
4. Balian JV. Accidental intraocular tobramycin injection: a case report. *Ophthalmic Surg.* 1983;14:353–354.
5. Judson PH. Aminoglycoside macular toxicity after subconjunctival injection. *Arch Ophthalmol.* 1989;107:1282–1283.
6. Pardines FH, Tapia-Quijada H, Hueso-Abancens JR. A case of aminoglycosides induced retinal toxicity treated with megadoses of steroids and an intravitreal dexamethasone implant (Ozurdex). *Arch Soc Esp Oftalmol.* 2016;91(6):288–291.
7. Campochiaro PA, Conway BP. Aminoglycoside toxicity – a survey of retinal specialists. *Arch Ophthalmol.* 1991;109:946–950.

8. Spalton DJ, Hitchings RA, Hunter PA. *Atlas of Clinical Ophthalmology*. 3rd ed. London: Mosby, Elsevier; 2005.

Drug: Trimethoprim

1. Arola O, Peltonen R, Rossi T. Arthritis, uveitis, and Stevens-Johnson syndrome induced by trimethoprim. *Lancet*. 1998;351(9109):1102.
2. Gilroy N, Gottlieb T, Spring P, et al. Trimethoprim-induced aseptic meningitis and uveitis. *Lancet*. 1997;350(9071):112.
3. Kristinsson JK, Hannesson OB, Sveinsson O, et al. Bilateral anterior uveitis and retinal haemorrhages after administration of trimethoprim. *Acta Ophthalmol Scand*. 1997;75(3):314–315.
4. Pathak S, Power B. Bilateral acute anterior uveitis as a side effect of trimethoprim. *Eye*. 2007;21(2):252–253.
5. Tilden ME, Rosenbaum JT, Fraunfelder FT. Systemic sulfonamides as a cause of bilateral, anterior uveitis. *Arch Ophthalmol*. 1991;109:67–69.

Drug: Amphotericin B

1. Li PK, Lai KN. Amphotericin B-induced ocular toxicity in cryptococcal meningitis. *Br J Ophthalmol*. 1989;73:397–398.
2. Bae JH, Lee SC. Intravitreal liposomal amphotericin B for treatment of endogenous candida endophthalmitis. *Jpn J Ophthalmol*. 2015;59(5):346–352.
3. Bell RW, Ritchey JP. Subconjunctival nodules after amphotericin B injection. *Arch Ophthalmol*. 1973;90:402–404.
4. Garcia-Valenzuela E, Song D. Intracorneal injection of amphotericin B for recurrent fungal keratitis and endophthalmitis. *Arch Ophthalmol*. 2005;123:1721–1723.
5. Sharma B, Kataria P, Anand R, et al. Efficacy profile of intracameral amphotericin B. The often forgotten step. *Asia-Pac J Ophthalmol*. 2015;4(6):360–366.
6. Payne JF, Keenum DG, Sternberg Jr P, et al. Concentration intravitreal amphotericin B in fungal endophthalmitis. *Arch Ophthalmol*. 2010;128(12):1546–1550.

Drug: Griseofulvin

1. Delman M, Leubuscher K. Transient macular edema due to griseofulvin. *Am J Ophthalmol*. 1963;56:658.

Drug: Voriconazole

1. Voriconazole. 2018 Retrieved from http://www.pdr.net.
2. Hariprasad SM, Mieler WF, Holz ER, et al. Determination of vitreous, aqueous, and plasma concentration of orally administered voriconazole in humans. *Arch Ophthalmol*. 2004;122:42–47.
3. Holmes NE, Trevillyan JM, Kidd SE, et al. Locally extensive angio-invasive Scedosporium prolificans infection following resection for squamous cell lung carcinoma. *Med Mycol Case Rep*. 2013;2:98–102.
4. Palamar M, Egrilmez S, Yilmaz SG, et al. Does topical voriconazole trigger dysplastic changes on the ocular surface? *J Chemother*. 2015;27(2):111–113.

5. Bayhan GI, Garipardic M, Karaman K, et al. Voriconazole-associated visual disturbances and hallucinations. *Cutan Ocul Toxicol*. 2016;35(1):80–82.
6. Kadikoy H, Barkmeier A, Peck B, et al. Persistent photopsia following course of oral voriconazole. *J Ocul Pharmacol Th*. 2010;26(4):387–389.
7. Laties AM, Fraunfelder FT, Tomaszewski K, et al. Long-term visual safety of voriconazole in adult patients with paracoccidioidomycosis. *Clin Ther*. 2010;32(13):2207–2217.
8. Cheng MP, Paquette K, Lands LC, et al. Voriconazole inhibition of vitamin A metabolism: Are adverse events increased in cystic fibrosis patients? *Pediatr Pulm*. 2010;45(7):661–666.

Drug: Clofazimine

1. Kaur I, Ram J, Kumar B, et al. Effect of clofazimine on eye in multibacillary leprosy. *Indian J Lepr*. 1990;62(1):87–90.
2. Craythorn JM, Swartz M, Creel DJ. Clofazimine-induced bull's-eye retinopathy. *Retina*. 1986;6:50–52.
3. Cunningham CA, Friedberg DN, Carr RE. Clofazimine-induced generalized retinal degeneration. *Retina*. 1990;10(2):131–134.
4. Forester DJ, Causey DM, Rao NA. Bull's eye retinopathy and clofazimine (letter). *Ann Int Med*. 1992;116(10):876–877.
5. Agarwal A. Clofazimine retinopathy: toxic diseases affecting the pigment epithelium and retina. In: *Gass' Atlas of Macular Diseases*. 5th ed. US: Elsevier Health Sciences; 2011:764.
6. Kasturi N, Srinivasan R. Clofazimine-induced premaculopathy in a vitiliginous patient. *J Pharmacol Pharmacother*. 2016;7(3):149–151.

Drug: Dapsone

1. Daneshmend TK, Homeida M. Dapsone-induced optic atrophy and motor neuropathy. *BMJ*. 1981;283:311.
2. Kenner DJ, Holt K, Agnello R, et al. Permanent retinal damage following massive dapsone overdose. *Br J Ophthalmol*. 1980;64:741–744.
3. Alexander TA, Raju R, Kuriakose T, et al. Presumed DDS ocular toxicity. *Indian J Ophthalmol*. 1989;37:150–151.
4. Chakrabarti M, Suresh PN, Namperumalsamy P. Bilateral macular infarction due to diaminodiphenyl sulfone (4,4′ DDS) toxicity. *Retina*. 1999;19(1):83–84.
5. Brandt F, Adiga RB, Pradhan H. Lagophthalmos and posterior synechias during treatment of leprosy with diaminodiphenylsulfone. *Klin Monatsbl Augenheilkd*. 1984;184:28–31.
6. Chalioulias K, Mayer E, Darvay A, et al. Anterior ischemic optic neuropathy associated with dapsone. *Eye*. 2006;20(8):943–945.
7. Hanuschk D, Kozyreff A, Tafzi N, et al. Acute visual loss following dapsone-induced methemoglobinemia and hemolysis. *Clin Toxicol (Phila)*. 2015;53(5):489–492.
8. Dapsone. 2018 Retrieved from http://www.pdr.net.

Drugs: Chloroquine phosphate, hydroxychloroquine sulfate

1. Easterbrook M. Is corneal decompensation of antimalarial any indication of retinal toxicity? *Can J Ophthalmol.* 1990;25(5):249–251.
2. Beebe WE, Abbott RL, Fung WE. Hydroxychloroquine crystals in the tear film of a patient with rheumatoid arthritis. *Am J Ophthalmol.* 1986;101:377–378.
3. Marmor MF. Despite plaquenil dosing recommendations, retinal toxicity remains. *Ocular Surgery News US Edition.* 2018.
4. Melles RB, Marmor MF. Pericentral retinopathy and racial differences in hydroxychloroquine toxicity. *Ophthalmology.* 2015;122(1):110–116.
5. Lee DH, Melles RB, Joe SG, et al. Pericentral hydroxychloroquine retinopathy in Korean patients. *Ophthalmology.* 2015;122(6):1252–1256.
6. Ahn SJ, Joung J, Lim HW, et al. Optic coherence tomography protocols for screening of hydroxychloroquine retinopathy in Asian patients. *Am J Ophthalmol.* 2017;184:11–18.
7. Rosenbaum JT, Trune DR, Barkhuizen A, et al. Ocular, aural, and oral manifestations. In: *Dubois' Lupus Erythematosus and Related Syndromes.* 8th ed. Elsevier; 2012:393–400.
8. Hobbs HE, Sorsby A, Freedman A. Retinopathy following chloroquine therapy. *Lancet.* 1959;2(7107):478–780.
9. Marmor MF, Carr RE, Easterbrook M, et al. Recommendations on screening for chloroquine and hydroxychloroquine retinopathy: a report by the. *American Academy of Ophthalmology.* 2002;109(7):1377–1382.
10. Osadchy A, Ratnapalan T, Koren G. Ocular toxicity in children exposure in utero to antimalarial drugs: review of the literature. *J Rheumatol.* 2011;38(12):2504–2508.
11. Wittbrodt ET. Drugs and myasthenia gravis. *Arch Int Med.* 1997;157:399–408.
12. Cumming RG, Mitchell P. Medications and cataract: The Blue Mountain Eye Study. *Ophthalmology.* 1998;105(9):1751–1758.
13. Leung LS, Neal JW, Wakelee HA, et al. Rapid onset of retinal toxicity from high-dose hydroxychloroquine given for cancer therapy. *Am J Ophthalmol.* 2015;160(4):799–805.
14. Marmor MF, Kellner U, Lai TYY, et al. American Academy of Ophthalmology Statement: Recommendations on screening for chloroquine and hydroxychloroquine retinopathy (2016 Revision). *Ophthalmology.* 2016;124(3):28–29.
15. Melles RB, Marmor MF. The risk of toxic retinopathy in patients on long-term hydroxychloroquine therapy. *JAMA Ophthalmol.* 2014;132:1453–1460.
16. Pham BH, Marmor MF. Sequential changes in hydroxychloroquine retinopathy up to 20 years after stopping the drug: implications for mild vs. severe toxicity. *Retina.* 2019;39:492–501.

Drug: Mefloquine hydrochloride

1. Palmer KJ, Holliday SM, Brogden RN. Mefloquine: a review of its antimalarial activity pharmacokinetic properties and therapeutic efficacy. *Drugs.* 1993;45(3):430–475.
2. Mefloquine. 2018 Retrieved from http://www.pdr.net.
3. Walker RA, Colleaux KM. Maculopathy associated with mefloquine (Lariam) therapy for malaria prophylaxis. *Can J Ophthalmol.* 2007;42:125–126.
4. Jain M, Nevin RL, Ahmed I. Mefloquine-associated dizziness, diplopia, and central serous chorioretinopathy: a case report. *J Med Case Rep.* 2016;10(1):305.
5. De Mendonca Melo M, Martinez Ciriano JP, van Genderen PJJ. Narrow vision after view-broadening travel. *J Travel Med.* 2008;15(4):278–280.
6. Fujii T, Kaku K, Jelinek T, et al. Malaria and mefloquine prophylaxis use among Japan Ground Self-Defense Force personnel deployed in East Timor. *J Travel Med.* 2007;14(4):226–232.
7. Schneider C, Adamcova M, Jick SS, et al. Use of anti-malarial drugs and the risk of developing eye disorders. *Travel Med Infect Dis.* 2014;12(1):40–47.
8. Adamcova M, Schaerer MT, Bercaru I, et al. Eye disorders reported with the use of mefloquine (Lariam) chemoprophylaxis – a drug safety database analysis. *Travel Med Infect Dis.* 2015;13(5):400–408.

Drug: Quinine sulfate

1. Grant WM, Schuman JS. Effects on the eyes and visual system from chemicals, drugs, metals and minerals, plants, toxins and venoms; also, systemic side effects from eye medications. In: *Toxicology of the Eye.* 4th ed. Springfield, IL: Charles C. Thomas; 1993.
2. Waddell K. Blindness from quinine as an antimalarial (letter). *Trans Roy Soc Trop Med Hygiene.* 1996;89(4):331–332.
3. Boland MD, Roper SMB, Henry JA. Complications of quinine poisoning. *J Ir Med Assoc.* 1974;67:46–47.
4. Zahn JR, Brinton GF, Norton E. Ocular quinine toxicity followed by electroretinogram, electro-oculogram, and pattern visually evoked potential. *Am J Optom Physiol Optics.* 1981;58:492–498.
5. Su D, Robson AG, Xu D, et al. Quinine toxicity: multimodal retinal imaging and electroretinography findings. *Retin Cases Brief Rep.* 2017;11(suppl 1):S102–S106.
6. Hustead JD. Granulomatous uveitis and quinidine hypersensitivity. *Am J Ophthalmol.* 1991;112(4):461–462.
7. Segal A, Aisemberg A, Ducasse A. Quinine transitory myopia and angle-closure glaucoma. *Bull Soc Ophtalmol Fr.* 1983;83:247–249.
8. Schuman JS. Acute bilateral transitory myopia associated with open angle glaucoma. In: Epstein DL, Allingham RR, Schuman JS, eds. *Chandler and Grant's Glaucoma.* 4th ed. Baltimore: Williams and Wilkens; 1997:341.
9. Canning CR, Hague S. Ocular quinine toxicity. *Br J Ophthalmol.* 1988;72:23–26.
10. Knox DL, Palmer CA, English F. Iris atrophy after quinine amblyopia. *Arch Ophthalmol.* 1966;76:359–362.
11. Traill A, Patmaraj R, Zamir E. Quinine iris toxicity. *Arch Ophthalmol.* 2007;125:430.

12. Smidt D, Torpet LA, Nauntofte B, et al. Associations between oral and ocular dryness, labial and whole salivary flow rates, systemic diseases and medications in a sample of older people. *Community Dent Oral.* 2011;39(3):276–288.
13. Worden AN, Frape DL, Shephard NW. Consumption of quinine hydrochloride in tonic water. *Lancet.* 1987;1:271–272.
14. Quinine sulfate. (2018). Retrieved from http://www.pdr.net.
15. Spalton DJ, Hitchings RA, Hunter PA. *Atlas of Clinical Ophthalmology.* 3rd ed. London: Mosby Elsevier; 2005.

Drug: Metronidazole

1. Putnam D, Fraunfelder FT, Dreis M. Metronidazole and optic neuritis. *Am J Ophthalmol.* 1991;112(6):737.
2. Snavely SR, Hodges GR. The neurotoxicity of antibacterial agents. *Ann Intern Med.* 1984;101:92–104.
3. Kafadar I, Moustafa F, Yalcin K, et al. A rare adverse effect of metronidazole. *Pediatr Emer Care.* 2013;29(6):751–752.
4. McGrath NM, Kent-Smith B, Franzco DM. Reversible optic neuropathy due to metronidazole. *Clin Experiment Ophthalmol.* 2007;35(6):585–586.
5. Bouraoui R, Limaiem R, Bouladi M, et al. Effets secondaires neuro-ophtalmologiques due traitment par metronidazole chez l'enfant: a propos de deux cas. *Arch Pediatr.* 2016;23(2):167–170.
6. Lee SU, Jung IE, Kim HJ, et al. Metronidazole-induced combined peripheral and central vestibulopathy. *J Neurol Sci.* 2016;365:31–33.
7. Etxeberria A, Lonneville S, Rutgers MP, et al. Metronidazole-cerebellopathy associated with peripheral neuropathy, downbeat nystagmus, and bilateral ocular abduction deficit. *Rev Neurol. (Paris).* 2012;168(2):192–195.
8. Grinbaum A, Ashkenazi I, Avni I, et al. Transient myopia following metronidazole treatment for trichomonas vaginalis. *JAMA.* 1992;267(4):511–512.
9. Kirkham G, Gott J. Oculogyric crisis associated with metronidazole. *BMJ.* 1986;292:174.
10. Turnbull AMJ. Severe bilateral anterior uveitis secondary to giardiasis, initially misdiagnosed as a side effect of metronidazole. *Eye (Lond).* 2013;27(10):1225–1226.
11. Cantu JM, Garcia-Cruz D. Midline facial defect as a teratogenic effect of metronidazole. *Birth Defects.* 1982;18:85–88.

Drug: Suramin sodium

1. Hemady RK, Sinibaldi VJ, Eisenberger MA. Ocular symptoms and signs associated with suramin sodium treatment for metastatic cancer of the prostate. *Am J Ophthalmol.* 1996;121(3):291–296.
2. Teich SA, Handwerger S, Mathur-Wagh U, et al. Toxic keratopathy associated with suramin therapy. *N Engl J Med.* 1986;314:1455–1456.
3. Holland EJ, Stein CA. Palestine AG, et al. Suramin keratopathy. *Am J Ophthalmol.* 1988;106:216–220.

Drug: Cycloserine

1. Weaver DT, Bartley GB. Cyclosporine-induced trichomegaly. *Am J Ophthalmol.* 1990;109(2):239.

Drug: Ethambutol hydrochloride

1. Kim KL, Park SP. Visual function test for early detection of ethambutol induced ocular toxicity at the subclinical level. *Cutan Ocul Toxicol.* 2016;35(3):228–232.
2. Kakisu Y, Adachi-Usami E, Mizota A. Pattern of electroretinogram and visual evoked cortical potential in ethambutol optic neuropathy. *Doc Ophthalmol.* 1988;67:327–334.
3. Bouffard MA, Nathavitharana RR, Yassa DS, et al. Retreatment with ethambutol after toxic optic neuropathy. *J Neuro-Ophthalmol.* 2017;37:40–42.
4. Ethambutol hydrochloride. (2018). Retrieved from http://www.pdr.net.
5. Guerra R, Casu L. Hydroxocobalamin for ethambutol-induced optic neuropathy. *Lancet.* 1981;2:1176.
6. Heng JE, Vorwerk CK, Lessell E, et al. Ethambutol is toxic to retinal ganglion cells via excitotoxic pathway. *Invest Ophthalmol Vis Sci.* 1999;40(1):190–196.
7. Melamud A, Kosmorsky GS, Lee MS. Ocular ethambutol toxicity. *Mayo Clin Proc.* 2003;78:1409–1411.

Drug: Ethionamide

1. Ethionamide. (2018). Retrieved from http://www.pdr.net.

Drug: Isoniazid

1. Neunhöffer H, Gold A, Hoerauf H, et al. Isolated ocular Harisch-Herxheimer reaction after initiating tuberculostatic therapy in a child. *Int Ophthalmol.* 2014;34(3):675–677.
2. Kim Y-K, Hwang J-M. Serial retinal nerve fiber layer changes in patients with toxic optic neuropathy associated with antituberculosis pharmacotherapy. *J Ocul Pharmacol Ther.* 2009;25(6):531–535.
3. Dompeling E, Schut E, Vles H, et al. Diplopia and strabismus convergens mimicking symptoms of tuberculous meningitis as side-effects of isoniazid. *Eur J Pediatr.* 2004;163:503–504.
4. Honegger H, Genee E. Disturbances of accommodation in association with treatment with tuberculostatics. *Klin Monatsbl Augenheilkd.* 1969;155:361–380.
5. Neff TA. Isoniazid toxicity – lactic acidosis and keratopathy. *Chest.* 1971;59:245–248.
6. Gan NY, Teoh SC. Isoniazid-related bilateral choroidal effusions. *Eye.* 2010;24:1408–1409.

Drug: Rifabutin

1. Fraunfelder FW, Rosenbaum JT. Drug-induced uveitis. *Drug Safety.* 1997;17(3):197–207.
2. Shafran SD, Deschênes J, Miller M, et al. For the MAC study group of the Canadian HIV trials network. Uveitis and pseudojaundice during a regimen of clarithromycin, rifabutin, and ethambutol. *N Engl J Med.* 1994;330:438–439.

3. Chaknis MJ, Brooks SE, Mitchell KT, et al. Inflammatory opacities of the vitreous in rifabutin-associated uveitis. *Am J Ophthalmol.* 1996;122(4):580–582.

4. Jacobs DS, Piliero PJ, Kuperwaser MG, et al. Acute uveitis associated with rifabutin use in patients with human immunodeficiency virus infection. *Am J Ophthalmol.* 1994;118:716–722.

5. Smith JA, Mueller BU, Nussenblatt RB, et al. Corneal endothelial deposits in children positive for human immunodeficiency virus receiving rifabutin prophylaxis for *Mycobacterium avium* complex bacteremia. *Am J Ophthalmol.* 1999;127(2):164–169.

6. Mazzotta C, Traversi C, Nuti E, et al. Rifabutin corneal deposits in a patient with acquired immunodeficiency syndrome: in vivo confocal microscopy investigation. *Eur J Ophthalmol.* 2009;19(3):481–483.

7. Williams K, Ilari L. Persistent corneal endothelial deposits associated with rifabutin therapy for Crohn's disease. *Cornea.* 2010;29(6):706–707.

8. Jones DF, Irwin AE. Discoloration of intraocular lens subsequent to rifabutin use. *Arch Ophthalmol.* 2002;120:1211–1212.

9. Ponjavic V, Gränse L, Bengtsson-Stigma E, et al. Retinal dysfunction and anterior segment deposits in a patient treated with rifabutin. *Act Ophthalmol Scand.* 2002;80:553–556.

Drug: Rifampin

1. Girling DJ. Ocular toxicity due to rifampicin. *BMJ.* 1976;1:585.

2. Lyons RW. Orange contact lenses from rifampin. *N Engl J Med.* 1979;300:372–373.

3. Fraunfelder FT. Orange tears. *Am J Ophthalmol.* 1980;89:752.

FURTHER READING
Broxyquinoline and diiodohydroxyquinoline

Baumgartner G, Gawel MJ, Kaeser HE, et al. Neurotoxicity of halogenated hydroxyquinolines: clinical analysis of cases reported outside Japan. *J Neurol Neurosurg Psychiatry.* 1979;42:1073–1083.

Committee on Drugs. 1989–. Clioquinol (iodochlorhydroxyquin, vioform) and iodoquinol (diiodohydroxyquin): blindness and neuropathy. *Pediatrics.* 1990;86(5):797–798.

Guy-Grand B, Basdevant A, Soffer M. Oxyquinoline neurotoxicity. *Lancet.* 1983;1(8331):993.

Hanakago R, Uono M. Clioquinol intoxication occurring in the treatment of acrodermatitis enteropathica with reference to SMON outside of Japan. *Clin Toxicol.* 1981;18:1427–1434.

Hansson O, Herxheimer A. Neurotoxicity of oxyquinolines. *Lancet.* 1980;2:1253–1254.

Kono R. Review of subacute myelo-optic neuropathy (SMON) and studies done by the SMON research commission. *Jpn J Med Sci Biol.* 1975;28(suppl):121.

Oakley GP. The neurotoxicity of the halogenated hydroxyquinolines. *JAMA.* 1973;225:395–397.

Ricoy JR, Ortega A, Cabello A. Subacute myelo-optic neuropathy (SMON). First neuro-pathological report outside Japan. *J Neurol Sci.* 1982;53:241–251.

Rose FC, Gawel M. Clioquinol neurotoxicity: an overview. *Acta Neurol Scand.* 1984;70(suppl 100):137–145.

Shibasaki H, Kakigi R, Ohnishi A, et al. Peripheral and central nerve conduction in subacute myelo-optic neuropathy. *Neurology.* 1982;32:1186–1189.

Shigematsu I. Subacute Myelo-Optic Neuropathy (SMON) and clioquinol. *Jpn J Med Sci Biol.* 1975;28(suppl):35–55.

Sturtevant FM. Zinc deficiency acrodermatitis enteropathica, optic atrophy SMON, and 5,7-dihalo-8-quinolinols. *Pediatrics.* 1980;65:610–613.

Tjälve H. The aetiology of SMON may involve an interaction between clioquinol and environmental metals. *Med Hypotheses.* 1984;15:293–299.

Emetine hydrochloride

Lasky MA. Corneal response to emetine hydrochloride. *Arch Ophthalmol.* 1950;44:47–52.

Porges N. Tragedy in compounding (Letter). *J Am Pharm Assoc Pract Pharm.* 1948;9:593.

Torres Estrada A. Ocular lesions caused by emetine. *Bol Hosp Oftal NS Luz (Mex).* 1944;2:145. (*Am J Ophthalmol.* 1945;28:1060).

Diethylcarbamazine citrate

Bird AC, El-Sheikh H, Anderson J, et al. Visual loss during oral diethylcarbamazine treatment for Onchocerciasis. *BMJ.* 1979;2:46.

Bird AC, El-Sheikh H, Anderson J, et al. Changes in visual function and in the posterior segment of the eye during treatment of onchocerciasis with diethylcarbamazine citrate. *Br J Ophthalmol.* 1980;64:191–200.

Dadzie KY, Bird AC. Ocular findings in a double-blind study of ivermectin versus diethylcarbamazapine versus placebo in the treatment of onchocerciasis. *Br J Ophthalmol.* 1987;71:78–85.

Hawking F. Diethylcarbamazine and new compounds for treatment of filariasis. *Adv Pharmacol Chemother.* 1979;16:129–194.

Jones BR, Anderson J, Fuglsang H. Effects of various concentrations of diethylcarbamazine citrate applied as eye drops in ocular onchocerciasis, and the possibilities of improved therapy from continuous non-pulsed delivery. *Br J Ophthalmol.* 1978;62:428–439.

Taylor HR, Greene BM. Ocular changes with oral and transepidermal diethylcarbamazine therapy of onchocerciasis. *Br J Ophthalmol.* 1981;65:494–502.

Mepacrine hydrochloride

Abbey EA, Lawrence EA. The effect of Atabrine suppressive therapy on eyesight in pilots. *JAMA.* 1946;130:786.

Ansdell VE, Common JD. Corneal changes induced by mepacrine. *J Trop Med Hyg.* 1979;82:206–207.

Blumenfeld NE. Staining of the conjunctiva and cornea. *Vestn Oftalmol.* 1946;25:39.

Carr RE, Henkind P, Rothfield N, et al. Ocular toxicity of antimalarial drugs: long term follow-up. *Am J Ophthalmol.* 1968;66:738–744.

Chamberlain WP, Boles DJ. Edema of cornea precipitated by quinacrine (Atabrine). *Arch Ophthalmol.* 1946;35:120–134.

Dame LR. Effects of Atabrine on the visual system. *Am J Ophthalmol.* 1946;29:1432–1434.

Evans RL, Khalid S, Kinney JL. Antimalarial psychosis revisited. *Arch Dermatol.* 1984;120:765–767.

Ferrera A. Optic neuritis from high doses of Atebrin. *Rass Intal Ottalmol.* 1943;12:123.

Granstein RD, Sober AJ. Drug-and heavy metal-induced hyperpigmentation. *J Am Acad Dermatol.* 1981;5:1–18.

Koranda FC. Antimalarials. *J Am Acad Dermatol.* 1981;4:650–655. In: Sokol RJ, Lichenstein PK, Farrell MK, eds. Quinacrine hydrochloride yellow discoloration of the skin in children. *Pediatrics.* 1982;69:232–233.

Piperazine

Bomb BS, Bebi HK. Neurotoxic side-effects of piperazine. *Trans R Soc Trop Med Hyg.* 1976;70:358.

Brown HW, Chan KF, Hussey KL. Treatment of enterobiasis and ascariasis with piperazine. *JAMA.* 1956;161:515–520.

Combes B, Damon A, Gottfried E. Piperazine (Antepar) neurotoxicity report of case probably due to renal insufficiency. *N Engl J Med.* 1956;254:223–237.

Mezey P. The role of piperazine derivates in the pathogenesis of cataract. *Klin Monatsbl Augenheilkd.* 1967;151:885–887.

Mossmer A. On the effectiveness, dosage, and toxic effects of piperazine preparations. *Med Mschr.* 1956;10:517–526.

Neff L. Another severe psychological reaction to side effect of medication in an adolescent. *JAMA.* 1966;197:218–219.

Rouher F, Cantat MA. Instructive observation of an ocular paralysis after taking piperazine. *Bull Soc Franc Ophthalmol.* 1962;75:460–465.

Thiabendazole

Drugs for parasitic infections. *Med Lett Drugs Ther.* 1982;24:12.

Fink AI, MacKay CJ, Cutler SS. Sicca complex and cholestatic jaundice in two members of a family caused by thiabendazole. *Trans Am Ophthalmol Soc.* 1978;76:108–115.

Fraunfelder FT. Interim report: National Registry of Drug-Induced Ocular Side Effects. *Ophthalmology.* 1979;86:126–130.

Fraunfelder FT, Meyer SM. Ocular toxicology update. *Aust J Ophthalmol.* 1984;12:391–394.

Robinson HJ, Stoerk HC, Graessle O. Studies on the toxicologic and pharmacologic properties of Thiabendazole. *Toxicol Appl Pharmacol.* 1965;7:53–63.

Amikacin sulfate

Jackson TL, Williamson TH. Amikacin retinal toxicity. *Br J Ophthalmol.* 1999;83:1199–1200.

Piguet B, Chobaz C, Grounauer PA. Toxic retinopathy caused by intravitreal injection of amikacin and vancomycin. *Klin Monatsbl Augenheilkd.* 1996;208:358–359.

Seawright AA, Bourke RD, Cooling RJ. Macula toxicity after intravitreal amikacin. *Austral New Zealand J Ophthalmol.* 1996;24:143–146.

Verma L, Arora R, Sachdev MS. Macular infarction after intravitreal injection of amikacin. *Can J Ophthalmol.* 1993;28:241–243.

Amoxicillin, ampicillin, nafcillin sodium, piperacillin, ticarcillin monosodium

Argov Z, Brenner T, Abramsky O. Ampicillin may aggravate clinical and experimental myasthenia gravis. *Arch Neurol.* 1986;43:255–256.

Brick DC, West C, Ostler HB. Ocular toxicity of subconjunctival nafcillin. *Invest Ophthalmol Vis Sci.* 1979;18(suppl):132.

Johnson AP, Scoper SV, Woo FL, et al. Azlocillin levels in human tears and aqueous humor. *Am J Ophthalmol.* 1985;99:469–472.

Kaeser HE. Drug-induced myasthenic syndromes. *Acta Neurol Scand.* 1984;70(suppl 100):39–47.

Azithromycin, clarithromycin, clindamycin, erythromycin

Aslan Bayhan S, Bayhan HA, Colgecen E, et al. Effects of topical acne treatment on the ocularsurface in patients with acne vulgaris. *Cont Lens Anterior Eye.* 2016;39(6):431–434.

Dorrell L, Ellerton C, Cottrell DG, et al. Toxicity of clarithromycin in the treatment of Mycobacterium avium complex infection in a patient with AIDS. *J Antimicrob Chemother.* 1994;34:605–606.

Flavia Monteagudo Paz A, Francisco Silvestre Salvador J, Latorre Martinez N, et al. Allergic contact dermatitis caused by azithromycin in an eye drop. *Contact Dermatitis.* 2011;64:300–301.

Kaeser HE. Drug-induced myasthenic syndromes. *Acta Neurol Scand.* 1984;70(suppl 100):39–47.

Lazar D, Rahim U, Ramee E. Ophthalmic erythromycin chronologically linked to acute Pancreatitis. *Ochsner J.* 2013;13(3):429–430.

Lund Kofoed M, Oxholm A. Toxic epidermal necrolysis due to erythromycin. *Contact Dermatitis.* 1985;13:273.

May EF, Calvert PC. Aggravation of myasthenia gravis by erythromycin. *Ann Neurol.* 1990;28:577–579.

Oral erythromycins. *Med Lett Drugs Ther.* 1985;27:1.

Tate Jr GW, Martin RG. Clindamycin in the treatment of human ocular toxoplasmosis. *Canad J Ophthalmol.* 1977;12:188–195.

Tole S, Speckert M, Campbell DM. Newborn with bilateral eyelid swelling, rash and erythema. *Paediatr Child Health.* 2017;22(5):243–244.

Tranos P, Nasr MB, Asteriades S, et al. Bilateral diffuse iris atrophy after the use of oral clarithromycin. *Cutan Ocul Toxicol.* 2014;33(1):79–81.

Tyagi AK, Kayarkar VV, McDonnell PJ. An unreported side effect of topical clarithromycin when used successfully to treat Mycobacterium avium-intracellulare keratitis. *Cornea.* 1999;18:606–607.

Zitelli BJ, Howrie DL, Altman H, et al. Erythromycin-induced drug interactions. An illustrative case and review of the literature. *Clin Pediat.* 1987;26:117–119.

Bacitracin

Kaeser HE. Drug-induced myasthenic syndromes. *Acta Neurol Scand.* 1984;70(suppl 100):39–47.

McQuillen MP, Cantor HE, O'Rourke JR. Myasthenic syndrome associated with antibiotics. *Arch Neurol.* 1968;18:402–415.

Petroutsos G, Guimaraes R, Giraud J, et al. Antibiotics and corneal epithelial wound healing. *Arch Ophthalmol.* 1983;101(11):1775–1778.

Small GA. Respiratory paralysis after a large dose of intraperitoneal polymyxin B and bacitracin. *Anesth Analg.* 1964;43:137–139.

Benzathine benzylpenicillin (benzathine G penicillin)

Alarcón-Segovia D. Drug-induced antinuclear antibodies and lupus syndromes. *Drugs.* 1976;12:69–77.

Crews SJ. Ocular adverse reactions to drugs. *Practitioner.* 1977;219:72–77.

Katzman B, Lu LW, Tiwari RP, et al. Pseudotumor cerebri: an observation and review. *Ann Ophthalmol.* 1981;13:887–892.

Laroche J. Modification of color vision by certain medications. *Ann Oculist.* 1967;200:275–286.

Robertson Jr CR. Hallucinations after penicillin injection. *Am J Dis Child.* 1985;139:1074–1075.

Schmitt BD, Krivit W. Benign intracranial hypertension associated with a delayed penicillin reaction. *Pediatrics.* 1969;43:50–53.

Snavely SR, Hodges GR. The neurotoxicity of antibacterial agents. *Ann Intern Med.* 1984;101:92–104.

Tseng SC, Maumenee AE, Stark WJ, et al. Topical retinoid treatment for various dry-eye disorders. *Ophthalmology.* 1985;92:717–727.

Cefaclor, cefadroxil, cefalexin (cephalexin), cefazolin sodium, cefditoren pivoxil, cefoperazone sodium, cefotaxime, cefotetan disodium, cefoxitin sodium, cefradine, ceftazidime, ceftizoxime sodium, ceftriaxone sodium, cefuroxime, cefuroxime axetil

Ballingall DLK, Turpie AGG. Cephaloridine toxicity. *Lancet.* 1967;2:835–836.

Berrocal AM, Schuman JS. Subconjunctival cephalosporin anaphylaxis. *Ophthalmic Surg Las.* 2001;32(1):79–80.

Campochiaro PA, Green R. Toxicity of intravitreous ceftazidime in primate retina. *Arch Ophthalmol.* 1992;110:1625–1629.

Green ST, Natarajan S, Campbell JC. Erythema multiforme following cefotaxime therapy. *Postgrad Med J.* 1986;62:415.

Jenkins CD, McDonnell PJ, Spalton DJ. Randomized single blind trial to compare the toxicity of subconjunctival gentamicin and cefuroxime in cataract surgery. *Br J Ophthalmol.* 1990;74:734–738.

Kannangara DW, Smith B, Cohen K. Exfoliative dermatitis during cefoxitin therapy. *Arch Intern Med.* 1982;142:1031–1032.

Kramann C, Pitz S, Schwenn O, et al. Effects of intraocular cefotaxime on the human corneal Endothelium. *J Cataract Refract Surg.* 2001;27:250–255.

Murray DL, Singer DA, Singer AB, et al. Cefaclor – a cluster of adverse reactions. *N Engl J Med.* 1980;303:1003.

Okumoto M, Smolin G, Grabner G, et al. In vitro and in vivo studies on cefoperazone. *Cornea.* 1983;2:35.

Taylor R, Ward MK. Cephaloridine encephalopathy. *BMJ.* 1981;283:409–410.

Villada JR, Ubaldo V, Javaloy J, et al. Severe anaphylactic reaction after intracameral antibiotic administration during cataract surgery. *J Refract Surg.* 2005;31:620–624.

Chloramphenicol

Abrams SM, Degnan TJ, Vinciguerra V. Marrow aplasia following topical application of chloramphenicol eye ointment. *Arch Intern Med.* 1980;140:576–577.

Brodsky E, Biger Y, Zeidan Z, et al. Topical application of chloramphenicol eye ointment followed by fatal bone marrow aplasia. *Isr J Med Sci.* 1989;25:54.

Bron AJ, Leber G, Rizk SN, et al. Ofloxacin compared with chloramphenicol in the management of external ocular infection. *Br J Ophthalmol.* 1991;75(11):675–679.

Chalfin J, Putterman AM. Eyelid skin depigmentation. *Ophthalmic Surg.* 1980;11:194–196.

De Sevilla TF, Alegre J, Vallespi T, et al. Adult pure red cell aplasia following topical ocular chloramphenicol. *Br J Ophthalmol.* 1990;74:640.

Diamond J, Leeming J. Chloramphenicol eye drops: a dangerous drug? *Practitioner.* 1995;239:608–611.

Doona M, Walsh JB. Use of chloramphenicol as topical eye medication: time to cry halt? *BMJ.* 1995;310:1217–1218.

Durosinmi MA, Ajayi AA. A prospective study of chloramphenicol induced aplastic anemia in Nigerians. *Trop Geogr Med.* 1993;45(4):159–161.

Godel V, Nemet P, Lazar M. Chloramphenicol optic neuropathy. *Arch Ophthalmol.* 1980;98:1417–1421.

Isenberg SJ. The fall and rise of chloramphenicol. *J Am Assoc Pediatr Ophthalmol Strab.* 2003;7(5):307–308.

Issaragrisil S, Piankijagum A. Aplastic anemia following administration of ophthalmic chloramphenicol: report of a case and review of the literature. *J Med Assoc Thai.* 1985;68:309–312.

Kushwaha KP, Verma RB, Singh YD, et al. Surveillance of drug induced diseases in children. *Indian J Pediatr.* 1994;61(4):357–365.

Lamda PA, Sood NN, Moorthy SS. Retinopathy due to chloramphenicol. *Scot Med J.* 1968;13:166–169.

Leone R, Ghiotto E, Conforti A, et al. Potential interaction between warfarin and ocular chloramphenicol (letter). *Ann Pharmacother.* 1999;33(1):114.

Liphshitz I, Loewenstein A. Anaphylactic reaction following application of chloramphenicol eye ointment. *Br J Ophthalmol.* 1991;75:64.

McGuinness R. Chloramphenicol eye drops and blood dyscrasia. *Med J Austral*. 1984;140:383.

McWhae JA, Chang J, Lipton JH. Drug-induced fatal aplastic anemia following cataract surgery. *Can J Ophthalmol*. 1992;27(6):313–315.

Sah SP, Raj GA, Rijal S, et al. Clinical-haematological and management profile of aplastic anaemia – a first series of 118 cases from Nepal. *Singapore Med J*. 1999;40(7):451–454.

Smith JR, Wesselingh S, Coster DJ. It is time to stop using topical chloramphenicol. *Aust NZ J Ophthalmol*. 1997;25(1):83–88.

Walker S, Diaper C, Bowman R, et al. Lack of evidence for systemic toxicity following topical chloramphenicol use. *Eye*. 1998;12:875–879.

Wiholm BE, Kelly JP, Kaufman D, et al. Relation of aplastic anaemia to use of chloramphenicol eye drops in two international case-control studies. *BMJ*. 1998;316:666.

Wilson III FM. Adverse external ocular effects of topical ophthalmic medications. *Surv Ophthalmol*. 1979;24:57–88.

Wilson WR, Cockerill III FR. Tetracyclines, chloramphenicol, erythromycin, and clindamycin. *Mayo Clin Proc*. 1983;58:92–98.

Ciprofloxacin, sparfloxacin, tosufloxacin

Alhabshan RN, Mansour TN. Association between oral fluoroquinolone use and lateral canthal tendon rupture: case report. *Orbit*. 2018;37(5):358–360.

Eiferman RA, Snyder JP, Nordquist RE. Ciprofloxacin microprecipitates and macroprecipitates in human corneal epithelium. *J Cataract Refract Surg*. 2001;27:1701–1702.

Kanellopoulos AJ, Miller F, Wittpenn JR. Deposition of topical ciprofloxacin to prevent re-epithelialization of a corneal defect. *Am J Ophthalmol*. 1994;117:258–259.

Moore B, Safani M, Keesey J. Ciprofloxacin exacerbation of myasthenia gravis? Case report. *Lancet*. 1988;1:882.

Motolese E, D'Aniello B, Addabbo G. Toxic optic neuropathy after administration of quinolone Derivative. *Boll Oculist*. 1990;69:1011–1013.

Stevens D, Samples JR. Fluoroquinolones for the treatment of microbial infections. *J Toxicol Cut Ocular Toxicol*. 1994;13(4):275–277.

Wilhelmus KR, Hyndiuk RA, Caldwell DR, et al. 0.3% Ciprofloxacin ophthalmic ointment in the treatment of bacterial keratitis. *Arch Ophthalmol*. 1993;111:1210–1218.

Winrow AP, Supramaniam G. Benign intracranial hypertension after ciprofloxacin administration. *Arch Dis Child*. 1990;65:1165–1166.

Demeclocycline hydrochloride, doxycycline, minocycline hydrochloride, oxytetracycline, tetracycline hydrochloride

Brothers DM, Hidayat AA. Conjunctival pigmentation associated with tetracycline medication. *Ophthalmology*. 1981;88:1212–1215.

Edwards TS. Transient myopia due to tetracycline. *JAMA*. 1963;186:175–176.

Friedman DI, Gordon LK, Egan RA, et al. Doxycycline and intracranial hypertension. *Neurology*. 2004;62:2297–2298.

Kaeser HE. Drug-induced myasthenic syndromes. *Acta Neurol Scand*. 1984;70(suppl 100):39–47.

Krejci L, Brettschneider I, Triska J. Eye changes due to systemic use of tetracycline in pregnancy. *Ophthalmic Res*. 1980;12:73–77.

Messmer E, Font RL, Sheldon G, et al. Pigmented conjunctival cysts following tetracycline/minocycline therapy. Histochemical and electron microscopic observations. *Ophthalmology*. 1983;90(12):1462–1468.

Morrison VL, Herndier BG, Kikkawa DO. Tetracycline-induced green conjunctival pigment deposits. *Br J Ophthalmol*. 2005;89:1372–1373.

Tabbara KF, Cooper H. Minocycline levels in tears of patients with active trachoma. *Arch Ophthalmol*. 1989;107:93–95.

Gatifloxacin, levofloxacin, moxifloxacin hydrochloride, norfloxacin, ofloxacin

Bettink-Remeijer MW, Brouwers K, van Langenhove L, et al. Uveitis-like syndrome and iris transillumination after the use of oral moxifloxacin. *Eye*. 2009;23:2260–2262.

Das S, Mondal S. Oral levofloxacin-induced optic neuritis progressing in loss of vision. *Ther Drug Monit*. 2012;34(2):124–125.

Gallelli L, Del Negro S, Naty S, et al. Levofloxacin-induced taste perversion, blurred vision and dyspnoea in a young woman. *Clin Drug Invest*. 2004;24:487–489.

Kamiya K, Kitahara M, Shimizu K. Corneal deposits after topical tosufloxacin in a patient with poor tear secretion. *Cornea*. 2009;28(1):114–115.

Konishi M, Yamada M, Mashima Y. Corneal ulcer associated with deposits of norfloxacin. *Am J Ophthalmol*. 1998;125(2):258–260.

Kovoor TA, Kim AS, McCulley JP, et al. Evaluation of the corneal effects of topical ophthalmic fluoroquinolones using in vivo confocal microscopy. *Eye Contact Lens*. 2004;30:90–94.

Moxifloxacin (Avelox). *Can Adverse Reaction Newslett*. 2002;12:3.

Gentamicin sulfate

Conway BP, Campochiaro PA. Macular infarction after endophthalmitis treated with vitrectomy and intravitreal gentamicin. *Arch Ophthalmol*. 1986;104:367–371.

Davison CR, Tuft SJ, Dart JKG. Conjunctival necrosis after administration of topical fortified aminoglycosides. *Am J Ophthalmol*. 1991;111:690–693.

De Maio R, Oliver GL. Recovery of useful vision after presumed retinal and choroidal toxic effects from gentamicin administration. *Arch Ophthalmol*. 1994;112(6):736–738.

Litwin AS, Pimenides D. Toxic anterior segment syndrome after cataract surgery secondary to subconjunctival gentamicin. *J Cataract Refract Surg*. 2012;38(12):2196–2197.

Lowenstein A, Esther Z, Yafa V, et al. Retinal toxicity of gentamicin after subconjunctival injection performed adjacent to thinned sclera. *Ophthalmology.* 2001;108:759–764.

Minor LB. Gentamicin-induced bilateral vestibular hypofunction. *JAMA.* 1998;279(7):541–544.

Nauheim R, Nauheim J, Merrick NY. Bulbar conjunctival defects associated with gentamicin. *Arch Ophthalmol.* 1987;105:1321.

Schatz H, McDonald HR. Acute ischemic retinopathy due to gentamicin injection. *JAMA.* 1986;256:1725–1726.

Stern GA, Schemmer GB, Farber RD, et al. Effect of topical antibiotic solutions on corneal epithelial wound healing. *Arch Ophthalmol.* 1983;101:644–647.

Waltz K. Intraocular gentamicin toxicity. *Arch Ophthalmol.* 1991;109:911.

Kanamycin sulfate

D'Amico DJ, Caspers-Velu L, Libert J, et al. Comparative toxicity of intravitreal aminoglycoside antibiotics. *Am J Ophthalmol.* 1985;100:264–275.

Finegold SM. Kanamycin. *Arch Intern Med.* 1959;104:15–29.

Finegold SM. Toxicity of kanamycin in adults. *Ann NY Acad Sci.* 1966,132:942–956.

Freemon FR, Parker Jr RL, Greer M. Unusual neurotoxicity of kanamycin. *JAMA.* 1967;200:410–411.

Kaeser HE. Drug-induced myasthenic syndromes. *Acta Neurol Scand.* 1984;70(suppl 100):39–47.

Linezolid

Carallo CE, Paull AE. Linezolid-induced optic neuropathy. *Med J Aust.* 2002;177:332.

De Vriese AS, Van Coster R, Smet J, et al. Linezolid-induced inhibition of mitochondrial protein synthesis. *Clin Infect Dis.* 2006;42:1111–1117.

Ferry T, Ponceau B, Simon M, et al. Possibly linezolid-induced peripheral and central neurotoxicity: report of four cases. *Infection.* 2005;33(3):151–154.

Frippiat F, Derue G. Causal relationship between neuropathy and prolonged linezolid use. *Clin Infect Dis.* 2004;39(3):439.

Frippiat F, Bergiers C, Michel C, et al. Severe bilateral neuritis associated with prolonged linezolid therapy. *J Antimicrob Chemother.* 2004;53(6):1114–1115.

Fraunfelder FT, Fraunfelder FW. Toxic optic nerve neuropathies. In: Russell Gabbedy, Ben Davie, eds. *Ocular Disease: Mechanisms and Management.* China: Saunders; 2010:257–361.

Hernandez PC, Llinarea TF, Climent GE, et al. Peripheral and optic neuropathy associated to linezolid in multidrug resistant Mycobacterium bovis infections. *Medicinia Clinica.* 2005;124(20):797–798.

McKinley SH, Foroozan R. Optic neuropathy associated with linezolid treatment. *J Neuroophthalmol.* 2005;25:18–21.

Rucker JC, Hamilton SR, Bardenstein D, et al. Linezolid-associated toxic optic neuropathy. *Neurology.* 2006;66:595–598.

Saijio T, Hayashi K, Yamada H, et al. Linezolid-induced optic neuropathy. *Am J Ophthalmol.* 2005;139(6):1114–1116.

Nalidixic acid

Drugs that cause psychiatric symptoms. *Med Lett Drugs Ther* 1986;28:81.

Gedroyc W, Shorvon SD. Acute intracranial hypertension and nalidixic acid therapy. *Neurology.* 1982;32:212–215.

Granstrom G, Santesson B. Unconsciousness after one therapeutic dose of nalidixic acid. *Acta Med Scand.* 1984;216:237.

Haut J, Haye C, Legras M, et al. Disturbances of color perception after taking nalidixic acid. *Bull Soc Ophthalmol Fr.* 1972;72:147–149.

Katzman B, Lu LW, Tiwari RP, et al. Pseudotumor cerebri: an observation and review. *Ann Ophthalmol.* 1981;13:887–892.

Kilpatrick C, Ebeling P. Intracranial hypertension in nalidixic acid therapy. *Med J Aust.* 1982;1:252.

Lane RJ, Routledge PA. Drug-induced neurological disorders. *Drugs.* 1983;26:124–147.

Mukherjee A, Dutta P, Lahiri M, et al. Benign intracranial hypertension after nalidixic acid overdose in infants. *Lancet.* 1990;335:1602.

Riyaz A, Abbobacker CM, Streelatha PR. Nalidixic acid induced pseudotumor cerebri in children. *J Indian Med Assoc.* 1998;96(10):308–314.

Rubinstein A. LE-like disease caused by nalidixic acid. *N Engl J Med.* 1979;301:1288.

Safety of antimicrobial drugs in pregnancy. *Med Lett Drugs Ther.* 1985;27:93.

Wall M. Idiopathic intracranial hypertension. *Neurol Clin.* 1991;9:73–95.

Neomycin sulfate

Baldinger J, Weiter JJ. Diffuse cutaneous hypersensitivity reaction after dexamethasone/polymyxin B/neomycin combination eyedrops. *Ann Ophthalmol.* 1986;18:95–96.

Fisher AA. Topical medications which are common sensitizers. *Ann Allergy.* 1982;49:97–100.

Fisher AA, Adams RM. Alternative for sensitizing neomycin topical medications. *Cutis.* 1981;28:491.

Kaeser HE. Drug-induced myasthenic syndromes. *Acta Neurol Scand.* 1984;70(suppl 100):39–47.

Kaufman HE. Chemical blepharitis following drug treatment. *Am J Ophthalmol.* 1983;95:703.

Kruyswijk MR, van Driel LM, Polak BC, et al. Contact allergy following administration of eyedrops and eye ointments. *Doc Ophthalmol.* 1979;48:251–253.

Wilson II FM. Adverse external ocular effects of topical ophthalmic medications. *Surv Ophthalmol.* 1979;24:57–88.

Nitrofurantoin

Mesaros MP, Seymour J, Sadjadpour K. Lateral rectus muscle palsy associated with nitrofurantoin (Macrodantoin). *Am J Ophthalmol.* 1982;94:816–817.

Nitrofurantoin. *Med Lett Drugs Ther.* 1980;22:36.

Penn RG, Griffin JP. Adverse reactions to nitrofurantoin in the United Kingdom, Sweden, and Holland. *BMJ.* 1982;284:1440–1442.

Pringle E, Ho H, O'Sullivan E, et al. Reversible bilateral optic disc swelling in a renal patient treated with nitrofurantoin. *NDR Plus*. 2008;1(5):344–345.

Sharma DB, James A. Benign intracranial hypertension associated with nitrofurantoin therapy. *BMJ*. 1974;4:771.

Toole JF, Parrish MD. Nitrofurantoin polyneuropathy. *Neurology*. 1973;23:554–559.

Wasserman BN, Chronister TE, Stark BI, et al. Ocular myasthenia and nitrofurantoin. *Am J Ophthalmol*. 2000;130:531–533.

Polymyxin B sulfate

Baldinger J, Weiter JJ. Diffuse cutaneous hypersensitivity reaction after dexamethasone/polymyxin B/neomycin combination eyedrops. *Ann Ophthalmol*. 1986;18:95–96.

Francois J, Mortiers P. The injurious effects of locally and generally applied antibiotics on the Eye. *T Geneeskd*. 1976;32:139.

Hudgson P. Adverse drug reactions in the neuromuscular apparatus. *Adverse Drug React Acute Poisoning Rev*. 1982;1:35.

Kaeser HE. Drug-induced myasthenic syndromes. *Acta Neurol Scand*. 1984;70(suppl 100):39–47.

Koenig A, Ohrloff C. Influence of local application of Isoptomax eye drops on neuromuscular transmission. *Klin Monatsbl Augenheilkd*. 1981;179:109–112.

Lane RJ, Routledge PA. Drug-induced neurological disorders. *Drugs*. 1983;26:124–147.

Stern GA, Schemmer GB, Farber RD, et al. Effect of topical antibiotic solutions on corneal epithelial wound healing. *Arch Ophthalmol*. 1983;101:644–647.

Sulfacetamide sodium, sulfadiazine, sulfafurazole (sulfisoxazole), sulfamethizole, sulfamethoxazole, sulfanilamide, sulfasalazine, sulfathiazole

Bovino JA, Marcus DF. The mechanism of transient myopia induced by sulfonamide therapy. *Am J Ophthalmol*. 1982;94:99–102.

Chirls IA, Norris JW. Transient myopia associated with vaginal sulfanilamide suppositories. *Am J Ophthalmol*. 1984;98:120–121.

Fajardo RV. Acute bilateral anterior uveitis caused by sulfa drugs. In: Saari KM, ed. *Uveitis Update*. Amsterdam: Excerpta Medica; 1984:115–118.

Flach AJ, Peterson JS, Mathias CG. Photosensitivity to topically applied sulfisoxazole ointment.

Evidence for a phototoxic reaction. *Arch Ophthalmol*. 1982;100:1286–1287.

Genvert GI, Cohen EJ, Donnenfeld ED, et al. Erythema multiforme after use of topical sulfacetamide. *Am J Ophthalmol*. 1985;99:465–468.

Hook SR, Holladay JT, Prager TC, et al. Transient myopia induced by sulfonamides. *Am J Ophthalmol*. 1986;101:495–496.

Mackie BS, Mackie LE. Systemic lupus erythematosus – dermatomyositis induced by sulphacetamide eyedrops. *Aust J Dermatol*. 1979;20:49–50.

Northrop CV, Shepherd SM, Abbuhl S. Sulfonamide-induced iritis. *Am J Emerg Med*. 1996;14(6):577–579.

Riley SA, Flagg PJ, Mandal BK. Contact lens staining due to sulphasalazine. *Lancet*. 1986;1:972.

Vanheule BA, Carswell F. Sulphasalazine-induced systemic lupus erythematosus in a child. *Eur J Pediatr*. 1983;140:66–68.

Telithromycin

Nieman RB, Sharma K, Edelber H, et al. Telithromycin and myasthenia gravis. *Clin Infect Dis*. 2003;37:1579.

Shi J, Montay G, Bhargava VO. Clinical pharmacokinetics of telithromycin, the first ketolide antibacterial. *Clin Pharmacokinet*. 2005;44(9):915–934.

Vuorio A, Rajaratnam R. Telithromycin and visual disturbances. *TABU*. 2009;2:44–47.

Wellington K, Noble S. Telithromycin. *Drugs*. 2004;64(15):1683–1694.

Tobramycin

American Academy of Ophthalmology. Corneal toxicity with antibiotic/steroid-soaked collagen shields. *Clinical Alert*. 1990;11:1.

Caraffini S, Assalve D, Stingeni L, et al. Allergic contact conjunctivitis and blepharitis from tobramycin. *Contact Dermatitis*. 1995;32(3):186–187.

Davison CR, Tuft SJ, Dart KG. Conjunctival necrosis after administration of topical fortified aminoglycosides. *Am J Ophthalmol*. 1991;111:690–693.

McCartney CF, Hatley LH, Kessler JM. Possible tobramycin delirium. *JAMA*. 1982;247:1319.

Pflugfelder SC, Murchison JF. Corneal toxicity with an antibiotic/steroid-soaked collagen shield (letter). *Arch Ophthalmol*. 1993;111(1):18.

Wilhelmus KR, Gilbert ML, Osato MS. Tobramycin in ophthalmology. *Surv Ophthalmol*. 1987;32(2):111–122.

Trimethoprim

Chandler MJ. Recurrence of phototoxic skin eruption due to trimethoprim. *J Infect Dis*. 1986;153(5):1001.

Nwokolo C, Byrne L, Misch KJ, et al. Toxic epidermal necrolysis occurring during treatment with trimethoprim alone. *Br Med J*. 1988;296:970.

Penmetcha M. Drug points: Trimethoprim induced erythema multiforme. *Br Med J (Clin Res Ed)*. 1987;295(6597):556.

Amphotericin B

Brod RD, Flynn HW, Clarkson JG. et al. Endogenous candida endophthalmitis. Management without intravenous amphotericin B. *Ophthalmology*. 1990;97:666–674.

Doft BH, Weiskopf J, Nilsson-Ehle I, et al. Amphotericin clearance in vitrectomized versus nonvitrectomized eyes. *Ophthalmology*. 1985;92:1601–1605.

Foster CS, Lass JH, Moran-Wallace K, et al. Ocular toxicity of topical antifungal agents. *Arch Ophthalmol*. 1981;99:1081–1084.

Lavine JB, Binder PS, Wickham MG. Antimicrobials and the corneal endothelium. *Ann Ophthalmol.* 1979;11:1517–1528.

O'Day DM, Head WS, Robinson RD, et al. Intraocular penetration of systemically administered antifungal agents. *Curr Eye Res.* 1985;4:131–134.

O'Day DM, Smith R, Stevens JB. Toxicity and pharmacokinetics of subconjunctival amphotericin B. *Cornea.* 1991;10(5):411–417.

Griseofulvin

Alarcón-Segovia D. Drug-induced antinuclear antibodies and lupus syndromes. *Drugs.* 1976;12:69–77.

Epstein JH, Wintroub BU. Photosensitivity due to drugs. *Drugs.* 1985;30:41–57.

Madhok R, Zoma A, Capell H. Fatal exacerbation of systemic lupus erythematosus after treatment with griseofulvin. *BMJ.* 1985;291:249–250.

Voriconazole

Denning DW, Griffiths CE. Muco-cutaneous retinoid – effects and facial erythema related to the novel triazole agent voriconazole. *Clin Exp Dermatol.* 2001;26:648–653.

FDA Antiviral Drugs Advisory Committee. Briefing Document for Voriconazole (Oral and Intravenous Formulations). 2001.

Herbrecht R, Denning DW, Patterson TF, et al. Open Randomized Comparison of Voriconazole and Amphotericin-B Followed by other Licensed Antifungal Therapy for Primary Therapy of Invasive Aspergillosis. *Presented at the 4th Interscience Conference on Antimicrobial Agents and Chemotherapy.* Chicago, IL; 2001.

Mounier A, Agard E, Douma I, et al. Macular toxicity and blind spot enlargement during a treatment by voriconazole: a case report. *Eur J Ophthalmol.* 2018;28(4):NP11–NP14.

Rubenstein M, Levy ML, Metry D. Voriconazole-induced retinoid-like photosensitivity in children. *Pediatr Dermatol.* 2004;21:675–678.

Tomaszewski K, Purkins L. *Visual Effects with Voriconazole (A-639).* Chicago, IL: Presented at: Program and abstracts of the 41st Interscience Conference on Antimicrobial Agents and Chemotherapy; 2001:16–19.

Clofazimine

Font RL, Sobol W, Matoba A. Polychromatic corneal and conjunctival crystals secondary to clofazimine therapy in a leper. *Ophthalmology.* 1989;96(3):311–315.

Granstein RD, Sober AJ. Drug and heavy metal-induced hyperpigmentation. *J Am Acad Dermatol.* 1981;5:1–18.

Mieler WF, Williams GA, Williams DF, et al. *Systemic Therapeutic Agents Retinal Toxicity.* New Orleans, LA: American Academy of Ophthalmology Instruction Course; 2004.

Moore VJ. A review of side effects experienced by patients taking clofazimine. *Lepr Rev.* 1983;54:327–335.

Ohman L, Wahlberg I. Ocular side effects of clofazimine. *Lancet.* 1975;2:933–934.

Walinder PE, Gip L, Stempa M. Corneal changes in patients treated with clofazimine. *Br J Ophthalmol.* 1976;60:526–528.

Dapsone

Daneshmend TK. The neurotoxicity of dapsone. *Adverse Drug React Acute Poisoning Rev.* 1984;3:43–58.

Homeida M, Babikr A, Daneshmend TK. Dapsone-induced optic atrophy and motor neuropathy. *BMJ.* 1980;281:1180.

Leonard JN, Tucker WF, Fry L. et al. Dapsone and the retina. *Lancet.* 1982;1:453.

Seo MS, Yoon KC, Park YG. Dapson maculopathy. *Korean J Ophthalmol.* 1997;11:70–73.

Chloroquine phosphate, hydroxychloroquine sulfate

Ahn SJ, Ryu SJ, Joung JY, et al. Choroidal thinning associated with hydroxychloroquine retinopathy. *Am J Ophthalmol.* 2017;183:56–64.

Marmor MF. Efficient and effective screening for hydroxychloroquine toxicity. *Am J Ophthalmol.* 2013;155(3):413–414.

Marmor MF. The demise of the bull's eye (screening for hydroxychloroquine retinopathy). *Retina.* 2016;36(10):1803–1805.

Maturi RK, Minzhong Y, Weleber RG. Multifocal electroretinographic evaluation of long-term hydroxychloroquine users. *Arch Ophthalmol.* 2004;122:973–981.

Mavrikakis I, Sfikakis PP, Mavrikakis E, et al. The incidence of irreversible retinal toxicity in patients treated with hydroxychloroquine. *Ophthalmology.* 2003;110:1321–1326.

Michaelides M, Stover NB, Francis PJ. et al. Retinal toxicity associated with hydroxychloroquine and chloroquine: risk factors, screening, and progression despite cessation of therapy. *Arch Ophthalmol.* 2011;129(1):30–39.

Mititelu M, Wong BJ, Brenner M, et al. Progression of hydroxychloroquine toxic effects after drug therapy cessation. *JAMA Ophthalmol.* 2013;131(9):1187–1197.

Robertson JE, Fraunfelder FT. Hydroxychloroquine retinopathy. *JAMA.* 1986;255:403.

Selvaag E. Vitiligolike depigmentation: possible side effect during chloroquine antimalarial therapy. *J Toxicol Cut Ocular Toxicol.* 1997;16:5–8.

Shroyer NF, Lewis RA, Lupski JR. Analysis of the ABCR (ABCA4) gene in 4-aminoquinoline retinopathy: is retinal toxicity by chloroquine and hydroxychloroquine related to Stargardt disease? *Am J Ophthalmol.* 2001;131:761–766.

Stern EM, et al. Highly accelerated onset of hydroxychloroquine macular retinopathy. *Ochsner J.* 2017;17(3):280–283.

Mefloquine hydrochloride

Borruat FX, Nater B, Robyn L, et al. Prolonged visual illusions induced by mefloquine (lariam): a case report. *J Travel Med.* 2001;8:148–149.

Lobel HO, Bernard KW, Williams SL, et al. Effectiveness and tolerance of long-term malaria prophylaxis with mefloquine. *JAMA.* 1991;3:361–364.

Shlim DR. Severe facial rash associated with mefloquine. *Correspondence. JAMA.* 1991;13:2560.

Suriyamongkol V, Timsaad S, Shanks GD. Mefloquine chemoprophylaxis of soldiers on the Thai-Cambodian border. *Southeast Asian J Trop Med Pub Health.* 1991;22:515–518.

Van den Enden E, Van Gompel A, Colebunders R, et al. Meflo-quine-induced Stevens-Johnson syndrome (letter). *Lancet.* 1991;337(8742):683.

Quinine sulfate

Brinton GS, Norton EW, Zahn JR, et al. Ocular quinine toxic-ity. *Am J Ophthalmol.* 1980;90:403–410.

Dyson EH, Proudfoot AT, Bateman DN. Quinine amblyopia: is current management appropriate? *Clin Toxicol.* 1985-1986;23:571.

Dyson EH, Proudfoot AT, Prescott LF, et al. Death and blind-ness due to overdose of quinine. *BMJ.* 1985;291:31–33.

Fisher CM. Visual disturbances associated with quinidine and quinine. *Neurology.* 1981;31:1569–1571.

Fong LP, Kaufman DV, Galbraith JE. Ocular toxicity of qui-nine. *Med J Austr.* 1984;41:528–529.

Friedman L, Rothkoff L, Zaks U. Clinical observations on qui-nine toxicity. *Ann Ophthalmol.* 1980;12:641.

Gangitano JL, Keltner JL. Abnormalities of the pupil and visu-al-evoked potential in quinine amblyopia. *Am J Ophthalmol.* 1980;89:425–430.

Horgan SE, Williams RW. Chronic retinal toxicity due to qui-nine in Indian tonic water (letter). *Eye.* 1995;9(Pt 5):637–638.

Kaeser HE. Drug-induced myasthenic syndromes. *Acta Neurol Scand.* 1984;70(suppl 100):39–47.

Rheeder P, Sieling WL. Acute, persistent quinine-induced blindness. A case report. *So Afr Med J.* 1991;79:563–564.

Metronidazole

Chen KT, Twu SJ, Chang HJ. et al. Outbreak of Stevens-John-son syndrome/toxic epidermal necrolysis associated with mebendazole and metronidazole use among Filipino labor-ers in Taiwan. *Am J Public Health.* 2003;93:489–492.

Czeizel AE, Rockenbauer M. A population-based case-control teratologic study of oral metronidazole treatment during pregnancy. *Br J Obstetrics Gyn.* 1998;105:322–327.

DeBleecker JL, Leroy BP, Meire VI. Reversible visual deficit and corpus callosum lesions due to metronidazole toxicity. *Eur Neurol.* 2005;53:93–95.

Dunn PM, Stewart-Brown S, Peel R. Metronidazole and the fetal alcohol syndrome. *Lancet.* 1979;2:144.

Kuriyama A, Jackson JL, Doi A, et al. Metronidazole-induced central nervous system toxicity: a systematic review. *Clin Neuropharmacol.* 2011;34(6):241–247.

Metronidazole hydrochloride (Flagyl IV). *Med Lett Drugs Ther.* 1981;23:13.

Schentag JJ, Ziemniak JA, Greco JM, et al. Mental confusion in a patient treated with metronidazole – a concentration-related effect? *Pharmacotherapy.* 1982;2:384–387.

Suramin sodium

Adverse effects of antiparasitic drugs. *Med Lett Drugs Ther.* 1982;24:12.

Thylefors B, Rolland A. The risk of optic atrophy following suramin treatment of ocular onchocerciasis. *Bull World Health Organ.* 1979;57(3):479–480.

Tryparsamide

LeJeune JR. Les oligo-elements et chelateurs. *Bull Soc Belge Ophthalmol.* 1972;160:241.

Sloan LL, Woods AC. Effect of tryparsamide on the eye. *Am J Syph.* 1936;20:583–613.

Cycloserine

Drugs that cause psychiatric symptoms. *Med Lett Drugs Ther.* 1986;28:81.

Ethambutol hydrochloride

Behbehani RS, Affel EL, Sergott RC, et al. Multifocal ERG in ethambutol associated visual loss. *Br J Ophthalmol.* 2005;89:976–982.

Dette TM, Spitznas M, Gobbels M, et al. Visually evoked cortical potentials for early detection of optic neuritis in ethambutol therapy. *Fortschritte der Ophthalmologie.* 1991;88(5):546–548.

Dotti MT, Plewnia K, Cardaioli E, et al. A case of ethambu-tol-induced optic neuropathy harbouring the primary mitochondrial LHON mutation at nt 11778. *J Neurol.* 1998;245(5):302–303.

Ezer N, Benedetti A, Darvish-Zargar M, et al. Incidence of ethambutol-related visual impairment during treatment of active tuberculosis. *Int J Tuberc Lung Dis.* 2013;17(4):447–455.

Hennekes R. Clinical ERG findings in ethambutol intoxi-cation. *Graefe's Arch Clin Exp Ophthalmol.* 1982;218:319–321.

Joubert PH, Strobele JG, Ogle CW, et al. Subclinical impair-ment of colour vision in patients receiving ethambutol. *Br J Clin Pharmacol.* 1986;21:213–216.

Kaimbo WK, Bifuko ZA, Longo MB, et al. Color vision in 42 Congolese patients with tuberculosis receiving ethambutol treatment. *Bull Soc Belge D Ophthalmol.* 2002;284:57–61.

Karmon G. Bilateral optic neuropathy due to combined ethambutol and isoniazid treatment. *Ann Ophthalmol.* 1979;11:1013–1017.

Karnik AM, Al-Shamali MA, Fenech FF. A case of ocular toxic-ity to ethambutol – An idiosyncratic reaction? *Postgrad Med J.* 1985;61:811–813.

Kim KL, Park SP. Visual function test for early detection of ethambutol induced ocular toxicity at the subclinical level. *Cutan Ocul Toxicol.* 2016;35(3):228–232.

Kim YK, Hwang JM. Serial retinal nerve fiber layer changes in patients with toxic optic neuropathy associated with antituberculosis pharmacotherapy. *J Ocul Pharmacol Ther.* 2009;25(6):531–535.

Kozak SF, Inderlied CB, Hsu HY, et al. The role of copper on ethambutol's antimicrobial action and implications for eth-ambutol-induced optic neuropathy. *Diagn Microbiol Infect Dis.* 1998;30(2):83–87.

Kumar A, Sandramouli S, Verma L, et al. Ocular etham-butol toxicity: is it reversible? *J Clin Neuro-Ophthalmol.* 1993;13(1):15–17.

Leibold JE. The ocular toxicity of ethambutol and its relation to dose. *Ann NY Acad Sci.* 1966;135:904–909.

Levy M, Rigaudiere F, de Lauzanne A, Koehl B, et al. Ethambutol-related impaired visual function in children less than 5 years of age treated for mycobacterial infection. *Pediatr Infect Dis J.* 2015;34(4):346–350.

Libershteyn Y. Ethambutol/linezolid toxic optic neuropathy. *Optom Vis Sci.* 2016;93(2):211–217.

Lu PG, Kung NH, Van Stavern GP. Ethambutol optic neuropathy associated with enhancement at the optic chiasm. *Can J Ophthalmol.* 2017;52(5):e178–e181.

Salmon JF, Carmichael TR, Welsh NH. Use of contrast sensitivity measurement in the detection of subclinical ethambutol toxic optic neuropathy. *Br J Ophthalmol.* 1987;71:192–196.

Seth V, Khosla PK, Semwal OP, et al. Visual evoked responses in tuberculous children on ethambutol therapy. *Indian Pediatr.* 1991;28(7):713–727.

Sivakumaran P, Harrison AC, Marschner J, et al. Ocular toxicity from ethambutol: a review of four cases and recommended precautions. *N Z Med J.* 1998;111(1077):428–430.

Song W, Shancheng S. The rare ethambutol-induced optic neuropathy: a case-report and literature review. *Medicine (Baltimore).* 2017;96(2):e5889.

Srivastava AK, Goel UC, Bajaj S, et al. Visual evoked responses in ethambutol induced optic neuritis. *J Assoc Physicians India.* 1997;45:847–849.

Trau R, Salu P, Jonckheere P, et al. Early diagnosis of myambutol (ethambutol) ocular toxicity by electrophysiological examination. *Bull Soc Belge Ophtalmol.* 1981;193:201–212.

Tsai RK, Lee YH. Reversibility of ethambutol optic neuropathy. *J Ocular Pharm Therap.* 1997;13(5):473–477.

Yang HK, Park MJ, Lee JH, et al. Incidence of toxic optic neuropathy with low-dose ethambutol. *Int J Tuberc Lung Dis.* 2016;20(2):264–264.

Yen MY. Ethambutol retinal toxicity: an electrophysiologic study. *J Formos Med Assoc.* 2000;99:630–634.

Yiannikas C, Walsh JC, McLeod JG. Visual evoked potentials in the detection of subclinical optic toxic effects secondary to ethambutol. *Arch Neurol.* 1983;40:645–648.

Ethionamide

Argov Z, Mastaglia FL. Drug-induced peripheral neuropathies. *BMJ.* 1979;1:663–666.

Drugs that cause psychiatric symptoms. *Med Lett Drugs Ther.* 1986;28:81.

Fox W, Robinson DK, Tall R, et al. A study of acute intolerance to ethionamide, including a comparison with prothionamide, and of the influence of a vitamin B complex additive in prophylaxis. *Tubercule.* 1969;50:125–143.

Michiels J. Noxious effects of systemic medications on the visual apparatus. *Bull Soc Belge Ophtalmol.* 1972;160:515–516.

Isoniazid

Alarcón-Segovia A. Drug-induced antinuclear antibodies and lupus syndromes. *Drugs.* 1976;12:69–77.

Bomb BS, Purohit SD, Bedi HK. Stevens-Johnson syndrome caused by isoniazid. *Tubercle.* 1976;57:229–230.

Boulanouar A, Abdallah E, el Bakkali M, et al. Severe toxic optic neuropathies caused by isoniazid. Apropos of 3 cases. *J Francais d'Ophtalmol.* 1995;18(3):183–187.

Gonzalez-Gay MA, Sanchez-Andrade A, Aguero JJ. et al. Optic neuritis following treatment with isoniazid in a hemodialyzed patient. *Nephron.* 1993;63(3):360.

Karmon G, Savir H, Zevin D, et al. Bilateral optic neuropathy due to combined ethambutol and isoniazid treatment. *Ann Ophthalmol.* 1979;11:1013–1017.

Kass I, Mandel W, Cohen H, et al. Isoniazid as a cause of optic neuritis and atrophy. *JAMA.* 1957;164:1740–1743.

Keeping JA, Searle SWA. Optic neuritis following isoniazid therapy. *Lancet.* 1955;2:278.

Kiyosawa M, Ishikawa S. A case of isoniazid-induced optic neuropathy. *Neuro-Ophthalmology.* 1981;2:67.

Kratka W. Isoniazid and ocular tuberculosis. *Arch Ophthalmol.* 1955;54:330–334.

Nair KG. Optic neuritis due to INH complicating tuberculous meningitis. *J Assoc Physicians India.* 1976;24:263–264.

Renard G, Morax PV. Optic neuritis in the course of treatment of tuberculosis. *Ann Oculist.* 1977;210:53.

Stratton MA. Drug-induced systemic lupus erythematosus. *Clin Pharm.* 1985;4:657–663.

Sutton PH, Beattie PH. Optic atrophy after administration of isoniazid with PAS. *Lancet.* 1955;1:650–651.

Zuckerman BD, Lieberman TW. Corneal rust ring. *Arch Ophthalmol.* 1960;63:254–2E65.

Rifabutin

Arevalo JF, Freeman WR. Corneal endothelial deposits in children positive for human immunodeficiency virus receiving rifabutin prophylaxis for *Mycobacterium avium* complex bacteremia. *Am J Ophthalmol.* 1999;127:164–169.

Awotesu O, Missotten T, Pitcher MC, et al. Uveitis in a patient receiving rifabutin for Crohn's disease. *J Roy Soc Med.* 2004;97:440–441.

Bhagat N, Read RW, Narsing RA, et al. Rifabutin-associated hypopyon uveitis in human immunodeficiency virus-negative immunocompetent individuals. *Ophthalmology.* 2001;108:750–752.

Brogden RN, Fitton A. Rifabutin: a review of its antimicrobial activity pharmacokinetic properties and therapeutic efficacy. *Drugs.* 1994;47(6):983–1009.

Dunn AM, Tizer K, Cervia JS. Rifabutin-associated uveitis in a pediatric patient. *Pediatr Infect Dis J.* 1995;3(14):246–247.

Frank MO, Graham MB, Wispelway B. Rifabutin and uveitis. *New Engl J Med.* 1994;24:868.

Fuller JD, Stanfield LE, Craven DE. Rifabutin prophylaxis and uveitis (letter). *N Engl J Med.* 1994;330(18):1315–1316.

Mahboobi H, Mysliwiec TJ, Greene AM, et al. Corneal deposits secondary to rifabutin. *Clin Exp Optom.* 2016;99(6):597–600.

Nichols CW. *Mycobacterium avium* complex infection, rifabutin, and uveitis: is there a connection? *Clin Infect Dis.* 1996;22(suppl 1):S43–S49.

Saran BR, Maguire AM, Nichols C, et al. Hypopyon uveitis in patients with acquired immunodeficiency syndrome treated for systemic *Mycobacterium avium* complex infection with rifabutin. *Arch Ophthalmol.* 1994;112:1159–1165.

Skolik S, Willermain F, Caspers LE. Rifabutin-associated panuveitis with retinal vasculitis in pulmonary tuberculosis. *Ocul Immunol Inflamm.* 2005;13:483–485.

Tseng AL, Walmsley SL. Rifabutin-associated uveitis. *Ann Pharmaco Ther*. 1995;29:1149–1155.

Vaudaux JD, Guex-Crosier Y. Rifabutin-induced cystoid macular oedema. *J Antimicrob Chemother*. 2002;49:421–422.

Rifampin

Bolan G, Laurie RE, Broome CV. Red man syndrome: Inadvertent administration of an excessive dose of rifampin to children in a day-care center. *Pediatrics*. 1986;77:633–635.

Calissendorff B. Melanotropic drugs and retinal functions. *Acta Ophthalmol*. 1976;54:118–128.

Cayley FE, Majumdar SK. Ocular toxicity due to rifampicin. *BMJ*. 1976;1:199–200.

Darougar S, Jones BR, Viswalingam N, et al. Topical therapy of hyperendemic trachoma with rifampicin, oxytetracycline, or spiramycin eye ointments. *Br J Ophthalmol*. 1980;64:37–42.

Grosset J, Leventis S. Adverse effects of rifampin. *Rev Infect Dis*. 1983;5(suppl 3):440–450.

Mangi RJ. Reactions to rifampin. *N Engl J Med*. 1976;294:113.

Mirsaeidi M, Schraufnagel D. Rifampin induced angioedema: a rare but serious side effect. *Braz J Infect Dis*. 2014;18(1):102–103.

Nyirenda R, Gill GV. Stevens-Johnson syndrome due to rifampicin. *BMJ*. 1977;2:1189.

Thioacetazone (amithiozone)

Mame-Thierna D, On S, Thierno-Nydiaye S, et al. Lyell syndrome in Senegal: responsibility of thiacetazone. *Ann Dermatol Venereol*. 2001;128:1305–1307.

Ravindran P, Joshi M. Dermatological hypersensitivity to thiacetazone. *Indian J Chest Dis*. 1974;16:58–60.

Sahi SP, Chandra K. Thiacetazone-induced Stevens-Johnson syndrome: a case report. *Indian J Chest Dis*. 1974;16:124–125.

Sarma OA. Reactions to thiacetazone. *Indian J Chest Dis*. 1976;18:51–55.

CHAPTER 5

Drugs Affecting the Central Nervous System

CLASS: ANALEPTICS

Generic Name:
Gabapentin.

Proprietary Names:
Active-PAC with Gabapentin, Gralise, Horizant, Neurontin.

Primary Use
This antiepileptic drug is used in refractory seizure patients.

Ocular Side Effects

Systemic administration – oral

Certain
1. Decreased vision
2. Nystagmus
3. Diplopia
4. Visual hallucinations
5. Color vision defect
6. Contrast sensitivity – reduced
7. Visual evoked potential – abnormal
8. Pattern electroretinogram (ERG) – abnormal

Probable
1. Myasthenia gravis – aggravated
   a. Diplopia
   b. Ptosis
   c. Paresis of extraocular muscles

Possible
1. Eyelids or conjunctiva
   a. Conjunctivitis
   b. Erythema multiforme
2. Macular edema

Clinical Significance
Gabapentin's most common ocular side effect is a decrease in central vision. The effect may be zigzag lines, a crowding of central letters on Snellen testing, or decreased vision. The median onset of these symptoms is 4 days. Browne reported an incidence of nystagmus at 11% and diplopia at 6%.[1] The *Physicians' Desk Reference* (PDR) reported incidences of diplopia at 1–6%.[2] Conjunctivitis occurred in 1.2% over placebo controls. All ocular side effects are reversible. This drug may aggravate myasthenia with worsening of ptosis.

Gabapentin may have toxic effects on the neurotransmitter function of the optic nerve.[3,4] Kim et al described a case of bilateral macular edema due to gabapentin; however, the patient was also on oral methylprednisolone.[5] There are 7 cases of macular edema associated with this drug in the spontaneous reports.

Generic Name:
Lamotrigine.

Proprietary Names:
Lamictal, Lamictal CD, Lamictal ODT, Lamictal XR, Subvenite.

Primary Use
This is an antiepileptic drug believed to suppress seizures by inhibiting the release of excitatory neurotransmitters.

Ocular Side Effects
Systemic administration – oral
Certain
1. Diplopia
2. Decreased vision
3. Nystagmus

Probable
1. Visual hallucinations
2. Blepharospasms
3. Eyelid blinking – excessive
4. Oculogyric crisis
5. Drug reaction with eosinophilia and systemic symptoms (DRESS syndrome)
   a. Acute posterior multifocal placoid pigment epitheliopathy

Possible
1. Eyelids or conjunctiva
   a. Edema
   b. Conjunctivitis
2. Photophobia
3. Uveitis

Conditional/unclassified
1. Visual field changes – primarily generalized constriction
2. Uveal effusion
3. Acute myopia

Clinical Significance
Lamotrigine is mainly an add-on drug used when current antiepileptic drugs are ineffective, which confuses its adverse effect profile. In placebo-controlled clinical trials, 2 of its 5 most common side effects were ocular, with 22% of patients having diplopia and 15% having decreased vision compared with controls.[1] Betts et al noted that less than 5% had nystagmus.[2] Alkawi et al reported a case of downbeat nystagmus.[3] The *Physicians' Desk Reference* (PDR) states incidence rates of 5–49% for diplopia, 4–25% for decreased vision, 2–4.9% for visual impairment, and 2–4.9% for nystagmus.[4]

Blepharospasm and involuntary blinking are well documented.[5–9]

Of interest is a few reports of a rare ocular side effect associated with DRESS syndrome, a systemic hypersensitivity reaction due to a drug that involves a number of organ systems. Acute posterior multifocal pigment epitheliopathy may occur.[10–12] Some cases are associated with anterior or panuveitis.

Veerapandiyan et al reported 4 cases of oculogyric crisis.[13] In this series, the mode was 4 days with 75% of patients less than 11 years old. All patients had positive dechallenge if put on a reduced dosage or stopped the drug. There are 41 additional cases of oculogyric crisis in the spontaneous reporting systems.

Visual hallucinations have also been reported.[14] The PDR states the incidence rate is 0.1–1%.[4] Decreasing the dosage may significantly decrease most or all ocular side effects. Yang et al found that Asians had more severe cutaneous reactions to this class of drugs than non-Asians.[15]

Generic Name:
Pregabalin.

Proprietary Names:
Lyrica, Lyrica CR.

Primary Use
A structural analog of gamma aminobutyric acid (GABA) used in various pain management, including diabetes and herpes zoster. Also used in the treatment of seizures and fibromyalgia.

Ocular Side Effects
Systemic administration – oral
Certain
1. Decreased vision
2. Diplopia
3. Nonrapid eye movement sleep (enhanced)

Probable
1. Periocular edema

Possible
1. May aggravate or cause ocular sicca
2. Extraocular muscles – abnormal movements
3. Oculogyric crisis

Clinical Significance
This drug is used so often with other medications that a drug profile as to adverse effects is difficult. About 1% of patients discontinue pregabalin due to visual complaints.[1] This was mainly due to decreased vision or visual impairment. The *Physicians' Desk Reference* (PDR) states that the incidence of decreased vision is 0.5–12% with severe visual impairment at 1–5%.[2] The cause of the decreased vision is obscure; however, the drug affects nerve transmission. It is not unusual for this to occur within a few days after starting the medication. Decreased vision may resolve even if the drug is continued.[2] Since this drug is a known producer of xerostomia, in all probability, it may cause or aggravate ocular sicca. Diplopia occurred in 5% of controls but occurred in 14% of those on pregabalin.[3] The PDR states an incidence of 0.5–12%.[2] Pregabalin causes enhanced nonrapid eye movement sleep.[4]

Generic Name:
Vigabatrin.

Proprietary Name:
Sabril.

Primary Use
Antiepileptic drug effective for refractory epilepsy, generalized tonic-clonic seizures, and infantile spasms. Also used short-term for drug dependency.

Ocular Side Effects
Systemic administration – oral

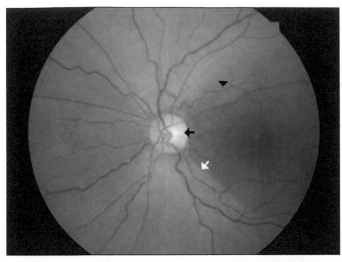

FIG. 5.1 Vigabatrin-induced retinal nerve fiber layer loss. The black *arrow* indicates temporal disc pallor, the white *arrow* represents the demarcation between atrophic and nonaffected nerve fiber layer, and the black *triangle* shows the telltale change in superficial light reflex aligning along the course of the exposed small vessel of the atrophic macula.[19]

Certain

1. Decreased vision
2. Visual field defects – may be irreversible
   a. Concentric peripheral constriction
   b. Variable visual field defects
   c. Scotoma
3. Retina
   a. Peripheral atrophy
   b. Retinal nerve fiber layer (RNFL)
      i. Increases in thickness
      ii. Progresses with therapy
      iii. Loss (Fig. 5.1)
   c. Surface wrinkling retinopathy
   d. Hypopigment spots
4. Contrast sensitivity – reduced
5. Optic atrophy
6. Color vision defect
7. Abnormal electroretinogram (ERG) and electrooculogram (EOG)

Possible

1. Eyelid edema
2. Nystagmus

Clinical Significance

Major changes in the overview of ocular toxicology of this drug have occurred since US Food and Drug Administration (FDA) approval in 2009. This has occurred since the FDA mandated vigabatrin drug registry and the phase IV vigabatrin vision study.[1,2] Although many unanswered questions exist, clearly the frequency and severity of ocular side effects are less than thought, although long-term use is still unclear. Prior studies did not have visual fields done before starting vigabatrin. With no baseline visual fields, a 37% abnormal field rate was found, whereas with baseline visual fields only a 2% new abnormal field rate was found.[3] Visual field studies are difficult for the majority of these patients due to their disease affecting their ability to perform these tests. Therefore the *Physicians' Desk Reference* (PDR) black box warning has been omitted, lowering the age from 17 years old to 10 years old for acceptable use, and "required" eye examinations have been changed to "recommended."[4] Based on current data in the United States, it takes months to years for toxicity to surface in a clinically meaningful manner, so questions still remain.[3]

The only "certain" side effect, based on a 1-year study, is a significant increase in the RNFL, which regression analysis confirmed to progress with duration of vigabatrin exposure.[2] Although the cause is unknown, Foroozan suggested that this might be caused by intra-axonal and intracellular edema.[3]

Vigabatrin has been available for 2 decades; however, the potential for ocular side effects makes it one of the more controversial drugs with regard to ocular safety issues. Some countries have banned its use. This drug is often indispensable for adults with refractory epilepsy, but as of yet there are no good data as to incidence of ocular side effects after many years of exposure.

Much was published before Foroozan's article—many with other conclusions. Lawden's editorial based on the work of Krauss et al and others showed that vigabatrin, not epilepsy or other nervous system diseases, causes these ocular changes.[5,6] Visual field defects may occur after a few months to years after starting the drug. They are bilateral and range from a localized nasal defect of 30 to 40 degrees in eccentricity and may extend to complete concentric contraction. Clayton et al point out, using optic coherence tomography (OCT), that nerve fiber layer thinning in the nasal superior 30 degrees may occur before any visual field abnormality.[7] Besch et al has shown vigabatrin toxicity goes undetected by the patient because there is usually sparing of the temporal fields bilaterally up to 60 degrees eccentricity, which allows for lack of awareness.[8] In rare instances, central vision can be involved. Johnson et al deny reversibility of visual field loss; however, visual acuity, color vision, and ERG amplitude loss may be reversible if recognized early in patients with minimal or no field loss.[9] Best et al studied patients on the drug alone or in combination with other antiepileptic drugs for a minimum of 5 years.[10] This was in patients who elected to continue the medication for good seizure control. All patients had unequivocal visual field defects. They found only 1 in 16 had progression, and the range of follow-up was 18–43 months. Arndt et al felt that visual field changes were enhanced if the patients were also on valproate.[11] Graniewski-Wijnands et al showed some recovery of EOG and ERG but no change in visual fields once the drug was discontinued.[12] Berezina et al reported on the use of vigabatrin in the management of cocaine abusers.[13] Treatment with vigabatrin for 3 months or less did not show significant visual field changes.

The incidence of visual field defects was 2% at 6 months.[14] There is evidence to suggest that this is dose related, more common in males, and more progressive with increased light exposure in mice; but the time of onset varies greatly.[15] Conway et al felt maximum daily dosage was the simplest, most-reliable indicator of visual field changes.[16] Some cases occur as soon as 1 month after starting the drug, and other cases have occurred after 6 or more years of treatment. The mechanism behind the visual field defects could be related to impairment of the highly GABA-ergic amacrine cells in the retina. Histopathological studies in animals show a microvacuolation in myelin sheaths of white matter when exposed to vigabatrin. How these alterations affect the visual field in patients receiving vigabatrin is not known. Frisén et al, Viestenz et al, Buncic et al, and Rebolleda et al have described optic nerve pallor and atrophy secondary to vigabatrin.[17–20] It is felt that there is a toxic effect on the axons of the retinal ganglion cells, resulting in various degrees of optic atrophy. Most often, this atrophy occurs nasally.

The primary retinal side effects are peripheral atrophy and nerve fiber bundle defects. Choi et al have shown RNFL defects correlating with visual field constriction.[21] Outer retinal dysfunction should be present if visual field changes are present. Banin et al suggested that vigabatrin impairs not only peripheral cones but also foveal cones based on ERG amplitudes.[22] These changes are usually irreversible; however, there are rare reports of some reversibility.[23] Other retinal effects include abnormal macular light reflexes, surface wrinkling retinopathy, and narrowing of the arterial tree.

The EOG is possibly a more sensitive and specific diagnostic tool than ERG for drug-related retinal effects. Wild et al felt OCT of the RNFL thickness could efficiently identify this drug's damage in adults and children unable to perform perimetry.[24] It may also be helpful in cases where the question of toxic damage is equivocal. Lawthorn et al, Moseng et al, Kjellström et al, and Foroozan have shown peripapillary or RNFL thickness attenuation with OCT.[3,25–27] They both concur that OCT has a role in following vigabatrin toxicity in selected patients. The nerve fiber layer thinning is characteristic and seems to be a useful biomarker to identify toxicity. Hovath et al described a single case in a 7-year-old child who developed a retinal dystrophy while on vigabatrin.[28]

The PDR has published guidelines for following these patients.[4]

CLASS: ANOREXIANTS

Generic Names:

1. Amfetamine (amphetamine); 2. dextroamfetamine sulfate (dexamphetamine); 3. methamfetamine hydrochloride (methamphetamine).

Proprietary Names:

1. Adzenys, Adzenys XR, Dyanavel XR, Evekeo; 2. Dexedrine, Dexedrine Spansule, DextroStat, Liquadd, ProCentra, Zenzedi; 3. Desoxyn.

Street Names:

1-3. Crank, diet pills, speed, uppers, ups.

Primary Use

These sympathomimetic amines are used in the management of exogenous obesity. These are also effective in the management of narcolepsy and in the management of minimal brain dysfunction in children. They are also used off-label as recreational drugs. This may be oral, intravenous, intramuscular, subcutaneous, smoke inhalation, insufflation, nasal, rectal, or vaginal.

Ocular Side Effects

Systemic administration – oral

Certain

1. Decreased vision
2. Pupils
   a. Mydriasis – may precipitate acute glaucoma
   b. Decreased reaction to light
3. Increase in critical flicker frequency
4. Visual hallucinations
5. Color vision defect – objects have blue tinge (amphetamine)

Probable

1. May aggravate or cause ocular sicca
2. Photosensitivity

Possible

1. Ocular teratogenic effects (methamphetamine)
2. Oculogyric crisis (dextroamphetamine sulfate)
3. Eyelids and conjunctiva – edema

Off-label use – depending on method of administration (see text)

Certain

1. Decreased vision
2. Cornea
   a. Keratitis
   b. Ulceration
3. Conjunctivitis

Probable

1. Retina
   a. Venous thrombosis
   b. Intraretinal hemorrhages
   c. Ischemic changes
   d. Arterial narrowing
   e. Vasculitis
   f. Central or branch vein occlusion
2. Optic nerve
   a. Ischemic changes
   b. Optic atrophy

Possible

1. Crystalline retinopathy

2. Episcleritis
3. Scleritis
4. Endophthalmitis

Clinical Significance

Ocular side effects due to these sympathomimetic amines are dependent on purity of the product, method of administration, and length of use. Use of these drugs in a legal format—orally—may cause mydriasis with potential for acute glaucoma. Decreased vision is not uncommon but seldom is a problem. These drugs can cause edema anywhere on the body. Because these drugs cause xerostomia, ocular sicca may also be caused or aggravated. Hallucination is well documented with these mind-altering drugs. Ocular consequences of these drugs may be minimal or severe.[1,2] Isaak et al and McKeever et al pointed out that retinal emboli, endophthalmitis, scleritis, and episcleritis may occur with intravenous use.[3,4] Chuck et al described recurrent corneal ulcers in a patient with chronic methamphetamine abuse, much like the "crack eye syndrome" resulting from the smoked form of cocaine.[5] This same ocular pattern is evident secondary to the smoked form of methamphetamine, known as "ice." Several hours after methamphetamine was applied to the nose of a young female, she developed decreased vision and intraretinal hemorrhages. This was felt to be due to a sudden increase in blood pressure caused by the drug.[6] Wijaya et al described a similar case of methamphetamine applied once nasally to a 35-year-old male with a unilateral acute loss of vision, with resultant ischemic optic neuropathy.[7] Shaw et al described a patient who developed amaurosis fugax and retinal vasculitis 36 hours after nasal exposure to methamphetamine on the same side as the nasal drug exposure.[8] Kumar et al described a 48-year-old male who snorted methamphetamine several times per week for many years and who developed bilateral crystalline retinopathy without visual loss.[9] No change was seen after a 1-year follow-up.

Hertle et al reported a case of "paradoxically" improved nystagmus, binocular function, and visual acuity in a child with retinal dystrophy and congenital nystagmus while taking Dexedrine (dextroamphetamine sulfate).[10] Fogel et al described reversible eye findings after accidental poisoning of an 11-month-old infant.[11]

Generic Names:

1. Benzfetamine hydrochloride (benzphetamine); 2. diethylpropionate hydrochloride (amfepramone); 3. phendimetrazine tartrate; 4. phentermine hydrochloride.

Proprietary Names:

1. Didrex, Regimex; 2. Depletite #2, Durad, Radtue, Tenuate, Tenuate Dospan; 3. Bock-Arate, Bontril, Bontril PDM, Bontril SR, Melfiat 105 Unicelles, Prelu-2, Stabec-1, X-Trozine, X-Trozine L.A.; 4. Adipex-P, Atti-Plex P, Atti-Plex P Spansule, Fastin, Ionamin, Lomaira, Pro-Fast, Suprenza, Tara-8.

Primary Use

These sympathomimetic amines are used in the treatment of exogenous obesity.

Ocular Side Effects

Systemic administration – oral

Certain

1. Decreased vision
2. Visual hallucinations
3. Eyelids or conjunctiva
   a. Allergic reactions
   b. Erythema
   c. Urticaria
4. Increased critical flicker fusion frequency (amfepramone)

Probable

1. Mydriasis – weak
2. Irritation
   a. Photophobia
   b. Pain
   c. Burning sensation

Possible

1. Decreased accommodation
2. Diplopia

Conditional/unclassified

1. Acute glaucoma
2. Optic neuritis (phentermine)
3. Posterior subcapsular cataracts (phentermine, amfepramone)
4. Vasoplastic amaurosis fugax (amfepramone)

Clinical Significance

Ocular side effects due to these sympathomimetic amines are rare and seldom of clinical significance. All proven side effects, especially decreased vision, are reversible or resolve even while remaining on the drug. These drugs have the ability to cause sympathetic stimulation; therefore mydriasis and acute narrow-angle glaucoma may occur.[1] However, Grewal and a search of the spontaneous reporting systems found no well-documented cases of these drugs causing narrow-angle glaucoma.[2]

In premarketing trials, phendimetrazine had the most prominent sympathetic actions, including decreased vision (1–10%).[1] Posterior subcapsular cataracts have been reported in patients receiving phentermine or amfepramone, but a cause-and-effect relationship has not been proven. Evans reported a unilateral, reversible, ocular, migraine-type aura with a positive dechallenge but no rechallenge in a patient on amfepramone.[3]

Patients had "paradoxical" improvement of congenital nystagmus and binocular function while taking diethylpropionate or with amfepramone.[4]

There is a single report of possible phendimetrazine-induced central retinal vein occlusion occurring 2 days after the drug was started.[5]

CLASS: ANTIANXIETY DRUGS

Generic Names:

1. Alprazolam; 2. chlordiazepoxide; 3. clonazepam; 4. clorazepate dipotassium; 5. diazepam; 6. flurazepam hydrochloride; 7. lorazepam; 8. midazolam hydrochloride; 9. oxazepam; 10. temazepam; 11. triazolam.

Proprietary Names:

1. Niravam, Xanax, Xanax XR; 2. Librium; 3. Ceberclon, Klonopin; 4. Gen-Xene, Tranxene, Tranxene SD, Tranxene T-Tab; 5. Acudial, Diastat, Dizac, Valium; 6. Dalmane; 7. Ativan; 8. Versed; 9. Serax; 10. Restoril; 11. Halcion.

Primary Use

These benzodiazepine derivatives are effective in the management of psychoneurotic states manifested by anxiety, tension, or agitation. They are also used as adjunctive therapy in the relief of skeletal muscle spasms and as preoperative medications.

Ocular Side Effects

Systemic administration – intramuscular, intravenous, or oral

Certain

1. Decreased vision
2. Risk factor for causing intraoperative floppy iris syndrome (IFIS)
3. Visual hallucinations
4. Abnormal electrooculogram (EOG) (diazepam)

Probable

1. Eyelids or conjunctiva
   a. Allergic reactions
   b. Erythema

c. Conjunctivitis – nonspecific
d. Blepharospasm (lorazepam)
e. Edema
2. Decreased corneal reflex (clorazepate, diazepam)
3. Extraocular muscles
  a. Nystagmus – horizontal or gaze evoked
  b. Decreased spontaneous movements
  c. Abnormal conjugate deviations
  d. Jerky pursuit movements
  e. Decreased saccadic movements
  f. Oculogyric crises
  g. Paresis
4. Decreased depth perception (chlordiazepoxide)
5. Color vision defect (lorazepam, oxazepam)
6. Photophobia

Possible
1. Pupils
  a. Mydriasis (rare)
  b. Decreased reaction to light
  c. Miosis (midazolam)
  d. May precipitate acute glaucoma
2. Diplopia
3. Decreased accommodation
4. Lacrimation
5. Irritation
  a. Pain
  b. Burning sensation
6. Loss of eyelashes or eyebrows (clonazepam)

Conditional/unclassified
1. Brown lens opacification (diazepam)
2. Retinopathy (clonazepam)
3. Visual field defects (diazepam)

Ocular teratogenic effects
Probable
1. Increased incidences strabismus (diazepam)
2. Epicanthal folds (oxazepam, diazepam)
3. "Slant eyes" (oxazepam, diazepam)

Clinical Significance
Benzodiazepine derivatives are often used in combination with other drugs, so clear-cut drug-induced ocular side effects are difficult to determine. However, ocular side effects are seldom of clinical importance, and most are reversible. Of greatest clinical interest is that this group of drugs, on a statistical basis (p value < 0.001), can cause IFIS.[1] At therapeutic dosage levels, these drugs may cause decreased corneal reflex, decreased accommodation, decreased depth perception, and abnormal extraocular muscle movements. Speeg-Schatz et al and others have shown that a single dosage in susceptible individuals can cause phorias, diplopia, and fusional impairment.[2] There are cases in the spontaneous reports where diplopia was severe enough to require discontinuing the drug. All drugs in this class appear to cross-react as if allergic conjunctivitis because they have the metabolite desmethyldiazepam, a probable antigen, in common. This may give a type I immune reaction. Typically, the allergic conjunctivitis occurs within 30 minutes of taking the drug, with the peak reaction occurring within 4 hours and subsiding in 1–2 days. Symptoms include decreased vision, photophobia, burning, tearing, and a foreign body sensation. Contact lens wearers have confused this adverse drug effect with poorly fitted lenses. To what degree these benzodiazepine derivatives cause pupillary dilatation is uncertain. There are cases in the literature, and the *Physicians' Desk Reference* (PDR) confirms that patients may develop a narrow-angle attack after receiving 1 of these drugs.[3-5] In the spontaneous reporting systems, most of these drugs have case reports of precipitating narrow-angle glaucoma, but it is rare and the cases are poorly documented. However, it is common enough that there is a "possible" association. These benzodiazepines do not have antimuscarinic actions, so causation for precipitation is unknown, whereas in narrow-angle glaucoma, most are not contraindicated; however, according to the PDR, alprazolam, clorazepate, clonazepam, diazepam, and lorazepam are.[5] The report of maculopathy secondary to gazing into a bright video camera light in 2 patients taking triazolam may or may not be a drug-enhanced photopic effect.[6]

Diazepam taken over many years has been reported to cause the lens to become brown or in high dosage (100 mg) to cause significant visual field loss.[7,8]

Generic Names:
1. Carisoprodol; 2. meprobamate.

Proprietary Names:
1. Soma, Vanadom; 2. Miltown, Tranmep.

Primary Use
These drugs are used to treat skeletal muscle spasms. In addition, meprobamate is used as a psychotherapeutic sedative in the treatment of nervous tension, anxiety, and simple insomnia.

Ocular Side Effects
Systemic administration – oral
Probable
1. Decreased accommodation

2. Decreased vision
3. Diplopia
4. Paresis of extraocular muscles
5. Eyelids or conjunctiva
   a. Allergic reactions
   b. Edema
   c. Urticaria
6. Random ocular movements

Possible
1. Mydriasis
2. Decreased corneal reflex
3. Visual fields
   a. Constriction
   b. Enlargement
4. Irritation
   a. Edema
   b. Burning sensation
5. Nystagmus
6. Eyelids or conjunctiva
   a. Erythema multiforme
   b. Exfoliative dermatitis

Clinical Significance
Significant ocular side effects due to these drugs are uncommon and transitory. At normal dosage levels, decreased accommodation, diplopia, and paralysis of extraocular muscles may only rarely be found. Carisoprodol has been associated with acute porphyria attacks, and this association needs to be considered if acute photophobia or eyelid reactions occur.

CLASS: ANTICONVULSANTS

Generic Names:
1. Divalproex sodium (valproate semisodium); 2. valproate sodium; 3. valproic acid.

Proprietary Names:
1. Depakote, Depakote ER; 2. Depacon; 3. Depakene.

Primary Use
These anticonvulsants are used to treat epilepsy and bipolar disease and to prevent migraine headaches.

Ocular Side Effects
Systemic administration – intravenous or oral
Certain
1. Decreased vision
2. Diplopia
3. Nystagmus
4. Oscillopsia
5. Visual hallucinations

Probable
1. Mydriasis (valproate semisodium)
2. Irritation
   a. Pain
   b. Photophobia
   c. Conjunctivitis
3. May aggravate or cause ocular sicca

Possible
1. Lacrimal gland
   a. Dacryoadenitis
   b. Enlargement
2. Pigmentary retinal dystrophies – visual field decline
3. Decreased thickness of peripapillary retinal nerve fiber layer

Conditional/unclassified
1. Pseudotumor cerebri

Ocular teratogenic effects – fetal anticonvulsant syndrome (Fig. 5.2)
Certain
1. Myopia
2. Hypoplastic front – orbital edges
3. Proptosis
4. Poliosis
5. Epicanthus
6. Shallow orbitals
7. Septo-optic dysplasia
8. Coloboma

Clinical Significance
These drugs appear to have identical adverse ocular side effects. The *Physicians' Desk Reference* (PDR) estimates incidences of nystagmus, decreased vision, conjunctivitis, ocular pain, and ocular sicca at 1.1–5% and diplopia at 16%.[1]

There may be an idiosyncratic susceptibility in some patients characterized by various forms of diplopia, oscillopsia, impaired vergence mechanisms, vertical nystagmus, or abnormalities of the vestibulo-ocular reflex. Other side effects include ocular motor abnormalities involving pursuit and gaze-holding patterns. Bhalla et al concluded that these drugs play a role in pigment retinal dystrophies, including retinitis pigmentosa, with a decline in vision and visual fields if they are used on a long-term basis.[2] Clemson et al reported 2 patients taking valproic acid for retinitis pigmentosa and developing visual field loss.[3] Dereci et al, using optic coherence tomography measurements, found that the average and superior peripapillary retinal nerve fiber layer thickness was reduced in children on monotherapy with valproic

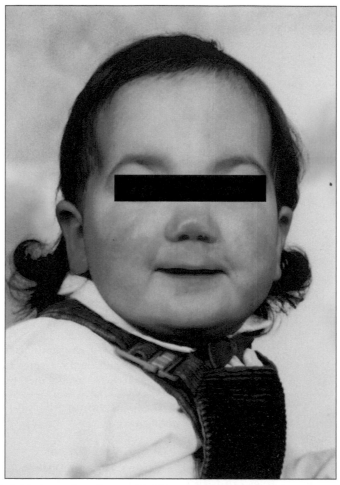

FIG. 5.2 Craniofacial features of a 1.5-year-old child exposed in utero to both sodium valproate and carbamazepine. She has cherubic facies, a tall forehead, broad nasal root and flat nasal bridge, blunt nasal tip, smooth philtrum, and thin vermilion border to the upper lip.[8]

acid compared with healthy children.[4] Based on psychophysical testing, Bayer et al felt that valproic acid had no effect on retinal function.[5] The issue if valproate can cause mydriasis is complicated. According to the FDA, mydriasis was most often reported in patients who were 30 to 39 years old, taking this drug for less than 1 month, also taking quetiapine, and experiencing pain. Two-thirds were female. The incidence of the mydriasis was 0.18%.[6] There are 69 cases in the spontaneous reports of mydriasis being caused by this drug, but this is unproven because in the same series 46 cases of miosis were reported.

Lyons et al described bilateral dacryoadenitis and salivary gland enlargement in a 7-year-old child after 3 months on valproic acid.[7]

Valproic acid has many ocular teratogenic effects, especially myopia.[8] Glover et al reviewed the "fetal anticonvulsant syndrome."[9] Boyle et al reported decreased corneal sensation and severe dry eyes in a child with a fetal valproate syndrome.[10] Although pseudotumor cerebri has been associated with these drugs, this remains unproven. Jackson et al reported 4 cases of coloboma, and recent cases in the literature support choroidal-retinal colobomas may be part of the fetal valproate syndrome.[11]

Generic Names:

1. Ethosuximide; 2. methsuximide.

Proprietary Names:

1. Zarontin; 2. Celontin.

Primary Use

These succinimides are effective in the management of petit mal seizures.

Ocular Side Effects

Systemic administration – oral
Probable

1. Decreased vision
2. Photophobia
3. Myopia (ethosuximide)
4. Periorbital edema (methsuximide)
5. Eyelids or conjunctiva
   a. Hyperemia
   b. Allergic reactions
   c. Edema (methsuximide)
6. Visual hallucinations

Possible

1. Myasthenia gravis – aggravated
   a. Diplopia
   b. Paresis of extraocular muscles
   c. Ptosis
2. Eyelids or conjunctiva
   a. Lupoid syndrome
   b. Erythema multiforme
   c. Exfoliative dermatitis

Clinical Significance

Methsuximide induces ocular side effects more frequently than ethosuximide. All adverse ocular reactions other than those due to anemias or dermatologic conditions are reversible after discontinuation of the drug. This group of drugs can trigger systemic lupus erythematosus by producing antinuclear antibodies. They may also aggravate myasthenia gravis.

Generic Name:

Ethotoin.

Proprietary Name:

Peganone.

Primary Use

This hydantoin is effective in the management of psychomotor and grand mal seizures.

Ocular Side Effects

Systemic administration – oral
Certain

1. Nystagmus
2. Photophobia

3. Eyelids or conjunctiva
   a. Allergic reactions
   b. Conjunctivitis – nonspecific
   c. Edema
   d. Urticaria

Probable

1. Diplopia

Possible

1. Eyelids or conjunctiva
   a. Lupoid syndrome
   b. Erythema multiforme
   c. Exfoliative dermatitis
   d. Lyell syndrome

Clinical Significance

Ocular side effects are seen more frequently with mephenytoin than with ethotoin and are reversible either by decreasing the dosage or discontinuing use of the drug. As with phenytoin, nystagmus may persist for some time after the drug is stopped. Mephenytoin has been implicated in inducing systemic lupus erythematosus by producing antinuclear antibodies. Corneal or lens opacities and myasthenic neuromuscular blocking effect have not been proven as drug related.

Generic Name:

Phenytoin.

Proprietary Names:

Cerebyx, Dilantin, Dilantin-125, Phenytek.

Primary Use

This hydantoin is effective in the prophylaxis and treatment of chronic epilepsy.

Ocular Side Effects

Systemic administration – intramuscular, intravenous, or oral
Certain

1. Decreased vision
2. Nystagmus – downbeat, horizontal, or vertical
3. Diplopia
4. Visual sensations
   a. Glare phenomenon – objects appear to be covered with white snow
   b. Flashing lights
   c. Oscillopsia
   d. Photophobia
5. Color vision defect
   a. Objects have white tinge
   b. Colors appear faded

6. External ophthalmoplegia
7. Abnormal electroretinogram (ERG)

Probable
1. Pupils
   a. Mydriasis
   b. Decreased reaction to light
2. Decreased accommodation
3. Decreased convergence
4. Visual hallucinations
5. Myasthenia gravis
   a. Diplopia
   b. Ptosis
   c. Paresis of extraocular muscles

Possible
1. Papilledema secondary to pseudotumor cerebri
2. Cataracts (long-term therapy)
3. Eyelids or conjunctiva
   a. Allergic reactions
   b. Ulceration
   c. Purpura
   d. Lupoid syndrome
   e. Erythema multiforme
   f. Exfoliative dermatitis
   g. Lyell syndrome
4. Pain

Ocular teratogenic effects (fetal hydantoin syndrome)
Probable
1. Hypertelorism
2. Ptosis
3. Epicanthal fields
4. Strabismus
5. Retinal coloboma

Possible
1. Glaucoma
2. Optic nerve or iris hypoplasia
3. Retinoschisis
4. Trichomegaly
5. Abnormal lacrimal system
6. Congenital glaucoma

Clinical Significance

Most ocular side effects due to phenytoin are reversible and often will decrease in extent or disappear with reduction in dosage. Phenytoin toxicity may be manifested as a syndrome of vestibular, cerebellar, and/or ocular abnormalities. The ocular findings are most notably nystagmus and diplopia. Nystagmus-induced phenytoin toxicity is directly related to the blood levels of the drug. Fine nystagmus may occur even at therapeutic dosages, but coarse nystagmus is indicative of a toxic state. Downbeat- and unidirectional-gaze paretic nystagmus have also been reported. Instances of nystagmus persisting for 20 months or longer after discontinued use of phenytoin have been reported. Paralysis of extraocular muscles is uncommon, reversible, and primarily found in toxic states. However, in the spontaneous reporting systems, diplopia was the most commonly reported adverse ocular side effect, with almost 400 possible cases. Remler et al have reported an idiosyncratic response in patients on carbamazepine and phenytoin with an increase in incidences of vertical and horizontal diplopia with or without oscillopsia.[1] This appears to be a central effect on the vergence centers and/or the vestibulo-ocular reflex. A prodrome of ocular or systemic "discomfort" frequently occurred before the onset of these changes. Color vision changes are complex with various manifestations, including frosting or white tinges on objects, decreased brightness, or specific color loss. Benign intracranial hypertension in a patient with a seizure disorder has been confirmed with phenytoin rechallenge. Bar et al and Mathers et al reported cases of presenile cataracts in patients on prolonged hydantoin therapy at toxic levels of phenytoin or with concomitant phenobarbital ingestion.[2,3]

Phenytoin, alone or in combination, has a 2–3 times greater risk for delivering a child with congenital defects. Ocular abnormalities are not unusual in these deformities.

Generic Name:

Topiramate.

Proprietary Names:

Qudexy XR, Topamax, Topamax Sprinkle, Topiragen, Trokendi XR.

Primary Use

Topiramate is a novel drug used to treat patients with various types of epilepsy and migraine headaches. It is used off-label as a "magic" weight reducer, in bipolar disorder, and in clinical depression.

Ocular Side Effects
Systemic administration – oral
Certain
1. Decreased vision
2. Acute glaucoma – primarily bilateral
   a. Increased bilateral intraocular pressure
   b. Anterior chamber shallowing (Fig. 5.3)

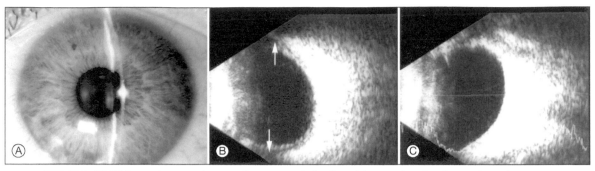

FIG. 5.3 **(A)** Slit lamp photography revealing severe shallowing of the anterior chamber and anterior convexity of lens–iris diaphragm secondary to topiramate. **(B)** B-scan ultrasound study at presentation revealed shallow choroidal effusions bilaterally (effusion narrowed). **(C)** Resolution of effusion occurred within 1 week of topiramate cessation.[17]

   c. Suprachoroidal effusions
   d. Ocular hyperemia
   e. Uveitis
   f. Mydriasis
   g. Visual field defects
   h. Pain
3. Acute myopia (up to 6–8.5 diopters)
4. Nystagmus
5. Decreased accommodation
6. Palinopsia

Possible
 1. Visual field changes – cause unknown
 2. Blepharospasm
 3. Oculogyric crisis
 4. Diplopia
 5. Periorbital edema
 6. Scleritis
 7. Papilledema secondary to pseudotumor cerebri
 8. Electroretinogram (ERG) changes
 9. Myokymia
10. Macular striae

Ocular teratogenic effects
Possible
1. Ocular malformations

Clinical Significance
Banta et al first reported a case of uveal effusion and secondary angle-closure glaucoma associated with topiramate.[1] This has now developed into a well-recognized syndrome.[2] This usually occurs within the first 2 weeks after starting topiramate therapy. In some cases, it develops within hours after increasing the dosage. Almost all cases are bilateral. The syndrome may include the typical findings of acute glaucoma, including acute ocular pain, headache, nausea and vomiting, pupillary changes, hyperemia, corneal edema, cataract, retinal and vascular changes, visual field defect, and blindness, if not recognized soon enough. Suprachoroidal effusions have been reported by Rhee et al and others and should be looked for as the cause of the glaucoma.[3] These effusions cause a forward rotation of the ciliary processes with angle closure. A few cases of scleritis have been reported, although glaucoma-induced hyperemia may mimic or mask the signs of scleritis. Effusions along with acute pressure elevation may cause uveitis. Jabbarpoor Bonyadi et al reported a severe uveitis resulting in hypopyon formation.[4]

Topiramate is a sulfa drug, a class that is known to cause transient myopia. Acute myopia up to 8.5 diopters may occur in a matter of hours after starting this drug; however, it may take a number of weeks to resolve once the drug is discontinued. Causation is not fully known but includes lenticular swelling, forward rotation of the iris and lens diaphragm, ciliary body swelling causing increased curvature of the lens surface, and spasms of accommodation.

Palinopsia is a persistence of visual images after the initial stimulus has been removed. It may include echoing, ghosting, multiple images, smearing, streaming, trailing, or vibrating of the initial image.[5] Enough cases in the literature and spontaneous reports with positive dechallenge and rechallenge data make this a "certain" adverse ocular side effect.[6–9] Many drugs can cause this side effect, including some used in conjunction with topiramate. Yun et al, in a series of 9 cases, found that palinopsia occurred at dosages as low as 25 mg twice a day.[5] Symptoms were often worse in the early morning or late evening. In all of the reported cases, symptoms either improved or stopped on decreasing the dosage, and all symptoms stopped when the drug was discontinued. Some patients accepted this side effect and continued the topiramate or another drug that also causes palinopsia.

Diplopia and nystagmus are seen primarily in high dosages, and the mechanism is unknown. However, other neurologic muscular defects, such as myokymia, oculogyric crisis, and blepharospasms, have been reported. Foroozan et al reported a single case of homonymous hemianopia.[10] There are a few cases of visual field changes with long-term use of this drug without any history of glaucoma.[11] We have personally seen this and have no explanation and agree with the Australian Therapeutic Goods Administration's (TGA) precaution regarding visual field defects. The following has been added to the product information for topiramate recommendations: "[H]ealth-care professionals should advise patients and caregivers of this issue and educate them regarding the signs and symptoms of visual field defects. Patients should be instructed to seek immediate medical attention if any problems are suspected."[12] Vaphaiades et al reported a single case of bilateral pigmentary retinopathy possibly due to this drug.[13] There are no spontaneous case reports of this. Tsui et al reported a case of ERG changes possibly due to topiramate.[14] Animal work supports this possibility.

Gualtieri et al described a case of bilateral macular striae radiating from both fovea with a cellophane-like reflex.[15] Vision was hand motion in the right eye and count fingers in the left eye. Topiramate was discontinued, and oral steroids were started. Vision returned to 6/6 in both eyes within 3 days, and the rest of the ocular examination was normal. Çerman et al reported a case-controlled study that showed accommodation lag in patients on this drug, which may account for the visual symptoms while on it.[16]

Recommendations[2]
1. The patient should stop the medication in concert with the prescribing physician because dropping the drug by as little as 50 mg may exacerbate the preexisting systemic disease.
2. Institute maximum medical therapy for glaucoma, including topical ocular cycloplegic drugs, along with topical beta blockers and oral pressure–lowering drugs.
3. Laser iridotomy or peripheral iridectomy are probably not beneficial, as they do not resolve the suprachoroidal effusions.

4. Topical ocular miotics are probably contraindicated because they may precipitate a relative papillary block.

Generic Name:
Zonisamide.

Proprietary Name:
Zonegran.

Primary Use
This sulfonamide derivative is used as a broad-spectrum antiepileptic medication. Off-label uses include migraine headache prophylaxis and weight loss.

Ocular Side Effects
Systemic administration – oral
Certain
1. Decreased vision
2. Diplopia
3. Nystagmus

Probable
1. Acute glaucoma (rare)
   a. Increased intraocular pressure
   b. Anterior chamber shallowing
   c. Suprachoroidal effusions
   d. Ocular hyperemia
   e. Uveitis
   f. Mydriasis
   g. Visual field defects
   h. Pain
2. Acute myopia (rare)
3. Visual hallucinations

Possible
1. Eyelids or conjunctiva
   a. Chemosis
   b. Congestion
2. Palinopsia

Clinical Significance
Numerous cases in the spontaneous reports and data in the package inserts support the side effects of diplopia (6% incidence) and nystagmus (4% incidence) secondary to zonisamide.[1] Weppner et al reported the first case of extraocular restricted eye movements, which included diplopia, inability to abduct the left eye, dysmetria, and horizontal nystagmus, after off-label use of zonisamide.[2] Symptoms slowly resolved after discontinuing the drug.

This sulfonamide derivative can probably cause most of the sulfonamide ocular side effects. Probably the most significant, but rare, are choroidal effusions and secondary narrow-angle glaucoma.[3] There are 8 possible cases of this in the spontaneous reports. We were personally involved in a case of bilateral acute glaucoma secondary to uveal effusion, which mimicked the classic syndrome caused by topiramate. Acute myopic shift also probably occurs as a rare side effect.[3] There are 6 cases in the spontaneous reports. The decreased vision may be, in rare instances, secondary to the drug being secreted in the tears, which can be associated with hyperemia, chemosis, and photophobia.

Akman et al reported a series of complex visual hallucinations secondary to zonisamide that completely resolved when the drug was discontinued.[4] Palinopsia has been reported with this class of drugs.[5,6]

Hypersensitivity and cross-hypersensitivity with other sulfonamides have been reported.

CLASS: ANTIDEPRESSANTS

Generic Names:

1. Amitriptyline hydrochloride; 2. clomipramine hydrochloride; 3. doxepin hydrochloride; 4. trimipramine maleate.

Proprietary Names:

1. Elavil, EnovaRX, Equipto Amitriptyline, Vanatrip; 2. Anafranil; 3. Prudoxin, Silenor, Sinequan, Zonalon; 4. Surmontil.

Primary Use

These tertiary amine tricyclic antidepressants are used in the treatment of psychoneurotic anxiety or depressive reactions.

Ocular Side Effects
Systemic administration – oral or topical
Certain
1. Decreased vision

Probable
1. Mydriasis – potential acute glaucoma
2. May aggravate or cause ocular sicca
3. Decreased accommodation
4. Decreased contact lens tolerance
5. Suppression of rapid eye movement in sleep (clomipramine)

Possible
1. Blepharospasm
2. Extraocular muscles
   a. Diplopia

b. Oculogyric crises
c. Nystagmus – horizontal or rotary – toxic states
d. Paresis – toxic states

Conditional/unclassified
1. Acute macular neuroretinopathy (amitriptyline/atomoxetine)
2. Upbeat nystagmus
3. Congenital ocular abnormalities

Clinical Significance
Adverse ocular reactions due to these tricyclic antidepressants are seldom of major clinical importance. Ocular anticholinergic effects are the most frequent and include blurred vision (which may require decreasing the dosage), disturbance of accommodation, and mydriasis. Blurred vision occurs early, at an occurrence of at least 10% with each of these drugs.[1] Blurred vision may interfere with fusion therapy, thereby causing diplopia. This may regress even if on the same dosage. The package inserts for these drugs recommend caution in patients with narrow chamber angles due to mydriasis, which may cause acute glaucoma.[1] They also warn of contact lens intolerance due to potential ocular sicca.[1,2]

Kupfer et al have shown that clomipramine suppresses rapid eye movement (REM) during sleep.[3] Osborne et al reported a case of upbeat nystagmus after stopping amitriptyline.[4] Shah et al reported 3 cases of acute macular neuroretinopathy with the use of 2 oral norepinephrine reuptake inhibitors (amitriptyline/atomoxetine).[5] Berard et al reported some evidence of congenital ocular abnormalities occurring with the use of each of these drugs during pregnancy.[6]

Generic Names:

1. Amoxapine; 2. desipramine hydrochloride; 3. imipramine hydrochloride; 4. nortriptyline hydrochloride.

Proprietary Names:

1. Asendin; 2. Norpramin; 3. Tofranil, Tofranil-PM; 4. Aventyl, Pamelor.

Primary Use

These secondary amine tricyclic antidepressants and tranquilizers are effective in the relief of symptoms of mental depression.

Ocular Side Effects
Systemic administration – oral
Certain
1. Decreased vision

Probable

1. Mydriasis – potential acute glaucoma
2. May aggravate or cause ocular sicca
3. Decreased accommodation
4. Decreased contact lens tolerance
5. Visual hallucinations

Possible

1. Photosensitivity
2. Intraoperative floppy iris syndrome (IFIS) (imipramine)
3. Increase blink rate

Clinical Significance

Adverse ocular reactions due to these tricyclic antidepressants are seldom of major clinical importance. Ocular anticholinergic effects are the most frequent and include decreased vision (which may require decreasing the dosage), disturbance of accommodation, and mydriasis. Decreased vision occurs early, at an occurrence of at least 10% with each of these drugs.[1] Decreased vision may interfere with fusion, thereby causing diplopia. This may regress even if on the same dosage. The package inserts for these drugs recommend caution in narrow chamber angles due to possible mydriasis.[1] They also warn of contact lens intolerance due to potential ocular sicca.[1]

The clinician needs to be aware that tricyclic antidepressants potentiate the systemic blood pressure elevation from topical ocular epinephrine preparations.

Gupta et al reported 3 cases of floppy lid syndrome in patients on imipramine.[2] They felt imipramine led to chronic blockage of α-1 adrenoceptors of the papillary dilator muscle, which possibly caused atrophy of the iris stroma and may have led to the occurrence of IFIS.

Recommendation

Roberts et al recommended sun-blocking ocular protection for patients placed on imipramine because it is a photosensitizer for the lens with peak absorption above that which the cornea filters out.[3] They recommended that when working outside, patients on this drug should consider wearing ultraviolet (UV)–blocking glasses that protect to at least 320 nm.

Generic Names:

1. Atomoxetine; 2. duloxetine; 3. venlafaxine hydrochloride.

Proprietary Names:

1. Strattera; 2. Cymbalta, Irenka; 3. Effexor, Effexor XR.

Primary Use

Serotonin–norepinephrine reuptake inhibitor (SNRI) antidepressants affecting muscarinic, histamine H, and alpha-adrenergic receptors.

Ocular Side Effects

Systemic administration – oral
Certain

1. Decreased vision
2. Mydriasis

Probable

1. Acute glaucoma

Possible

1. May aggravate or cause ocular sicca
2. Eyelids
   a. Edema
   b. Blepharospasm
   c. Blink rate increased (atomoxetine, duloxetine)
3. Cataracts
4. Visual hallucinations
5. Conjunctivitis
6. Photophobia

Conditional/unclassified

1. Horner's syndrome
2. Acute macular neuropathy (atomoxetine)

Clinical Significance

This group of drugs rarely causes significant ocular side effects. Initially decreased vision and occasional accommodation changes occur, but seem to clear with time. Decreased vision occurs at an incidence of 3–6%.[1]

These drugs have weak or minimal anticholinergic effects; however, in already compromised chamber angles, unilateral and often bilateral acute angle-closure glaucoma has been seen with all 3 of these drugs.[2-10] Wicinski et al recently reviewed the associated between SNRIs and acute-angle glaucoma.[11] They pointed out the complexity of the possible mechanism of causation and reviewed published cases with each of these 3 drugs This is probably in relation to the 1–3% incidence rate of mydriasis.[1]

Acute macular neuroretinopathy has been reported with atomoxetine; however, we are not aware of any other reports.[12]

These drugs have been implicated in neurotransmission side effects. Blink rate changes were unaffected with venlafaxine.[13] However, an increase has been reported with atomoxetine and duloxetine via spontaneous reporting systems. Blepharospasms have been reported by Reif et al and in spontaneous reports with all 3 drugs.[14] Diplopia is a rare and unproven side effect.

Chou et al reported an increase in cataracts in almost all patients on long-term antidepressants.[15]

These drugs cause xerostomia, so they probably cause ocular sicca as well.[16] The cause of late onset of conjunctivitis (3%) is unknown.[1]

There are numerous reports of periocular and eyelid edema of unknown cause.

Generic Name:
Bupropion hydrochloride.

Proprietary Names:
Alpenzin, Budeprion SR, Budeprion XL, Buproban, Forfivo XL, Wellbutrin, Wellburtin SR, Wellbutrin XL, Zyban.

Primary Use
Oral aminoketone class of antidepressants used in the management of severe depression and in smoking cessation.

Ocular Side Effects
Systemic administration – oral
Certain
1. Decreased vision
2. Visual hallucinations
3. Mydriasis – weak

Possible
1. Myopia
2. Diplopia
3. May aggravate or cause ocular sicca
4. Eyelids or conjunctiva
   a. Edema
   b. Photosensitivity
5. Periorbital edema
6. Mydriasis – may precipitate acute glaucoma
7. Uveal effusion

Clinical Significance
Very few ocular side effects have been reported due to bupropion. Most are reversible with few sequelae. Bupropion is chemically completely unrelated to other antidepressants. Bupropion only has a quarter of the anticholinergic ocular effects that the tricyclic antidepressants have.[1] Decreased vision occurring shortly after taking bupropion may occur in up to 15% of patients. This seldom requires stopping the drug. This drug may well be a weak mydriatic and rarely has been associated

with bilateral acute narrow-angle glaucoma.[2] Bilateral angle-closure glaucoma secondary to uveal effusions was attributed to this drug, and 11 spontaneous reports of this syndrome support this.[3] Up to 27% of patients in phase III trials had xerostomia. This is a signal that this drug can cause ocular sicca with its associated signs and symptoms.

Generic Names:
1. Carbamazepine; 2. oxcarbazepine.

Proprietary Names:
1. Carbatrol, Epitol, Equetro, Tegretol, Tegretol-XR, Teril; 2. Oxtellar XR, Trileptal.

Primary Use
Carboxamide anticonvulsants also used as mood stabilizers.

Ocular Side Effects
Systemic administration – oral
Certain
1. Extraocular muscles
   a. Diplopia
   b. Downbeat or horizontal nystagmus
   c. Oculogyric crises
   d. Decreased spontaneous movements
2. Decreased vision
3. Visual hallucinations
4. Photosensitivity, increased glare
5. Color vision defect – decreased blue perception (carbamazepine)
6. Decreased accommodation
7. Decreased convergence
8. Mydriasis (weak)

Probable
1. Eyelids
   a. Edema
   b. Urticaria
   c. Blepharoclonus

Possible
1. Myasthenia gravis - aggravated (carbamazepine)
   a. Diplopia
   b. Ptosis
   c. Paresis of extraocular muscles
2. May aggravate or cause ocular sicca
3. Eyelids or conjunctiva
   a. Pain
   b. Lupoid syndrome
   c. Erythema multiforme

d. Exfoliative dermatitis
e. Lyell syndrome

Conditional/unclassified
1. Cataracts
   a. Punctate cortical
   b. Anterior and posterior subcapsular
2. Retinal pigmentary change
3. Corneal metaplasia

Ocular teratogenic effects
Probable
1. Anophthalmos
2. Microphthalmos
3. Optic disc coloboma
4. Optic nerve hypoplasia

Clinical Significance
One of the most common side effects due to these drugs is ocular, with transitory diplopia being the most frequent, followed by decreased vision, and a "heavy feeling in the eyes." Both drugs are structurally similar, with a 25–30% cross reactivity. Carbamazepine, when compared with oxcarbazepine, has a higher frequency and severity of drug interactions.[1] Ocular adverse reactions are reversible, usually disappear as the dosage is decreased, and may spontaneously clear even without reduction of the drug dosage. A toxic syndrome may occur as an acute phenomenon with downbeat nystagmus, confusion, drowsiness, and ataxia. The *Physicians' Desk Reference* (PDR) stated incidences of carbamazepine versus oxcarbazepine of decreased vision, 5–6% versus 1–4%; diplopia, 12% versus 4%; nystagmus, incidence unknown versus 2%; and xerostomia, 8% versus 3% (indicated high likelihood of ocular sicca).[2] Bayer et al pointed out that patients complain of increased glare and have a blue color deficiency.[3] Carbamazepine may also cause the ocular effects of lupus erythematosus. Carbamazepine can be recovered in the tears, and this method has been advocated to test for blood levels as a noninvasive technique in the pediatric age group.

The cataractogenic potential of this drug is still open to debate. Although Neilsen et al first postulated this association, this has not been proven.[4] Neilsen et al reported 2 patients with retinotoxicity attributed to long-term therapeutic use of carbamazepine, and although there have been a few spontaneous reports, there is no proven association.[4] This drug interacts with multiple other drugs causing visual side effects, such as bilateral acute-angle closure secondary to uveal effusions associated with flucloxacillin and carbamazepine. Toxic reactions in overdosage situations

possibly cause dilated, sluggish, or nonreactive pupils and papilledema. There are several reports of a fetal carbamazepine syndrome, which may include ocular abnormalities.[5,6]

Recommendations
The pharmaceutical company that manufactures carbamazepine recommends that before starting the drug, use caution in glaucoma or other conditions associated with increased intraocular pressure. Baseline and periodic eye examinations, including slit lamp, fundoscopy, and tonometry, are recommended.

Generic Names:
1. Citalopram hydrobromide; 2. escitalopram oxalate; 3. fluoxetine hydrochloride; 4. fluvoxamine maleate; 5. paroxetine hydrochloride; 6. sertraline hydrochloride.

Proprietary Names:
1. Celexa; 2. Lexapro; 3. Prozac, Prozac Weekly, Sarafem, Selfemra; 4. Generic only; 5. Brisdelle, Paxil, Paxil CR, Pexeva; 6. Zoloft.

Primary Use
These selective inhibitors of serotonin reuptake are used as antidepressants.

Ocular Side Effects
Systemic administration – oral
Certain
1. Decreased vision
2. Photophobia
3. May aggravate or cause ocular sicca
4. Increased intraocular pressure (minimal)
5. Non-REM (NREM) during sleep

Probable
1. Pupil
   a. Mydriasis
   b. Anisocoria
2. Oculogyric crisis
3. Abnormal ocular sensations (paroxetine)

Possible
1. Conjunctivitis – nonspecific
2. Diplopia
3. Eyelids
   a. Tics
   b. Rash
   c. Urticaria
   d. Edema
4. Inability to cry

5. Optic nerve
   a. Neuritis
   b. Ischemic optic neuropathy
6. Cataracts

Conditional/unclassified
1. Activation of ocular herpes (fluoxetine)
2. Papilledema secondary to pseudotumor cerebri
3. Maculopathy (sertraline)

Clinical Significance
This group of selective serotonin reuptake inhibitors (SSRIs) is one of the most commonly prescribed antidepressant drugs in the world because of its favorable safety profile. Although ocular side effects are few and rare, they may be of clinical importance. Costagliola et al, in a 20-patient, double-blind crossover study, showed that all 20 patients had subclinical intraocular pressure elevations within 2 hours of oral ingestion.[1,2] Some pressures remained elevated for up to 8 hours. This was also found with other SSRI drugs such as citalopram, fluvoxamine, paroxetine, and sertraline.[3,4] Although the authors cannot prove an association, they implied causation. Although rare, the mydriasis effect of these drugs may precipitate narrow-angle glaucoma.[5-8] Clinical trials against placebo showed that decreased vision and xerostomia may be significant. Kocer et al confirmed this in a smaller study.[9]

There are several positive rechallenge cases of this class of drugs causing photophobia. Schenck et al have shown that fluoxetine can cause extensive, prominent eye movements during NREM sleep.[10] In 1 case, this continued for 19 months after the drug was discontinued. Although diplopia, ptosis, and nystagmus have been seen, it is hard to prove a direct cause-and-effect relationship because these patients are often on multiple drugs. Armitage et al reported that fluoxetine could cause these findings because it causes increased availability of serotonin with secondary dopaminergic effects.[11] Wakeno et al described 3 patients who, after discontinuing paroxetine, developed abnormal ocular sensations with abnormal eye movement.[12] This occurred within 2–6 days after the drug was stopped, and in all cases, the abnormal sensation disappeared as soon as the drug was restarted. Etminan et al in a nested case-control study showed a possible association of this group of drugs and cataract formation.[13] The risk was highest with fluvoxamine and venlafaxine. Erie et al, in a large epidemiologic study with controls, showed an increased risk of cataract surgery in patients on this class of drugs.[14] Both Etminan et al and Erie et al pointed out that they could not rule out smoking or secondhand smoke as a contributing factor.[13,14] SSRIs probably have a weak mydriatic effect. This may be unilateral, as Barrett reported, and we confirmed this with several additional spontaneous reports.[15]

There are 3 cases of bilateral maculopathy after sertraline ingestion.[16-18] Times to onset were 2 weeks, 4 months, and 1 year. Macular appearances were similar, and after stopping the medication, little visual improvement occurred. Spontaneous reports of macular problems were primarily only with sertraline. This commonly prescribed drug has been on the market for nearly 3 decades, and with only a few cases reported without a typical fundus pattern, this association is suspect.

Optic neuropathy has been reported in the literature and in spontaneous reports; causation is difficult to prove.[19]

Generic Names:
1. Isocarboxazid; 2. phenelzine sulfate; 3. tranylcypromine sulfate.

Proprietary Names:
1. Marplan; 2. Nardil; 3. Parnate.

Primary Use
These monoamine oxidase inhibitors are used in the symptomatic relief of reactive or endogenous depression.

Ocular Side Effects
Systemic administration – oral
Certain
1. Decreased vision
2. Visual hallucinations (phenelzine)

Possible
1. Mydriasis – weak (primarily overdose)
2. Extraocular muscles
   a. Diplopia
   b. Nystagmus (phenelzine, tranylcypromine)
   c. Strabismus
3. Myasthenia gravis
   a. Diplopia
   b. Ptosis
   c. Paresis of extraocular muscles
4. Photophobia
5. Color vision defect – red-green defect
6. Visual field defects (tranylcypromine)

Clinical Significance
Ocular side effects due to these monoamine oxidase inhibitors are reversible and usually insignificant. All

of these drugs may cause decreased vision, which only rarely requires stopping of the drug. Pupillary reactions occur primarily in overdose situations. Nystagmus has been associated with phenelzine or tranylcypromine, and visual hallucinations have been associated with phenelzine therapy.

Generic Name:
Maprotiline hydrochloride.

Proprietary Name:
Ludiomil.

Primary Use
This tetracyclic antidepressant is used in the treatment of depression.

Ocular Side Effects
Systemic administration – oral
Certain
1. Decreased vision

Probable
1. Mydriasis – may precipitate acute glaucoma
2. May aggravate or cause ocular sicca
3. Decreased accommodation
4. Decreased contact lens tolerance
5. Visual hallucinations

Possible
1. Photosensitivity

Conditional/unclassified
1. Palinopsia
2. Illusory visual spread

Clinical Significance
Adverse ocular reactions due to this tetracyclic antidepressant are seldom of major clinical significance. Anticholinergic effects are the most frequent and include decreased vision (which may require decreasing the dosage), disturbance of accommodation, and mydriasis. Decreased vision occurs early and at an incidence rate of 4%.[1] Decreased vision may interfere with fusion, thereby causing diplopia. This may regress even on the same dosage.

The package insert for this drug recommends caution in patients with narrow chambers, as mydriasis may cause acute glaucoma.[1] It also warns of contact lens intolerance due to potential ocular sicca.[1]

Kadoi et al reported bilateral angle-closure glaucoma with no light perception in both eyes in a 71-year-old

female.[2] Her depression was treated with maprotiline, clotiazepam, and alprazolam. Visual hallucinations are usually associated with drug overdosage. Myoclonus can be seen in other muscles, so one can expect to see this in periocular muscles as well. Terao et al reported a case of visual perseveration on maprotiline; however, the patient was also on levomepromazine, which may increase the plasma levels of maprotiline.[3]

Generic Name:
Methylphenidate hydrochloride.

Proprietary Names:
Aptensio XR, Concerta, Cotempla XR, Daytrana, Metadate CD, Metadate ER, Methylin, Methylin ER, QuilliChew ER, Quillivant, Quillivant XR, Relexxii, Ritalin, Ritalin LA, Ritalin SR.

Primary Use
This piperidine derivative is used in the treatment of mild depression and in the management of children with hyperkinetic syndrome.

Ocular Side Effects
Systemic administration – oral
Certain
1. Decreased vision

Probable
1. Mydriasis – weak
2. Oculogyric crisis
3. Visual hallucinations

Possible
1. Posterior subcapsular cataract
2. Extraocular muscle disorders
3. Accommodation – abnormal

Systemic administration – intravenous
Certain
1. Talc retinopathy (Fig. 5.4)
   a. Small yellow-white emboli
   b. Neovascularization – late
   c. Retinal hemorrhages
2. Decreased vision
3. Tractional retinal detachment

Clinical Significance
Ocular side effects due to methylphenidate are rare, reversible, and seldom clinically significant except for possible lens changes. Duman et al, in a case-controlled series, found 5 posterior subcapsular cataracts with

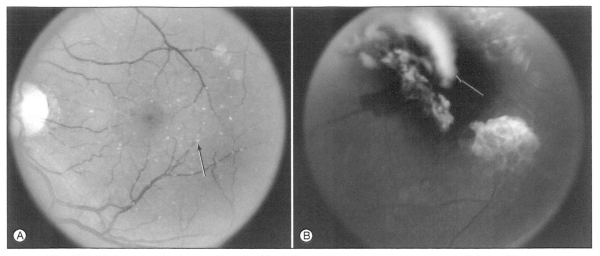

FIG. 5.4 **(A)** A red-free fundus photograph of the left eye shows numerous intravascular talc particles in the macula (*arrow*). **(B)** Fluorescein angiography of the left eye demonstrates leakage of dye from peripheral retinal neovascularization in the superotemporal periphery (*arrow*).[7]

clear nuclei in patients 6–17 years old taking methylphenidate for attention deficit hyperactivity disorder.[1] All 5 patients were taking the drug for over 1 year. Bartlik et al also reported a case that had the same lens changes and some evidence of increased density with increased length of exposure.[2] This "possible" side effect may even be "probable" because the cataracts seem to all be posterior subcapsular.

The methylphenidate package insert points out that some commercial products containing this drug are contraindicated in glaucoma patients.[3] However, as pointed out by Dunman et al, this drug only has a weak anticholinergic effect and seldom causes acute glaucoma.[1] In the spontaneous reports there are only 3 possible cases of acute glaucoma and 31 cases of elevated intraocular pressure. There are a few cases, however, in the literature including glaucoma and cataracts.[2-5]

There are 156 cases of diplopia or eye movement disorders, 35 cases of abnormal accommodation, 78 cases of mydriasis, and 27 cases of oculogyric crisis in the spontaneous reports. Although extraocular muscle abnormalities and diplopia have been reported, this possible side effect is hard to evaluate because these findings are increased in patients for whom this drug is prescribed.

Methylphenidate tablets intended for oral use have been used by drug addicts, who crush the tablets and inject the drug intravenously. The filler in the tablet is insoluble talc, cornstarch, or various binders and lodges in the retina and other tissues as emboli.[6] These glistening refractile particles in the retina, which are fairly stationary, may cause visual symptoms, and neovascularization may form in time.

Recommendations
1. Children on the drug for over 2 years should be examined for lens changes.
2. Intraocular pressure should be taken at the same time as the lens examination.

Generic Name:
Trazodone hydrochloride.

Proprietary Names:
Desyrel, Oleptro, Oleptro E-R.

Primary Use
This triazolopyridine derivative is used in the treatment of depression.

Ocular Side Effects
Systemic administration – oral
Certain
1. Decreased vision
2. Visual image
   a. Objects have sheen, metallic ghost images, bright shiny lights
   b. Palinopsia
3. Mydriasis – weak

Possible
1. Irritation
2. May aggravate or cause ocular sicca
3. Aggravation of acute glaucoma
4. Eyelids or conjunctiva
   a. Allergic reactions
   b. Erythema
   c. Blepharoconjunctivitis
   d. Photosensitivity
5. Diplopia

Conditional/unclassified
1. Increased blink rate

Clinical Significance

Ocular side effects due to trazodone occur only occasionally and are reversible with decreased dosage or discontinued drug use. Palinopsia has been well documented by Hughes et al.[1] Occasionally, patients will complain of a sheen on objects, metallic ghost images, bright shiny lights, or strobe light–type effects. Copper et al reported a case of trazodone causing an increased blink rate.[2] Trazodone possibly aggravated angle-closure glaucoma, as reported by Pae et al.[3] The *Physicians' Desk Reference* (PDR) cautions the use of this drug in closed-angle glaucoma due to its weak mydriatic effect.[4] It is well documented that this drug can xerostomia; therefore it may also aggravate or cause ocular sicca. The incidence of ocular sicca is 0–1.0%.[4] Spontaneous case reports include changes in refraction and transient problems with accommodation.

CLASS: ANTI–MULTIPLE SCLEROSIS DRUGS

Generic Name:
Fingolimod.

Proprietary Name:
Gilenya.

Primary Use
Sphingosine 1-phosphage receptor inhibitor used to reduce the frequency of multiple sclerosis exacerbations.

Ocular Side Effects
Systemic administration – oral
Certain
1. Decreased vision
2. Metamorphopsia

3. Macula
   a. Edema
   b. Color changes in appearance
   c. Leakage – fluorescein angiography
4. Intraretinal cysts
5. Retinal elevation

Probable
1. Retinal hemorrhages

Possible
1. Branch retinal vein occlusion

Conditional/unclassified
1. May increase aqueous flow
2. Conjunctival lymphoma

Clinical Significance

Fingolimod is the first FDA–approved oral drug for the management of relapsing forms of multiple sclerosis. Fingolimod-associated macular edema (FAME) has been well documented with positive dechallenge and rechallenge data.[1] The incidence is variable and dependent on the dosage. In pooled data, at 0.5 mg, the incidence is 0.3% and at 1.25 mg, the incidence is 1.2%.[1] These incidences increase significantly in patients with uveitis and diabetes. The macular edema developed within the first 3–4 months. Late cases may occur even after a year of therapy.[1] Presentation may be asymptomatic to metamorphopsia, decreased vision, and central vision loss. In FAME, 25% of the time the macular edema is bilateral. Compared with some other drug-related macular edema, with this drug there appears to be intramacular leakage on fluorescein angiography. Jain et al confirmed intraretinal cysts characteristic of cystoid macular edema in FAME patients.[2] Minuk et al and Afshar et al have reported cystoid macular edema.[3,4] Khimani et al reported a case, possibly due to this drug, in which the retinal fluid was subretinal with a central serous appearance and an absence of cystic intraretinal changes.[5] The case had both positive dechallenge and rechallenge. There are over 1000 suspected cases of FAME in the spontaneous reports and literature. The edema usually resolved after stopping the drug.

There are multiple cases in the literature and spontaneous reports of possible exacerbation of ocular herpes simplex and zoster with fingolimod exposure.[6] A few cases of possible secondary drug-induced retinal hemorrhages or retinal vascular occlusion have been reported.[7–10] Christopher et al reported a possible conjunctival lymphoma secondary to this drug.[11]

Recommendations[2]

1. Baseline ophthalmic examination, including dilated fundus examination. Consider macular contact lens to evaluate macular thickening. Consider baseline optical coherence tomography (OCT) in patients with uveitis, diabetic retinopathy, recent cataract surgery, or optic nerve pallor. Consider fluorescein angiography in patients with diabetic retinopathy or suspect macular edema.
2. Teach patients Amsler grid testing for home use.
3. Repeat ophthalmic examination at 3–4 months. With any macular abnormality, decreased best corrected visual acuity, visual symptoms, or abnormal Amsler grid, consider ordering OCT and/or fluorescein angiography.
4. Follow-up examinations at 6 months, then annually, but sooner if any visual changes. More frequent examinations should probably be done in patients with diabetes or a history of uveitis.
5. Advise patients to avoid starting fingolimod within 3 months of an intraocular surgery or preexisting macular edema.
6. Sergotti suggested that in some patients, varicella zoster antibody titers may be obtained and vaccinations given if levels are low or absent.[12]

CLASS: ANTIPSYCHOTIC DRUGS

Generic Name:
Amisulpride.

Proprietary Names:
Amazeo, Amipride, Amival, Solian, Soltus, Sulpitac, Sulprix, Socian.

Primary Use
Antipsychotic used to treat schizophrenia.

Ocular Side Effects
Systemic administration – oral
Probable
1. Decreased vision
2. Accommodative spasms
3. Oculogyric crisis

Possible
1. Eyelid blinking movements

Clinical Significance
All side effects are transitory and often do not occur with reduction in dosage.[1] Oculogyric crisis has been reported in the literature, and there are over 35 cases in the spontaneous reports.[2] Lin et al reported involuntary, frequent eye blinking movements.[3] This resolved with reduction in dosage of amisulpride. Barrett et al reported various eye muscle effects due to this drug in a placebo-controlled trial.[4]

Generic Name:
Aripiprazole.

Proprietary Names:
Abilify, Abilify Discmelt, Abilify Maintena, Aristada.

Primary Use
Aripiprazole is a partial dopamine agonist of a second generation of antipsychotics. The drug has antidepressant properties and is used to treat schizophrenia, bipolar disorder, and clinical depression.

Ocular Side Effects
Systemic administration – intramuscular or oral
Certain
1. Decreased vision

Probable
1. Oculogyric crisis

Possible
1. Myopia
2. Photophobia
3. Mydriasis
4. Diplopia
5. Blepharospasm

Conditional/unclassified
1. Chorioretinopathy

Clinical Significance
Although decreased vision may occur early after taking aripiprazole, with an incidence of 3–8%, it is rarely a reason to discontinue the drug.[1] There are almost 200 cases of oculogyric crisis in the spontaneous reports and literature.[2-4] On average, this side effect occurs after about 8 months of therapy. This side effect may be associated with blepharospasm and/or myopia. Myopia has been reported in 13 spontaneous reports and in the literature.[5-10] Other possible side effects are rare, primarily occur after 5 months, and are unproved. Matsuo et al felt that this drug may be a weak cause of intraoperative floppy iris syndrome.[11] This drug may be a weak mydriatic and may cause acute glaucoma. Shen et al reported a single case, and there are 7 unproven

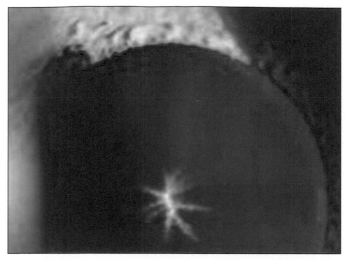

FIG. 5.5 Anterior lens stellate cataracts related to chlorpromazine.[15]

cases in the spontaneous reports.[12] Faure et al reported a case of chorioretinopathy, and there are 4 unproven cases in the spontaneous reports.[13]

Generic Names:

1. Chlorpromazine hydrochloride; 2. fluphenazine hydrochloride; 3. perphenazine; 4. prochlorperazine; 5. promethazine hydrochloride; 6. thiethylperazine; 7. thioridazine hydrochloride.

Proprietary Names:

1. Thorazine, Sonazine; 2. Prolixin, Prolixin Decanoate; 3. Trilafon; 4. Compazine, Compro; 5. Anergan-50, Pentazine, Phenadoz, Phenergan, Prometh, Promethegan; 6. Torecan; 7. Mellaril.

Primary Use

These phenothiazines are used in the treatment of depressive, involutional, senile, or organic psychoses and various forms of schizophrenia. Some of the phenothiazines are also used as adjuncts to anesthesia, as antiemetics, and in the treatment of tetanus.

Ocular Side Effects

Systemic administration – intramuscular, intravenous, oral, or rectal suppository

Not all of the ocular side effects listed have been reported for each phenothiazine.

Certain

1. Decreased vision
2. Decrease or paralysis of accommodation
3. Night blindness
4. Color vision defect
   a. Red-green defect
   b. Objects have yellow or brown tinge
   c. Colored haloes around lights
5. Cornea
   a. Pigmentary deposits – epithelium, deep stroma, and endothelium
   b. Punctate keratitis
6. Pupils – variable, dependent on which drug
   a. Mydriasis
   b. Miosis
   c. Decreased reaction to light
7. Oculogyric crises
8. Lens (worse with chlorpromazine; seen with most others if long-term)
   a. Subcapsular dust-like granular deposits – whitish to yellowish brown in pupillary area (early)
   b. Stellate anterior cortical changes (late) (Fig. 5.5)
9. Visual hallucinations
10. Nystagmus
11. Jerky pursuit movements
12. Photophobia
13. Eyelids or conjunctiva
    a. Allergic reactions
    b. Edema
    c. Hyperpigmentation
    d. Photosensitivity
    e. Blepharospasm
14. Abnormal electroretinogram (ERG) or electrooculogram (EOG)

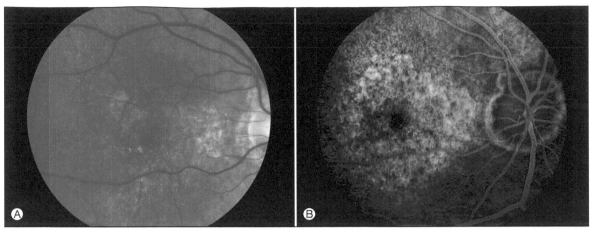

FIG. 5.6 **(A)** Retinal pigment epithelial atrophy from systemic thioridazine. **(B)** Fluorescein angiogram of widespread bull's-eye changes from systemic thioridazine.[15]

Probable

1. Retina (rare – long-term therapy) (Fig. 5.6)
   a. Pigmentary changes
   b. Edema
2. Visual fields
   a. Scotomas – annular, central, or paracentral
   b. Constriction
3. May aggravate or cause ocular sicca
4. Horner's syndrome
5. Toxic amblyopia
6. Myasthenia gravis
   a. Diplopia
   b. Ptosis
   c. Paresis of extraocular muscles
7. Ocular teratogenic effects

Possible

1. Optic atrophy
2. Papilledema
3. Myopia

Conditional/unclassified

1. Intraoperative floppy iris syndrome (IFIS) – weak

Retrobulbar injections – chlorpromazine
Probable

1. Acute periorbital inflammation
   a. Chemosis
   b. Blepharoptosis
   c. Edema may involve the face and neck
2. Neurotrophic corneal ulcers
3. Chronic orbital inflammation with fibrosis

Clinical Significance

As a class, phenothiazines are some of the most widely used drugs in the practice of medicine. The most commonly prescribed drug in this group is chlorpromazine. This medication has been so thoroughly investigated that over 10,000 publications have been written on this drug alone. Even so, these drugs are remarkably safe. Their overall rate of side effects is estimated at only 3%. However, if patients are on phenothiazine therapy for a number of years, a 30% rate of ocular side effects has been reported. If therapy continues over 10 years, the rate of ocular side effects increases to nearly 100%. Side effects are dose and drug dependent, with the most significant side effects reported with chlorpromazine because this drug is the most often prescribed. These drugs in very high dosages can cause significant ocular adverse effects within a few days, whereas the same reactions usually would take many years to develop in the normal dosage range. Each phenothiazine has the potential to cause ocular side effects, although it is not likely to cause all of those mentioned. Pinpointing the toxic effects to a specific phenothiazine is difficult because most of these patients are taking more than 1 drug. The most common adverse ocular effect with this group of drugs is decreased vision, probably due to anticholinergic interference. In chronic therapy, chlorpromazine, can cause pigmentary deposits in or on the eye, with multiple reports claiming that other phenothiazines can cause this as well. These deposits are first seen on the lens surface in the pupillary aperture, later near Descemet's membrane or corneal endothelium, and only in rare cases in the corneal epithelium. Pigmentary changes in the cornea seem to be reversible, but lens deposits may be permanent. Lens deposits are described as not interfering with vision (pseudocataracts). A report by Isaac et al clearly showed an increased incidence of cataract surgery in patients taking these drugs,[1] and an anterior capsular opacity seems characteristic in long-term therapy.[2-5] Matsuo et al reported that an incomplete IFIS may rarely occur.[6]

Retinopathy, optic nerve disease, and blindness are exceedingly rare at the recommended dosage levels, and then they are almost exclusively found in patients on long-term therapy. A phototoxic process has been postulated to be involved in both the increased ocular pigmentary deposits and the retinal degeneration. These groups of drugs with piperidine side chains (thioridazine has been removed from the market) have a greater incidence of causing retinal problems than the phenothiazine derivatives with aliphatic side chains (chlorpromazine), which has had relatively little retinal toxicity reported. Power et al reported a patient taking fluphenazine for 10 years who developed bilateral maculopathy after 2 minutes of unprotected welding arc exposure.[7] Lee et al described bilateral maculopathy after 10 years of exposure to fluphenazine without increased light exposure.[8] The phenothiazines combine with ocular and dermal pigment and are only slowly released. This slow release has, in part, been given as the reason for the progression of adverse ocular reactions even after use of the drug is discontinued.

Retrobulbar injections of chlorpromazine with or without alcohol have been used to control ocular pain. Most reports are various degrees of inflammation and edema, some requiring temporary tarsorrhaphy to a case involving forehead, cheek, and ipsilateral eyelids.[9] Cotliar et al reported a case of secondary diffuse orbital fibrosis probably due to retrobulbar chlorpromazine.[10] Hauck et al reported a case of neurotrophic corneal ulcer felt to be due to chlorpromazine causing neurosensory denervation of the cornea.[11] Kuruvilla et al described systemic chlorpromazine side effects with retrobulbar injection.[12]

Recommendations

1. Photo-induced skin eruptions are well known, especially with chlorpromazine. Pigmentation-induced photosensitivity can be blocked in part by sunglasses that block out ultraviolet radiation up to 400 nm.
2. This is also true for possible lens-induced changes.
3. Avoid bright light when possible.
4. Functional visual disturbances are primarily metabolic and therefore if detected early should be reversible.[13]

5. Contact lens use while on promethazine may precipitate acute glaucoma.[14]

Generic Names:
1. Clozapine; 2. loxapine, 3. olanzapine.

Proprietary Names:
1. Clozaril, FazaClo, Versacloz; 2. Adasuve, Loxitane; 3. Zyprexa, Zyprexa Intramuscular, Zyprexa Relprevv, Zyprexa Zydis.

Primary Use
These antipsychotic drugs are used in the treatment of schizophrenia and various mental conditions.

Ocular Side Effects
Systemic administration – oral
Certain
1. Decreased vision
2. Oculogyric crisis
3. Photosensitivity

Probable
1. Decreased accommodation
2. Mydriasis – may precipitate acute glaucoma
3. May aggravate or cause ocular sicca (clozapine)

Possible
1. Visual hallucinations
2. Eyelids or conjunctiva
   a. Edema
   b. Chemosis
   c. Ptosis
   d. Blepharospasm
3. Intraoperative floppy iris syndrome (IFIS)

Conditional/unclassified
1. Pigmentation – conjunctival, lens, retinal
2. Nystagmus (clozapine)
3. Cataract (clozapine)

Clinical Significance
Most all ocular side effects are uncommon and fully reversible. The most common are anticholinergic effects of decreased vision and decreased accommodation. These occur early and may clear without changes in medication. Clozapine may cause the highest incidence of decreased vision at 5%.[1] Oculogyric crisis has been seen with all 3 drugs; Gardner et al estimate an incidence of about 1.8%.[2] This may occur after the first dose, but usually within the first few months.[3] There is a delayed form that may occur after

many years of therapy. This appears to be more common if the patient is on multiple other antipsychotic medications.

Mydriasis occurs rarely and has been implicated in causing narrow-angle glaucoma.[4] Miosis has also been observed and is in numerous spontaneous reports with all 3 drugs.[1,5,6]

Ceylan et al reported clozapine may induce a dry eye syndrome with morphologic alterations in the cornea secondary to its anticholinergic and antidopaminergic actions.[7] Balibey et al reported ocular sicca after long-term olanzapine use.[8]

Matsuo et al reported this class of drugs possibly causes a mild form of IFIS.[9]

There have been rare reports of conjunctival, iris, or retinal pigmentary changes attributed to these drugs. This is difficult to evaluate because some patients may have been on chlorpromazine prior to this. Choy et al, however, describe an unusual bilateral pigment dispersion in full-thickness cornea and the anterior lens surface with a decrease in vision.[10]

Alam et al reported a single case of possible cataract formation in a 28-year-old patient associated with clozapine that required surgery.[11]

Generic Names:
1. Droperidol; 2. haloperidol.

Proprietary Names:
1. Inapsine; 2. Haldol, Haldol Decanoate.

Primary Use
These butyrophenone derivatives are used in the management of acute and chronic schizophrenia and manic depressive, involutional, senile, organic, and toxic psychoses. Droperidol is also used as an adjunct to anesthesia and as an antiemetic.

Ocular Side Effects
Systemic administration – intramuscular, intravenous, or oral
Certain
1. Decreased vision
2. Oculogyric crises
3. Visual hallucinations

Probable
1. Acute glaucoma
2. Decrease or paralysis of accommodation (weak)
3. Pupils (weak)
   a. Mydriasis (haloperidol)
   b. Miosis (rare)

Possible
1. Eyelids or conjunctiva
   a. Allergic reactions
   b. Photosensitivity
   c. Edema
   d. Blepharospasm
2. Decreased intraocular pressure (weak)
3. Cataracts
4. Myopia (haloperidol)
5. Corneal decompensation (haloperidol with multiple drugs)
6. Intraoperative floppy iris syndrome (IFIS) – incomplete
7. Nystagmus

Clinical Significance
Most ocular side effects due to these drugs are transient, reversible, and quite rare. Although, on occasion, significant bilateral pupillary dilation occurs due to haloperidol, seldom does this cause acute glaucoma. This is more likely if that patient is on other concomitant anticholinergic drugs.[1] Myopia is rarely associated with the use of haloperidol. This is possibly secondary to drug-induced hyponatremia.[2] There is a report by Nishida et al that patients on multiple tranquilizing drugs, including haloperidol, may experience damage to the endothelium and give a clinical picture of bilateral bullous keratopathy.[3] Stopping the drugs allows for the corneas to return to normal. The decreased intraocular pressure due to these drugs is not a sufficient amount to be of clinical value. Uchida et al reported a case with positive rechallenge of haloperidol causing the visual outlines of small objects or patterns to appear increasingly vivid, with the effects lasting for 1 hour after taking the drug.[4] Isaac et al reported a 3.5 times increased risk of cataract extraction in patients on haloperidol, either currently taking the drug or exposed to the drug 2–5 years before extraction. This study included controlling other suspected risk factors.[5] Honda suggested that these drugs have been associated with the onset of subcapsular cataracts after long-term therapy.[6] Long-term therapy seems reasonable as to cataractogenesis. Cataract extraction incidences without more data on the length of treatment make data on cataractogenesis "possible." These appear as subepithelial changes near the equator. Histologically, they appear as large, round balloon cells without proliferation of lens epithelium. Nystagmus is listed in the *Physicians' Desk Reference* (PDR), but the incidence is unknown.[1]

Matsuo et al described a patient on long-term haloperidol and another on haloperidol plus other antipsychotic drugs who developed incomplete IFIS.[7]

Generic Name:
Lithium carbonate.

Proprietary Names:
Eskalith, Eskalith CR, Lithobid.

Primary Use
This lithium salt is used in the management of the manic phase of manic-depressive psychosis.

Ocular Side Effects
Systemic administration – oral
Certain
1. Decreased vision
2. Nystagmus
   a. Horizontal
   b. Vertical
   c. Downbeat
3. Extraocular muscles
   a. Oculogyric crises
   b. Decreased spontaneous movements
   c. Lateral conjugate deviations
   d. Jerky pursuit movements
   e. Oscillopsia
4. Eyelids or conjunctiva
   a. Conjunctivitis – nonspecific
   b. Edema
5. Irritation
   a. Lacrimation
   b. Photophobia
   c. Burning sensation
   d. Decreased lacrimation
6. Decreased accommodation
7. Visual hallucinations
8. Pseudotumor cerebri
   a. Papilledema
   b. Visual field defect
9. Abnormal electrooculogram (EOG) or visual evoked potential (VEP)

Probable
1. Myasthenia gravis – aggravated
   a. Diplopia
   b. Ptosis
   c. Paresis of extraocular muscles
2. May aggravate or cause ocular sicca

Possible
1. Cornea and conjunctiva – fine lithium deposits
2. Exophthalmos – thyroid eye disease
3. Loss of eyelashes or eyebrows
4. Decreased dark adaptation

Clinical Significance
Lithium salts have been widely used for decades, and lithium intoxication is common because therapeutic blood levels have a narrow range before toxicity occurs. Lithium therapy is mainly prophylactic, with therapy lasting years to decades. The review article by Fraunfelder et al is probably the definitive work on the effects of lithium on the visual system.[1]

Lithium affects many areas of the visual system, including direct effects on the central nervous system and on endocrine glands, leading to ocular effects. In general, the ocular side effects of lithium are reversible on withdrawal of the drug or lowering of the dosage. However, other side effects, such as downbeat nystagmus, can be permanent. Decreased vision is probably the most common side effect experienced by patients taking lithium, but is seldom significant enough to require the cessation of therapy. Usually with time, even while keeping the same dosage, decreased vision will disappear. Decreased vision, however, can be a signal of pending problems, such as pseudotumor cerebri. In most cases, patients who develop pseudotumor cerebri have been taking lithium for many years.

Lithium can cause various forms of nystagmus, the most characteristic being downbeat. This can occur at therapeutic dosage ranges of lithium and may be the only adverse drug effect. Although some patients have a full recovery after stopping or reducing the dosage of lithium, it may develop into irreversible downbeat nystagmus. If downbeat nystagmus occurs, one needs to reevaluate the risk–benefit ratio of lithium therapy. Lithium can also cause extraocular muscle abnormalities, especially vertical or lateral far-gaze diplopia. In therapeutic dosages, Gooding et al have shown no effect of lithium on smooth pursuit eye tracking performance.[2] Diplopia in any patient taking lithium may require a workup for myasthenia gravis, especially if associated with ptosis. Ptosis can occur alone. Oculogyric crises have been reported primarily in patients also taking haloperidol.

Thyroid-related eye disease in various forms secondary to hypothyroidism or hyperthyroidism has been seen in patients receiving lithium therapy. Although this is uncommon, exophthalmos has occurred. Lithium is secreted in the tears and may cause an irritative forum of conjunctivitis, causing epiphora. However, with time many patients complain of xerostomia at about the same time as ocular sicca. Lithium has been reported to cause corneal and conjunctival deposits, but the documentation for this is limited. Lithium can cause a decrease in accommodation, which may occur in up to 10% of patients. However, this primarily occurs in young patients and is rare in older patients. In general, this side effect is minimal and usually resolves after a few months, even while taking the drug. Etminan et al, in a case-control study, showed that lithium use in the elderly increased the risk of injurious motor vehicle accidents.[3]

Generic Name:
Pimozide.

Proprietary Name:
Orap.

Primary Use
This diphenylbutylpiperidine derivative is used for suppression of motor and vocal tics of Tourette syndrome.

Ocular Side Effects
Systemic administration – oral
Certain
1. Decreased vision
2. Decreased accommodation
3. Visual hallucinations
4. Oculogyric crisis

Possible
1. Eyelids
   a. Erythema
   b. Edema
2. May aggravate or cause ocular sicca
3. Photophobia

Clinical Significance
Up to 20% of patients on this drug have some form of visual disturbance shortly after starting pimozide.[1] Between 2.7% and 4% of these visual side effects have been rated as severe.[1] These side effects are mainly decreased vision and decreased accommodation. Most all ocular side effects are reversible. This drug has a 5% incidence of xerostomia and therefore can probably aggravate ocular sicca.[1] A 1% incidence of photophobia has also been reported.[1]

Generic Name:
Quetiapine fumarate.

Proprietary Names:
Seroquel, Seroquel XR.

Primary Use
This drug belongs to a chemical class of dibenzothiazephine derivatives used in the management of bipolar mania or in schizophrenia.

Ocular Side Effects
Systemic administration – oral
Certain
1. Decreased vision

Probable
1. Intraoperative floppy iris syndrome (IFIS)
2. May aggravate or cause ocular sicca – weak
3. Myasthenia gravis – aggravated
   a. Diplopia
   b. Ptosis
   c. Paresis of extraocular muscles
4. Visual hallucinations
5. Oculogyric crisis

Possible
1. Cataracts
2. Acute glaucoma
3. Frequent blinking
4. Extraocular muscles – rapid-eye-movement sleep behavior disorders
5. Photopsia (high dose)

Clinical Significance
Ocular side effects attributed to quetiapine are rare, transitory, and infrequent. Ocular sicca is "probable" because xerostomia is one of the most frequent systemic side effects of this drug, with an incidence of 7–44%.[1] Because this drug has caused lens changes in dogs and is an inhibitor of cholesterol biosynthesis, there has been interest as to the cataractogenic potential of this drug. Valibhai et al have reported a clinically suspect case.[2] Large postmarketing surveillance studies have not found a higher incidence of cataracts. The lack of a characteristic pattern led to the conclusion, at worse, that the drug has a very weak cataractogenic potential. However, there are 356 cases in the spontaneous reports of lens changes associated with quetiapine use.

There are a few reports in the literature and spontaneous reports of rapid blinking and rapid-eye-movement sleep behavior disorder.[3,4] Rocke et al reported that this drug, as with other psychotropics, may cause acute glaucoma.[5] Eight similar cases were found in the spontaneous reports. IFIS was confirmed in a prospective study, as well as in a clinical report.[6,7] Hazra et al reported photopsias after high-dose quetiapine.[8] Ghosh et al reported a case of oculogyric crisis.[9] There are an additional 81 cases in the spontaneous reports. Yong et al reported a case of retinal vein occlusion, and there are 11 cases of vein occlusions in the spontaneous reports.[10]

Recommendations

The manufacturer recommends that any patient receiving chronic treatment be examined at the initiation of treatment and then twice yearly for lens changes. Fraunfelder recommended only having patients examined as per the guidelines established by the American Academy of Ophthalmology, regardless of whether or not the patient is on quetiapine.[11] In a letter to the editor, Gaynes preferred more frequent examinations, but in reply, Fraunfelder did not concur.[12,13]

Generic Name:

Risperidone.

Proprietary Names:

Risperdal, Risperdal Consta, Risperdal M-Tab.

Primary Use

Serotonin–dopamine antagonist used in the management of schizophrenia, bipolar disorders, dementia-related psychosis, and autistic disorders.

Ocular Side Effects

Systemic administration – intramuscular or oral
Certain
1. Decreased vision

Probable
1. Photophobia
2. Edema
   a. Eyelid
   b. Periorbital
3. Ocular erythema
4. Intraoperative floppy iris syndrome (IFIS)
5. Cataracts
6. Oculogyric crisis

Possible
1. Blepharospasm
2. May aggravate or cause ocular sicca

Clinical Significance

This drug has been available for over 25 years. The World Health Organization has it on a list of essential medicines due to its safety and effectiveness. Ocular side effects are rare and seldom require stopping the drug. Early in the start of treatment decreased vision, photophobia, ocular erythema, and lid edema may occur (1–7%).[1] These typically regress with time. Gardner et al projected the incidence of these second-generation antipsychotic drugs causing oculogyric crisis at 1.8%.[2] There are cases of oculogyric crisis that persist unless the medication is stopped.[3] Numerous reports in the literature have also suggested other reversible extraocular muscle abnormalities causing diplopia.

Ford et al was one of the first to report the risk of IFIS during cataract surgery.[4] This was followed by Health Canada and the pharmaceutical manufacturer sending out a health advisory warning physicians of this "possible" or "probable" side effect.[5]

The issue of this drug causing cataracts is complex because schizophrenic patients already have an increased risk of developing cataracts. However, with increased dose and duration of this drug, it still appears to be a weak cataractogenic drug, especially in women.[6-9]

Generic Name:

Thiothixene.

Proprietary Name:

Navane.

Primary Use

This thioxanthene derivative is used in the management of schizophrenia.

Ocular Side Effects

Systemic administration – oral
Certain
1. Decreased vision
2. Oculogyric crises
3. Mydriasis
4. Cornea
   a. Fine particulate deposits
   b. Keratitis
5. Lens
   a. Fine particulate deposits
   b. Stellate cataracts

Probable
1. Decrease or paralysis of accommodation
2. Eyelids or conjunctiva
   a. Allergic reactions
   b. Photosensitivity
   c. Edema
   d. Urticaria
3. May aggravate or cause ocular sicca
4. Acute glaucoma

Possible
1. Retinal pigmentary changes

Clinical Significance

In short-term therapy, ocular side effects due to this drug are reversible and usually insignificant. This drug has anticholinergic effects, and if on a concomitant antiparkinsonian drug, can worsen or cause acute glaucoma; therefore it should be used with caution in patients with narrow chamber angles.[1] This may also account for the occasional patient who gets decreased vision and mydriasis. The incidence of xerostomia is 10%, so ocular sicca may also be aggravated or occur.[1] In long-term therapy, cases of corneal or lens deposits or lens pigmentation have been reported. Retinal pigmentary changes are exceedingly rare and only occur with long-term therapy. This is also a strong photosensitizing drug.

CLASS: DEPRESSANTS

Generic Name:
Alcohol (ethanol, ethyl alcohol).

Proprietary Name:
Generic only.

Primary Use

This colorless liquid is used as a solvent, an antiseptic, a beverage, and as a nerve block in the management of certain types of intractable pain.

Ocular Side Effects
Systemic administration – acute intoxication
Certain
1. Extraocular muscles
   a. Phorias
   b. Diplopia
   c. Nystagmus – various types, including downbeat nystagmus
   d. Convergent strabismus
   e. Decreased convergence
   f. Jerky pursuit movements
   g. Decreased spontaneous movements
2. Pupils
   a. Mydriasis
   b. Decreased reaction to light
   c. Anisocoria
3. Tear film
   a. Alcohol secreted in the tears
   b. Increased osmolarity
   c. Shortened tear film break-up time
   d. Ocular surface disease
4. Decreased vision
5. Decreased accommodation
6. Color vision defect
   a. Blue-yellow or red-green defect
   b. Objects have blue tinge
7. Decreased dark adaptation
8. Decreased intraocular pressure – transitory
9. Constriction of visual fields
10. Decreased depth perception
11. Decreased optokinetic and peripheral gaze nystagmus
12. Visual hallucinations
13. Prolonged glare recovery
14. Ptosis (unilateral or bilateral)
15. Impaired oculomotor coordination
16. Toxic amblyopia
17. Abnormal electroretinogram (ERG), visual evoked potential (VEP) or critical flicker fusion
18. Choroidal thickness – increased

Systemic administration – chronic intoxication
Certain
1. Extraocular muscles
   a. Paralysis
   b. Jerky pursuit movements
2. Downbeat nystagmus
3. Decreased accommodation
4. Pupils
   a. Miosis
   b. Decreased or absent reaction to light
5. Decreased vision
6. Visual fields
   a. Papillomacular scotomas
   b. Abnormal static perimetry
   c. Abnormal kinetic perimetry
7. Color vision defect – red-green defect
8. Oscillopsia
9. Lacrimation
10. Decreased intraocular pressure – transitory
11. Visual hallucinations

Possible
1. Optic nerve
   a. Neuritis
   b. Temporal pallor
2. Corneal deposits (arcus senilis)
3. Toxic amblyopia
4. Cataracts
5. Macular degeneration – early onset
6. May aggravate or cause ocular sicca

Ocular teratogenic effects (fetal alcohol syndrome)
Certain
1. Retinal blood vessels – increased tortuosity

2. Decreased vision
3. Optic nerve – hypoplasia
4. Palpebral fissure – horizontal shortening
5. Ptosis
6. Strabismus (convergent or divergent)
7. Abnormalities of anterior chamber angles
8. Secondary glaucoma
9. Duane retraction syndrome
10. Cornea
    a. Decreased polymegathism
    b. Decreased hexagonality

Local ophthalmic use or exposure – retrobulbar injection

Certain
1. Irritation
   a. Hyperemia
   b. Pain (acute)
   c. Edema
2. Keratitis
3. Paresis of extraocular muscles
4. Nystagmus
5. Ptosis
6. Corneal ulceration
7. Decreased vision
8. Eyelids – depigmentation
9. Ocular anesthesia

Inadvertent ocular exposure

Certain
1. Irritation
   a. Lacrimation
   b. Hyperemia
   c. Pain
   d. Edema
   e. Burning sensation
2. Keratitis
3. Corneal necrosis or opacities (prolonged exposure)

Clinical Significance

Consumption of alcoholic beverages leads to a host of well-known ocular side effects. Acute intoxication may result in nystagmus, a finding used by law enforcement personnel to screen for inebriated motor-vehicle operators. Pupil abnormalities, ptosis, and strabismus are also well-known effects of inebriation. Also reported are temporary corneal clouding and a methanol-like loss of vision associated with alcohol-induced metabolic acidosis. Kang et al pointed out that acute consumption of ethanol significantly increases the mean subfoveal choroidal thickness for the first 60 minutes.[1] This decreases over the next 120 minutes. Chronic alcoholism leads to malnutrition in severe cases, with resultant ocular sicca or toxic amblyopia. Wang et al, in a literature review, pointed out that there was no consistent evidence supporting a major role of moderate alcohol consumption in the development or progression of any common eye diseases.[2] Various types of cataracts have been reported to be more common in heavy users of ethanol, but data from various studies suggest that moderate alcohol ingestion may reduce the need for cataract surgery.[3] Knudtson et al showed no effect—increase or decrease—of alcohol use on the risk of age-related macular degeneration.[4] It is suspected that alcoholics are also more prone to infectious keratitis. Adams et al reported an approximate 20% increase in the odds of early-onset age-related macular degeneration.[5] You et al, using meta-analysis, reported that alcohol ingestion may be a significant risk factor in causing ocular sicca.[6]

Kim et al has shown that oral alcohol is secreted in human tears.[7] This causes hyperosmolarity, shortened tear film break-up time, and ocular surface disease. This process is probably aggravated in those who abuse alcohol. Inadvertent splashes of alcoholic beverage onto the eye surface are a frequent occurrence and result in irritation of the conjunctiva and cornea, but there are no reports of permanent damage. Most distilled alcoholic beverages are 40% alcohol by volume, but concentrations up to 75% are available commercially in the United States. In the photorefractive keratectomy procedure, ophthalmic surgeons use concentrations of less than 40% alcohol to remove corneal epithelium. It has been shown that the duration of application of 20% alcohol is important to corneal epithelial cell survival. A 30-second or less application allows cell survival, whereas a 60-second application may lead to cell death. There is a spontaneous report of an adverse event in which alcohol was placed in the anterior chamber during cataract surgery, resulting in permanent endothelial damage.

Children born with fetal alcohol syndrome have multiple orbital and ocular structural abnormalities.

Recommendations

1. Inadvertent ocular splashes of high concentrations of ethanol should be treated with routine irrigation, and patients should be followed for the development of corneal abrasion or ulceration.
2. The ocular side effects of retrobulbar alcohol injections are many, and thus the use of alcohol in cases of blind and painful eyes should be considered if evisceration or enucleation is not possible.

3. The neuro-ophthalmic side effects of acute ethanol intoxication are usually reversed within 24 hours. Chronic use of alcohol will have less untoward ocular effects if the diet is supplemented with vitamins.

Generic Name:
Methanol.

Synonyms:
Methyl alcohol, wood alcohol, wood spirits.

Proprietary Names/Products Containing:
Found in automobile engine cleaners, antifreeze, deicers, and paint/stain removers.

Primary Use
Known as *wood alcohol,* methanol was once produced by the distillation of wood. It is now produced synthetically. Methanol is the simplest alkyl alcohol. It is used primarily as a solvent and as an antifreeze. It is also found in several cleaners and is used to denature ethanol. Methanol occurs in small amounts naturally in the environment.

Ocular Side Effects
Topical ocular exposure
Possible
1. Irritation

Systemic exposure
Certain
1. Blindness
2. Decreased vision
3. Optic disc
   a. Hyperemia
   b. Atrophy
   c. Cupping
4. Visual field defects
5. Decreased pupil reactions
6. Color vision defect

Clinical Significance
Many unfortunate accidents involving the consumption of methanol have been recorded in the literature. Methanol is often used to denature ethanol for industrial uses, and as its odor is milder and sweeter than ethanol, its presence in denatured alcohol is difficult to detect. People may accidentally consume methanol while consuming what they believe to be unadulterated ethanol. A report of multiple victims of methanol toxicity in Port Moresby, Papua New Guinea, showed that a dose-related response exists with ocular effects ranging from none to blindness.[1] With consumption of higher volumes, vision loss often precedes death. Rarely, significant systemic toxicity may occur via percutaneous or inhalational exposure.

Temporary reactions to systemic methanol exposure include peripapillary edema, optic disc hyperemia, diminished papillary reactions, and central scotoma. Permanent ocular abnormalities include decreased visual acuity, blindness, optic disc pallor, disc cupping, attenuation or sheathing of arterioles, diminished papillary reaction to light, and visual field defects.[2] Zakharov et al pointed out that long-term follow-up is necessary because long-term sequelae may occur.[3] Magnetic resonance imaging (MRI) studies have shown one location of neurologic damage from methanol to be in the putamen.[4] Pathologic studies revealed that methanol probably damages mitochondria in the photoreceptors.[5] Moschos et al reported on OCT and electrophysiologic tests, which supports the hypothesis that methanol affects photoreceptors, Müller cells, and the retrolaminar portion of the optic nerve.[6]

Recommendations
1. People who are suspected to have ingested methanol need immediate care, preferably in an intensive care unit setting. Treatment of systemic methanol poisoning consists of trying to prevent the metabolism of methanol to formaldehyde, which then is converted to formic acid. Formic acid inhibits cytochrome oxidase, a key protein in the production of adenosine triphosphate (ATP) within mitochondria, and its formation is thought to precipitate the neurologic side effects of methanol consumption. Peak concentrations of methanol occur within an hour of ingestion. A latent period occurs while the methanol is converted to formic acid, and a metabolic acidosis ensues. Visual loss often precedes the potentially fatal side effects of the formic acidosis. To block the metabolism toward formic acid, competitive inhibition of alcohol dehydrogenase may be achieved by giving the patient ethanol or fomepizole (which does not cause inebriation).
2. Hemodialysis may enhance the elimination of methanol and its metabolic by-products, allowing improved chances of recovery.
3. Desai et al have shown that the degree of acidosis at presentation appears to determine the final vision.[7] They found early presentation did not significantly change the visual outcome, especially in severe poisoning.
4. Bansal et al suggested autologous bone marrow–derived stem cells as therapy for this entity.[8]

CLASS: GENITOURINARY TRACT DRUGS

Generic Names:
1. Fesoterodine fumarate; 2. solifenacin succinate; 3. oxybutynin chloride.

Proprietary Names:
1. Toviaz; 2. VESIcare; 3. Ditropan, Ditropan XL, Gelnique, Oxytrol.

Primary Use
Oral muscarinic antagonists used to treat overactive bladder with symptoms of urgency and frequency.

Ocular Side Effects
Systemic administration – oral
Certain
1. Decreased vision
2. Mydriasis
3. Decreased accommodation amplitude
4. May aggravate or cause ocular sicca
5. Decreased tear film break-up time (oxybutynin)

Probable
1. Acute glaucoma
2. Extraocular muscles
   a. Esophoria
   b. Esotropia
3. Decreased contact lens tolerance secondary to ocular sicca (oxybutynin)

Clinical Significance
Ocular side effects from these drugs are seldom a reason to stop the drug. Decreased vision occurs with solifenacin succinate in 3.8–4.2% of patients and 1–9.6% with oxybutynin chloride.[1,2] Altan-Yaycioglu et al emphasized that oxybutynin may have more ocular side effects, especially those affect the lacrimal glands, with significant effects on tear film break-up times, than other drugs in this class.[3] Acar et al found that 4 mg/day fesoterodine fumarate caused a decrease in accommodation with a 0.6-diopter decrease after 30 days and 1.0-diopter decrease after 90 days.[4] They also found statistically significant mydriasis. Altan-Yaycioglu et al confirmed both the mydriatic (maximum of 20% change) and accommodative (found in 7% of patients) effects with oxybutynin use.[3] Although this class of drugs has no effect on intraocular pressure, the dilation effect can precipitate narrow-angle glaucoma.[5] The same is true in causing esophoria and esotropia.[6]

A major side effect with both drugs is xerostomia; therefore it is not surprising for ocular sicca to be an occasional complaint. Xerostomia occurred at an incidence rate of 0.3–1.6% in clinical trials with solifenacin succinate.[2] Sekeroglu et al found short-term solifenacin succinate had no effect on Schirmer 1 tests or tear break-up time; however, patients had more significant ocular surface symptoms than controls.[7] Altan-Yaycioglu et al found significant sicca effects with oxybutynin.[3] The *Physicians' Desk Reference* (PDR) warns that oxybutynin use may affect contact lens users.[1] They report keratoconjunctivitis at a rate of 1–4.9%.

CLASS: PSYCHEDELIC DRUGS

Generic Names:
1. Dronabinol (tetrahydrocannabinol, THC); 2. hashish; 3. marihuana (marijuana, cannabis).

Proprietary Name:
1. Marinol, Syndros; 2. Generic only; 3. Generic only.

Street Names:
1. The one; 2. bhang, charas, gram, hash, keif, black Russian; 3. ace, Acapulco gold, baby, Belyando sprue, boo, brown weed, bush, cannabis, charas, dank, dope, gage, ganja, grass, green, gungeon, hay, hemp, herb, home grown, jay, joint, kick sticks, kryptonite, lid, locoweed, Mary Jane, Mexican green, MJ, muggles, OJ (opium joint), Panama red, pot, rainyday woman, reefer, roach, rope, sinsemilla, stick, tea, twist, weed, wheat.

Primary Use
These psychedelic drugs are occasionally used as cerebral sedatives for muscle spasms, chronic pain, and nausea and are narcotics commonly available for medical and recreational use. Dronabinol is also medically indicated for the treatment of nausea and vomiting associated with chemotherapy.

Ocular Side Effects
Systemic administration – inhalation or oral
Certain
1. Visual hallucinations
2. Color vision defect
   a. Objects have yellow or violet tinge
   b. Colored flashing lights
   c. Heightened color perception
3. Nystagmus
4. Irritation
   a. Hyperemia
   b. Conjunctivitis
   c. Photophobia (variable)
   d. Burning sensation

5. Decreased accommodation
6. Decreased dark adaptation
7. Decreased vision
8. Blepharospasm
9. Decreased intraocular pressure
10. Decreased lacrimation
11. Pupils – early
    a. Miosis
    b. Anisocoria
12. Extraocular muscles
    a. Increased phorias
    b. Intermittent tropia
    c. Diplopia
    d. Some changes in tracking
13. Binocular depth inversion – reduced
14. Blinking impairment
15. Increased retinal circulation
16. Visual spatial summation – decreased
17. Decreased corneal endothelial cell count

Possible
1. Ganglion cell dysfunction

Clinical Significance
Marijuana is the most widely used illicit drug in the United States and one of the oldest recorded medicines in the world. The oral form, dronabinol, is largely unappealing to the addict and therefore has a very low abuse potential with few, if any, ocular side effects. The *Physicians' Desk Reference* (PDR) lists the incidence of conjunctivitis at 0.3–1%.[1] Levi et al as well as Laffi et al found vision disturbances lasting 24 hours after marijuana use.[2,3] Alterations included depth perception, sensorial disconnection when talking with people, intermittent light phenomena, strobe-like effects, bright spots flickering randomly in high frequency, and alteration of the sensory perception of one's external environment. Ocular side effects due to these drugs are transient and seldom of clinical importance. However, Steimetz et al and Kowal et al have shown that probable irreversible disruption of classic eye blink may occur in heavy users.[4,5]

Semple et al, using binocular depth inversion testing, discovered persistent sensory visual abnormalities in chronic marijuana users.[6] There is some evidence that marijuana decreases basal lacrimal secretion, decreases photosensitivity, increases dark adaptation, increases color-match limits, and increases Snellen visual acuity. Huestegge et al have shown defects in visual spatial working memory in cannabis users.[7] Possibly in some, within the first 5–15 minutes on these drugs, some pupillary constriction may occur. However, most do not show pupillary constriction, and to date,

no long-term pupillary effect is noted. Conjunctival hyperemia is not uncommon and is more pronounced at 15 minutes after exposure.

The cannabinols found in marijuana can lower intraocular pressure by an average of 25%, but the effect only lasts 3–4 hours. There is significant variation in the individual response to these drugs, as well as diminished response with time. Most patients on these drugs for glaucoma control cannot use it for prolonged periods due to lack of glaucoma control. Isolated cannabinols, which lower intraocular pressure, have the complicating factor that one cannot separate the central nervous system high from its ocular pressure–lowering effect, so their value clinically is quite limited. Few patients are able to use marijuana for long-term control of their glaucoma and remain functional in the workplace. These drugs are occasionally used medically, but have no long-term value in clinical ophthalmology.

Polat et al found significant decreased corneal endothelial cell counts in chronic cannabinoid users.[8] Cell morphology was not changed.

Schwitzer et al showed an association with cannabis use and ganglion cell dysfunction.[9] Lyons et al, in an accompanying editorial, felt this has yet to be fully proven.[10]

Generic Names:
1. Lysergic acid diethylamide (LSD), lysergide; 2. mescaline; 3. psilocybin.

Proprietary Name:
1. Generic only; 2. Generic only; 3. Generic only.

Street Names:
1. Acid, barrels, big d, blotter acid, blue acid, brown dots, California sunshine, crackers, cubes, cupcakes, grape parfait, green domes, Hawaiian sunshine, Lucy in the sky with diamonds, micro dots, purple barrels, purple haze, purple ozolone, sunshine, the animal, the beast, the chief, the hawk, the ticket, trips, twenty-five, yellow dimples, windowpane; 2. buttons, cactus, mesc, peyote, the bad seed, topi; 3. Magic mushroom, shrooms.

Primary Use
Illicit psychedelic and psychotomimetic drugs that may be both natural and synthetic products.

Ocular Side Effects
Systemic administration – intravenous or oral
Certain
1. Visual hallucinations
   a. Image distortion

b. Color intensification
c. Geometric figure
d. False perception of movement
e. Afterimages
2. Spontaneous recurrence of abnormal visual perception after discontinuation of the drug (LSD)
a. Transitory
b. Long-term
c. Permanent
3. Palinopsia – visual perversion of recently seen objects (LSD)
a. Acute
b. Permanent
4. Color vision defect – heightened color perception
5. Pupils
a. Mydriasis
b. Anisocoria
c. Decreased or absent reaction to light
6. Decreased accommodation
7. Decreased dark adaptation
8. Decreased vision
9. Abnormal electroretinogram (ERG), visual evoked potential (VEP), and depressed critical flicker fusion
10. Photophobia

Topical ocular application – liquid LSD
Conditional/unclassified
1. Cornea
a. Melting
b. Scarring
c. Severe pannus
2. Conjunctiva – scarring

Ocular teratogenic effects
Possible
1. Cataract
2. Iris coloboma
3. Ocular dysplasia
4. Microphthalmos
5. Corneal opacities
6. Persistent hyperplastic primary vitreous
7. Retinal dysplasia
8. Optic disc hypoplasia
9. Optic nerve coloboma
10. Anophthalmia

Clinical Significance
Ocular side effects due to these drugs are very common. Some claim true visual hallucinations seldom occur with these drugs, but rather a complicated visual experience results from a drug-induced perceptual disturbance. Perception changes include alterations in colors and shapes. Halpern et al reviewed the literature on "hallucinogen persisting perception disorder," also known as *flashbacks*.[1] They are uncommon, but can persist for months or even many years. Some have persisted for 20 years plus. Lysergide (LSD) is 100 times more potent than psilocybin, which in turn is 4000 times more potent than mescaline. The visual side effects noted are therefore due to LSD and then, to a lesser degree, to the other drugs. A large number of cases of sun gazing–induced macular damage has been reported in persons using these drugs. Abraham first reported irreversible impairment of color discrimination.[2] Kawasaki et al reported 3 patients who had persistent palinopsia after LSD ingestion.[3] These prolonged afterimages lasted 3-plus years after being off the drug.

There is a case of liquid LSD splashed into 1 eye of a 20-year-old patient in the spontaneous reports. The cornea had significant melt with a resultant marked pannus. A conjunctival flap was necessary to save the globe. The eye was permanently disabled.

Lo et al described a case of LSD-impregnated blotting paper inserted into the inferior fornices of both eyes causing "kissing" ulcerations and corneal opacities.[4]

Generic Name:
Phencyclidine.

Proprietary Name:
Generic only.

Street Names:
Angel dust, angel's mist, busy bee, crystal, DOA, goon, hog/horse tranquilizer, love boat, lovely mist, monkey tranquilizer, PCP, peace pill, rocket fuel, sheets, super weed, tac, tic.

Primary Use
This nonbarbiturate anesthetic was removed from the market because of postoperative psychiatric disturbances; however, it is still available on the illicit drug market.

Ocular Side Effects
Systemic administration – inhalation or nasal
Certain
1. Extraocular muscles
a. Nystagmus – horizontal, rotary, or vertical
b. Diplopia
c. Jerky pursuit movements
2. Pupils
a. Miosis
b. Decreased reaction to light

3. Decreased vision
4. Visual hallucinations
5. Ptosis
6. Oculogyric crises
7. Decreased corneal reflex
8. Drug found in vitreous body
9. Decreased blink rate

Conditional/unclassified
1. Increased intraocular pressure

Clinical Significance

Even with relatively low doses (5 mg), phencyclidine may give a characteristic type of nystagmus in which vertical, horizontal, and rotary eye movements occur in sudden bursts. In addition, this drug may produce hallucinations and visual defects, including distortion of body image and substitution of fairytale characters. Acute toxic reactions can last up to a week after a single dose, although some mental effects can linger for more than a month. These effects may keep recurring in sudden episodes while the patient is apparently recovering. A state of sensory blockade or a blank stare in which the eyes remain conjugate and open but with little or no spontaneous movement is characteristic of phencyclidine coma.

Cox et al found this drug regularly in the vitreous humor of persons in nontoxic states.[1] However, its concentration in the postmortem state was too variable to have interpretative value.

CLASS: SEDATIVES AND HYPNOTICS

Generic Names:

1. Amobarbital; 2. butabarbital sodium; 3. butalbital; 4. methohexital sodium; 5. methylphenobarbital (mephobarbital); 6. pentobarbital sodium; 7. phenobarbital; 8. primidone; 9. secobarbital sodium.

Proprietary Names:

1. Amytal; 2. Butisol; 3. Multi-ingredient preparations only; 4. Brevital; 5. Mebaral; 6. Nembutal; 7. Luminal; 8. Mysoline; 9. Seconal.

Street Names:

1–9. Barbs, bluebirds, blues, tooies, yellow jackets.

Primary Use

These barbituric acid derivatives vary primarily in duration and intensity of action and are used as central nervous system depressants, hypnotics, sedatives, and anticonvulsants.

Ocular Side Effects
Systemic administration (primarily excessive dosage or chronic use) – intramuscular, intravenous, oral, or rectal
Certain
1. Eyelids
   a. Ptosis
   b. Blepharoclonus
2. Pupils
   a. Mydriasis
   b. Miosis (coma)
   c. Decreased reaction to light
   d. Hippus
3. Extraocular muscles
   a. Decreased convergence
   b. Paresis
   c. Jerky pursuit movements
   d. Random ocular movements
   e. Vertical gaze palsy
4. Oscillopsia
5. Nystagmus
   a. Downbeat, gaze-evoked, horizontal, jerk, or vertical
   b. Depressed or abolished optokinetic, latent, positional, voluntary, or congenital nystagmus
6. Decreased vision
7. Color vision defect – objects have yellow or green tinge
8. Visual hallucinations
9. Eyelids or conjunctiva
   a. Allergic reactions
   b. Conjunctivitis – nonspecific
   c. Edema
   d. Photosensitivity
   e. Urticaria
10. Decreased accommodation (primidone)
11. Abnormal electroretinogram (ERG), visual evoked potential (VEP), or critical flicker fusion

Possible
1. May aggravate or cause ocular sicca
2. Optic nerve disorders (chronic use)
   a. Retrobulbar or optic neuritis
   b. Papilledema
   c. Optic atrophy
3. Visual fields
   a. Scotomas
   b. Constriction

Ocular teratogenic effects (primidone)
Possible
1. Optic atrophy
2. Ptosis
3. Hypertelorism
4. Epicanthus
5. Strabismus

Clinical Significance
New classes of drugs are generally replacing these short- and long-acting barbiturates; however, phenobarbital is still widely used. Numerous adverse ocular side effects have been attributed to barbiturate usage, yet nearly all significant ocular side effects are in acute barbiturate poisoning or habitual users. Few toxic ocular reactions are found due to barbiturate usage at therapeutic dosages or on short-term therapy. The most common ocular abnormalities are disturbances of ocular movement, such as decreased convergence, paresis of extraocular muscles, or nystagmus. The pupillary response to barbiturate intake is quite variable, so this sign has questionable clinical value. Phenobarbital has the most frequently reported ocular side effects; however, all barbiturates may produce some adverse ocular effects. Chronic barbiturate users have a "tattle-tale" ptosis and blepharoclonus. Normally, a tap on the glabella area of the head produces a few eyelid blinks, but in the barbiturate addict, the response will be a rapid fluttering of the eyelids.[1] Bilateral blindness or decreased vision after barbiturate-induced coma usually returns to normal vision. There are a few reports, however, of permanent blindness. Optic neuropathy with complete recovery in a 12-year-old boy from chronic phenobarbital medication was a unique case.[2] The barbiturates do not appear to have teratogenic effects, except possibly primidone. Primidone has been shown to be associated with acute attacks of porphyria. Acute onset of severe photophobia and/or lid reactions is an indicator of ocular porphyria.

This class of drugs may cause xerostomia, so ocular sicca can probably occur. Marino et al reported such a case.[3]

Generic Name:
Chloral hydrate.

Proprietary Names:
Aquachloral, NocTec, Novo-Chlorhydrate, Somnos, Somnote.

Primary Use
This nonbarbiturate sedative-hypnotic is effective in the treatment of insomnia. It is not approved by the FDA, but is available in the United States and some other countries.

Ocular Side Effects
Systemic administration – oral or suppository
Certain
1. Decreased vision
2. Pupils
   a. Mydriasis – toxic states
   b. Miosis
3. Visual hallucinations
4. Ptosis
5. Decreased convergence
6. Eyelids or conjunctiva
   a. Allergic reactions
   b. Hyperemia
   c. Edema
7. Lacrimation
8. Irritation
9. Nystagmus
10. Extraocular muscles – toxic states
    a. Paresis
    b. Jerky pursuit movements

Clinical Significance
Whereas the more serious ocular side effects due to chloral hydrate occur at excessive dosage levels, decreased convergence, miosis, and occasionally ptosis are seen at recommended therapeutic dosages. The ptosis may be unilateral. Lilliputian hallucinations (in which objects appear smaller than their actual size) are said to be almost characteristic for chloral hydrate–induced delirium. Mydriasis only occurs in toxic states. Chloral hydrate frequently can cause lid edema with or without dermatitis. Ocular hyperemia and chemosis of the conjunctiva may also be seen. Although this drug has fallen from use due to newer, safer drugs, it is still occasionally being used. West et al, Burnett et al, and Wilson et al have reported its safety in pediatric ophthalmology.[1–3]

REFERENCES
Drug: Gabapentin
1. Browne T. Efficacy and safety of gabapentin. In: Chadwick D, ed. *New Trends in Epilepsy Management: the Role of Gabapentin.* London: Royal Society of Medicine Service; 1993:47–58.
2. Gabapentin. Retrieved from http://www.pdr.net; 2018.
3. Hilton EJ, Hosking SL, Betts T. The effect of antiepileptic drugs on visual performance. *Seizure.* 2004;13:113–128.
4. Steinhoff BJ, Freudenthaler N, Paulus W. The influence of established and new antiepileptic drugs on visual

perception. A placebo-controlled, double-blind, single-dose study in healthy volunteers. *Epilepsy Res.* 1997;29:35–47.

5. Kim JY, Kim DG, Kim SH, et al. Macular edema after gabapentin. *Korean J Ophthalmol.* 2016;30(2):153–155.

Drug: Lamotrigine

1. Schachter SC. A multicenter, placebo-controlled evaluation of the safety of lamotrigine (Lamictal) as add-on therapy in outpatients with partial seizures. Presented at the 1992 Annual Meeting of the American Epilepsy Society. Seattle; 1992.

2. Betts T, Goodwin G, Withers RM, et al. Human safety of lamotrigine. *Epilepsia.* 1991;32(suppl 1):S17–S21.

3. Alkawi A, Kattah JC, Wyman K. Downbeat nystagmus as a result of lamotrigine toxicity. *Epilepsy Res.* 2005;63:85–88.

4. Lamotrigine. Retrieved from http://www.pdr.net; 2018.

5. Kim DG, Oh SH, Kim OJ. A case of lamotrigine-induced excessive involuntary eye blinking. *J Clin Neurol.* 2007;3(2):93–95.

6. Das KB, Harris C, Smyth DP, et al. Unusual side effects of lamotrigine therapy. *J Child Neurol.* 2003;18:479–480.

7. Sotero de Menezes MA, Rho JM, Murphy P, et al. Lamotrigine-induced tic disorder: report of five pediatric cases. *Epilepsia.* 2000;41(7):862–867.

8. Alkin T, Onur E, Ozerdem A. Co-occurrence of blepharospasm, tourettism and obsessive-compulsive symptoms during lamotrigine treatment. *Prog Neuropsychopharmacol Biol Psychiatry.* 2007;31(6):1339–1340.

9. Verma A, Miller P, Carwile ST, et al. Lamotrigine-induced blepharospasm. *Pharmacotherapy.* 1999;19(7):877–880.

10. Acute posterior multifocal placoid pigment epitheliopathy associated with drug reaction with eosinophilia and systemic symptoms syndrome. *JAMA Ophthalmol.* 2017;135(2):169–171.

11. Hsu CT, Harlan JB, Goldberg MF, et al. Acute posterior multifocal placoid pigment epitheliopathy associated with a systemic necrotizing vasculitis. *Retina.* 2003;23(1):64–68.

12. Schauer P, Salaun N, Bazin S, et al. DRESS syndrome with bilateral panuveitis, elevated intraocular pressure, and HHV-6 reactivation: a case report. *J Fr Ophthalmol.* 2006;29(6):659–664.

13. Veerapandiyan A, Gallentine WB, Winchester SA, et al. Oculogyric crisis secondary to lamotrigine overdosage. *Epilepsia.* 2011;52(3):e4–e6.

14. Huber B, Hilgemann C. Hallucinosis using lamotrigine. *Nervenarzt.* 2009;80(2):202–204.

15. Yang CY, Dao RL, Lee TJ, et al. Severe cutaneous adverse reactions to antiepileptic drugs in Asians. *Neurology.* 2011;77:2025–2033.

Drug: Pregabalin

1. Owen RT. Pregabalin: its efficacy, safety and tolerability profile in generalized anxiety. *Drugs Today.* 2007;43(9):601–610.

2. Pregabalin. Retrieved from http://www.pdr.net; 2018.

3. Arroyo S, Anhut H, Kugler AR, et al. Pregabalin add-on treatment: a randomized, double-blind, placebo-controlled, dose-response study in adults with partial seizures. *Epilepsia.* 2004;45(1):20–27.

4. Kubota T, Fang J, Meltzer LT, et al. Pregabalin enhances nonrapid eye movement sleep. *J Pharmacol Exp Ther.* 2001;299(3):1095–1105.

Drug: Vigabatrin

1. Pellock JM, Faught E, Foroozan R, et al. Registry initiated to characterize vision loss associated with vigabatrin therapy. *Epilepsy Behav.* 2011;22:710–717.

2. Sergott RC, Johnson CA, Laxer KD, et al. Retinal structure and function in vigabatrin-treated adult patients with refractory complex partial seizures. *Epilepsia.* 2016;57(10):1634–1642.

3. Foroozan R. Vigabatrin: lessons learned from the United States experience. *J Neuroophthalmol.* 2018;38:442–450.

4. Vigabatrin. Retrieved from http://www.pdr.net; 2018.

5. Krauss GL, Johnson MA, Miller NR. Vigabatrin-associated retinal cone system dysfunction. *Neurology.* 1998;50:614–618.

6. Lawden MC. Vigabatrin, tiagabine, and visual fields. *J Neurol Neurosurg Psychiatry.* 2003;74:286.

7. Clayton LM, Devile M, Punte T, et al. Patterns of peripapillary retinal nerve fiber layer thinning in vigabatrin-exposed individuals. *Ophthalmology.* 2012;119(10):2152–2160.

8. Besch D, Schiefer U, Eter N, et al. Modeling the topography of absolute defects in patients exposed to the anti-epileptic drug vigabatrin and in normal subjects using automated static suprathreshold perimetry of the entire 80° visual field. *Graefes Arch Clin Exp Ophthalmol.* 2011;249:1333–1343.

9. Johnson MA, Krauss GL, Miller NR, et al. Visual function loss from vigabatrin: effect of stopping the drug. *Neurology.* 2000;55:40–45.

10. Best JL, Acheson JF. The natural history of vigabatrin associated visual field defects in patients electing to continue their medication. *Eye.* 2005;19:41–44.

11. Arndt CF, Derambure P, Defoort-Dhellemmes S, et al. Outer retinal dysfunction in patients treated with vigabatrin. *Neurology.* 1999;52:1205–1208.

12. Graniewski-Wijnands HS, Van Der Torren K. Electro-ophthalmological recovery after withdrawal from vigabatrin. *Doc Ophthalmol.* 2002;104:189–194.

13. Berezina TL, Khouri AS, Winship MD, et al. Visual field and ocular safety during short-term vigabatrin treatment in cocaine abusers. *Am J Ophthalmol.* 2012;154:326–332.

14. Wilton LV, Stephens MD, Mann RD. Interim report of the incidence of visual field defects in patients on long term vigabatrin therapy. *Pharmacoepidemiol Drug Saf.* 1999;8:S9–S14.

15. Yang J, Naumann MC, Tsai YT, et al. Vigabatrin-induced retinal toxicity is partially mediated by signaling in rod and cone photoreceptors. *PLoS ONE.* 2012;7(8):e43889.

16. Conway M, Cubbidge RP, Hosking SL. Visual field severity indices demonstrate dose-dependent visual loss from vigabatrin therapy. *Epilepsia.* 2008;49(1):108–116.

17. Frisén L, Malmgren K. Characterization of vigabatrin-associated optic atrophy. *Acta Ophthalmol Scand.* 2003;81:466–473.
18. Viestenz A, Viestenz A, Mardin CV. Vigabatrin-associated bilateral simple optic nerve atrophy with visual field constriction. A case report and a survey of the literature. *Ophthalmologe.* 2003;100:402–405.
19. Buncic RJ, Westall CA, Panton CM, et al. Characteristic retinal atrophy with secondary "inverse" optic atrophy identifies vigabatrin toxicity in children. *Ophthalmology.* 2004;11:1935–1942.
20. Rebolleda G, García Pérez JL, Muñoz Negrete FJ, et al. Vigabatrin toxicity in children. *Ophthalmology.* 2005;112:1322–1323.
21. Choi HJ, Kim DM. Visual field constriction associated with vigabatrin: retinal nerve fiber layer photographic correlation. *J Neurol Neurosurg Psychiatry.* 2004;75:1395.
22. Banin E, Shclev RS, Obolensky A, et al. Retinal function abnormalities in patients treated with vigabatrin. *Arch Ophthalmol.* 2003;121:811–816.
23. Fledelius HC. Vigabatrin-associated visual field constriction in a longitudinal series. Reversibility suggested after drug withdrawal. *Acta Ophthalmol Scand.* 2003;81:41–45.
24. Wild JM, Robson CR, Jones AL, et al. Detecting vigabatrin toxicity by imaging of the retinal nerve fiber layer. *Invest Ophthalmol Vis Sci.* 2006;47:917–924.
25. Lawthom C, Smith PE, Wild JM. Nasal retinal nerve fiber layer attenuation: a biomarker for vigabatrin toxicity. *Ophthalmology.* 2009;116:565–571.
26. Moseng L, Saeter M, Morch-Johnsen GH, et al. Retinal nerve fibre layer attenuation: clinical indicator for vigabatrin toxicity. *Acta Ophthalmol.* 2011;89(5):452–458.
27. Kjellström U, Andreasson S, Ponjavic V. Attenuation of the retinal nerve fibre layer and reduced retinal function assessed by optic coherence tomography and full-field electroretinography in patients exposed to vigabatrin medication. *Acta Ophthalmol.* 2014;92(2):149–157.
28. Horvath GA, Stockler-Ipsiroglu S, Aroichane M, et al. Eye findings in SSADH deficiency. *Mol Genet Metab.* 2012;105(3):325.

Drugs: Amfetamine (amphetamine), dextroamfetamine sulfate (dexamphetamine), methamfetamine hydrochloride (methamphetamine)

1. Thrasher DL, Von Derau K, Burgess J. Health effects from reported exposure to methamphetamine labs: a poison center-based study. *J Med Tox: Official J Am College Med Tox.* 2009;5(4):200–204.
2. Hazin R, Cadet JL, Kahook MY, et al. Ocular manifestations of crystal methamphetamine use. *Neurotox Res.* 2009;15(2):187–191.
3. Isaak BL, Liesegang TJ. Conjunctival and episcleral injection in drug abuse. *Ann Ophthalmol.* 1983;15:806–807.
4. McKeever RG, Lange J, Vearrier D, et al. Ocular ischemic syndrome associated with repeated intravenous injection of cocaine and methamphetamine. *Clin Toxicol.* 2016;54(4):379–380.

5. Chuck RS, Williams JM, Goldberg MA, et al. Recurrent corneal ulcerations associated with smokeable methamphetamine abuse. *Am J Ophthalmol.* 1996;121(5):571–572.
6. Wallace RT, Brown GC, Benson W, et al. Sudden retinal manifestations of intranasal cocaine and methamphetamine abuse. *Am J Ophthalmol.* 1992;114:158–160.
7. Wijaya J, Salu P, Leblanc A, et al. Acute unilateral visual loss due to a single intranasal methamphetamine abuse. *Bull Soc Belge Ophtalmol.* 1999;271:19–25.
8. Shaw Jr HE, Lawson JG, Stulting RG. Amaurosis fugax and retinal vasculitis associated with methamphetamine inhalation. *J Clin Neuroophthalmol.* 1985;5:169–176.
9. Kumar RL, Kaiser PK, Lee MS. Crystalline retinopathy from nasal ingestion of methamphetamine. *Retina.* 2005;26(7):823–824.
10. Hertle RW, Maybodi M, Bauer RM, et al. Clinical and oculographic response to Dexedrine in a patient with rod–cone dystrophy, exotropia, and congenital aperiodic alternating nystagmus. *Binocul Vis Strabismus Q.* 2001;16:259–264.
11. Fogel S, Lesage F, Cheron G. Intoxication involontaire aux amphetamines chez un nourrisson de 11 mois. *Arch Pediatr.* 2016;23(8):820–822.

Drugs: Benzfetamine hydrochloride (benzphetamine), diethylpropionate hydrochloride (amfepramone), phendimetrazine tartrate; 4. phentermine hydrochloride

1. Benzfetamine hydrochloride, diethylpropionate hydrochloride, phendimetrazine tartrate, phentermine hydrochloride. 2018. Retrieved from http://www.pdr.net.
2. Grewal DS, Goldstein DA, Khatana AK, et al. Bilateral angle closure following use of a weight loss combination agents containing topiramate. *J Glaucoma.* 2015;24(5):e132–e136.
3. Evans RW. Monocular visual aura with headache: retinal migraine? *Headache.* 2000;40:603–604.
4. Hertle RW, Maybodi M, Mellow SD, et al. Clinical and oculographic response to Tenuate Dospan (diethylpropionate) in a patient with congenital nystagmus. *Am J Ophthalmol.* 2002;133:159–160.
5. Cho AR, Yoon YH. Central retinal vein occlusion noted 2 days after use of phendimetrazine as an appetite suppressant. *JAMA Ophthalmol.* 2016;134(4):463–464.

Drugs: Alprazolam, chlordiazepoxide, clonazepam, clorazepate dipotassium, diazepam, flurazepam hydrochloride, lorazepam, midazolam hydrochloride, oxazepam, temazepam, triazolam

1. Chatziralli IP, Peponis V, Parikakis E, et al. Risk factors for intraoperative floppy iris syndrome: a prospective study. *Eye.* 2016;30:1039–1044.
2. Speeg-Schatz C, Giersch A, Boucart M, et al. Effects of lorazepam on vision and oculomotor balance. *Binocul Vis Strabismus Q.* 2001;16:99–104.

3. Kadoi C, Hayasaka S, Tsukamoto E, et al. Bilateral angle closure glaucoma and visual loss precipitated by antidepressant and antianxiety agents in a patient with depression. *Ophthalmologica*. 2000;214:360–361.

4. Avalos-Franco N, Castellar-Cerpa J, Santos-Bueso E, et al. Angle closure secondary to use of lorazepam in patient with myopia magna. *Arch Soc Esp Oftalmol*. 2015;90(12):588–592.

5. Alprazolam, chlordiazepoxide, clonazepam, clorazepate dipotassium, diazepam, flurazepam hydrochloride, lorazepam, midazolam hydrochloride, oxazepam, temazepam, triazolam. (2018). Retrieved from http://www.pdr.net.

6. Miyagawa M, Hayasaka S, Noda S. Photic maculopathy resulting from the light of a video camera in patients taking triazolam. *Ophthalmologica*. 1994;208(3):145–146.

7. Pau H. Braune scheibenförmige einlagerungen in die lines nach langzeitgabe von Diazepam (Valium). *Klin Monatsbl Augenheilkd*. 1985;187:219–220.

8. Elder MJ. Diazepam and its effects on visual fields. *Aust NZ J Ophthalmol*. 1992;20:267–270.

Drugs: Divalproex sodium (valproate semisodium), valproate sodium, valproic acid

1. Divalproex sodium, valproic acid, valproate sodium. 2018. Retrieved from http://www.pdr.net.

2. Bhalla S, Joshi D, Bhullar S, et al. Long-term follow-up for efficacy and safety of treatment of retinitis pigmentosa with valproic acid. *Br J Ophthalmol*. 2013;97:895–899.

3. Clemson CM, Tzekov R, Krebs M, et al. Therapeutic potential of valproic acid for retinitis pigmentosa. *Br J Ophthalmol*. 2011;95(1):89–93.

4. Dereci S, Koca T, Akcam M, et al. An evaluation of peripapillary retinal nerve fiber layer thickness in children with epilepsy receiving treatment of valproic acid. *Pediatr Neurol*. 2015;53(1):53–57.

5. Bayer AU, Thiel HJ, Zrenner E, et al. Color vision tests for early detection of antiepileptic drug toxicity. *Neurology*. 1997;48(5):1394–1397.

6. Depakote and mydriasis – from FDA reports. 2018. Retrieved from http://www.ehealthme.com/ds/depakote/mydriasis/.

7. Lyons C. Bilateral subacute lacrimal gland enlargement mimicking dacryoadenitis in a 7-year-old boy: a rare adverse effect of valproic acid (sodium valproate). *J AAPOS*. 2017;21(3):257–258.

8. Panigrahi I, Kalra J. Anti-epileptic drug therapy: an overview of fetal effects. *J Ind Med Assoc*. 2011;109(2):108–110.

9. Glover SJ, Quinn AG, Barter P, et al. Ophthalmic findings in fetal anticonvulsant syndrome. *Ophthalmology*. 2002;109:942–947.

10. Boyle NJ, Clark MP, Figueiredo F. Reduced corneal sensation and severe dry eyes in a child with fetal valproate syndrome. *Eye*. 2001;15:661–662.

11. Jackson A. Ocular coloboma and foetal valproate syndrome: four further cases and a hypothesis for aetiology. *Clin Dysmorphol*. 2014;23(2):74–75.

Drug: Phenytoin

1. Remler BF, Leigh J, Osorio I, et al. The characteristics and mechanisms of visual disturbance associated with anticonvulsant therapy. *Neurology*. 1990;40:791–796.

2. Bar S, Feller N, Savir N. Presenile cataracts in phenytoin-treated epileptic patients. *Arch Ophthalmol*. 1983;101:422–425.

3. Mathers W, Kattan H, Earll J, et al. Development of presenile cataracts in association with high serum levels of phenytoin. *Ann Ophthalmol*. 1987;19:291–292.

Drug: Topiramate

1. Banta JT, Hoffman K, Budenz DL, et al. Presumed topiramate-induced bilateral acute angle-closure glaucoma. *Am J Ophthalmol*. 2001;132:112–114.

2. Fraunfelder FW, Fraunfelder FT, Keates EU. Topiramate-associated acute bilateral secondary angle-closure glaucoma. *Ophthalmology*. 2004;111:109–111.

3. Rhee DJ, Goldbery MJ, Parrish RK. Bilateral angle-closure glaucoma and ciliary body swelling from topiramate. *Arch Ophthalmol*. 2001;119:1721–1723.

4. Jabbarpoor Bonyadi MH, Soheilian R, Soheilian M. Topiramate-induced bilateral anterior uveitis associated with hypopyon formation. *Ocul Immunol Inflamm*. 2011;19(1):86–88.

5. Yun SH, Lavin PJ, Schatz MP, et al. Topiramate-induced palinopsia: a case series and review of the literature. *J Neuroophthalmol*. 2015;35(2):148–151.

6. Evans RW. Reversible palinopsia and the Alice in Wonderland syndrome associated with topiramate use in migraineurs. *Headache*. 2006;46:815–817.

7. Belcastro V, Cupini LM, Corbelli I, et al. Palinopsia in patients with migraine: a case-control study. *Cephalalgia*. 2011;31(9):999–1004.

8. Fontenelle LF. Topiramate-induced palinopsia. *J Neuropsychiatry Clin Neurosci*. 2008;20(2):249–250.

9. Sierra-Hidalgo F, de Pablo-Fernandez E. Palinopsia induced by topiramate and zonisamide in a patient with migraine. *Clin Neuropharmacol*. 2013;36(2):63–64.

10. Foroozan R, Buono LM. Foggy visual field defect. *Survey Ophthalmol*. 2003;48:447–451.

11. Haque S, Shaffi M, Tang KC. Topiramate associated non-glaucomatous visual field defects. *J Clin Neurosci*. 2016;31:210–213.

12. Medicines Safety Update. *TGA*. 2014;5(6).

13. Vaphiades MS, Mason J. Foggy visual field defect [letter]. *Survey Ophthalmol*. 2004;4:266–297.

14. Tsui I, Casper D, Chou CL, et al. Electronegative electroretinogram associated with topiramate toxicity and vitelliform maculopathy. *Doc Ophthalmol*. 2008;116(1):57–60.

15. Gualtieri W, Janula J. Topiramate maculopathy. *Int Ophthalmol*. 2013;33(1):103–106.

16. Çerman E, Turhan SA, Eraslan M, et al. Topiramate and accommodation: does topiramate cause accommodative dysfunction. *Can J Ophthalmol*. 2017;52(1):20–25.

17. Craig JE, Ong TJ, Louis DL, et al. Mechanism of topiramate-induced acute-onset myopia and angle closure glaucoma. *Am J Ophthalmol*. 2004;137:193–195.

Drug: Zonisamide

1. Zonisamide. 2018. Retrieved from http://www.pdr.net.
2. Weppner JL, Raiser SN, Diamond PT. Functional decline secondary to progressive ataxia, dizziness and diplopia: the increasing role of the inpatient rehabilitation service in the evaluation and management of undiagnosed neurologic conditions: a case report. *PM R.* 2016;8(9S):S277.
3. Weiler DL. Zonisamide-induced angle closure and myopic shift. *Optom Vis Sci.* 2015;92(2):e46–e51.
4. Akman CI, Goodkin HP, Rogers DP, et al. Visual hallucinations associated with zonisamide. *Pharmacotherapy.* 2003;23:93–96.
5. Pomeranz HD, Lessell S. Palinopsia in the absence of drugs or cerebral disease. *Neurology.* 2000;54:855–859.
6. Sierra-Hidalgo F, de Pablo-Fernandez E. Palinopsia induced by topiramate and zonisamide in a patient with migraine. *Clin Neuropharmacol.* 2013;36:63–64.

Drugs: Amitriptyline hydrochloride, clomipramine hydrochloride, doxepin hydrochloride, trimipramine maleate

1. Amitriptyline hydrochloride, clomipramine hydrochloride, doxepin hydrochloride, trimipramine maleate. 2018. Retrieved from http://www.pdr.net.
2. Taavola H. Amitriptyline and dry eyes: an ADR overlooked in labelling. *WHO Pharmaceuticals Newsletter.* 2017;5:14.
3. Kupfer DJ, Pollock BG, Perel JM, et al. Effect of pulse loading with clomipramide on EEG sleep. *Psychiatry Res.* 1994;54(2):161–175.
4. Osborne SF, Vivian AJ. Primary position upbeat nystagmus associated with amitriptyline use. *Eye.* 2004;18(1):106.
5. Shah SP, Goren JF, Lazzara MD, et al. Acute macular neuroretinopathy associated with the use of norepinephrine reuptake inhibitors: a case series and OCT findings. *Retin Cases Brief Rep.* 2013;7(2):146–149.
6. Berard A, Zhao JP, Sheehy O. Antidepressant use during pregnancy and the risk of major congenital malformations in a cohort of depressed pregnant women: an updated analysis of the Quebec Pregnancy Cohort. *BMJ Open.* 2017;7(1):e013372.

Drugs: Amoxapine, desipramine hydrochloride, imipramine hydrochloride, nortriptyline hydrochloride

1. Amoxapine, desipramine hydrochloride, imipramine hydrochloride, nortriptyline hydrochloride. 2018. Retrieved from http://www.pdr.net.
2. Gupta A, Srinivasan R. Floppy iris syndrome with oral imipramine: a case series. *Indian J Ophthalmol.* 2012;60(2):136–138.
3. Roberts JE, Reme CE, Dillon J, et al. Bright light exposure and the concurrent use of photosensitizing drugs. *N Engl J Med.* 1992;326(22):1500–1501.

Drugs: Atomoxetine, duloxetine, venlafaxine hydrochloride

1. Atomoxetine, duloxetine, venlafaxine. 2018. Retrieved from http://www.pdr.net.

2. Shifera AS, Leoncavallo A, Sherwood M. Probable association of an attack of bilateral acute angle-closure glaucoma with duloxetine. *Ann Pharmacother.* 2014;48(7):936–939.
3. Botha VE, Bhikoo R, Merriman M. Venlafaxine-induced intraocular pressure rise in a patient with open angle glaucoma. *Clin Exp Ophthalmol.* 2016;44(8):734–735.
4. Aragona M, Inghilleri M. Increased ocular pressure in two patients with narrow angle glaucoma treated with venlafaxine. *Clin Neuropharmacol.* 1998;21(2):130–131.
5. Duarte AL, Silva SE, Melo A. *Acute Angle Closure Glaucoma Induced by Duloxetine.* Copenhagen, Denmark: 10th European Glaucoma Society Congress; 2012.
6. Ezra DG, Storoni M, Whitefield LA. Simultaneous bilateral acute angle closure glaucoma following venlafaxine treatment. *Eye (Lond).* 2006;20(1):128–129.
7. Guzman MH, Thiagalingam S, Ong PY, et al. Bilateral acute angle closure caused by supraciliary effusions associated with venlafaxine intake. *Med J Aust.* 2005;182(3):121–123.
8. Lam YWF. Probable association between duloxetine, acute angle-closure glaucoma. *Ophthalmologica.* 2007;221(6):388–394.
9. Ng B, Sanbrook GMC, Malouf AJ, et al. Venlafaxine and bilateral acute angle closure glaucoma. *Med J Aust.* 2002;176(5):241.
10. Turcotte S, Fredette MJ. Angle closure glaucoma associated with venlafaxine treatment. Abstracts from the 2012 European Association for Vision and Eye Research Conference.
11. Wicinski M, Kaluzny BJ, Liberski S, et al. Association between serotonin-norepinephrine reuptake inhibitors and acute angle closure: what is known? *Surv Ophthalmol.* 2019;64:185–194.
12. Shah SP, Goren JF, Lazzara MD, et al. Acute macular neuroretinopathy associated with the use of norepinephrine reuptake inhibitors: a case series and OCT findings. *Retin Cases Brief Rep.* 2013;7(2):146–149.
13. Semlitsch HV, Saletu B, Binder GA, et al. Acute effects of the novel antidepressant venlafaxine on cognitive event-related potentials (P300), eye blink rate and mood in young healthy subjects. *Int Clin Psychopharmacol.* 1993;8(3):155–166.
14. Reif A, Pfuhlmann B. Venlafaxine and reversible blepharoedema. *Int J Neuropsychopharmacol.* 2002;5(4):413–414.
15. Chou PH, Chu CS, Chen YH, et al. Antidepressants and risk of cataract development: a population-based, nested case-control study. *J Affect Disord.* 2017;215:237–244.
16. Kocer E, Kocer A, Özsütcü M, et al. Dry eye related to commonly used new antidepressants. *J Clin Psychopharmacol.* 2015;35(4):411–413.

Drug: Bupropion hydrochloride

1. Van Wyck Fleet J, Manberg PJ, Miller LL, et al. Overview of clinically significant adverse reactions to bupropion. *J Clin Psychiatry.* 1983;44(5 Pt 2):191–196.
2. Murphy RM, Bakir B, O'Brien C, et al. Drug-induced bilateral secondary angle-closure glaucoma: a literature synthesis. *J Glaucoma.* 2016;25(2):e99–e105.

3. Takusagawa HL, Hunter RS, Jue A, et al. Bilateral uveal effusion and angle-closure glaucoma associated with bupropion use. *Arch Ophthalmol.* 2012;130(1):120–122.

Drugs: Carbamazepine, oxcarbazepine

1. Kalis MM, Huff NA. Oxcarbazepine, an antiepileptic agent. *Clin Ther.* 2001;23(5):680–700.
2. Carbamazepine, oxcarbazepine. 2018. Retrieved from http://www.pdr.net.
3. Bayer A, Thiel HJ, Zrenner E, et al. Sensitive physiologic perceptual tests for ocular side effects of drugs exemplified by various anticonvulsants. *Ophthalmologe.* 1995;92:182–190.
4. Neilsen NV, Syversen K. Possible retinotoxic effect of carbamazepine. *Acta Ophthalmol.* 1986;64:287–290.
5. Glover SJ, Quinn AG, Barter P, et al. Ophthalmic findings in fetal anticonvulsant syndrome(s). *Ophthalmology.* 2002;109:942–947.
6. Sutcliffe AG, Jones RB, Woodruff G. Eye malformations associated with treatment with carbamazepine during pregnancy. *Ophthalmic Genet.* 1998;19:59–62.

Drugs: Citalopram hydrobromide, escitalopram oxalate, fluoxetine hydrochloride, fluvoxamine maleate, paroxetine hydrochloride, sertraline hydrochloride

1. Costagliola C, Mastropasqua L, Steardo L, et al. Fluoxetine oral administration increases intraocular pressure. *Br J Ophthalmol.* 1996;80:678.
2. Costagliola C, Parmeggiani F, Sebastiani A. SSRIs and intraocular pressure modifications: evidence, therapeutic implications and possible mechanisms. *CNS Drugs.* 2004;18:475–484.
3. Jiménez-Jiménez FJ, Ortí-Pareja M, Zurdo JM. Aggravation of glaucoma with fluvoxamine. *Ann Pharmacother.* 2001;35:1565–1566.
4. Eke T, Carr S. Acute glaucoma, chronic glaucoma, and serotoninergic drugs. *Br J Ophthalmol.* 1998;82:976–977.
5. Ahmad S. Fluoxetine and glaucoma. *DICP Ann Pharmacother.* 1991;25:436.
6. Sierra-Rodriguez MA, Saenz-Frances F, Santos-Bueso E, et al. Chronic angle-closure glaucoma related to paroxetine treatment. *Semin Ophthalmol.* 2013;28(4):244–246.
7. Ho HY, Kam KW, Young AL, et al. Acute angle closure glaucoma after sertraline. *Gen Hosp Psychiatry.* 2013;35(5):575e1–575e2.
8. AlQuorain S, Alfaraj S, Alshahrani M. Bilateral acute closed angle glaucoma associated with the discontinuation of escitalopram: a case report. *Open Access Emerg Med.* 2016;8:61–65.
9. Kocer E, Kocer A, Özsütcü M, et al. Dry eye related to commonly used new antidepressants. *J Clin Psychopharmacol.* 2015;35(4):411–413.
10. Schenck CH, Mahowald MW, Kim SW, et al. Prominent eye movements during NREM sleep and REM sleep behavior disorder associated with fluoxetine treatment of depression and obsessive-compulsive disorder. *Sleep.* 1992;15(3):226–235.

11. Armitage R, Trivedi M, Rush AJ. Fluoxetine and oculomotor activity during sleep in depressed patients. *Neuropsychopharmacology.* 1995;12(2):159–165.
12. Wakeno M, Kato M, Takekita Y, et al. A series of case reports on abnormal sensation on eye movement associated with paroxetine discontinuation. *Inter Clin Psychopharmacol.* 2006;21(4):A29–A30.
13. Etminan M, Mikelberg FS, Brophy JM. Selective serotonin reuptake inhibitors and the risk of cataracts. *Ophthalmology.* 2010;117(6):1251–1255.
14. Erie JC, Brue SM, Chamberlain AM, et al. Selective serotonin reuptake inhibitor use and increased risk of cataract surgery: a population-based, case-control study. *Am J Ophthalmol.* 2014;158(1):192–197.
15. Barrett J. Anisocoria associated with selective serotonin reuptake inhibitors. *BMJ.* 1994;309:1620.
16. Sener EC, Kiratli H. Presumed sertraline maculopathy. *Acta Ophthalmol Scand.* 2001;79(4):428–430.
17. Ewe SY, Abell RG, Vote BJ. Bilateral maculopathy associated with sertraline. *Australas Psychiatry.* 2014;22(6):573–575.
18. Mason 3rd JO, Patel SA. Bull's eye maculopathy in a patient taking sertraline. *Retin Cases Brief Rep.* 2015;9(2):131–133.
19. Lochhead J. SSRI-associated neuropathy. *Eye (Lond).* 2015;29(9):1233–1235.

Drug: Maprotiline hydrochloride

1. Maprotiline hydrochloride. 2018. Retrieved from http://www.pdr.net.
2. Kadoi C, Hayasaka S, Tsukamoto E, et al. Bilateral angle closure glaucoma and visual loss precipitated by antidepressant and antianxiety agents in a patient with depression. *Ophthalmologica.* 2000;214(5):360–361.
3. Terao HH, Nakamura J. Visual perseveration: a new side effect of maprotiline. *Acta Psychiatr Scand.* 2000;101(6):476–477.

Drug: Methylphenidate hydrochloride

1. Duman NS, Duman R, Gökten ES, et al. Lens opacities in children using methylphenidate hydrochloride. *Cutan Ocul Toxicol.* 2017;36(4):362–365.
2. Bartlik B, Harmon G. Use of methylphenidate in a patient with glaucoma and attention-deficit hyperactivity disorder: a clinical dilemma. *Arch Gen Psychiatry.* 1997;54:188–189.
3. Kimko HC, Cross JT, Abernethy DR. Pharmacokinetics and clinical effectiveness of methylphenidate. *Clin Pharmacokinet.* 1999;37:457–470.
4. Allen D, Vasavada A. Cataract and surgery for cataract. *BMJ.* 2006;333:128–132.
5. Lu CK, Kuang TM, Chou JC. Methylphenidate (Ritalin)-associated cataract and glaucoma. *J Chin Med Assoc.* 2006;69(12):589–590.
6. Atlee Jr WE. Talc and cornstarch emboli in eyes of drug abusers. *JAMA.* 1972;219(1):49–51.
7. Sharma MC, Ho AC. Macular fibrosis associated with talc retinopathy. *Am J Ophthalmol.* 1999;128(4):517–519.

Drug: Trazodone hydrochloride

1. Hughes MS, Lessell S. Trazodone-induced palinopsia. *Arch Ophthalmol.* 1990;108:399–400.
2. Copper MD, Dening TR. Excessive blinking associated with combined antidepressants. *BMJ.* 1986;293:1243.
3. Pae CU, Lee CU, Lee SJ, et al. Association of low dose trazodone treatment with aggravated angle-closure glaucoma. *Psychiatry Clin Neurosci.* 2003;57(1):127–129.
4. Trazodone hydrochloride. 2018. Retrieved from http://www.pdr.net.

Drug: Fingolimod

1. Zarbin MA, Jampol LM, Jager RD, et al. Ophthalmic evaluations in clinical studies of fingolimod (FTY720) in multiple sclerosis. *Ophthalmology.* 2013;120(7):1432–1439.
2. Jain N, Tariq Bhatti M. Fingolimod-associated macular edema: incidence, detection, and management. *Neurology.* 2012;78(9):672–680.
3. Minuk A, Belliveau MJ, Almeida DR, et al. Fingolimod-associated macular edema: resolution by sub-tenon injection of triamcinolone with continued fingolimod use. *JAMA Ophthalmol.* 2013;131(6):802–803.
4. Afshar AR, Fernandes JK, Patel RD, et al. Cystoid macular edema associated with fingolimod use for multiple sclerosis. *JAMA Ophthalmol.* 2013;131(1):103–107.
5. Khimani KS, Foroozan R. Central serous chorioretinopathy associated with fingolimod treatment. *J Neuroophthalmol.* 2018;38(3):337–338.
6. Ayers MC, Conway DS. A case of presumed herpes keratouveitis in a patient treated with fingolimod. *Mult Scler J Exp Transl Clin.* 2016;2.
7. Gallego-Pinazo R, Espana-Gregori E, Casanova B, et al. Branch retinal vein occlusion during fingolimod treatment in a patient with multiple sclerosis. *J Neuroophthalmol.* 2011;31(3):292–293.
8. Bhatti MT, Freedman SM, Mahmoud TH. Fingolimod therapy and macular hemorrhage. *J Neuroophthalmol.* 2013;33(4):370–372.
9. Ueda N, Saida K. Retinal hemorrhages following fingolimod treatment for multiple sclerosis: a case report. *BMC Ophthalmol.* 2015;15:135.
10. Sia PI, Aujla JS, Chan WO, et al. Fingolimod-associated retinal hemorrhages and Roth spots. *Retina.* 2018;38(10):e80–e81.
11. Christopher KL, Elner VM, Demirci H. Conjunctival lymphoma in a patient on fingolimod for relapsing-remitting multiple sclerosis. *Ophthalmic Plast Reconstr Surg.* 2017;33(3):e73–e75.
12. Sergott RC. Oral MS medication may increase risk of macular edema in some patients. *Ocular Surgery News US Edition.* 2011.

Drug: Amisulpride

1. Stratos AA, Peponis VG, Portaliou DM, et al. Secondary pseudomyopia induced by amisulpride. *Optom Vis Sci.* 2011;88(11):1380–1382.
2. Nebhinani N, Suthar N. Oculogyric crisis with atypical antipsychotics: a case series. *Indian J Psychiatry.* 2017;59(4):499–501.
3. Lin CL, Yeh CB, Wan FJ, et al. Amisulpride related tic-like symptoms in an adolescent schizophrenic. *Prog Neuropsychopharmacol Biol Psychiatry.* 2006;30(1):144–146.
4. Barrett SL, Bell R, Watson D, et al. Effects of amisulpride, risperidone and chlorpromazine on auditory and visual latent inhibition, prepulse inhibition, executive function and eye movements in healthy volunteers. *J Psychopharmacol.* 2004;18(2):156–172.

Drug: Aripiprazole

1. Aripiprazole. 2018. Retrieved from http://www.pdr.net.
2. Bhachech JT. Aripiprazole-induced oculogyric crisis (acute dystonia). *J Pharmacol Pharmacother.* 2012;3(3):279–281.
3. Rizzo R, Gulisano M, Cali PV. Oculogyric crisis: a rare extrapyramidal side effect in the treatment of Tourette syndrome. *Eur Child Adolesc Psychiatry.* 2012;21(10):591–592.
4. Suhar N, Nebhinani N. Aripiprazole-induced neck dystonia and oculogyric crisis. *Asian J Psychiatr.* 2018;31:94–95.
5. Kaya H, Dilbaz N, Okay T, et al. Aripiprazole induced acute myopia: a case report. *Klinik Psikofarmakoloji Bulteni.* 2009;19(suppl 1):147–148.
6. Nair AG, Nair AG, George RJ, et al. Aripiprazole induced transient myopia: A case report and review of literature. *Cutan Ocul Toxicol.* 2012;31(1):74–76.
7. Selvi Y, Atli A, Aydin A, et al. Aripiprazole-related acute transient myopia and diplopia. A case report. *J Clin Psychopharmacol.* 2011;31(2):249–250.
8. Gunes M, Demir S, Bulut M, et al. Acute unilateral myopia induced by add-on aripiprazole: a case report. *Klinik Psikofarmakol Bulteni.* 2016;26(1):68–71.
9. Karadoğ H, Acar M, Özdel K. Aripiprazole induced acute transient bilateral myopia: a case report. *Balkan Med J.* 2015;32(2):230–232.
10. Praveen Kumar KV, Chiranjeevi P, Alam MS. Aripiprazole-induced transient myopia: a rare entity. *Indian J Ophthalmol.* 2018;66(1):130–131.
11. Matsuo M, Sano I, Ikeda Y, et al. Intraoperative floppy-iris syndrome associated with use of antipsychotic drugs. *Can J Ophthalmol.* 2016;51(4):294–296.
12. Shen E, Farukhi S, Schmutz M, et al. Acute angle-closure glaucoma with aripiprazole in the setting of plateau iris configuration. *J Glaucoma.* 2018;27(2):e40–e43.
13. Faure C, Audo I, Zeitz C, et al. *Doc Ophthalmol.* 2015;131:35–41.

Drugs: Chlorpromazine hydrochloride, fluphenazine hydrochloride, perphenazine, prochlorperazine, promethazine hydrochloride, thiethylperazine, thioridazine hydrochloride

1. Isaac NE, Walker AM, Jick H, et al. Exposure to phenothiazine drugs and risk of cataract. *Arch Ophthalmol.* 1991;109(2):256–260.

2. Webber SK, Domniz Y, Sutton GL, et al. Corneal deposition after high-dose chlorpromazine hydrochloride therapy. *Cornea*. 2001;20(2):217–219.

3. Leung AT, Cheng AC, Chan WM, et al. Chlorpromazine-induced refractile corneal deposits and cataract. *Arch Ophthalmol*. 1999;117(12):1662–1663.

4. Siddall JR. Ocular toxic changes associated with chlorpromazine and thioridazine. *Can J E Ophthalmol*. 1966;1(3):190–198.

5. Rasmussen K, Kirk L, Faurbye A. Deposits in the lens and cornea of the eye during long-term chlorpromazine medication. *Acta Psychiatr Scand*. 1976;53(1):1–6.

6. Matsuo M, Sano I, Ikeda Y, et al. Intraoperative floppy-iris syndrome with use of antipsychotic drugs. *Can J Ophthalmol*. 2016;51(4):294–296.

7. Power WJ, Travers SP, Mooney DJ, et al. Welding arc maculopathy and fluphenazine. *Br Ophthalmol*. 1991;75(7):433–455.

8. Lee MS, Fern AI. Fluphenazine and its toxic maculopathy. *Ophthalmic Res*. 2004;36(4):237–239.

9. McCulley TJ, Kersten RC. Periocular inflammation after retrobulbar chlorpromazine (thorazine) injection. *Ophthal Plast Reconst Surg*. 2006;22(4).283–285.

10. Cotliar JM, Shields CL, Meyer DR. Chronic orbital inflammation and fibrosis after retrobulbar alcohol and chlorpromazine injections in a patient with choroidal melanoma. *Ophthal Plast Reconstr Surg*. 2008;24(5):410–411.

11. Hauck MJ, Lee HH, Timoney PJ, et al. Neurotrophic corneal ulcer after retrobulbar injection of chlorpromazine. *Ophthal Plast Reconstr Surg*. 2012;28(3):e74–e76.

12. Kuruvilla R, Sahu PD, Meltzer MA. Systemic update of chlorpromazine after delivery via retrobulbar injection. *Arch Ophthalmol*. 2012;130(10):1348–1349.

13. Scholz RT, Sunness JS. Dark adaptation abnormalities and recovery in acute thioridazine toxicity. *Retin Cases Brief Rep*. 2014;8(1):45–49.

14. Promethazine hydrochloride. 2018. Retrieved from http://www.pdr.net.

15. Kanski JJ. *Clinical Diagnosis in Ophthalmology*. London: Elsevier Mosby; 2006.

Drugs: Clozapine, loxapine, olanzapine

1. Clozapine. 2018. Retrieved from http://www.pdr.net.

2. Gardner DM, Abidi S, Ursuliak Z, et al. Incidence of oculogyric crisis and long-term outcomes with second-generation antipsychotics in a first-episode psychosis program. *J Clin Psychopharmacol*. 2015;35(6):715–718.

3. Rosenhagen MC, Schmidt U, Winkelmann J, et al. Olanzapine-induced oculogyric crisis. *J Clin Psychopharmacol*. 2006;26(4):431.

4. Achiron A, Aviv U, Mendel L, et al. Acute angle closure glaucoma precipitated by olanzapine. *Int J Geriatr Psychiatry*. 2015;30(10):1101–1102.

5. Olanzapine. 2018. Retrieved from http://www.pdr.net.

6. Loxapine. 2018. Retrieved from http://www.pdr.net.

7. Ceylan E, Ozer MD, Yilmaz YC, et al. The ocular surface side effects of an anti-psychotic drug Clozapine. *Cutan Ocul Toxicol*. 2016;35(1):62–66.

8. Balibey H, Balikci A, Ates A. Keratoconjunctivitis sicca due to antipsychotic use. *Eur Psychiatry*. 2013;28(suppl 1):2355.

9. Matsuo M, Sano I, Ikeda Y, et al. Intraoperative floppy-iris syndrome associated with use of antipsychotic drugs. *Can J Ophthalmol*. 2016;51(4):294–296.

10. Choy BN, Ng AL, Shum JW, et al. Anti-psychotic agents related ocular toxicity. *Medicine (Baltimore)*. 2016;95(15):e3360.

11. Alam MS, Praveen Kumar KV. Clozapine-induced cataract in a young female. *J Pharmacol Pharmacother*. 2016;7(4):184–186.

Drugs: Droperidol, haloperidol

1. Droperidol, haloperidol. 2018. Retrieved from http://www.pdr.net.

2. Mendelis PS. *Haldol (haloperidol) hyponatremia*. ADR Highlights; 1981.

3. Nishida K, Ohashi Y, Kinoshita S, et al. Endothelial decompensation in a schizophrenic patient receiving long-term treatment with tranquilizers. *Cornea*. 1992;11(5):475–478.

4. Uchida H, Suzuki T, Watanabe K, et al. Antipsychotic-induced paroxysmal perceptual alteration. *Am J Psychiatr*. 2003;160:2243–2244.

5. Isaac NE, Walker AM, Jick H, et al. Exposure to phenothiazine drugs and risk of cataract. *Arch Ophthalmol*. 1991;109(2):256–260.

6. Honda S. Drug-induced cataract in mentally ill subjects. *Jpn J Clin Ophthalmol*. 1974;28:521.

7. Matsuo M, Sano I, Ikeda Y, et al. Intraoperative floppy-iris syndrome associated with use of antipsychotic drugs. *Can J Ophthalmol*. 2016;51(4):294–296.

Drug: Lithium carbonate

1. Fraunfelder FT, Fraunfelder FW, Jefferson JW. Monograph: the effects of lithium on the human visual system. *J Toxicol Cut Ocular Toxicol*. 1992;11:97–169.

2. Gooding DC, Iacono WG, Katsanis J, et al. The association between lithium carbonate and smooth pursuit eye tracking among first-episode patients with psychotic affective disorders. *Psychophysiology*. 1993;30:3–9.

3. Etminan M, Hemmelgarn B, Delaney JA, et al. Use of lithium and the risk of injurious motor vehicle crash in elderly adults: case-control study nested within a cohort. *BMJ*. 2004;328:895–896.

Drug: Pimozide

1. Pimozide. 2018. Retrieved from http://www.pdr.net.

Drug: Quetiapine fumarate

1. Quetiapine fumarate. 2018. Retrieved from http://www.pdr.net.

2. Valibhai F, Phan NB, Still DJ, et al. Cataracts and quetiapine. *Am J Psychiatry*. 2001;158:966.
3. George M, Haasz M, Coronado A, et al. Acute dyskinesia, myoclonus, and akathisia in an adolescent male abusing quetiapine via nasal insufflation: a case study. *BMC Pediatr*. 2013;13:187.
4. Tan L, Zhou J, Liang B, et al. A case of quetiapine-induced rapid eye movement sleep behavior disorder. *Biol Psychiatry*. 2016;79(5):e11–e12.
5. Rocke JR, O'Day R, Roydhouse TC. Angle closure glaucoma secondary to psychotropic medications. *Australasian Med J*. 2017;10(7):581–586.
6. Bhatziralli IP, Peponis V, Parikakis E, et al. Risk factors for intraoperative floppy iris syndrome: a prospective study. *Eye*. 2016;30(8):1039–1044.
7. Bilgin B, Ilhan D, Cetinkaya A, et al. Intraoperative floppy iris syndrome associated with quetiapine. *Eye*. 2013;27(5):673.
8. Hazra M, Culo S, Mamo D. High-dose quetiapine and photopsia. *J Clin Pyschopharmacol*. 2006;26(5):546–547.
9. Ghosh S, Bhutan D. Oculogyric crisis with quetiapine: a case report. *14th World Congress of Psychiatry*. 2008;894. abstr:P-01–168.
10. Yong KC, Kah TA, Ghee YT, et al. Branch retinal vein occlusion associated with quetiapine fumarate. *BMC Ophthalmol*. 2011;11(1):24.
11. Fraunfelder FW. Twice-yearly exams unnecessary for patients taking quetiapine. *Am J Ophthalmol*. 2004;138:870–871.
12. Gaynes BI. Twice-yearly exams unnecessary for patients taking quetiapine [comment]. *Am J Ophthalmol*. 2005;140:348–349.
13. Fraunfelder FW Twice-yearly exams unnecessary for patients taking quetiapine [author's reply]. *Am J Ophthalmol*. 2005;140:349.

Drug: Risperidone

1. Risperidone. 2018. Retrieved from http://www.pdr.net.
2. Gardner DM, Abidi S, Ursuliak Z, et al. Incidence of oculogyric crisis and long-term outcomes with second-generation antipsychotics in a first-episode psychosis program. *J Clin Psychopharmacol*. 2015;35(6):715–718.
3. Gourzis P, Polychronopoulos P, Argyriou AA, et al. Quetiapine successfully treating oculogyric crisis induced by antipsychotic drugs. *J Clin Neurosci*. 2007;14(4):396–398.
4. Ford RL, Sallam A, Towler HM. Intraoperative floppy iris syndrome associated with risperidone Intake. *Eur J Ophthalmol*. 2011;21(2):210–211.
5. Lau C. Risperidone – or paliperidone-containing products – intraoperative floppy iris syndrome (IFIS) – for healthcare professions. *Internet Document*; 2013. Available from http://healthycanadians.gc.ca.
6. Souza VB, Moura Filho FJ, Souza FG, et al. Cataract occurrence in patients treated with antipsychotic drugs. *Rev Bras Psiquiatr*. 2008;30(3):222–226.
7. Dsouza MC. Could risperidone have caused the cataract?: a case report and review of literature. *J Res Psychiatr Behav Sci*. 2015;1(1):25–26.
8. Laties AM, Flach AJ, Baldycheva I, et al. Cataractogenic potential of quetiapine versus risperidone in the long-term treatment of patients with schizophrenia or schizoaffective disorder: a randomized, open-label, ophthalmologist-masked, flexible-dose, non-inferiority trial. *J psychopharmacol*. 2015;29(1):69–79.
9. US Food and Drug Administration (FDA). *Risperidone and cataract*. Internet Document; 2017. Available from http://www.eheathme.com/ds/risperidone/cataract.

Drug: Thiothixene

1. Thiothixene. 2018. Retrieved from http://www.pdr.net.

Drug: Alcohol (ethanol, ethyl alcohol)

1. Kang HM, Woo YJ, Koh HJ, et al. The effect of consumption of ethanol on subfoveal choroidal thickness in acute phase. *Br J Ophthalmol*. 2016;100(3):383–388.
2. Wang S, Wang JJ, Wong TY. Alcohol and eye disease. *Surv Ophthalmol*. 2008;53(5):512–525.
3. Kanthan GL, Mitchell P, Burlutsky G, et al. Alcohol consumption and the long-term incidence of cataract and cataract surgery: the blue mountain eye study. *Am J Ophthalmol*. 2010;150(3):434–440.
4. Knudtson MD, Klein R, Klein BE. Alcohol consumption and the 15-year cumulative incidence of age-related macular degeneration. *Am J Ophthalmol*. 2007;143(6):1026–1029.
5. Adams MKM, Chong E, Williamson E, et al. 20/20 – alcohol and age-related macular degeneration. *Am J Epidemiol*. 2012;176:289–298.
6. You YS, Qu NB, Yu XN. Alcohol consumption and dry eye syndrome: a Meta-analysis. *Int J Ophthalmol*. 2016;9(10):1487–1492.
7. Kim JH, Kim JH, Nam WH, et al. Oral alcohol administration disturbs tear film and ocular surface. *Ophthalmology*. 2012;119(5):965–971.

Drug: Methanol

1. Naraqi S, Dethlefs RF, Slobodniuk RA, et al. An outbreak of acute methyl alcohol intoxication. *Aust N Z J Med*. 1979;9(1):65–68.
2. Dethlefs R, Naragi S. Ocular manifestations and complications of acute methyl alcohol Intoxication. *Med J Aust*. 1978;4(10):483–485.
3. Zakharov S, Pelclova D, Diblik P, et al. Long-term visual damage after acute methanol poisonings: longitudinal cross-sectional study in 50 patients. *Clin Toxicol (Phila)*. 2015;53(9):884–892.
4. Onder F, Ilker S, Kansu T, et al. Acute blindness and putaminal necrosis in methanol Intoxication. *Int Ophthalmol*. 1998-1999;22(2):81–84.
5. Seme MT, Summerfelt P, Neitz J, et al. Differential recovery of retinal function after mitochondrial inhibition by methanol intoxication. *Invest Ophthalmol Vis Sci*. 2001;42(3):834–841.

6. Moschos MM, Gouliopoulos NS, Rouvas A, et al. Vision loss after accidental methanol intoxication: a case report. *BMC Res Notes.* 2013;6:479.

7. Desai T, Sudhalkar A, Vyas U, et al. Methanol poisoning: predictors of visual outcomes. *JAMA Ophthalmol.* 2013;131(3):358–364.

8. Bansal H, Chaparia Y, Agrawal A, et al. Reversal of methanol-induced blindness in adults by autologous bone marrow-derived stem cells: a case series. *J Stem Cells.* 2015;10(2):127–139.

Drugs: Fesoterodine fumarate, solifenacin succinate, oxybutynin chloride

1. Oxybutynin chloride. 2018. Retrieved from http://www.pdr.net.

2. Solifenacin succinate. 2018. Retrieved from http://www.pdr.net.

3. Altan-Yaycioglu R, Yaycioglu O, Aydin Akova Y, et al. Ocular side-effects of tolterodine and oxybutynin, a single-blind prospective randomize trial. *Br J Clin Pharmacol.* 2005;59(5):588–592.

4. Acar DE, Acar U, Ozdemir O, et al. The short-term and long term adverse ocular effects of fesoterodine fumarate. *Cutan Ocul Toxicol.* 2016;35(3):181–184.

5. Sung VC, Corridan PG. Acute-angle closure glaucoma as a side effect of oxybutynin. *Br J Urol.* 1998;81(4):634–635.

6. Wong EY, Harding A, Kowal L. Oxybutynin-associated esotropia. *J AAPOS.* 2007;11(6):624–625.

7. Sekeroglu MA, Hekimoglu E, Tasci Y, et al. Ocular surface changes following oral anticholinergic use for overactive bladder. *Cutan Ocul Toxicol.* 2016;35(3):218–221.

Drugs: Dronabinol (tetrahydrocannabinol, THC), hashish, marihuana (marijuana, cannabis)

1. Dronabinol. 2018. Retrieved from http://www.pdr.net.

2. Levi L, Miller NR. Visual illusions associated with previous drug abuse. *F Clin Neuro-ophthalmol.* 1990;10:103–110.

3. Laffi GL, Safran AB. Persistent visual changes following hashish consumption. *Br J Ophthalmol.* 1993;77:601–602.

4. Steinmetz AB, Edwards CR, Vollmer JM, et al. Examining the effects of former cannabis use on cerebellum-dependent eyeblink conditioning in humans. *Psychopharmacol.* 2012;221(1):133–141.

5. Kowal MA, Colzato LS, Hommel B. Decreased spontaneous eye blink rates in chronic cannabis users: evidence for striatal cannabinoid-dopamine interactions. *PLoS ONE.* 2011;6(11):e26662.

6. Semple DM, Ramsden F, McIntosh AM. Reduced binocular depth inversion in regular cannabis users. *Pharmacol Biochem Behav.* 2003;25:789–793.

7. Huestegge L, Kunert HJ, Radach R. Long-term effects of cannabis on eye movement control reading. *Psychopharmacol.* 2010;209(1):77–84.

8. Polat N, Cumurcu B, Cumurcu T, et al. Corneal endothelial changes in long-term cannabinoid users. *Cutan Ocul Toxicol.* 2018;37(1):19–23.

9. Schwitzer T, Schwan R, Albuisson E, et al. Association between regular cannabis use and ganglion cell dysfunction. *JAMA Ophthalmol.* 2017;135(1):54–60.

10. Lyons CJ, Robson AG. *JAMA Ophthalmol.* 2017;135(1):60–61.

Drugs: Lysergic acid diethylamide (LSD), lysergide, mescaline, psilocybin

1. Halpern JH, Pope HG. Hallucinogen persisting perception disorder: what do we know after 50 years? *Drug Alcohol Depend.* 2003;69:109–119.

2. Abraham HD. A chronic impairment of colour vision in users of LSD. *Br J Psychiatry.* 1982;140:518–520.

3. Kawasaki A, Purvin V. Persistent palinopsia following ingestion of lysergic acid diethylamide (LSD). *Arch Ophthalmol.* 1996;114:47–50.

4. Lo D, Cobbs L, Chua M, et al. "Eye Dropping" – a case report of transconjunctival lysergic acid diethylamide drug abuse. *Cornea.* 2018;37(10):1324–1325.

Drug: Phencyclidine

1. Cox D, Jufer Phipps RA, Levine B, et al. Distribution of phencyclidine into vitreous humor. *J Anal Toxicol.* 2007;31(8):537–539.

Drugs: Amobarbital, butabarbital sodium, butalbital, methohexital sodium, methylphenobarbital (mephobarbital), pentobarbital sodium, phenobarbital, primidone, secobarbital sodium

1. Hamburger E. Identification and treatment of barbiturate abusers. *JAMA.* 1965;193:143–144.

2. Homma K, Wakakura M, Ishikawa S. A case of phenobarbital-induced optic neuropathy. *Neuroophthalmology.* 1989;9(6):357–359.

3. Marino D, Malandrini A, Rocchi R, et al. Transient "sicca syndrome" during phenobarbital treatment. *Neurol Sci.* 2011;300(1–2):164.

Drug: Chloral hydrate

1. West SK, Griffiths B, Shariff Y, et al. Utilisation of an outpatient sedation unit in paediatric ophthalmology: safety and effectiveness of chloral hydrate in 1509 sedation episodes. *Br J Ophthalmol.* 2013;97(11):1437–1442.

2. Burnett HF, Lambley R, West SK, et al. Cost-effectiveness analysis of clinic-based chloral hydrate sedation versus general anaesthesia for paediatrtic ophthalmological procedures. *Br J Ophthalmol.* 2015;99(11):1565–1570.

3. Wilson ME, Karaoui M, Al Djasim L, et al. The safety and efficacy of chloral hydrate sedation for pediatric ophthalmic procedures: a retrospective review. *J Pediatr Ophthalmol Strabismus.* 2014;51(3):154–159.

FURTHER READING

Gabapentin

Boneva N, Brenner T, Argov Z. Gabapentin may be hazardous in myasthenia gravis. *Muscle Nerve.* 2000;23:1204–1208.

Goa KL, Sorkin EM. Gabapentin. A review of its pharmacological properties and clinical potential in epilepsy. *Drugs*. 1993;46(3):409–427.

Scheschonka A, Beuche W. Treatment of post-herpetic pain in myasthenia gravis: exacerbation of weakness due to gabapentin. *Pain*. 2003;104:423–424.

Lamotrigine

Goa KL, Ross SR, Chrisp P. Lamotrigine. *Drugs*. 1993;46:152–176.

Kolomeyer AM, Kodati S. Lamotrigine-induced tubulointerstitial nephritis and uveitis-atypical Cogan syndrome. *Eur J Ophthalmol*. 2016;26(1):e14–e16.

Lee AR, Sharma S, Mahmoud TH. Tubulointerstitial nephritis and uveitis syndrome with a primary presentation of acute posterior multifocal placoid epitheliopathy. *Retin Cases Brief Rep*. 2017;11(2):100–103.

Woodcock IR, Taylor LE, Ruddle JB, et al. Acute bilateral myopia caused by lamotrigine-induced uveal effusions. *J Paediatr Child Health*. 2017;53(10):1013–1014.

Pregabalin

Ekinci AS, Ciftci S, Cavus B, et al. Could pregabalin cause oculomotor symptoms in lower dose? A case with down beat nystagmus as a side effect. *Acta Neurol Belg*. 2017;117(3):777–778.

Hounnou P, Nicoucar K. Delayed onset of rotary self-motion perception, dysdiadochokinesia and disturbed eye pursuit caused by low-dose pregabalin. *BMJ Case Rep*. 2014;2014.

Parsons B, Sanin L, Yang R, et al. Efficacy and safety of pregabalin in patients with spinal cord injury: a pooled analysis. *Curr Med Res Opin*. 2013;29(12):1675–1683.

Vigabatrin

Blackwell N, Hayllar J, Kelly G. Severe persistent visual field constriction associated with vigabatrin. Patients taking vigabatrin should have regular visual field testing (letter, comment). *BMJ*. 1997;314:180–181.

Fecarotta CM. Vigabatrin and visual field loss in children. *Rev Ophthalmol*. 2014.

Harding GF. Severe persistent visual field constriction associated with vigabatrin. *BMJ*. 1998;316:232–233.

Koul R, Chacko A, Ganesh A, et al. Vigabatrin associated retinal dysfunction in children with Epilepsy. *Arch Dis Child*. 2001;85:469–473.

Mackenzie R, Klistorner A. Severe persistent visual field constriction associated with vigabatrin. Asymptomatic as well as symptomatic defects occur with vigabatrin (letter; comment). *BMJ*. 1998;314:233.

Nousiainin I, Kalviainen R, Mantyjarvi M. Color vision in epilepsy patients treated with vigabatrin or carbamazepine monotherapy. *Ophthalmology*. 2000;107:884–888.

Origlieri C, Geddie B, Karwoski B, et al. Optical coherence tomography to monitor vigabatrin toxicity in children. *J AAPOS*. 2016;20(2):136–140.

Riikonen R, Rener-Primec Z, Carmant L, et al. Does vigabatrin treatment for infantile spasms cause visual field defects?

An international mulicentre study. *Dev Med Child Neurol*. 2015;57(1):60–67.

Westall CA, Wright T, Cortese F, et al. Vigabatrin retinal toxicity in children with infantile spasms: an observational cohort study. *Neurology*. 2014;83(24):2262–2268.

Wright T, Kumarappah A, Stavropoulos A, et al. Vigabatrin toxicity in infancy is associated with retinal defect in adolescence: a prospective observational study. *Retina*. 2017;37(5):858–866.

Amfetamine (amphetamine), dextroamfetamine sulfate (dexamphetamine), methamfetamine hydrochloride (methamphetamine)

Acute drug abuse reactions. *Med Lett Drugs Ther*. 1985;27:77.

D'Souza T, Shraberg D. Intracranial hemorrhage associated with amphetamine use. *Neurology*. 1981;31:922–923.

Kim YT, Kwon DH, Chang Y. Impairments of facial emotion recognition and theory of mind in methamphetamine users. *Psychiatry Res*. 2011;186(1):80–84.

Limaye SR, Goldberg MH. Septic submacular choroidal embolus associated with intravenous drug abuse. *Ann Ophthalmol*. 1982;14:518–522.

Lowe T, Cohen DJ, Detlor J. Stimulant medications precipitate Tourette's syndrome. *JAMA*. 1982;247:1729–1731.

Rouher F, Cantat MA. Anorexic medications and retinal venous thromboses. *Bull Soc Ophtalmol Fr*. 1962;62:65–71.

Smart JV, Sneddon JM, Turner P. A comparison of the effects of chlorphentermine, diethylpropion, and phenmetrazine on critical flicker frequency. *Br J Pharmacol*. 1967;30:307–316.

Vesterhauge S, Peitersen E. The effects of some drugs on the caloric induced nystagmus. *Adv Otorhinolaryngol*. 1979;25:173–177.

Yung A, Agnew K, Snow J, et al. Two unusual cases of toxic epidermal necrolysis. *Australas J Dermatol*. 2002;43:35–38.

Benzfetamine hydrochloride (benzphetamine), diethylpropionate hydrochloride (amfepramone), phendimetrazine tartrate, phentermine hydrochloride

Chan JW. Acute nonarteritic ischaemic optic neuropathy after phentermine. *Eye*. 2005;19:1238–1239.

Smart JV, Sneddon JM, Turner P. A comparison of the effects of chlorphentermine, diethylpropion, and phenmetrazine on critical flicker frequency. *Br J Pharmacol*. 1967;30:307–316.

Alprazolam, chlordiazepoxide, clonazepam, clorazepate dipotassium, diazepam, flurazepam hydrochloride, lorazepam, midazolam hydrochloride, oxazepam, temazepam, triazolam

Berlin RM, Conell LJ. Withdrawal symptoms after long-term treatment with therapeutic doses of flurazepam: a case report. *Am J Psychiatry*. 1983;140:488–490.

Gatzonis Karadimas P, Gatzonis Bouzas EA. Clonazepam associated retinopathy. *Eur J Ophthalmol*. 2003;13:813–815.

Laegreid L, Olegård R, Walström J, et al. Teratogenic effects of benzodiazepine use during Pregnancy. *J Pediatr*. 1989;114:126–131.

Laroche J, Laroche C. Modification of colour vision. *Ann Pharm Fr.* 1977;35(5–6):173–179.

Lutz EG. Allergic conjunctivitis due to diazepam. *Am J Psychiatry.* 1975;132(5):548.

Marttila JK, Hammel RJ, Alexander B, et al. Potential untoward effects of long-term use of flurazepam in geriatric patients. *J Am Pharm Assoc.* 1977;17:692–695.

Nelson LB, Ehrlich S, Calhoun JH, et al. Occurrence of strabismus in infants born to drug-dependent women. *Am J Dis Child.* 1987;141:175–178.

Noyes Jr R, Clancy J, Coryell WH, et al. A withdrawal syndrome after abrupt discontinuation of alprazolam. *Am J Psychiatry.* 1985;142:114–116.

Sandyk R. Orofacial dyskinesia associated with lorazepam therapy. *Clin Pharm.* 1986;5:419–421.

Tyrer PJ, Seivewright N. Identification and management of benzodiazepine dependence. *Postgrad Med J.* 1984;60(suppl 2):41–46.

Vital-Herne J, Brenner R, Lesser M. Another case of alprazolam withdrawal syndrome. *Am J Psychiatry.* 1985;142:1515.

Watanabe Y, Kawada A, Ohnishi Y, et al. Photosensitivity due to alprazolam with positive oral photochallenge test after 17 days administration. *J Am Acad Dermatol.* 1999;40.832–833.

Carisoprodol, meprobamate

Barret LG, Vincent FM, Arsac PL, et al. Internuclear ophthalmoplegia in patients with toxic coma. Frequency, prognostic value, diagnostic significance. *J Toxicol Clin Toxicol.* 1983;20:373–379.

Edwards JG. Adverse effects of antianxiety drugs. *Drugs.* 1981;22:495–514.

Hermans G. Les Psychotropes. *Bull Soc Belge Ophtalmol.* 1972;160:15–85.

Divalproex sodium (valproate semisodium), valproate sodium, valproic acid

Bayer AU, Thiel HJ, Zrenner E, et al. Color vision tests for early detection of antiepileptic drug toxicity. *Neurology.* 1997;48(5):1394–1397.

Bellman MH, Ross EM. Side effects of sodium valproate. *BMJ.* 1977;1:1662.

Gosala Raja Kukkuta S, Srinivas M, Raghunandan N, et al. Reversible vertical gaze palsy in sodium valproate toxicity. *J Neuroophthalmol.* 2013;33(2):202–203.

McMahon CL, Braddock SR. Septo-optic dysplasia as a manifestation of valproic acid embryopathy. *Teratology.* 2001;64:83–86.

Scullica L, Trombetta CJ, Tuccari G. Toxic effect of valproic acid on the retina. Clinical and experimental investigation. In: Blodi F, et al., ed. *Acta XXV Concilium Ophthalmologicum. Proceedings of the XXVth International Congress of Ophthalmology.* Vol. 2. Rome: Kugler & Ghedini Publishers; 1986.

Uddin S. Drug-induced pseudotumor cerebri. *Clin Neuropharmacol.* 2003;26:236–238.

Yang CY, Dao RL, Lee TJ, et al. Severe cutaneous adverse reactions to antiepileptic drugs in Asians. *Neurology.* 2011;77(23):2025–2033.

Ethosuximide, methsuximide

Alarcón-Segovia D. Drug-induced antinuclear antibodies and lupus syndrome. *Drugs.* 1976;12:69–77.

Beghi E, DiMascio R, Tognoni G. Adverse effects of anticonvulsant drugs – a critical review. *Adverse Drug React Acute Poisoning Rev.* 1986;5:63–86.

Drugs for epilepsy. *Med Lett Drugs Ther.* 1983;25:83.

Millichap JG. Anticonvulsant drugs. Clinical and electroencephalographic indications, efficacy and toxicity. *Postgrad Med.* 1965;37:22–34.

Taaffe A, O'Brien C. A case of Stevens-Johnson syndrome associated with the anti-convulsants sulthiame and ethosuximide. *Br Dent J.* 1975;138:172–174.

Ethotoin

Alarcón-Segovia D. Drug-induced antinuclear antibodies and lupus syndromes. *Drugs.* 1976;12:69–77.

Hermans G. Les anticonvulsivants. *Bull Soc Belge Ophtalmol.* 1972;160:89–96.

Phenytoin

Bartoshesky LE, Bhan I, Nagpaul K, et al. Severe cardiac and ophthalmologic malformations in an infant exposed to diphenylhydantoin in utero. *Pediatrics.* 1982;69:202–203.

Bayer A, Thiel HJ, Zrenner E, et al. Sensitive physiologic perceptual tests for ocular side effects of drugs exemplified by various anticonvulsants. *Pediatrics.* 1995;92(2):182–190.

Bayer A, Zrenner E, Thiel HJ, et al. *Retinal disorders induced by anticonvulsant drugs.* Sedona, Arizona: Third Congress International Society of Ocular Toxicology; 1992:11.

Boles DM. Phenytoin ophthalmoplegia. *S Afr Med J.* 1984;65:546.

Glover SJ, Quinn AG, Barter P, et al. Ophthalmic findings in fetal anticonvulsant syndrome. *Ophthalmology.* 2002;109:942–947.

Herishanu Y, Osimani A, Louzoun Z. Unidirectional gaze paretic nystagmus induced by phenytoin intoxication. *Am J Ophthalmol.* 1982;94:122–123.

Kalanie H, Niakan E, Harati Y, et al. Phenytoin-induced intracranial hypertension. *Neurology.* 1986;36:443.

Lachapelle P, Blain L, Quigley MG, et al. The effect of diphenylhydantoin on the electroretinogram. *Doc Ophthalmol.* 1990;73:359–368.

Puri V, Chaudhry N. Total external ophthalmoplegia induced by phenytoin: a case report and review of literature. *Neurol India.* 2004;52:386–387.

Rizzo M, Corbett J. Bilateral internuclear ophthalmoplegia reversed by naloxone. *Arch Neurol.* 1983;40:242–243.

Shores MM, Sloan KL. Phenytoin-induced visual disturbances misdiagnosed as alcohol withdrawal. *Psychosomatics.* 2002;43:336–355.

Wittbrodt ET. Drugs and myasthenia gravis: an update. *Arch Intern Med.* 1997;157:399–408.

Topiramate

Chen TC, Chao CW, Sorkin JA. Topiramate induced myopic shift and angle closure glaucoma. *Br J Ophthalmol.* 2003;87:648–649.

DaCosta J, Younis S. Topiramate-induced maculopathy in IgG4-related disease. *Drug Health Patient Saf.* 2016;8:59–63.

Dhar SK, Sharma V, Kapoor G, et al. Topiramate induced bilateral anterior uveitis with choroidal detachment and angle closure glaucoma. *Med J Armed Forces India.* 2015;71(1):88–91.

Hulihan J. *Important drug warning [letter]*; 2003. Retrieved from: http://www.fda.gov/medwatch/SAFETY/2001/topamax_deardoc.PDF.

Mansoor Q, Jain S. Bilateral angle-closure glaucoma following oral topiramate therapy. *Acta Ophthalmol Scand.* 2005;83:627–628.

Medeiros FA, Zhang XY, Bernd AS, et al. Angle-closure glaucoma associated with ciliary body detachment in patients using topiramate. *Arch Ophthalmol.* 2003;121:282–284.

Rapoport Y, Benegas N, Kuchtey RW, et al. Acute myopia and angle closure glaucoma from topiramate in a seven-year-old: a case report and review of the literature. *BMC Pediatr.* 2014;14:96.

Sakai H, Morine-Shiniyo S, Shinzato M, et al. Uveal effusion in primary angle-closure glaucoma. *Ophthalmology.* 2005;112:413–419.

Sankar PS, Pasquale LR, Grosskreutz CL. Uveal effusion and secondary angle-closure glaucoma associated with topiramate use. *Arch Ophthalmol.* 2001;119:1210–1211.

Sen HA, O'Halloran HS, Lee WB. Topiramate-induced acute myopia and retinal striae. *Arch Ophthalmol.* 2001;119:775–777.

Thambi L, Leonard KP, Chambers W, et al. Topiramate-associated secondary angle-closure glaucoma: a case series. *Arch Ophthalmol.* 2002;120:1108.

Yeung TL, Li PS, Li KK. Presumed topiramate retinopathy: a case report. *J Med Case Rep.* 2016;10:210.

Zhao K, Spiegel JH. Topiramate-induced unilateral ptosis. *Otolaryngol – Head Neck Surg.* 2012;147(suppl 2):P130.

Zonisamide

Majeres KD, Suppes TA. Cautionary note when using zonisamide in youths: a case report of association with toxic epidermal necrolysis. *J Clin Psychiatry.* 2004;65:1720.

Amitriptyline hydrochloride, clomipramine hydrochloride, doxepin hydrochloride, trimipramine maleate

Beal MF. Amitriptyline ophthalmoplegia. *Neurology.* 1982;32:1409.

Botter PA, Sunier A. The treatment of depression in geriatrics with Anafranil. *J Int Med Res.* 1975;3:345.

Delaney P, Light R. Gaze paresis in amitriptyline overdose. *Ann Neurol.* 1981;9:513.

Donhowe SP. Bilateral internuclear ophthalmoplegia from doxepin overdose. *Neurology.* 1984;34:259.

Horstl H, Pohlmann-Eden B. Amplitudes of somatosensory evoked potentials reflect cortical hyperexcitability in antidepressant-induced myoclonus. *Neurology.* 1990;40:924–926.

Hotson JR, Sachdev HS. Amitriptyline: another cause of internuclear ophthalmoplegia with coma. *Ann Neurol.* 1982;12:62.

Hughes IW. Adverse reactions in perspective, with special reference to gastrointestinal side-effects of clomipramine (Anafranil). *J Int Med Res.* 1973;1:440.

LeWitt PA. Transient ophthalmoparesis with doxepin overdosage. *Ann Neurol.* 1981;9:618.

Schenck CH, Mahowald MW, Kim SW, et al. Prominent eye movements during NREM sleep and REM sleep behavior disorder associated with fluoxetine treatment of depression and obsessive-compulsive disorder. *Sleep.* 1992;15(3):226–235.

Spector RH, Schnapper R. Amitriptyline-induced ophthalmoplegia. *Neurology.* 1981;31:1188–1190.

Amoxapine, desipramine hydrochloride, imipramine hydrochloride, nortriptyline hydrochloride

Barnes FF. Precipitation of mania and visual hallucinations by amoxapine hydrochloride. *Compr Psychiatry.* 1982;23:590–592.

Hunt-Fugate AK, Zander J, Lesar TS. Adverse reactions due to dopamine blockade by amoxapine. *Pharmacotherapy.* 1984;4:35–39.

Karson CN. Oculomotor signs in a psychiatric population: a preliminary report. *Am J Psychiatry.* 1979;136:1057–1060.

Pulst SM, Lombroso CT. External ophthalmoplegia, alpha and spindle coma in imipramine overdose: case report and review of the literature. *Ann Neurol.* 1983;14:587–590.

Steele TE. Adverse reactions suggesting amoxapine-induced dopamine blockade. *Am J Psychiatry.* 1982;139:1500–1501.

Von Knorring L. Changes in saliva secretion and accommodation width during short-term administration of imipramine and zimelidine in healthy volunteers. *Int Pharmacopsych.* 1981;16:69–78.

Vonvoigtlander PF, Kolaja GJ, Block EM. Corneal lesions induced by antidepressants: a selective effect upon young Fischer 344 rats. *J Pharmacol Exp Ther.* 1982;222:282–286.

Walter-Ryan WG, Kern 3rd EE, Shirriff JR, et al. Persistent photoaggravated cutaneous eruption induced by imipramine. *JAMA.* 1985;254:357–358.

Atomoxetine, duloxetine, venlafaxine hydrochloride

Gonzalez-Martin-Moro J, Gonzalez-Lopez JJ, Zarallo-Gallardo J, et al. Intraoperative floppy iris syndrome after treatment with duloxetine: coincidence, association, or causality? *Arch Soc Esp Oftalmol.* 2015;90(2):94–96.

McInnis CP, Haynor DR, Francis CE. Horner syndrome in fibromuscular dysplasia without carotid dissection. *Can J Ophthalmol.* 2016;51(2):e53–e55.

Bupropion hydrochloride

Fayyazi Bordbar MR, Jafarzadeh M. Bupropion-induced diplopia in an Iranian patient. *Iran J Psychiatry Behav Sci.* 2011;5(2):136–138.

Kojima G, Tamai A, Karino S, et al. Bupropion-related visual hallucinations in a veteran with posttraumatic stress disorder and multiple sclerosis. *J Clin Psychopharmacol.* 2013;33(5):717–719.

Korkmaz S. Visual hallucinations associated with bupropion use: a case report. *Klinik Psikofarmakologi Bulteni.* 2012;22(2):187–189.

Carbamazepine, oxcarbazepine

Atalay E, Tamcelik N, Capar O. High intraocular pressure after carbamazepine and gabapentin intake in a pseudoexfoliative patient. *J Glaucoma.* 2014;23(8):574–576.

Bayer A, Thiel HJ, Zrenner E, et al. Disorders of color perception and increased glare sensitivity in phenytoin and carbamazepine therapy: Ocular side effects of anticonvulsants. *Nervenarzt.* 1995;66:89–96.

Breathnach SM, McGibbon DH, Ive FA, et al. Carbamazepine ("Tegretol") and toxic epidermal necrolysis: report of three cases with histopathological observations. *Clin Exp Dermatol.* 1982;7:585–591.

Chan KCY, Sachdev N, Wells AP. Bilateral acute angle closure secondary to uveal effusions associated with flucloxacillin and carbamazepine. *Br J Ophthalmol.* 2008;92(3):428–430.

Chang YS, Huang FC, Tseng SH, et al. Erythema multiforme, Stevens-Johnson syndrome, and toxic epidermal necrolysis: acute ocular manifestations, causes and management. *Cornea.* 2007;26(2):123–129.

Chrousos GA, Cowdry R, Schuelein M, et al. Two cases of downbeat nystagmus and oscillopsia associated with carbamazepine. *Am J Ophthalmol.* 1987;103:221–224.

Delafuente JC. Drug-induced erythema multiforme: a possible immunologic pathogenesis. *Drug Intell Clin Pharm.* 1985;19:114–117.

Goldman MJ, Shultz-Ross RA. Adverse ocular effects of anticonvulsants. *Psychosomatics.* 1993;34:154–158.

Gualtieri CT, Evans RW. Carbamazepine-induced tics. *Dev Med Child Neurol.* 1984;26:546–548.

Kinoshita A, Kitaoka T, Oba K, et al. Bilateral drug-induced cataract in patient receiving anticonvulsant therapy. *Jpn J Ophthalmol.* 2004;48:81–82.

Kulkantrakorn K, Tassaneeyakul W, Tiamkao S, et al. HLA-B* 1502 strongly predicts carbamazepine-induced Stevens-Johnson syndrome and toxic epidermal necrolysis in Thai patients with neuropathic pain. *Pain Pract.* 2012;12(3):202–208.

Kurian MA, King MD. Antibody positive myasthenia gravis following treatment with carbamazepine – a chance association? *Neuropediatrics.* 2003;34:276–277.

Mullally WJ. Carbamazepine-induced ophthalmoplegia. *Arch Neurol.* 1982;39:64.

Noda S, Umezaki H. Carbamazepine-induced ophthalmoplegia. *Neurology.* 1982;32:1320.

Ponte CD. Carbamazepine-induced thrombocytopenia, rash and hepatic dysfunction. *Drug Intel Clin Pharm.* 1983;17:642–644.

Rasmussen M. Carbamazepine and myasthenia gravis. *Neuropediatrics.* 2004;35:259.

Silverstein FS, Parrish MA, Johnston MV. Adverse behavioral reactions in children treated with carbamazepine (Tegretol). *J Pediatr.* 1982;101:785–787.

Smith H, Newton R. Adverse reactions to carbamazepine managed by desensitization. *Lancet.* 1985;1:785.

Sullivan JB, Rumack BH, Peterson RG. Acute carbamazepine toxicity resulting from overdose. *Neurology.* 1981;31:621–624.

Tedeschi G, Gasucci G, Allocca S, et al. Neuro-ocular side effects of carbamazepine and phenobarbital in epileptic patients as measured by saccadic eye movements analysis. *Epilepsia.* 1989;30(1):62–66.

West J, Burke JP, Stachan I. Carbamazepine, epilepsy, and optic nerve hypoplasia. *Br J Ophthalmol.* 1990;74:511.

Wheller SD, Ramsey RE, Weiss J. Drug-induced downbeat nystagmus. *Ann Neurol.* 1982;12:227–228.

Yang CY, Dao RL, Lee TJ, et al. Severe cutaneous adverse reactions to antiepileptic drugs in Asians. *Neurology.* 2011;77(23).2025–2033.

Citalopram hydrobromide, escitalopram oxalate, fluoxetine hydrochloride, fluvoxamine maleate, paroxetine hydrochloride, sertraline hydrochloride

Anonymous. SSRIs and increased intraocular pressure. *Aust Adverse Drug React Bull.* 2001;20:3.

Arias Palomero A, Infantes Molina EJ, Lopez Arroquia E, et al. Uveal effusion induced by escitalopram. *Arch Soc Esp Oftalmol.* 2015;90(7):327–330.

Beasley CM, Koke SC, Nilsson ME, et al. Adverse events and treatment discontinuations in clinical trials of fluoxetine in major depressive disorder: an updated meta-analysis. *Clin Ther.* 2000;22:1319–1330.

Cunningham M, Cunningham K, Lydiard RB. Eye tics and subjective hearing impairment during fluoxetine therapy. *Am J Psychiatry.* 1990;147:947–948.

Heiligenstein JH, Faries DE, Rush AJ, et al. Latency to rapid eye movement sleep as a predictor of treatment response to fluoxetine and placebo in non-psychotic depressed outpatients. *Psychiatry Res.* 1994;52(3):327–329.

Holguin-Lew JC. "When I want to cry I can't": inability to cry following SSRI treatment. *Rev Colomb Psiquiatr.* 2013;42(4):304–310.

Ozkul Y, Bozlar S. Effects of Fluoxetine on habituation of pattern reversal visually evoked potentials in migraine prophylaxis. *Headache.* 2002;42:582–587.

Isocarboxazid, phenelzine sulfate, tranylcypromine sulfate

Drugs for psychiatric disorders. *Med Lett Drugs Ther.* 1983;25:45.

Drugs that cause photosensitivity. *Med Lett Drugs Ther.* 1986;28:51.

Kaeser HE. Drug-induced myasthenic syndromes. *Acta Neurol Scand.* 1984;70(suppl 100):39–47.

Kaplan RF, Feinglass NG, Webster W, et al. Phenelzine overdose treated with dantrolene sodium. *JAMA.* 1986;255(5):642–644.

Shader RI, Greenblatt DJ. The reappearance of a monoamine oxidase inhibitor. *J Clin Psychopharmacol.* 1999;19(2):105–106.

Thomann P, Hess R. Toxicology of antidepressant drugs. *Handb Exp Pharmacol.* 1980;55:527.

Weaver KE. Amoxapine overdose. *J Clin Psychiatry.* 1985;46:545.

Zaratzian VL. Psychotropic drugs – neurotoxicity. *Clin Toxicol.* 1980;17:231–270.

Maprotiline hydrochloride

Albala AA, Weinberg N, Allen SM. Maprotiline-induced hypnopompic hallucinations. *J Clin Psychiatry.* 1983;44(4):149–150.

Forstl H, Pohlmann-Eden B. Amplitudes of somatosensory evoked potentials reflect cortical hyperexcitability in antidepressant-induced myoclonus. *Neurology.* 1990;40(6):924–926.

Oakley AM, Hodge L. Cutaneous vasculitis from maprotiline. *Aust NZJ Med.* 1985;15(2):256–257.

Park J, Proudfoot AT. Acute poisoning with maprotiline hydrochloride. *BMJ.* 1977;1(6076):1573.

Methylphenidate hydrochloride

Acute drug abuse reactions. *Med Lett Drugs Ther.* 1985;27:77.

Bluth LL, Hanscom TA. Retinal detachment and vitreous hemorrhages due to talc emboli. *JAMA.* 1981;246:980.

Bucci MP, Stordeur C, Septier M, et al. Oculomotor abnormalities in children with attention-deficit/hyperactivity disorder are improved by methylphenidate. *J Child Adolesc Psychopharmacol.* 2017;27(3):274–280.

Gross-Tsur V, Joseph A, Shalev RS. Hallucinations during methylphenidate therapy. *Neurology.* 2004;63:753–754.

Gunby P. Methylphenidate abuse produces retinopathy. *JAMA.* 1979;241:546.

James ER. The etiology of steroid cataract. *J Ocul Pharmacol Ther.* 2007;23:403–420.

Lederer Jr CM, Sabates FN. Ocular findings in the intravenous drug abuser. *Ann Ophthalmol.* 1982;14:436–438.

Methylphenidate (Ritalin) and other drugs for treatment of hyperactive children. *Med Lett Drugs Ther.* 1977;19:53.

Porfirio MC, Giana G, Giovinazzo S, et al. Methylphenidate-induced visual hallucinations. *Neuropediatrics.* 2011;42(1):30–31.

Schoenberger SD, Argarwal A. Images in clinical medicine. Talc retinopathy. *N Engl J Med.* 2013;368(9):852.

Tse DT, Ober RR. Talc retinopathy. *Am J Ophthalmol.* 1980;90:624–640.

Trazodone hydrochloride

Ban TA, Lehmann HE, Amin M, et al. Comprehensive clinical studies with trazodone. *Curr Ther Res.* 1973;15:540–551.

Damlouji NF, Ferguson JM. Trazodone-induced delirium in bulimic patients. *Am J Psychiatry.* 1984;141:434–435.

Ford HE, Jenike MA. Erythema multiforme associated with trazodone therapy: case report. *J Clin Psychiatry.* 1985;46:294–295.

Hassan E, Miller DD. Toxicity and elimination of trazodone after overdose. *Clin Pharm.* 1985;4:97–100.

Kraft TB. Psychosis following trazodone administration. *Am J Psychiatry.* 1983;140:1383–1384.

Rongioletti F, Rebora A. Drug eruption from trazodone. *J Am Acad Dermatol.* 1986;14:274–275.

Fingolimod

Tedesco-Silva H, Pescovitz MD, Cibrik D, et al. FTY720 Study Group. Randomized controlled trial of FTY720 vs MMF in de novo renal transplantation. *Transplantation.* 2006;82(12):1689–1697.

Aripiprazole

Keck PE, Calabrese JR, McQuade RD, et al. A randomized, double-blind, placebo-controlled 26-week trial of aripiprazole in recently manic patients with bipolar I disorder. *J Clin Psychiatry.* 2006;67(4):626–637.

Mazza M, Squillacioti MR, Pecora RD, et al. Beneficial acute antidepressant effects of aripiprazole as an adjunctive treatment or monotherapy in bipolar patients unresponsive to mood stabilizers: results from a 16-week open-label trial. *Expert Opin Pharmacother.* 2008;9(18):3145–3149.

Chlorpromazine hydrochloride, fluphenazine hydrochloride, perphenazine, prochlorperazine, promethazine hydrochloride, thiethylperazine, thioridazine hydrochloride

Ball WA, Caroff SN. Retinopathy, tardive dyskinesia and low-dose thioridazine. *Am J Psychiatry.* 1986;143(2):256–257.

Cook FF, Davis RG, Russo Jr LS. Internuclear ophthalmoplegia caused by phenothiazine Intoxication. *Arch Neurol.* 1981;38(7):465–466.

Deluise VP, Flynn JT. Asymmetric anterior segment changes induced by chlorpromazine. *Ann Ophthalmol.* 1981;13(8):953–955.

Eicheubaum JW, D'Amico RA. Corneal injury by a thorazine spansule. *Ann Ophthalmol.* 1981;13(2):199–200.

Hamilton JD. Thioridazine retinopathy within the upper dosage limit. *Psychosomatics.* 1985;26(10):823–824.

Kaeser HE. Drug-induced myasthenic syndromes. *Acta Neurol Scand.* 1984;70(suppl 100):39–47.

Lam RW, Remick RA. Pigmentary retinopathy associated with low-dose thioridazine treatment. *Can Med Assoc J.* 1985;132(7):737.

Marmor HF. Is thioridazine retinopathy progressive? Relationship of pigmentary changes to visual function. *Br J Ophthalmol.* 1990;74(12):739–742.

Miyata M, Imai H, Ishikawa S, et al. Changes in human electroretinography associated with thioridazine administration. *Acta Ophthalmol.* 1980;181:175–180.

Ngen CC, Singh P. Long-term phenothiazine administration and the eye in 100 Malaysians. *Br J Psychiatry.* 1988;152:278–281.

Phua YS, Patel DV, McGhee CN. In vivo confocal microstructural analysis of corneal endothelial changes in a patient on long-term chlorpromazine therapy. *Graefes Arch Clin Exp Ophthalmol*. 2005;243(7):721–723.

Toshida H, Uesugi Y, Ebihara N, et al. In vivo observations of a case of chlorpromazine deposits in the cornea using an HRT II rostock corneal module. *Cornea*. 2007;26(9):1141–1143.

Clozapine, loxapine, olanzapine

Arora T, Maharshi V, Rehan HS, et al. Blepharospasm: an uncommon adverse effect caused by long-term administration of olanzapine. *J Basic Clin Physiol Pharmacol*. 2017;28(1):85–87.

Borovik AM, Bosch MM, Watson SL. Ocular pigmentation association with clozapine. *Med J Aust*. 2009;190(4):210–211.

Duggal HS, Mendhekar DN. Clozapine-induced tardive dystonia (blepharospasm). *J Neuropsychiatry Clin Neurosci*. 2007;19(1):86–87.

Kuppili PP, Nebhinani N, Jain S, et al. Olanzapine associated palpebral edema: an uncommon adverse effect of a commonly prescribed drug. *Asian J Psychiatr*. 2018;36:60–61.

Praharaj SK, Sarkar S, Sinha VK. Olanzapine-induced tardive oculogyric crisis. *J Clin Psychopharmacol*. 2009;29(6):604–606.

Takaki M, Mizuki Y, Miki T. Blonanserin improved dystonia induced by risperidone or olanzapine in two patients with schizophrenia. *J Neuropsychiatry Clin Neurosci*. 2014;26(2):E14.

Visscher AJ, Cohen D. Periorbital oedema and treatment-resistant by hypertension as rare side effects of clozapine. *Aust NZ J Psychiat*. 2011;45(12):1097–1098.

Droperidol, haloperidol

Andrus PF. Lithium and carbamazepine. *J Clin Psychiatry*. 1984;45:525.

Drugs that cause photosensitivity. *Med Lett Drugs Ther*. 1986;28:51.

Isaac NE, Walker AM, Jick H, et al. Exposure to phenothiazine drugs and risk of cataract. *Arch Ophthalmol*. 1991;109:256–260.

Jhee SS, Zarotsky V, Mohaupt SM, et al. Delayed onset of oculogyric crisis and torticollis with intramuscular haloperidol. *Ann Pharmacother*. 2003;37:1434–1437.

Konikoff F, Kuritzky A, Jerushalmi Y, et al. Neuroleptic malignant syndrome induced by a single injection of haloperidol. *BMJ*. 1984;289:1228–1229.

Laties AM. Ocular toxicology of haloperidol. In: Leopold IH, Burns RP, eds. *Symposium on Ocular Therapy*. 9th ed. New York: John Wiley & Sons; 1976:87–95.

Patton Jr CM. Rapid induction of acute dyskinesia by droperidol. *Anesthesiology*. 1975;43:126–127.

Selman FB, McClure RF, Helwig H. Loxapine succinate: a double-blind comparison with haloperidol and placebo in schizophrenics. *Curr Ther Res*. 1976;19:645–652.

Shapiro AK. More on drug-induced blurred vision. *Am J Psychiatry*. 1977;134:1449.

Lithium carbonate

Brenner R, Cooper TB, Yablonski ME, et al. Measurement of lithium concentrations in human tears. *Am J Psychiatry*. 1982;139:678–679.

Corbett JJ, Jacobson DM, Thompson HS, et al. Downbeat nystagmus and other ocular motor defects caused by lithium toxicity. *Neurology*. 1989;39:481–487.

Deleu D, Ebinger G. Lithium-induced internuclear ophthalmoplegia. *Clin Neuropharmacol*. 1989;12:224–226.

Dry J, Aron-Rosa A, Pradalier A. Onset of exophthalmos during treatment with lithium carbonate. *Biological Hyperthyroidism Therapie*. 1974;29:701–708.

Emrich HM, Zihl J, Raptis C, et al. Reduced dark-adaptation: An indication of lithium's neuronal action in humans. *Am J Psychiatry*. 1990;147:629–631.

Fenwick PB, Robertson R. Changes in the visual evoked potential to pattern reversal with lithium medication. *Electroencephalogr Clin Neurophysiol*. 1983;55:538–545.

Fraunfelder FT. Lithium carbonate therapy and macular degeneration. *JAMA*. 1983;249:2389.

Fraunfelder FT, Meyer S. Ocular toxicity of antineoplastic agents. *Ophthalmology*. 1983;90:1–3.

Halmagyi GM, Lessell I, Curthoys IS, et al. Lithium-induced downbeat nystagmus. *Am J Ophthalmol*. 1989;107:664–679.

Halmagyi GM, Rudge P, Gresty MA, et al. Downbeating nystagmus – a review of 62 cases. *Arch Neurol*. 1983;40:777–784.

Levine S, Puchalski C. Pseudotumor cerebri associated with lithium therapy in two patients. *J Clin Psychiatry*. 1990;51:251–253.

Levy DL, Dorus E, Shaughnessy R, et al. Pharmacologic evidence for specificity of pursuit dysfunction to schizophrenia. Lithium carbonate associated with abnormal pursuit. *Arch Gen Psychiatry*. 1985;42:335–341.

Pakes G. Eye irritation and lithium carbonate. *Arch Ophthalmol*. 1980;98:930.

Sandyk R. Oculogyric crisis induced by lithium carbonate. *Eur Neurol*. 1984;23:92–94.

Saul RF, Hamburger HA, Selhorst JB. Pseudotumor cerebri secondary to lithium carbonate. *JAMA*. 1985;253:2869–2870.

Slonim R, McLarty B. Sixth cranial nerve palsy – unusual presenting symptom of lithium toxicity? *Can J Psychiatry*. 1985;30:443–444.

Thompson CH, Baylis PH. Asymptomatic Grave's disease during lithium therapy. *Postgrad Med J*. 1986;62:295–296.

Ullrich A, Adamczyk J, Zihl J, et al. Lithium effects on ophthalmological electrophysiological parameters in young healthy volunteers. *Acta Psychiatr Scand*. 1985;72:113–119.

Pimozide

Morris PA, MacKenzie DH, Masheter HC. A comparative double blind trial of pimozide and fluphenazine in chronic schizophrenia. *Br J Psychiatry*. 1970;117:683–684.

Taub RN, Baker MA. Treatment of metastatic malignant melanoma with pimozide. *Lancet*. 1979;1:605.

Quetiapine fumarate

Brown GC, Brown MM, Fischer DH. Photopsias: a key to diagnosis. *Ophthalmology.* 2015;122(10):2084–2094.

Nasrallah HA, Dev V, Rak I, et al. *Safety update with quetiapine and lenticular examinations: experience with 300,000 patients [poster]. Acapulco, Mexico.* Presented at the Annual Meeting of the American College of Neuropsychopharmacology; 1999.

Shahzad S, Suleman M-I, Shahab H, et al. Cataract occurrence with antipsychotic drugs. *Psychosomatics.* 2002;43:354–359.

Risperidone

Graovac M, Ruzic K, Rebic J, et al. The influence of side effect of antipsychotic on the course of treatment in adolescent. *Psychiatr Danub.* 2010;22(1):108–111.

Thiothixene

Drugs for psychiatric disorders. *Med Lett Drugs Ther.* 1983;25:45.

Drugs that cause photosensitivity. *Med Lett Drugs Ther.* 1986;28:51.

Eberlein-Konig B, Bindl A, Przybilla B. Phototoxic properties of neuroleptic drugs. *Dermatology.* 1997;194:131–135.

McNevin S, MacKay M. Chlorprothixene-induced systemic lupus erythematosus. *J Clin Psychopharmacol.* 1982;2:411–412.

Alcohol (ethanol, ethyl alcohol)

Al-Faran MF, Al-Omar OM. Retrobulbar alcohol injection in blind painful eyes. *Ann Ophthalmol.* 1990;22:460–462.

Dreiss AK, Winkler von Mohrenfels C, Gabler B, et al. Laser epithelial keratomileusis (LASEK): histological investigation for vitality of corneal epithelial cells after alcohol exposure. *Klin Monatsbl Augenheilkd.* 2002;219:365–369.

Garber JM. Steep corneal curvature: a fetal alcohol syndrome landmark. *J Am Optom Assoc.* 1984;55:595–598.

Hsu HY, Piva A, Sadun AA. Devastating complication from alcohol cauterization of recurrent Rathke cleft cyst: case report. *J Neurosurg.* 2004;100:1087–1090.

Kondo M, Ogino N. An accidental irrigation of the anterior chamber with ethanol during cataract surgery. *Jpn J Clin Ophthalmol.* 1989;43:1851–1853.

Leibowitz HM, Ryan W, Kupferman A, et al. The effect of alcohol intoxication on inflammation of the cornea. *Arch Ophthalmol.* 1985;103:723–725.

Lindblad BE, Hakansson N, Philipson B, et al. Alcohol consumption and risk of cataract extraction: a prospective cohort study of women. *Ophthalmology.* 2007;114:680–685.

Reisin I, Reisin LH, Aviel E. Corneal melting in a chronic contact lens wearer. *CLAO J.* 1996;22:146–147.

Roncone DP. Xerophthalmia secondary to alcohol-induced malnutrition. *Optometry.* 2006;77:124–133.

Shiono T, Asano Y, Hashimoto T, et al. Temporary corneal edema after acute intake of alcohol. *Br J Ophthalmol.* 1987;71:462–465.

Stein HA, Stein RM, Price C, et al. Alcohol removal of the epithelium for excimer laser ablation: outcomes analysis. *J Cataract Refract Surg.* 1997;23:1160–1163.

Yanagawa Y, Kiyozumi T, Hatanaka K, et al. Reversible blindness associated with alcoholic ketoacidosis. *Am J Ophthalmol.* 2004;137:775–777.

Methanol

Barceloux DG, Bond GR, Krenzelok EP, et al. American Academy of Clinical Toxicology practice guidelines on the treatment of methanol poisoning. *J Toxicol Clin Toxicol.* 2002;40(4):415–416.

Brent J, McMartin K, Phillips S, et al. Fomepizole for the treatment of methanol poisoning. *N Engl J Med.* 2001;344(6):424–429.

Eells JT, Henry MM, Summerfelt P, et al. Therapeutic photobiomodulation for methanol-induced retinal toxicity. *Proc Natl Acad Sci USA.* 2003;100(6):3439–3444.

Nurieva O, Diblik P, Kuthan P, et al. Progressive chronic retinal axonal loss following acute methanol-induced optic neuropathy: four-year prospective cohort study. *Am J Ophthalmol.* 2018;191:100–115.

Tanrivermis Sayit A, Aslan K, Elmali M, et al. Methanol-induced toxic optic neuropathy with diffusion weighted MRI findings. *Cutan Ocul Toxicol.* 2016;35(4):337–340.

Fesoterodine fumarate, solifenacin succinate, oxybutynin chloride

Sekeroglu MA, Hekimoglu E, Petricli IS, et al. The effect of oral solifenacin succinate treatment on intraocular pressure: glaucoma paradox during overactive bladder treatment. *Int Urogynecol J.* 2014;25(11):1479–1482.

Turkoglu AR. Changes in intraocular pressure and tear secretion in patients given 5 mg solifenacin for the treatment of overactive bladder. *Int Urogynecol J.* 2017;28(5):777–781.

Vardy MD, Mitcheson HD, Samuels TA, et al. Effects of solifenacin on overactive bladder symptoms, symptom bother and other patient-reported outcomes: results from VIBRANT – a double-blind, placebo-controlled trial. *Int J Clin Pract.* 2009;63(12):1702–1714.

Dronabinol (tetrahydrocannabinol, THC), hashish, marihuana (marijuana, cannabis)

Flach AJ. Delta-9-tetrahydrocannabinol (THC) in the treatment of end-stage open-angle glaucoma. *Trans Am Ophthalmol Soc.* 2002;100:215–222.

Fried PA. Marihuana use by pregnant women and effects on offspring: an update. *Neurobehav Toxicol Teratol.* 1982;4:451–452.

Gaillard MC, Borruat FX. Persisting visual hallucinations and illusions in previously drug-addicted patients. *Klin Monatsbl Augenheilkd.* 2003;220:176–178.

Green K. Marijuana and the eye – a review. *J Toxicol Cut Ocular Toxicol.* 1982;1:3.

Green K, Roth M. Ocular effects of topical administration of delta 9-tetrahydrocannabinol in man. *Arch Ophthalmol.* 1982;100:265–267.

Jay WM, Green K. Multiple-drop study of topically applied 1% delta 9-tetrahydrocannabinol in human eyes. *Arch Ophthalmol.* 1983;101:591–593.

Mazow ML, Garrett III CW. Intermittent esoktropia secondary to marihuana smoking. *Binocular Vis.* 1988;3:219.

Merritt JC, Perry DD, Russell DN, et al. Topical delta 9-tetrahydrocannabinol in hypertensive glaucomas. *J Pharm Pharmacol.* 1981;33:40–41.

Poster DS, Penta JS, Bruno S, et al. Delta 9-tetrahydrocannabinol in clinical oncology. *JAMA.* 1981;245:2047–2051.

Qazi QH, Mariano E, Milman DH, et al. Abnormal fetal development linked to intrauterine exposure to marijuana. *Dev Pharmacol Ther.* 1985;8:141–148.

Schwartz RH. Marijuana: a crude drug with a spectrum of underappreciated toxicity. *Pediatrics.* 1984;73:455–458.

Tomida I, Pertwee RG, Azuara-Blanco A. Cannabinoids and glaucoma. *Br J Ophthalmol.* 2003;88:708–713.

Treffert DA, Joranson DE. Delta 9-tetrahydrocannabinol and therapeutic research legislation for cancer patients. *JAMA.* 1983;249:1469–1472.

Weinberg D, Lande A, Hilton N, et al. Intoxication from accidental marijuana ingestion. *Pediatrics.* 1983;71:848–850.

Zhan G, Cmaras CB, Palmber PF, et al. Effect of marijuana on aqueous humor dynamics in a glaucoma patient. *J Glaucoma.* 2005;14:175–177.

Lysergic acid diethylamide (LSD), lysergide, mescaline, psilocybin

Abraham HD. Visual phenomenology of the LSD flashback. *Arch Gen Psychiatry.* 1983;40:884–889.

Abraham HD, Duffy FH. EEG coherence in post-LSD visual hallucinations. *Psychiatry Res.* 2001;107:151–163.

Fohlmeister C, Gertsner W, Ritz R, et al. Spontaneous excitations in the visual cortex: stripes, spirals, rings, and collective bursts. *Neurol Comput.* 1995;7:905–914.

Gaillard MC, Borruat FX. Persisting visual hallucination and illusion in previously drug-addicted patients. *Klin Monatsbl Augenheilkd.* 2003;220:176–178.

Gouzoulis-Mayfrank E, Thelen B, Maier S, et al. Effects of the hallucinogen psilocybin on covert orienting of visual attention in humans. *Neuropsychobiology.* 2002;45:205–212.

Kaminer Y, Hrecznyj B. Lysergic acid diethylamide-induced chronic visual disturbances in an adolescent. *J Nervous Mental Dis.* 1991;179:173–174.

Krill AE, Wieland AM, Ostfeld AM. The effect of two hallucinogenic agents on human retinal function. *Arch Ophthalmol.* 1960;64:724–733.

Lerner AG, Sufman E, Kodesh A, et al. Risperidone-associated, benign transient visual disturbances in schizophrenic patients with a past history of LSD abuse. *Isr J Psychiatry Relat Sci.* 2002;39:57–60.

Levi L, Miller NR. Visual illusions associated with previous drug abuse. *J Clin Neuroophthalmol.* 1990;10:103–110.

Margolis S, Martin L. Anophthalmia in an infant of parents using LSD. *Ann Ophthalmol.* 1980;12:1378–1381.

Sunness JS. Persistent afterimages (palinopsia) and photophobia in a patient with a history of LSD use. *Retina.* 2004;24:805.

Phencyclidine

Acute drug abuse reactions. *Med Lett Drugs Ther.* 1985;27:77.

Corales RL, Maull KI, Becker DP. Phencyclidine abuse mimicking head injury. *JAMA.* 1980;243:2323–2324.

McCarron MM, Schulze BW, Thompson GA, et al. Acute phencyclidine intoxication: incidence of clinical findings in 1,000 cases. *Ann Emerg Med.* 1981;10:237–242.

Pearlson GD. Psychiatric and medical syndromes associated with phencyclidine (PCP) abuse. *Johns Hopkins Med J.* 1981;148:25–33.

Amobarbital, butabarbital sodium, butalbital, methohexital sodium, methylphenobarbital (mephobarbital), pentobarbital sodium, phenobarbital, primidone, secobarbital sodium

Alpert JN. Downbeat nystagmus due to anticonvulsant toxicity. *Ann Neurol.* 1978;4:471–473.

Amarenco P, Royer I, Guillevin L. Ophthalmoplegia externa in barbiturate poisoning. *Presse Med.* 1984;13:2453.

Clarke RSJ, Fee JH, Dundee JW. Hypersensitivity reactions to intravenous anaesthetics. In: Watkins J, Ward A, eds. *Adverse Response to Intravenous Drugs.* New York: Grune & Stratton; 1978:41–47.

Crosby SS, Murray KM, Marvin JA, et al. Management of Stevens-Johnson syndrome. *Clin Pharm.* 1986;5:682–689.

Martin E, Thiel T, Joeri P, et al. Effect of pentobarbital on visual processing in man. *Hum Brain Mapp.* 2000;10:132–139.

Müller E, Huk W, Pauli E, et al. Maculo-papillary branch retinal artery occlusions following the Wada test. *Graefes Arch Clin Exp Ophthalmol.* 2000;238:715–718.

Murphy DF. Anesthesia and intraocular pressure. *Anesth Analg.* 1985;64:520–530.

Nakame Y, Okuma T, Takahashi R, et al. Multi-institutional study on the teratogenicity and fetal toxicity of antiepileptic drugs: a report of a collaborative study group in Japan. *Epilepsia.* 1980;21:663–680.

Raitta C, Karhunen U, Seppäläinen AM, et al. Changes in the electroretinogram and visual evoked potentials during general anesthesia. *Graefes Arch Clin Exp Ophthalmol.* 1979;211:139–144.

Tedeschi G, Bittencourt PR, Smith AT, et al. Specific oculomotor deficits after amylobarbitone. *Psychopharmacology (Berl).* 1983;79:187–189.

Tseng SC, Maumenee AE, Stark WJ, et al. Topical retinoid treatment for various dry-eye disorders. *Ophthalmology.* 1985;92:717–727.

Wallar PH, Genstler DE, George CC. Multiple systemic and periocular malformations associated with the fetal hydantoin syndrome. *Ann Ophthalmol.* 1978;10:1568–1572.

Chloral hydrate

Goldstein JII. Effects of drugs on cornea, conjunctiva, and lids. *Int Ophthalmol Clin.* 1971;11(2):13 34

Hermans G. Les psychotropes. *Bull Soc Belge Ophtalmol.* 1972;160:15–85.

Lane RJ, Routledge PA. Drug-induced neurological disorders. *Drugs.* 1983;26:124–147.

Levy DL, Lipton RB, Holzman PS. Smooth pursuit eye movements: effects of alcohol and chloral hydrate. *J Psychiatr Res.* 1981;16:1–11.

Lubeck MJ. Effects of drugs on ocular muscles. *Int Ophthalmol Clin.* 1971;11(2):35–62.

Margetts EL. Chloral delirium. *Psychiatr Q.* 1950;24:278–279.

Mowry JB, Wilson GA. Effect of exchange transfusion in chloral hydrate overdose. *Vet Human Toxicol.* 1983;25(suppl 1):15.

Varadaraj V, Munoz B, Karaoui M, et al. Effect of chloral hydrate sedation on intraocular pressure in a pediatric population. *Am J Ophthalmol.* 2018;194:126–133.

CHAPTER 6

Drugs Affecting the Autonomic Nervous System

CLASS: STIMULANTS

Generic Name:
Nicotine.

Primary Use
This drug is a stimulant of the autonomic ganglia. It is a highly toxic alkaloid that dramatically stimulates neurons and ultimately blocks synaptic transmission. It is important medically because of its presence in tobacco smoke from cigarettes, cigars, and pipes. Nonsmokers are also affected due to secondhand smoke.

Ocular Side Effects
Systemic Administration – inhalation
Certain
1. Decreased vision
2. Age-related macular degeneration
3. Cataracts
4. Uveitis
5. Diabetic retinopathy – worsens
6. Color vision defect
7. Vascular changes
    a. Decreased retinal flow
    b. Decreased choroidal flow
    c. Decreased perfusion pressure
8. Toxicity
    a. Neurosensory retina
    b. Pigment epithelium
    c. Macula

Probable
1. Aggravates ocular inflammatory disease
2. Cystoid macular edema – increase in uveitis
3. Graves' ophthalmopathy

Possible
1. Dacryoliths
2. Corneal endothelial loss

Clinical Significance
Clearly smoking and secondhand smoke have significant ocular side effects. Decreased vision may occur, as well as retinal, macular, lens, and corneal tear film effects. Vision may be permanently affected, including blindness. Blindness is 4 times more common in older people who smoke versus nonsmokers.[1] Cigarette smoking is a major risk factor for developing ocular artery thickness and atherosclerosis. It also causes microvasculature changes that interfere with vision. Besides direct toxicity to ocular tissue, many changes are secondary to decreased blood flow to the retina, choroid, and fovea.[2-4]

Possibly of greatest clinical importance is its effect on the macula. Data suggest that in smokers, macular degeneration occurs 5 years earlier, is 3 times more common, and is 5.5 times more common in those over 80 years old.[5-12] Toxicity to the neurosensory retina and/or pigment epithelium can occur.[13,14]

Ocular inflammation may be harder to control in smokers, and cystoid macular edema increases in smokers with uveitis. Diabetic retinopathy incidence and progression are significantly worse due to low birth weight children in smoking mothers. Color vision changes, especially in the red and green perception, may occur.[15-17]

Chronic smokers have twice the incidence of primary nuclear sclerotic cataracts versus nonsmokers. Toxic effects of smoke on the external eye are poorly understood, but smoke aggravates ocular sicca and has an increased risk of corneal ulcers in contact lens wearers.

Smokers with Graves' disease have increased ocular complications compared with nonsmokers.[18]

There is a possibility of smoking causing corneal endothelial damage and dacryolithiasis.[19,20]

REFERENCES
Drug: Nicotine
1. Nicotine. 2018. Retrieved from https://en.wikipedia.org/wiki/Nicotine.
2. Wimpissinger B, Resch H, Berish F, et al. Response of choroidal blood flow to carbogen breathing in smokers and non-smokers. *Br J Ophthalmol.* 2004;88:776–781.
3. Hara K. Effects of cigarette smoking on ocular circulation chronic effect on choroidal circulation. *Nippon Ganka Gakkai Zasshi.* 1991;95:939–943.
4. Steigerwalt Jr RD, Laurora G, Incandela L, et al. Ocular and orbital blood flow in cigarette smokers. *Retina.* 2000;20:394–397.
5. Age-Related Eye Disease Study Research Group (AREDS). Risk factors associated with age-related macular degeneration. A case-control study in the age-related eye disease study: age-Related Eye Disease Study Report Number 3. *Ophthalmology.* 2000;107:2224–2232.
6. Age-Related Eye Disease Study Research Group (AREDS). A randomized, placebo-controlled, clinical trial of high-dose supplementation with vitamins C and E, beta carotene, and zinc for age-related macular degeneration and vision loss: AREDS report no. 8. *Arch Ophthalmol.* 2001;119:1417–1436.
7. Khan JC, Thurlby DA, Shahid H, et al. Smoking and age-related macular degeneration: the number of pack years of cigarette smoking is a major determinant of risk for both geographic atrophy and choroidal neovascularization. *Br J Ophthalmol.* 2006;90:75–80.
8. Chakravarthy U, Wong TY, Fletcher A, et al. Clinical risk factors for age-related macular degeneration: a systematic review and meta-analysis. *BMC Ophthalmol.* 2010;10:31.
9. Chakravarthy U, Augood C, Bentham GC, et al. Cigarette smoking and age-related macular degeneration in the EUREYE Study. *Ophthalmology.* 2007;114:1157–1163.
10. Mitchell P, Wang JJ, Smith W, Leeder SR. Smoking and the 5-year incidence of age-related maculopathy: the Blue Mountains Eye Study. *Arch Ophthalmol.* 2002;120:1357–1363.
11. Klein R, Cruickshanks KJ, Nash SD, et al. The prevalence of age-related macular degeneration and associated risk factors. *Arch Ophthalmol.* 2010;128:750–758.
12. SanGiovanni JP, Chew EY, Clemons TE, et al. The relationship of dietary carotenoid and vitamin A, E, and C intake with age-related macular degeneration in a case-control study: AREDS report no. 22. *Arch Ophthalmol.* 2007;125:1225–1232.
13. Patil AJ, Gramajo AL, Sharma A, et al. Effects of benzo(e)pyrene on the retinal neurosensory cells and human microvascular endothelial cells in vitro. *Curr Eye Res.* 2009;34:672–682.
14. Sharma A, Neekhra A, Gramajo AL, et al. Effects of Benzo(e)pyrene, a toxic component of cigarette smoke, on human retinal pigment epithelial cells in vitro. *Invest Ophthalmol Vis Sci.* 2008;49:5111–5117.
15. Lin P, Loh AR, Margolis TP, et al. Cigarette smoking as a risk factor for uveitis. *Ophthalmology.* 2010;117(3):585–590.
16. Moss SE, Klein R, Klein BE. Cigarette smoking and ten-year progression of diabetic retinopathy. *Ophthalmology.* 1996;103(9):1438–1442.
17. Thorne JE, Daniel E, Jabs DA, et al. Smoking as a risk factor for cystoid macular edema complicating intermediate uveitis. *Am J Ophthalmol.* 2008;145:841–846.
18. Xing L, Ye L, Zhu W, et al. Smoking was associated with poor response to intravenous steroids therapy in Graves' ophthalmopathy. *Br J Ophthalmol.* 2015;99(12):1683–1691.
19. Golabchi K, Abahi MA, Salehi A, et al. The effects of smoking on corneal endothelial cells: a cross-sectional study on a population from Isfahan, Iran. *Cutan Ocul Toxicol.* 2018;37(1):9–14.
20. Mishra K, Hu KY, Kamal S, et al. Dacryolithiasis: a review. *Ophthalmic Plast Reconstr Surg.* 2017;33(2):83–89.

FURTHER READING
Nicotine
Boonman ZF, de Keizer RJ, Watson PG. Smoking delays the response to treatment in episcleritis and scleritis. *Eye.* 2005;19:949–955.
El-Shazly AAE, Farweez YAT, Elzankalony YA, et al. Effect of smoking on macular function and structure in active smokers versus passive smokers. *Retina.* 2018;38(5):1031–1040.
Galor A, Feuer W, Kempen JH, et al. Adverse effects of smoking on patients with ocular inflammation. *Br J Ophthalmol.* 2010;94(7):848–853.

CHAPTER 7

Analgesics, Narcotic Antagonists, and Drugs Used to Treat Arthritis

CLASS: DRUGS USED TO TREAT GOUT

Generic Name:
Allopurinol sodium.

Proprietary Names:
Aloprim, Lopurin, Zyloprim.

Primary Use
This potent xanthine oxidase inhibitor is primarily used in the treatment of chronic hyperuricemia.

Ocular Side Effects
Systemic administration – intravenous or oral
Certain
1. Decreased vision
2. Cataracts (Fig. 7.1)
3. Eyelids or conjunctiva
   a. Allergic reactions
   b. Erythema
   c. Conjunctivitis – nonspecific
   d. Edema
   e. Photosensitivity
   f. Ulceration
   g. Urticaria
   h. Purpura

Possible
1. Crystalline maculopathy

Clinical Significance
The only side effects of major clinical importance are the lens changes associated with prolonged use of this drug. Lerman et al implicated the role of ultraviolet radiation as the instigator of this process.[1] Garbe et al performed a large-scale population-based epidemiologic study showing that patients taking a cumulative dose of more than 400 g of allopurinol for longer than 3 years were associated with a twofold increased risk for cataract surgery.[2] This type of study is rare for ophthalmology, but it gives definitive proof of an association between allopurinol and cataract formation. Leske et al implicated the gout medications as second only to steroids as a major risk factor in cataractogenesis.[3] The lens changes seen with allopurinol are anterior and posterior capsular changes with anterior subcapsular vacuoles. With time, wedge-shaped anterior and posterior cortical haze occurs. This may progress to dense posterior subcapsular opacities. Although a few cases of macular changes are reported in the literature and in the spontaneous reports, to date there is no clear-cut association between allopurinol and macular changes. Cheah et al reported bilateral perifoveal deposits and maculopathy changes in a 33-year-old woman after 6 months of allopurinol therapy.[4] Optical coherence tomography showed hyper-reflective intraretinal crystals in both eyes. There are no other cases reported, including spontaneous reports, of this kind or crystal deposits in any other ocular tissue. Almost 90% of allopurinol systemic drug side effects are skin related. Because the eyelids have some of the thinnest skin on the body, eyelid changes occur.

Recommendations
1. Patients taking allopurinol should wear ultraviolet-blocking glasses. This is especially true in occupations and hobbies with increased sunlight exposure. Ultraviolet-blocking lenses should decrease the incidence of lens changes and eyelid changes secondary to the photosensitivity effects of this drug.
2. Patients should probably have an ophthalmic examination every 2 years.

Generic Name:
Colchicine.

Proprietary Names:
ColiGel, Colcrys, Mitigare.

Primary Use
This alkaloid is used in the prophylaxis and treatment of acute gout. It is also used for treating familial Mediterranean fever, Behçet disease, rheumatoid arthritis, and primary cholangitis.

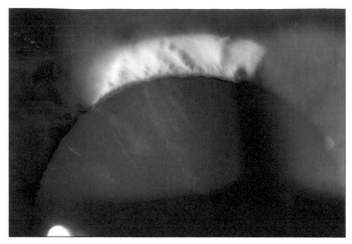

FIG. 7.1 Allopurinol-induced cataracts.[5]

Ocular Side Effects
Systemic administration – oral or topical
Certain
1. Reduction or inhibition of fibrosis
   a. Delays wound healing
   b. Enhances filtration surgery success

Probable
1. Inhibition of mitosis and migration of epithelial cells with delayed healing
   a. Dellen
   b. Corneal erosion
   c. Corneal ulcers
   d. Conjunctival wound, i.e. strabismus surgery

Possible
1. Papilledema – toxic states
2. Decreased vision – toxic states

Inadvertent ocular exposure
Certain
1. Decreased vision
2. Conjunctival hyperemia
3. Corneal clouding

Clinical Significance
Ocular side effects secondary to colchicine, although rare, have clinical importance. Alster et al and Biedner et al both warned that cessation of colchicine should be considered in patients who have corneal ulcers, dellen, corneal or conjunctival epithelial defects, or any ocular wounds that are refractory to conventional treatment.[1,2] Although these complications are probably colchicine side effects, most of the proof comes in part from animal data. Vignes et al described a case of colchicine-induced intracranial hypertension.[3] Dickenson et al described a case of bilateral eyelid necrosis secondary to pseudomonal septicemia brought on by colchicine-induced neutropenia.[4] Optic nerve changes have been found in animals, but to date there are no cases in the spontaneous reports.

CLASS: ANTIRHEUMATIC DRUGS

Generic Names:
1. Adalimumab; 2. etanercept; 3. infliximab.

Proprietary Names:
1. Cyltezo, Humira; 2. Enbrel; 3. Inflectra, Remicade, Renflexis.

Primary Use
These drugs block the activity of tumor necrosis factor (TNF). These drugs are primarily used in the management of various arthritic diseases and Crohn's disease.

Ocular Side Effects
Systemic administration – intravenous or subcutaneous
Probable
1. Uveitis (etanercept)

Possible
1. Optic or retrobulbar neuritis
2. May aggravate or cause ocular sicca

3. Sarcoidosis
    a. Orbital
    b. Uveitis
4. Uveitis (infliximab)

Conditional/unclassified

1. Scleritis
2. Episcleritis
3. Cornea infiltrates – peripheral
4. Retinal vascular abnormalities (infliximab)
5. Intranuclear ophthalmoplegia
6. Visual field loss
7. Orbital myositis
8. Orbital cellulitis

Intravitreal injections (infliximab)
Certain

1. Vision decreased
2. Panuveitis
3. Cystoid macular edema
4. Abnormal electroretinogram (ERG)
5. Visual fields – decreased

Clinical Significance

The reports in the *Physicians' Desk Reference* (PDR), literature, and spontaneous reports are primarily decreased vision, uveitis, and ocular sicca.[1] All of these are seen with the diseases that these drugs are treating; therefore a clear profile of visual side effects is at this time suspect. Because these drugs can cause xerostomia, they may aggravate ocular sicca. Cataracts, although mentioned, are probably associated with the steroids used to control the disease. Of interest is optic neuritis. Smith et al reported 60 cases of etanercept and optic neuritis.[2] Symptoms develop within 1–14 months after starting therapy, with a mean development time of 9.5 months. Nine patients had positive dechallenge, and 3 had positive rechallenge. Tauber et al and Noguera-Pons et al also reported an association of this drug with optic neuritis.[3,4] Foroozan et al, Mejico, ten Tusscher et al, Strong et al, and Tran et al suggested an association of optic or retrobulbar neuritis with infliximab usage.[5-9] Chung et al reported 2 cases of optic neuritis associated with adalimumab use.[10] Winthrop et al in a retrospective, population-based cohort study of 61,227 patients did not find a higher incidence of optic neuritis among anti-TNF alpha therapy.[11] It is unproven whether these drugs cause optic neuritis. Positive rechallenge data suggest perhaps a small subset may be hypersensitive to these drugs.

The question of whether these drugs cause intraocular inflammation is confused by the fact that the diseases that the drugs are used to treat can also cause uveitis. There are 2 cases in the literature and spontaneous reports where uveitis occurred each time etanercept was started and cleared each time the drug was stopped.[12] Taban et al reported a case of positive double rechallenge of etanercept exacerbating anterior uveitis.[13] Lim et al, in a review of 59 cases of uveitis, found that 43 were associated with etanercept, 14 with infliximab, and 2 with adalimumab.[14] They concluded that etanercept is associated with a significantly higher rate of uveitis than other TNF inhibitors and that uveitis may be more drug specific than class specific. Hashkes et al reported sarcoid-related uveitis occurring during etanercept therapy.[15]

Data suggest that this class of drugs may cause autoimmune diseases such as sarcoid and lupus. Orbital sarcoid-like granulomatosis and sarcoid uveitis possibly due to adalimumab injections have been reported.[16]

Although there are a few reports in the literature of retinal abnormalities occurring shortly after starting infliximab, compounding factors makes one suspect normal background noise.

Although some suggest etanercept as a treatment for scleritis, There are 3 cases in the spontaneous reports where this drug was implicated as causing or exacerbating scleritis. Because the disease that these drugs are used to treat can also cause scleritis, at this time a drug-induced effect is only suspect. Reports of these drugs causing systemic vasculitis and suppression of the hemopoietic systems possibly support occasional reports of retinal vascular abnormalities and vitreous hemorrhage.

Single cases of possible retinal toxicity causing visual field changes with etanercept, orbital myositis, and orbital cellulitis have been reported.[17-19]

Low-dosage intravitreal infliximab injections in humans were not well tolerated.[20]

Internuclear ophthalmoplegia was associated with a single dose of adalimumab.[21] Peripheral corneal infiltrates were associated in a single case after subcutaneous adalimumab treatment.[22]

Generic Name:
Auranofin.

Proprietary Name:
Ridaura.

Primary Use
This heavy metal is used in the treatment of active rheumatoid arthritis and nondisseminated lupus erythematosus.

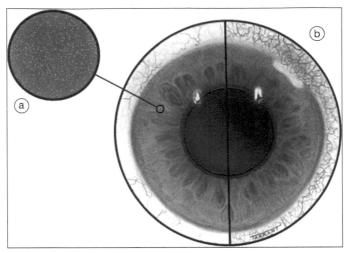

FIG. 7.2 **(A)** Dust-like or glittering purple granules and **(B)** marginal keratitis related to systemic auranofin use.[5]

Ocular Side Effects
Systemic administration – oral
Certain

1. Red, violet, purple, or brown-gold deposits (Fig. 7.2)
   a. Eyelids
   b. Conjunctiva
   c. Cornea
   d. Surface of lens
2. Eyelids or conjunctiva
   a. Allergic reactions
   b. Hyperemia
   c. Erythema
   d. Blepharoconjunctivitis
   e. Edema
   f. Photosensitivity
   g. Symblepharon
   h. Urticaria
   i. Purpura
3. Photophobia
4. Cornea
   a. Keratitis
   b. Ulceration
   c. Stromal melting
5. Iris and ciliary body
   a. Hyperemia
   b. Inflammation
   c. Cells and flare

Possible

1. Myasthenia gravis
   a. Diplopia
   b. Ptosis
   c. Paresis or paralysis of extraocular muscles

2. Nystagmus
3. May activate
   a. Herpes infections
   b. Guillain-Barré syndrome

Clinical Significance

Patients taking auranofin may show 1 of 2 patterns of ocular chrysiasis. The more common pattern is where gold salts are deposited in the conjunctiva, all layers of the cornea, and the crystalline lens. Gold deposition in the cornea may take a Hudson-Stähli line distribution or a vortex distribution, not unlike Fabry disease. The gold deposits tend to be increased in areas of corneal scarring. Deep corneal deposition is usually in the posterior half of the cornea and denser inferiorly, whereas the superior cornea and perilimbal areas are more often spared. Lopez et al, using confocal microscopy, found gold deposits most frequently in the anterior and mid-corneal stroma.[1] Lens deposits of gold are much less frequent than corneal deposits and are of little to no clinical importance. These deposits are reversible after stopping gold therapy, but may take 3–12 months, and in some cases many years, to resolve. Visual acuity is unaffected, and deposition of gold in the cornea or lens is not an indication for cessation of therapy. In general, at least 1 g of gold ingested is needed before corneal changes are seen. In total dosages of 1.5 g, 40–80% of patients will have gold deposition in the cornea. Whereas lens deposits have previously been considered rare, 55% of patients on daily dosages over 1 g for 3 or more years have been reported to develop lens deposits. Corneal deposits may be seen as early as 1 month after starting therapy. It has been suggested that gold deposits in the cornea and lens are secondary to metal from the aqueous fluid or perilimbal blood vessels.

The second variant of ocular chrysiasis is much less common. This type presents as an inflammatory response secondary to gold, including corneal ulceration, subepithelial white perilimbal infiltrates, brush-like perilimbal stromal vascularization, and interstitial keratitis.[2,3] Corneal ulceration is more often marginal, crescent shaped, and possibly 2–3 mm in length. This response is felt to be an idiosyncratic allergic reaction, may be unilateral or bilateral, and is an indication in most patients to stop therapy. Zamir et al pointed out that in patients presenting with marginal keratitis, this variant of chrysiasis should be considered.[4] Stopping gold therapy along with looking for systemic toxicity is often warranted. Patients must be continuously followed because stromal inflammation may recur even after gold is stopped.

Generic Names:
1. Celecoxib; 2. etodolac.

Proprietary Names:
1. Celebrex; 2. Lodine, Lodine XL.

Primary Use
These nonsteroidal anti-inflammatory drugs are selective inhibitors of cyclooxygenase-2 (COX-2) and are used in various forms in the treatment of arthritis, acute pain, and dysmenorrhea.

Ocular Side Effects
Systemic administration – oral
Certain
1. Decreased vision
2. Conjunctivitis

Possible
1. Eyelids or conjunctiva
   a. Stevens-Johnson syndrome
   b. Toxic epidermal necrolysis
2. May aggravate or cause ocular sicca

Conditional/unclassified
1. Visual field defects
   a. Orange spots
   b. Central scotomas
   c. Scintillating scotoma
2. Temporary blindness
3. Teichopsia
4. Retinal venous occlusions

Clinical Significance
The side effects mentioned are extremely rare. Fraunfelder et al reported that these COX-2 inhibitors can cause decreased vision and conjunctivitis with multiple cases of positive rechallenge.[1] The onset may occur within a few hours to days, and if the drug is discontinued, it resolves within 72 hours. Meyer et al made known a possible association of thrombotic events in selected patients.[2] These findings include central retinal vein or other retinal venous occlusions. Recchia et al reviewed 111 consecutive retinal venous occlusion patients with 321 controls and could not find a significantly higher rate of retinal venous occlusive disease in COX-2 inhibitor users.[3] Meyer et al pointed out that the US Food and Drug Administration strongly associates the use of COX-2 inhibitors with Stevens-Johnson syndrome and toxic epidermal necrolysis.[2] Coulter et al reported a case of temporary blindness and another with bilateral jelly-bean-shaped loss of central vision.[4,5] Lund et al reported a case of orange spots in both visual fields.[6] All signs and symptoms are fully reversible. The mechanism of action is postulated as inhibition of synthesis of prostaglandins that control blood flow. Also, most of these drugs are sulfonamides with known drug-induced transient myopia. These drugs may cause xerostomia and therefore may aggravate or cause ocular sicca.[7]

Generic Name:
Fenoprofen calcium.

Proprietary Names:
Nalfon, Profeno.

Primary Use
This nonsteroidal anti-inflammatory drug is used in the management of rheumatoid arthritis.

Ocular Side Effects
Systemic administration – oral
Certain
1. Decreased vision
2. Eyelids or conjunctiva
   a. Erythema
   b. Conjunctivitis – nonspecific
   c. Edema
   d. Urticaria

Possible
1. Diplopia
2. Optic nerve toxicity
3. Visual field defects
   a. Scotomas – centrocecal or paracentral

b. Enlarged blind spot
c. Constriction
4. May aggravate or cause ocular sicca

Clinical Significance

Ocular side effects are seldom of clinical significance with fenoprofen. The most common adverse event is decreased vision (2.2%).[1] Skin lesions associated with the use of this drug require stopping the drug and obtaining dermatologic consultation because a small number go on to develop severe systemic disease. Again, as with others in this group of drugs, there may be a rare idiosyncratic optic nerve response that may be associated with the use of this drug. There are cases in the spontaneous reports of a unilateral or bilateral decrease in visual acuity ranging from 20/80 to 20/200 after 6 months of therapy. Visual fields may show various types of scotoma. If the medication is stopped, the visual acuity usually returns to normal in 1–3 months. However, it has taken over 8 months for color vision to return. It is not possible to state a positive cause-and-effect relationship between optic nerve toxicity and this drug. It may be prudent, however, to stop the medication if optic nerve pathology occurs until causation can be established.[2] This drug can cause xerostomia and therefore may aggravate or cause ocular sicca.[1]

Generic Name:
Flurbiprofen.

Proprietary Names:
Ansaid, Ocufen.

Primary Use
Systemic
This nonsteroidal anti-inflammatory drug is used in the treatment of rheumatoid arthritis.

Ophthalmic
Flurbiprofen is used for the inhibition of intraoperative miosis.

Ocular Side Effects
Systemic administration – oral
Possible
1. Decreased vision
2. Eyelids or conjunctiva
   a. Erythema
   b. Conjunctivitis – nonspecific
   c. Urticaria
3. Diplopia
4. May aggravate or cause ocular sicca
5. Nystagmus (overdose)

Conditional/unclassified
1. Optic neuritis

Local ophthalmic use or exposure – topical ocular application
Certain
1. Antimiotic
2. Irritation
   a. Hyperemia
   b. Burning sensation
3. Cornea
   a. Punctate keratitis
   b. Delayed wound healing

Probable
1. May aggravate herpes infections
2. Increased ocular or periocular bleeding

Clinical Significance

Ocular side effects secondary to systemic administration of this drug are infrequent. Whereas side effects reported with other nonsteroidal anti-inflammatory drugs must be looked for, to date there are no cases of optic neuritis or pseudotumor cerebri in the spontaneous reports. Generally, short-term therapy with ophthalmic flurbiprofen has been well tolerated; the most frequent adverse reactions have been mild transient stinging and burning on instillation. Flurbiprofen has been shown to inhibit corneal scleral wound healing, decrease leukocytes in tears, and increase complications of herpetic keratitis. Flurbiprofen is one of the more potent nonsteroidal anti-inflammatory drugs and can interfere with thrombocyte aggregation. This may cause intraoperative bleeding as a rare event. This is more common if the patient is already on anticoagulants. Flurbiprofen has been reported to possibly cause xerostomia and ocular sicca.[1]

Generic Name:
Ibuprofen.

Proprietary Names:
Advil, Advil Children's, Advil Infants', Advil Junior Strength, Advil Migraine, Caldolor, Children's Ibuprofen, ElixSure IB, EnovaRX, Genpril, Ibren, IBU, Midol, Midol Cramps and Body Aches, Motrin, Motrin Children's, Motrin IB, Motrin Infants', Motrin Junior Strength, Motrin Migraine Pain, PediaCare Children's Pain Reliever/Fever Reducer IB, PediaCare Infants' Pain Reliever/Fever Reducer IB, Samson-8, Toxicology Saliva Collection.

Primary Use

This antipyretic analgesic is used in the treatment of rheumatoid arthritis and osteoarthritis.

Ocular Side Effects

Systemic administration – oral

Certain

1. Decreased vision – transitory
2. Edema
   a. Orbital
   b. Periorbital
   c. Eyelids
3. Cornea – vortex keratopathy
4. Photophobia

Probable

1. Diplopia
2. Color vision defect
   a. Red-green defect
   b. Colors appear faded
3. Abnormal visual sensations
   a. Moving mosaic of colored lights
   b. Shooting streaks
4. Abnormal electroretinogram (ERG) or visual evoked potential (VEP)
5. Visual hallucinations
6. Eyelids or conjunctiva
   a. Erythema
   b. Conjunctivitis – nonspecific

Possible

1. May aggravate or cause ocular sicca
2. Optic or retrobulbar neuritis
3. Myopia
4. Papilledema secondary to pseudotumor cerebri
5. Toxic amblyopia
6. Macular edema
7. Myokymia
8. Oculogyric crisis

Clinical Significance

Ibuprofen is one of the largest-selling antiarthritic drugs in the world. Adverse ocular events are rare and seldom a reason to stop the drug. Orbital or periorbital edema make up 50% of the ocular cases in the spontaneous reports, with over 5600 cases, and eyelid edema makes up 30%, with over 3300 cases. This appears to be an underrecognized likely side effect. Cases with a positive drug rechallenge include transient decreased vision, refractive error changes, diplopia, photophobia, ocular sicca, and decrease in color vision. A typical vortex keratopathy with deposition limited to the corneal epithelium has been described.[1] Once the drug was stopped, this resolved within 3 weeks. Although ocular sicca has been attributed to this drug, one suspects that this in part is secondary to the drug being in the tears and aggravating an already dry eye. Ocular sicca, however, is probably the most common ocular complaint in patients with rheumatoid arthritis, which is a major disease that this drug is used for. Nicastro described 3 young females who were long-term ibuprofen users, who possibly developed macular edema with vision in the 20/30 to 20/50 range.[2] Once the drug was stopped, vision returned to 20/20. Reversible toxic amblyopia has been reported.[3,4] Myokymia has been reported primarily in younger females after 1 month of drug exposure.[5]

This drug can cause other central nervous system (CNS) changes, including aseptic meningitis, with secondary effects on the visual system. If ibuprofen is not discontinued, permanent visual loss may result. For a drug so commonly used in combination with other drugs, it is not possible to implicate this drug specifically. However, many of the cases are outside the usual multiple sclerosis age group and occur shortly after starting this medication. Patients on this drug should therefore be told to stop this medication if a sudden decrease in vision occurs. If there is an unexplained decrease in vision that occurs while on ibuprofen, tests to rule out optic nerve abnormalities should be considered. There may be a rare idiosyncratic optic nerve response associated with the use of this drug. The typical sequence is that after a few months of therapy, a unilateral or bilateral marked decrease in visual acuity occurs, with vision receding to the 20/80 to 20/200 range. Visual fields may show various types of scotomas. If the medication is stopped, visual acuity usually returns to normal in 1–3 months, but it may take up to 8 months for color vision to return to normal.

Ibuprofen, as well as other nonsteroidal anti-inflammatories, may possibly cause pseudotumor cerebri. This is more common if used in combination with other antiarthritic drugs, which can also induce this side effect.

A postoperative, bilateral orbital, and periorbital ecchymosis has been reported.[6]

Generic Name:

Indomethacin (indometacin).

Proprietary Names:

Indocin, Indocin SR, Indo-Lemmon, Indomethegan G, Tivorbex.

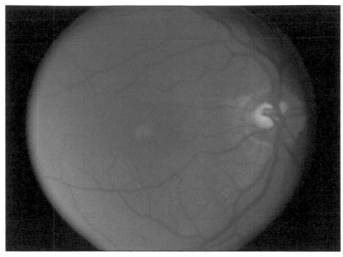

FIG. 7.3 Indomethacin-induced macular pigment mottling.[6]

Primary Use
Systemic
This nonsteroidal anti-inflammatory drug is a methyl-ated indole derivative used as an antipyretic, analgesic, or anti-inflammatory drug in the treatment of rheuma-toid arthritis, rheumatoid spondylitis, and degenerative joint disease.

Ophthalmic
Indomethacin has been advocated for the treatment of cystoid macular edema or to enhance mydriasis pre-operatively at cataract surgery. It has also been advo-cated in the management of symptoms due to corneal scars, edema, erosions, or postrefractory surgery pain.

Ocular Side Effects
Systemic administration – intravenous, oral, or rectal
Certain
1. Decreased vision
   a. Transitory – early
   b. Significant – long-term use
2. Conjunctiva and cornea
   a. Irritation
   b. Keratitis
   c. Corneal deposits
   d. Corneal erosions
3. Abnormal electroretinogram (ERG) or electroocculo-gram (EOG) – long-term use

4. Color vision defect – blue or yellow defect – long-term use
5. Retina or macula – long-term use
   a. Edema
   b. Degeneration – retinal pigment epithelium, perifoveal, and perimacular
   c. Pigment mottling (Fig. 7.3)

Possible
1. Edema
   a. Periorbital
   b. Orbit
   c. Eyelids
2. Pseudotumor cerebri
   a. Papilledema
   b. Visual field changes
   c. 6th-nerve palsy
3. Photosensitivity
4. Optic neuritis

Local ophthalmic use or exposure – topical ocular application
Certain
1. Burning sensation
2. Superficial punctate keratitis
3. Eyelids
   a. Edema
   b. Erythema
   c. Contact dermatitis

4. Decreased miosis during intraocular surgery (weak)
5. Local anesthesia

Possible
1. Cornea – long-term use
   a. Ulceration
   b. Descemetocele
   c. Perforation

Clinical Significance

Indomethacin has been used for over 5 decades with few significant ocular side effects unless the drug is used for prolonged periods in high doses. Its most serious side effect is retinal pigmentary changes, with macular atrophy and a waxy disc.[1,2] This is associated with depressed ERG and constricted visual fields. Although decreased vision may occur after starting this drug, seldom is it of clinical significance. The drug is probably secreted in the tears, thereby causing corneal deposits, irritation, and occasionally keratitis. Pseudotumor cerebri and optic neuritis have been reported with indomethacin use.

Keratorefractive surgery has brought topical ocular indomethacin back into clinical use, in large part because it has fewer side effects than steroids. Its main use is as a local anesthetic, showing less damage to the corneal epithelium in the immediate postoperative period.[3] Sheehan et al reported a case of possible acute asthma due to topical ocular indomethacin.[4] Gueudry et al reported 8 patients who developed corneal ulceration, descemetocele, or perforation after topical ocular 0.1% indomethacin 3–4 times daily, primarily after clear cornea cataract extraction.[5] Most patients were on other topical ocular medications as well. They stated, "even though our study does not prove a causal relationship between the use of indomethacin and the development of corneal complications, their onsets were temporally associated with the start of NSAIDs use."

Generic Name:
Ketoprofen.

Proprietary Names:
Active-Ketoprofen 5%, Orudis, Oruvail.

Primary Use

This nonsteroidal anti-inflammatory drug with antipyretic and analgesic properties is used in the treatment of rheumatoid arthritis, osteoarthritis, ankylosing spondylitis, and gout.

Ocular Side Effects
Systemic administration – oral or topical
Probable
1. Edema
   a. Periorbital
   b. Orbital
   c. Eyelids
2. Photosensitivity
3. Irritation
   a. Hyperemia
   b. Pain
   c. Conjunctivitis
4. Visual hallucinations

Possible
1. Decreased vision
2. May aggravate the following disease
   a. Ocular sicca
   b. Myasthenia gravis
   c. Herpes infections
3. Pseudotumor cerebri

Conditional/unclassified
1. Paresis or paralysis of extraocular muscles

Clinical Significance

Ketoprofen rarely causes ocular problems. It may be an underrecognized cause of periorbital, eyelid, and orbital edema; this development is probably time delayed.[1] There are almost 1000 unsubstantiated cases of ocular and periocular edema from ketoprofen in the spontaneous reports. This may be possible because there is a 2% incidence of peripheral edema associated with this drug.[1] The drug may be secreted in the tears, causing superficial irritation, conjunctivitis, and ocular sicca.[2] It is also a photosensitizing drug so it may cause photophobia.[3,4] Ketoprofen has been associated with precipitating cholinergic crises. There is 1 report of precipitating a cholinergic crisis in a patient with myasthenia gravis.[5] Ketoprofen has been associated with herpes simplex activation, both ocularly and systemically, and pseudotumor cerebri.[6]

Generic Name:
Naproxen sodium.

Proprietary Names:
Aflaxen, Aleve, Aleve Arthritis, All Day Relief, Anaprox, Anaprox DS, EC-Naprosyn, EnovaRX, Equipto Naproxen, Naprelan, Naprosyn, Walgreens Naproxen Sodium.

Primary Use

This antipyretic analgesic is used in the treatment of rheumatoid arthritis, osteoarthritis, and ankylosing spondylitis.

Ocular Side Effects

Systemic administration – oral

Certain

1. Edema
   a. Periorbital
   b. Eyelids
   c. Orbital
2. Decreased vision
3. Papilledema secondary to pseudotumor cerebri
4. Eyelids or conjunctiva
   a. Allergic reactions
   b. Erythema
   c. Conjunctivitis – nonspecific

Probable

1. Photosensitivity
2. Corneal opacities – verticillata pattern

Possible

1. Color vision defect – objects have green or red tinge
2. Optic or retrobulbar neuritis

Conditional/unclassified

1. Cornea – peripheral ulcerations

Clinical Significance

With increased use of this nonsteroidal anti-inflammatory drug, more adverse ocular effects have been reported. Naproxen is a much underrecognized cause of ophthalmic edema. There are almost 5000 unsubstantiated cases in the spontaneous reports of periorbital, eyelid, or orbital edema. This makes up 77% of all of the cases in the spontaneous reports due to naproxen. This may be reasonable because systemic edema occurs in up to 12% and severe acute angioedema in up to 1% of patients.[1] Eyelid edema may occur even after a few dosages and may clear within a few days after stopping the drug. Although some patients complain of decreased vision, this is seldom a significant finding and occurs in only about 3% of patients.[1] In rare instances, it is possible that this drug can cause optic or retrobulbar neuritis; however, this has not been proven, although this class of drugs can cause numerous CNS side effects. Typically, patients with optic or retrobulbar neuritis have been on the drug for about a year before this side effect is seen. There are rare cases in the spontaneous reports of this occurring after only a few months of therapy. The drug should be discontinued until an etiology of the neuritis has been established. This may be a possible side effect and seems to be more common in patients with renal disease, on multiple other drugs, or with autoimmune disease. Pseudotumor cerebri seems to be well documented to occur with naproxen. Well-described aseptic meningitis is seen with this drug with secondary effects on the visual system. Whether or not this drug causes anterior or posterior cataracts is unknown, but there is neither pattern nor proof to date of a cause-and-effect relationship. Whorl-like corneal opacities have been associated with the use of naproxen, and there are several cases of peripheral corneal ulcerations in the spontaneous reports.[2] This drug is one of the more potent photosensitizing nonsteroidal anti-inflammatory drugs. Ultraviolet light–blocking lenses may be indicated in selected patients. Fincham reported a case of exacerbation of glaucoma, which may be secondary to naproxen.[3]

Generic Name:

Piroxicam.

Proprietary Name:

Feldene.

Primary Use

This nonsteroidal anti-inflammatory drug is used in the treatment of osteoarthritis and rheumatoid arthritis.

Ocular Side Effects

Systemic administration – oral

Certain

1. Irritation
   a. Lacrimation
   b. Hyperemia
   c. Burning sensation
2. Decreased vision
3. Eyelids, conjunctiva, and periocular
   a. Erythema
   b. Conjunctivitis – nonspecific
   c. Photosensitivity
   d. Edema
4. Visual hallucinations

Possible

1. Optic neuritis
2. Loss of eyelashes or eyebrows
3. May aggravate or cause ocular sicca

Systemic Side Effects

Systemic administration–oral

Possible

1. Alopecia

Clinical Significance

Piroxicam is one of the most widely prescribed nonsteroidal anti-inflammatory drugs and appears to have no serious ocular side effects except a questionable optic neuritis, which is described by Fraunfelder et al.[1] Piroxicam is one of the few nonsteroidal anti-inflammatory drugs with which pseudotumor cerebri has not been reported. Ocular side effects are infrequent and usually transient. This drug is a strong photosensitizer, and ultraviolet light–blocking lenses may be indicated. Patients who are allergic to thimerosal have a high prevalence of piroxicam photosensitivity.[2]

One of the most common ocular side effects in the spontaneous reports on this drug is eyelid and orbital edema. Although not mentioned in the *Physicians' Desk Reference* (PDR), it does state that this drug may cause fluid retention.[3]

This drug may cause xerostomia and therefore it may also aggravate or cause ocular sicca.[3]

CLASS: MILD ANALGESICS

Generic Name:
Acetaminophen (paracetamol).

Proprietary Names:
Acephen, Aceta, Actamin, Adult Pain Relief, Anacin Aspirin Free, Apra, Children's Acetaminophen, Comtrex Sore Throat Relief, ED-APAP, ElixSure Fever/Pain, Feverall, Genapap, Genebs, Goody's Back & Body Pain, Infantaire, Liquid Pain Relief, Little Fevers, Mapap, Mapap Arthritis Pain, Mapap Infants, Mapap Junior, Nortemp, Ofirmev, Pain & Fever, Pain and Fever, Pain Relief, Pain Relief Extra Strength, Pain Reliever, Panadol, PediaCare Children's Fever Reducer/Pain Reliever, PediaCare Children's Smooth Metls Fever Reducer/Pain Reliever, PediaCare Infant's Fever Reducer/Pain Reliever, Pediaphen, Pharbetol, Q-Pap, Q-Pap Extra Strength, Silapap, Triaminic Fever Reducer and Pain Reliever, Triaminic Infant Fever Reducer and Pain Reliever, Tylenol, Tylenol 8 Hour, Tylenol Arthritis Pain, Tylenol Children's, Tylenol CrushableTablet, Tylenol Extra Strength, Tylenol Infants Pain + Fever, Tylenol Infants', Tylenol Junior Strength, Tylenol Sore Throat, XS No Aspirin, XS Pain Reliever.

Primary Use
This para-aminophenol derivative is used in the control of fever and mild pain.

Ocular Side Effects
Systemic administration – intravenous, oral, or rectal
Certain
1. Color vision defect – objects have yellow tinge
2. Visual hallucinations

3. Green or chocolate discoloration of subconjunctival or retinal blood vessels
4. Pupils
   a. Mydriasis – toxic states
   b. Decreased reaction to light – toxic states

Probable
1. Eyelids or conjunctiva
   a. Allergic reactions
   b. Erythema
   c. Conjunctivitis – nonspecific
   d. Edema
   e. Urticaria

Possible
1. Decreased vision

Clinical Significance
Ocular side effects due to this analgesic are extremely rare except in toxic states. Data in the spontaneous reports suggest that adverse reactions have occurred at quite low doses, implying a drug idiosyncrasy, a peculiar sensitivity, or just a chance event not related to the drug. Although not mentioned in the *Physicians' Desk Reference* (PDR), the most common adverse ocular event, with over 4500 cases in the spontaneous reports, is periorbital and eyelid edema. This may be real because the PDR reports both angioedema and peripheral edema due to this drug.[1] Toxic responses, mostly self-inflicted, have been reported due to acetaminophen. In chronic therapy, this drug can produce sulfhemoglobinemia, which accounts for the greenish- or chocolate-color change in the subconjunctival or retinal blood vessels.[2]

Confusion in naming this drug is brought on because it is called acetaminophen in the United States and paracetamol in some other countries.

Generic Name:
Aspirin (acetylsalicylic acid [ASA]).

Proprietary Names:
Anacin Adult Low Strength, Aspergum, Aspir-Low, Aspir-Trin, Aspirtab, Bayer Advanced Aspirin, Bayer Aspirin, Bayer Aspirin Extra Strength, Bayer Aspirin Plus, Bayer Aspirin Regimen, Bayer Children's Aspirin, Bayer Extra Strength, Bayer Extra Strength Plus, Bayer Genuine Aspirin, Bayer Low Dose Aspirin Regimen, Bayer Womens Aspirin, Bufferin, Bufferin Extra Strength, Bufferin Low Dose, DURLAZA, Ecotrin, Genacote, Halfprin, MiniPrin, Safety Coated Aspirin, St. Joseph Adult Low Strength, St. Joseph Aspirin.

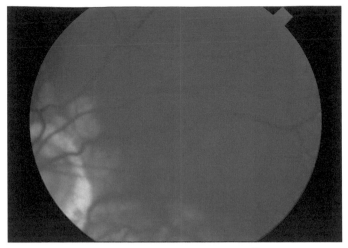

FIG. 7.4 Subretinal hemorrhage.[23]

Primary Use

This salicylate is used as an antipyretic analgesic in the management of gout, acute rheumatic fever, rheumatoid arthritis, subacute thyroiditis, and renal calculi.

Ocular Side Effects
Systemic administration – oral
Certain

1. Decreased vision
2. Myopia – transient
3. Drug secreted in tears
   a. May aggravate or cause ocular sicca
   b. Superficial punctate keratitis
4. Eyelids, conjunctiva, and periorbital
   a. Allergic reactions
   b. Conjunctivitis – nonspecific
   c. Edema – increased if on additional nonsteroidal anti-inflammatories
   d. Urticaria
   e. Purpura
5. Reduces photodynamic therapy with verteporfin

Possible

1. Increased bleeding
   a. Retinal bleeding (Fig. 7.4)
   b. Posttrauma
   c. Neovascularization
2. Improves ocular sicca via anti-inflammatory effect

Conditional/unclassified

1. Cataract – weak cataractogenesis
2. Macular degeneration – exacerbated

Toxic states
Certain

1. Color vision defect
   a. Red-green defect
   b. Objects have yellow tinge
2. Paresis or paralysis of extraocular muscles
3. Diplopia
4. Visual hallucinations
5. Decreased intraocular pressure
6. Nystagmus
7. Pupils
   a. Mydriasis
   b. Decreased or absent reaction to light
8. Visual field defects
   a. Scotomas
   b. Constriction
   c. Hemianopsia
   d. Scintillating scotomas
9. Papilledema
10. Retinal edema
11. Subconjunctival or subretinal hemorrhages (see Fig. 7.4)
12. Toxic amblyopia

Inadvertent ocular exposure or self-mutilation
Certain

1. Conjunctiva and cornea
   a. Edema
   b. Keratitis
   c. Ulceration
   d. Vascularization

Clinical Significance

ASA is one of the most commonly ingested medications in the world. This drug rarely causes ocular problems at normal dosages; however, at higher dosages problems may become clinically significant. This drug can be secreted in the tears, so transient decreased vision, aggravation of ocular sicca, and a keratitis can occur. In rare instances, transient myopia can take place. There are well-documented cases in the spontaneous reports with multiple rechallenge data that ASA may cause decreased vision lasting 3–4 weeks even after 1 dose. Idiosyncratic or hypersensitivity reactions do occur. Those most susceptible to this are middle-aged females and those with asthma, chronic urticaria, rhinitis, or a history of nasal polyps. These hypersensitivity reactions may involve many organ systems, but from the ocular viewpoint, they mainly involve allergic ocular reactions. It has been suggested that corneal donors on high doses of ASA may have the potential for cytotoxic concentrations of the drug to the donor graft endothelium.

Two major studies, the Beaver Dam study and the European Eye study, both have implicated ASA as a possible cofactor in the causation of macular degeneration.[1,2] The Beaver Dam Study showed no effect after 5 years of ASA use; however, 10 years of regular ASA use was associated with a small but statistically significant increase in the risk of incident late and neovascular age-related macular degeneration (AMD).[1] The European study showed that the frequent use of ASA was associated with early AMD and wet late AMD, and the odds ratio increased with increasing frequency and consumption.[2] Both groups stated that further evaluations of these findings are warranted. More recent studies dispute that ASA has an influence on causing or progressing both dry and wet forms of AMD as well as diabetic retinopathy.[3-7]

This drug increases bleeding time, decreases platelet adhesiveness, and can cause hypoprothrombinemia. It can irreversibly prevent platelet aggregation for the 10-day life span of the affected platelet. Conjunctival or retinal bleeds from a clinical perspective are larger in patients on ASA, and clearly bleeding at ocular surgery is prolonged. Regardless of this, there is significant disagreement among ocular surgeons about whether or not ASA should be stopped before ocular surgery; however, most surgeons do not stop ASA.[8,9] Parkin et al pointed out that some oculoplastic surgeons, where appropriate, will limit ASA use preoperatively and immediately postoperatively.[10] The use of ASA in exudative AMD is usually not contraindicated. Wilson et al found ASA protective for choroidal neovascularization in AMD patients.[11]

When used in diabetes, Banerjee et al found no increase in the onset of first-time vitreous hemorrhages.[12]

There are almost 4000 spontaneous case reports of periorbital or eyelid edema associated with ASA use. Berges-Gimeno et al showed that this was only true if the patient was on more than 1 nonsteroidal anti-inflammatory drug.[13]

Ranchod et al have shown that patients taking ASA require more photodynamic therapy (verteporfin) and have poorer outcomes than those who are not taking ASA.[14] They felt that this was possibly due to ASA's effect on the inhibition of platelet aggregation and that it thereby diminishes the effectiveness of photodynamic therapy.

The role of ASA in the causation of ocular sicca is confusing. Two Beaver Dam studies, as well as Smidt et al, have shown that ASA can cause dry eyes.[1,15-17] Foong et al and Tong et al found the opposite.[18,19] In the Singapore Malay eye study of 3280 persons based on a questionnaire, 2.5% of participants on ASA had symptomatic dry eye, whereas 6.5% were symptomatic without ASA.[18] They concluded that, first, ASA is secreted in tears and may have a direct anti-inflammatory effect on the ocular surface; second, there may be a direct effect on the lacrimal gland by inhibiting the release of lysosomal hydrolases or β-hexosaminidase into the tear film; and, third, ASA may systemically suppress cyclooxegenase-2 (COX-2) in the immune system. Therefore there is disagreement; in the end, ASA may play a role in the evaporative form (mechanical effect – crystals in the tear film) of dry eye, making sicca worse, while possibly being of value in the inflammatory form of dry eye.[20]

Toxicity can occur from increased dosages to control pain, cross-sensitivity, additive effects with other nonsteroidal anti-inflammatory drugs, suicide attempts, and other drugs that allow ASA to pass more easily through the blood–brain barrier. ASA in toxic states affects the occipital visual cortex, causing transitory blindness lasting from 3–24 hours, dilated pupils (which react to light), narrow retinal vascular tree, color vision problems, nystagmus, and optic nerve atrophy. Cases of scintillating scotoma, diplopia, papilledema, color vision defects, pupillary changes, and visual field problems may rarely occur. Christen et al suggested a small increased risk in cataracts with chronic ASA use.[21]

Sacca et al pointed out the safety of 1–3% ASA collyrium on the eye for treatment of allergic conjunctivitis.[22] However, as in self-mutilation, the "crushed" tablets can cause mechanical abrasions, leading to ulceration, secondary infection, and even loss of the eye. ASA needs to be considered in any self-mutilation ocular case.

Generic Names:
1. Codeine; 2. dextropropoxyphene.

Proprietary Names:
1. Multi-ingredient preparations only; 2. Darvon.

Primary Use
These mild analgesics are used for the relief of mild to moderate pain. Codeine is also used as an antitussive drug.

Ocular Side Effects
Systemic administration – oral
Certain
1. Pupils
    a. Miosis – acute and toxic states
    b. Pinpoint pupils – initial
    c. Mydriasis – withdrawal
2. Decreased vision – withdrawal
3. Eyelid or conjunctival edema (codeine)
4. Extraocular muscles
    a. Strabismus
    b. Diplopia

Possible
1. Myopia (codeine)
2. Visual hallucinations
3. May aggravate or cause ocular sicca (dextropropoxyphene)
4. Lacrimation – withdrawal states
5. Urticaria (codeine)

Conditional/unclassified
1. Optic atrophy – toxic states (dextropropoxyphene)

Clinical Significance
Codeine and dextropropoxyphene seldom cause significant ocular side effects. Whereas codeine may cause miosis, dextropropoxyphene does so only in overdose situations. Visual disturbances are usually insignificant. Cases in the spontaneous reports implicate codeine in causing transient myopia. Bergmanson et al reported that Darvocet-N, a compound containing dextropropoxyphene and acetaminophen, caused reduced tear secretion, which resulted in soft contact lens dehydration and corneal epithelial abrasion.[1] Weiss reported bilateral optic atrophy possibly associated with an overdose of Darvon, a compound containing dextropropoxyphene, aspirin, and caffeine.[2] Other contributing factors in this patient may have been acidosis, hypokalemia, or hypoxia. Cases of transient internuclear ophthalmoplegia have been reported, but it is difficult to prove a cause-and-effect relationship.[3,4] Intravenous

naloxone, however, caused the ophthalmoplegia to return to normal.

CLASS: NARCOTIC ANTAGONISTS

Generic Name:
Naltrexone hydrochloride.

Proprietary Names:
Depade, ReVia, Vivitrol.

Primary Use
This narcotic antagonist is used primarily in the management of narcotic-induced respiratory depression.

Ocular Side Effects
Systemic administration – intramuscular or oral
Certain
1. Miosis
2. Visual hallucinations – withdrawal states
3. Lacrimation – withdrawal states

Probable
1. Eyelids or conjunctiva
    a. Allergic reactions
    b. Erythema
    c. Photosensitivity
    d. Urticaria
2. Irritation
    a. Photophobia
    b. Pain
    c. Edema
    d. Burning sensation

Possible
1. Decreased vision
2. Pseudoptosis
3. Mydriasis – if a recent narcotic user

Clinical Significance
Although ocular side effects due to this narcotic antagonist are common, they have little clinical significance other than as a screening test to discover narcotic users. This drug may produce either a miosis or no effect on the pupils when administered to non-addicts, but in addicts they cause mydriasis. Vivid visual hallucinations are seen both as an adverse ocular reaction and as a withdrawal symptom. Because up to 5% of patients may have secondary xerostomia, naltrexone may also aggravate or cause ocular sicca.[1]

CLASS: STRONG ANALGESICS

Generic Name:
Diacetylmorphine (diamorphine, heroin).

Proprietary Name:
Generic only.

Street Names:
Boy, brother, brown sugar, caballo, ca-ca, crap, h, harry, horse, junk, poison, scag, schmeck, shit, smack, stuff, tecata.

Primary Use
This potent narcotic analgesic is administered preoperatively and postoperatively and in the terminal stage of cancer for the relief of severe pain.

Ocular Side Effects
Systemic administration – epidural, inhalation, intramuscular, intrathecal, intravenous, oral, or subcutaneous
Certain
1. Pupils
   a. Miosis
   b. Pinpoint pupils – toxic states
   c. Absence of reaction to light
   d. Mydriasis – withdrawal states
   e. Anisocoria – withdrawal states
2. Decreased accommodation
3. Irritation
   a. Lacrimation
   b. Photophobia
4. Eyelids or conjunctiva
   a. Hyperemia
   b. Erythema
   c. Edema
   d. Urticaria
   e. Decreased blink rate
5. Ocular motility
   a. Esotropia (on withdrawal)
   b. Exotropia

Probable
1. Intranuclear ophthalmoplegia (toxic)

Possible
1. Horner's syndrome
   a. Ptosis
   b. Increased sensitivity to sympathetic drugs

Ocular teratogenic effects
Probable
1. Strabismus

Clinical Significance
Heroin can cause pupillary changes, which are often used to identify probable users. Ocular irritation and conjunctival changes are common.

There are various extraocular muscle abnormalities due to toxic states of this drug, but mainly during withdrawal.[1-5] There is typically full recovery when the drug is discontinued. Firth and Kowal et al have well documented that esotropia with double vision occurs with heroin withdrawal, and its use can cause intermittent or persistent exotropia.[4,6] Sutter et al described a case where diplopia occurred within hours after taking heroin and cleared within 4 days.[2] Exotropia may be more common with toxic states and esotropia on withdrawal. Awareness of these ocular side effects is essential to avoid neurologic referrals.

Heroin addiction has been associated with bacterial and fungal endophthalmitis, probably due to contaminated intravenous administration and impurities on an embolus basis. If undiagnosed and incompletely treated, these indirect drug-related entities can result in permanent loss of vision. Horner's syndrome has been reported in chronic addicts. Withdrawal of diacetylmorphine in the addict may cause excessive tearing, irregular pupils, and decreased accommodation.

In opiate-dependent mothers, primarily on methadone, Gill et al estimated at least a 10-fold increase over the general population of ocular strabismus.[7]

Generic Name:
Fentanyl.

Proprietary Names:
ABSTRAL, Actiq, Duragesic, Fentora, IONSYS, Lazanda, Sublimaze, SUBSYS.

Primary Use
A phenylpiperidine synthetic opiate agonist used in anesthesia and for chronic pain.

Ocular Side Effects
Systemic administration – oral or transdermal
Certain
1. Decreased vision

Probable
1. Pupils
   a. Miosis (primary intravenous)
   b. Mydriasis (toxic states)
2. Visual hallucinations
3. Oculogyric crisis

Possible
1. Extraocular muscles
    a. Ptosis
    b. Diplopia
    c. Abnormal movements
2. Eyelids or conjunctiva
    a. Edema
    b. Periorbital edema

Conditional/unclassified
1. Elevated intraocular pressure

Systemic Side Effects
Systemic administration – intravenous
Possible
1. Sneezing reflex

Clinical Significance

Fentanyl may be 75–100 times more toxic than morphine. Ocular side effects associated with fentanyl use are rare and seldom of clinical significance. Decreased vision may occur early, but is transitory and seldom of clinical importance. Pupillary changes, although rare, can cause miosis at around a 1% rate if the drug is given intravenously. Given orally, this is a rare event and may be dose dependent. In suicide attempts mydriasis has occurred. Transdermal fentanyl causes hallucinations in 3–10% of patients.[1] In spontaneous reports, oculogyric crisis was reported in a higher frequency than with most other drugs. Although this drug rarely affects extraocular or intraocular muscles, pharmacologically one might expect a decrease in accommodation or convergence. An unusual suspected effect of reverse ocular dripping has been reported.[2] This consisted of cyclic involuntary conjugate upward ocular movements, followed by a tonic phase, followed by a downward movement to the primary position.

Ahn et al report that when fentanyl is given as a preoperative sedation, increased sneezing may occur.[3]

Generic Names:

1. Hydromorphone hydrochloride (dihydromorphinone); 2. oxymorphone hydrochloride.

Proprietary Names:

1. Dilaudid, Dilaudid-HP, Exalgo, Simplist Dilaudid; 2. Numorphan, Opana.

Primary Use

These hydrogenated ketones of morphine are used for the relief of moderate to severe pain.

Ocular Side Effects
Systemic administration – intramuscular, intranasal, intravenous, oral, or sublingual
Certain
1. Decreased vision
2. Decreased accommodation
3. Pupils
    a. Miosis
    b. Pinpoint pupils – toxic states
    c. Mydriasis – hypoxic states
4. Eyelids or conjunctiva
    a. Allergic reactions
    b. Urticaria
    c. Contact dermatitis

Probable
1. Extraocular muscles
    a. Nystagmus
    b. Diplopia
2. Visual hallucinations

Clinical Significance

Although not uncommon, adverse ocular effects due to these drugs are rarely significant. All ocular side effects are reversible and transitory. Difficulty in focusing is probably the most frequent complaint. These drugs cause xerostomia and ocular sicca in up to 2% of patients.[1]

Shah et al described diffuse retinal ischemia with permanent count-fingers vision in a patient after 8 episodes over a 1-month period of abuse with crushed extended-release oxymorphone taken intravenously.[2] A similar case was reported by Aseem et al.[3]

Generic Name:

Meperidine hydrochloride (pethidine).

Proprietary Names:

Demerol, Meperitab.

Primary Use

This phenylpiperidine narcotic analgesic is used for the relief of pain, as a preoperative medication, and to supplement surgical anesthesia.

Ocular Side Effects
Systemic administration – intramuscular, intravenous, oral, or subcutaneous
Probable
1. Pupils
    a. Miosis
    b. Mydriasis – toxic reaction
    c. Decreased reaction to light (overdose)

2. Decreased intraocular pressure – minimal
3. Decreased vision
4. Eyelids or conjunctiva
   a. Allergic reactions
   b. Erythema
   c. Urticaria
5. Visual hallucinations

Possible
1. Nystagmus
2. Ocular signs of drug-induced Parkinson disease
   a. Paresis or paralysis of extraocular muscles
   b. Ptosis
   c. Diplopia

Inadvertent ocular exposure – dust
Certain
1. Blepharitis
2. Conjunctivitis – nonspecific

Clinical Significance
None of the ocular side effects due to pethidine are of major clinical importance, and all are transitory. Miosis is uncommon at therapeutic dosages and seldom significant. Mydriasis and decreased pupillary light reflexes are seen only in acute toxicity or in long-term addicts. Decrease in intraocular pressure is minimal. Ocular side effects, such as blepharitis or conjunctivitis, have been seen secondary to pethidine dust.

Generic Name:
Methadone hydrochloride.

Proprietary Names:
Dolophine, Methadose.

Street Names:
Dolly, doses, juice, meth.

Primary Use
This synthetic analgesic is useful in the treatment of chronic painful conditions and in the detoxification treatment of patients dependent on heroin or other morphine-like drugs.

Ocular Side Effects
Systemic administration – intramuscular (rare), intravenous, or oral
Certain
1. Pupils
   a. Miosis

   b. Pinpoint pupils – toxic states
   c. Mydriasis – withdrawal states
2. Talc retinopathy (intravenous)
3. Decreased vision
4. Decreased spontaneous eye movements

Probable
1. Eyelids
   a. Urticaria
   b. Edema

Ocular teratogenic effects
Possible
1. May aggravate or cause ocular sicca
2. Extraocular muscles
   a. Diplopia
   b. Nystagmus
   c. Strabismus
3. Cerebral visual impairment
4. Visual evoked potential – reduced

Clinical Significance
Methadone seldom causes significant ocular side effects. Miosis is uncommon, but may occur at therapeutic dosages. In severe toxic states, there may be "pinpoint" pupils. Talc emboli, appearing as small white glistening dots in the macular area, have been reported in addicts who intravenously inject oral medications that contain talc as filler.[1] A case of cortical blindness, apparently secondary to anoxia, has been reported in a child who experienced severe respiratory depression.[2] Nelson et al and Gill et al reported the incidence of strabismus in infants of methadone-dependent mothers to be at least 10 times greater than that seen in the general population.[3,4] Yoo et al confirmed this at an incidence of 2–3 times higher than average.[5]

Infants born of drug-misusing mothers prescribed methadone in their pregnancy may be at risk for a wide range of visual problems.[6,7] Hamilton summarized their data: "We cannot be certain whether the visual abnormalities described are secondary to substitute methadone, ongoing illicit maternal opiate and/or benzodiazepine misuse, pharmacologic drugs (including oral morphine solution and/or phenobarbitone) used to treat neonatal abstinence syndrome, or other unidentified factors."[6] McGlone et al showed abnormal visual electrophysiology in infants born to drug-misusing mothers prescribed maintenance methadone.[8] It persisted to 6 months of age and was associated with abnormal clinical visual assessment.

Methadone may impair driving.[9] However, other studies have found driving to be safe if the patient is screened, including urine tests, for other drugs.[10–12] This is only for oral methadone because both intramuscular and intravenous methadone cause sedation.

Withdrawal states with ocular side effects include mydriasis, photophobia, and epiphora.[13]

Generic Names:

1. Morphine sulfate; 2. opium.

Proprietary Names:

1. Arymo ER, Astramorph PF, Avinza, DepoDur, Duramorph, Duramorph PF, Infumorph, Kadian, Morphabond, MS Contin, Oramorph SR, RMS, Roxanol, Roxanol-T; 2. Generic only.

Street Names:

1. M, morf, white stuff; 2. Joy plant, pen yan, skee.

Primary Use

These opioids are used for the relief of severe pain. Morphine is the alkaloid that gives opium its analgesic action.

Ocular Side Effects
Systemic administration – intramuscular, oral, rectal, or subcutaneous
Certain

1. Pupils
   a. Miosis
   b. Pinpoint pupils – toxic states
   c. Mydriasis – withdrawal or extreme toxic states
   d. Irregularity – withdrawal states
2. Decreased vision
3. Extraocular muscles
   a. Diplopia
   b. Nystagmus
   c. Decreased convergence
4. Decreased accommodation
5. Decreased intraocular pressure
6. Visual hallucinations
7. Lacrimation
   a. Increased – withdrawal states
   b. Decreased
8. Eyelids or conjunctiva
   a. Allergic reactions
   b. Conjunctivitis – nonspecific
   c. Urticaria
   d. Pruritus
9. Color vision defect – mainly blues and yellows (addicts)
10. Pain
11. Ptosis (opium)

Possible

1. Myopia
2. May aggravate or cause ocular sicca
3. Accommodative spasm

Systemic administration – epidural or intravenous
Certain

1. Vertical nystagmus

Ocular teratogenic effects
Probable

1. Increased incidence of strabismus

Local ophthalmic use or exposure – morphine
Certain

1. Miosis
2. Increased intraocular pressure
3. Anesthesia

Clinical Significance

These narcotics seldom cause significant ocular side effects, and all proven drug-induced toxic effects are transitory. Miosis is the most frequent ocular side effect and is commonly seen at therapeutic dosage levels. Up to 10% of patients on these drugs have xerostomia; therefore they may also have ocular sicca.[1] Ocular side effects reported in long-term addicts may include color vision or visual field changes that may be due to vitamin deficiency rather than to the drug itself. Withdrawal of morphine or opium in the addict may cause excessive tearing, irregular pupils, decreased accommodation, and diplopia. Epidural and intravenous opioids have been reported to cause vertical nystagmus.[2,3] Castano et al reported that intravenous morphine could cause eyelid pruritus.[4]

Gill et al reported that the incidence of strabismus in infants of opiate-dependent mothers is at least 10 times greater than that seen in the general population.[5]

Generic Name:

Pentazocine.

Proprietary Name:

Talwin.

Primary Use

This benzomorphan narcotic analgesic is used for the relief of pain, as a preoperative medication, and to supplement surgical anesthesia.

Ocular Side Effects
Systemic administration – intramuscular, intravenous, or subcutaneous
Certain
1. Miosis
2. Decreased vision
3. Visual hallucinations

Probable
1. Nystagmus
2. Diplopia
3. Lacrimation – abrupt withdrawal states
4. Decreased accommodation
5. Eyelids or conjunctiva
   a. Erythema
   b. Conjunctivitis – nonspecific
   c. Edema
6. Decreased spontaneous eye movements

Possible
1. Oculogyric crisis

Clinical Significance

Ocular side effects due to pentazocine are usually insignificant and reversible. Miosis is the most frequent and is seen routinely even at suggested dosage levels. Although visual complaints are seldom of major consequence, diplopia may be incapacitating. Vivid visual hallucinations, some of which are threatening, have been reported with this drug.[1] Once pentazocine is discontinued, the hallucinations cease. Burstein et al reported oculogyric crisis possibly related to this drug.[2]

REFERENCES
Drug: Allopurinol sodium
1. Lerman S, Megaw JM, Gardner K. Allopurinol therapy and human cataractogenesis. *Am J Ophthalmol.* 1982;94:141–146.
2. Garbe E, Suissa S, LeLorier J. Exposure to allopurinol and the risk of cataract extraction in elderly patients. *Arch Ophthalmol.* 1998;116:1652–1656.
3. Leske MC, Chylack LT, Wu S. The lens opacities case-control study. Risk factors for cataract. *Arch Ophthalmol.* 1991;109:244–251.
4. Cheah CK, Vijaya Singham N, Gun SC. A case report on allopurinol induced crystalline maculopathy. *Int J Rheum Dis.* 2017;20(12):2253–2255.
5. Fraunfelder FT. Allopurinol-induced cataracts [photograph]. Portland (OR): Casey Eye Institute; Oregon Health & Science University:c1990. 1 photograph: color.

Drug: Colchicine
1. Alster Y, Varssano D, Loewenstein A, et al. Delay of corneal wound healing in patients treated with colchicine. *Ophthalmology.* 1997;104:118–119.
2. Biedner BZ, Rothkoff L, Friedman L, et al. Colchicine suppression of corneal healing after strabismus surgery. *Br J Ophthalmol.* 1977;61:496–497.
3. Vignes S, Vidailhet M, Dormont D, et al. Pseudotumorous presentation of neuro-Behçet: role of the withdrawal of colchicine. *Revue de Medecine Interne.* 1998;19(1):55–59.
4. Dickenson AJ, Yates J. Bilateral eyelid necrosis as a complication of pseudomonal septicaemia. *Br J Oral Maxillofac Surg.* 2002;40:175–176.

Drugs: Adalimumab, etanercept, infliximab
1. Adalimumab etanercept. *infliximab;* 2018. Retrieved from http://www.pdr.net.
2. Smith JR, Levinson RD, Holland GN, et al. Differential efficacy of tumor necrosis factor inhibition in the management of inflammatory eye disease and associated rheumatic disease. *Arthritis Care Res.* 2001;45:252–257.
3. Tauber T, Daniel D, Barash J, et al. Optic neuritis associated with etanercept therapy in two patients with extended oligoarticular juvenile idiopathic arthritis. *Rheumatology.* 2005;44:405.
4. Noguera-Pons R, Borrás-Blasco J, Romero-Crespo I, et al. Optic neuritis with concurrent etanercept and isoniazid therapy. *Ann Pharmacother.* 2005;39:2131–2135.
5. Foroozan R, Buono LM, Sergott RC, et al. Retrobulbar optic neuritis associated with infliximab. *Arch Ophthalmol.* 2002;120:985–987.
6. Mejico LJ. Infliximab-associated retrobulbar optic neuritis. *Arch Ophthalmol.* 2004;122:793–794.
7. ten Tusscher MP, Jacobs PJ, Busch MJ, et al. Bilateral anterior toxic neuropathy and the use of infliximab. *BMJ.* 2003;326:579.
8. Strong BYC, Erny BC, Herzenberg H, et al. Retrobulbar optic neuritis associated with infliximab in a patient with Crohn disease. *Ann Intern Med.* 2004;140:677–678.
9. Tran TH, Milea D, Cassoux N, et al. Optic neuritis associated with infliximab. *J Fr Ophthalmol.* 2005;28:201–204.
10. Chung JH, Van Stavern GP, Frohman LP, et al. Adalimumab-associated optic neuritis. *J Neurol Sci.* 2006;244:133–136.
11. Winthrop KL, Chen L, Fraunfelder FW, et al. Initiation of anti-TNF therapy and the risk of optic neuritis: from the safety assessment of biologic therapy (SABER) study. *Am J Ophthalmol.* 2013;155(1):183–189.
12. Reddy AR, Backhouse OC. Does etanercept induce uveitis? *Br J Ophthalmol.* 2003;87:925.
13. Taban M, Dupps WJ, Mandell B, et al. Etanercept (enbrel)-associated inflammatory eye disease: case report and review of the literature. *Ocul Immunol Inflamm.* 2006;14:145–150.
14. Lim LL, Fraunfelder FW, Rosenbaum JT. Do tumor necrosis factor inhibitors cause uveitis? A registry-based study. *Arthritis Rheum.* 2007;56(10):3248–3252.

15. Hashkes PJ, Shajrawi I. Sarcoid-related uveitis occurring during etanercept therapy. *Clin Exp Rheumatol.* 2003;21:645–646.
16. Wladis EJ, Tarasen AJ, Roth ZJ, et al. Orbital sarcoid-like granulomatosis after inhibition of tumor necrosis factor-α. *Ophthal Plast Reconstr Surg.* 2016;32(2):e30–e32.
17. Clifford LJ, Rossiter JD. Peripheral visual field loss following treatment with etanercept. *Br J Ophthalmol.* 2004;88:842.
18. Caramaschi P, Carletto A, Biasi D, et al. Orbital myositis in rheumatoid arthritis patient during etanercept treatment. *Clin Exp Rheumotol.* 2003;21:136–137.
19. Roos JCP, Ostor AJK. Orbital cellulitis in a patient receiving infliximab for ankylosing spondylitis. *Am J Ophthalmol.* 2006;141:767–769.
20. Giganti M, Beer PM, Lemanski N, et al. Adverse events after intravitreal infliximab (remicade). *Retina.* 2010;30:71–80.
21. Drury J, Hickman SJ. Internuclear ophthalmoplegia associated with anti-TNFα medication. *Strabismus.* 2015;23(1):30–32.
22. Matet A, Daruich A, Beydoun T, et al. Systemic adalimumab induced peripheral corneal infiltrates: a case report. *BMC Ophthalmol.* 2015,15:57.

Drug: Auranofin
1. Lopez JD, Benitez del Castillo JM, Lopez CD, et al. Confocal microscopy in ocular chrysiasis. *Cornea.* 2003;22:573–575.
2. Arffa RC. Drugs and metals. In: Arffa RC, ed. *Grayson's Diseases of the Cornea.* 3rd ed. St Louis: Mosby; 1991:617–631.
3. McCormick SA, DiBartolomeo AG, Raju VK, et al. Ocular chrysiasis. *Ophthalmology.* 1985;92:1432–1435.
4. Zamir E, Read RW, Affeldt JC. Gold induced interstitial keratitis. *Br J Ophthalmol.* 2001;85:1386–1387.
5. Kanski JJ. *Clinical Diagnosis in Ophthalmology.* London: Mosby Elsevier; 2006.

Drugs: Celecoxib, etodolac
1. Fraunfelder FW, Solomon J, Mehelas TJ. Ocular adverse effects associated with cyclooxygenase-2 inhibitors. *Arch Ophthalmol.* 2006;124:277–278.
2. Meyer CH, Mennel S, Schmidt JC, et al. Adverse effects of cyclooxygenase-2 inhibitors on ocular vision. *Arch Ophthalmol.* 2006;124:1368.
3. Recchia FM, Chen E, Li C, et al. Use of COX-2 inhibitors in patients with retinal venous occlusive disease. *Retina.* 2008;28:134–137.
4. Coulter DM, Clark DW. Disturbance of vision by COX-2 inhibitors. *Expert Opin Drug Saf.* 2004;3:607–614.
5. Coulter DM, Clark DW. Visual disturbances with COX-2 inhibitors. *Prescr Update.* 2004;25:8–9.
6. Lund BC, Neiman RF. Visual disturbance associated with celecoxib. *Pharmacotherapy.* 2001;21:114–115.
7. Celecoxib etodolac. 2018. Retrieved from http://www.pdr.net.

Drug: Fenoprofen calcium
1. Fenoprofen calcium. 2018. Retrieved from http://www.pdr.net.

2. Fraunfelder FT, Samples JR, Fraunfelder FW. Possible optic nerve side effects associated with nonsteroidal anti-inflammatory drugs. *J Toxicol Cutan Ocul Toxicol.* 1994;13(4):311–316.

Drug: Flurbiprofen
1. Flurbiprofen. 2018. Retrieved from http://www.pdr.net.

Drug: Ibuprofen
1. Szmyd L, Perry HD. Keratopathy associated with the use of naproxen. *Am J Ophthalmol.* 1985;99:598.
2. Nicastro NJ. Visual disturbances associated with over-the-counter ibuprofen in three patients. *Ann Ophthalmol.* 1989;29:447–450.
3. Ravi S, Keat AC, Keat EC. Colitis caused by non-steroidal anti-inflammatory drugs. *Postgrad Med J.* 1986;62:773–776.
4. Clements D, Williams GT, Rhodes J. Colitis associated with ibuprofen. *BMJ.* 1990;301:987.
5. Ibuprofen and eye twitch – from FDA reports. ; 2018. Retrieved from http://www.ehealthme.com.
6. Nasiri J, Zamani F. Periorbital ecchmyosis (raccoon eye) and orbital hematoma following endoscopic retrograde cholangiopancreatography. *Case Rep Gastroenterol.* 2017;11(1):134–141.

Drug: Indomethacin (indometacin)
1. Burns CA. Indomethacin, reduced retinal sensitivity, and corneal deposits. *Am J Ophthalmol.* 1968;66:825–835.
2. Henkes HE, van Lith GH, Canta LR. Indomethacin retinopathy. *Am J Ophthalmol.* 1972;73:846–856.
3. Badalá F, Fiorett M, Macrí A. Effect of topical 0.1% indomethacin solution versus 0.1% fluorometholone acetate on ocular surface and pain control following laser subepithelial keratomileusis (LASEK). *Cornea.* 2004;23:550–553.
4. Sheehan GJ, Kutzner MR. Acute asthma attack due to ophthalmic Indocin. *Ann Int Med.* 1989;111:337–338.
5. Gueudry J, Lebel H, Muraine M. Severe corneal complications associated with topical indomethacin use. *Br J Ophthalmol.* 2010;94(1):133–134.
6. Fraunfelder FT. *Indomethacin-induced macular pigment mottling [photograph].* Portland, OR: Casey Eye Institute, Oregon Health & Science University; ©1990. 1 photograph: color.

Drug: Ketoprofen
1. Ketoprofen. 2018 Retrieved from http://www.pdr.net.
2. Umez-Eronini EM. Conjunctivitis due to ketoprofen. *Lancet.* 1978;2:737.
3. Alomar A. Ketoprofen photodermatitis. *Contact Dermatitis.* 1985;12:112–113.
4. Le Coz CJ, Bottlaender A, Scrivener JN, et al. Photocontact dermatitis from ketoprofen and tiaprofenic acid: cross-reactivity study in 12 consecutive patients. *Contact Dermatitis.* 1998;38(5):245–252.
5. McDowell IFW, McConnell JB. Cholinergic crisis in myasthenia gravis precipitated by ketoprofen. *BMJ.* 1985;291:1094.

6. Larizza D, Colombo A, Lorini R, et al. Ketoprofen causing pseudotumor cerebri in Bartter's syndrome. *N Engl J Med.* 1979;300:796.

Drug: Naproxen sodium
1. Naproxen sodium. 2018. Retrieved from http://www.pdr.net.
2. Szmyd Jr L, Perry HD. Keratopathy associated with the use of naproxen. *Am J Ophthalmol.* 1985;99:598.
3. Fincham JE. Exacerbation of glaucoma in an elderly female taking naproxen sodium: a case report. *J Geriatr Drug Ther.* 1989;3:139–143.

Drug: Piroxicam
1. Fraunfelder FT, Samples JR, Fraunfelder FW. Possible optic nerve side effects associated with nonsteroidal anti-inflammatory drugs. *J Toxicol Cut Ocular Toxicol.* 1994;13(4):311–316.
2. Varela P, Amorim I, Sanches M, et al. Photosensitivity induced by piroxicam. *Acta Med. Portuguesa.* 1998;11(11):997–1001.
3. Piroxicam. 2018. Retrieved from http://www.pdr.net.

Drug: Acetaminophen (paracetamol)
1. Acetaminophen. 2018. Retrieved from http://www.pdr.net.
2. Kneezel LD, Kitchens CS. Phenacetin-induced sulfhemoglobinemia: report of a case and review of the literature. *Johns Hopkins Med J.* 1976;139:175–177.

Drug: Aspirin (acetylsalicylic acid)
1. Klein R, Klein BE, Linton KL. Prevalence of age-related maculopathy: the Beaver Dam Eye Study. *Ophthalmology.* 1992;99(6):933–943.
2. de Jong PT, Chakravarthy U, Rahu M, et al. Associations between aspirin use and aging macula disorder: the European eye study. *Ophthalmology.* 2012;11:112–118.
3. Michalska-Malecka K, Regucka A, Spiewak D, et al. Does the use of acetylsalicylic acid have an influence on our vision? *Clin Interv Aging.* 2016;11:1567–1574.
4. Buitendijk GHS, Schauwvlieghe AME, Vingerling JR, et al. Antiplatelet and anticoagulant drugs do not affect visual outcome in neovascular age-related macular degeneration in the BRAMD trial. *Am J Ophthalmol.* 2018;187:130–137.
5. De Jong PT, Wang JJ, Fletcher AE. Aspirin use and aging macular disorder. *JAMA Ophthalmol.* 2014;132(1):9–10.
6. Small KW, Garabetian CA, Shaya FS. Macular degeneration and aspirin use. *Retina.* 2017;37:1630–1635.
7. Shi Y, Tham YC, Cheung N, et al. Is aspirin associated with diabetic retinopathy? The Singapore Epidemiology of Eye Disease (SEED) study. *PLoS One.* 2017;12(4):e0175966.
8. Assia EI, Raskin T, Kaiserman I, et al. Effect of aspirin intake on bleeding during cataract surgery. *J Cataract Refract Surg.* 1998;24:1243–1246.
9. Kokolakis S, Zafirakis P, Livir-Rallatos G, et al. Aspirin intake and bleeding during cataract surgery. *J Cataract Refract Surg.* 1999;25:301–302.

10. Parkin B, Manners R. Aspirin and warfarin therapy in oculoplastic surgery. *Br J Ophthalmol.* 2000;84:1426–1427.
11. Wilson HL, Schwartz DM, Bhatt HR, et al. Statin and aspirin therapy are associated with decreased rates of choroidal neovascularization among patients with age-related macular degeneration. *Am J Ophthalmol.* 2004;137:615–624.
12. Banerjee S, Denniston AK, Gibson JM, et al. Does cardiovascular therapy affect the onset and recurrence of preretinal and vitreous haemorrhage in diabetic eye disease? *Eye.* 2004;18:821–825.
13. Berges-Gimeno MP, Stevenson DD. Nonsteroidal anti-inflammatory drug-induced reactions and desensitization. *J Asthma.* 2004;41(4):375–384.
14. Ranchod TM, Guercio JR, Ying G-S, et al. Effect of aspirin therapy on photodynamic therapy with verteporfin for choroidal neovascularization. *Retina.* 2008;28:711–716.
15. Klein BE, Howard KP, Gangnon RE, et al. Long-term use of aspirin and age-related macular degeneration. *JAMA.* 2012;308(23):2469–2478.
16. Klein R, Klein BE, Jensen SC, et al. The five-year incidence and progression of age-related maculopathy: the Beaver Dam Eye Study. *Ophthalmology.* 1997;104(1):7–21.
17. Smidt D, Torpet LA, Nauntofte B, et al. Associations between oral and ocular dryness, labial and whole salivary flow rates, systemic diseases and medications in a sample of older people. *Community Dent Oral Epidemiol.* 2011;39:276–288.
18. Foong AW, Saw SM, Loo JL, et al. Rationale and methodology for a population-based study of eye diseases in Malay people: the Singapore Malay eye study (SiMES). *Ophthalmic Epidemiol.* 2007;14:25–35.
19. Tong L, Wong TY. Aspirin and dry eye? *Ophthalmology.* 2009;116(1):167–168.
20. Fraunfelder FT, Sciubba JJ, Mathers WD. The role of medications in causing dry eye. *J Ophthalmol.* 2012;2012:285851.
21. Christen WG, Ajani UA, Schaumberg DA, et al. Aspirin use and risk of cataract in posttrial follow-up of physicians' health study I. *Arch Ophthalmol.* 2001;119:405–412.
22. Sacca SC, Cerqueti PM, et al. Topical use of aspirin in allergic conjunctivitis. *Bull Ocul.* 1988;67(suppl 4):193–196.
23. Chak M, Williamson TH. Spontaneous suprachoroidal haemorrhage associated with high myopia and aspirin. *Eye.* 2003;17:525–527.

Drugs: Codeine, dextropropoxyphene
1. Bergmanson JP, Rios R. Adverse reaction to painkiller in Hydrogel lens wearer. *Am Optom Assoc.* 1981;52:257–258.
2. Weiss IS. Optic atrophy after propoxyphene overdose. Report of a case. *Ann Ophthalmol.* 1982;14:586–587.
3. El-Mallakh RS. Internuclear ophthalmoplegia with narcotic overdosage. *Ann Neurol.* 1986;20:107.
4. Rizzo M, Corbett J. Bilateral internuclear ophthalmoplegia reversed by naloxone. *Arch Neurol.* 1983;40:242–243.

Drug: Naltrexone hydrochloride
1. Naltrexone hydrochloride. 2018. Retrieved from http://www.pdr.net.

Drug: Diacetylmorphine (diamorphine, heroin)
1. Mattoo SK, Mahajan S, Nebhinani N, et al. Diplopia with dextropropoxyphene withdrawal. *Gen Hosp Psychiatry*. 2013;35(1):100–101.
2. Sutter FK, Landau K. Heroin and strabismus. *Swiss Med Wkly*. 2003;133:293–294.
3. Firth AY. Heroin withdrawal as a possible cause of acute concomitant esotropia in adults. *Eye*. 2001;15:189–192.
4. Kowal L, Mee JJ, Nadkarni S, et al. Acute esotropia in heroin withdrawal: a case series. *Binocul Vis Strabismus Q*. 2003;18:163–166.
5. Burian HM, Miller JE. Committant convergent strabismus with acute onset. *Am J Ophthalmol*. 1958;45:55–64.
6. Firth AY. Heroin and diplopia. *Addiction*. 2005;100:46–50.
7. Gill AC, Oei J, Lewis NL, et al. Strabismus in infants of opiate-dependent mothers. *Acta Paediatr*. 2003;92:379–385.

Drug: Fentanyl
1. Jeal W, Benfield P. Transdermal fentanyl: a review of its pharmacological properties and therapeutic efficacy in pain control. *Drugs*. 1997;53(1):109–138.
2. Kitagawa N, Sakurai M. Drug-induced reverse ocular dripping. *BMJ Case Rep*. 2014;2014 Sep 29.
3. Ahn ES, Mills DM, Meyer DR, et al. Sneezing reflex associated with intravenous sedation and periocular anesthetic injection. *Am J Ophthalmol*. 2008;146(1):31–35.

Drugs: Hydromorphone hydrochloride (dihydromorphinone), oxymorphone hydrochloride
1. Hydromorphone hydrochloride, oxymorphone hydrochloride. 2018. Retrieved from http://www.pdr.net.
2. Shah RJ, Cherney EF. Diffuse retinal ischemia following intravenous crushed oxymorphone abuse. *JAMA Ophthalmol*. 2014;132(6):780–781.
3. Aseem F, Zamora BG, Kauffman L, et al. Bilateral exudative retinal detachments due to thrombotic microangiopathy associated with intravenous abuse of Opana ER. *Am J Ophthalmol Case Rep*. 2018;11:72–74.

Drug: Methadone hydrochloride
1. Murphy SB, Jackson WB, Pare JA. Talc retinopathy. *Can J Ophthalmol*. 1978;13:152–156.
2. Ratcliffe SC. Methadone poisoning in a child. *BMJ*. 1963;1:1056–1070.
3. Nelson LB, Ehrlich S, Calhoun JH, et al. Occurrence of strabismus in infants born to drug-dependent women. *Am J Dis Child*. 1987;141:175–178.
4. Gill AC, Oei J, Lewis NL, et al. Strabismus in infants of opiate-dependent mothers. *Acta Paediatr*. 2003;92:379–385.
5. Yoo SH, Jansson LM, Park HJ. Sensorimotor outcomes in children with prenatal exposure to methadone. *J AAPOS*. 2017;21(4):316–321.

6. Hamilton R, McGlone L, MacKinnon JR, et al. Ophthalmic, clinical and visual electrophysiological findings in children born to mothers prescribed substitute methadone in pregnancy. *Br J Ophthalmol*. 2010;94:696–700.
7. Gupta M, Mulvihill AO, Lascaratos G, et al. Nystagmus and reduced visual acuity secondary to drug exposure in utero: long-term follow up. *J Ped Ophthalmol Strab*. 2012;49(1):58–63.
8. McGlone L, Hamilton R, McCulloch DL, et al. Visual outcome in infants born to drug-misusing mothers prescribed methadone in pregnancy. *Br J Ophthalmol*. 2014;98:238–245.
9. Giacomuzzi SM, Ertl M, Vigl A, et al. Driving capacity of patients treated with methadone and slow-release oral morphine. *Addiction*. 2005;100(7):1027.
10. Reece AS. Experience of road and other trauma by the opiate dependent patient: a survey report. *Subst Abuse Treat Prev Policy*. 2008;3:10.
11. *Methadone and driving article abstracts: brief literature review*. Institute for Metropolitan Affairs: Roosevelt University; 2008.
12. Ford C, Barnard J, Bury J, et al. *Guidance for the Use of Methadone for the Treatment of Opioid Dependence in Primary Care*. Royal College of General Practitioners; 2018. Retrieved from http://www.rcgp.org.uk/PDF/drug_meth guidance.pdf.
13. Methadone withdrawal symptoms. *Michael's House Drug and Alcohol Treatment Centers*; 2018. Retrieved from https://www.michaelshouse.com/methadone-addiction/withdrawal-symptoms/.

Drugs: Morphine sulfate, opium
1. Morphine sulfate. 2018. Retrieved from http://www.pdr.net.
2. Fish DJ, Rosen SM. Epidural opioids as a cause of vertical nystagmus. *Anesthesiology*. 1990;73:785–786.
3. Henderson RD, Wijdicks EF. Downbeat nystagmus associated with intravenous patient-controlled administration of morphine. *Anesth Analg*. 2000;91:691–692.
4. Castano G, Lyons CJ. Eyelid pruritus with intravenous morphine. *J Am Assoc Pediatr Ophthalmol Strabismus*. 1999;3(1):60.
5. Gill AC, Oei J, Lewis NL, et al. Strabismus in infants of opiate-dependent mothers. *Acta Paediatr*. 2003;92:379–385.

Drug: Pentazocine
1. Jones KD. A novel side-effect of pentazocine. *Br J Clin Pract*. 1975;29:218.
2. Burstein AH, Fullerton T. Oculogyric crisis possibly related to pentazocine. *Ann Pharm*. 1993;27(7–8):874–876.

FURTHER READING

Allopurinol sodium

Fraunfelder FT, Hanna C, Dreis MW, et al. Cataracts associated with allopurinol therapy. *Am J Ophthalmol*. 1982;94:137–140.
Fraunfelder FT, Lerman S. Allopurinol and cataracts. *Am J Ophthalmol*. 1985;99:215–216.

Jick H, Brandt DE. Allopurinol and cataracts. *Am J Ophthalmol.* 1984;98:355–358.

Laval J. Allopurinol and macular lesions. *Arch Ophthalmol.* 1968;80:415.

Lerman S, Megaw JM, Gardner K. Allopurinol therapy and human cataractogenesis. *Am J Ophthalmol.* 1982;94:141–146.

Pennell DJ, Nunan TO, O'Doherty MJ, et al. Fatal Stevens-Johnson syndrome in a patient on captopril and allopurinol. *Lancet.* 1984;1:463.

Pinnas G. Possible association between macular lesions and allopurinol. *Arch Ophthalmol.* 1968;79:786–787.

Colchicine

Arroyo MP, Saunders S, Yee H, et al. Toxic epidermal necrolysis-like reaction secondary to colchicines overdose. *Br J Dermatol.* 2004;150:581–588.

Estable JJ. The ocular effect of several irritant drugs applied directly to the conjunctiva. *Am J Ophthalmol.* 1948;31:837–844.

Heaney D, Derghazarian CB, Pineo GF, et al. Massive colchicine overdose: a report on the toxicity. *Am J Med Sci.* 1976;271:233–238.

Leibovitch I, Alster Y, Lazer M, et al. Corneal wound healing in a patient treated with colchicine for familial Mediterranean fever. *Rheumatology.* 2003;42(8):1021–1022.

Naidus RM, Rodvien R, Mielke Jr CH. Colchicine toxicity. A multisystem disease. *Arch Intern Med.* 1977;137:394–396.

Stapczynski JS, Rothstein RJ, Gaye WA, et al. Colchicine overdose: report of two cases and review of the literature. *Ann Emerg Med.* 1981;10:364–369.

Adalimumab, etanercept, infliximab

Bleumink BS, terBorg EJ, Ramselaar CG, et al. Etanercept-induced subacute cutaneous lupus erythematosus. *Rheumatology.* 2001;40:1317–1319.

Chan JW, Castellanos A. Infliximab and anterior optic neuropathy: case report and review of the literature. *Graefes Arch Clin Exp Ophthalmol.* 2010;248(2):283–287.

Farukhi FI, Bollinger K, Ruggieri P, et al. Infliximab-associated third nerve palsy. *Arch Ophthalmol.* 2006;124:1055–1057.

Fonollosa A, Artaraz J, Les I, et al. Sarcoid intermediate uveitis following etanercept treatment: a case report and review of the literature. *Ocul Immunol Inflamm.* 2012;20(1):44–48.

Gaujoux-Viala C, Giampietro C, Gaujoux T, et al. Scleritis: a paradoxical effect of etanercept? Etanercept-associated inflammatory eye disease. *J Rheumatol.* 2012;39(2):233–239.

Hernandez-Illas M, Tozman E, Fulcher SF, et al. Recombinant human tumor necrosis factor receptor Fc fusion protein (etanercept): experience as a therapy for sight-threatening scleritis and sterile corneal ulceration. *Eye Contact Lens.* 2004;30:2–5.

Kakkassery V, Mergler S, Pleyer U. Anti-TNF-alpha treatment: a possible promoter in endogenous uveitis observational report on six patients: occurrence of uveitis following etanercept treatment. *Curr Eye Res.* 2010;35(8):751–760.

Koizumi K, Poulaki V, Doehmen S, et al. Contribution of TNF-alpha to leukocyte adhesion, vascular leakage, and apoptotic cell death in endotoxin-induced uveitis in vivo. *Invest Ophthalmol Vis Sci.* 2003;44:2184–2191.

Le Garrec J, Marcelli C, Mouriaux F. Can tumor necrosis factor inhibitors induce sclera-uveitis? *J Fr Ophthalmol.* 2009;32(7):511.

Li SY, Birnbaum AD, Goldstein DA. Optic neuritis associated with adalimumab in the treatment of uveitis. *Ocul Immunol Inflamm.* 2010;18(6):475–481.

Papadia M, Herbort CP. Infliximab-induced demyelination causes visual disturbance mistaken for recurrence of HLA-B27-related uveitis. *Ocul Immunol Inflamm.* 2010;18(6):482–484.

Pulido JS, Pulido JE, Michet CJ, et al. More questions than answers: a call for a moratorium on the use of intravitreal infliximab outside of a well-designed trial. *Retina.* 2010;30(1):1–5.

Rajaraman RT, Kimura Y, Li S, et al. Retrospective case review of pediatric patients with uveitis treated with infliximab. *Ophthalmology.* 2006;113:308–314.

Reiff A, Takei S, Sadeghi S, et al. Etanercept therapy in children with treatment-resistant uveitis. *Arthritis Rheum.* 2001;44:1411–1415.

Rosenbaum JT. Effect of etanercept on iritis in patients with ankylosing spondylitis. *Arthritis Rheum.* 2004;50:3736–3737.

Scheinfeld N. A comprehensive review and evaluation of the side effects of the tumor necrosis factor alpha blockers etanercept, infliximab and adalimumab. *J Dermatol Treat.* 2004;15:280–294.

Song WK, Cho AR, Yoon YH. Highly suspected primary intraocular lymphoma in a patient with rheumatoid arthritis treated with etanercept: a case report. *BMC Ophthalmol.* 2018;18(1):156.

Swale VJ, Perrett CM, Denton CP. Etanercept-induced systemic lupus erythematosus. *Clin Exp Dermatol.* 2003;28:604–607.

Tiliakos AN, Tiliakos NA. Ocular inflammatory disease in patients with rheumatoid arthritis taking etanercept: is discontinuation of etanercept necessary? *J Rheumatol.* 2003;30:2727.

Wang F, Wang NS. Etanercept therapy–associated acute uveitis: a case report and literature review. *Clin Exp Rheumatol.* 2009;27:838–839.

Yokobori S, Yokota H, Yamamoto Y. Pediatric posterior reversible leukoencephalopathy syndrome and NSAID-induced acute tubular interstitial nephritis. *Pediatr Neurol.* 2006;34(3):245–247.

Young JD, McGwire BS. Infliximab and reactivation of cerebral toxoplasmosis. *N Engl J Med.* 2005;353:1530–1531.

Zierhut M. Ocular cicatricial pemphigoid induced by adalimumab. *Invest Ophthalmol Vis Sci.* 2017;58(8).

Auranofin

Bron A, McLendon B, Camp A. Epithelial deposition of gold in the cornea in patients receiving systemic therapy. *Am J Ophthalmol.* 1979;88:354–360.

Dick D, Raman D. The Guillain-Barré syndrome following gold therapy. *Scand J Rheumatol.* 1982;11:119–120.

Fam AG, Paton TW, Cowan DH. Herpes zoster during gold therapy. *Ann Intern Med.* 1981;94:712–713.

Gottlieb NL, Major JC. Ocular chrysiasis correlated with gold concentrations in the crystalline lens during chrysotherapy. *Arthritis Rheum.* 1978;21:704–708.

Kincaid MC, Green WR, Hoover RE, et al. Ocular chrysiasis. *Arch Ophthalmol.* 1982;100:1791–1794.

Moore AP, Williams AC, Hillenbrand P. Penicillamine-induced myasthenia reactivated by gold. *BMJ.* 1984;288:192–193.

Segawa K. Electron microscopy of the trabecular meshwork in open-angle glaucoma associated with gold therapy. *Glaucoma.* 1981;3:257.

Weidle EG. Lenticular chrysiasis in oral chrysotherapy. *Am J Ophthalmol.* 1987;103:240–241.

Celecoxib, etodolac

Coulter DM, Clark DW, Savage RL. Celecoxib, rofecoxib, and acute temporary visual impairment. *BMJ.* 2003;327:1214–1215.

Cyclooxygenase-2 inhibitors: reports of visual disturbances. *WHO Pharmaceuticals Newsletter.* 2004;3:4.

Fenoprofen calcium

Bigby M, Stern R. Cutaneous reactions to nonsteroidal anti-inflammatory drugs: a review. *J Am Acad Dermatol.* 1985;12:866–876.

Treusch PJ, Woelke BJ, Leichtman D, et al. Agranulocytosis associated with fenoprofen. *JAMA.* 1979;241:2700–2701.

Flurbiprofen

Bergamini MVW. Pharmacology of flurbiprofen, a nonsteroidal anti-inflammatory drug. *Int Ophthalmol Rep.* 1981;6:2.

Feinstein NC. Toxicity of flurbiprofen sodium. *Arch Ophthalmol.* 1988;106:311.

Flurbiprofen – an ophthalmic, 1987 Flurbiprofen – an ophthalmic NSAID. *Med Lett Drugs Ther.* 1987;29:58.

Gimbel HV. The effect of treatment with topical nonsteroidal anti-inflammatory drugs with and without intraoperative epinephrine on the maintenance of mydriasis during cataract surgery. *Ophthalmology.* 1989;96(5):585–588.

Romano A, Pietrantonio F. Delayed hypersensitivity to flurbiprofen. *J Int Med.* 1997;241(1):81–83.

Samples JR. Sodium flurbiprofen for surgically induced miosis and the control of inflammation. *J Toxicol Cut Ocular Toxicol.* 1989;8(2):163–166.

Trousdale MD, Dunkel EC, Nesburn AB. Effect of flurbiprofen on herpes simplex keratitis in rabbits. *Invest Ophthalmol Vis Sci.* 1980;19:267–270.

Ibuprofen

Asherov J, Schoenberg A, Weinberger A. Diplopia following ibuprofen administration. *JAMA.* 1982;248:649.

Bernstein HN. Some iatrogenic ocular diseases from systemically administered drugs. *Int Ophthalmol Clin.* 1970;10:553–619.

Collum LM, Bowen DI. Ocular side-effects of ibuprofen. *Br J Ophthalmol.* 1971;55:472–477.

Court H, Streete P, Volans GN. Acute poisoning with ibuprofen. *Human Toxicol.* 1983;2:381–384.

Dua HS, Forrester JV. The corneoscleral limbus in human corneal epithelial wound healing. *Am J Ophthalmol.* 1990;110:646–656.

Fraunfelder FT. Interim report: national registry of possible drug-induced ocular side effects. *Ophthalmology.* 1980;87:87–90.

Hamburger HA, Beckman H, Thompson R. Visual evoked potentials and ibuprofen (Motrin) toxicity. *Ann Ophthalmol.* 1984;16:328–329.

Melluish JW, Brooks CD, Ruoff G, et al. Ibuprofen and visual function. *Arch Ophthalmol.* 1975;93:781–782.

Palmer CA. Toxic amblyopia from ibuprofen. *BMJ.* 1972;3:765.

Palungwachira P, Palungwachira P, Ogawa H. Localized periorbital edema induced by ibuprofen. *J Dermatol.* 2005;32:969–971.

Quinn JP, Weinstein RA, Caplan LR. Eosinophilic meningitis and ibuprofen therapy. *Neurology.* 1984;34:108–109.

Tullio CJ. Ibuprofen-induced visual disturbance. *Am J Hosp Pharm.* 1981;38:1362.

Indomethacin (indometacin)

Carr RE, Siegel IM. Retinal function in patients treated with indomethacin. *Am J Ophthalmol.* 1973;75:302–306.

Fraunfelder FT, Samples JR, Fraunfelder FW. Possible optic nerve side effects associated with nonsteroidal anti-inflammatory drugs. *J Toxicol Cut Ocular Toxicol.* 1994;13(4):311–316.

Frucht-Pery J, Levinger S, Zauberman H. The effect of topical administration of indomethacin on symptoms in corneal scars and edema. *Am J Ophthalmol.* 1991;112(2):186–190.

Frucht-Pery J, Siganos CS, Solomon A, et al. Topical indomethacin solution versus dexamethasone solution for treatment of inflamed pterygium and pinguecula: a prospective randomized clinical study. *Am J Ophthalmol.* 1999;127:148–152.

Gimbel HW. The effect of treatment with topical nonsteroidal anti-inflammatory drugs with and without intraoperative epinephrine on the maintenance of mydriasis during cataract surgery. *Ophthalmology.* 1989;96(5):585–588.

Gomez A, Florido JF, Quiralte J, et al. Allergic contact dermatitis due to indomethacin and diclofenac. *Contact Dermatitis.* 2000;43:59.

Graham CM, Blach RK. Indomethacin retinopathy: case report and review. *Br J Ophthalmol.* 1988;72:434–438.

Katz IM. Indomethacin. *Ophthalmology.* 1981;88:455–458.

Katzman B, Lu L, Tiwari RP, et al. Pseudotumor cerebri: an observation and review. *Ann Ophthalmol.* 1981;13:887–892.

Palimeris G, Koliopoulos J, Velissaropoulos P. Ocular side effects of indomethacin. *Ophthalmologica.* 1972;164:339–353.

Procianoy RS, Garcia-Prats JA, Hittner HM, et al. Use of indomethacin and its relationship to retinopathy of prematurity in very low birth weight infants. *Arch Dis Child.* 1980;55:362–364.

Rich LF. Toxic drug effects on the cornea. *J Toxicol Cut Ocular Toxicol.* 1982;1(4):267–297.

Toler SM. Oxidative stress plays an important role in the pathogenesis of drug-induced retinopathy. *Exp Biol Med.* 2004;229:607–615.

Yoshizumi MO, Schwartz S, Peterson M. Ocular toxicity of topical indomethacin eye drops. *J Toxicol.* 1991;10(3):201–206.

Ketoprofen

Fraunfelder FT, Samples JR, Fraunfelder FW. Possible optic nerve side effects associated with nonsteroidal anti-inflammatory drugs. *J Toxicol Cut Ocular Toxicol.* 1994;13(4):311–316.

Naproxen sodium

Fraunfelder FT. Interim report: national registry of possible drug-induced ocular side effects. *Ophthalmology.* 1979;86:126–130.

Fraunfelder FT, Samples JR, Fraunfelder FW. Possible optic nerve side effects associated with nonsteroidal anti-inflammatory drugs. *J Toxicol Cut Ocular Toxicol.* 1994;13(4):311–316.

Harry DJ, Hicks H. Naproxen hypersensitivity. *Hosp Form.* 1983;18:648.

Mordes JP, Johnson MW, Soter NA. Possible naproxen associated vasculitis. *Arch Intern Med.* 1981;140:985.

Shelley WB, Elpern DJ, Shelley ED. Naproxen photosensitization demonstrated by challenge. *Cutis.* 1986;38:169–170.

Svihovec J. Anti-inflammatory analgesics and drugs used in gout. In: Dukes MNG, ed. *Meyler's Side Effects of Drugs.* 9th ed. Amsterdam: Excerpta Medica; 1980:152.

Piroxicam

Duró JC, Herrero C, Bordas X. Piroxicam-induced erythema multiforme. *J Rheumatol.* 1984;11:554–555.

Halasz CL. Photosensitivity to the nonsteroidal anti-inflammatory drug piroxicam. *Cutis.* 1987;39:37–39.

Roujeau JC, Phlippoteau C, Koso M, et al. Sjögren-like syndrome after drug-induced toxic epidermal necrolysis. *Lancet.* 1985;1:609–611.

Stern RS, Bigby M. An expanded profile of cutaneous reactions to nonsteroidal anti-inflammatory drugs. Reports to a specialty-based system for spontaneous reporting of adverse reactions to drugs. *JAMA.* 1984;252:1433–1437.

Vasconcelos C, Magina S, Quirino P, et al. Cutaneous drug reactions to piroxicam. *Contact Dermatitis.* 1998;39(3):145.

Acetaminophen (paracetamol)

Blanca-Lopez N, Haroun-Diaz E, Ruano FJ, et al. Acetyl salicylic acid challenge in children with hypersensitivity reactions to nonsteroidal anti-inflammatory drugs differentiates between cross-intolerant and selective responders. *J Allergy Clin Immunol Pract.* 2018;6(4):1226–1235.

Gérard A, Roche G, Presles O, et al. Drug-induced Lyell's syndrome. Nine cases. *Therapie.* 1982;37:475–480.

Johnson DA. Drug-induced psychiatric disorders. *Drugs.* . 1981;22:57–69.

Kashihara M, Danno K, Miyachi Y, et al. Bullous pemphigoid-like lesions induced by phenacetin. Report of a case and an immunopathologic study. *Arch Dermatol.* 1984;120:1196–1199.

Krenzelok EP, Best L, Manoguerra AS. Acetaminophen toxicity. *Am Hosp Pharm.* 1977;34:391–394.

Malek-Ahmadi P, Ramsey M. Acute psychosis associated with codeine and acetaminophen: a case report. *Neurobehav Toxicol Teratol.* 1985;7:193–194.

Neetans A, Martin J, Rubbens MC, et al. Possible iatrogenic action of phenacetin at the levels of the visual pathway. *Bull Soc Belge Ophthalmol.* 1977;178:65–76.

Aspirin (acetylsalicylic acid)

Basu PK, Matuk Y, Kapur BM, et al. Should corneas from donors receiving a high dose of salicylate be used as grafts: an animal experimentation. *Exp Eye Res.* 1984;39:393–400.

Benawra R, Mangurten HH, Duffell DR. Cyclopia and other anomalies following maternal ingestion of salicylates. *Pediatrics.* 180;96:1069–1071.

Black RA, Bensinger RE. Bilateral subconjunctival hemorrhage after acetylsalicylic acid overdose. *Ann Ophthalmol.* 1982;14:1024–1025.

Cheng H. Aspirin and cataract. *Br J Ophthalmol.* 1992;76:257–258.

Chew EY, Klein ML, Murphy RP, et al. Effects of aspirin on vitreous/preretinal hemorrhage in patients with diabetes mellitus. *Arch Ophthalmol.* 1995;113:52–55.

Cumming RG, Mitchell P. Medications and cataract. The Blue Mountains Eye Study. *Ophthalmology.* 1999;105:1751–1757.

Early Treatment Diabetic Retinopathy Study Research Group. Early Treatment Diabetic Retinopathy Study Research Group. Effects of aspirin treatment on diabetic retinopathy. *Ophthalmology.* 1991;98(1991):757–765.

Ganley JP, Geiger JM, Clement JR, et al. Aspirin and recurrent hyphema after blunt ocular trauma. *Am J Ophthalmol.* 1983;96:797–801.

Kageler WV, Moake JL, Garcia CA. Spontaneous hyphema associated with ingestion of aspirin and alcohol. *Am J Ophthalmol.* 1976;82:631–634.

Lumme P, Laatikainen LT. Risk factors for intraoperative and early postoperative complications in extracapsular cataract surgery. *Eur J Ophthalmol.* 1994;4:151–158.

Makeia A-L, Lang H, Korpela P. Toxic encephalopathy with hyperammonaemia during high-dose salicylate therapy. *Acta Neurol Scand.* 1980;61:146–156.

Moss SE, Klein R, Klein BE. Prevalence of and risk factors for dry eye syndrome. *Arch Ophthalmol.* 2000;118(9):1264–1268.

Moss SE, Klein R, Klein BE. Long-term incidence of dry eye in an older population. *Optom Vis Sci.* 2008;85(8):668–674.

Ong-Tone L, Paluck EC, Hart-Mitchell RD. Perioperative use of warfarin and aspirin in cataract surgery by Canadian Society of Cataract and Refractive Surgery members: survey. *J Cataract Refract Surg.* 2005;31:991–996.

Paris GL, Waltuch GF. Salicylate-induced bleeding problem in ophthalmic plastic surgery. *Ophthalmic Surg.* 1982;13:627–629.

Price KS, Thompson DM. Localized unilateral periorbital edema induced by aspirin. *Ann Allergy Asthma Immunol.* 1997;79:420–422.

Ruocco V, Pisani M. Induced pemphigus. *Arch DeKrmatol Res.* 1982;274:123–140.

Schachat AP. Can aspirin be used safely for patients with proliferative diabetic retinopathy? *Arch Ophthalmol.* 1992;110:180.

Smidt D, Torpet LA, Nauntofte B, et al. Associations between oral and ocular dryness, labial and whole salivary flow rates, systemic diseases and medications in a sample of older people. *Community Dent Oral Epidemiol.* 2011;39:276–288.

Tilanus MA, Vaandrager W, Cuyper MH, et al. Relationship between anticoagulant medication and massive intraocular hemorrhage in age-related macular degeneration. *Graefes Arch Clin Exp Ophthalmol.* 2000;238:482–485.

Valentic JP, Leopold IH, Dea FJ. Excretion of salicylic acid into tears following oral administration of aspirin. *Ophthalmology.* 1980;87:815–820.

Codeine, dextropropoxyphene

Leslie PJ, Dyson EH, Proudfoot AT. Opiate toxicity after self poisoning with aspirin and codeine. *BMJ.* 1986;292:96.

Mattoo SK, Mahajan S, Nebhinani N, et al. Diplopia with dextropropoxyphene withdrawal. *Gen Hosp Psychiatry.* 2013;35(1):100–101.

Ostler HB, Conant MA. Groundwater J. Lyell's disease, the Stevens-Johnson syndrome, and exfoliative dermatitis. *Trans Am Ophthalmol Otolaryngol.* 1970;74:1254–1265.

Ponte CD. A suspected case of codeine-induced erythema multiforme. *Drug Intell Clin Pharm.* 1983;17:128–130.

Wall R, Linford SM, Akhter MI. Addiction to distalgesic (dextropropoxyphene). *BMJ.* 1980;280:1213–1214.

Naltrexone hydrochloride

Bellini C, Bacaini M, D'Egidio P, et al. Naloxone anisocoria: a noninvasive inexpensive test for opiate addiction. *Int J Clin Pharm Res.* 1982;11:55.

Drago F, Aguglia E, Dal Bello A, et al. Ocular instillation of naloxone increases intraocular pressure in morphine-addicted patients: a possible test for detecting misuse of morphine. *Experimentia.* 1985;41:266–267.

Fanciullacci M, Boccuni M, Pietrini U, et al. The naloxone conjunctival test in morphine addiction. *Eur J Pharmacol.* 1980;61:319–320.

Jasinski DR, Martin WR, Haertzen C. The human pharmacology and abuse potential of N-allylnoroxymorphone (naloxone). *J Pharmacol Exp Ther.* 1967;157(2):420–426.

Martin WR. Opioid antagonists. *Pharmacol Rev.* 1967;19:463–521.

Nomof N, Elliott HW, Parker KD. The local effect of morphine, nalorphine, and codeine on the diameter of the pupil of the eye. *Clin Pharmacol Ther.* 1968;9:358–364.

Diacetylmorphine (diamorphine, heroin)

Alinlari A, Hashem B. Effect of opium addiction on intraocular pressure. *Glaucoma.* 1985;7:69.

Caradoc-Davies TH. Opiate toxicity in elderly patients. *BMJ.* 1981;283:905–906.

Cosgriff TM. Anisocoria in heroin withdrawal. *Arch Neurol.* 1973;29:200–201.

Crandall DC, Leopold IH. The influence of systemic drugs on tear constituents. *Ophthalmology.* 1979;86:115–125.

Dally S, Thomas G, Mellinger M. Loss of hair, blindness and skin rash in heroin addicts. *Vet Human Toxicol.* 1982;24(suppl):62.

Gómez Manzano C, Fueyo J, Garcés JM, et al. Internuclear ophthalmopathy associated with opiate overdose. *Med Clin. (Barc).* 1990;94:637.

Hawkins KA, Bruckstein AH, Guthrie TC. Percutaneous heroin injection causing heroin syndrome. JAMA 1977l237:1963–1964.

Hogeweg M, De Jong PT. Candida endophthalmitis in heroin addicts. *Doc Ophthalmol.* 1983;55:63–71.

Rathod NH, De Alarcon R, Thomson IG. Signs of heroin usage detected by drug users and their parents. *Lancet.* 1967;2:1411–1414.

Salmon JF, Partridge BM, Spalton DJ. Candida endophthalmitis in a heroin addict: a case report. *Br J Ophthalmol.* 1983;67:306–309.

Siepser SB, Magargal LE, Augsburger JJ. Acute bilateral retinal microembolization in a heroin addict. *Ann Ophthalmol.* 1981;13:699–702.

Tarr KH. Candida endophthalmitis and drug abuse. *Aust J Ophthalmol.* 1980;8:303–305.

Vastine DW, Horsley W, Guth SB, et al. Endogenous candida endophthalmitis associated with heroin use. *Arch Ophthalmol.* 1976;94:1805.

Hydromorphone hydrochloride (dihydromorphinone), oxymorphone hydrochloride

Acute drug abuse reactions. *Med Lett Drugs Ther.* 1985;27:77.

De Cuyper C, Goeteyn M. Systemic contact dermatitis from subcutaneous hydromorphone. *Contact Dermatitis.* 1992;27(4):220–223.

Katcher J, Walsh D. Opioid-induced itching: morphine sulfate and hydromorphone hydrochloride. *J Pain Symptom Manage.* 1999;17(1):70–72.

Meperidine hydrochloride (pethidine)

Bron AJ. Vortex patterns of the corneal epithelium. *Trans Ophthalmol Soc UK.* 1973;93:455–472.

Carlson VR. Individual pupillary reactions to certain centrally acting drugs in man. *J Pharmacol Exp Ther.* 1957;121:501–506.

Goetting MG, Thirman MJ. Neurotoxicity of meperidine. *Ann Emerg Med.* 1985;14:1007–1009.

Hovland KR. Effects of drugs on aqueous humor dynamics. *Int Ophthalmol Clin.* 1971;11(2):99–119.

Johnson DA. Drug-induced psychiatric disorders. *Drugs.* 1981;22:57–69.

Lubeck MJ. Effects of drugs on ocular muscles. *Int Ophthalmol Clin.* 1971;11(2):35–62.

Waisbren BA, Smith MB. Hypersensitivity to meperidine. *JAMA.* 1978;239:1395.

Methadone hydrochloride

Linzmayer L, Fischer G, Grunberger J. Pupillary diameter and papillary reactions in heroin dependent patients and in patients participating in a methadone and morphine replacement program. *Weiner Medizinische Wochenschrift.* 1997;147(3):67–69.

Rothenberg S, Peck EA, Schottenfeld S, et al. Methadone depression of visual signal detection performance. *Pharmacol Biochem Behav.* 1979;11:521–527.

Rothenberg S, Schottenfeld S, Gross K, et al. Specific oculomotor deficit after acute methadone. I. Saccadic eye movements. *Psychopharmacology (Berl).* 1980;67:221–227.

Rothenberg S, Schottenfeld S, Selkoe D, et al. Specific oculomotor deficit after acute methadone. II. Smooth pursuit eye movements. *Psychopharmacology (Berl).* 1980;67:229–234.

Morphine sulfate, opium

Aminlari A, Hashem B. Effect of opium addiction on intraocular pressure. *Glaucoma.* 1965;7:69.

Andersen PT. Alopecia areata after epidural morphine. *Anesth Analg.* 1984;63:1142.

Crandall DC, Leopold IH. The influence of systemic drugs on tear constituents. *Ophthalmology.* 1979;86:115–125.

Murphy DF. Anesthesia and intraocular pressure. *Anesth Analg.* 1985;64:520–530.

Shelly MP, Park GR. Morphine toxicity with dilated pupils. *BMJ.* 1984;289:1071–1072.

Stevens RA, Sharrock NE. Nystagmus following epidural morphine. *Anesthesiology.* 1991;74:390–391.

Ueyama H, Nishimura M, Tashiro C. Naloxone reversal of nystagmus associated with intrathecal morphine [letter]. *Anesthesiology.* 1992;76:153.

Pentazocine

Belleville JP, Dorey F, Bellville JW. Effects of nefopam on visual tracking. *Clin Pharmacol Ther.* 1979;26:457–463.

Davidson SI. Reports of ocular adverse reactions. *Trans Ophthalmol Soc UK.* 1973;93:495–510.

Gould WM. Central nervous disturbance with pentazocine. *BMJ.* 1972;1:313–314.

Martin WR. Opioid antagonists. *Pharmacol Rev.* 1967;19:463–521.

CHAPTER 8

Drugs Used in Anesthesia

CLASS: ADJUNCTS TO ANESTHESIA

Generic Name:
Hyaluronidase.

Proprietary Names:
Amphadase, Hydase, Hylenex, Vitrase.

Primary Use
This enzyme is added to local anesthetic solutions to enhance the effect of infiltrative anesthesia. It has also been used in paraphimosis, lepromatous nerve reactions, and the management of carpal tunnel syndrome.

Ocular Side Effects
Local ophthalmic use or exposure – retrobulbar or subconjunctival injection
Certain
1. Eyelids, conjunctiva, and orbit
   a. Allergic reactions
   b. Conjunctivitis – follicular
   c. Edema (Fig. 8.1)
   d. Toxic reaction
2. Irritation
3. Myopia (subconjunctival)
4. Astigmatism (subconjunctival)
5. Decreased length of action of local anesthetics
6. Increased frequency of local anesthetic reactions

Probable
1. May spread infection
2. May spread tumor
3. Decreases local anesthetic toxicity to adjacent extraocular muscles and nerves

Conditional/unclassified
1. Cystoid macular edema
2. Orbital inflammatory disease

Clinical Significance
Adverse ocular reactions due to periocular injection of hyaluronidase are either quite rare or masked by postoperative surgical reactions. Subconjunctival injection of this drug causes myopia and astigmatism secondary to changes in the corneal curvature. This is a transitory phenomenon, with recovery occurring within 2–6 weeks. Irritative or allergic reactions are often stated to be due to impurities in the preparation, because pure hyaluronidase is felt to be nontoxic. However, a number of reports suggest allergic reactions to hyaluronidase and not some other cause. These reports included orbital inflammation, orbital cellulitis, and choroidal effusion and proptosis.[1-4] Zamora-Alejo et al reported 7 cases where they felt that postoperative periorbital edema was due to a type A toxic reaction to hyaluronidase.[5] They felt this was a dose-dependent toxicity rather than a hypersensitivity reaction. Minning reported allergic reactions secondary to retrobulbar hyaluronidase.[6] This occurred as an acute process simulating an expulsive choroidal or retrobulbar hemorrhage. Massive retrobulbar, peribulbar, and intraorbital swelling may occur. Cases similar to this are in the spontaneous reports. Hyaluronidase decreases the duration of action of local anesthetic drugs by allowing them to diffuse out of the tissue more rapidly. Brown et al and Jehan et al pointed out that hyaluronidase may be important in decreasing or preventing damage from local anesthetics on adjacent extraocular muscles and nerves.[7-9] This may occur, in part, by diffusion of the anesthetic, thereby decreasing the anesthetic concentration adjacent to muscle tissue. Miller has not found this to be true because he has not seen restrictive diplopia in over 7000 ocular procedures without using hyaluronidase.[10] Ortiz-Perez et al described 2 patients with orbital inflammation after hyaluronidase and zoledronic acid retrobulbar injection.[11]

Some side effects of the local anesthetic are probably more frequent when it is used with hyaluronidase because its absorption rate is increased. Infection or tumor cells may be allowed to spread as well, based on the same mechanism. A prospective double-blind study that suggested that cystoid macular edema is possibly caused by the use of hyaluronidase is of clinical importance. To date, these data are not completely accepted, and some of these cases may be secondary to inadvertent intraocular injection.[12] If the patient is on heparin or if there is associated bleeding in the area of injection, the effect of hyaluronidase may be decreased because both human serum and heparin inhibit this drug.

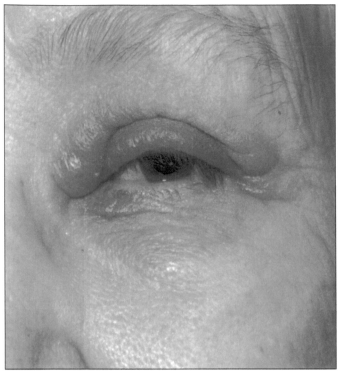

FIG. 8.1 Mild to moderate periorbital edema associated with itching after otherwise uncomplicated phacoemulsification in the left eye related to hyaluronidase usage.[13]

Generic Names:
1. Hyoscine butylbromide (scopolamine butylbromide); 2. hyoscine hydrobromide (scopolamine hydrobromide); 3. hyoscine methobromide (methscopolamine).

Proprietary Names:
1. Buscopan; 2. Transderm Scop, Isopto Hyoscine; 3. Pamine.

Primary Use
Systemic
These quaternary ammonium derivatives are used as preanesthetic medications to decrease bronchial secretions, as sedatives and antispasmodics, and in the prophylaxis of motion sickness.

Ophthalmic
Ocular hyoscine is used for mydriasis and cycloplegia in diagnostic procedures and in the treatment of iridocyclitis.

Ocular Side Effects
Systemic administration – intramuscular, intravenous, oral, subcutaneous, or transdermal
Certain
1. Mydriasis – may precipitate acute glaucoma
2. Decreased accommodation
3. Decreased vision
4. May aggravate or cause ocular sicca
5. Visual hallucinations
6. Decreased tear lysozymes
7. Impairment of saccadic eye movements (intramuscular injection)

Local ophthalmic use or exposure – topical ocular application
Certain
1. Decreased vision
2. Mydriasis – may precipitate acute glaucoma
3. Decreased accommodation
4. Eyelids or conjunctiva
   a. Allergic reactions

b. Conjunctivitis – follicular
c. Eczema
5. Irritation
   a. Hyperemia
   b. Photophobia
   c. Edema
6. Increased intraocular pressure
7. May aggravate or cause ocular sicca
8. Visual hallucinations

Systemic absorption or finger-to-eye cross-contamination from topical application to the skin
Certain
1. Pupils
   a. Mydriasis – may precipitate acute glaucoma
   b. Anisocoria
   c. Absent reaction to light – toxic states
2. Decreased accommodation
3. Decreased vision
4. May aggravate or cause ocular sicca
5. Visual hallucinations
6. Nystagmus

Systemic Side Effects
Local ophthalmic use or exposure – topical ocular application
Certain
1. Psychosis
2. Agitation
3. Confusion
4. Hostility
5. Amnesia
6. Ataxia
7. Vomiting
8. Urinary incontinence
9. Somnolence
10. Fever
11. Vasodilation

Clinical Significance
Although ocular side effects from systemic administration of these drugs are common, they are reversible and seldom serious. Occasionally, patients on scopolamine have aggravated ocular sicca problems due to decreased tear production. This is the only autonomic drug that has been reported to cause decreased tear lysozymes. Mydriasis and paralysis of accommodation are intended ocular effects resulting from topical ophthalmic application of hyoscine, but may also occur from oral administration. This drug may elevate the intraocular pressure in open-angle glaucoma and can precipitate angle-closure glaucoma. Allergic reactions are not uncommon after topical ocular application. Transient impairment of ocular accommodation, including decreased vision and mydriasis, has also been reported after the application of transdermal hyoscine patches.[1] Several case reports of unilateral dilated pupils with associated decreased vision and acute glaucoma have been published, and inadvertent finger-to-eye contamination has been shown to be the cause.[2-5]

Systemic side effects from topical ophthalmic use of hyoscine have been reported infrequently and are similar to those seen secondary to topical ophthalmic atropine. Toxic psychosis, however, especially in the elderly or visually impaired, has been reported in the literature and spontaneous reports.[6-9]

Generic Name:
Succinylcholine chloride (suxamethonium chloride).

Proprietary Names:
Anectine; Quelicin.

Primary Use
This neuromuscular blocking drug is used as an adjunct to general anesthesia to obtain relaxation of skeletal muscles.

Ocular Side Effects
Systemic administration – intramuscular or intravenous
Certain
1. Extraocular muscles
   a. Eyelid retraction (initial – lasting up to 5 minutes)
   b. Enophthalmos (initial – lasting up to 5 minutes)
   c. Globe rotates inferiorly
   d. Paralysis (initial – lasting up to 5 minutes)
   e. Adduction of abducted eyes (initial – lasting up to 5 minutes)
   f. Alters forced duction tests (initial – lasting up to 20 minutes)
2. Intraocular pressure
   a. Increased (lasting 20–30 seconds)
   b. Decreased (late)
3. Ptosis
4. Diplopia
5. Eyelids or conjunctiva
   a. Allergic reactions
   b. Erythema
   c. Edema
   d. Urticaria

Conditional/unclassified
1. Precipitates acute glaucoma

Clinical Significance

All ocular side effects due to succinylcholine are transitory. The importance of the possible side effects of this drug effect on the "open" eye is an ongoing debate. Some feel a transient contraction of extraocular muscles may cause 5–15 mmHg of intraocular pressure elevations within 20–30 seconds or increased choroidal blood flow after succinylcholine is given, lasting from 1-4 minutes.[1] Although this short-term elevation of intraocular pressure has little or no effect in the normal or glaucomatous eye, it has the potential to cause expulsion of the intraocular contents in a surgically opened or perforated globe. McGoldrick considers the drug safe in human "open" eyes with the benefits far outweighing the "unproven" risks.[2] There are at least 20 publications taking either side of this argument, with most recommending avoiding this drug in an "open" eye. This may require anesthesiologists to use a drug that they are not as familiar with, and the overall risk of this may be greater than that of using succinylcholine. Chidiac suggested an algorithm that asks 2 questions with a total of 3 answers to help with the decision on whether or not to use this drug (see "Recommendations" section).[3] Brinkley et al concur with this methodology.[4] Eldor et al reported 2 cases of this drug inducing acute glaucoma.[5]

Extraocular muscle contraction induced by succinylcholine may cause lid retraction or an enophthalmos. This may cause the surgeon to misjudge the amount of resection needed in ptosis procedures. Eyelid retraction may be due to a direct action on Müller's muscle. Both eyelid retraction and enophthalmos seldom last for over 5 minutes after drug administration. Succinylcholine may cause abnormal forced duction tests up to 20 minutes after the drug is administered.

Prolonged respiratory paralysis may follow administration of succinylcholine during general anesthesia in patients with recent exposure to topical ocular echothiophate, anticholinesterase insecticides, or in those with cholinesterase deficiency. Oral clonidine, thiopentone, and mivacurium have been suggested to minimize succinylcholine ocular pressure effects on the eye.[6–8]

Recommendations[3]

Recommendations for use in the open globe are as follows:
1. If intubation is easy, avoid using succinylcholine chloride.
2. If intubation is difficult, ask if the eye is viable or not:
   a. If the eye is viable, then use succinylcholine.
   b. If the eye is not viable, then use fiber-optic laryngoscopy.

CLASS: GENERAL ANESTHESIA

Generic Name:
Ether (anesthetic ether).

Proprietary Name:
Generic only.

Primary Use

This potent inhalation anesthetic, analgesic, and muscle relaxant is used during induction of general anesthesia.

Ocular Side Effects

Systemic administration – inhalation
Certain
1. Pupils – dependent on plane of anesthesia
   a. Mydriasis – reactive to light (initial)
   b. Miosis – reactive to light (deep level of anesthesia)
   c. Mydriasis – nonreactive to light (coma)
2. Extraocular muscles – dependent on plane of anesthesia
   a. Slow oscillations (initial)
   b. Eccentric placement of globes (initial)
   c. Concentric placement of globes (coma)
3. Irritation
4. Conjunctival hyperemia
5. Lacrimal secretion – dependent on plane of anesthesia
   a. Increased (initial)
   b. Decreased (coma)
   c. Abolished (coma)
6. Decreased intraocular pressure
7. Decreased vision
8. Cortical blindness

Inadvertent ocular exposure
Certain
1. Irritation
   a. Hyperemia
   b. Edema
2. Punctate keratitis
3. Corneal opacities

Clinical Significance

Adverse ocular reactions due to ether are common, reversible, and seldom of clinical importance other than in the determination of the plane of anesthesia. Ether decreases intraocular pressure, probably on the basis of increasing outflow facility. Ether vapor is an irritant to all mucous membranes, including the conjunctiva. In addition, ether vapor has a vasodilator property. Permanent corneal opacities have been reported due to direct contact of liquid ether with the cornea. Blindness after induction of general anesthesia is probably due to asphyxia-related cerebral cortical damage.

Generic Name:
Ketamine hydrochloride.

Proprietary Name:
Ketalar.

Primary Use
This intravenous nonbarbiturate anesthetic is used for short-term diagnostic or surgical procedures. It may also be used as an adjunct to anesthesia. Orally, it is taken for refractory major depression.

Ocular Side Effects
Systemic administration – intramuscular, intravenous, or oral
Certain
1. Decreased vision
2. Extraocular muscles
   a. Abnormal conjugate deviations
   b. Random ocular movements
   c. Diplopia
   d. Horizontal nystagmus
3. Postsurgical visually induced "emergence reactions"
4. Visual hallucinations
5. Distortion of visual perception

Probable
1. Increased intraocular pressure – minimal (deep level of anesthesia)

Possible
1. Corneal edema – rare
2. Tunnel vision
3. Lacrimation

Conditional/unclassified
1. Optic neuritis
2. Blindness – transient

Clinical Significance
All ocular side effects due to ketamine are transient and reversible. After ketamine anesthesia, diplopia may persist for up to 30 minutes during the recovery phase and may be particularly bothersome to some patients. "Emergence reactions" occur in 12% of patients and may consist of various psychological manifestations from pleasant dream-like states to irrational behavior. The incidence of these reactions is increased by visual stimulation as the drug is wearing off. El'kin et al showed inadequate evaluation of size, shape, and velocity in visual perception for the first 24 hours postanesthesia.[1] Fine et al reported 3 cases of transient blindness after ketamine anesthesia lasting about half an hour, with complete restoration of sight and no apparent sequelae.[2] This is thought to be a toxic cerebral-induced phenomenon or an anoxic insult. The effect of ketamine on intraocular pressure is somewhat confusing, with various authors obtaining different results. Intraocular pressure is probably not elevated in the first 8–10 minutes after the drug is administered; however, after that time, there may be increased muscle tone with a resultant increase in intraocular pressure. Drayna et al found that at dosages of 4 mg/kg or less, no clinically meaningful levels of increased intraocular pressure are reached at any point in time.[3] Fantinati et al reported a case of bilateral optic neuritis after a general anesthesia possibly induced by ketamine.[4] Ketamine is also used as a recreational drug for its psychedelic effect, and abusers may develop visual hallucinations, coarse horizontal nystagmus, abnormal conjugate eye deviations, and diplopia.

Starte et al reported a case of bilateral corneal edema in the 20/200 to 20/400 range after oral ketamine for at least 8 months.[5] The drug was stopped, and the patient had Descemet's stripping in 1 eye with improvement. The drug was restarted, and the edema recurred. The drug was stopped again, and the bilateral edema progressively improved. There is an additional case of suspected corneal edema due to ketamine in the spontaneous reports.

Generic Name:
Nitrous oxide.

Proprietary Name:
Generic only.

Primary Use
This inhalation anesthetic and analgesic is used in dentistry, in the second stage of labor in pregnancy, and during induction of general anesthesia.

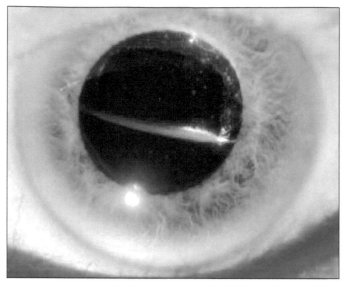

FIG. 8.2 Vitreous cavity approximately 50% full of gas.[11]

Ocular Side Effects
Systemic administration – inhalation
Certain

1. Nitrous oxide general anesthesia – in patients undergoing retinal surgery with intravitreal gas injection (Fig. 8.2)
   a. Decreased vision
   b. Acute glaucoma
   c. Central retinal artery occlusion
   d. Optic atrophy
   e. Pupillary block
2. Pupils – dependent on plane of anesthesia
   a. Mydriasis – reactive to light (initial)
   b. Miosis – reactive to light (deep level of anesthesia)
   c. Mydriasis – nonreactive to light (coma)
3. Intraocular pressure
   a. Increased during anesthesia
   b. Decreased immediately postanesthesia
4. Decreased vision
5. May aggravate or cause ocular sicca
6. Abnormal electroretinogram (ERG) or visual evoked potential (VEP)
7. Cortical blindness

Probable

1. Mydriasis (direct contact with eye)

Clinical Significance

The key side effect of nitrous oxide anesthesia is its effect on remaining vitreous intraocular gas during retinal detachment surgery. The remaining intravitreal gas bubble can absorb nitrogen from nitrous oxide from the bloodstream, causing the intravitreal bubble to expand. This rapid expansion of the bubble can cause a dramatic increase in intraocular pressure.[1-3] This then may cause all the sequelae of acute glaucoma if it goes unrecognized during or after surgery. Whereas most gases will absorb within 10 days, Lee reports the onset of this complication at 3–7 days, and Seaberg et al at 42 days postanesthesia.[4,5] If intraocular gases are present, nitrous oxide anesthesia is contraindicated, and patients should be instructed to wear identifying bracelets (Fig. 8.3) until the gas bubble is absorbed. There are multiple cases of irreversible blindness secondary to increased intraocular pressure in patients with intraocular gas who went under nitrous oxide inhalation anesthesia.[3,5-7]

Pupillary changes due to nitrous oxide are common; however, other than aiding in determination of the anesthetic plane, they are seldom of importance. Braksick et al described a case of unilateral mydriasis that developed 12+ hours after inhalation of nitric oxide for pulmonary hypertension.[8] There was a possible leak of the drug around the face mask with exposure to the left eye. The authors postulated a mechanism that induced smooth muscle relaxation with resultant mydriasis.

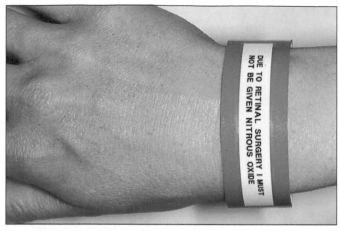

FIG. 8.3 Wristband worn by patient after retinal surgery using intraocular gas.[7]

Nitrous oxide, as well as other anesthetics, produces the transitory effect of decreased basal-tear production during general anesthesia. Although decreased vision or blindness after induction of general anesthesia is quite rare, this phenomenon is more frequent with nitrous oxide than with most other general anesthetics. Visual loss is probably secondary to asphyxia-related cerebral cortical damage.

Fenwick et al and Raitta et al have studied the electrophysiologic effects of nitrous oxide on the eye.[9,10]

Generic Name:
Propofol.

Proprietary Names:
Diprivan, Fresenius Propoven.

Primary Use
This short-acting sedative-hypnotic is used in the induction and maintenance of anesthesia or sedation.

Ocular Side Effects
Systemic administration – intravenous
Certain
1. Extraocular muscles
   a. Diplopia
   b. Palsy
   c. Paresis
   d. External ophthalmoplegia
2. Inability to open eyes
3. Eyelids
   a. Rash
   b. Edema
4. Decreased intraocular pressure

Probable
1. Decreased vision
2. Nystagmus
3. Oculogyric crisis

Accidental direct ocular exposure
Certain
1. Intense ocular burning
2. Temporary blindness
3. Keratitis

Clinical Significance
Propofol is an intravenous medication that can cause transitory visual complications. To date, none of the reported events have been permanent.

Reilly et al first reported a 50% decrease in intraocular pressure due to propofol.[1] Yamada et al showed that during surgery, while in lateral decubitus position, the lower dependent eye had a significant increase in intraocular pressure under sevoflurane, but not under propofol.[2]

One of the more unusual side effects is that after patients have recovered from anesthesia (i.e. respond to verbal commands and have a return of muscular power), they are unable to open their eyes either spontaneously or in response to a command for 3–20 minutes. This may include the transitory loss of all ocular or periocular muscle movements. Decreased vision can occur, but it is usually inconsequential. Exposure-associated keratitis occurs due to lack of eyelid control and restriction of Bell phenomena. Nystagmus has been reported, but it is difficult to prove a cause-and-effect relationship. Neel et al reported that with a single, low-dose bolus of intravenous sedation before cataract surgery, there was a moderate reduction in intraocular pressure.[3]

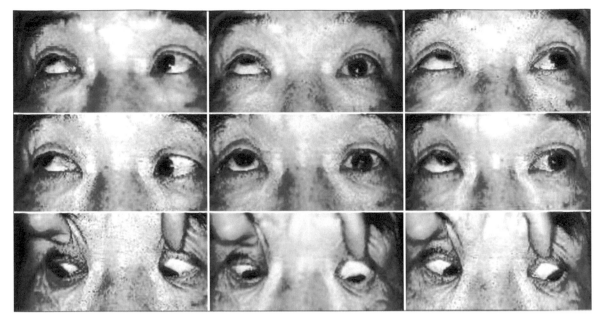

FIG. 8.4 Results of motility examination 6 months after cataract surgery show a right hypertropia in primary position, increasing to right gaze, and decreasing to left gaze.[4]

Size et al reported oculogyric crisis due to propofol, and there are 34 additional cases in the spontaneous reports.[4]

Reddy reported that as an anesthetist, he inadvertently got this liquid drug on his eyes and experienced intense burning for several minutes until his eye could be irrigated.[5] He could not continue giving the anesthetic, as he was experiencing a complete loss of vision. Ameen had a similar experience but could continue and eventually developed a keratitis, which resolved without sequelae.[6]

CLASS: LOCAL ANESTHETICS

Generic Names:
1. Bupivacaine hydrochloride; 2. chloroprocaine hydrochloride; 3. lidocaine; 4. mepivacaine hydrochloride; 5. prilocaine; 6. procaine hydrochloride.

Proprietary Names:
1. Marcaine, Sensorcaine, Sensorcaine MPF; 2. Nescaine, Nescaine-MPF; 3. 7T Lido, Akten, Anastia, AneCream, Anestacon, Aspercreme with Lidocaine, Astero, CidalEaze, EnovaRX, Glydo, LidaMantle, LIDO-K, Lidocare, Lidoderm, LidoDose, Lidomar, LidoRx, Lidosense 4, Lidozion, LMX 4, LMX 4 with Tegaderm, LMX 5, Mento-Caine, Numbonex, Professional DNA Collection Kit, RectaSmoothe, RectiCare, Senatec, Solupak, Tranzarel, VacuStim Silver, Xylocaine, Xylocaine MPF, Xylocaine Viscous, Zilactin-L, Zingo, ZTlido; 4. Carbocaine, Isocaine, Polocaine, Polocaine MPF, Scandonest Plain; 5. Citanest Plain; 6. Novocain.

Primary Use
These amides or esters of para-aminobenzoic acid are used in infiltrative, epidural block, as well as peripheral or sympathetic nerve block anesthesia or analgesia.

Ocular Side Effects
Systemic administration – epidural, infiltration, intracaudal, intradermal, intramuscular, intraspinal, intrathecal, intravenous, perineural, topical, transdermal, or urethral
Certain
1. Extraocular muscles
   a. Paresis or paralysis (Fig. 8.4)
   b. Diplopia
   c. Nystagmus
   d. Jerky pursuit movements – toxic states
   e. Abnormal doll's head movements – toxic states
2. Decreased vision
3. Horner's syndrome
   a. Miosis
   b. Ptosis
4. Pupils
   a. Mydriasis – toxic states
   b. Anisocoria – toxic states

5. Color vision defect (lidocaine)
6. Visual hallucinations (lidocaine)

Probable
1. Retinal hemorrhages (caudal block)
2. Macular edema
3. Photosensitivity

Local ophthalmic use or exposure – parabulbar or retrobulbar injection (bupivacaine, lidocaine, mepivacaine, procaine)
Certain
1. Decreased or loss of vision – temporary
2. Paresis or paralysis of extraocular muscles, including contralateral 6th nerve (see Fig. 8.4)
3. Decreased intraocular pressure
4. Eyelids or conjunctiva
   a. Allergic reactions
   b. Hyperemia
   c. Blepharoconjunctivitis
   d. Edema
   e. Urticaria
   f. Blepharoclonus
5. Pain – dependent in part on temperature of solution

Possible
1. Eyelids or conjunctiva – exfoliative dermatitis

Conditional/unclassified
1. Orbital inflammation

Inadvertent topical intraocular injection – anterior or posterior segment
Certain
1. Vision loss
2. Corneal edema
3. Endothelial cell loss
4. Increased intraocular pressure (transitory)
5. Uveitis
6. Hypotony
7. Decreased pupillary function
8. Pigment dispersion syndrome
9. Cataracts
10. Chronic Descemet's membrane wrinkling

Inadvertent ocular exposure (lidocaine)
Certain
1. Pupils
   a. Mydriasis
   b. Absence of reaction to light
2. Decreased vision
3. Superficial punctate keratitis

Systemic side effects
Local ophthalmic use or exposure – retrobulbar injection
Certain
1. Convulsion
2. Apnea
3. Cardiac arrest
4. Methemoglobin (prilocaine)

Clinical Significance
Spinal, caudal, epidural, and extradural injections of local anesthetics rarely cause ocular side effects. The most common ocular adverse event is an extraocular nerve palsy or paralysis. This may start with or without a headache followed by a weakness of the 6th nerve, although the 3rd and 4th nerves may also be involved. This may occur as soon as 2 hours after the spinal injection or up to 3 weeks later. Recovery usually occurs in 3 days to 3 weeks, but has required up to 18 months. Acute bilateral central scotomas, possibly due to hypotension or macular ischemia, have been reported. These side effects were more common decades ago when the purity of some products was in doubt or before the detergents used to clean equipment were found to be toxic.

Regional anesthesia has caused ocular adverse events, but it is difficult to rule out mechanical (speed of injection, bolus effect, increased local pressure) emboli from a toxic effect. Case reports include diplopia after a dental procedure, bilateral transient blindness during hand surgery, and permanent uniocular blindness after a dental extraction.[1-3]

Adverse events secondary to retrobulbar or peribulbar injections of anesthetics are seldom of clinical importance. However, problems may arise secondary to injections into the optic nerve sheath or nerve itself. Irreversible ischemic changes secondary to pressure effects that impede ocular blood flow, direct toxicity to muscle, or needle-induced trauma may occur. Myotoxic effects of local anesthetics, which could cause degeneration and subsequent regeneration of extraocular muscles, could explain some cases of postoperative diplopia and ptosis. Han et al stated that persistent diplopia postretrobulbar anesthesia is due to drug myotoxicity or from direct trauma.[4] Transient loss of vision is practically routine from retrobulbar injections of lidocaine or procaine. There have been occasional reports of cardiopulmonary arrest or grand mal seizures after the retrobulbar administration of bupivacaine, lidocaine, mepivacaine, or procaine. Warming the anesthetic before injection was found by Ursell et al to decrease the iatrogenic pain of the injection.[5]

Inadvertent intraocular injection of a local anesthetic into the anterior chamber is a rare but potentially devastating event. Instances of toxicity to the corneal endothelial cell secondary to local anesthesia have recently increased due to the use of intracameral anesthesia. Judge et al has reviewed this in animals.[6] Shah et al, along with others, pointed out that if one uses preservative-free 1% xylocaine (lidocaine), then the endothelium is not adversely affected during phacoemulsification.[7] Eggeling et al concurred that lidocaine at 1% appears safe.[8] Dance et al pointed out that some patients allergic to "caines" do not react adversely to preservative-free lidocaine.[9] Lee et al confirmed that intracameral 1% lidocaine causes pupillary dilation in the eyes that are difficult to dilate.[10] Higher concentrations of local anesthetics are toxic to the lens and cornea epithelium. Inadvertent intraocular injection of lidocaine has been reported to cause cataracts. Pigment dispersion is common, and much of this may be mechanical due to the firehose effect of a fluid under pressure being forced out through a small-gauge needle. The resultant stream has a shearing effect on the tissue it comes into contact with. Pupillary function is often decreased, and even absent, partially due to acute secondary glaucoma, synechiae, or a direct drug effect. The spectrum of injury is broad; however, if the posterior segment is not involved and chronic glaucoma is avoided, the prognosis may be good with corneal surgery. The outcome of inadvertent local anesthetic injected into the posterior segment is often dependent on the direct effect of the penetration trauma. Although a double perforation may have a better prognosis than a single perforation, an injection through the pars plana may be devoid of significant effects other than the acute rise in intraocular pressure. The immediate effect of the injection is a marked increase in intraocular pressure, with or without pupillary dilation, corneal edema, or loss of vision. All of these effects are transitory because there appear to be no significant long-term toxic effects of the local anesthetic on the retina or optic nerve. The chief concern is control of the acute rise in pressure, which may be severe enough to cause central retinal venous or arterial occlusion. Next are the problems from retinal perforation, vitreous adhesion, or retinal detachment. Lemagne et al reported a case of Purtscher-like retinopathy with a retrobulbar injection of a local anesthetic.[11] The exudates and hemorrhages disappeared, but a localized paracentral scotoma and afferent pupillary defect were permanent.

Numerous systemic reactions from topical ocular applications of local anesthetics have been reported. Many of these occur in part from the fear of the impending procedure or possibly an oculocardiac reflex. Side effects reported include syncope, convulsions, and anaphylactic shock.

Local anesthetics applied to the eye are seldom of importance except with multiple repeat exposures. After chronic exposure, marked anterior segment changes occur, including blindness. Kumar reported that even a single instillation of lignocaine caused significant corneal damage.[12]

CLASS: THERAPEUTIC GASES

Generic Name:
Carbon dioxide.

Proprietary Name:
Generic only.

Primary Use
This odorless, colorless gas is used as a respiratory stimulant to increase cerebral blood flow and in the maintenance of acid–base balance.

Ocular Side Effects
Systemic administration – extreme concentrations
Certain
1. Decreased vision
2. Decreased convergence
3. Decreased accommodation
4. Decreased dark adaptation
5. Photophobia
6. Visual fields
   a. Constriction
   b. Enlarged blind spot
7. Color vision defect – objects have yellow tinge
8. Retinal vascular engorgement
9. Pupils
   a. Mydriasis
   b. Absence of reaction to light
10. Visual hallucinations
11. Diplopia
12. Abnormal conjugate deviations
13. Papilledema
14. Increased intraocular pressure
15. Ptosis
16. Decreased corneal reflex
17. Proptosis
18. Decreased ability to detect coherent motion

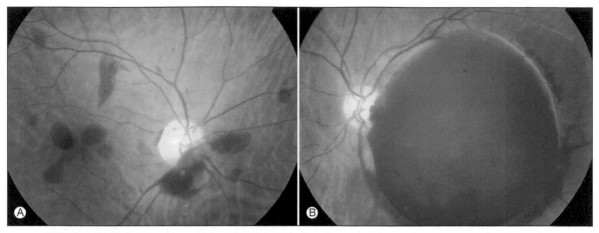

FIG. 8.5 **(A)** Right eye with multiple retinal, intraretinal, and preretinal hemorrhages surrounding the optic nerve head and the posterior pole. **(B)** An extensive premacular subhyaloid hemorrhage involving the left macular region due to oxygen-ozone therapy.[5]

Clinical Significance

Although ocular side effects due to carbon dioxide are numerous, they are rare, and nearly all significant findings are in toxic states. Transient elevation of intraocular pressure has been reported in the inhalation of 10% carbon dioxide. It is of interest in evaluating "sick building syndrome" that the percentage of CO_2 in the air may be correlated with ocular stinging and discomfort.[1,2] Yang reported that a 2.5% rise in CO_2 in the air may cause temporary impairment of the ability to detect coherent motion.[3] Recently, with the discovery of "astronaut ophthalmic syndrome," it has been hypothesized that genetic factors influence the ocular side effects associated with the 1-carbon metabolic pathway.[4]

Generic Names:

1. Oxygen; 2. oxygen-ozone.

Proprietary Name:

1. Generic only; 2. Generic only.

Primary Use

This colorless, odorless, and tasteless gas is used in inhalation anesthesia and in hypoxia. Oxygen-ozone (O_2O_3) is used as intradiscal injections for the treatment of lumbar sciatic pain peridurally and lumbar disc herniation.

Ocular Side Effects

Systemic administration – inhalation
Certain

1. Retinal vascular changes
   a. Constriction
   b. Spasms
   c. Hemorrhages (oxygen-ozone) (Fig. 8.5)
2. Decreased vision
3. Visual field constriction
4. Retrolental fibroplasia – in newborns or young infants
5. Heightened color perception
6. Retinal detachment
7. Abnormal electroretinogram (ERG)
8. Decreased dark adaptation
9. Myopia
10. Cataracts – nuclear

Clinical Significance

Toxic ocular effects due to oxygen are more prominent in premature infants, but may be found in any age group under hyperbaric oxygen therapy. Otherwise, ocular side effects secondary to oxygen therapy are rare. Whereas ocular changes due to retrolental fibroplasia are irreversible, most other side effects are transient after use of oxygen is discontinued.[1] Permanent bilateral blindness probably due to 80% oxygen during general anesthesia has been reported. It has been suggested that in susceptible people, severe retinal vasoconstriction or even direct retinal toxicity may occur from oxygen therapy.[2] Bilateral retinal hemorrhages with permanent partial visual loss have been reported secondary to a sudden increase in cerebrospinal fluid pressure after an excessive volume of oxygen was used in a myelogram contrast study.[3] A slow increase in myopia after prolonged hyperbaric oxygen has been seen in premature infants and adults. In addition, oxidative damage to the lens proteins has been postulated as a cause of nuclear cataracts in patients exposed to hyperbaric oxygen treatments.[4]

In a single case report, Giudice et al described O_2O_3 injected spinal disc infiltration causing bilateral retinal hemorrhage.[5]

REFERENCES

Drug: Hyaluronidase

1. Halliday L, Sia PI, Durkin S, et al. Atypical case of hyaluronidase allergy with orbital compartment syndrome and visual loss. *Clin Exp Ophthalmol.* 2018;46(5):563–564.
2. Raichura ND, Alam MS, Jaichandran VV, et al. Hyaluronidase allergy mimicking orbital cellulitis. *Orbit.* 2018;37(2):149–153.
3. Park S, Lim LT. Orbital inflammation secondary to a delayed hypersensitivity reaction to sub-tenon's hyaluronidase. *Orbit.* 2014;29(2):57–58.
4. Murphy T, O'Reilly P. A case of choroidal effusion with dramatic proptosis during cataract surgery. *Irish J Med Sci.* 2018;187(suppl 1):S9.
5. Zamora-Alejo K, Moore S, Leatherbarrow B, et al. Hyaluronidase toxicity: a possible cause of postoperative periorbital inflammation. *Clin Exp Ophthalmol.* 2013;41(2):122–126.
6. Minning CA. Hyaluronidase allergy simulating expulsive choroidal hemorrhage. Case reports. *Arch Ophthalmol.* 1994;112:585–586.
7. Brown SM, Brooks SE, Mazow ML, et al. Cluster diplopia cases after periocular anesthesia without hyaluronidase. *J Cataract Refract Surg.* 1999;25:1245–1249.
8. Brown SM, Coats DK, Collins ML, et al. Second cluster of strabismus cases after periocular anesthesia without hyaluronidase. *J Cataract and Refract Surg.* 2001;27:1872–1875.
9. Jehan FS, Hagan III JC, Whittaker TJ, et al. Diplopia and ptosis following injection of local anesthesia without hyaluronidase. *J Cataract Refract Surg.* 2001;27:1876–1879.
10. Miller RD. Hyaluronidase and diplopia. *J Cataract Refract Surg.* 2000;26:478–480.
11. Ortiz-Perez S, Fernandez E, Molina JJ, et al. Two cases of drug-induced orbital inflammatory disease. *Orbit.* 2011;30(1):37–39.
12. Kraff MC, Sanders DR, Jampol LM, et al. Effect of retrobulbar hyaluronidase on pseudophakic cystoid macular edema. *Am Intra-Ocular Implant Soc J.* 1983;9:184–185.
13. Eberhart AH, Weiler CR, Erie JC. Angioedema related to the use of hyaluronidase in cataract surgery. *Am J Ophthalmol.* 2004;138:142–143.

Drugs: Hyoscine butylbromide (scopolamine butylbromide), hyoscine hydrobromide (scopolamine hydrobromide), hyoscine methobromide (methscopolamine)

1. Firth AY. Visual side-effects from transdermal scopolamine (hyoscine). *Dev Med Child Neurol.* 2006;48:137–138.
2. Fraunfelder FT. Transdermal scopolamine precipitating narrow-angle glaucoma. *N Engl J Med.* 1982;307:1079.
3. Lin YC. Anisocoria from transdermal scopolamine. *Paediatr Anaesth.* 2001;11:626–627.
4. Namill MB, Suelflow JA, Smith JA. Transdermal scopolamine delivery system (Transderm-V) and acute angle-closure glaucoma. *Ann Ophthalmol.* 1983;15:1011–1012.
5. Price BH. Anisocoria from scopolamine patches. *JAMA.* 1985;253:1561.
6. Kortabarria RP, Duran JA, Chaco JR. Toxic psychosis following cycloplegic eyedrops, DICP. *Ann Pharmacother.* 1990;24:708–709.
7. MacEwan GW, Remick RA, Noone JA. Psychosis due to transdermally administered scopolamine. *Can Med Assoc J.* 1985;133:431–432.
8. Rubner O, Kummerhoff PW, Haase H. An unusual case of psychosis caused by long-term administration of a scopolamine membrane patch. Paranoid hallucinogenic and delusional symptoms. *Nervenarzt.* 1997;68(1):77–79.
9. Seenhauser FN, Schwarz NP. Toxic psychosis from transdermal scopolamine in a child. *Lancet.* 1986;2:1033.

Drug: Succinylcholine chloride (suxamethonium chloride)

1. Robinson R, White M, McCann P, et al. Effect of anaesthesia on intraocular blood flow. *Br J Ophthalmol.* 1991;75:92–93.
2. McGoldrick KE. The open globe: is an alternative to succinylcholine necessary? *J Clin Anesthesia.* 1993;5(1):1–4.
3. Chidiac EJ. Succinylcholine and the open globe: question unanswered. *Anesthesiology.* 2004;100:1035–1036.
4. Brinkley JR, Henrick A. Role of extraocular pressure in open globe injury. *Anesthesiology.* 2004;100:1036.
5. Eldor J, Admoni M. Acute glaucoma following nonophthalmic surgery. *Isr J Med Sci.* 1989;25:293–294.
6. Polarz H, Bohrer H, Fleischer F, et al. Effects of thiopentone/suxamethonium on intraocular pressure after pretreatment with alfentanil. *Eur J Clin Pharmacol.* 1992;43(3):311–313.
7. Polarz H, Bohrer H, Martin E, et al. Oral clonidine premedication prevents the rise in intraocular pressure following succinylcholine administration. *Germ J Ophthalmol.* 1993;2(2):97–99.
8. Chiu CL, Lang CC, Wong PK, et al. The effect of mivacurium pretreatment on intraocular pressure changes induced by suxamethonium. *Anaesthesia.* 1998;53(5):501–505.

Drug: Ketamine hydrochloride

1. El'kin IO, Verbuk AM, Egorov VM. Comparative characterization of changes in visual perception after ketamine and brietal anesthesia in children. *Anesteziol Reanimatol.* 2000;1:17–19.

2. Fine J, Weissman J, Finestone SC. Side effects after ketamine anesthesia: transient blindness. *Anesth Analg.* 1974;53:72–74.

3. Drayna PC, Estrada C, Wang W, et al. Ketamine sedation is not associated with clinically meaningful elevation of intraocular pressure. *Am J Emerg Med.* 2012;30(7):1215–1218.

4. Fantinati S, Casarotto R. Bilateral retrobulbar neuritis after general anesthesia. *Ann Ophthalmol.* 1988;114:649.

5. Starte JM, Fung AT, Kerdraon YA. Ketamine-associated corneal edema. *Cornea.* 2012;31(5):572–574.

Drug: Nitrous oxide

1. Smith RB, Carl B, Linn Jr JG, et al. Effect of nitrous oxide on air in vitreous. *Am J Ophthalmol.* 1974;78:314–317.

2. Stinson III TW, Donion Jr JV. Interaction of intraocular air and sulfur hexafluoride with nitrous oxide: a computer simulation. *Anesthesiology.* 1982;56:385–388.

3. Lockwood AJ, Yang YF. Nitrous oxide inhalation anaesthesia in the presence of intraocular gas can cause irreversible blindness. *Br Dent J.* 2008;204(5):247–248.

4. Lee EJ. Use of nitrous oxide causing severe visual loss 37 days after retinal surgery. *Br J Anaesth.* 2004;93:464–466.

5. Seaberg RR, Freeman WR, Goldbaum MH, et al. Permanent postoperative vision loss associated with expansion of intraocular gas in the presence of nitrous oxide-containing anesthetic. *Anesthesiology.* 2002;97:1309–1310.

6. Boucher MC, Meyers E. Effects of nitrous oxide anesthesia on intraocular air volume. *Can J Ophthalmol.* 1983;18:246–247.

7. Hart RH, Vote BJ, Borthwick JH, et al. Loss of vision caused by expansion of intraocular perfluoropropane (C_3F_8) gas during nitrous oxide anesthesia. *Am J Ophthalmol.* 2002;134:761–763.

8. Braksick SA, Wijdicks EF. Moisture and mydriasis. *Pract Neurol.* 2014;14(3):187–188.

9. Fenwick PB, Stone SA, Bushman J, et al. Changes in the pattern reversal visual evoked potential as a function of inspired nitrous oxide concentration. *Electroencephalogr Clin Neurophysiol.* 1984;57:178–183.

10. Raitta C, Karhunen U, Seppäläinen AM, et al. Changes in the electroretinogram and visual evoked potentials during general anaesthesia. *Graefes Arch Clin Exp Ophthalmol.* 1979;211:139–144.

11. Yang YF, Herber L, Rüschen RJ, et al. Nitrous oxide anaesthesia in the presence of intraocular gas can cause irreversible blindness. *BMJ.* 2002;325:532–533.

Drug: Propofol

1. Reilly CS, Nimmo WS. New intravenous anaesthetics and neuromuscular blocking drugs. A review of their properties and clinical use. *Drugs.* 1987;34(1):98–135.

2. Yamada MH, Takazawa T, Iriuchijima N, et al. Changes in intraocular pressure during surgery in the lateral decubitus position under sevoflurane and propofol anesthesia. *J Clin Monit Comput.* 2016;30:869–874.

3. Neel S, Deitch R, Moorthy SS, et al. Changes in intraocular pressure during low dose intravenous sedation with propo-

fol before cataract surgery. *Br J Ophthalmol.* 1995;79:1093–1097.

4. Size MH, Rubin JS, Patel A. Acute dystonic reaction to general anesthesia with propofol and ondansetron: a graded response. *Ear Nose Throat J.* 2013;92(1):e16–e18.

5. Reddy MB. Can propofol cause keratitis? *Anaesthesia.* 2002;57:183–208.

6. Ameen H. Can propofol cause keratitis? *Anaesthesia.* 2001;56:1017–1018.

Drugs: Bupivacaine hydrochloride, chloroprocaine hydrochloride, lidocaine, mepivacaine hydrochloride, prilocaine, procaine hydrochloride

1. Walker M, Drangsholt M, Czartoski TJ, et al. Dental diplopia with transient abducens palsy. *Neurology.* 2004;63:2449–2450.

2. Sawyer RJ, von Schroeder H. Temporary bilateral blindness after acute lidocaine toxicity. *Anesth Analg.* 2002;95:224–226.

3. Rishiraj B, Epstein JB, Fine D, et al. Permanent vision loss in one eye following administration of local anesthesia for a dental extraction. *Int J Oral Maxillofac Surg.* 2005;34:220–223.

4. Han SK, Kim JH, Hwang JM. Persistent diplopia after retrobulbar anesthesia. *J Cataract Refract Surg.* 2004;30:1248–1253.

5. Ursell PG, Spalton DJ. The effect of solution temperature on the pain of peribulbar anesthesia. *Ophthalmology.* 1996;103(5):839–841.

6. Judge AJ, Najafi K, Lee DA, et al. Corneal endothelial toxicity of topical anesthesia. *Ophthalmology.* 1997;104:1373–1379.

7. Shah AR, Diwan RP, Vasavada AR, et al. Corneal endothelial safety of intracameral preservative-free 1% xylocaine. *Indian J Ophthalmol.* 2004;52:133–138.

8. Eggeling P, Pleyer U, Hartmann C, et al. Corneal endothelial toxicity of different lidocaine concentrations. *J Cataract Refract Surg.* 2000;6:1403–1408.

9. Dance D, Basti S, Koch DD. Use of preservative-free lidocaine for cataract surgery in a patient allergic to "caines." *J Cataract Refract Surg.* 2005;31:848–850.

10. Lee JJ, Moster MR, Henderer JD, et al. Pupil dilation with intracameral 1% lidocaine during glaucoma filtering surgery. *Am J Ophthalmol.* 2003;136:201–203.

11. Lemagne JM, Michiels X, Van Causenbroeck S, et al. Purtscher-like retinopathy after retrobulbar anesthesia. *Ophthalmology.* 1990;97(7):859–861.

12. Kumar A. Diffuse epithelial keratopathy following a single instillation of topical lignocaine: the damaging drop. *Cutan Ocul Toxicol.* 2016;35(2):173–175.

Drug: Carbon dioxide

1. Hempel-Jorgensen A, Kjaergaard SK, Molhave L. Integration in human eye irritation. *Int Arch Occup Environ Health.* 1997;69(4):289–294.

2. Kjaergaard S, Pedersen OF, Molhave L. Sensitivity of the eyes to airborne irritant stimuli: influence of individual characteristics. *Int Arch Occup Environ Health.* 1992;47(1):45–50.

3. Yang Y, Sun C, Sun M. The effect of moderately increased CO$_2$ concentration on perception of coherent motion. *Aviation Space Environ Med.* 1997;68(3):187–191.
4. Zwart SR, Gibson CR, Gregory JF, et al. Astronaut ophthalmic syndrome. *FASEB J.* 2017;31:3746–3756.

Drugs: Oxygen, oxygen-ozone

1. Kalina RE, Karr DJ. Retrolental fibroplasia. *Ophthalmology.* 1982;89:91–95.
2. Ashton N. Oxygen and the retinal vessels. *Trans Ophthalmol Soc UK.* 1980;100:359–362.
3. Oberman J, Cohn N, Grand MG. Retinal complications of gas myelography. *Arch Ophthalmol.* 1979;97:1905–1906.
4. Palmquist BM, Philipson B, Barr PO. Nuclear cataract and myopia during hyperbaric oxygen therapy. *Br J Ophthalmol.* 1984;68:113–117.
5. Giudice GL, Valdi F, Gismondi M, et al. Acute bilateral vitreo-retinal hemorrhages following oxygen-ozone therapy for lumbar disk herniation. *Am J Ophthalmol.* 2004;138:175–177.

FURTHER READING

Hyaluronidase

Ahluwalia HS, Lukaris A, Lane CM. Delayed allergic reaction to hyaluronidase: a rare sequel to cataract surgery. *Eye.* 2003;17:263–266.
Barton D. Side reactions to drugs in anesthesia. *Int Ophthalmol Clin.* 1971;11(2):185.
Hagan III JC, Whittaker TJ, Byars SR. Diplopia cases after periocular anesthesia without hyaluronidase. *J Cataract Refract Surg.* 1999;25:1560–1561.
Roper DL, Nisbet RM. Effect of hyaluronidase on the incidence of cystoids macular edema. *Ann Ophthalmol.* 1978;10:1673–1678.
Salkie ML. Inhibition of wydase by human serum. *Can Med Assoc. J.* 1979;121:845.
Singh D. Subconjunctival hyaluronidase injection producing temporary myopia. *J Cataract Refract Surg.* 1995;21(4):477–478.
Taylor IS, Pollowitz JA. Little known phenomenon. *Ophthalmology.* 1984;91:1003.
Treister G, Romano A, Stein R. The effect of subconjunctivally injected hyaluronidase on corneal refraction. *Arch Ophthalmol.* 1969;81:645–649.

Hyoscine butylbromide (scopolamine butylbromide), hyoscine hydrobromide (scopolamine hydrobromide), hyoscine methobromide (methscopolamine)

Gleiter CH, Antonin KH, Brodrick T, et al. Transdermal scopolamine and basal acid secretion. *N Engl J Med.* 1984;311:1378.
Goldfrank L, Flomenbaum N, Lewin N, et al. Anticholinergic poisoning. *J Toxicol Clin Toxicol.* 1982;19:17–25.
McBride WG, Vardy PN, French J. Effects of scopolamine hydrobromide on the development of the chick and rabbit embryo. *Aust I Biol Sci.* 1982;35:173–178.
Namborg-Petersen B, Nielsen MM, Thordal C. Toxic effect of scopolamine eye drops in children. *Acta Ophthalmol.* 1984;62:485–488.
Oliva GA, Bucci MP, Fioravanti R. Impairment of saccadic eye movements by scopolamine treatment. *Percept Motor Skills.* 1993;76(1):159–167.
Rengstorff RN, Doughty CB. Mydriatic and cycloplegic drugs: a review of ocular and systemic complications. *Am J Optom Physiol Optics.* 1982;59:162–177.

Succinylcholine chloride (suxamethonium chloride)

Cook JH. The effect of suxamethonium on intraocular pressure. *Anaesthesia.* 1981;36:359–365.
France NK, France TD, Woodburn Jr JD, et al. Succinylcholine alteration of the forced duction test. *Ophthalmology.* 1980;87:1282–1287.
Goldstein JH, Gupta MK, Shah MD. Comparison of intramuscular and intravenous succinylcholine on intraocular pressure. *Ann Ophthalmol.* 1981;13:173–174.
Indu B, Batra YK, Puri GD, et al. Nifedipine attenuates the intraocular pressure response to intubation following succinylcholine. *Can J Anesthesiol.* 1989;36:269–272.
Kelly RE, Dinner M, Turner LS, et al. Succinylcholine increases intraocular pressure in the human eye with the extraocular muscles detached. *Anesthesiology.* 1993;79:948–952.
Lingua RW, Feuer W. Intraoperative succinylcholine and the postoperative eye alignment. *J Pediatr Ophthalmol Strabismus.* 1992;29(3):167–170.
Metz HS, Venkatesh B. Succinylcholine and intraocular pressure. *J Pediatr Ophthalmol Strabismus.* 1981;18:12–14.
Meyers EF, Singer P, Otto A. A controlled study of the effect of succinylcholine self-taming on intraocular pressure. *Anesthesiology.* 1980;53:72–74.
Mindel JS, Raab EL, Eisenkraft JB, et al. Succinylcholine-induced return of the eyes to the basic deviation. *Ophthalmology.* 1980;87:1288–1295.
Moreno RJ, Kloess P, Carlson DW. Effect of succinylcholine on the intraocular contents of open globes. *Ophthalmology.* 1991;98:636–638.
Nelson LB, Wagner RS, Harley RD. Prolonged apnea caused by inherited cholinesterase deficiency after strabismus surgery. *Am J Ophthalmol.* 1983;96:392–393.
Vachon CA, Warner DO, Bacon DR. Succinylcholine and the open globe. *Anesthesiology.* 2003;99:220–223.

Ether (anesthetic)

Murphy DF. Anesthesia and intraocular pressure. *Anesth Analg.* 1985;64:530.

Ketamine hydrochloride

Ausinsch B, Rayburn RL, Munson ES, et al. Ketamine and intraocular pressure in children. *Anesth Analg.* 1976;55:773–775.
Crandall DC, Leopold IH. The influence of systemic drugs on tear constituents. *Ophthalmology.* 1979;86(1):115–125.
Drugs that cause psychiatric symptoms. *Med Lett Drugs Ther.* 1986;28:81.
MacLennan FM. Ketamine tolerance and hallucinations in children. *Anaesthesia.* 1982;37:1214–1215.
Meyers EF, Charles P. Prolonged adverse reactions to ketamine in children. *Anesthesiology.* 1979;49:39–40.

Shaw IH, Moffett SP. Ketamine and video nasties. *Anaesthesia.* 1990;45:422.

Whitwam JG. Adverse reactions to intravenous agents: side effects. In: Thorton JA, ed. *Adverse Reactions to Anaesthetic Drugs.* New York: Elsevier; 1981:47–57.

Nitrous oxide

Crandall DC, Leopold IN. The influence of systemic drugs on tear constituents. *Ophthalmology.* 1979;86:115–125.

Fu AR, McDonald HR, Eliott D, et al. Complications of general anesthesia using nitrous oxide in eyes with preexisting gas bubbles. *Retina.* 2002;22:569–574.

Lane GA, Nahrwold ML, Tait AR, et al. Anesthetics as teratogens: nitrous oxide is fetotoxic, xenon is not. *Science.* 1980;210:899–901.

Mostafa SM, Wong SH, Snowdown SL, et al. Nitrous oxide and internal tamponade during vitrectomy. *Br J Ophthalmol.* 1991;75(12):726–728.

Sebel PS, Flynn PJ, Ingram DA. Effect of nitrous oxide on visual, auditory and somatosensory evoked potentials. *Br J Anaesth.* 1984;56:1403–1407.

Vote BJ, Hart RH, Worsley DR, et al. Visual loss after use of nitrous oxide gas with general anesthetic in patients with intraocular gas still persistent up to 30 days after vitrectomy. *Anesthesiology.* 2002;97:1305–1308.

Wolf GE, Capuano C, Hartung J. Effect of nitrous oxide on gas bubble volume in the anterior chamber. *Arch Ophthalmol.* 1985;103:418–419.

Propofol

Kumar CM, McNeela BJ. Ocular manifestation of propofol allergy. *Anaesthesia.* 1989;44:266.

Lenart SB, Garrity JA. Eye care for patients receiving neuromuscular blocking agents or propofol during mechanical ventilation. *Am J Crit Care.* 2000;9:188–191.

Marsch SC, Schaefer HG. External ophthalmoplegia after total intravenous anaesthesia. *Anaesthesia.* 1994;49(6):525–527.

Marsch SC, Schaefer HG. Problems with eye opening after propofol anesthesia. *Anesth Analg.* 1990;70:127–128.

Bupivacaine hydrochloride, chloroprocaine hydrochloride, lidocaine, mepivacaine hydrochloride, prilocaine, procaine hydrochloride

Anderson NJ, Woods WD, Terry K, et al. Intracameral anesthesia. *Arch Ophthalmol.* 1999;117:225–232.

Antoszyk AN, Buckley EG. Contralateral decreased visual acuity and extraocular palsies following retrobulbar anesthesia. *Ophthalmology.* 1986;93:462–465.

Breslin CW, Nershenfeld S, Motolko M. Effect of retrobulbar anesthesia on ocular tension. *Can J Ophthalmol.* 1983;18:223–225.

Carruthers JD, Sanmugasunderan S, Mills K, et al. The efficacy of topical corneal anesthesia with 0.5% bupivacaine eyedrops. *Can J Ophthalmol.* 1995;30(5):264–266.

Cohen RG, Hartstein M, Ladav M, et al. Ocular toxicity following topical application of anesthetic cream to the eyelid skin. *Ophthalmic Surg Lasers.* 1996;27:374–377.

Duker JS, Belmont JB, Benson W, et al. Inadvertent globe perforation during retrobulbar and peribulbar anesthesia. Patient characteristics, surgical management, and visual outcome. *Ophthalmology.* 1991;98(4):519–526.

Eltzschig H, Rohrbach M, Hans Schroeder T. Methaemoglobinaemia after peribulbar blockade: an unusual complication in ophthalmic surgery. *Br J Ophthalmol.* 2000;84:439.

Gild WM, Posner KL, Caplan RA, et al. Eye injuries associated with anesthesia. A closed claims analysis. *Anesthesiology.* 1992;76:204–208.

Gills JP. Effect of lidocaine on lens epithelial cells. *J Cataract Refract Surg.* 2004;30:1152–1153.

Haddad R. Fibrinous iritis due to oxybuprocaine. *Br J Ophthalmol.* 1989;73:76–77.

Kim T, Holley GP, Lee JH, et al. The effects of intraocular lidocaine on the corneal endothelium. *Ophthalmology.* 1998;105(1):125–130.

Lincoff H, Zweifach P, Brodie S, et al. Intraocular injection of lidocaine. *Ophthalmology.* 1985;92:1587–1591.

Meyer D, Hamilton RC, Gimbel HV. Myasthenia gravis-like syndrome induced by topical ophthalmic preparations. A case report. *J Clin Neuroophthalmol.* 1992;12(3):210–212.

Mukherji S, Esakowitz L. Orbital inflammation after sub-Tenon's anesthesia. *J Cataract Refract Surg.* 2005;31:2221–2223.

Salama H, Farr AK, Guyton DL. Anesthetic myotoxicity as a cause of restrictive strabismus after scleral buckling surgery. *Retina.* 2000;20:478–482.

Sprung J, Haddox JD, Maitra-D'Cruze AM. Horner's syndrome and trigeminal nerve palsy following epidural anaesthesia for obstetrics. *Can J Anaesthesia.* 1991;38(6):767–771.

Sullivan KL, Brown GC, Forman AR, et al. Retrobulbar anesthesia and retinal vascular obstruction. *Ophthalmology.* 1983;90:373–377.

Wittpenn JR, Rapoza P, Sternberg Jr P, et al. Respiratory arrest following retrobulbar anesthesia. *Ophthalmology.* 1986;93:867–870.

Carbon dioxide

Dumont L, Mardirosoff C, Dumont C, et al. Bilateral mydriasis during laparoscopic surgery. *Acta Anaesthesiologica Belgica.* 1998;49(1):33–37.

Freedman A, Sevel D. The cerebro-ocular effects of carbon dioxide poisoning. *Arch Ophthalmol.* 1966;76:59–65.

Lincoff A, Lincoff H, Solorzano C, et al. Selection of xenon gas for rapidly disappearing retinal tamponade. *Arch Ophthalmol.* 1982;100:996–997.

Podlekareva D, Pan Z, Kjaergaard S, et al. Irritation of the human eye mucous membrane caused by airborne pollutants. *Int Arch Occup Environ Health.* 2002;75:359–364.

Sevel D, Freedman A. Cerebro-retinal degeneration due to carbon dioxide poisoning. *Br J Ophthalmol.* 1967;51:475–482.

Sieker NO, Nickam JB. Carbon dioxide intoxication: the clinical syndrome, its etiology and management, with particular reference to the use of mechanical respirators. *Medicine.* 1956;35:389–423.

Wolbarsht ML, George GS, Kylstra J, et al. Speculation on carbon dioxide and retrolental fibroplasias. *Pediatrics.* 1983;71:859–860.

Oxygen, oxygen-ozone

Campbell PB, Bull MJ, Ellis F, et al. Incidence of retinopathy of prematurity in a tertiary newborn intensive care unit. *Arch Ophthalmol.* 1983;101:1686–1688.

Fisher AB. Oxygen therapy. Side effects and toxicity. *Am Rev Respir Dis.* 1980;122:61–69.

Gallin-Cohen PF, Podos SM, Yablonski ME. Oxygen lowers intraocular pressure. *Invest Ophthalmol Vis Sci.* 1980;19:43–48.

Handelman IL, Robertson JE, We Leber RG, et al. Retinal toxicity of therapeutic agents. *J Toxicol Cut Ocular Toxicol.* 1983;2:131.

Lyne AJ. Ocular effects of hyperbaric oxygen. *Trans Ophthalmol Soc UK.* 1978;98:66–68.

Nissenkorn I, Yassur Y, Mashkowski D, et al. Myopia in premature babies with and without retinopathy of prematurity. *Br J Ophthalmol.* 1983;67:170–173.

CHAPTER 9

Gastrointestinal Drugs

CLASS: DRUGS USED TO TREAT ACID PEPTIC DISORDERS

Generic Names:

1. Cimetidine; 2. ranitidine hydrochloride.

Proprietary Names:

1. Acid Reducer, Major Acid Reducer, Tagamet, Tagamet HB; 2. Acid Reducer, Ranitidine, Taladine, Wal-Zan, Zantac, Zantac 150, Zantac 75.

Primary Use

These histamine H_2 receptor antagonists are used in the treatment of duodenal ulcers.

Ocular Side Effects

Systemic administration – intramuscular, intravenous, or oral

Certain

1. Visual hallucinations
2. Eyelids or conjunctiva
   a. Hyperemia
   b. Erythema
   c. Conjunctivitis – nonspecific

Probable

1. Decreased vision
2. Pupils – toxic states
   a. Mydriasis – may precipitate acute glaucoma
   b. Decreased reaction to light

Possible

1. Color vision defect
2. Myopia
3. Immune modulation (cimetidine) (Fig. 9.1A)
4. Nystagmus (ranitidine)
5. Photophobia
6. Photosensitivity reactions

Clinical Significance

Adverse ocular effects secondary to these drugs are uncommon. Transient myopia, yellow or pink tinge to objects, and sicca-like symptoms are all possibly drug related. Visual hallucinations have occurred, particularly with high doses in elderly patients with renal impairment[1] All adverse ocular reactions are transient and disappear with withdrawal of drug therapy. There is a debate on whether or not these drugs cause changes in intraocular pressure. The case by Dobrilla et al, along with cases in the spontaneous reports, suggest that in rare instances, this class of drugs may be associated with changes in intraocular pressure.[2] However, data by Feldman et al and Garcia-Rodríguez et al do not support this.[3,4] If these drugs do cause pressure elevation, it is in all likelihood in predisposed eyes and is a rare event. Gardner et al showed that a combination of astemizole and ranitidine caused increased blood–retinal barrier permeability in patients with diabetic retinopathy.[5] Butragueño Laiseca et al reported a case of downbeat nystagmus due to ranitidine in a 3-month-old.[6] Shields et al reported improvement of diffuse conjunctival papillomatosis in an 11-year-old child after starting cimetidine (Fig. 9.1B).[7]

CLASS: ANTACIDS

Generic Name:

Bismuth subsalicylate.

Proprietary Names:

Bismatrol, Diotame, Kaopectate, Kapectolin, Kola-Pectin, Pepto-Bismol.

Primary Use

Bismuth salts are primarily used as antacids.

Ocular Side Effects

Systemic administration – oral

Probable

1. Eyelids or conjunctiva – blue discoloration
2. Corneal deposits
3. Visual hallucinations – toxic states

Local ophthalmic use or exposure – topical ocular application or ocular shield

Probable

1. Eyelids or conjunctiva – contact dermatitis

Clinical Significance

Adverse ocular reactions to bismuth preparations are quite rare and seldom of clinical significance except in

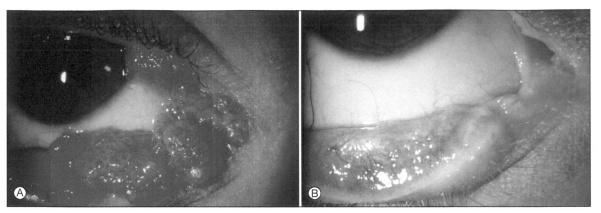

FIG. 9.1 **(A)** Patient with recurrent conjunctival papillomatosis nonresponsive to biopsy, cryotherapy, or mitomycin C treatment. **(B)** Resolution of papillomas after systemic cimetidine administration.[7]

toxic states. Bismuth-containing corneal deposits have been documented.[1]

Bismuth is used for its bacteriostasis on skin lesions. It is used in some eye ointments and can rarely cause allergic reactions.[2]

Recommendation[3]

Packing orbital exenteration with bismuth-containing material, where exposed to large surface areas or long periods of exposure, may cause significant local and systemic neurotoxicity.

CLASS: ANTIEMETICS

Generic Name:
Metoclopramide.

Proprietary Names:
Metozolv; Reglan.

Primary Use

This orthopramide is used as adjunctive therapy in roentgen-ray examination of the stomach and duodenum, for the prevention and treatment of irradiation sickness, and as an antiemetic.

Ocular Side Effects
Systemic administration – intramuscular, intravenous, or oral
Certain
1. Extraocular muscles
   a. Oculogyric crises
   b. Diplopia

   c. Paresis
   d. Nystagmus
   e. Strabismus

Probable
1. Decreased vision
2. Eyelids or conjunctiva
   a. Edema
   b. Urticaria

Possible
1. Mydriasis – may precipitate acute glaucoma
2. Photophobia
3. Color vision defect

Clinical Significance

Ocular side effects secondary to metoclopramide are rare, but the drug can produce acute dystonic reactions, particularly in children. This includes transitory oculogyric crises, inability to close the eyelids, nystagmus, and various extraocular muscle abnormalities. These dystonic reactions usually occur within 36 hours of starting treatment and subside within 24 hours of stopping the drug. There are approximately 2200 cases of oculogyric crisis in the spontaneous reports.

Sudheera et al, in a randomized, double-blind, placebo-controlled study of 60 patients, showed that metoclopramide did not significantly change intraocular pressure during anesthesia or tracheal intubation.[1]

Generic Name:
Ondansetron hydrochloride.

Proprietary Names:

Zofran, Zofran ODT, Zuplenz.

Primary Use

This 5-HT3 receptor antagonist is used as an antiemetic for patients on chemotherapy and postoperatively.

Ocular Side Effects

Systemic administration – intramuscular or oral

Probable

1. Decreased vision
2. Oculogyric crisis
3. May aggravate or cause ocular sicca

Clinical Significance

Decreased vision occurs shortly after taking ondansetron and is fully reversible and of minimal clinical importance. Oculogyric crisis is reported in the literature.[1-3] An additional 74 cases are in the spontaneous reports. There is 1 report of postoperative blindness lasting 1 minute with full recovery.[4] This drug can cause xerostomia, so it probably aggravates ocular sicca.

CLASS: ANTILIPIDEMIC DRUGS

Generic Names:

1. Atorvastatin calcium; 2. fluvastatin sodium; 3. lovastatin; 4. pitavastatin; 5. pravastatin sodium; 6. rosuvastatin calcium; 7. simvastatin.

Proprietary Names:

1. Lipitor; 2. Lescol; 3. Altoprev, Mevacor; 4. Livalo; 5. Pravachol; 6. Crestor; 7. Zocor.

Primary Use

These inhibitors of 3-hydroxy-3-methylglutaryl-coenzyme A (HMG-CoA) reductase are used to treat patients with hypercholesterolemia by lowering total cholesterol and low-density lipoprotein (LDL) cholesterol while increasing high-density lipoprotein (HDL) cholesterol. Fluvastatin and lovastatin are also indicated for preventing coronary atherosclerosis.

Ocular Side Effects

Systemic administration – oral

Probable

1. Decreased rate of choroidal neovascularization
2. Type 2 diabetes retinopathy
   a. Reduced severity of hard exudates
   b. Reduced subfoveal lipid migration
   c. Reduced clinically significant macula edema

3. Intraocular pressure
   a. Decreases
   b. Reduced risk of open-angle glaucoma
4. Diplopia

Possible

1. Myasthenia gravis
   a. Diplopia
   b. Ptosis
   c. Paresis of extraocular muscles
2. Decreased vision
3. Eyelids or conjunctiva
   a. Erythema multiforme
   b. Decreased xanthelasma
4. External ophthalmoplegia (reversible)
5. Ptosis
6. Decreased incidence of uveitis
7. Cataracts - increased risk if taken with erythromycin

Conditional/unclassified

1. May aggravate or cause ocular sicca

Clinical Significance

This group of medications, commonly called the *statins*, is one of the largest groups of prescription drugs in the world. Although there are millions of patients on long-term therapy with these drugs and multiple peer-review articles on their effects on the eye, little concrete data are available. There are no "certain" visual side effects, although some patients may complain of a decrease in vision from an unknown cause. This is not statistically significant compared with a placebo in phase III trials. The side effects more likely, although still only "possible," are ptosis, diplopia, and muscle paralysis. Fraunfelder et al described 71 cases of possible diplopia associated with the use of HMG-CoA reductase inhibitors, with 31 having positive dechallenge tests and 2 positive rechallenge tests.[1] Years later, Fraunfelder et al described possible drug-induced myositis from statin therapy causing cases of diplopia, blepharoptosis, and ophthalmoplegia.[2] Presumably the skeletal extraocular muscles develop myositis, leading to these adverse events. Purvin et al showed that statins can also exacerbate myasthenia gravis. There are spontaneous reports of statins associated with reversible external ophthalmoplegia with an unknown mechanism.[3]

There are numerous peer-review papers on both sides on whether or not these drugs are cataractogenic. It has been suggested that they are possibly weakly cataractogenic, but Cumming et al, along with others, have shown no clear association of a cataractogenic effect.[4] Klein et al have reported that these drugs decrease the incidence of nuclear sclerosis of aging.[5] In a retrospective cohort study, Leuschen et al showed an increased risk of cataracts with statin users compared with nonusers.[6] Another debate is if these drugs impede the development of age-related maculopathy. Several authors feel there is a plausible explanation to support a potential role of anticholesterol drugs, especially the statins, to protect against age-related maculopathy. A study by McGwin et al showed that statins may increase the risk of age-related maculopathy.[7] A single case of pitavastatin-associated bull's-eye maculopathy has been reported.[8] Wilson et al have shown a decreased rate of choroidal neovascularization in age-related maculopathy when patients are on statins.[9] Klein et al pooled these findings in a perspective editorial.[5] Nagaoka et al have shown an increase in blood velocity and blood flow in retinal arteries and veins, an increase in plasma nitrites/nitrates, and a decrease in intraocular pressure probably due to an increase in nitric oxide.[10] Gupta et al have reported that in patients on atorvastatin with type 2 diabetes and dyslipidemia, statins reduced the severity of hard exudates and subfoveal lipid migration in clinically significant macular edema.[11] McGwin et al suggest that long-term use of statins may be associated with a reduced risk of open-angle glaucoma, especially in patients with cardiovascular disease and lipid disease.[12] Yunker et al did a retrospective nested case-control study that suggests a decreased incidence of uveitis using statins.[13] This is supported by Borkar et al.[14] The longer the duration of use, the lower the incidence of uveitis. The questions of the effect of statins on cataracts, age-related maculopathy, type 2 diabetes, retinopathy, and glaucoma need additional confirmation to determine causation.

CLASS: ANTISPASMODICS

Generic Names:
1. Atropine; 2. homatropine.

Proprietary Names:
1. Atropen, Atropine Care, Atropine sulfate Ansyr plastic syringe, Atropisol, Isopto Atropine, Ocu-Tropine; 2. Topical ocular multi-ingredient preparations only.

Primary Use
Systemic
These anticholinergic drugs are used in the management of gastrointestinal tract spasticity, peptic ulcers, hyperactive carotid sinus reflex, and Parkinson disease; in the treatment of dysmenorrhea; and to decrease secretions of the respiratory tract.

Ophthalmic
These topical anticholinergic mydriatic and cycloplegic drugs are used in refractions, semi-occlusive therapy, accommodative spasms, and uveitis.

Ocular Side Effects
Systemic administration – intramuscular, intravenous, oral, or rectal
Certain
1. Decreased vision
2. Mydriasis – may precipitate acute glaucoma
3. Decreased accommodation
4. Photophobia
5. Micropsia
6. May aggravate or cause ocular sicca
7. Visual hallucinations
8. Color vision defect – objects have red tinge

Local ophthalmic use or exposure – topical ocular application
Certain
1. Decreased vision
2. Decreased accommodation
3. Irritation
   a. Hyperemia
   b. Photophobia
   c. Pain
   d. Edema
4. Mydriasis
   a. Possible precipitated acute glaucoma
   b. Possible elevated intraocular pressure
5. Eyelids or conjunctiva
   a. Allergic reactions
   b. Blepharoconjunctivitis – follicular and/or papillary
6. Micropsia
7. May aggravate or cause ocular sicca
8. Visual hallucinations

Local ophthalmic use or exposure – subconjunctival injection
Probable
1. Brawny scleritis
2. Conjunctival necrosis (Fig. 9.2)
3. Ocular pigment dispersion syndrome (chronic atropine use)

Systemic Side Effects
Local ophthalmic use or exposure – topical ocular application
Certain
1. Agitation

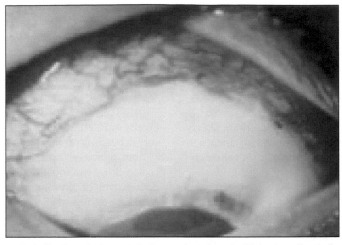

FIG. 9.2 Conjunctival necrosis from subconjunctival injection of atropine.[4]

2. Confusion
3. Psychosis
4. Delirium
5. Ataxia
6. Hostility
7. Fever
8. Xerostomia
9. Vasodilation
10. Dysarthria
11. Tachycardia
12. Convulsion
13. Cardiac dysrhythmias

Possible

1. Central anticholinergic syndrome

Clinical Significance

Atropine and homatropine have essentially the same ocular side effects whether they are administered systemically or by topical ocular application. Systemic administration causes fewer and less severe ocular side effects because significantly smaller amounts of the drug reach the eye. Mydriasis is of greatest ocular concern from systemic anticholinergics. Data in the spontaneous reports support the fact that acute glaucoma occurs more commonly unilaterally and only very rarely is it precipitated bilaterally.

Topical ocular atropine and homatropine have the same ocular effects. The action of homatropine's cycloplegic and mydriatic actions are more rapid and of shorter duration than those of atropine. Irritation or allergic reactions of the eyelids or conjunctiva are the most frequent occurrences, followed by increased light sensitivity. Conjunctival papillary hypertrophy usually suggests a hypersensitivity reaction, whereas a follicular response suggests a toxic or irritative reaction to these drugs. However, as with systemic exposure, the effect on the pupil and ciliary body with resultant elevation in intraocular pressure, with or without the precipitation of acute glaucoma, is of greatest concern. Gizzi et al reported a case of bilateral pigment dispersion syndrome after many years use of bilateral topical atropine for congenital cataracts.[1]

Atropine, but not homatropine, is said to produce a greater pupillary response in patients with Down syndrome. Permanent, fixed, dilated pupils may result from chronic atropinization or large doses of atropine used in resuscitation. Geyer et al discussed the disagreement of whether long-term atropinization postkeratoplasty can cause irreversible mydriasis.[2]

Unilateral atropinization during visual immaturity may cause amblyopia if used inappropriately.[3] Seo et al and cases in the spontaneous reports support that subconjunctival atropine injection may cause necrosis of the sclera and conjunctiva.[4]

Systemic reactions may occur after ocular instillation of these anticholinergic drugs, particularly in children or elderly patients. Symptoms of systemic toxicity include dryness of the mouth and skin, flushing, fever, rash, thirst, tachycardia, irritability, hyperactivity, ataxia, confusion, somnolence, visual hallucinations, and delirium. These reactions have been observed most frequently after the use of atropine. Rarely, convulsions, coma, and death have occurred after ocular instillation of atropine in infants and children, primarily if the solution form was used. Mydriasis due to atropine can be distinguished by applying topical ocular 1.0% pilocarpine, which will not constrict the pupil if atropine is present.

Generic Names:
1. Dicyclomine hydrochloride (dicycloverine); 2. glycopyrrolate (glycopyrronium bromide); 3. mepenzolate bromide; 4. propantheline bromide; 5. tolterodine tartrate.

Proprietary Names:
1. Antispas, Bentyl, Byclomine, Dibent, Di-Spaz, Dilomine; 2. Cuvposa, Glycate, GLYRX-PF, Lonhala Magnair, Robinul, Robinul Forte, Seebri Neohaler; 3. Cantil; 4. Pro-banthine; 5. Detrol, Detrol LA, Unidet.

Primary Use
Systemic
These anticholinergic drugs are effective in the management of gastrointestinal tract spasticity and peptic ulcers. Tolterodine is used for overactive bladder and urinary incontinence.

Topical
Glycopyrrolate is used for hyperhidrosis.

Ocular Side Effects
Systemic administration – inhalation, intramuscular, intravenous, or oral
Certain
1. Decreased vision
2. Mydriasis – may precipitate acute glaucoma
3. Decreased accommodation
4. Photophobia
5. Diplopia
6. Color vision defect – colored flashing lights (propantheline)

Probable
1. May aggravate or cause ocular sicca

Systemic administration – topical (glycopyrrolate)
Probable
1. Mydriasis
2. Decreased accommodation

Inadvertent ocular exposure
Certain

1. Pupils
   a. Mydriasis
   b. Absence of reaction to light

Possible
1. Decreased accommodation

Clinical Significance
Ocular side effects due to these anticholinergic drugs vary depending on the drug. Adverse ocular reactions are seldom significant and are reversible. None of the preceding drugs has more than 10–15% of the anticholinergic activity of atropine. The most frequent ocular side effects are decreased vision, mydriasis, decreased accommodation, and photophobia. Although these effects are not uncommon with some of these drugs, rarely are they severe enough to modify the use of the drug. The weak anticholinergic effect of these drugs seldom aggravates open-angle glaucoma; however, it has the potential to precipitate acute glaucoma attacks. Some of these drugs, especially tolterodine, may increase tear film breakup time. All of these drugs can cause xerostomia and therefore are suspect in causing or aggravating ocular sicca. There are over 400 reports of ocular sicca associated with tolterodine in the spontaneous reports. Two cases of unilateral pupillary dilatation were seen in patients who inadvertently got antiperspirants containing propantheline on their fingers and transferred it to their eyes.[1]

Glycopyrrolate cream is applied to the axilla for hair removal. The thinness of the skin in this area may allow for systemic absorption, causing mydriasis and accommodative failure in susceptible patients.[2–5]

CLASS: GASTROINTESTINAL AND URINARY TRACT STIMULANTS

Generic Name:
Bethanechol chloride.

Proprietary Names:
Duvoid, Myotonachol, Urecholine.

Primary Use
This quaternary ammonium parasympathomimetic drug is effective in the management of postoperative abdominal distention and nonobstructive urinary retention.

Ocular Side Effects
Systemic administration – oral
Certain
1. Irritation
   a. Lacrimation

b. Hyperemia
c. Burning sensation
d. Pruritus
2. Decreased accommodation
3. Miosis

Clinical Significance

Adverse ocular reactions due to bethanechol are unusual, but they may continue long after use of the drug is discontinued. Some advocate use of this drug in the treatment of Riley Day syndrome and ocular pemphigoid because the drug is associated with an increase in lacrimal secretion.

Generic Name:

Carbachol.

Proprietary Names:

Carbostat, Isopto Carbachol, Miostat.

Primary Use

Systemic

This quaternary ammonium parasympathomimetic drug is effective in the management of postoperative intestinal atony and urinary retention.

Ophthalmic

This topical or intraocular drug is used for open-angle glaucoma.

Ocular Side Effects

Systemic administration – oral
Certain

1. Decreased accommodation

Local ophthalmic use or exposure – topical ocular application
Certain

1. Miosis
2. Decreased vision
3. Decreased intraocular pressure
4. Accommodative spasm
5. Eyelids or conjunctiva
   a. Allergic reactions
   b. Hyperemia
   c. Conjunctivitis – follicular
   d. Pemphigoid-like lesion with symblepharon and shortening of the fornices
6. Irritation
   a. Lacrimation
   b. Pain
7. Blepharoclonus

8. Myopia
9. Retinal detachment
10. Color vision defect – objects have yellow tinge
11. Cataract formation
12. Myokymia

Possible

1. Night blindness

Local ophthalmic use or exposure – intracameral injection
Certain

1. Miosis
2. Corneal edema
3. Decreased vision
4. Anterior chamber – cells and flare (increased after cataract surgery)
5. Decreases macular thickness and volume (early postoperatively)

Systemic Side Effects

Local ophthalmic use or exposure – topical ocular application
Probable

1. Headaches – frontal
2. Dizziness
3. Vomiting
4. Diarrhea
5. Stomach pain
6. Intestinal cramps
7. Bradycardia
8. Arrhythmia
9. Hypotension
10. Syncope
11. Asthma – may aggravate
12. Salivation increase
13. Perspiration increase
14. Bronchospasm
15. Generalized muscle weakness

Clinical Significance

In general, systemic reactions to carbachol are rare, usually occurring only after excessive use of the medication. Probably the most frequent ocular side effect due to carbachol is a decrease in vision secondary to miosis or accommodative spasms. In the younger age groups, transient drug-induced myopia also may occur. Follicular conjunctivitis often occurs after long-term therapy, but this in general is of limited clinical significance. Some of the topical ocular side effects may be aggravated or caused by the benzalkonium chloride preservative. Enhancement of cataract formation is probably common to all miotics after many years of exposure. Miotics can induce retinal detachments, but probably only in eyes with preexisting retinal pathology.[1] This topical ocular medication may be one of the more toxic drugs on the corneal epithelium. Roberts showed increased cells and flare post–cataract surgery due to carbachol by delaying the reestablishment of the blood–aqueous barrier after surgery, causing a more prolonged inflammatory process.[2] Phillips et al suggested that intraocular carbachol postsurgery did not play a role in increasing post–capsular opacification.[3] Pekel et al found decreased macular thickness and volume but no change in retinal vessel caliber early in the postoperative cataract removal surgery using intracameral carbachol.[4]

If there are abrasions of the conjunctiva or corneal epithelium, care must be taken not to apply topical ocular carbachol because this enhances absorption and increases the incidences of systemic side effects.

Recommendation

Remove contact lenses before application of the eye drop because benzalkonium chloride is the preservative. Also, microabrasion allows greater intraocular concentrations of the drug.

REFERENCES

Drugs: Cimetidine, ranitidine hydrochloride

1. Agarwal SK. Cimetidine and visual hallucinations. *JAMA.* 1978;240:214.
2. Dobrilla G, Felder M, Chilovi F, et al. Exacerbation of glaucoma associated with both cimetidine and ranitidine. *Lancet.* 1982;1:1078.
3. Feldman F, Cohen MM. Effect of histamine-2 receptor blockade by cimetidine on intraocular pressure in humans. *Am J Ophthalmol.* 1982;93:351–355.
4. García-Rodríguez LA, Mannino S, Wallander MA, et al. A cohort study of the ocular safety of anti-ulcer drugs. *Br J Clin Pharmacol.* 1996;42:213–216.
5. Gardner TW, Eller AW, Fribert TR, et al. Antihistamines reduce blood-retinal barrier permeability in Type I (insulin-dependent) diabetic patients with nonproliferative retinopathy. *Retina.* 1995;15(2):134–140.
6. Butragueño Laiseca L, Toledo del Castillo B, Rodriguez Jiminez C, et al. Downbeat nystagmus due to ranitidine in a pediatric patient. *Eur J Paediatr Neurol.* 2017;21(4):682–684.
7. Shields CL, Lally MR, Singh AD, et al. Oral cimetidine (Tagamet) for recalcitrant, diffuse conjunctival papillomatosis. *Am J Ophthalmol.* 1999;128:362–364.

Drug: Bismuth subsalicylate

1. Fischer FP. Bismuthiase secondaire de la cornee. *Ann Oculist* (Paris). 1950;183:615.
2. Wictorin A, Hansson C. Allergic contact dermatitis from a bismuth compound in an eye ointment. *Contact Derm.* 2001;24:318.
3. Chen Y, Psaltis A, Curragh D, et al. Neurotoxicity secondary to bismuth iodoform paraffin paste packing in an orbital exenteration cavity. *Ophthalmic Plast Reconstr Surg.* 2018;34(2):179–180.

Drug: Metoclopramide

1. Sudheera KS, Bhardwaj N, Yaddanapudi S. Effect of intravenous metoclopramide on intraocular pressure: a prospective, randomized, double-blind, placebo-controlled study. *J Postgrad Med.* 2008;54(3):195–198.

Drug: Ondansetron hydrochloride

1. Size MH, Rubin JS, Patel A. Acute dystonic reaction to general anesthesia with Propofol and ondansetron: a graded response. *Ear Nose Throat J.* 2013;92(1):E16–E18.
2. Macachor JD, Kurniawan M, Loganathan SB. Ondansetron-induced oculogyric crisis. *Eur J Anaesthesiol.* 2014;31(12):712–713.
3. Plumb J, Thomas R, Weaver N. Oculogyric crisis in a child after administration of ondansetron. *Clin Toxicol.* 2015;53(7):662.
4. Cherian A, Maguire M. Transient blindness following intravenous ondansetron. *Anaesthesia.* 2005;60(9):938–939.

Drug: Atorvastatin calcium, fluvastatin sodium, lovastatin, pitavastatin, pravastatin sodium, rosuvastatin calcium, simvastatin

1. Fraunfelder FW, Fraunfelder FT, Edwards R. Diplopia and HMG-CoA reductase inhibitors. *J Toxicol Cut Ocular Toxicol.* 1999;18:319–321.
2. Fraunfelder FW, Richards AB. Diplopia, blepharoptosis, and ophthalmoplegia and 3-hydroxy-3-methylglutaryl-CoA reductase inhibitor use. *Ophthalmology.* 2008;115:2282–2285.
3. Purvin V, Kawasaki A, Smith KH, et al. Statin-associated myasthenia gravis: report of 4 cases and review of the literature. *Medicine.* 2006;85:82–85.
4. Cumming RG, Mitchell P. Medications and cataract: the blue mountains eye study. *Ophthalmology.* 1998;105:1751–1758.
5. Klein BE, Klein R, Lee KE, et al. Statin use and incident nuclear cataract. *JAMA.* 2006;295:2752–2758.
6. Leuschen J, Mortensen EM, Frei CR, et al. Association of statin use with cataracts: a propensity score-matched analysis. *JAMA Ophthalmol.* 2013;131(11):1427–1434.
7. McGwin Jr G, Owsley C, Curcio CA, et al. The association between statin use and age related Maculopathy. *Br J Ophthalmol.* 2003;87:1121–1125.
8. Iverson S. Bull's eye maculopathy secondary to pitavastatin (Livalo). *Invest Ophthalmol Vis Sci.* 2016;57(12):5391.

9. Wilson HL, Schwartz DM, Bhatt HR, et al. Statin and aspirin therapy are associated with decreased rates of choroidal neovascularization among patients with age-related macular degeneration. *Am J Ophthalmol.* 2004;137:615–624.

10. Nagaoka T, Takahashi A, Sato E, et al. Effect of systemic administration of simvastatin on retinal circulation. *Arch Ophthalmol.* 2006;124:665–670.

11. Gupta A, Gupta V, Thapar S, et al. Lipid-lowering drug atorvastatin as an adjunct in the management of diabetic macular edema. *Am J Ophthalmol.* 2004;137:675–682.

12. McGwin Jr G, McNeal S, Owsley C, et al. Statins and other cholesterol lowering medication and the presence of glaucoma. *Arch Ophthalmol.* 2004;122:822–826.

13. Yunker JJ, McGwin Jr G, Read RW. Statin use and ocular inflammatory disease risk. *J Ophthalmic Inflamm Infect.* 2013;3(1):8.

14. Borkar DS, Tham VM, Shen E, et al. Association between statin use and uveitis: results from the Pacific Ocular Inflammation Study. *Am J Ophthalmol.* 2015;159(4):707–713.

Drugs: Atropine, homatropine

1. Gizzi C, Mohamed-Noriega J, Murdoch I. A case of bilateral pigment dispersion syndrome following many years of uninterrupted treatment with atropine 1% for bilateral congenital cataracts. *J Glaucoma.* 2017;26(10):e225–e228.

2. Geyer O, Rothkoff L, Lazar M. Atropine in keratoplasty for keratoconus. *Cornea.* 1991;10(5):372–373.

3. Morrison DG, Palmer NJ, Sinatra RB, et al. Severe amblyopia of the sound eye resulting from atropine therapy combined with optical penalization. *J Pediatr Ophthalmol Strabismus.* 2005;42:52–53.

4. Seo KY, Kim CY, Lee JH, et al. Amniotic membrane transplantation for necrotizing conjunctival ulceration following subconjunctival atropine injection. *Br J Ophthalmol.* 2002;86(11):1316–1317.

Drugs: Dicyclomine hydrochloride (dicycloverine), glycopyrrolate (glycopyrronium bromide), mepenzolate bromide, propantheline bromide, tolterodine tartrate

1. Nissen SN, Nielsen PG. Unilateral mydriasis after use of propantheline bromide in an antiperspirant. *Lancet.* 1977;2:1134.

2. Izadi S, Choudhary A, Newman W. Mydriasis and accommodative failure from exposure to topical glycopyrrolate used in hyperhidrosis. *J Neuroophthalmol.* 2006;26(3):232–233.

3. Panting KJ, Alkali AS, Newman WD, et al. Dilated pupils caused by topical glycopyrrolate for hyperhidrosis. *Br J Dermatol.* 2007;158(1):187–188.

4. Williams L, Sharma V, Downes T. *Minerva. BMJ.* 2008;336:52.

5. Williams SG, Staudenmeier J. Hallucinations with tolterodine. *Psychiatr Serv.* 2004;55(11):1318–1319.

Drug: Carbachol

1. Beasley H, Fraunfelder FT. Retinal detachments and topical ocular miotics. *Ophthalmology.* 1979;86:95–98.

2. Roberts CW. Intraocular miotics and postoperative inflammation. *J Cat Refractive Surg.* 1993;19(6):731–734.

3. Phillips B, Crandall AS, Mamalis N, et al. Intraoperative miotics and posterior capsular opacification following phacoemulsification with intraocular lens insertion. *Ophthalmic Surg Lasers.* 1997;28(11):911–914.

4. Pekel G, Yagci R, Acer S, et al. Effect of intracameral carbachol in phacoemulsification surgery on macular morphology and retinal vessel caliber. *Cutan Ocul Toxicol.* 2015;34(1):42–45.

FURTHER READING

Cimetidine, ranitidine hydrochloride

De Giacomo C, Maggiore G, Scotta MS. Ranitidine and loss of colour vision in a child. *Lancet.* 1984;2:47.

Hoskyns BL. Cimetidine withdrawal. *Lancet.* 1977;1:254–255.

Bismuth subsalicylate

Cohen EL. Conjunctival hemorrhage after bismuth injection. *Lancet.* 1945;1:627.

Goas JY, Borsotti JP, Missoum A, et al. Encephalopathie myoclinique par le sous-nitrate de Bismuth. Une observation recente. *Nouv Presse Med.* 1981;10:3855.

Supino-Viterbo V, Sicard C, Risvegliato M, et al. Toxic encephalopathy due to ingestion of bismuth salts: clinical and ERG studies of 45 patients. *J Neurol Neurosurg Psychiatry.* 1977;40:748–752.

Zurcher K, Krebs A. *Cutaneous Side Effects of Systemic Drugs.* Basel: S. Karger; 1980:302.

Metoclopramide

Berkman N, Frossard C, Moury F. Oculogyric crises and metoclopramide. *Bull Soc Ophthalmol Fr.* 1981;81:153–155.

Bui NB, Marit G, Noerni B. High-dose metoclopramide in cancer chemotherapy-induced nausea and vomiting. *Cancer Treat Rep.* 1982;66:2107–2108.

Hyser CL, Drake Jr ME. Myoclonus induced by metoclopramide therapy. *Arch Intern Med.* 1983;143:2201–2202.

Kofoed PE, Kamper J. Extrapyramidal reactions caused by antiemetics during cancer chemotherapy. *J Pediatr.* 1984;105:852–853.

Laroche J, Laroche C. Etude de l'action d'un 4e groupe de medicaments sur la discrimination des couleurs et recapitulation des resultats acquis. *Ann Pharm Fr.* 1980;38:323–331.

Terrin BN, McWilliams NB, Maurer HM. Side effects of metoclopramide as an antiemetic in childhood cancer chemotherapy. *J Pediatr.* 1984;104:138–140.

Atorvastatin calcium, fluvastatin sodium, lovastatin, pitavastatin, pravastatin sodium, rosuvastatin calcium, simvastatin

Cartwright MS, Jeffery DR, Nuss GR, et al. Statin-associated exacerbation of myasthenia gravis. *Neurology.* 2004;63:2188.

Ertas FS, Ertas NM, Gulec S, et al. Unrecognized side effect of statin treatment: unilateral blepharoptosis. *Ophthal Plast Reconstr Surg.* 2006;22:222–224.

Fong DS, Poon KY. Recent statin use and cataract surgery. *Am J Ophthalmol.* 2012;153:222–228.

Hall NF, Gale CR, Syddall H, et al. Risk of macular degeneration in users of statins: cross sectional study. *BMJ.* 2001;323:375–376.

Klein R, Klein BE. Do statins prevent age-related macular degeneration? *Am J Ophthalmol.* 2004;137:747–749.

Klein R, Klein BE, Tomany SC, et al. Relation of statin use to the 5-year incidence and progression of age-related maculopathy. *Arch Ophthalmol.* 2003;121:1151–1155.

Leung DY, Li FC, Kwong YY, et al. Simvastatin and disease stabilization in normal tension glaucoma: a cohort study. *Ophthalmology.* 2010;117:471–476.

McCarty CA, Mukesh BN, Guymer RH, et al. Cholesterol-lowering medication reduces the risk of age-related maculopathy progression. *Let Med J Aust.* 2001;175:340.

McGwin Jr G, Modjarrad K, Hall TA, et al. 3-Hydroxy-3-methylglutaryl coenzyme a reductase inhibitors and the presence of age-related macular degeneration in the cardiovascular health study. *Arch Ophthalmol.* 2006;124:33–37.

Stein JD, Newman-Casey PA, Talwar N, et al. The relationship between statin use and open-angle glaucoma. *Ophthalmology.* 2012;119:2074–2081.

Tan JS, Mitchell P, Rochtchina E, et al. Statins and the long-term risk of incident age-related macular degeneration: the blue mountains eye study. *Am J Ophthalmol.* 2007;143:685–687.

van Leeuwen R, Vingerling JR, Hofman A, et al. Cholesterol lowering drugs and risk of age related maculopathy: prospective cohort study with cumulative exposure measurement. *BMJ.* 2003;363:255–256.

Atropine, homatropine

Arnold RW, Goinet E, Hickel J, et al. Duration and effect of single-dose atropine: paralysis of accommodation in penalization treatment of functional amblyopia. *Binocul Vis Strabismus Q.* 2004;19:81–86.

Chhabra A, Mishra S, Kumar A, et al. Atropine-induced lens extrusion in an open eye surgery. *Pediatr Anaesth.* 2006;16:59–62.

Decraene T, Goossens A. Contact allergy to atropine and other mydriatic agents in eye drops. *Contact Derm.* 2001;45:309–310.

Gooding JM, Nolcomb MC. Transient blindness following intravenous administration of atropine. *Anesth Analg.* 1977;56:872–873.

Merli GJ, Weitz H, Martin JH, et al. Cardiac dysrhythmias associated with ophthalmic atropine. *Arch Intern Med.* 1986;116:45–47.

O'Brien D, Haake MW, Braid B. Atropine sensitivity and serotonin in mongolism. *J Dis Child.* 1960;100:873–874.

Panchasara A, Mandavia D, Anovadiya AP, et al. Central anticholinergic syndrome induced by single therapeutic dose of atropine. *Curr Drug Saf.* 2012;7(1):35–36.

Sanitato JJ, Burke MJ. Atropine toxicity in identical twins. *Ann Ophthalmol.* 1983;15:380–382.

The Pediatric Eye Disease Investigator Group. A randomized trial of atropine vs patching for treatment of moderate amblyopia in children. *Arch Ophthalmol.* 2002;120:268–278.

The Pediatric Eye Disease Investigator Group. A randomized trial of atropine regimens for treatment of moderate amblyopia in children. *Ophthalmology.* 2004;111:2076–2085.

Tran T. Accidental atropine eye drop ingestion leading to anticholinergic toxidrome. *Ochsner J.* 2016;16(3):411.

Verma NP. Drugs as a cause of fixed, dilated pupils after resuscitation. *JAMA.* 1986;255:3251.

von Noorden GK. Amblyopia caused by unilateral atropinization. *Ophthalmology.* 1981;88:131–133.

Wark NJ, Overton JH, Marian P. The safety of atropine premedication in children with Down's syndrome. *Anaesthesia.* 1983;38:871–874.

Wilhelm H, Wilhelm B, Schiefer U. Mydriasis caused by plant content. *Fortschr Ophthalmol.* 1991;88(5):588–591.

Wilson II FM. Adverse external ocular effects of topical ophthalmic medications. *Surv Ophthalmol.* 1979;24:57–88.

Wright BD. Exacerbation of a kinetic seizure by atropine eye drops. *Br J Ophthalmol.* 1992;76(3):179–180.

Yung M, Herrema I. Persistent mydriasis following intravenous atropine in a neonate. *Paediatr Anaesth.* 2000;10:438–440.

Dicyclomine hydrochloride (dicycloverine), glycopyrrolate (glycopyrronium bromide), mepenzolate bromide, propantheline bromide, tolterodine tartrate

Altan-Yaycioglu R, Yaycioglu O, Aydin-Akova Y, et al. Ocular side-effects of tolterodine and oxybutynin, a single-blind prospective randomized trial. *Br J Clin Pharmacol.* 2005;59:588–592.

Brown DW, Gilbert GD. Acute glaucoma in patient with peptic ulcer. *Am J Ophthalmol.* 1953;36:1735–1736.

Cholst M, Goodstein S, Bernes C. Glaucoma in medical practice, danger of use of systemic antispasmodic drugs in patients predisposed to or having glaucoma. *JAMA.* 1958;166:1276–1280.

Henry DA, Langman MJS. Adverse effects of anti-ulcer drugs. *Drugs.* 1981;21:444–459.

Hufford AR. Bentyl hydrochloride: successful administration of a parasympatholytic antispasmodic in glaucoma patients. *Am J Dig Dis.* 1952;19:257–258.

Jaroudi M, Fadi M, Farah F, et al. Glycopyrrolate induced bilateral angle closure glaucoma after cervical spine surgery. *Middle East Afr J Ophthalmol.* 2013;20(2):182–184.

Leung DL, Kwong YY, Lam DS. Ocular side-effects of tolterodine and oxybutynin, a single-blind prospective randomized trial. *Br J Clin Pharmacol.* 2005;60:668.

McHardy G, Brown DC. Clinical appraisal of gastrointestinal antispasmodics. *South Med J.* 1952;45:1139–1144.

Mody MV, Keeney AH. Propantheline (Pro-Banthine) bromide in relation to normal and glaucomatous eyes: effects on intraocular tension and pupillary size. *JAMA.* 1955;159:113–114.

Schwartz N, Apt L. Mydriatic effect of anticholinergic drugs used during reversal of nondepolarizing muscle relaxants. *Am J Ophthalmol.* 1979;88:609–612.

Varssano D, Rothman S, Haas K, et al. The mydriatic effect of topical glycopyrrolate. *Graefes Arch Clin Exp Ophthalmol.* 1996;234(3):205–207.

Bethanechol chloride

Crandall DC, Leopold IH. The influence of systemic drugs on tear constituents. *Ophthalmology.* 1979;86:115–125.

Perritt RA. Eye complications resulting from systemic medications. *Ill Med J.* 1960;117:423–424.

Carbachol

Beasley H, Borgmann AR, McDonald TO, et al. Carbachol in cataract surgery. *Arch Ophthalmol.* 1968;80:39–41.

Crandall DC, Leopold IH. The influence of systemic drugs on tear constituents. *Ophthalmology.* 1979;86:115–125.

Fraunfelder FT. Corneal edema after use of carbachol. *Arch Ophthalmol.* 1979;97:975.

Hesse RJ, Smith AD, Roberts AD, et al. The effect of carbachol combined with intraoperative viscoelastic substances on postoperative IOP response. *Ophthalmic Surg.* 1988;19:224.

Hung PT, Hsieh JW, Chiou GC. Ocular hypotensive effects of N-demethylated carbachol on open angle glaucoma. *Arch Ophthalmol.* 1982;100:262–264.

Krejci L, Harrison R. Antiglaucoma drug effects on corneal epithelium. A comparative study in tissue culture. *Arch Ophthalmol.* 1970;81:766–769.

Monig H, Bruhn HD, Meissner A, et al. Kreislaufkollaps durch carbachol-haltige augentropgen. *Dtsch Med Wochenschr.* 1989;114(47):1860.

Olson RJ, Kolodner H, Riddle P, et al. Commonly used intraocular medications and the corneal endothelium. *Arch Ophthalmol.* 1980;98:2224–2226.

Pape LG, Forbes M. Retinal detachment and miotic therapy. *Am J Ophthalmol.* 1978;85:558–566.

Vaughn ED, Hull DS, Green K. Effect of intraocular miotics on corneal endothelium. *Arch Ophthalmol.* 1978;96:1897–1900.

CHAPTER 10

Cardiac, Vascular, and Renal Drugs

CLASS: DRUGS USED TO TREAT MIGRAINE

Generic Names:

1. Ergometrine maleate (ergonovine); 2. ergotamine tartrate; 3. methylergometrine (methylergonovine maleate).

Proprietary Names:

1. Ergotrate; 2. Ergomar; 3. Methergine.

Primary Use

These ergot alkaloids and derivatives are effective in the management of orthostatic hypertension migraine or other vascular types of headaches and as oxytocic drugs.

Ocular Side Effects

Systemic administration – intramuscular, intravenous, or oral
Certain

1. Decreased vision
2. Miosis (ergotamine)
3. Eyelids or conjunctiva
   a. Allergic reactions
   b. Erythema
   c. Edema

Probable

1. Retinal vascular disorders
   a. Spasms
   b. Constriction
   c. Stasis
   d. Thrombosis
   e. Occlusion
2. Visual fields
   a. Scotomas
   b. Hemianopsia
3. Color vision defect
   a. Red-green defect
   b. Objects have red tinge
4. Visual hallucinations
5. Decreased dark adaptation

Possible

1. Decreased intraocular pressure – minimal
2. Decreased accommodation
3. Eyelids or conjunctiva – lupoid syndrome

Clinical Significance

Ocular side effects due to these ergot alkaloids are rare, but patients on standard therapeutic dosages can develop significant adverse ocular effects. This is probably due to an unusual susceptibility, sensitivity, or preexisting disease that is exacerbated by the ergot preparations. Increased ocular vascular complications have been seen in patients with a preexisting occlusive peripheral vascular disease, especially in dosages higher than normal. Crews reported a healthy 19-year-old patient in whom a standard therapeutic injection of ergotamine apparently precipitated a central retinal artery occlusion.[1] Borooah et al reported a prolonged cilioretinal artery spasm leading to a permanent retinal disturbance in a 31-year-old postpartum patient after receiving ergometrine during delivery.[2] Gupta et al reported a bilateral ischemic optic neuritis that may have been due to ergotamine.[3] Merhoff et al reported a case with possible drug-induced central scotoma, retinal vasospasms, and retinal pallor.[4] Heider et al reported the case of a long-term ergotamine user who developed reversible decreased vision with decreased sensitivity in the central 30° in his visual field.[5] Sommer et al described a 31-year-old male who developed bilateral ischemic optic neuropathy after administration of ergotamine tartrate and macrolides.[6] Mieler reported a 19-year-old female who received ergot alkaloids to control postpartum hemorrhage and had a toxic retinal reaction, including bilateral cystoid macular edema, central retinal vein occlusion, papillitis, and optic disc pallor.[7] Ahmad described a case of ergometrine given intravenously that unmasked a previously "cured" myasthenia gravis.[8] According to Creze et al, methylergometrine-induced cerebral vasospasm may have caused transitory cortical blindness.[9] There are sporadic reports of cataracts in the literature, but these are rare, and it is difficult to prove a cause-and-effect relationship.

CLASS: ANTIANGINAL DRUGS

Generic Names:

1. Amlodipine besylate; 2. diltiazem hydrochloride; 3. nifedipine; 4. verapamil hydrochloride.

Proprietary Names:

1. Norvasc; 2. Cardizem, Cardizem CD, Cardizem LA, Cardizem XT, Cartia XT, Dilacor XR, Dilt-CD, Diltzac, Taztia XT, Teczem, Tiazac; 3. Adalat, Adalat CC, Afeditab CR, Nifediac CC, Nifedical XL, Procardia, Procardia XL; 4. Calan, Calan SR, Cover-HS, Isoptin, Isoptin SR, Verelan, Verelan PM.

Primary Use

These various calcium channel blockers are used in the treatment of vasospastic angina, chronic stable angina, and hypertension.

Ocular Side Effects

Systemic administration – oral

Probable

1. Decreased vision – transient
2. Eyelids or conjunctiva
   a. Chemosis
   b. Erythema
   c. Conjunctivitis – nonspecific
   d. Photosensitivity
   e. Edema
   f. Urticaria
   g. Purpura
3. Nystagmus – rotary (nifedipine, verapamil)
4. Periorbital edema
5. Visual hallucinations

Possible

1. Irritation
   a. Lacrimation
   b. Photophobia (nifedipine)
   c. Pain
2. Eyelids or conjunctiva – erythema multiforme
3. Aggravates myasthenia gravis (verapamil)

Conditional/unclassified

1. Blepharospasm
2. May make open-angle glaucoma more difficult to manage

Systemic Side Effects

Systemic administration – oral

Possible

1. May cause cardiac arrhythmias when used with topical ocular glaucoma medication

Clinical Significance

Ocular side effects are uncommon, reversible, and seldom of enough clinical importance to stop the drug. Decreased vision, chemosis, and eyelid and periorbital edema appear to be the most common. A unique finding with amlodipine besylate was a unilateral inferior extensive dependent conjunctival chemosis with onset occurring 3–4 months after starting the drug.[1,2] This chemosis was totally reversible within 6–8 months once the drug was discontinued.

The area of clinical interest is in the management of glaucoma. Intraocular pressure does not appear to be affected by calcium channel blockers, although there are questionable data that glaucoma patients may be more difficult to control on these drugs. Muskens et al, in a subset of 3842 participants with an average 6.5-year follow-up, suggested that the use of calcium channel antagonists is associated with open-angle glaucoma.[3]

Overall, although there are a number of scattered reports of ocular vascular effects, it is difficult to implicate this class of drugs, which is used in a population with significant vascular disease. Verapamil has been implicated in worsening myasthenia gravis because of the drug's inhibition of potassium outflow from cells at the motor endplate.[4]

There is increasing evidence that topical ocular beta blockers given to patients who are on calcium channel blockers may, in rare cases, result in an arrhythmia. This has been suggested in 4 separate literature reports and in 5 spontaneous reports.[5–8.] The proposed mechanism is that each drug acts in a different way to decrease the heart rate, so the effects may be additive, causing an arrhythmia.

Recommendation

Be aware that oral calcium channel blockers may interact with topical ocular beta blockers, causing cardiac arrhythmias.

Generic Name:

Amyl/butyl nitrite.

Proprietary Name:

Generic only.

Street Names:

Ames, aroma of men, banapple gas, liquid gold, liquid rush, locker room, poppers, ram and thrust, rush.

Primary Use

This short-acting nitrite antianginal drug is effective in the treatment of acute attacks of angina pectoris. It is used illegally to enhance orgasms.

Ocular Side Effects
Systemic administration – inhalation
Certain
1. Vision loss
   a. Transitory
   b. Permanent
2. Subfovea (Fig. 10.1)
   a. Fuzziness – optical coherence tomography (OCT)
   b. Vitelliform lesions
   c. Detachment
   d. Microholes
3. Mydriasis – transitory
4. Color vision defect
   a. Objects have yellow tinge
   b. Colored haloes around objects – mainly blue or yellow
5. Intraocular pressure
   a. Initially increased – momentarily
   b. Decreased – transient
6. Visual hallucinations
7. Eyelids or conjunctiva – allergic reactions

Conditional/unclassified
1. Optic neuritis

Local ophthalmic use or exposure – inadvertent contact with liquid
Certain
1. Eyelids – erythema
2. Irritation – stinging pain
3. Cornea and conjunctiva
   a. Sloughing of epithelial
   b. Limbal ischemia
   c. Edema

Clinical Significance
This drug has been used as a "club" drug and aphrodisiac since the 1970s. Possibly due to changes in chemical composition, significant ocular side effects have now been seen. This drug is made by multiple manufacturers and is sold as a liquid in glass vials. Although multiple names are associated with this illicit drug, the most common is "poppers" because you "pop" off the cap of the vial to inhale its contents. The classic ocular history is a sudden onset of disruption of central vision occurring shortly after inhalation. Hundreds of cases of maculopathy in the literature and spontaneous reports have confirmed a "certain" association.[1-4] Vignal-Clermont et al first reported this syndrome; however, recent clinical phenotypes have been reported by Van Bol et al to better

define this ocular side effect.[5,6] In their retrospective series of 39 patients, they discovered 3 phenotypes based primarily on OCT analysis:
1. Subfoveal disturbance of the ellipsoid layer – A "fuzzy" aspect of the ellipsoid layer in patients taking the drug for 2 years or less. Vision was not worse than 20/30, and about half returned to normal within 2 years after stopping the drug. Fundus autofluorescence (FAF) images in most all of these patients were normal.
2. Vitelliform-like lesion – Fundus examination showed bilateral yellow foveal spots, with OCT showing subfoveal detachment with hyperreflective areas of thickening extending from the ellipsoid layer to the external limiting membrane. FAF often showed a central area of mildly increased autofluorescence. Visual acuity decreased up to 20/60. Use of "poppers" was at least once a week for 2–15 years. Whereas some recovered visual acuity after stopping the drug (no structural recovery), most did not show significant recovery.
3. Microhole – Rarely seen and not as well studied (only 4 patients). Usually seen as an asymmetric, well-defined, subfoveal defect of the ellipsoid layer. Vision may be normal to 20/30 and may occur after only 1 drug exposure.

Rewbury et al found that the cause of this side effect is isopropyl nitrite.[7]

The use of "poppers" in Australia involves at least 60% of the homosexual population.[8] Romanelli et al also found that the nonmedical use of this drug is primarily in the homosexual population.[9]

Amyl nitrite ordinarily causes a slight rise of <3 mm of mercury for several seconds followed by a fall in intraocular pressure for only 10–20 minutes. This decrease in pressure is felt to be secondary to a fall in blood pressure. Fledelius reported a case of optic neuritis with irreversible loss of vision after amyl nitrite inhalation.[10]

These drugs, when used as recreational drugs, can come into contact with the eye in a liquid form. Mearza et al showed that anterior injury can be extensive, but heals without complication in time.[11]

Generic Names:
1. Flecainide acetate; 2. procainamide hydrochloride.

Proprietary Names:
1. Tambocor; 2. Procanbid, Pronestyl, Pronestyl SR.

Primary Use
These primary amine analogs of lidocaine are used in the treatment of resistant ventricular arrhythmia.

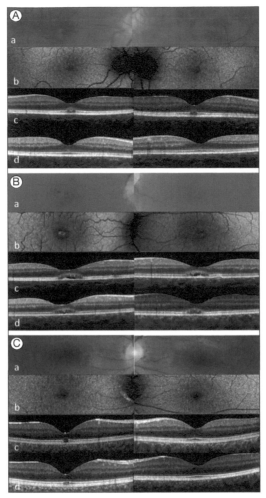

FIG. 10.1 **(A)** Case of subfoveal disturbance of the ellipsoid layer with decreased central vision (20/30 in both eyes) 48 hours after a single trial of poppers. Fundus photographs (a) demonstrate a subtle yellowish lesion in both fovea corresponding to a normal autofluorescent signal on fundus autofluorescence (FAF) (b). The spectral-domain optical coherence tomography (SD-OCT) (c) at baseline shows a subfoveal area of disturbance of the reflectivity of the ellipsoid layer. Five months after exposure, visual acuity recovered to 20/16 in both eyes, and a complete resolution of the foveal changes is observed on SD-OCT (d). **(B)** Case of vitelliform-like lesion with bilateral central scotoma and a vision of 20/60 in both eyes in a context of heavy poppers use (two to three times a week for 4 years). Fundus photographs (a) showing bilateral yellow spots with subtle pigmentary clumping, corresponding to an area of enhanced autofluorescent signal surrounded by a ring of reduced autofluorescence on FAF (b). SD-OCT at presentation (c), showing bilateral subfoveal detachment with a hyperreflective area of thickening extending from the ellipsoid layer to the external limiting membrane. A total of 24 months later, vision remains stable, and only a partial regression of the foveal changes is noticed on SD-OCT despite drug cessation (d). **(C)** Case of microhole with 20/20 vision and symptoms of metamorphopsia occurring after a single trial of poppers. Fundus photographs (a), autofluorescence (b), and SD-OCT (c) at presentation. A well-defined defect at the level of the ellipsoid layer is demonstrated on the right side. Five months later, a partial resolution of this defect is highlighted on SD-OCT (d).[6]

Ocular Side Effects
Systemic administration – intramuscular, intravenous, or oral
Certain
1. Decreased vision (flecainide)
2. Various visual sensations (flecainide)
   a. "Spots before eyes"
   b. Peripheral bright or flashing lights
   c. Photophobia
   d. pain
3. Rectus muscle (flecainide)
   a. Spasms
   b. Pain
   c. Diplopia
4. Corneal deposits (flecainide)
5. Nystagmus (flecainide)
6. Visual hallucinations (flecainide)
7. Eyelids or conjunctiva
   a. Erythema
   b. Edema
   c. Urticaria (flecainide)
   d. Loss of eyelashes or eyebrows
   e. Irritation
   f. Photosensitivity (procainamide)

Possible
1. Myasthenia gravis (procainamide)
   a. Diplopia
   b. Ptosis
   c. Paresis of extraocular muscles
2. Eyelids or conjunctiva
   a. Lupoid syndrome
   b. Exfoliative dermatitis (flecainide)
   c. Lupus erythematosus
3. Visual hallucinations (procainamide)

Conditional/unclassified
1. Scleritis

Clinical Significance
There are little data on ocular side effects from this class of drugs other than with flecainide. Gentzkow et al, as well as others, have stated that the most common side effects of flecainide are visual disturbances, with decreased vision occurring in about 30% of patients.[1] Ikäheimo et al found that decreased vision occurred in 10.5% of patients in their series.[2] This was only in lateral gaze and lasted only for a few seconds. Decreased accommodation with nonspecific visual symptoms such as "spots before eye," peripheral bright lights, and photophobia also occur. Well-documented cases of intermittent diplopia, rectus muscle spasms, decreased depth perception, and nystagmus are in the

literature and spontaneous reports. These can be dose dependent and resolve at lower dosages. Skander et al reported painful lateral rectus muscle spasms.[3] Moller et al reported 2 patients on flecainide who developed superficial gray whorl corneal deposits.[4] Ikäheimo et al found brownish epithelial deposits in a thin horizontal linear pattern in the inferior cornea.[2] This occurred in 14.5% of their patients, but did not appear to be dose or time related. High-pressure liquid chromatography suggested these are due to flecainide and peptide corneal deposition. Stopping the drug resulted in corneal clearing over a 3-month period. All ocular signs and symptoms are reversible either at decreased dosages or when the drug is discontinued.

Turgeon et al described a case of procainamide-induced lupus, which presented first with scleritis.[5] Nichols et al reported a case of severe retinal vaso-occlusive disease secondary to procainamide-induced lupus.[6]

Generic Name:
Nicorandil.

Proprietary Names:
Angedil, Aprior, Dancor, Ikorel, Nikoran, Nitorubin, PCA, Sigmart.

Primary Use
Nicorandil is a vasodilatory drug used to treat angina.

Ocular Side Effects
Systemic administration – oral
Probable
1. Corneal ulceration
2. Conjunctival ulceration
3. Abnormal vision

Possible
1. Increased risk of age-related macular degeneration
2. Oculomotor palsy

Clinical Significance
Nicorandil is available around the world, but not in the United States. It is associated with ulceration throughout the mucous membranes of the body, and perhaps this is unique to this class of drug. Oral, anal, perianal, perivulval, vulvovaginal, penile, gastrointestinal, colonic, peristomal, and skin ulcerations are now well recognized. Eye ulcerations with nicorandil appear logical, as the eye is also part of the mucous membranes of the body.[1–4] The average age of patients who develop ocular ulcerations is over 75 years, and advanced age may be contributory to the risk of developing ocular ulcerations from nicorandil.[5] The

mechanism is not known. Fortunately, all case reports indicate that, if recognized, withdrawing nicorandil will lead to resolution of the drug-related conjunctival or corneal ulceration.

Klein et al, in their Beaver Dam Eye Study, suggested that all vasodilators have a modest association in the early onset of age-related macular degeneration.[6] Jeong et al described an acute intractable headache with reversible limited unilateral ocular movements in all positions of gaze.[7] This was accompanied by ptosis and sluggish pupillary reaction to light on the same side.

Generic Name:
Nitroglycerin.

Proprietary Names:
Deponit, Gonitro, Minitran, Nitrek, Nitro Bid, Nitro-Dur, Nitro-Time, Nitrodisc, Nitrolingual, NitroMist, Nitropress, Nitroquick, Nitrostat, Nitrotab, Rectiv, Transdermal-NTG, Tridil.

Primary Use
This short-acting trinitrate vasodilator is effective in the treatment of acute attacks of angina pectoris.

Ocular Side Effects
Systemic administration – intravenous, oral, sublingual, topical, or transdermal
Certain
1. Vasodilatation – transitory
   a. Conjunctiva
   b. Retina

Probable
1. Decreased vision – transitory
2. Color vision defect – colored haloes around lights, mainly yellow or blue
3. Eyelids – allergic reactions
4. Precipitated visual auras

Possible
1. Increased risk of age-related macular degeneration
2. Eyelids – exfoliative dermatitis
3. Pseudotumor cerebri (intravenous)

Clinical Significance
Oral nitroglycerin appears to have few significant ocular side effects. However, recently Klein et al, in their Beaver Dam Eye Study, showed a modest association between vasodilators (nitroglycerin in particular) and early onset of age-related macular degeneration.[1] The *Physicians' Desk Reference* (PDR) states that on rare occasions sublingual nitroglycerin can cause transient blurring of vision.[2] Bánk and Afridi et al described cases where nitroglycerin-induced migraines started with a visual aura.[3,4] Employees manufacturing this drug have reported acute intoxication with transient visual loss followed by a severe headache.[5] Ohar et al suggested an association of pseudotumor cerebri with intravenous nitroglycerin.[6] Inadvertent ocular exposure to nitroglycerin-containing pastes has caused conjunctival injection, mydriasis, and eyelid reactions.[7]

CLASS: ANTIARRYTHMIC DRUGS

Generic Name:
Amiodarone hydrochloride.

Proprietary Names:
Cordarone, Nexterone, Pacerone.

Primary Use
This benzofuran derivative is effective in the treatment of various arrhythmias.

Ocular Side Effects
Systemic administration – intravenous or oral
Certain
1. Visual changes
   a. Photophobia
   b. Decreased vision
   c. Glare
   d. Halos around light – most prominent at night
2. Cornea
   a. Deposits – grayish or golden brown – epithelium vortex keratopathy (Fig. 10.2)
   b. Epithelial erosion
   c. Decreased sensation
   d. Reduction keratocyte density
   e. Endothelial deposits
   f. Clearing of deposits may signal decrease serum drug levels
   g. Keratitis
3. Eyelids or conjunctiva
   a. Yellow-brown or gray deposits
   b. Blepharoconjunctivitis
   c. Photosensitivity reactions
   d. May aggravate or cause ocular sicca
   e. Photosensitivity
4. Lens
   a. Anterior subcapsular small yellow-white punctuate opacities
   b. Cortical changes

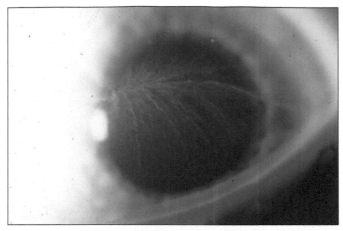

FIG. 10.2 Amiodarone whorl-like pattern of golden-brown deposits in the anterior cornea.[18]

c. Intraocular lenses – brown discoloration
5. Drug found in the tears

Possible
1. Optic neuropathy
   a. Visual loss
   b. Disc edema
   c. Disc hemorrhage
   d. Optic nerve pallor (Fig. 10.3)
   e. Visual field defects
2. Loss of eyelashes or eyebrows
3. Thyroid eye disease
   a. Hypothyroid ocular signs
   b. Hyperthyroid ocular signs
4. Pseudotumor cerebri

Clinical Significance

Amiodarone was first introduced in the 1960s, and its most frequent drug-induced side effects are ocular. These side effects, especially in the anterior segment, are dose and time dependent. Corneal microdeposits due to amiodarone occur in all patients who are using the drug long term. The corneal epithelial whorl-like drug-related deposition is indistinguishable from that due to drugs such as quinacrine, indomethacin, and chlorpromazine. The keratopathy may reach a steady state with no progression even with continued drug use, or a decrease may indicate a low serum drug level.[1] The usual pattern for corneal deposition initially, in stage 1, is a horizontal, irregular, branching line near the junction of the mid and outer one-third of the cornea.[2] In stage 2, this increases so that there are 6–10 branches,

with an increase in length and curve superiorly. Any increase in the number of branches constitutes stage 3. Stage 4 is the whorl-like pattern with clumping deposits. The deposits may be seen as early as 2 weeks after starting the drug, but in general the visible keratopathy develops in most patients within weeks after initiation of amiodarone therapy and reaches its peak within 3–6 months. Patients taking 100–200 mg per day have only minimal or even no visible corneal deposits. At dosages of 400 mg or more, almost all patients will show corneal deposits. Once the drug is stopped, most deposits completely regress in 3–7 months, but this may take up to 2 years. In patients using soft contact lenses, the keratopathy is significantly less. Visual changes due to these deposits are uncommon, but on occasion they are severe enough to stop the drug. Patient complaints consist of photophobia, hazy vision, or colored haloes around lights. Occasionally, a patient may complain that bright lights, especially headlights at night, will cause a significant glare problem. Frings et al found that topical ocular heparin enhances clearing of amiodarone-induced corneal verticillata.[3] Keratitis sicca has been reported because the drug is secreted in tears, which may aggravate borderline sicca cases or enhance the evaporative form of sicca. A probable autoimmune reaction can occur, which is associated with xerostomia, ocular sicca, peripheral neuropathy, and pneumonitis. Slate-gray periocular skin pigmentation or blue skin discoloration has been seen secondary to photosensitivity reactions. Corneal ulcerations can rarely occur during treatment with amiodarone. Flach et al first described subtle anterior subcapsular lens opacities in

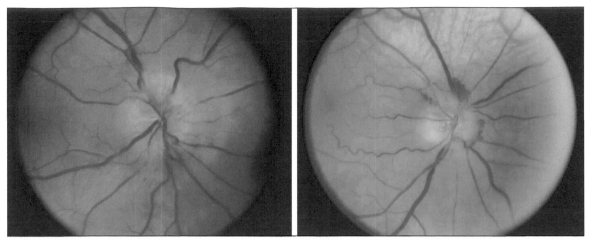

FIG. 10.3 Optic nerve with presumed amiodarone-induced optic neuropathy.[19]

patients taking amiodarone long term.[4] These changes primarily occur in the pupillary area and are yellow-white, loosely packed deposits that rarely interfere with vision. The location of the deposits suggests a photosensitizing effect of amiodarone on the lens. Cumming et al reported increased cortical cataracts.[5]

Does amiodarone cause optic neuropathy? It is not known if this is simply a variant of nonarteritic ischemic optic neuropathy (NAION), in which swelling of the disc is prolonged, or if amiodarone is an independent risk factor of NAION. Regardless, from a practical point of view, one may need to practice defensive medicine because the legal system has determined a relationship between amiodarone and NAION in a number of cases. Scientific data (along the guidelines of Murphy et al) are necessary to determine whether a relationship exists or not.[6] However, some feel amiodarone optic neuropathy is possibly characterized by an insidious onset and slower progression, which often has bilateral visual loss and protracted disc swelling. NAION may be characterized as an acute, unilateral visual loss that is usually complete at onset with resolution of disc edema over several weeks. Optic nerve swelling and peripapillary nerve-fiber layer hemorrhages tend to persist for several months in amiodarone-induced optic neuropathy, whereas in NAION these usually resolve more quickly. After discontinuation of amiodarone, visual acuity and visual field defects tend to stabilize. Purvin et al have recently recommended a systemic approach with well-defined diagnostic criteria to help the clinician manage these patients (Table 10.1).[7]

TABLE 10.1
Management of Patients Taking Amiodarone[7]

	Disc Edema	Management
Group I	Simultaneous and bilateral; further tests to rule out increased intracranial pressure giant cell arteritis	If other tests are negative, strongly consider discontinuation of amiodarone
Group II	Unilateral atypical NAION; insidious onset of symptoms, relatively mild optic nerve dysfunction, generous cup-to-disc ratio in fellow eye, prolonged disc edema	Strongly consider discontinuation of amiodarone
Group III	Unilateral typical NAION; immediate onset of disc edema, crowded contralateral disc, moderate to substantial defects of optic nerve dysfunction, no systemic symptoms of amiodarone	Continuation of amiodarone may be appropriate

In a literature review of 296 reports of possible optic neuropathy, Passman et al found that the mean duration of amiodarone therapy before vision loss was 9 months (range 1–84 months).[8] Insidious onset of amiodarone-associated optic neuropathy (44%) was the most common presentation, and nearly one-third were asymptomatic. Optic disc edema was present in 85% of cases. After drug cessation, 58% had improved visual acuity, 21% were unchanged, and 21% had further decreased visual acuity. Legal blindness (<20/200) was noted in at least 1 eye in 20% of cases. There are hundreds of cases in the literature and spontaneous reports of unilateral and bilateral suspected amiodarone optic neuropathy, some with permanent blindness.[9,10] Cheng et al, in a nationwide retrospective population-based cohort study, concluded that there was a higher risk of optic neuropathy in patients treated with amiodarone, especially males and possibly patients on a longer duration of treatment.[11] Mindel et al, in a letter to the editor, did not concur with some of their findings.[12] Cheng et al then responded that their methodology and conclusions were valid.[13]

Although the mechanism of amiodarone optic neuropathy, or even if it occurs, is unknown, ultrastructural changes in the human optic nerve illustrate a primary lipidosis. Selective accumulation of intracytoplasmic lamellar inclusions in large optic nerve axons may mechanically or biochemically decrease axoplasmic flows. Resultant optic nerve head edema may persist as long as transport is inhibited (perhaps as long as several months after discontinuation of amiodarone, which has a half-life of up to 100 days). There is no documented evidence that this drug causes human retinal damage, although intracytoplasmic granulations have been found in the retinal pigment epithelium and choroid, as well as the ciliary body, iris, cornea, conjunctiva, and lens. This drug is a photosensitizing drug, and, in selected cases, sunglasses that block ultraviolet (UV) rays from the sunlight to 400 nm may be considered for eyelid and lens changes.

Is amiodarone optic neuropathy real? Our bias, based in part by informal discussions with neuro-ophthalmologists, is "probable/possible." Still, a "certain" association is lacking. Mindel, however, using surveys from many databases, disagrees.[14] However, the *Physicians' Desk Reference* (PDR) does mention optic neuropathy under "Contraindications/Precautions."[15] Wang et al support a positive association.[16] Recently Fasler et al did a comprehensive review and outlined that controversy still exists.[17] The overall emphasis was that if in doubt, "amiodarone treatment should be stopped if there is an alternative solution to control arrhythmia."

Recommendations
1. Baseline ophthalmic examination before or shortly after starting amiodarone.
2. If any visual disturbances occur while on the drug, the patient should see an ophthalmologist.
3. If there is any suggestion of an optic neuropathy, discuss with the patient and their physician the possibility of using alternative medication, or obtain an informed consent as to the possible ocular side effects if amiodarone therapy is continued.
4. Carry out ophthalmic examinations on an annual basis.
5. In patients with photosensitizing side effects, consider UV-blocking lenses.
6. In children, it is especially important to get informed consent and to stress to the parent the difficulty in getting accurate vision and visual fields, which may delay diagnosis and limit the ability to follow progression accurately. In young children, the inability to do these tests require regular 3-month optic disc examinations.

Generic Name:
Digoxin.

Proprietary Names:
Digitek, Lanoxin, Lanoxin Pediatric.

Primary Use
This cardiac glycoside is primarily used for arrhythmias, heart failure, and abortions.

Ocular Side Effects
Systemic administration – intravenous or oral
Certain
1. Visual changes
   a. Decreased vision
      i. Near
      ii. Distance
   b. Photopsia
   c. Glare
2. Dyschromatopsia
   a. Primarily xanthopsia
   b. Cyanopsia
   c. Chloropsia
3. Visual hallucinations
4. Electroretinogram (ERG)
   a. Photopic
   b. Scotopic
5. Visual fields
   a. Central scotoma
   b. Pericentral scotoma

Probable
1. Mydriasis
2. Diplopia

Possible
1. Colored vitreous floaters
2. Monolateral paresis of superior oblique muscle

Clinical Significance

Digoxin toxicity is most often determined by cardiac and noncardiac symptoms; however, some feel that ocular side effects such as blurred or decreased vision are more specific.[1] Also, because pacemakers may mask cardiac signs and symptoms, ocular findings are important. The ophthalmologic tests that are considered most useful to support a diagnosis of digoxin intoxication are photopic and scotopic ERG seeking b-wave delayed implicit time and decreased b-wave amplitude.[2]

Although dyschromatopsia was felt to be a classic finding, especially xanthopsia, more recent testing has found that dyschromatopsia has a high incidence in the elderly, so formal color vision testing may have limited value.[3] Visual hallucinations may be an early sign of digoxin toxicity or even an isolated symptom.[4]

Visual symptoms may occur at therapeutic doses, in part due to narrow therapeutic-to-toxic blood levels.[5,6] Toxic visual effects include blurred vision, dim vision, hazy vision, misty vision, snowy vision, flashing lights, scintillating lights, moving spots and shapes, diplopia, and pain on ocular movement.[7] In a series of 179 patients with suspected digoxin toxicity, 95% had visual complaints, with decreased ability to read and hazy vision being the most common.[8] Visual effects may, in extremely rare cases, include blindness.[9] Mydriasis and diplopia are well documented.[1] Ross described 2 patients, 1 with positive rechallenge, who had monolateral superior oblique paresis after taking digoxin.[10]

Ocular side effects may occur hours, days, months, or even years after starting digoxin. They may resolve within days, months, or years if the dosage is reduced or the drug is discontinued.[1] Although most all are completely reversible, full reversibility of central scotoma is uncertain.[7]

One of the more complete overviews of digoxin visual effects is by Piltz et al.[7] They pointed out that "while cardiac, gastrointestinal, and neuromuscular symptoms are commonly encountered in digoxin toxicity, visual dysfunction is frequently the reason for presentation to the doctor. The ophthalmologist or neurologist may therefore be the first physician consulted with digitalis toxicity." Digoxin toxicity is a potentially life-threatening disorder.

Generic Name:
Disopyramide phosphate.

Proprietary Names:
Norpace, Norpace CR.

Primary Use
This anticholinergic drug is indicated for suppression and prevention of recurrence of cardiac arrhythmias.

Ocular Side Effects
Systemic administration – oral
Certain
1. Decreased vision
2. Eyelids or conjunctiva
   a. Erythema
   b. Conjunctivitis – nonspecific
   c. Photosensitivity
3. Mydriasis – may precipitate acute glaucoma
4. Decreased accommodation

Probable
1. May aggravate or cause ocular sicca
2. Visual hallucinations

Clinical Significance
The anticholinergic effects of disopyramide can cause blurred vision and fluctuation of visual acuity by up to 28%. Because this drug can cause mydriasis, there are cases in the literature and the spontaneous reports of acute glaucoma occurring shortly after or up to 3 weeks after the patient started taking the medication.[1,2] Disopyramide can cause xerostomia (32%) and is therefore suspect in also aggravating or causing ocular sicca.[3]

Generic Name:
Methacholine chloride.

Proprietary Name:
Provocholine.

Primary Use
Systemic
This quaternary ammonium parasympathomimetic drug is primarily used in diagnostic testing.

Ophthalmic
This topical drug is used in the management of acute glaucoma and in the diagnosis of Adie pupil.

Ocular Side Effects
Systemic administration – inhalation
Certain
1. Decreased accommodation
2. Lacrimation

Local ophthalmic use or exposure – topical ocular application
Certain
1. Pupils
   a. No effect – normal pupil
   b. Miosis – Adie pupil
2. Decreased intraocular pressure
3. Eyelids or conjunctiva
   a. Allergic reactions
   b. Hyperemia
4. Myopia
5. Blepharoclonus
6. Lacrimation

Systemic Side Effects
Local ophthalmic use or exposure – retrobulbar injection
Certain
1. Nausea
2. Vomiting
3. Heart block
4. Incontinence
5. Cardiac arrest

Clinical Significance
Topical ocular application of methacholine causes a number of ocular side effects, but all are reversible and have minimal clinical importance. Whereas miosis normally occurs with topical ocular 10% methacholine solutions, no effect is seen with 2.5% solutions, except in patients with Adie pupil or familial dysautonomia.

Generic Names:
1. Oxprenolol hydrochloride; 2. propranolol hydrochloride.

Proprietary Names:
1. Captol, Corbeton, Coretal, Laracor, Kerpin, Slow-Pren, Slow-Trasicor, Tevacor, Trasacor, Trasicor, Trasidex, Trasitensin; 2. Hemangeol, Inderal, Inderal LA, Inderal XL, InnoPran XL.

Primary Use
Systemic
These beta-adrenergic blocking drugs are effective in the management of angina pectoris, certain arrhythmias, hypertrophic subaortic stenosis, pheochromocytoma, and certain hypertensive states.

Ophthalmic
Used in the management of thyrotoxic lid retraction and in glaucoma therapy.

Ocular Side Effects
Systemic administration – intravenous or oral
Certain
1. Decreased vision
2. Diplopia – transient
3. Visual hallucinations
4. Eyelids or conjunctivitis
   a. Allergic reactions
   b. Erythema
   c. Conjunctivitis – nonspecific
   d. Urticaria
   e. Purpura
   f. Pemphigoid lesion
   g. May aggravate or cause ocular sicca
5. Irritation
   a. Lacrimation
   b. Photophobia
   c. Pain

Probable
1. Decreased intraocular pressure
2. Myasthenia gravis
   a. Diplopia
   b. Ptosis
   c. Paresis of extraocular muscles

Possible
1. Decreased accommodation
2. Exophthalmos – withdrawal states
3. Eyelids or conjunctiva
   a. Lupoid syndrome
   b. Erythema multiforme
   c. Exfoliative dermatitis
4. Inflammatory pseudotumor – intraocular

Conditional/unclassified
1. Pseudotumor cerebri

Local ophthalmic use or exposure – topical ocular application
Certain
1. Local anesthetic effect (propranolol)
2. Irritation
   a. Hyperemia
   b. Pain
   c. Burning sensation
3. Decreased intraocular pressure
4. Miosis

Clinical Significance
Adverse ocular side effects due to these drugs are usually insignificant and transient. Dennis et al reviewed

a series of patients with side effects from oral beta blockers.[1] The visual side effect (changes in vision) was the fifth most common of all systemic complaints. As with all beta-adrenergic blocking drugs, one needs to be aware of the possibility of sicca-like syndrome. There are many cases in the literature and spontaneous reports to implicate these drugs in causing an ocular sicca-like syndrome, probably on the basis of decreased lacrimation. This often appears as a sudden onset of ocular sicca with conjunctival hyperemia shortly after starting the drug. From cases in the spontaneous reports, one of the most bothersome side effects is transient diplopia with an unknown cause. This may resolve even if these drugs are continued. Yeomans et al described a case where propranolol may have caused an inflammatory lymphoid process of the iris and ciliary body, which resolved without treatment when propranolol was discontinued.[2] Although propranolol is structurally similar to practolol, to date there has been no oculocutaneous syndrome associated with this drug. Glasman et al showed that systemic propranolol caused a clinically significant reduction in an infant's refractive error and anisometropia.[3]

Topical ocular use of these drugs has little clinical application, although it has been advocated for thyrotoxic lid retraction and glaucoma therapy. Propranolol given topically on the eye has a local anesthetic effect.

Generic Name:
Quinidine gluconate or sulfate.

Proprietary Names:
Quinaglute, Quinora.

Primary Use
This isomer of quinine is effective in the treatment and prevention of atrial, nodal, and ventricular arrhythmias.

Ocular Side Effects
Systemic administration – intramuscular, intravenous, or oral
Certain
1. Decreased vision

Possible
1. Color vision defect – red-green defect
2. Eyelids or conjunctiva
   a. Allergic reactions
   b. Hyperpigmentation
   c. Photosensitivity
   d. Edema
   e. Urticaria

   f. Lupoid syndrome
3. Anterior granulomatous uveitis
4. Visual hallucinations
5. May aggravate or cause ocular sicca
6. Myasthenia gravis
   a. Diplopia
   b. Ptosis
   c. Paresis of extraocular muscles
7. Corneal deposits

Conditional/unclassified
1. Night blindness
2. Optic neuritis

Clinical Significance
Ocular side effects possibly associated with quinidine are rare, and many are not well proven. Although decreased vision has been reported in the literature and spontaneous reports, this is seldom a significant problem and is reversible. There are reports of optic neuritis, constricted visual fields, mydriasis, scotomas, night blindness, ocular sicca, photophobia, and toxic amblyopia, but a cause-and-effect relationship has not been proven. Zaidman reported fine gray epithelial opacities in a whorl-type pattern resembling those of chloroquine in a patient on quinidine for 2 years.[1] These disappeared 2 months after stopping the drug. There is only 1 such case in the spontaneous reports. We are aware of 9 cases of uveitis associated with this drug. This is probably an allergic or type I or II hypersensitivity reaction characterized by keratic precipitates, flare, and cells in the anterior chamber. Koeppe nodules and elevation of intraocular pressure have been reported.[2-5] Five of the 9 cases were bilateral. Although there are no rechallenge data, patients improved rapidly with treatment when the drug was discontinued. Edeki et al showed that this drug blocks the action of the cytochrome P450 enzyme CYPZD6, which metabolizes timolol.[6] Higher plasma levels of this beta blocker have therefore occurred. Higginbotham reviewed this in an ophthalmic editorial.[7]

CLASS: ANTIHYPERTENSIVE DRUGS

Generic Names:
1. Acebutolol; 2. atenolol; 3. carvedilol; 4. labetalol hydrochloride; 5. metoprolol tartrate; 6. nadolol; 7. pindolol.

Proprietary Names:
1. Sectral; 2. Tenormin; 3. Coreg, Coreg CR; 4. Normodyne, Trandate; 5. Kapspargo, Lopressor, Toprol, Toprol XL; 6. Corgard; 7. Visken.

Primary Uses
Systemic
These adrenergic blockers are used in the management of mild to severe hypertension, myocardial infarction, and chronic stable angina pectoris.

Ophthalmic
These adrenergic blockers are used in the treatment of elevated intraocular pressure.

Ocular Side Effects
Systemic administration – intravenous or oral
Certain
1. Decreased vision
2. Visual hallucinations
3. Irritation (labetalol, metoprolol)
   a. Photophobia
   b. Pain

Probable
1. Eyelids or conjunctiva
   a. Hyperemia (metoprolol)
   b. Erythema
   c. Blepharoconjunctivitis (metoprolol)
   d. Urticaria (labetalol, metoprolol)
   e. Purpura (metoprolol)
   f. Eczema (metoprolol)
2. May aggravate or cause ocular sicca

Possible
1. Decreased intraocular pressure – minimal
2. Myasthenia gravis
   a. Diplopia
   b. Ptosis
   c. Paresis of extraocular muscles
3. Enhances migraine scotoma
4. Eyelids or conjunctiva – lupoid syndrome (acebutolol, labetalol)
5. Floppy lid syndrome (carvedilol, labetalol)

Local ophthalmic use or exposure – topical ocular application
Certain
1. Decreased intraocular pressure
2. Irritation
   a. Lacrimation
   b. Burning sensation
3. Keratitis
4. Local anesthetic effect
5. May aggravate or cause ocular sicca
6. Blepharoconjunctivitis (nadolol)

Systemic Side Effects
Local ophthalmic use or exposure – topical ocular application
Possible
1. Bradycardia
2. Hypotension

Clinical Significance
Not all of the listed ocular side effects have been associated with each of the beta blockers. All appear to cause transitory minor visual disturbances, probably decrease tear production, cause ocular sicca, and possibly enhance migraine ocular scotoma. Carvedilol use may require lubricants in contact lens users.[1] If a muscle imbalance or diplopia occurs, then an evaluation for myasthenia gravis may be necessary. These drugs can cause vivid visual hallucinations that are dosage dependent and may disappear at lower dosages. When these drugs are given systemically, rarely do they cause a lowering of intraocular pressure; if they do, it is usually only minimal.

Topically applied medication may cause sicca symptoms, decreased tear film break-up times, corneal anesthesia, and ocular irritation. Systemic side effects from these topical ophthalmic beta blockers appear to be minimal; measurements of plasma concentrations of these ocularly applied drugs were below those levels known to induce systemic beta-blockade. Regardless, one must be aware that some of these drugs have been associated with systemic beta blocker side effects after topical ocular application.

Generic Names:
1. Alfuzosin hydrochloride; 2. doxazosin mesylate; 3. silodosin; 4. tamsulosin hydrochloride; 5. terazosin hydrochloride.

Proprietary Names:
1. Uroxatral; 2. Cardura, Cardura XL; 3. Rapaflo; 4. Flomax; 5. Hytrin.

Primary Use
These alpha-adrenergic antagonists are used to treat benign prostatic hyperplasia, and most also treat hypertension.

Ocular Side Effects
Systemic administration – oral
Certain
1. Intraoperative floppy iris syndrome (IFIS)
   a. Flaccid iris stroma
   b. Progressive miosis during intraocular surgery

c. May impede pharmacologic induced mydriasis
2. Anterior chamber
   a. Depth decreased
   b. Volume decreased
   c. Width decreased
3. Decreased thickness of iris dilator muscle (Fig. 10.4)
4. Decreased pupil size

Probable
1. Decreased vision
2. Choroidal detachment

Possible
1. Decreased iris pigment (chronic use)
2. Rebound uveitis
3. Macular edema
4. Increased intraocular pressure – 1-day postop
5. Conjunctivitis

Conditional/unclassified
1. Entropion

Clinical Significance
IFIS was first associated with tamsulosin as reported by Chang et al.[1] The US Food and Drug Administration (FDA) has declared IFIS and alpha-adrenergic antagonists a class drug effect. Data suggest that 86% of patients have some degree of IFIS at surgery on tamsulosin, whereas only 15% on taking alfuzosin; therefore there may be a marked difference of causation of IFIS due to various alpha-adrenergic antagonists.[2] Spontaneous reports and cases in the literature tend to show that tamsulosin has the most frequent ocular side effects; however, almost all of the listed side effects here have been reported with all of these alpha-adrenergic antagonists.

The onset of IFIS after starting any of these drugs may be only a matter of days and may even have a lifelong effect on the iris. Shah et al reported a case of IFIS 2 days after starting tamsulosin.[3] Bell et al studied 96,000 older men who had cataract surgery over a 5-year period, and those taking tamsulosin had a 2.3 times higher serious complication rate at cataract surgery than the control group.[4] Although IFIS usually occurs during cataract extraction, it has also been reported after trabeculectomy.[5,6] Panagis et al suggested that IFIS

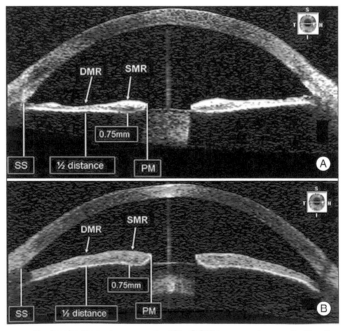

FIG. 10.4 Slit lamp–optical coherence tomography (SL-OCT) images demonstrating the standardized positions where iris thickness was measured. Iris thinning at the dilator muscle region (DMR) in a patient on tamsulosin **(A)** when compared with an age-matched control. **(B)** *PM,* Pupillary margin; *SMR,* sphincter muscle region; *SS,* sclera spur.[18]

may develop because of iris vascular dysfunction, and the iris vasculature may have structural in addition to nutritive functions.[6] Santaella et al found cadaver eyes of patients on tamsulosin exhibited decreased iris dilator thickness compared with controls.[7]

Martin-Moro et al reported in a small observational series that patients on long-term tamsulosin may demonstrate iris hypochromia.[8] Santaella et al noted increased incidence of IFIS in lightly pigmented iris but pointed out a long-term study is necessary to prove this.[7]

Yuksel et al documented the effects of tamsulosin or doxazosin on the anterior segment.[9] They felt that the surgeon should be aware of the decrease in anterior chamber depth, volume, and width. Gonzalez-Martin-Moro et al, in a large retrospective cohort study, showed a statistically significant increase in rebound uveitis and macular edema compared with the control group of normal preoperative cataract patients.[10] This, however, may not be due to the drug and may instead be due to the increased trauma at the time of surgery.

There are 10 cases of unilateral spontaneous choroidal detachments associated with tamsulosin use. Two cases were without surgery.[11,12] Shapiro et al had a postsurgery patient develop a choroidal detachment on tamsulosin.[13] When tamsulosin was stopped, the choroidal detachment resolved, but it recurred when terazosin was started. Terazosin was then stopped, and there was complete resolution. Saw palmetto (an herbal product), which is known to act as an alpha-adrenoreceptor antagonist, was then started, and the choroidal attachment recurred. In all but 1 of these 10 cases, the choroidal detachment resolved when the drug was stopped. It is possible that there was shorter follow-up in the 1 case and therefore we do not know the full outcome.

In a retrospective review, Bonnell et al reported that patients on tamsulosin after cataract surgery were 2.8 times more likely to experience a 10 mmHg intraocular pressure increase than the controls and were 3.8 times more like to experience a spike of over 30 mmHg.[14] This is possibly due to the increased trauma dealing with IFIS at surgery.

Waqar et al reported a case of tamsulosin's effect on Müller's muscle, which contributed to an entropion occurring.[15]

Kelly et al reported an unusual case with positive rechallenge of chronic bilateral conjunctivitis when taking this drug.[16] When the drug was stopped, there was complete resolution. When rechallenged, pruritus, pain, and scleral injection developed after approximately 20 minutes.

Recommendations[1,17]

1. Stopping tamsulosin before cataract surgery probably does not lessen the rate or severity of IFIS, although not all agree.
2. If atropine is used for surgery, be aware that stopping the alpha blocker may cause acute urinary retention.
3. Patients with early cataracts and benign prostatic hyperplasia (BPH) who have not started BPH treatment, should start finasteride (Proscar), dutasteride (Avodart), or a non-subtype-selective antagonist, i.e. alfuzosin (Uroxatral), doxazosin (Cardura), or terazosin (Hytrin), in place of tamsulosin, which has a much higher incidence of IFIS than these 3 do.
4. In some, if not most, this class of drugs has a lifelong potential to cause IFIS.

Generic Names:

1. Captopril; 2. enalapril.

Proprietary Names:

1. Capoten; 2. Epaned, Vasotec.

Primary Use

These angiotensin-converting enzyme (ACE) inhibitors are used in the management of hypertension.

Ocular Side Effects

Systemic administration – intravenous or oral

Certain

1. Decreased vision
2. Eyelids
   a. Edema
   b. Brown discoloration
   c. Blepharoconjunctivitis
   d. Urticaria
   e. Pemphigoid lesion
3. Conjunctivitis
4. Photosensitivity
5. Visual hallucinations

Possible

1. Eyelids or conjunctiva – lupoid syndrome
2. May aggravate or cause ocular sicca

Clinical Significance

The ACE inhibitors have a much higher incidence than most drugs of causing edema that includes the eye and orbit.[1–3] This is often associated with a facial urticaria. Edema may occur within 2 months of starting the drug or 1–5 years after drug exposure. This resolves once the drug is discontinued. Conjunctivitis is the most common ocular adverse event. Ocular photosensitivity reactions are rare. Wizemann reported a case of necrotizing blepharitis as the first clinical signal of captopril-induced agranulocytosis.[4] Balduf et al reported an unusual case of acute epiphora and rhinorrhea, usually unilateral but could alternate from side to side, which ceased when captopril was discontinued.[5]

Generic Name:
Clonidine hydrochloride.

Proprietary Names:
Catapres, Catapres-TTS, Duraclon, Kapvay.

Primary Use
Systemic
This alpha-adrenergic agonist is used in the management of hypertension.

Ophthalmic
Topical ocular clonidine has been used investigationally to reduce intraocular pressure.

Ocular Side Effects
Systemic administration – epidural, oral, or percutaneous
Certain
1. Decreased vision
2. Eyelids or conjunctiva
   a. Edema
   b. Urticaria
3. Irritation – burning sensation
4. Visual hallucinations
5. Abnormal electrooculogram (EOG)

Probable
1. May aggravate or cause ocular sicca
2. Decreased intraocular pressure

Conditional/unclassified
1. Pemphigoid

Local ophthalmic use or exposure – topical ocular application
Certain
1. Decreased vision
2. Decreased intraocular pressure
3. Eyelids or conjunctiva
   a. Irritation – burning sensation
   b. Edema
   c. Urticaria

4. Miosis
5. Follicular conjunctivitis
6. Corneal epithelial apoptosis

Possible
1. May aggravate or cause ocular sicca

Systemic Side Effects
Local ophthalmic use or exposure – topical ocular application
Probable
1. Hypotension

Clinical Significance
Ocular side effects associated with systemic clonidine have been inconsequential and cease after discontinuation of the drug. Clonidine-induced visual hallucinations may resolve with continued drug usage. Because systemic clonidine has been reported to cause vulval pemphigoid, one should be alert for ocular signs of pemphigoid. Ocular sicca has been reported, as well as xerostomia.[1] Topical ocular clonidine has been found to reduce intraocular pressure up to 30%, while reducing systemic blood pressure up to 10%. The eye drops are moderately well tolerated and produce miosis in the treated and contralateral eye. Fan et al reported corneal epithelial apoptosis secondary to low-dose topical ocular clonidine.[2]

Generic Name:
Diazoxide.

Proprietary Names:
Hyperstat, Proglycem.

Primary Use
This nondiuretic benzothiadiazine derivative is used in the emergency treatment of malignant hypertension.

Ocular Side Effects
Systemic administration – oral
Certain
1. Lacrimation

Possible
1. Eyelids or conjunctiva
   a. Allergic reactions
   b. Erythema
2. Decreased vision
3. Oculogyric crisis

Conditional/unclassified
1. Optic nerve infarction
2. Transient lens changes

Clinical Significance
Ocular side effects due to diazoxide are uncommon except for increased lacrimation, which occurs in up to 20% of patients taking this drug. In some instances, the lacrimation continued long after discontinued use of diazoxide. The cause of this unusual phenomenon is unknown. Cove et al reported (along with a case in the spontaneous reports) blindness secondary to hypotension from a rapid decrease of blood pressure in malignant hypertension, with presumed ischemia of the optic nerve.[1] An increase in eyelashes can occur with generalized hypertrichosis due to diazoxide.[2] The *Physicians' Desk Reference* (PDR) reported a transient cataract in an infant.[3] Lens changes have been described in beagle dogs.[4]

Generic Name:
Guanethidine monosulfate.

Proprietary Name:
Ismelin.

Primary Use
This adrenergic blocker is effective in the treatment of moderate to severe hypertension.

Ocular Side Effects
Systemic administration – intravenous or oral
Certain
1. Decreased vision
2. Irritation
   a. Hyperemia
   b. Edema
3. Horner's-like syndrome
   a. Miosis
   b. Ptosis

Possible
1. Decreased intraocular pressure
2. Photophobia

Clinical Significance
Ocular side effects from oral guanethidine are rare and seldom of clinical significance, although Brest et al reported an incidence of "blurring of vision" in 17% of patients taking 70 mg of this drug per day.[1] Some patients have a slight transitory ptosis, miosis, and conjunctival hyperemia. The drug is probably secreted in the tears.

Generic Name:
Hydralazine hydrochloride.

Proprietary Name:
Apresoline.

Primary Use
Systemic
This phthalazine derivative is effective in the management of essential or malignant hypertension, hypertensive complications of pregnancy, and hypertension associated with acute glomerulonephritis.

Ophthalmic
This is a new class of ocular hypotensive drugs.

Ocular Side Effects
Systemic administration – intramuscular, intravenous, or oral
Certain
1. Decreased vision
2. Irritation
   a. Lacrimation
   b. Photophobia
   c. Ocular pain
3. Eyelids or conjunctiva
   a. Allergic reactions
   b. Erythema
   c. Conjunctivitis – nonspecific
   d. Edema
   e. Urticaria

Probable
1. Periorbital edema

Possible
1. Colored flashing lights
2. Eyelids or conjunctiva – lupoid syndrome
3. Ischemic optic neuropathy

Local ophthalmic use or exposure – topical ocular application
Certain
1. Conjunctival hyperemia

Possible
1. Increased intraocular pressure – minimal

Clinical Significance
Ocular side effects due to hydralazine are reversible, transient, and seldom of clinical significance. A syndrome resembling systemic lupus erythematosus

associated with hydralazine therapy is generally considered a benign condition that resolves without permanent sequelae. Several patients with hydralazine-induced lupus syndrome with ocular manifestations, including retinal vasculitis, episcleritis, and exophthalmos, have been described. This drug, when used in the presence of increased intracranial pressure, may result in increased cerebral ischemia by lowering blood pressure.[1] This may result in visual defects.

Choi et al described a case in a 31-year-old patient with malignant hypertension after treatment with intravenous hydralazine and sublingual nifedipine followed by oral fosinopril and candesartan who developed relative hypotension, bilateral ischemic optic neuropathy, and optic atrophy with hand motion vision.[2] They also referenced other cases of this type.

Larsson et al studied topical ocular 0.1% hydralazine and found no clinically significant cardiovascular effects or significant ocular toxicity.[3] Mild to moderate conjunctival hyperemia and a small increase in intraocular pressure occurred in their series.

Generic Name:
Prazosin hydrochloride.

Proprietary Names:
Minipress, Minipress XL.

Primary Use
This quinazoline derivative is used in the treatment of hypertension.

Ocular Side Effects
Systemic administration – oral
Certain
1. Decreased vision
2. Eyelids or conjunctiva
   a. Erythema
   b. Conjunctivitis – nonspecific
   c. Edema
   d. Urticaria
3. Intraoperative floppy iris syndrome (IFIS)

Possible
1. May aggravate or cause ocular sicca
2. Visual hallucinations

Conditional/unclassified
1. Central serous retinopathy

2. Sclera – red discoloration

Clinical Significance
Of greatest concern with this drug is the causation of IFIS, an entity of progressive miosis during cataract surgery despite preoperative dilating medications.[1,2] There appears to be no benefit in stopping the drug before cataract surgery. Decreased vision occurs in some patients, primarily after the first dosage. Schachat reported 2 cases of retrobulbar optic neuritis possibly related to prazosin therapy. Spontaneous reports suggest that this drug can possibly cause ocular sicca. This seems reasonable because drying of the nose and mouth may occur (1–4%).[1] The very unusual finding of reddening of the sclera was reported by Carruthers.[3]

Generic Name:
Reserpine.

Proprietary Names:
Raudixin, Serpalan, Serpasil.

Primary Use
This indole alkaloid is used in the management of hypertension and agitated psychotic states.

Ocular Side Effects
Systemic administration – oral
Certain
1. Conjunctival hyperemia
2. Irritation - lacrimation

Probable
1. Color vision defect – objects have yellow tinge

Possible
1. Horner's syndrome
   a. Miosis
   b. Ptosis
   c. Increased sensitivity to topical ocular epinephrine preparations
2. Extraocular muscles
   a. Oculogyric crises
   b. Decreased spontaneous movements
   c. Abnormal conjugate deviations
   d. Jerky pursuit movements
3. Decreased vision
4. Decreased intraocular pressure
5. Mydriasis – may precipitate acute glaucoma

Clinical Significance

Due to significant systemic side effects, the use of reserpine has been markedly reduced in the United States and banned in the United Kingdom. Ocular conjunctival hyperemia is not uncommon with reserpine, but is of little clinical importance. This may or may not be associated with increased lacrimation. Occasionally, there may be a slight decrease in intraocular pressure. On rare occasions, mydriasis may cause acute glaucoma. Ocular side effects are otherwise rare, and nearly all are reversible. Shimohira et al have shown rapid eye movements during sleep in infants on reserpine who have neonatal jitteriness.[1]

CLASS: BRONCHODILATORS

Generic Name:
Albuterol (salbutamol).

Proprietary Names:
Accuneb, Proair HFA, ProAir RespiClick, Proventil, Proventil HFA, Proventil Repetabs, Respirol, Ventolin, Ventolin HFA, Volmax, VoSpire ER.

Primary Use
This sympathomimetic amine is primarily used as a bronchodilator in the symptomatic relief of bronchospasm. Also used in premature labor and to treat hyperkalemia.

Ocular Side Effects
Systemic administration – inhalant or intravenous
Certain
1. Decreased vision
2. Eyelids or conjunctiva
   a. Erythema
   b. Blepharoconjunctivitis
   c. Urticaria
3. Mydriasis – may precipitate acute glaucoma
4. Pain

Probable
1. Visual hallucinations
2. Eyelid edema
3. May aggravate or cause ocular sicca

Clinical Significance
Oral albuterol has no reported significant adverse ocular effects. This beta-agonist only has significant ocular side effects if delivered via a nebulizer with the drug coming into direct contact with the eye. Methods to prevent ocular contact should completely prevent all ocular effects. Albuterol can cause mydriasis and may increase intraocular pressure in predisposed narrow angles.[1] This drug is often given also in nebulized form with ipratropium and can induce angle-closure glaucoma by its parasympathetic inhibitory effect.[2,3] In a study by Kalra et al, both salbutamol and ipratropium were administered simultaneously via nebulizers without eye protection to patients with narrow angles, and transient angle closure occurred in 50%.[4] This effect was completely prevented when protective eye goggles were worn. Contact of this drug with the eye and eyelids may occasionally cause transitory irritation and/or ocular pain. Visual hallucinations have been reported only in children.[5] Albuterol can cause xerostomia in up to 3% of patients; therefore it can probably also aggravate or cause ocular sicca.[6] Sami et al pointed out that this drug can cause chronic eyelid edema.[7]

Generic Name:
Ipratropium.

Proprietary Names:
Atrovent, Atrovent HFA.

Primary Use
An inhaled anticholinergic drug used for its bronchodilation and antisecretory properties in chronic obstructive pulmonary disease and asthmatics.

Ocular Side Effects
Systemic administration – inhalation, nasal, or oral
Certain (more often from inadvertent exposure)
1. Decreased vision
2. Pupillary dilation (Fig. 10.5)
   a. Precipitates acute glaucoma
   b. Anisocoria
3. Decreased accommodation
4. Eyelids and conjunctiva
   a. May aggravate or cause ocular sicca
   b. Urticaria
   c. Edema
5. Irritation

Clinical Significance
This drug may be delivered to the eye via finger from the liquid, aerosol, or spray formulation, which may confuse reactions from systemic exposure. Decreased vision, decreased accommodation, and mydriasis are the most

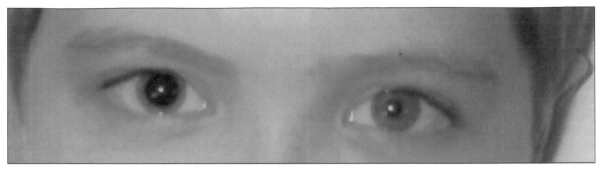

FIG. 10.5 Anisocoria after exposure to aerosol ipratropium.[3]

common ocular side effects seen. Anisocoria is clinically the most disturbing side effect because it may mimic an early sign of an impending neurologic emergency. A unilateral exposure to ipratropium is more often seen in the pediatric age group due to an ill-fitting face mask, in an intensive care setting, with a self-administered nebulizer, or misdirecting the inhaler.[1-4] There are reports of ipratropium-induced angle-closure glaucoma, some with salbutamol, but these are rare.[5-9] This drug dries all mucous membranes, including the eye. Direct conjunctival drug contact may result in irritation and hypersensitivity reactions. Other than acute glaucoma, all ocular side effects are transitory and reversible.

Inadvertent exposure, probably more often than systemic absorption, causes ocular side effects. These include mydriasis, pain, cycloplegia, decreased vision, conjunctivitis, acute glaucoma, and ocular sicca. These are transitory, except rare acute glaucoma. Contact lens wearers may require lubricating drops.[10]

CLASS: DIURETICS

Generic Names:
1. Chlorothiazide; 2. hydrochlorothiazide; 3. indapamide; 4. methyclothiazide; 5. metolazone.

Proprietary Names:
1. Diuril, Sodium Diuril; 2. Esidrix, Ezide, HydroDiuril, Microzide, Oretic, Zide; 3. Lozol; 4. Aquatensen, Enduron; 5. Zaroxolyn.

Primary Use
These thiazides or thiazide-like diuretics are effective in the maintenance therapy of edema associated with chronic congestive heart failure, essential hypertension, renal dysfunction, cirrhosis, pregnancy, premenstrual tension, and hormonal imbalance.

Ocular Side Effects
Systemic administration – intravenous or oral
Certain
1. Decreased vision
2. Myopia (Fig. 10.6)
3. Color vision defect (chlorothiazide)
   a. Xanthopsia
   b. Large yellow spots on white background
4. Eyelids or conjunctiva
   a. Allergic reactions
   b. Conjunctivitis – nonspecific
   c. Photosensitivity
   d. Urticaria
   e. Purpura
5. Visual hallucinations
6. Choroidal effusion
7. Increased anterior-posterior lens diameter
8. Shallow anterior chambers
9. Acute glaucoma

Possible
1. Retinal edema
2. May aggravate or cause ocular sicca
3. Decreased intraocular pressure – minimal
4. Decreased accommodation
5. Eyelids or conjunctiva – lupoid syndrome
6. Retinal phototoxic reaction

Clinical Significance
Ocular side effects due to these diuretics are rare, but occasionally are vision threatening. The most severe is the classic picture of sulfonamide-derived drugs, as outlined with topiramate, where acute glaucoma and myopia occur.[1-3] This is shown by the well-documented cases of unilateral or bilateral ciliary body edema or effusions, which produce anterior rotation of the ciliary body at the scleral spur, allowing laxity of the lens zonule and forward displacement of the iris lens diaphragm.

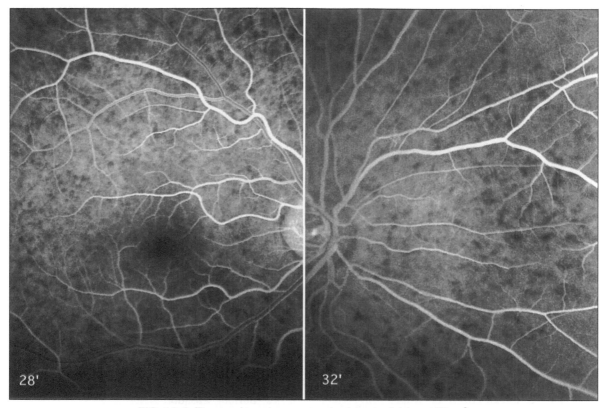

28'   32'

FIG. 10.6 Fluorescein angiogram showing islands of delayed filling.[6]

This increases the anteroposterior diameter of the lens, allowing for a shallowing of the anterior chamber with a resultant narrow angle. The cause of the ciliary body edema is unknown; however, Geanon et al described a case they felt was due to a hypersensitivity reaction.[4] Krieg et al showed that prostaglandins and eicosanoids are involved.[5]

Myopia can be explained by a similar mechanism. Blain et al, using angiography, showed diffuse choroidal thickness during indapamide-induced myopia.[6] Vegh et al reported indapamide-induced transient myopia with supraciliary effusion and suggested that ciliary muscle contraction and ciliary body edema may play a role in the pathomechanism.[7]

Sponsel et al reported a posterior subcapsular cataract after indapamide therapy; however, there are no other data to support this.[8] Miller et al described a case of transient oculomotor nerve palsy associated with thiazide-induced glucose intolerance.[9] Thiazide diuretics can also cause hypercalcemia, which may result in band keratopathy.

When thiazide diuretics are used in combination with carbonic anhydrase inhibitors, one should be alert for signs of hypokalemia. These diuretics are photosensitizers, and Hartzer et al showed that in tissue culture, hydrochlorothiazide will interact with ultraviolet-A (UV-A) radiation to produce toxic synergistic effects on human retinal pigment epithelium (RPE) cells.[10] In a case control study, de la Mamierre et al concluded that drug-induced phototoxicity (thiazide diuretics in long-term treatment) may be involved in causing more severe neovascularization in age-related macular degeneration.[11] Costagliola et al reported a case of suspected retinal phototoxicity caused by a UV tanning booth in a patient on hydrochlorothiazide.[12] Iacono et al reported macular edema secondary to hydrochlorothiazide treatment.[13]

Generic Name:

Furosemide.

Proprietary Names:

Delone, Lasix.

Primary Use

This potent sulfonamide diuretic is effective primarily in the treatment of hypertension complicated by congestive heart failure or renal impairment.

Ocular Side Effects

Systemic administration – intramuscular, intravenous, or oral

Certain

1. Decreased vision
2. Color vision defect – objects have yellow tinge
3. Eyelids or conjunctiva
   a. Allergic reactions
   b. Photosensitivity
   c. Urticaria
   d. Purpura
   e. Pemphigoid lesion
4. Visual hallucinations

Probable

1. Decreased intraocular pressure – minimal
2. Decreased contact lens tolerance

Possible

1. Eyelids or conjunctiva – lupoid syndrome
2. Acute glaucoma
3. Ocular teratologic effects

Clinical Significance

Furosemide has potent systemic side effects and is not commonly used. Ocular side effects are rare and seldom of significance. A single case of the well-known sulfa idiosyncratic reaction causing ciliary body effusions with resultant bilateral acute glaucoma has been reported.[1,2] There is a case in the spontaneous reports of a baby born blind after the mother took 40 mg of furosemide 3 times daily during her second trimester. Lee et al found little clinical or pharmacologic evidence of sulfa allergy causing life-threatening cross-reaction with furosemide.[3]

CLASS: OSMOTICS

Generic Name:

Glycerol (glycerin).

Proprietary Names:

Colace infant/child, Computer Eye Drops, Eye Lube-A, Fleet Bablax, Osmoglyn, Sani-Supp.

Primary Use

Systemic

This trihydric alcohol is a hyperosmotic drug used to decrease intraocular pressure in various acute glaucoma

and in preoperative intraocular procedures.

Ophthalmic

This topical trihydric alcohol is a hyperosmotic used to reduce corneal edema for diagnostic procedures, increased comfort, or improved vision.

Ocular Side Effects

Systemic administration – oral

Certain

1. Decreased intraocular pressure
2. Subconjunctival or retinal hemorrhages
3. Visual hallucinations
4. Decreased vision

Possible

1. Retinal tears
2. Expulsive hemorrhage

Local ophthalmic use or exposure – topical ocular application

Certain

1. Irritation
   a. Lacrimation
   b. Hyperemia
   c. Pain
   d. Burning sensation
2. Vasodilation
3. Subconjunctival hemorrhages

Possible

1. Corneal endothelial damage
2. Contact allergy

Clinical Significance

Systemic glycerin causes decreased intraocular pressure, which is an intended ocular response, and has surprisingly few other ocular effects. However, severe vitreal dehydration with resultant shrinkage of the vitreous body may possibly cause traction on the adjacent retina, resulting in a tear. This principle has been described with cerebral dehydration as causing intracranial hemorrhages. Severe dehydration from systemic or topical ocular administration can rupture fine vessels, causing local bleeds. In addition, visual hallucinations are thought to occur, probably due to cerebral dehydration. There have been reports of expulsive hemorrhages occurring during intraocular surgery due to strong osmotic drugs. The postulated mechanism is that a sudden drop in intraocular pressure may rupture sclerotic posterior ciliary arteries. Patients with renal, cardiovascular, or diabetic disease are more susceptible to serious systemic side effects, particularly if they are elderly and already somewhat dehydrated. Kalin et al reported percutaneous retrogasserian glycerol injection to control intractable pain, where inadvertent orbital injection caused proptosis and vision loss.[1] Mizuta et al reported a case of possible glycerol-induced asymmetry response to the inner ear, causing vertigo and a resultant vertical nystagmus.[2]

Generic Name:
Mannitol.

Proprietary Names:
Aridol, Osmitrol, Resectisol.

Primary Use
This hyperosmotic drug is used to decrease intraocular pressure in various acute glaucoma and in preoperative intraocular procedures. It is also used in the management of oliguria and anuria.

Ocular Side Effects
Systemic administration – intravenous
Certain
1. Decreased intraocular pressure
2. Increased aqueous flare
3. Decreased vision
4. Subconjunctival or retinal hemorrhages
5. Visual hallucinations
6. Eyelids or conjunctiva
   a. Edema
   b. Urticaria
7. Decreased global volume
8. Increased orbit volume
9. Protective endothelial cells during phacoemulsification
10. Increased choroidal thickness
11. Decreased axial length

Probable
1. Retinal tears
2. Expulsive hemorrhage

Clinical Significance
All visual side effects are probably secondary to dehydration. An increase in aqueous flare, but not cells, has been caused by mannitol, especially in the elderly. Severe vitreal dehydration with resultant shrinkage of the vitreous body may cause traction on the adjacent retina, resulting in a tear. This principle has also been described with cerebral dehydration causing intracranial hemorrhage. Expulsive hemorrhages have been reported to occur during surgery in which strong osmotic drugs were used. The postulated mechanism is the sudden decrease in intraocular pressure, which may

rupture sclerotic posterior ciliary arteries. Hasegawa et al described a case of temporary indented corneas at surgery after 900 mL of mannitol for cardiovascular surgery under general anesthesia.[1] Cardiovascular or renal disease may contraindicate use of isosorbide or mannitol. It has been suggested that these drugs open the blood–retinal barrier and may give drugs or chemicals greater access to the retina and central nervous system.

Weber et al determined that intravenous mannitol caused globe volume to decrease, while orbital volume increased.[2] These changes occurred during the time when intraocular pressure was normalized after the pressure-lowering effect of the drug. Hwang et al found that preoperative mannitolization decreased the postoperative endothelial corneal cell loss during phacoemulsification.[3] Caliskan et al found that mannitol infusion caused an increase in choroidal thickness and a decrease in axial length.[4]

CLASS: PERIPHERAL VASODILATORS

Generic Name:
Phenoxybenzamine hydrochloride.

Proprietary Name:
Dibenzyline.

Primary Use
This alpha-adrenergic blocking drug is used in the management of pheochromocytoma and sometimes in the treatment of vasospastic peripheral vascular disease other than the obstructive types.

Ocular Side Effects
Systemic administration – oral
Certain
1. Miosis
2. Ptosis
3. Conjunctival hyperemia
4. Decreased intraocular pressure – minimal

Possible
1. Posterior ischemic optic neuropathy

Clinical Significance
Although ocular side effects due to phenoxybenzamine are frequently seen, they are seldom clinically significant. Phenoxybenzamine is an alpha-adrenergic blocker, so it may cause miosis. Although this is rarely a problem, when it is associated with posterior subcapsular or central-lens changes, there may be a sudden decrease in vision. All adverse ocular reactions are reversible and transitory after discontinued drug use.

James et al described a unique case in which they felt phenoxybenzamine decreased autoregulation of vessels, which predisposed to venous engorgement causing edema of the optic nerve and surrounding tissue.[1] This, along with a prolonged prone position during surgery, may put patients on this drug at risk for developing posterior ischemic optic neuropathy.

CLASS: VASOPRESSORS

Generic Name:
Ephedrine sulfate.

Proprietary Names:
Akovaz, Corphedra.

Primary Use
Systemic
This sympathomimetic amine is effective as a vasopressor, a bronchodilator, and a nasal decongestant.

Ophthalmic
This topical sympathomimetic amine is used as a conjunctival vasoconstrictor.

Ocular Side Effects
Systemic administration – intramuscular, intravenous, or subcutaneous
Probable
1. Mydriasis – may precipitate acute glaucoma
2. Visual hallucinations
3. Decreased intraocular pressure

Possible
1. Acute macular neuroretinopathy
2. Transient myopia
3. Ciliochoroidal effusion

Local ophthalmic use or exposure – topical ocular application
Certain
1. Conjunctival vasoconstriction
2. Decreased vision
3. Eyelids or conjunctiva
   a. Allergic reactions
   b. Conjunctivitis – nonspecific
4. Irritation
   a. Lacrimation
   b. Rebound hyperemia
   c. Photophobia
5. Mydriasis – may precipitate acute glaucoma

6. Aqueous floaters – pigment debris
7. Decreased intraocular pressure – minimal

Clinical Significance
Ocular side effects from systemic administration of ephedrine are rare. O'Brien et al described an acute macular neuroretinopathy, possibly due to ephedrine.[1] Dark-red, outer retinal, wedge-shaped lesions surrounding all or part of the central macula, with normal vision but permanent paracentral scotomas, developed. This may be due to a direct retinal effect of the drug or an acute hypertensive effect. Lee et al described a case of −8.0 diopter with ciliochoroidal effusion in a 28-year-old patient on ephedrine and phendimetrazine for weight loss.[2] There was positive dechallenge without complication.

Topical ocular ephedrine is not currently used by most ophthalmologists. The currently used concentration is rarely sufficient to cause significant side effects other than the intended response of vasoconstriction. Repeated use of topical ocular ephedrine, however, may cause rebound conjunctival hyperemia or loss of the drug's vasoconstrictive effect. The *Physicians' Desk Reference* (PDR) states that "ephedrine is contraindicated in patients with closed-angle glaucoma."[3]

Generic Names:
1. Epinephrine; 2. norepinephrine bitartrate.

Proprietary Names:
1. Adrenaclick, Adrenalin, EpiPen, EpiPen Jr., Twinject, Twinject 0.3; 2. Levophed.

Primary Use
Systemic
This sympathomimetic amine is effective as a vasopressor, a bronchodilator, and a vasoconstrictor in prolonging the action of anesthetics.

Ophthalmic
Used in the management of open-angle glaucoma. Intracameral use for enhancing mydriasis primarily in intraoperative floppy iris syndrome.

Ocular Side Effects
Systemic administration – intracardiac, intramuscular, intravenous, nasal, or subcutaneous
Certain
1. Mydriasis – transitory – may precipitate angle-closure glaucoma
2. Color vision defect – transitory

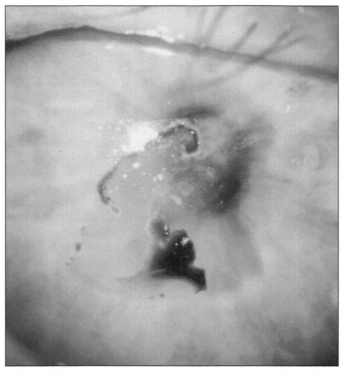

FIG. 10.7 Adrenochrome deposits in cornea from topical ocular epinephrine treatment.[10]

a. Red-green defect
b. Objects have green tinge
3. Upper eyelid elevation

Probable

1. Acute macular neuroretinopathy (epinephrine)
2. Increased aqueous production (epinephrine)
3. May precipitate an ocular vasoconstrictive vascular event (epinephrine)

Possible

1. Lacrimation (epinephrine)

Local ophthalmic use or exposure – topical ocular application or intracameral injection
Certain

1. Decreased intraocular pressure
2. Decreased vision
3. Mydriasis – may precipitate acute glaucoma
4. Eyelids or conjunctiva
   a. Allergic reactions
   b. Blepharoconjunctivitis – follicular
   c. Vasoconstriction (epinephrine)

d. Poliosis (epinephrine)
e. Cicatrizing conjunctivitis – pseudo-ocular pemphigoid (epinephrine)
f. Hyperplasia of sebaceous glands (epinephrine)
g. Loss of eyelashes or eyebrows (epinephrine)
h. Rebound hyperemia
5. Irritation
   a. Lacrimation
   b. Photophobia
   c. Pain
   d. Burning sensation
6. Adrenochrome deposits (epinephrine) (Fig. 10.7)
   a. Conjunctiva
   b. Cornea
   c. Nasolacrimal system (cast formation)
7. Cystoid macular edema (epinephrine)
8. Cornea (epinephrine)
   a. Superficial punctate keratitis
   b. Edema
9. Subconjunctival hemorrhages (epinephrine)
10. Paradoxical pressure elevation in open-angle glaucoma

11. Iris (epinephrine)
    a. Iritis
    b. Cysts
12. Black discoloration of soft contact lenses (epinephrine)
13. May aggravate herpes infections (epinephrine)
14. Narrowing or occlusion of lacrimal canaliculi (epinephrine)

Possible
1. Periorbital edema (epinephrine)

Systemic Side Effects
Local ophthalmic use or exposure – topical ocular application or intracameral injection (epinephrine)
Certain
1. Headache
2. Sweats
3. Syncope
4. Arrhythmia
5. Tachycardia
6. Palpitations
7. Hypertension
8. Ventricular extrasystole

Clinical Significance

Adverse events from systemic administration are heavily dose dependent or additive dependent on associated drug use. All events are rare because dosages used have been tested to be safe over time. O'Brien et al and Desai et al have reported cases of intravenous epinephrine causing acute macular neuroretinopathy.[1–3] Savino et al described 4 patients with severe visual loss after intranasal anesthetic with epinephrine injections.[4] The causes of the visual loss included retinal arterial occlusion and optic nerve ischemia, both of which the authors felt were due to secondary vasospasm induced by epinephrine. Narendran et al described a Purtscherlike retinopathy after a peribulbar anesthesia injection containing epinephrine and lidocaine.[5] There are cases of central retinal artery occlusion associated with epinephrine exposure.[6,7] Patients undergoing ocular surgery with halothane anesthesia may experience tachycardia and arrhythmia from supplemental injection of local anesthetics containing epinephrine, from topical ophthalmic administration, or from intracameral injection of epinephrine.

Norepinephrine causes few ocular side effects from systemic exposure, and those are transitory and reversible except in overdose situations. Jandrasits et al reported that high levels of circulating norepinephrine

have little impact on retinal vascular tone or retinal blood flow.[8]

In over 20% of patients, topical ocular epinephrine must be stopped after prolonged use because of ocular discomfort and rebound conjunctival hyperemia. Over 50% of patients develop reactive hyperemia with long-term use. Concomitant use of timolol and epinephrine therapy occasionally has an additive effect on reactive hyperemia, cardiac arrhythmia, or elevated blood pressure. Long-term topical ocular epinephrine preparations can cause cicatrizing conjunctivitis, which clinically or pathologically may be difficult to distinguish from ocular pemphigoid. This may include shortening of the fornices. Most epinephrine-induced macular edema is reversible, but lack of early detection may cause irreversible cystoid macular changes. Cystoid maculopathy may require more than 6 months to clear once the medication is discontinued. These changes occur more frequently in aphakic patients. This drug can cause conjunctival epidermalization, loss of eyelashes, blepharitis, and meibomianitis. Most ocular adverse reactions due to epinephrine resolve or significantly improve with discontinuation of the drug. However, adrenochrome deposits in the cornea or conjunctiva may be exceedingly slow to absorb. Adrenochrome deposits in the lacrimal ducts may cause obstruction with epiphora. There are data to suggest that long-term topical ocular or intracameral epinephrine may cause significant corneal edema. This primarily occurs in corneas with damaged epithelium, which allows for increased penetration of this drug to reach the endothelium.

Allergic epinephrine reactions occur, and Gutierrez Fernandez et al reported allergic contact conjunctivitis attributed to phenylephrine eye drops with cross-reaction between phenylephrine and epinephrine.[9] This was confirmed with prick tests.

Norepinephrine is seldom given topically because epinephrine is much more effective and potent. Ocular side effects from norepinephrine are transitory and minimal. Systemic side effects are less potent then epinephrine, but norepinephrine may have a greater effect on the elevation of blood pressure.

Generic Name:
Phenylephrine.

Proprietary Names:
4-Way Nasal, AH-chew D, AK-Dilate, Anu-Med, Children's nostril, Children's Sudafed PE, Hemorrhoidal, Little Remedies for Noses, Mydfrin, Neo-Synephrine, Neo-Synephrine Extra Strength, Neo-Synephrine Mild, Neofrin, Nostil, Ocu-Phrin, PediaCare Children's

Decongestant, Phenoptic, Prefin, Rectacaine, Relief, Rhinall, Sinex, Sudafed PE, Sudafed PE Children's Nasal Decongestant, Sudafed PE Congestion, Sudogest PE, Vazculep.

Primary Use
Systemic
This sympathomimetic amine is effective as a vasopressor and is used in the management of hypotension, shock, and tachycardia.

Ophthalmic
This topical sympathomimetic amine is used as a vasoconstrictor and a mydriatic.

Ocular Side Effects
Systemic administration – intramuscular, intravenous, nasal, oral, rectal, or subcutaneous
Certain
1. Acute glaucoma

Possible
1. Visual hallucinations
2. Facial and eyelid flushing

Local ophthalmic use or exposure – topical ocular application
Certain
1. Pupil
   a. Mydriasis – may decrease vision
   b. Rebound miosis
2. Intraocular pressure
   a. Precipitate acute glaucoma
   b. Transitory elevation of intraocular pressure – open angle
   c. Temporary decrease
3. Conjunctival vasoconstriction
4. Irritation
   a. Lacrimation
   b. Rebound hyperemia
   c. Photophobia
   d. Ocular pain
5. Cornea
   a. Punctate keratitis
   b. Edema
6. Eyelids or conjunctiva
   a. Allergic reactions
   b. Erythema
   c. Conjunctivitis – nonspecific
   d. Blepharospasm
   e. Eczema
   f. Palpebral fissure – increase in width
   g. Pseudo-ocular pemphigoid
   h. Periocular skin pallor (infants)
7. Aqueous floaters – pigment debris
8. Hydrogel keratoprosthesis
   a. Surface spoliation
   b. Internal deposition/coloration

Possible
1. Optic nerve – increases vaso-occlusive disease

Systemic Side Effects
Local ophthalmic use or exposure – topical ocular application
Certain
1. Hypertension
2. Myocardial infarct
3. Tachycardia
4. Subarachnoid hemorrhage
5. Cardiac arrest
6. Cardiac arrhythmia
7. Coronary artery spasm
8. Headache
9. Syncope

Probable
1. Pulmonary edema (premature infants)
2. Bronchoconstriction
3. Seizures
4. Feeding intolerance (neonates)

Conditional/unclassified
1. Renal failure (premature infants)

Clinical Significance
Phenylephrine is given systemically, primarily as sprays onto mucous membranes (nasal mucosa); therefore systemic side effects are essentially the same as for topical ocular exposure.

Ocular side effects due to topical ocular phenylephrine are usually of little significance unless it is used in neonates, 10% solutions, pledget applications, for prolonged periods, or with certain systemic medications. Phenylephrine used topically is one of the more toxic commercial drugs to the conjunctival and corneal epithelium. Soparkar et al have pointed out that even in low-concentration, over-the-counter ophthalmic decongestants, acute and chronic conjunctivitis can go unrecognized.[1] Unfortunately, signs and symptoms of these adverse effects of the drug may take 1–24 weeks to resolve. Although the drug is used for pupillary dilation, it may have a varied response on intraocular pressure. Initially, there may be a transitory decrease and later a transitory increase even with open angles. There may be no pressure change; or, in very rare instances, acute glaucoma may be precipitated. Pupillary dilatation lasting for prolonged periods has been reported, especially in patients on guanethidine. Mydriasis varies with iris pigmentation and depth of the anterior chamber. Blue irides and shallow anterior chambers produce the greatest mydriasis, and dark irides or deep chambers produce the least. A diminished mydriatic response has been seen after repeated use of phenylephrine. A 10% concentration of phenylephrine can cause significant keratitis and a reduction in the conjunctival PO_2, which may result in delayed wound healing by reducing aerobic metabolism of rapidly dividing cells. Blanching of the skin, particularly the lower eyelid, may occur secondary to topical ocular phenylephrine. After ophthalmic examination with a combination of phenylephrine and cyclopentolate in neonates, an increased risk of feeding intolerance may result, which could be due to the mydriatic drugs, the physical stress with applying eye medication, or a combination of these factors.[2] Pless et al described 4 patients with nonarteritic ischemic optic neuropathy who experienced acute worsening of visual function after instillation of phenylephrine for a dilated fundus examination.[3] Morrison et al pointed out the effects of topical ocular phenylephrine on hydrogel keratoprosthesis, promoting hydrogel cloudiness and surface deposits.[4] Chronic use of this drug may be one of the more common causes of contact dermatitis of the eyelids as per incidence of use. In fact, Villarreal reported that 93.5% of acute dermatitis from all eye drops was due to topical mydriatic drugs, primarily phenylephrine.[5]

Over 100 articles support the finding that topical ocular phenylephrine can cause, in rare instances, severe stress on the cardiovascular system and marked elevation of blood pressure. This was first reported by Fraunfelder et al, who reported 11 deaths.[6] Numerous additional terminal cases have been reported in the literature and spontaneous reports. Phenylephrine 10% should be used with caution or not at all in patients with cardiac disease, significant hypertension, aneurysms, and advanced arteriosclerosis. It also should be used with caution in the elderly and in patients on monoamine oxidase inhibitors, tricyclic antidepressants, or atropine. Similar findings were reported in 11 patients to whom 10% phenylephrine was applied to the eye in pledget form.[7] There have been a number of reports of topical ocular phenylephrine in concentrations of 10%, 5%, and 2.5% causing hypertension with pulmonary edema primarily in infants, but even in young children.[8-10]

Kim et al reported bronchoconstriction after topical ocular phenylephrine in premature infants.[11]

Numerous cases in the spontaneous reports and literature have associated unilateral and bilateral acute glaucoma with nasal sprays or solutions containing phenylephrine.[12,13] In a preterm infant, Berman et al postulated that 2.5% phenylephrine may have triggered a series of events to cause bilateral spontaneous pigment epithelial detachments.[14] Also, in infants, phenylephrine eye drops have been implicated in paralytic ileus and renal failure.[15,16]

REFERENCES

Drugs: Ergometrine maleate (ergonovine), ergotamine tartrate, methylergometrine (methyl-ergonovine maleate)

1. Crews SJ. Toxic effects on the eye and visual apparatus resulting from systemic absorption of recently introduced chemical agents. *Trans Ophthalmol Soc UK.* 1963;82:387–406.
2. Borooah S, Chadha V, Sutherland S. A case or permanent retinal disturbance postpartum following administration of ergometrine. *Can J Ophthalmol.* 2008;43(5):607–608.
3. Gupta DR, Strobos RJ. Bilateral papillitis associated with Cafergot therapy. *Neurology.* 1972;22:793–797.
4. Merhoff GC, Porter JM. Ergot intoxication. *Ann Surg.* 1974;180:773–779.
5. Heider W, Berninger T, Brunk G. Electroophthalmological and clinical findings in a case of chronic abuse of ergotamine. *Fortschr Ophthalmol.* 1986;83:539–541.
6. Sommer S, Delemazure B, Wagner M. Bilateral ischemic optic neuropathy secondary to acute ergotism. *J Fr Ophthalmol.* 1998;21(2):123–125.
7. Mieler WF. Systemic therapeutic agents and retinal toxicity. *Am Acad Ophthalmol.* 1997;15(12):5.
8. Ahmad S. Ergonovine: unmasking of myasthenia gravis. *Am Heart J.* 1991;121:1851.
9. Creze B. Transitory cortical blindness after delivery using Methergin. *Rev Fr Gynecol Obstet.* 1976;71:353.

Drugs: Amlodipine besylate, diltiazem hydrochloride, nifedipine, verapamil hydrochloride

1. Say AT, Shields CL, Bianciotto C, et al. Chronic conjunctival chemosis from amlodipine besylate (Norvasc). *Cornea.* 2011;30(5):604–607.
2. Kim KH, Kim WS. Chronic unilateral chemosis following the use of amlodipine besylate. *BMC Ophthalmol.* 2014;14:124.
3. Muskens RP, de Voogd S, Wolfs RC, et al. Systemic antihypertensive medication and incident open-angle glaucoma. *Ophthalmology.* 2007;114(12):2221–2226.
4. Swash M, Ingram DA. Adverse effect of verapamil in myasthenia gravis. *Muscle Nerve.* 1992;15:396–398.
5. Anastassiades CJ. Nifedipine and beta blocker drugs. *BMJ.* 1980;281:1251–1252.

6. Staffurth JS, Emery P. Adverse interaction between nifedipine and betablockade. *BMJ*. 1981;282:225.
7. Sinclair NI, Benzie JL. Timolol eye drops and verapamil – a dangerous combination. *Med J Aust*. 1983;1:549.
8. Pringle SD, MacEwen CJ. Severe bradycardia due to interaction of timolol eye drops and verapamil. *BMJ*. 1987;294:155–156.

Drug: Amyl/butyl nitrite

1. Gruener AM, Jeffries MAR, El Housseini Z, et al. Poppers maculopathy. *Lancet*. 2014;384:1606.
2. Isabelle Audo I, El Sanharawi M, Vignal-Clermont C, et al. Foveal damage in habitual poppers users. *Arch Ophthalmol*. 2011;129:703–708.
3. Pahlitzsch M, Mai C, Joussen AM, et al. Poppers maculopathy: complete restitution of macular changes in OCT after drug abstinence. *Semin Ophthalmol*. 2016;31:479–484.
4. Davies AJ, Kelly SP, Naylor SG, et al. Adverse ophthalmic reaction in poppers users: a case series of "poppers maculopathy." *Eye*. 2012;26:1479–1486.
5. Vignal-Clermont C, Audo I, Sahel JA, et al. Poppers-associated retinal toxicity. *N Engl J Med*. 2010;363:1583–1585.
6. Van Bol LB, Kurt RA, Keane PA, et al. Clinical phenotypes of poppers maculopathy and their links to visual and anatomic recovery. *Ophthalmology*. 2017;124(9):1425–1427.
7. Rewbury R, Hughes E, Purbrick R, et al. Poppers: legal highs with questionable contents? A case series of poppers maculopathy. *Br J Ophthalmol*. 2017;101:1530–1534.
8. Krilis M, Thompson J, Atik A, et al. 'Popper'-induced vision loss. *Drug Alcohol Rev*. 2013;32(3):333–334.
9. Romanelli F, Smith KM, Thornton AC, et al. Poppers: epidemiology and clinical management of inhaled nitrite abuse. *Pharmacotherapy*. 2004;24(1):69–78.
10. Fledelius HC. Irreversible blindness after amyl nitrite inhalation. *Acta Ophthalmol Scand*. 1999;77:719–721.
11. Mearza AA, Asaria RH, Little B. Corneal burn secondary to amyl nitrite. *Eye*. 2001;15:333–334.

Drugs: Flecainide acetate, procainamide hydrochloride

1. Gentzkow GD, Sullivan JY. Extracardiac adverse effects of flecainide. *Am J Cardiol*. 1984;53:101B–105B.
2. Ikäheimo K, Kettunen R, Mäntyjärvi M. Adverse ocular effects of flecainide. *Acta Ophthalmol Scand*. 2001;79:175–176.
3. Skander M, Issacs PE. Flecainide, ocular myopathy, and antinuclear factor. *BMJ*. 1985;291:450.
4. Moller HU, Thygesen K, Kruit PJ. Corneal deposits associated with flecainide. *BMJ*. 1991;302:506–507.
5. Turgeon PW, Slamovits TL. Scleritis as the presenting manifestation of procainamide-induced lupus. *Ophthalmology*. 1989;96:68–71.
6. Nichols CJ, Mieler WF. Severe retinal vaso-occlusive disease secondary to procainamide-induced lupus. *Ophthalmology*. 1989;96:1535–1540.

Drug: Nicorandil

1. Trechot P, Bazard MC, Petitpain N, et al. Conjunctival and corneal ulcerations: keep a sharp eye on nicorandil. *Br J Ophthalmol*. 2012;96(3):463–464.
2. Trechot F, Batta B, Petitpain N, et al. A case of nicorandil-induced unilateral corneal ulceration. *Int Wound J*. 2014;11(3):238–239.
3. Nikaido M, Miyamoto S, Iinuma S. Systemic ulcerative lesions in a patient with ischemic heart disease. *Gastroenterology*. 2014;147(6):e7–e8.
4. Campolmi N, Guy C, Cinotti E, et al. Cornea perforation: another side effect of nicorandil. *Cutan Ocul Toxicol*. 2014;33(2):96–98.
5. Fraunfelder FW, Fraunfelder FT. Conjunctival and corneal ulceration associated with nicorandil. *Cutan Ocul Toxicol*. 2014;33(2):120–121.
6. Klein R, Myers CE, Klein BEK. Vasodilators, blood pressure-lowering medications, and age-related macular degeneration: The Beaver Dam Eye Study. *Ophthalmology*. 2014;121(8):1604–1611.
7. Jeong SH, Kim H. Acute intractable headache and oculomotor nerve palsy associated with nicorandil: a case report. *Am J Emerg Med*. 2017;35(12):e3–e5.

Drug: Nitroglycerin

1. Klein R, Myers CE, Klein BEK. Vasodilators, blood pressure-lowering medications, and age-related macular degeneration: The Beaver Dam Eye Study. *Ophthalmology*. 2014;121(8):1604–1611.
2. Nitroglycerin. 2018. Retrieved from http://www.pdr.net.
3. Bánk J. Migraine with aura after administration of sublingual nitroglycerin tablets. *Headache*. 2001;41:84–87.
4. Afridi S, Kaube H, Goadsby PJ. Occipital activation in glyceryl trinitrate induced migraine with visual aura. *J Neurol Neurosurg Psychiatry*. 2005;76:1158–1160.
5. Casarett LJ, Doull J, Amdur M, et al. *Casarett and Doull's Toxicology: The Basic Science of Poisons*. 4th ed. New York: Pergamon Press; 1991.
6. Ohar JM, Fowler AA, Selhorst JB, et al. Intravenous nitroglycerin-induced intracranial hypertension. *Crit Care Med*. 1985;13:867–868.
7. McKenna KE. Allergic contact dermatitis from glyceryl trinitrate ointment. *Contact Derm*. 2000;42:246.

Drug: Amiodarone hydrochloride

1. Mehta S, Bunya VY, Orlin SE, et al. A significant drug–drug interaction detected through corneal examination: resolution of cornea verticillata while using amiodarone. *Cornea*. 2012;31(1):81–83.
2. Klingele TG, Alves LE, Rose EP. Amiodarone keratopathy. *Ann Ophthalmol*. 1984;16:1172–1176.
3. Frings A, Schargus M. Recovery from amiodarone-induced cornea verticillata by application of topical heparin. *Cornea*. 2017;36(11):1419–1422.
4. Flach AJ, Dolan BJ. Amiodarone-induced lens opacities: an 8-year follow-up study. *Arch Ophthalmol*. 1990;108:1668–1669.

5. Cumming RG, Mitchell P. Medications and cataract – the Blue Mountain Eye Study. *Ophthalmology*. 1998;105:1751–1757.
6. Murphy MA, Murphy JF. Amiodarone and optic neuropathy: the heart of the matter. *J Neuroophthalmol*. 2005;25(3):232–236.
7. Purvin V, Kawasaki A, Borruat F-X. Optic neuropathy in patients using amiodarone. *Arch Ophthalmol*. 2006;124:696–701.
8. Passman RS, Bennett CL, Purpura JM, et al. Amiodarone-associated optic neuropathy: a critical review. *Am J Med*. 2012;125:447–453.
9. Knudsen A. Short-term treatment with oral amiodarone resulting in bilateral optic neuropathy and permanent blindness. *BMJ Case Reports*. 2017.
10. Kervinen M, Falck A, Hurskainen M, et al. Bilateral optic neuropathy and permanent loss of vision after treatment with amiodarone. *J Cardiovasc Pharmacol*. 2013;62(4):394–396.
11. Cheng HC, Yeh HJ, Huang N, et al. Amiodarone-associated optic neuropathy. *Ophthalmology*. 2015;122(12):2553–2559.
12. Mindel JS, Bagiella E. Re: Cheng et al.: Amiodarone-associated optic neuropathy: a nationwide study. *Ophthalmology*. 2016;123(10):e58–e59.
13. Cheng HC, Yeh HJ, Huang N, et al. Reply. *Ophthalmology*. 2016;123(10):e59–e60.
14. Mindel JS. Absence of amiodarone-associated optic neuropathy. *Ophthalmology*. 2014;121(10):2074–2075.
15. Amiodarone hydrochloride. 2018. Retrieved from http://www.pdr.net.
16. Wang AG, Cheng HC. Amiodarone-associated optic neuropathy: clinical review. *Neuroophthalmology*. 2016;41(2):55–58.
17. Fasler K, Traber GL, Jaggi GP, et al. Amiodarone-associated optic neuropathy – a clinical criteria-based diagnosis? *Neuroophthalmology*. 2018;42(1):2–10.
18. Fraunfelder FT. Amiodarone Whorl-Like Pattern of Golden-Brown Deposits in the Anterior Cornea [Photograph]. Portland, OR: Casey Eye Institute, Oregon Health & Science University; ©1990. photograph: color.
19. Macaluso DC, Shults WT, Fraunfelder FT. Features of amiodarone optic neuropathy. *Am J Ophthalmol*. 1999;127:610–613.

Drug: Digoxin

1. Renard D, Rubil E, Voide N, et al. Spectrum of digoxin-induced ocular toxicity: a case report and literature review. *BMC Res Notes*. 2015;8:368.
2. Weleber RG, Shults WT. Digoxin retinal toxicity. Clinical and electrophysiological evaluation of a cone dysfunction syndrome. *Arch Ophthalmol*. 1981;99(9):1568–1572.
3. Lawrenson JG, Kelly C, Lawrenson AL, et al. Acquired colour vision deficiency in patients receiving digoxin maintenance therapy. *Br J Ophthalmol*. 2002;86(11):1259–1261.
4. Closson RG. Visual hallucinations as the earliest symptom of digoxin intoxication. *Arch Neurol*. 1983;40(6):386.

5. Horst HA, Kolenda KD, Duncker G, et al. Color vision deficiencies induced by subtoxic and toxic digoxin and digitoxin serum levels. *Med Klin*. 1988;83:541–547.
6. Duncker G, Kolenda KD, Schenk F. Digitalis-induced color vision deficiencies and therapeutic glycoside serum concentrations. *Fortschr Ophthalmol*. 1983;79:503–505.
7. Piltz JR, Wertenbaker C, Lance SE, et al. Digoxin Toxicity. Recognizing the varied visual presentations. *J Clin Neuroophthalmol*. 1993;13(4):275–280.
8. Lely AH, van Enter CHJ. Large scale digoxin intoxication. *Br Med J*. 1970;3:737–746.
9. Gelfand ML. Total blindness due to digitalis toxicity. *N Engl J Med*. 1956;254:1181–1182.
10. Ross JVM. Visual disturbances due to digitalis and similar preparations. *Am J Ophthalmol*. 1950;33:1438–1439.

Drug: Disopyramide phosphate

1. Ahmad S. Disopyramide: pulmonary complications and glaucoma. *Mayo Clin Proc*. 1990;65:1030–1031.
2. Trope GE, Hind VM. Closed-angle glaucoma in patients on disopyramide. *Lancet*. 1978;1:329.
3. Disopyramide phosphate. 2018. Retrieved from http://www.pdr.net.

Drugs: Oxprenolol hydrochloride, propranolol hydrochloride

1. Dennis KE, Froman D, Morrison AS, et al. Beta blocker therapy: identification and management of side effects. *Heart Lung*. 1991;20(5 Pt 1):459–463.
2. Yeomans SM, Knox DL, Green WR, et al. Ocular inflammatory pseudotumor associated with propranolol therapy. *Ophthalmology*. 1983;90:1422–1425.
3. Glasman P, Chandna A, Nayak H, et al. Propranolol and periocular capillary hemangiomas: assessment of refractive effect. *J Pediatr Ophthalmol Strabismus*. 2014;51(3):165–170.

Drug: Quinidine gluconate or sulfate

1. Zaidman GW. Quinidine keratopathy. *Am J Ophthalmol*. 1984;97:247–249.
2. Fraunfelder FW, Rosenbaum JT. Drug-induced uveitis: incidence, prevention and treatment. *Drug Safety*. 1997;1(3):197–207.
3. Spitzberg DH. Acute anterior uveitis secondary to quinidine sensitivity. *Arch Ophthalmol*. 1979;97:1993.
4. Hustead JD. Granulomatous uveitis and quinidine hypersensitivity. *Am J Ophthalmol*. 1991;112(4):461–462.
5. Caraco Y, Arnon R, Raveh D, et al. Quinidine-induced uveitis. *Isr J Med Sci*. 1992;28:741–743.
6. Edeki TI, He H, Wood AJ. Pharmacogenetic explanation for excessive β-blockade following timolol eye drops: potential for oral-ophthalmic drug interaction. *JAMA*. 1995;27:1611–1613.
7. Higginbotham EJ. Topical β-adrenergic antagonists and quinidine. *Arch Ophthalmol*. 1996;114:745–746.

Drugs: Acebutolol, atenolol, carvedilol, labetalol hydrochloride, metoprolol tartrate, nadolol, pindolol

1. Carvedilol. 2018. Retrieved from http://www.pdr.net.

Drugs: Alfuzosin hydrochloride, doxazosin mesylate, silodosin, tamsulosin hydrochloride, terazosin hydrochloride

1. Chang DF, Campbell JR. Intraoperative floppy iris syndrome associated with tamsulosin. *J Cataract Refract Surg.* 2005;31:664–673.
2. Blouin MC, Blouin J, Perreault S, et al. Intraoperative floppy-iris syndrome associated with alpha1-adrenoreceptors: comparison of tamsulosin and alfuzosin. *J Cataract Refract Surg.* 2007;33:1227–1234.
3. Shah N, Tendulkar M, Brown R. Should we anticipate intraoperative floppy iris syndrome (IFIS) even with very short history of tamsulosin? *Eye.* 2009;23:740.
4. Bell CM, Hatch WV, Fischer HD, et al. Association between tamsulosin and serious ophthalmic adverse events in older men following cataract surgery. *JAMA.* 2009;301(19):1991–1996.
5. Goseki T, Shimizu K, Ishikawa H, et al. Possible mechanism of intraoperative floppy iris syndrome: a clinicopathological study. *Br J Ophthalmol.* 2008;92(8):1156–1158.
6. Panagis L, Basile M, Friedman AH, et al. Intraoperative floppy iris syndrome. *Arch Ophthalmol.* 2010;128(11):1437–1441.
7. Santaella RM, Destafeno JJ, Stinnett SS, et al. The effect of α1-adrenergic receptor antagonist tamsulosin (Flomax) on iris dilator smooth muscle anatomy. *Ophthalmology.* 2010;117:1743–1749.
8. Martin-Moro JG, Sanz FG. Munoz-Negrete FJ. Tamsulosin and iris pigmentation (letter). *Ophthalmology.* 2010;117(12):2444–2445.
9. Yuksel N, Ozer MD, Takmaz T, et al. Anterior segment morphologic changes related to alpha-1 adrenergic receptor antagonist use. *Eur J Ophthalmol.* 2015;25(6):512–515.
10. Gonzalez-Martin-Moro J, Gonzalez-Lopez JJ, Gomez-Sanz F, et al. Impact of tamsulosin exposure on late complications following cataract surgery: a retrospective cohort study. *Int Ophthalmol.* 2014;34(4):761–766.
11. Kerimoglu H, Zengin N, Ozturk B, et al. Unilateral chemosis, acute onset myopia and choroidal detachment following the use of tamsulosin. *Acta Ophthalmol.* 2010;88(2):e20–e21.
12. Lubbers SM, Japing WJ. Unilateral choroidal detachment following the use of tamsulosin. *Can J Ophthalmol.* 2017;52(2):e75–e77.
13. Shapiro BL, Petrovic V, Lee SE, et al. Choroidal detachment following the use of tamsulosin (Flomax). *Am J Ophthalmol.* 2007;143(2):351–353.
14. Bonnell LN, SooHoo JR, Seibold LK, et al. One-day postoperative intraocular pressure spike after phacoemulsification cataract surgery in patients taking tamsulosin. *J Cataract Refract Surg.* 2016;42(12):1753–1758.
15. Waqar S, Simcock P. Lower lid entropion secondary to treatment with alpha-1a receptor antagonist: a case report. *J Med Case Rep.* 2010;4(77).
16. Kelly BT, Locke BA, Kelly KJ. Pseudoallergic conjunctivitis induced by tamsulosin, a selective alpha-1 adrenergic receptor antagonist. *J Allergy Clin Immunol Pract.* 2018.
17. Karmel M, Chang DF. The latest wisdom on managing floppy iris. *EyeNet.* 2009:25–27.
18. Prata TS, Palmiero PM, Angelilli A, et al. Iris morphologic changes related to alpha (1)-adrenergic receptor antagonists implications for intraoperative floppy iris syndrome. *Ophthalmology.* 2009;116:877–881.

Drugs: Captopril, enalapril

1. Gianos ME, Klaustermeyer WB, Kurohara M, et al. Enalapril induced angioedema. *Am J Emerg Med.* 1990;8:124–126.
2. Gonnering RS, Hirsch SR. Delayed drug-induced periorbital angioedema. *Am J Ophthalmol.* 1990;110(5):566–568.
3. Pillans PI, Coulter DM, Black P. Angioedema and urticaria with angiotensin converting enzyme inhibitors. *Euro J Clin Pharm.* 1996;51(2):123–126.
4. Wizemann A. Nekrotisierende blepharitis nach captopril-induzierter agranulozytose. *Klin Monatsbl Augenheilkd.* 1983;182:82–85.
5. Balduf M, Steinkraus V, Ring J. Captopril associated lacrimation and rhinorrhea. *BMJ.* 1992;305(6855):693.

Drug: Clonidine hydrochloride

1. Clonidine hydrochloride. 2018. Retrieved from http://www.pdr.net.
2. Fan D, Fan TJ. Clonidine induced apoptosis of human corneal epithelial cells through death receptors-mediated, mitochondria-dependent signaling pathway. *Toxicol Sci.* 2017;156(1):252–260.

Drug: Diazoxide

1. Cove DH, Seddon M, Fletcher RF, et al. Blindness after treatment for malignant hypertension. *BMJ.* 1979;2:245–246.
2. Burton JL, Schutt WH, Caldwell IW. Hypertrichosis due to diazoxide. *Br J Dermatol.* 1975;93:707–711.
3. Diazoxide. 2018. Retrieved from http://www.pdr.net.
4. Schiavo DM, Field WE, Vymetal FJ. Cataracts in beagle dogs given diazoxide. *Diabetes.* 1975;24:1041–1049.

Drug: Guanethidine monosulfate

1. Brest AN, Novack P, Kasparian H, et al. Guanethidine. *Dis Chest.* 1962;42:359–363.

Drug: Hydralazine hydrochloride

1. Hydralazine hydrochloride. 2018. Retrieved from http://www.pdr.net.
2. Choi J-H, Choi K-D, Kim JS, et al. Simultaneous posterior ischemic optic neuropathy, cerebral border zone infarction, and spinal cord infarction after correction of malignant hypertension. *J Neuro-Ophthalmol.* 2008;28(3):198–201.

3. Larsson LI, Maus TL, Brubaker RF, et al. Topically applied hydralazine: effects on systemic cardiovascular parameters, blood-aqueous barrier, and aqueous humor dynamics in normotensive humans. *J Ocul Pharmacol Ther.* 1995;11(2):145–156.

Drug: Prazosin hydrochloride

1. Prazosin hydrochloride. 2018. Retrieved from http://www.pdr.net.
2. Zhang Y, Shamie N, Daneshmand S. Assessment of urologists' knowledge on intraoperative floppy iris syndrome. *Urology.* 2016;97:40–45.
3. Carruthers SG. Adverse effects of α1-adrenergic blocking drugs. *Drug Safety.* 1994;11:12–20.

Drug: Reserpine

1. Shimohira M, Iwakawa Y, Kohyama J. Rapid-eye-movement sleep in jittery infants. *Early Him Dev.* 2002;66:25–31.

Drug: Albuterol (salbutamol)

1. Goldstein JB, Biousse V, Newman NJ. Unilateral pharmacologic mydriasis in a patient with respiratory compromise. *Arch Ophthalmol.* 1997;15:806.
2. Packe GE, Cayton RM, Mashhoudi N. Nebulised ipratropium bromide and salbutamol causing closed-angle glaucoma. *Lancet.* 1984;2:691.
3. Rho DS. Acute angle-closure glaucoma after albuterol nebulizer treatment. *Am J Ophthalmol.* 2000;130:123–124.
4. Kalra L, Bone MF. The effect of nebulized bronchodilator therapy on intraocular pressures in patients with glaucoma. *Chest.* 1988;93:739–741.
5. Khanna PB, Davies R. Hallucinations associated with the administration of salbutamol via a nebulizer. *BMJ.* 1986;292:1430.
6. Albuterol. 2018. Retrieved from http://www.pdr.net.
7. Sami MS, Soparker CN, Patrinely JR, et al. Eyelid edema. *Semin Plast Surg.* 2007;21(1):24–31.

Drug: Ipratropium

1. Woelfle J, Zielen S, Lentze MJ. Unilateral fixed dilated pupil in an infant after inhalation of nebulized ipratropium bromide. *J Pediatr.* 2000;136:423–424.
2. Bisquerra RA, Botz GH, Nates JL. Ipratropium-bromide–induced acute anisocoria in the intensive care setting due to ill-fitting face masks. *Respir Care.* 2005;50:1662–1664.
3. Weir RE, Whitehead DE, Zaidi FH, et al. Pupil blown by a puffer. *Lancet.* 2004;363:1853.
4. Han RC, Pearson A. A toddler with intermittent mydriasis. *BMJ.* 2016;355:i5083.
5. Ortiz-Rambla J, Hidalgo Mora JJ, Cascon-Ramon G, et al. Acute angle closure glaucoma and ipratropium bromide. *Med Clin.* 2005;124:795.
6. de Saint-Jean M, Bourcier T, Borderie V, et al. Acute closure-angle glaucoma after treatment with ipratropium bromide and salbutamol aerosols. *J Fr Ophthalmol.* 2000;23:603–605.

7. Lellouche N, Guglielminotti J, de Saint-Jean M, et al. Acute glaucoma in the course of treatment with aerosols of ipratropium. *Presse Med.* 1999;28:1017.
8. Lui P, Li Na, Liu Y, et al. Nebulized ipratropium bromide in fixed dilated pupil: three cases report and review of literature. *Int J Clin Exp Med.* 2016;9(7):14796–14800.
9. Kola M, Hacioglu D, Erdol H, et al. Bilateral acute angle closure developing due to use of ipratropium bromide and salbutamol. *Int Ophthalmol.* 2018;38(1):385–388.
10. Tafinlar. 2018. Retrieved from http://www.pdr.net.

Drugs: Chlorothiazide, hydrochlorothiazide, indapamide, methyclothiazide, metolazone

1. Fraunfelder FW, Fraunfelder FT, Keates EU. Topiramate-associated acute bilateral secondary angle-closure glaucoma. *Ophthalmology.* 2004;111:109–111.
2. Chen SH, Karanjia R, Chevrier RL, et al. Bilateral acute angle closure glaucoma associated with hydrochlorothiazide-induced hyponatraemia. *BMJ Case Rep.* 2014.
3. Murphy RM, Bakir B, O'Brien C, et al. Drug-induced bilateral secondary angle-closure glaucoma: a literature synthesis. *J Glaucoma.* 2016;25(2).e99–e105.
4. Geanon JD, Perkins TW. Bilateral acute angle-closure glaucoma associated with drug sensitivity to hydrochlorothiazide. *Arch Ophthalmol.* 1995;113:1231–1232.
5. Krieg PH, Schipper I. Drug-induced ciliary body oedema: a new theory. *Eye.* 1996;10(pt1):121–126.
6. Blain P, Paques M, Massin P, et al. Acute transient myopia induced by indapamide. *Am J Ophthalmol.* 2000;129(4):538–540.
7. Vegh M, Hari-Kovacs A, Rez K, et al. Indapamide-induced transient myopia with supraciliary effusion: case report. *BMC Ophthalmol.* 2013;13:58.
8. Sponsel WE, Rapoza PA. Posterior subcapsular cataract associated with indapamide therapy. *Arch Ophthalmol.* 1992;110:454.
9. Miller NR, Moses H. Transient oculomotor nerve palsy. Association with thiazide-induced glucose intolerance. *JAMA.* 1979;240:1887–1888.
10. Hartzer M, et al. Hydrochlorothiazide: increased human retinal epithelial cell toxicity following low-level UV-A irradiation. *ARVO Invest Ophthalmol Vis Sci Annual Meeting Abstract.* 1993;(Issue):3633–3640.
11. de la Marnierre E, Guigon B, Quaranta M, et al. Phototoxic drugs and age-related maculopathy. *J Fr Ophthalmol.* 2003;26:596–601.
12. Costagliola C, Menzione M, Chiosi F, et al. Retinal phototoxicity induced by hydrochlorothiazide after exposure to a UV tanning device. *Photochem Photobiol.* 2008;84(5):1294–1297.
13. Iacono P, Battaglia Parodi M, Bandello F. Macular edema associated with hydrochlorothiazide therapy. *Br J Ophthalmol.* 2011;95(7):1036–1037.

Drug: Furosemide

1. Boundaoui ON, Woodruff TE. Presumed furosemide-associated bilateral angle-closure glaucoma. *J Glaucoma.* 2016;25(8):e748–e750.

2. Fraunfelder FW, Fraunfelder FT, Keates EU. Topiramate, associated, acute, secondary angle-closure glaucoma. *Ophthalmology*. 2004;111(1):109–111.

3. Lee AG, Anderson R, Kardon RH, et al. Presumed "sulfa allergy" in patients with intracranial hypertension treated with acetazolamide or furosemide: cross-reactivity, myth or reality? *Am J Ophthalmol*. 2004;138: 114–118.

Drug: Glycerol (glycerin)

1. Kalin NS, Wulc AE, Piccone MR, et al. Visual loss after retrogasserian glycerol injection. *Am J Ophthalmol*. 1993;115(3):396–398.

2. Mizuta K, Furuta M, Ito Y, et al. A case of Meniere's disease with vertical nystagmus after administration of glycerol. *Auris Nasus Larynx*. 2000;27:271–274.

Drug: Mannitol

1. Hasegawa T, Matsui Y, Morita M. Dented corneas related to cardiovascular surgery under general anesthesia. *Graefes Arch Clin Exp Ophthalmol*. 2012;250(3):465–466.

2. Weber AC, Blandford AD, Costin BR, et al. Effect of mannitol on globe and orbital volumes in humans. *Eur J Ophthalmol*. 2018;28(2):163–167.

3. Hwang HS, Ahn YS, Cho YK. Preoperative mannitolization can decrease corneal endothelial cell damage after cataract surgery. *Curr Eye Res*. 2016;41(9):1161–1165.

4. Caliskan S, Ugurbas SC, Alpay A, et al. Changes in the choroidal thickness and axial length upon mannitol infusion in patients with asymmetric intraocular pressure. *J Glaucoma*. 2016;25(11):891–895.

Drugs: Phenoxybenzamine hydrochloride

1. James ML, Keifer JC. Posterior optic nerve ischemic neuropathy in the setting of phenoxybenzamine therapy after uneventful spinal fusion. *J Neurosurg Anesthesiol*. 2011;23(2):169–170.

Drug: Ephedrine sulfate

1. O'Brien DM, Farmer SG, Kalina RE, et al. Acute macular neuroretinopathy following intravenous sympathomimetics. *Retina*. 1989;9(4):281–286.

2. Lee W, Chang JH, Roh KW, et al. Anorexiant-induced transient myopia after myopic laser in situ keratomileusis. *J Cataract Refract Surg*. 2007;33:746–749.

3. Ephedrine sulfate. 2018. Retrieved from http://www.pdr.net.

Drug: Epinephrine, norepinephrine bitartrate

1. O'Brien DM, Farmer SG, Kalina RE, et al. Acute macular neuroretinopathy following intravenous sympathomimetics. *Retina*. 1989;9:281–286.

2. Desai UR, Sudhamathi K, Natarajan S. Intravenous epinephrine and acute macular neuroretinopathy. *Arch Ophthalmol*. 1993;111:1026–1027.

3. Wessel MM, Woodcome Jr HA, Borges O, et al. Acute macular neuroretinopathy following rhinosurgery. *Graefes Arch Clin Exp Ophthalmol*. 2013;251(11):2653–2655.

4. Savino PJ, Burde RM, Mills RP. Visual loss following intranasal anesthetic injection. *J Clin Neuro-Ophthalmol*. 1990;10(2):140–144.

5. Narendran S, Saravanan VR, Pereira M. Purtscher-like retinopathy: a rare complication of peribulbar anesthesia. *Indian J Ophthalmol*. 2016;64(6):464–466.

6. Lamichhane G, Gautam P. Central retinal arterial occlusion (CRAO) after phacoemulsification – a rare complication. *Nepal J Ophthalmol*. 2013;5(2):281–283.

7. Moon BG, Kim JG. A case of ophthalmic artery occlusion following subcutaneous injection of epinephrine mixed with lidocaine into the supratrochlear area. *Korean J Ophthalmol*. 2017;31(3):277–279.

8. Jandrasits K, Luksch A, Söregi G, et al. Effect of noradrenaline on retinal blood flow in healthy subjects. *Ophthalmology*. 2002;109:291–295.

9. Gutierrez Fernandez D, de la Varga Martinez R, Lasa Lucases EM, et al. Allergic contact conjunctivitis and cross-reaction between phenylephrine and epinephrine due to phenylephrine eye drops. *Ann Allergy Asthma Immunol*. 2016;117(5):564–565.

10. Krachmer JH, Palay DA. *Cornea Atlas*. 2nd ed. London: Mosby Elsevier; 2006.

Drug: Phenylephrine

1. Soparkar CN, Wilhelmus KR, Koch DD, et al. Acute and chronic conjunctivitis due to over-the-counter ophthalmic decongestants. *Arch Ophthalmol*. 1997;115(1): 34–38.

2. Hermansen MC, Hasan S. Abolition of feeding intolerance following ophthalmologic examination of neonates. *J Pediatr Ophthalmol Strabismus*. 1985;22(6):256–257.

3. Pless M, Friberg TR. Topical phenylephrine may result in worsening of visual loss when used to dilate pupils in patients with vaso-occlusive disease of the optic nerve. *Semin Ophthalmol*. 2003;18:218–221.

4. Morrison DA, Gridneva Z, Chirila TV, et al. Screening for drug-induced spoliation of the hydrogel optic of the AlphaCor artificial cornea. *Cont Lens Anterior Eye*. 2006;29:93–100.

5. Villarreal O. Reliability of diagnostic tests for contact allergy to mydriatic eyedrops. *Contact Derm*. 1998;38:150–154.

6. Fraunfelder FT, Scafidi AF. Possible adverse effects from topical ocular 10% phenylephrine. *Am J Ophthalmol*. 1978;85:447–453.

7. Fraunfelder FW, Fraunfelder FT, Jensvold B. Adverse systemic effects from pledgets of topical ocular phenylephrine 10%. *Am J Ophthalmol*. 2002;134:624–625.

8. Baldwin FJ, Morley AP. Intraoperative pulmonary oedema in a child following systemic absorption of phenylephrine eyedrops. *Br J Anaesth*. 2002;88:440–442.

9. Venkatakrishnan J, Jagadeesh V, Kannan R. Pulmonary edema following instillation of topical phenylephrine eyedrops in a child under general anesthesia. *Eur J Ophthalmol*. 2011;21(1):115–117.

10. Sbraglia F, Mores N, Garra R, et al. Phenylephrine eye drops in pediatric patients undergoing ophthalmic sur-

gery: incidence, presentation, and management of complications during general anesthesia. *Paediatr Anaesth.* 2014;24(4):400–405.

11. Kim HJ, Choi JG, Kwak KH. Bronchoconstriction following instillation of phenylephrine eye drops in premature infants with bronchopulmonary dysplasia: two cases report. *Korean J Anesthesiol.* 2015;68(6):613–616.

12. Khan MA, Watt LL, Hugkulstone CE. Bilateral acute angle-closure glaucoma after use of Fenox nasal drops. *Eye.* 2002;16:662–663.

13. Zenzen CT, Eliott D, Balok EM, et al. Acute angle-closure glaucoma associated with intranasal phenylephrine to treat epistaxis. *Arch Ophthalmol.* 2004;122:655–656.

14. Berman DH, Deutsch JA. Bilateral spontaneous pigment epithelial detachments in a premature neonate. *Arch Ophthalmol.* 1994;112(2):161–162.

15. Lim DL, Batilando M, Rajadurai VS. Transient paralytic ileus following the use of cyclopentolate-phenylephrine eyedrops during screening for retinopathy of prematurity. *J Paediatr Child Health.* 2003;39:318–320.

16. Shinomiya K, Kajima M, Tajika H, et al. Renal failure caused by eyedrops containing phenylephrine in a case of retinopathy of prematurity. *J Med Invest.* 2003;50.203–206.

FURTHER READING

Ergometrine maleate (ergonovine), ergotamine tartrate, methylergometrine (methylergonovine maleate)

Mindel JS, Rubenstein AE, Franklin B. Ocular ergotamine tartrate toxicity during treatment of Vacor-induced orthostatic hypotension. *Am J Ophthalmol.* 1981;92:492–496.

Wollensak J, Grajewski O. Bilateral vascular papillitis following ergotamine medication. *Klin Monatsbl Augenheilkd.* 1978;173:731–737.

Amlodipine besylate, diltiazem hydrochloride, nifedipine, verapamil hydrochloride

Beatty JF, Krupin T, Nichols PF, et al. Elevation of intraocular pressure by calcium channel Blockers. *Arch Ophthalmol.* 1984;102:1072–1076.

Coulter DM. Eye pain with nifedipine and taste disturbance with captopril, a mutually controlled study demonstrating a method of post marketing surveillance. *BMJ.* 1988;296:1086–1088.

Fang L, Turtschi S, Mozaffarieh M. The effect of nifedipine on retinal venous pressure of glaucoma patients with the Flammer-Syndrome. *Graefes Arch Clin Exp Ophthalmol.* 2015;253(6):935–939.

Friedland S, Kaplan S, Lahav M, et al. Proptosis and periorbital edema due to diltiazem treatment. *Arch Ophthalmol.* 1993;111:1027–1028.

Gubinelli E, Cocuroccia B, Girolomoni G. Subacute cutaneous lupus erythematosus induced by nifedipine. *J Cutan Med Surg.* 2003;7:243–246.

Harris A, Evans DW, Cantor LB, et al. Hemodynamic and visual function effects of oral nifedipine in patients with normal-tension glaucoma. *Am J Ophthalmol.* 1997;124(3):296–302.

Hockwin O, Dragomirescu V, Laser H, et al. Evaluation of the ocular safety of verapamil. Scheimpflug photography with densitometric image analysis of lens transparency in patients with hypertrophic cardiomyopathy subjected to long-term therapy with high doses of verapamil. *Ophthalmic Res.* 1984;16:264–275.

Indu B, Batra YK, Puri GD, et al. Nifedipine attenuates the intraocular pressure response to intubation following succinylcholine. *Can J Anesthes.* 1989;36:269–272.

Kelly SP, Walley TJ. Eye pain with nifedipine. *BMJ.* 1988;296:1401.

Kuykendall-Ivy T, Collier SL, Johnson SM. Diltiazem-induced hyperpigmentation. *Cutis.* 2004;73:239–240.

Manga P, Vythilingum S. Nifedipine: unstable angina. *S Afr Med J.* 1984;66:144.

Opie LH, White DA. Adverse interaction between nifedipine and beta-blockade. *BMJ.* 1980;281:1462.

Rainer G, Kiss B, Dallinger S, et al. A double masked placebo controlled study on the effect of nifedipine on optic nerve blood flow and visual field function in patients with open angle glaucoma. *Br J Clin Pharmacol.* 2001;52:210–212.

Roos JCP, Haridas AS. Prolonged mydriasis after inadvertent topical administration of the calcium channel antagonist amlodipine: implications for glaucoma drug development. *Cutan Ocul Toxicol.* 2015;34(1):84–87.

Scherschun L, Lee MW, Lim HW. Diltiazem-associated photodistributed hyperpigmentation: a review of 4 cases. *Arch Dermatol.* 2001;137:179–182.

Silverstone PH. Periorbital edema caused by nifedipine. *BMJ.* 1984;288:1654.

Tordjman K, Itosenthal T, Bursztyn M. Nifedipine-induced periorbital edema. *Am J Cardiol.* 1985;55:1445.

Amyl/butyl nitrite

Pece A, Patelli F, Milani P, et al. Transient visual loss after amyl isobutyl nitrite abuse. *Semin Ophthalmol.* 2004;19:105–106.

Flecainide acetate, procainamide hydrochloride

Cetnarowski AB, Rihn TL. Adverse reactions to tocainide and mexiletine. *Cardiovasc Rev Reports.* 1985;6:1335.

Clarke CW, el-Mahdi EO. Confusion and paranoia associated with oral tocainide. *Postgrad Med J.* 1985;61:79–81.

Hopson JR, Buxton AE, Rinkenberger RL, et al. Safety and utility of flecainide acetate in the routine care of patients with supraventricular tachyarrhythmias: results of a multicenter trial. The Flecainide Supraventricular Tachycardia Study Group. *Am J Card.* 1996;77(3):72A–82A.

Kaeser HE. Drug-induced myasthenic syndromes. *Acta Neurol Scand.* 1984;70:39–47.

Keefe DL, Kates RE, Harrison DC. New antiarrhythmic drugs: their place in therapy. *Drugs.* 1981;22:363–400.

Ramhamadany E, Mackenzie S, Ramsdale DR. Dysarthria and visual hallucinations due to flecainide toxicity. *Postgrad Med J.* 1986;62:61–62.

Smith AG. Drug-induced photosensitivity. *Adverse Drug React Bull.* 1989;136:508–511.

Vincent FM, Vincent T. Tocainide encephalopathy. *Neurology.* 1985;35:1804–1805.

Nicorandil

Colvin HS, Barakat T, Moussa O, et al. Nicorandil associated anal ulcers: an estimate of incidence. *Ann R Coll Surg Engl.* 2012;94(3):170–172.

Kamath S, Taylor M, Bhagwandas K. An unusual case of nicorandil-induced conjunctival erosions. *Clin Exp Dermatol.* 2012;37(6):681–682.

Ollagnier M, Guy C, Gain P. Cutaneous and corneal ulcerations under nicorandil: a case report. *Drug Safety.* 2008;31(10):897–898.

Phillippe C, Guy C, Gain P, et al. Corneal perforation induced by nicorandil: report of a case. *J Fr Ophthalmol.* 2009;32:1S125.

Reichert S, Antunes A, Trechot P, et al. Major aphthous stomatitis induced by nicorandil. *Eur J Dermatol.* 1997;7:132–133.

Smith VM, Lyon CC. Nicorandil: do the dermatological and gastrointestinal risks outweigh the benefits? *Br J Dermatol.* 2012;167(5):1048–1052.

Wang A, Chen F, Xie Y, et al. Protective mechanism of nicorandil on rat myocardial ischemia-reperfusion. *J Cardiovasc Med.* 2012;13(8):511–515.

Watson A, Al-Ozari O, Fraser A, et al. Nicorandil associated anal ulceration. *Lancet.* 2002;360:546–547.

Nitroglycerin

Purvin V, Dunn D. Nitrate-induced transient ischemic attacks. *South Med J.* 1981;74:1130–1131.

Robertson D, Stevens RM. Nitrates and glaucoma. *JAMA.* 1977;237:117.

Shorey J, Bhardwaj N, Loscalzo J. Acute Wernicke's encephalopathy after intravenous infusion of high-dose nitroglycerin. *Ann Intern Med.* 1984;101:500.

Sveska K. Nitrates may not be contraindicated in patients with glaucoma. *Drug Intell Clin Pharm.* 1985;19:361.

Wizemann AJ, Wizemann V. Organic nitrate therapy in glaucoma. *Am J Ophthalmol.* 1980;90:106–109.

Amiodarone hydrochloride

Banerjee S, James CB. Amiodarone and dysthyroid eye disease (letter). *Br J Ophthalmol.* 1996;80:851–852.

Ciancaglini M, Carpineto P, Zuppardi E, et al. In vivo confocal microscopy of patients with amiodarone-induced keratopathy. *Cornea.* 2001;20:368–373.

Cordon Lopez A, Muñoz Lopez A, Fernandez Jimenez S, et al. Acute intracranial hypertension during amiodarone infusion. *Crit Care Med.* 1985;13:688–689.

Dickerson EJ, Wolman RL. Sicca syndrome associated with amiodarone therapy. *BMJ.* 1986;293:510.

Erdurmus M, Selcoki Y, Yagci R, et al. Amiodarone-induced keratopathy: full-thickness corneal involvement. *Eye Contact Lens.* 2008;34(2):131–132.

Farwell AP, Abend SL, Huang SK, et al. Thyroidectomy for amiodarone induced thyrotoxicosis. *JAMA.* 1990;263:1526–1528.

Fikkers BG, Bogousslavsky J, Regli F, et al. Pseudotumor cerebri with amiodarone. *J Neurol Neurosurg Psychiatry.* 1986;49:606.

Fraunfelder FW, Fraunfelder FT. Scientific challenges in postmarketing surveillance of ocular adverse drug reactions. *Am J Ophthalmol.* 2007;143:145–149.

Hawthorne GC, Campbell NPS, Geddes JS, et al. Amiodarone-induced hypothyroidism. A common complication of prolonged therapy: a report of eight cases. *Arch Intern Med.* 1985;145:1016–1019.

Kaplan LJ, Cappaert WE. Amiodarone keratopathy. Correlation to dosage and duration. *Arch Ophthalmol.* 1982;100:601–602.

Katai N, Yokoyama R, Yoshimura N. Progressive brown discoloration of silicone intraocular lenses after vitrectomy in a patient on amiodarone. *J Cat Refract Surg.* 1999;25:451–452.

Mantyjarvi M, Tuppurainen K, Ikaheimo K. Ocular side effects of amiodarone. *Surv Ophthalmol.* 1998;42:360–366.

Mindel JM. Amiodarone and optic neuropathy – a medicolegal issue (editorial). *Surv Ophthalmol.* 1998;42:358–359.

Nagra PK, Forozoan R, Savino PJ, et al. Amiodarone induced optic neuropathy. *Br J Ophthalmol.* 2003;87:420–422.

Orlando RG, Dangel ME, Schaal SF. Clinical experience and grading of amiodarone keratopathy. *Ophthalmology.* 1984;91:1184–1187.

Roberts JE, Reme CE, Dillon J, et al. Exposure to bright light and the concurrent use of photosensitizing drugs. *New Engl J Med.* 1992;326(22):1500–1502.

Yagmur M, Okan O, Ersöz TR, et al. Confocal microscopic features of amiodarone keratopathy. *J Toxicol Cut Ocul Toxicol.* 2003;22:243–253.

Digoxin

Lawrenson JG, Kelly C, Lawrenson AL, et al. Acquired colour vision deficiency in patients receiving digoxin maintenance therapy. *Br J Ophthalmol.* 2002;86:1259–1261.

Mermoud A, Safran AB, de Stoutz N. Pain upon eye movement following digoxin absorption. *J Clin Neuroophthalmol.* 1992;12(1):41–42.

Disopyramide phosphate

Frucht J, Freimann I, Merin S. Ocular side effects of disopyramide. *Br J Ophthalmol.* 1984;68:890–891.

Keefe DL, Kates RE, Harrison DC. New antiarrhythmic drugs: their place in therapy. *Drugs.* 1981;22:363–400.

Schwartz JB, Keefe D, Harrison DC. Adverse effects of antiarrhythmic drugs. *Drugs.* 1981;21:23–45.

Wayne K, Manolas E, Sloman G. Fatal overdose with disopyramide. *Med J Aust.* 1980;1:231–232.

Methacholine chloride

Crandall DC, Leopold IH. The influence of systemic drugs on tear constituents. *Ophthalmology.* 1979;86:115–125.

Leopold IH. The use and side effects of cholinergic agents in the management of intraocular pressure. In: Drance

SM, Neufeld AH, eds. *Glaucoma: Applied Pharmacology in Medical Treatment*. New York: Grune & Stratton; 1984: 357–393.

Spaeth GL. The effect of autonomic agents on the pupil and the intraocular pressure of eyes treated with dexamethasone. *Br J Ophthalmol*. 1980;64:426–429.

Oxprenolol hydrochloride, propranolol hydrochloride

Almog Y, Monselise M, Almog C, et al. The effect of oral treatment with beta blockers on the tear secretion. *Metab Pediatr Syst Ophthalmol*. 1982;6:343–345.

Dollery CT, Bulpitt CJ, Daniel J, et al. Eye symptoms in patients taking propranolol and other hypotensive agents. *Br J Clin Pharmacol*. 1977;4:295–297.

Draeger J, Winter R. Corneal sensitivity and intraocular pressure. In: Krieglstein GK, Leydhecker W, eds. *Glaucoma Update II*. New York: Springer-Verlag; 1983:63–67.

Felminger R. Visual hallucinations and illusions with propranolol. *BMJ*. 1978;1:1182.

Holt PJ, Waddington E. Oculocutaneous reaction to oxprenolol. *BMJ*. 1975;2:539–540.

Kaeser HE. Drug-induced myasthenic syndromes. *Acta Neurol Scand*. 1984;70(suppl 100):39–47.

Knapp MS, Galloway NR. Ocular reactions to beta blockers. *BMJ*. 1975;2:557.

Lewis BS, Setzen M, Kokoris N. Ocular reaction to oxprenolol. A case report. *S Afr Med. J*. 1976;50:482–483.

Malm L. Propranolol as cause of watery nasal secretion. *Lancet*. 1981;1:1006.

Ohrstrom A, Pandolli M. Regulation of intraocular pressure and pupil size by β-blockers and epinephrine. *Arch Ophthalmol*. 1980;98:2182–2184.

Pecori-Giraldi J, et al. Topical propranolol in glaucoma therapy and investigations on the mechanism of action. *Glaucoma*. 1984;6:31.

Singer L, Knobel B, Itomem M. Influence of systemic administered beta blockers on tear secretion. *Ann Ophthalmol*. 1984;16:728–729.

Weber JC. Beta-adrenoreceptor antagonists and diplopia. *Lancet*. 1982;2:826–827.

Quinidine gluconate or sulfate

Fisher CM. Visual disturbances associated with quinidine and quinine. *Neurology*. 1981;31:1569–1571.

Hording M, Feldt-Rasmussen UF. Acute iridocyclitis with fever and liver involvement during quinidine therapy. *Ugeskr Laeger*. 1991;153(34):2362–2363.

Kaeser HE. Drug-induced myasthenic syndromes. *Acta Neurol Scand*. 1984;70(suppl 100):39–47.

Mahler R, Sissons W, Watters K. Pigmentation induced by quinidine therapy. *Arch Dermatol*. 1986;122:1062–1064.

Naschitz JE, Yeshurun D. Quinidine induced sicca syndrome. *J Toxicol Clin Toxicol*. 1983;20:367–371.

Wittbrodt ET. Drugs and myasthenia gravis: an update. *Arch Intern Med*. 1997;157:399–408.

Acebutolol, atenolol, carvedilol, labetalol hydrochloride, metoprolol tartrate, nadolol, pindolol

Almog Y, Monselise M, Almog C, et al. The effect of oral treatment with beta blockers on the tear secretion. *Metab Pediatr Syst Ophthalmol*. 1982;6:343–345.

Cervantes R, Hernandez HH, Frati A. Pulmonary and heart rate changes associated with nonselective beta blocker glaucoma therapy. *J Toxicol Cut Ocul Toxicol*. 1986;5:185–193.

Cocco G, et al. A review of the effects of β-adrenoceptor blocking drugs on the skin, mucosae and connective tissue. *Curr Ther Res*. 1982;31:362.

Kaul S, Wong M, Singh BN, et al. Nadolol and papilledema. *Ann Intern Med*. 1982;97:454.

Kumar KL, Cooney TG. Visual symptoms after atenolol therapy for migraine. *Ann Intern Med*. 1990;112(1):712–713.

Nielsen PG, Ahrendt N, Buhl H, et al. Metoprolol eyedrops 3%, a short-term comparison with pilocarpine and a five-month follow-up study. *Acta Ophthalmol*. 1982;60:347–352.

Perell H, Campbell DG, Vela A, et al. Choroidal detachment induced by a systemic beta blocker. *Ophthalmology*. 1988;95:410–411.

Petounis AD, Akritopoulos P. Influence of topical and systemic beta blockers on tear production. *Int Ophthalmol*. 1989;13:75–80.

Teicher A, Rosenthall T, Kissin E. Labetalol-induced toxic myopathy. *BMJ*. 1981;282(6):1824–1825.

Weber JC. Beta-adrenoreceptor antagonists and diplopia. *Lancet*. 1982;2:826–827.

Wittbrodt ET. Drugs and myasthenia gravis: an update. *Arch Intern Med*. 1997;157:399–408.

Alfuzosin hydrochloride, doxazosin mesylate, silodosin, tamsulosin hydrochloride, terazosin hydrochloride

Arshinoff SA. Modified SST-USST for tamsulosin-associated intraoperative floppy-iris syndrome. *J Cataract Refract Surg*. 2006;32:559–561.

Ingelheim Boehringer. Important safety on intraoperative floppy iris syndrome (IFIS). *Internet Document*. 2005. Available from: http://www.hc-sc.gc.ca.

Kershner RM. Intraoperative floppy iris syndrome associated with tamsulosin. *J Cataract Refract Surg*. 2005;31:2239–2241.

Lawrentschuk N, Blysma GW. Intraoperative "floppy iris" syndrome and its relationship to tamsulosin: a urologist's guide. *Br J Urol Int*. 2006;97:2–4.

Lin A, Steinert RF. Intraoperative floppy iris syndrome. Chapter 36. In: Levin LA, Albert DM, eds. *Ocular Disease: Mechanisms and Management*. Saunders; 2010.

Nguyen DQ, Sebastian RT, Philip J. Intraoperative floppy iris syndrome associated with Tamsulosin. *Br J Urol Int*. 2006;97:197.

Osher RH. Association between IFIS and flomax. *J Cataract Refract Surg*. 2006;32:547.

Parssinen O. The use of tamsulosin and iris hypotony during cataract surgery. *Acta Ophthalmol Scand*. 2005;83:624–626.

Schwinn DA, Afshari NA. Alpha 1-adrenergic antagonists and floppy iris syndrome: tip of the iceberg? *Ophthalmology.* 2005;112:2059–2060.

Yildirim A, Mehmet T, Yuksel H, et al. Diagnosis of malignant hypertension with ocular examination: a child case. *Semin Ophthalmol.* 2014;29(1):32–35.

Captopril, enalapril

Ahmad S. Enalapril and reversible alopecia. *Arch Intern Med.* 1991;151:404.

Carrington PR, Sanusi ID, Zahradka S, et al. Enalapril-associated erythema and vasculitis. *Cutis.* 1993;51(2):121–123.

Goodfield MJ, Millard LG. Severe cutaneous reactions to captopril. *BMJ.* 1985;290:1111.

Inman WH, Rawson NS, Wilton LV, et al. Postmarketing surveillance of enalapril I: results of prescription-event monitoring. *BMJ.* 1988;297:826–829.

Suarez M, Ho PW, Johnson ES, et al. Angioneurotic edema, agranulocytosis and fatal septicemia following captopril therapy. *Am J Med.* 1986;81:336–338.

Clonidine hydrochloride

Banner Jr W, Lund ME, Clawson L. Failure of naloxone to reverse clonidine toxic effect. *Am J Dis Child.* 1983;137:1170–1171.

Hodapp E, Kolker AE, Kass MA, et al. The effect of topical clonidine on intraocular pressure. *Arch Ophthalmol.* 1981;99:1208–1211.

Kosman ME. Evaluation of clonidine hydrochloride (Catapres). *JAMA.* 1975;233:174–176.

Krieglstein GK, Langham ME, Leydhecker W. The peripheral and central neural actions of clonidine in normal and glaucomatous eyes. *Invest Ophthalmol Vis Sci.* 1978;17:149–158.

Mathew PM, Addy DP, Wright N. Clonidine overdose in children. *Clin Toxicol.* 1981;18:169–173.

Petursson G, Cole R, Hanna C. Treatment of glaucoma using minidrops of clonidine. *Arch Ophthalmol.* 1984;102:1180–1181.

Van Joost TN, Faber WR, Manuel HR. Drug-induced anogenital pemphigoid. *Br J Dermatol.* 1980;102:715–718.

Diazoxide

Crandall DC, Leopold IH. The influence of systemic drugs on tear constituents. *Ophthalmology.* 1979;86:115–125.

Neary D, Thurston H, Pohl JE. Development of extrapyramidal symptoms in hypertensive patients treated with diazoxide. *BMJ.* 1973;3:474–475.

Thomson AE, Nickerson M, Gaskell P, et al. Clinical observations on an antihypertensive chlorothiazide analogue devoid of a diuretic activity. *Can Med Assoc J.* 1962;87:1306–1310.

Guanethidine monosulfate

Cant JS, Lewis DR. Unwanted pharmacological effects of local guanethidine in the treatment of dysthyroid upper lid retraction. *Br J Ophthalmol.* 1969;53:239–245.

Davidson SI. Reports of ocular adverse reactions. *Trans Ophthalmol Soc UK.* 1973;93:495–510.

Gloster J. Guanethidine and glaucoma. *Trans Ophthalmol Soc UK.* 1974;94:573–577.

Hoyng PF, Dake CL. The aqueous humor dynamics and biphasic response to intraocular pressure induced by guanethidine and adrenaline in the glaucomatous eye. *Graefes Arch Clin Exp Ophthalmol.* 1980;214:263–268.

Jones DE, Norton DA, Davies DJ. Control of glaucoma by reduced dosage guanethidine-adrenaline formulation. *Br J Ophthalmol.* 1979;63:813–816.

Krieglstein GK. The uses and side effects of adrenergic drugs in the management of intraocular pressure. In: Drance SM, Neufeld AH, eds. *Glaucoma: Applied Pharmacology in Medical Treatment.* New York: Grune & Stratton; 1984:255–276.

Wright P. Squamous metaplasia or epidermalization of the conjunctiva as an adverse reaction to topical medication. *Trans Ophthalmol Soc UK.* 1979;99:244–246.

Hydralazine hydrochloride

Crandall DC, Leopold IH. The influence of systemic drugs on tear constituents. *Ophthalmology.* 1979;86:115–125.

Doherty M, Maddison PJ, Grey RH. Hydralazine induced lupus syndrome with eye disease. *BMJ.* 1985;290:675.

Johansson M, Manhem P. SLE-syndrome with exophthalmos after treatment with hydralazine. *Lakartidningen.* 1975;72:153.

Mansilla-Tinoco R, Harland SJ, Ryan PJ, et al. Hydralazine, antinuclear antibodies, and the lupus syndrome. *BMJ.* 1982;284:936–939.

Peacock A, Weatherall D. Hydralazine-induced necrotising vasculitis. *BMJ.* 1981;282:1121–1122.

Singh S. Hydralazine-induced lupus. *South Med J.* 2006;99:6–7.

Prazosin hydrochloride

Chin DK, Ho AK, Tse CY. Neuropsychiatric complications related to use of prazosin in patients with renal failure. *BMJ.* 1986;293:1347.

Schachat A. Retrobulbar optic neuropathy associated with prazosin therapy. *Ophthalmology.* 1981;88(suppl 9):97.

Reserpine

Freedman DX, Benton AJ. Persisting effects of reserpine in man. *N Engl J Med.* 1961;264:529–533.

Fuldauer ML. Ocular spasm caused by reserpine. *Ned Tijdschr Geneeskd.* 1959;103:110.

Peczon JD, Grant WM. Sedatives, stimulants and intraocular pressure in glaucoma. *Arch Ophthalmol.* 1964;72:178–188.

Raymond LF. Ocular pathology in reserpine sensitivity: report of two cases. *J Med Soc NJ.* 1963;60:417–419.

Albuterol (salbutamol)

Basoglu OK, Emre S, Bacakoglu F, et al. Glaucoma associated with metered-dose bronchodilator therapy. *Respir Med.* 2001;95:844–845.

Shurman A, Passero MA. Unusual vascular reactions to albuterol. *Arch Intern Med.* 1984;144:1771–1772.

Ipratropium

Bond DW, Vyas H, Venning HE. Mydriasis due to self-administered inhaled ipratropium bromide. *Eur J Pediatr.* 2002;161:178.

Cabana MD, Johnson H, Lee CK, et al. Transient anisocoria secondary to nebulized ipratropium bromide. *Clin Pediatr.* 1999;38:318.

Iosson N. Nebulizer-associated anisocoria. *N Eng J Med.* 2006;354:e8.

Kizer KM, Bess DT, Bedfor N. Blurred vision from ipratropium bromide inhalation. *Am J Health Syst Pharm.* 1999;56:914.

Lust K, Livingstone I. Nebulizer-induced anisocoria. *Ann Intern Med.* 1998;128:327.

Chlorothiazide, hydrochlorothiazide, indapamide, methyclothiazide, metolazone

Beasley FJ. Transient myopia during trichlormethiazide therapy. *Ann Ophthalmol.* 1980;12:705.

Bergmann MT, Newman BL, Johnson Jr NC. The effect of a diuretic (hydrochlorothiazide) on tear production in humans. *Am J Ophthalmol.* 1985;99:473–475.

Blain P, Paques M, Massin P, et al. Acute transient myopia induced by indapamide. *Am J Ophthalmol.* 2000;129:538–540.

Grinbaum A, Ashkenazi I, Avni I. Drug induced myopia associated with treatment for gynecological problems. *Eur J Ophthalmol.* 1995;5(2):136–138.

Jampolsky A, Flom B. Transient myopia associated with anterior displacement of the crystalline lens. *Am J Ophthalmol.* 1953;36:81–89.

Klein BE, Klein R, Jensen SC, et al. Hypertension and lens opacities from the Beaver Dam Eye Study. *Am J Ophthalmol.* 1995;119:640–646.

Palmer FJ. Incidence of chlorthalidone-induced hypercalcemia. *JAMA.* 1978;239:2449.

Robinson HN, Morison WL, Hood AF. Thiazide diuretic therapy and chronic photosensitivity. *Arch Dermatol.* 1985;121:522–524.

Söylev MF, Green RL, Feldon SE. Choroidal effusion as a mechanism for transient myopia induced by hydrochlorothiazide and triamterene. *Am J Ophthalmol.* 1995;120(3):395–397.

Furosemide

Castel T, Gratacos R, Castro J, et al. Bullous pemphigoid induced by furosemide. *Clin Exp Dermatol.* 1981;6:635–638.

Davidson SI. Reports of ocular adverse reactions. *Trans Ophthalmol Soc UK.* 1973;93:495–510.

Peczon JD, Grant WM. Diuretic drugs in glaucoma. *Am J Ophthalmol.* 1968;66:680–683.

Zugerman C, La Voo EJ. Erythema multiforme caused by oral furosemide. *Arch Dermatol.* 1980;116:518–519.

Glycerol (glycerin)

Almog Y, Geyer O, Lazar M. Pulmonary edema as a complication of oral glycerol administration. *Ann Ophthalmol.* 1986;18:38–39.

Chang S, Abramson DH, Coleman DJ. Diabetic ketoacidosis with retinal tear. *Ann Ophthalmol.* 1977;9:1507–1510.

Goldberg MH, Koffler BH, Lemp MA, et al. The effects of topically applied glycerin on the human corneal endothelium. *Cornea.* 1982;1:39.

Hovland KR. Effects of drugs on aqueous humor dynamics. *Int Ophthalmol Clin.* 1971;11(2):99–119.

Mannitol

Chang S, Abramson DH, Coleman DJ. Diabetic ketoacidosis with retinal tear. *Ann Ophthalmol.* 1977;9:1507–1510.

Grabie MT, Gipstein RM, Adams DA, et al. Contraindications for mannitol in aphakic glaucoma. *Am J Ophthalmol.* 1981;91:265–267.

Lamb JD, Keogh JA. Anaphylactoid reaction to mannitol. *Can Anaesth Soc J.* 1979;26:435–436.

Mehra KS, Singh R. Lowering of intraocular pressure by isosorbide. *Arch Ophthalmol.* 1971;86:623–625.

Millay RH, Klein ML, Shults WT, et al. Maculopathy associated with combination chemotherapy and osmotic opening of the blood–brain barrier. *Am J Ophthalmol.* 1986;102:626–632.

Miyake Y, Miyake K, Maekubo K, et al. Increase in aqueous flare by a therapeutic dose of mannitol in humans. *Acts Soc Ophthalmol Jpn.* 1989;93:1149–1153.

Quon DK, Worthen DM. Dose response of intravenous mannitol on the human eye. *Ann Ophthalmol.* 1981;13:1392–1393.

Wood TO, Waltman SR, West C, et al. Effect of isosorbide on intraocular pressure after penetrating keratoplasty. *Am J Ophthalmol.* 1973;75:221–223.

Phenoxybenzamine hydrochloride

Potter DE, Rowland JM. Adrenergic drugs and intraocular pressure. *Gen Pharmacol.* 1981;12:1–13.

Ephedrine sulfate

Crandall DC, Leopold IH. The influence of systemic drugs on tear constituents. *Ophthalmology.* 1979;86:115–125.

Escobar JI, Karno M. Chronic hallucinosis from nasal drops. *JAMA.* 1982;247:1859–1860.

Epinephrine, norepinephrine bitartrate

Bealka N, Schwartz B. Enhanced ocular hypotensive response to epinephrine with prior dexamethasone treatment. *Arch Ophthalmol.* 1991;109:346–348.

Bigger JF. Norepinephrine therapy in patients allergic to or intolerant of epinephrine. *Ann Ophthalmol.* 1979;11:183–186.

Blondeau P, Cote M. Cardiovascular effects of epinephrine and dipivefrin in patients using timolol: a single-dose study. *Can J Ophthalmol.* 1984;19:29–32.

Brummett R. Warning to otolaryngologists using local anesthetics containing epinephrine: potential serious reactions occurring in patients treated with beta-adrenergic receptor blockers. *Arch Otolaryngol.* 1984;110:561.

Camras CB, Feldman SG, Podos SM, et al. Inhibition of the epinephrine-induced reduction of intraocular pressure by systemic indomethacin in humans. *Am J Ophthalmol.* 1985;100:169–175.

Edelhauser HF, Hyndiuk RA, Zeeb A, et al. Corneal edema and the intraocular use of epinephrine. *Am J Ophthalmol.* 1982;93:327–333.

Jay GT, Chow MS. Interaction of epinephrine and β-blockers. *JAMA.* 1995;274(23):1830.

Kacere RD, Dolan JW, Brubaker RF. Intravenous epinephrine stimulates aqueous formation in the human eye. *Invest Ophthalmol Vis Sci.* 1992;33(10):2861–2865.

Kaufman HE. Chemical blepharitis following drug treatment. *Am J Ophthalmol.* 1983;95:703.

Kerr CR, Hass I, Drance SM, et al. Cardiovascular effects of epinephrine and dipivalyl epinephrine applied topically to the eye in patients with glaucoma. *Br J Ophthalmol.* 1982;66:109–114.

Krejci L, Rezek P, Hoskovcova-Krejcova H. Effect of long-term treatment with antiglaucoma drugs on corneal endothelium in patients with congenital glaucoma: contact specular microscopy. *Glaucoma.* 1985;7:81.

Pollack IP, Rossi H. Norepinephrine in the treatment of ocular hypertension and glaucoma. *Arch Ophthalmol.* 1975;93:173–177.

Sasamoto K, Akagi Y, Kodama Y, et al. Corneal endothelial changes caused by ophthalmic drugs. *Cornea.* 1984;3:37–41.

Stewart R, Kimbrough RL, Martin PA, et al. Norepinephrine dipivalylate dose-response in ocular hypertensive subjects. *Ann Ophthalmol.* 1981;13:1279–1283.

Phenylephrine

Fraunfelder FT. Pupil dilation using phenylephrine alone or in combination with tropicamide. *Ophthalmology.* 1999;106(1):4.

Fraunfelder FT, Meyer SM. Possible cardiovascular effects secondary to topical ophthalmic 2.5% phenylephrine. *Am J Ophthalmol.* 1985;99:362–363.

Hanna C, Brainard J, Augspurger KD, et al. Allergic dermatoconjunctivitis caused by phenylephrine. *Am J Ophthalmol.* 1983;95:703–704.

Hermansen MC, Sullivan LS. Feeding intolerance following ophthalmologic examination. *Am J Dis Child.* 1985;139:367–368.

Isenberg SJ, Green BF. Effect of phenylephrine hydrochloride on conjunctival PO_2. *Arch Ophthalmol.* 1984;102:1185–1186.

Kumar SP. Adverse drug reactions in the newborn. *Ann Clin Lab Sci.* 1985;15:195–203.

Kumar V, Packer AJ, Choi WW. Hypertension following phenylephrine 2.5% ophthalmic drops. *Glaucoma.* 1985;7:131.

Kumar V, Schoenwald RD, Chien DS, et al. Systemic absorption and cardiovascular effects of phenylephrine eyedrops. *Am J Ophthalmol.* 1985;99:180–184.

Munden PM, Kardon RH, Denison CE, et al. Palpebral fissure responses to topical adrenergic drugs. *Am J Ophthalmol.* 1991;111:706–710.

Powers JM. Decongestant-induced blepharospasm and orofacial dystonia. *JAMA.* 1982;247:3244–3245.

Rafael M, Pereira F, Faria MA. Allergic contact blepharoconjunctivitis caused by phenylephrine associated with persistent patch test reaction. *Contact Derm.* 1997;39:143–144.

Ramsali MV, Kumar R, Koshy PG, et al. Subarachnoid hemorrhage in a patient following systemic absorption of phenylephrine eye drops. *J Anaesthesiol Clin Pharmacol.* 2018;34(3):423–424.

Resano A, Esteve C, Fernandez Benitez M. Allergic contact blepharoconjunctivitis due to phenylephrine eye drops. *J Invest Allerg Clin Immun.* 1999;9(1):55–57.

Wesley RE. Phenylephrine eyedrops and cardiovascular accidents after fluorescein angiography. *J Ocular Ther Surg.* 1983;2:212.

Whitson JT, Love R, Brown RH, et al. The effect of reduced eyedrop size and eyelid closure on the therapeutic index of phenylephrine. *Am J Ophthalmol.* 1993;115:357–359.

CHAPTER 11

Hormones and Drugs Affecting Hormonal Mechanisms

CLASS: ADRENAL CORTICOSTEROIDS

Generic Names:

1. Adrenal cortex injection; 2. beclomethasone dipropionate; 3. betamethasone dipropionate; 4. budesonide; 5. cortisone acetate; 6. dexamethasone; 7. fludrocortisone acetate; 8. fluorometholone; 9. fluticasone propionate; 10. hydrocortisone; 11. methylprednisolone; 12. prednisolone; 13. prednisone; 14. rimexolone; 15. triamcinolone acetonide.

Proprietary Names:

1. Generic only; 2. Beconase AQ, Qnasl, Qnasl Children's, QVAR; 3. Alphatrex, Beta 1 Kit, Beta Derm, Beta-Val, Betanate, Betatrex, Celestone, Del-Beta, Diprolene, Diprolene AF, Diprosone, Luxiq Foam, Maxivate, RRB Pak, Sernivo, Taclonex, Valisone; 4. Entocort EC, Pulmicort, Pulmicort Flexhaler, Pulmicort Respules, Rhinocort, Rhinocort Aqua, UCERIS; 5. Cortone; 6. AK-Dex, Baycadron, Cushing Syndrome Diagnostic, Decadron, DexPak Jr TaperPak, DexPak TaperPak, DEXYCU, DoubleDex, Hexadrol, Maxidex, Mymethasone, Ozurdex, Simplest Dexamethasone, Solurex, TaperDex, Zema-Pak, ZoDex, ZonaCort 11 Day, ZonaCort 7 Day; 7. Florinef; 8. Flarex, Fluor-Op, FML, FML Forte, FML Forte SOP; 9. ArmonAir RespiClick, Arnuity Ellipta, Cutivate, Flonase, Flonase Allergy Relief, Flonase Sensimist, Flovent Diskus, Flovent HFA, Veramyst, Xhance; 10. A-Hydrocort, Ala-Cort, Ala-Scalp, A-hydrocort, Anucort-HC, Anumed-HC, Anusol HC, Caldecort, Cetacort, Colocort, Cortaid, Cortaid Advanced, Cortaid Intensive Therapy, Cortalo, Cortef, Cortenema, Corticaine, Corticool, Cortifoam, Cortizone, Cortizone-10, Cortizone-10 Cooling Relief, Cortizone-10 Intensive Healing, Cortizone-10 Plus, Dermarest, Dricort, Dermarest Eczema, Encort, First-Hydrocortisone, Gly-Cort, GRx HiCort, Hemmorex-HC, Hemorrhoidal-HC, Hemril, Hi-Cor, Hycort, Hydro Skin, Hydrocortisone in Absorbase, Hydrocortone, Hydroskin, Hytone, Instacort, Lacticare HC, Locoid, Locoid Lipocream, MiCort-HC, Monistat Complete Care Instant Itch Relief Cream, Neosporin Eczema, NuCort, Nutracort, NuZon, Orabase HCA, Pandel, Penecort, Preparation H Hydrocortisone, Procto-Kit, Procto-Med HC, Procto-Pak, Protocort, Protocream-HC, Proctosert HC, Proctosol-HC, Protozone-HC, Rectacort HC, Rectasol-HC, Rederm, Sarnol-HC, Scalacort, Scalpicin Anti-Itch, Sitecort, Solu-Cortef, Sul-Cortef, Synacort, Texacort, Tucks HC, U-cort, Walgreens Intensive Healing, Westcort; 11. A-Methapred, Depmedalone-40, Depmedalone-80, Depo-Medrol, Medrol, Medrol Dosepak, Solu-Medrol; 12. AK-Pred, AsmallPred, Enconopred Plus; Inflamase Forte, Inflamase Mild, Medrol, Millipred, Millipred DP, Millipred DP 12-Day, Millipred DP 6 Day, Ocu-Pred A, Ocu-Pred Forte, Omnipred, Orapred, Orapred ODT, Pediapred, Pred Mild, Pred-Forte, Pred-Phosphate, Prednoral, Prelone, Veripred-20; 13. Deltasone, Predone, RAYOS, Sterapred, Sterapred DS; 14. Vexol; 15. Allernaze, Aristocort, Aristocort A, Aristocort HP, Aristospan, Arze-Ject-A, Azmacort, Cinalog, Cinolar, Flutex, Kenalog, Kenalog 10, Kenalog 40, Kenalog in Orabase, Nasocort, Nasocort AQ, Nasocort HFA, Oracort, Oralone, Pediaderm TA, Triacet, Triderm, Triamonide, Trianex, Triderm, Triesence, Zilretta.

Primary Use

Systemic

These corticosteroids are effective in the replacement therapy of adrenocortical insufficiency and in the treatment of inflammatory and allergic disorders. Nasal exhalation delivery systems (EDS) are used in the prophylaxis of asthma, allergic rhinitis, and nasal polyps.

Topical

These corticosteroids are effective for the relief of inflammatory and pruritic dermatoses.

Ophthalmic

Used in the treatment of ocular inflammatory and allergic disorders.

Ocular Side Effects
Systemic administration – articular, auricular, intramuscular, intravenous, nasal, oral, or rectal
Certain
1. Decreased vision
2. Posterior subcapsular cataracts (early – may be reversible)
3. Increased intraocular pressure
4. Decreased resistance to infection
5. Mydriasis – may precipitate acute glaucoma
6. Myopia
7. Exophthalmos
8. Papilledema secondary to pseudotumor cerebri
   a. Secondary to the drug
   b. Secondary to drug withdrawal
9. Myasthenic neuromuscular-blocking effect
   a. Diplopia
   b. Ptosis
   c. Paresis of extraocular muscles
10. Color vision defect
11. Delayed wound healing
12. Visual fields
    a. Scotomas
    b. Constriction
    c. Enlarged blind spot
    d. Glaucoma field defect
13. Visual hallucinations
14. Abnormal electroretinogram (ERG) or visual evoked potential (VEP)
15. Retina
    a. Edema
    b. Hemorrhage
    c. Central serous retinopathy
16. Translucent blue sclera
17. Eyelids or conjunctiva
    a. Hyperemia
    b. Edema
    c. "Rosacea-like" skin changes
18. Microcyst – nonpigment epithelium of ciliary body and pigment epithelium of iris
19. Subconjunctival hemorrhages
20. Decreased tear lysozymes
21. Toxic amblyopia
22. Retinopathy of prematurity – may increase

Possible
1. Eyelids or conjunctiva – Lyell syndrome
2. Permanent vision loss
3. Decreased risk of retinopathy of prematurity

Systemic administration – inhalant or topical
Certain
1. Increased intraocular pressure
2. Decreased resistance to infection
3. Eyelids or conjunctiva
   a. Photosensitivity
   b. Urticaria
   c. Purpura
   d. Telangiectasia
   e. Depigmentation
   f. Skin atrophy
4. Papilledema secondary to pseudotumor cerebri
5. Cataracts

Possible
1. May aggravate or cause ocular sicca

Local ophthalmic use or exposure – intralesional, retrobulbar injection, subconjunctival injection, subcutaneous injection, or topical ocular application
Certain
1. Increased intraocular pressure
2. Decreased resistance to infection
3. Delayed wound healing
4. Mydriasis – may precipitate acute glaucoma
5. Posterior subcapsular cataracts
6. Decreased vision
7. Enhances lytic action of collagenase
8. Decreased accommodation
9. Visual fields
   a. Scotomas
   b. Constriction
   c. Enlarged blind spot
   d. Glaucoma field defect
10. Color vision defect – colored haloes around lights
11. Eyelids or conjunctiva
    a. Allergic reactions
    b. Persistent erythema
    c. Hyperemia
    d. Telangiectasia
    e. Depigmentation
    f. Poliosis
    g. Scarring (subconjunctival injection)
    h. Fat atrophy (retrobulbar or subcutaneous injection)
    i. Skin atrophy (subcutaneous injection)
    j. Necrosis (subconjunctival injection)
    k. Ptosis (subconjunctival injection)
    l. Ulceration (subconjunctival injection)

12. Cornea
    a. Punctate keratitis
    b. Superficial corneal deposits
    c. Thickness – increase initially and then decrease
13. Irritation
    a. Lacrimation
    b. Photophobia
    c. Pain
    d. Burning sensation
    e. Anterior uveitis
14. Scleral
    a. Thickness
        i. Increased – initial
        ii. Decreased
    b. Blue color – transient
15. Central serous retinopathy
16. Proptosis (retrobulbar injections)
17. Granulomas
18. May aggravate the following diseases
    a. Herpes simplex
    b. Bacterial infection
    c. Fungal infections
    d. Scleromalacia perforans
    e. Corneal "melting" diseases
    f. Behçet disease
    g. Eales disease
    h. Presumptive ocular toxoplasmosis
    i. Facultative intraocular pathogens
19. Retinal embolic phenomenon

Probable
1. Cushing syndrome

Possible
1. Scleritis
2. May aggravate or cause ocular sicca

Local ophthalmic use or exposure – intraocular injection
Certain
1. Pain
2. Decreased vision
3. Cataracts
    a. Subcapsular
    b. All layers of the lens
4. Intraocular pressure
    a. Increased – initial
    b. Decreased
5. Retina
    a. Hemorrhage
    b. Degeneration

c. Necrosis
6. Ascending optic atrophy
7. Toxic amblyopia
8. Global atrophy
9. Endophthalmitis
    a. Sterile
    b. Enhances latent infections
    c. Pseudohypopyon (crystalline drug deposition)

Local ophthalmic use or exposure – intravitreal injection or periocular injection
Certain
1. Increased intraocular pressure
2. Decreased resistance to infection
3. Delayed wound healing
4. Mydriasis – may precipitate acute glaucoma
5. Posterior subcapsular cataracts
6. Decreased vision
7. Enhances lytic action of collagenase
8. Decreased accommodation
9. Visual fields
    a. Scotomas
    b. Constriction
    c. Enlarged blind spot
    d. Glaucoma field defect
10. Color vision defect – colored haloes around lights
11. Eyelids or conjunctiva
    a. Allergic reactions
    b. Persistent erythema
    c. Hyperemia
    d. Telangiectasia
    e. Depigmentation
    f. Poliosis
    g. Scarring
    h. Fat atrophy
    i. Skin atrophy
    j. Necrosis
    k. Ptosis (periocular injection)
12. Cornea
    a. Punctate keratitis
    b. Superficial corneal deposits
    c. Thickness – increases initially and then decreases
13. Irritation
    a. Lacrimation
    b. Photophobia
    c. Pain
    d. Burning sensation
    e. Anterior uveitis

14. Scleral
    a. Thickness
        i. Increased – initial
        ii. Decreased
    b. Blue color – transient
15. Toxic amblyopia
16. Granulomas
17. May aggravate the following diseases
    a. Herpes simplex
    b. Bacterial infections
    c. Fungal infections
    d. Scleromalacia perforans
    e. Corneal "melting" diseases
    f. Behçet disease
    g. Eales disease
    h. Presumptive ocular toxoplasmosis
    i. Enhances facultative intraocular pathogens
    j. Diabetes (periocular injection)
18. Retinal embolic phenomenon
19. Migration of injection into anterior chamber from vitreous
20. Crystalline maculopathy – triamcinolone insoluble crystals (intravitreal injection)

Ocular teratogenic effects
Certain
1. Cataracts

Clinical Significance
This group of medicines is one of the most commonly used in all of ophthalmology. There are over 1500 publications on ocular and periocular steroid complications, and these data alone could fill a textbook. This section is only a brief and incomplete review. Steroid ocular side effects may vary with age (younger lenses being more susceptible to changes), type of steroid (fluorinated compounds), increased fat atrophy, race (glaucoma is more common in Caucasians), and method of delivery (injections have a higher localized drug concentration, so there is an increased frequency and severity of local adverse events).

A large study clearly showed that oral and nasal spray steroids cause a statistically significant increase in cataract surgery in the elderly.[1] This study infers that we significantly underestimate the importance of steroids as a cofactor in cataractogenesis. Smeeth et al confirmed that high-dose inhaled steroids are associated with an increased risk of lens changes.[2] Jick et al, in a retrospective observational cohort study, found that in individuals above the age of 40 years old there was an increased risk of cataracts with inhaled steroids.[3] Wang et al, in a population-based cohort study over a

10-year period, found the same.[4] Lipworth found that although all inhaled steroids had increased risks of systemic side effects, fluticasone propionate exhibits greater dose-related systemic bioavailability, particularity at doses above 0.8 µg/dL.[5] All forms of drug delivery and methods of administration are associated with lens changes if the drug gets into the eye. It has been shown that 50% of patients using 800 drops of topical ocular 0.1% dexamethasone will develop some lens changes. Generally, steroid-induced posterior subcapsular cataracts are irreversible, but reversibility of cataracts in some early systemic steroid-induced changes of lenses, i.e. nephritic children, is possible. Cekiç et al have shown that single intravitreal triamcinolone injections can produce posterior subcapsular cataracts, whereas multiple injections result in all layers of the lens having opacity progression.[6] Thompson reported posterior subcapsular cataracts in 50% of patients; these are visually significant after 1 year with repeat intravitreal triamcinolone injections.[7]

Topical ocular corticosteroid-induced glaucoma may take a number of weeks to develop, and this occurs in about one-third of individuals. However, almost all those who are exposed to higher doses of topical ocular corticosteroids will develop some elevation in intraocular pressure if the drug is continued for more than 12 months. Inhaled steroids can cause or aggravate open-angle glaucoma, especially in patients with a family history of glaucoma.[8] Reports on various methods of injection, i.e. periorbital, intravitreal, and a host of others, confirm a strong association of injected corticosteroids with glaucoma.[9–11] Ideta et al reported permanent ptosis after a subtenon injection of triamcinolone.[12] Intractable glaucoma after intravitreal triamcinolone injections has been well documented.[13,14] Early, rapid rise of intraocular pressure may occur or be delayed even after more than 3 months.[14,15] Although individual variation to steroid exposure may be marked, steroid responders with elevated intraocular pressure secondary to topical ocular corticosteroids have more field loss than steroid nonresponders. Steroid-induced glaucoma patients will usually return to normal pressures after the drug is stopped. If optic damage has occurred, these patients can be confused easily with low-tension glaucoma patients. Rimexolone, a more recent topical ocular steroid, has the anti-inflammatory properties of the more potent steroids, but the glaucoma-inducing potential of midrange steroids, such as fluorometholone.[16]

Bangsgaard et al found that two-thirds of infants treated with standard glucocorticoid topical ocular protocols after congenital cataract surgery showed adrenal suppression.[17] This was directly associated with cumulative daily dosage of the eye drops. They recommended systemic assessment of adrenal function of those infants. Fatal complications have occurred.[18] Significant risk of adrenal axis suppression may occur.[19-21] Especially in younger individuals, care must be exercised as to the amount prescribed. Infants are the most vulnerable. Batton et al and Ehrenkranz felt there may be an association between increased retinopathy of prematurity and steroid exposure in infants.[22,23] The withdrawal of steroids can cause significant adverse effects in children, such as pseudotumor cerebri with severe visual loss after withdrawal.[24] Liu et al reported this reaction in adults as well.[25] Romano et al pointed out that primarily in infants and young children, periocular injections or topical ocular steroids in high dosages can cause severe systemic reactions of hypertension, Cushing syndrome, hypertensive encephalopathy, and death.[26,27]

The recent popularity of subconjunctival injections of steroids has been accompanied by additional ocular drug reactions. Subconjunctival injections of steroids placed over a diseased cornea or sclera can cause a thinning, and possibly a rupture, at the site of the injection. Zamir et al and Albini et al have shown that subconjunctival steroids in non-necrotizing anterior scleritis appear to be safe.[28,29] Periocular injections may produce sclerosing lipogranuloma.[30] Posterior subtenon injections may cause ptosis associated with orbital fat prolapse, cutaneous hypopigmentation, or retinal or choroidal vascular occlusion.[31-33] Feldman-Billard et al reported on a series of 25 patients with type 2 diabetes receiving subconjunctival or peribulbar injections of dexamethasone and found that this may induce a median doubling from baseline followed by a decrease in their blood glucose around 6 hours postinjection.[34] Intractable glaucoma can occur after subconjunctival depo-injections of steroids. The surgical removal of the steroids may be required to normalize the ocular pressure. Inadvertent intraocular steroid injections have caused blindness. This is probably due to the drug vehicle. Inadvertent intraocular depot injections are numerous and include a significant toxicity vehicle and the prolonged release of the steroid. Although triamcinolone acetonide appears to be the least toxic of the steroid medications with inadvertent vitreous injections, often vitrectomy is required to remove the depot steroid, prevent tract bands, and examine the penetration site. Pendergast et al reported a case of inadvertent depot betamethasone acetate and methasone sodium phosphate preserved with benzalkonium chloride that caused severe intraocular damage.[35] They felt that the preservative was the reason for the ocular changes. Some topical ocular steroids use benzalkonium chloride as a preservative, and it is contraindicated in contact lens wearers. The removal of depo steroids accidentally injected into the vitreous may be considered an emergency procedure. Keeping the patient prone before surgery to prevent the material from coming into contact with the macula is important.

Intravitreal triamcinolone is in common usage, and, especially in vitrectomized eyes, acute cluster or sediment will collect, especially in the posterior pole. These invariably resolve within a few months. Sarraf et al reported 13 patients (21 eyes) with insoluble triamcinolone components after triamcinolone intravitreal injections.[36] The crystal, although predominantly white, may be multicolored and on the superficial retinas, usually in the posterior pole, without obvious decrease in vision or retinal sequelae.

Multiple authors have implicated corticosteroids as causative factors in patients with central serous chorioretinopathy.[37,38] Nicholson et al, in a major review paper, concluded that the preponderance of the literature supports the existence of an association between glucocorticoids and central serous chorioretinopathy.[39] This may occur from oral, intranasal sprays, or intrajoint injections.[38,40] Carvalho-Recchia et al did a prospective case-controlled study that identified corticosteroids as significant risk factors for the development of acute exudative maculopathy.[41] Systemic steroids have been implicated in causing central serous chorioretinopathy when injected intravenously or epidurally.[42-44] In a retrospective population-based cohort study, the incidence of central serous chorioretinopathy per 10,000 person-years was 3.5 for those exposed to steroids (any method including ocular) versus 2.5 for the control group that was never exposed to steroids.[45] Steroids effect changes in almost all ocular structures. This has been reconfirmed by showing that steroids can cause microcysts of the iris pigment epithelium and of the ciliary body nonpigment epithelium. Corticosteroids have been implicated in causing an increased incidence of all forms of uveitis and endophthalmitis.[46,47]

The time required for onset of a major adverse effect from topical ocular steroids varies greatly. Effects to enhance epithelial herpes simplex may be days, whereas it may take years for posterior subcapsular cataracts to develop. Taravella et al have shown that topical ocular phosphate preparations can cause corneal band keratopathy, especially in patients with sicca.[48] Huige et al stated that topical ocular beta blockers enhance superficial stromal deposits of the phosphated forms of steroid eye drops.[49]

Fluticasone propionate is used as a new form of positive pressure delivery system (Optinose Exhalation Delivery System) that, in rare cases, may blow the drug and nasal contents up through the nasal lacrimal systems. Spontaneous reports suggest that if this goes unrecognized, it can lead to any side effects of topical ocular corticosteroids.

CLASS: ANDROGENS

Generic Name:
Danazol.

Proprietary Name:
Danocrine.

Primary Use
This synthetic androgen is used to treat pelvic endometriosis, fibrocystic breast disease, and hereditary angioedema.

Ocular Side Effects
Systemic administration – oral
Certain
1. Decreased vision
2. Eyelids or conjunctiva
   a. Erythema
   b. Edema
   c. Photosensitivity
   d. Urticaria
   e. Purpura
   f. Loss of eyelashes or eyebrows

Probable
1. Optic nerve
   a. Papilledema secondary to pseudotumor cerebri
   b. Pallor
   c. Atrophy
2. Visual field defects
3. Diplopia

Conditional/unclassified
1. Cataracts

Clinical Significance
Decreased vision, usually associated with headaches, is the most frequent ocular side effect reported secondary to danazol. This is reversible and may resolve while continuing to take the drug. There are multiple cases of pseudotumor cerebri with papilledema associated with this drug that were either published or in the spontaneous reports.[1,2] Only recently has a black box warning

been issued by the manufacturer.[3] Pseudotumor cerebri may occur while taking this medication or shortly after stopping it.[4-7] Causation is unknown, but may be due to danazol-induced weight gain, fluid retention, or cerebral venous thrombosis. There are not enough data to prove a positive association, but it seems probable. Presenile cataracts in young women treated with danazol have been found also in the absence of predisposed risk factors, but this is unsubstantiated.[8]

Generic Name:
Finasteride.

Proprietary Names:
Propecia, Proscar.

Primary Use
This synthetic analog of a gonadotropin-releasing hormone is given orally for the treatment of male pattern baldness.

Ocular Side Effects
Systemic administration – oral
Certain
1. Decreased vision
2. Pain
3. Tear film
   a. Increased debris
   b. Abnormal tear meniscus – decreased, irregular
   c. Tear film break-up time – decreased
4. Eyelids
   a. Edema
   b. Injection
   c. Metaplasia meibomian gland orifices
   d. Lipid secretion abnormal

Probable
1. Intraoperative floppy iris syndrome (IFIS)
2. May aggravate or cause ocular sicca

Conditional/unclassified
1. Retinal vascular accidents
2. Central serous macular edema
3. Anterior subcapsular cataracts

Clinical Significance
Recently finasteride has been added to the list of probable risk factors for causing IFIS.[1] Issa et al were the first to recognize this association, followed by Wong et al and Chatziralli et al.[1-4] These data all came from retrospective studies and therefore may require more confirmation.

Finasteride, like all antiandrogen drugs, has been shown to cause changes in the human meibomian gland and ocular surface. Krenzer et al showed that patients taking antiandrogen treatment compared with age-related controls had increased tear film debris, abnormal tear meniscus, irregular posterior lid margins, conjunctival tarsal injection, and orifice metaplasia of the meibomian gland and abnormal secretions.[5] They also noted increased tear film break-up times with increased light sensitivity, ocular pain, and decreased vision. This drug can probably cause ocular sicca. The second most commonly reported adverse ocular side effect in the spontaneous reports is ocular sicca, and it has been confirmed animal models.[6] However, there is no mention of this in the manufacturer's clinical trials.[7] Krenzer et al and Check et al have both suggested this as an ocular side effect of finasteride.[5,8]

Finasteride has been implicated in systemic vascular incidents, and a few reports implicate the eye, including central serous macular edema.[9] There have been 2 reports of bilateral anterior subcapsular cataracts.[3,10]

Generic Name:

Leuprolide acetate (leuprorelin acetate).

Proprietary Names:

Eligard, Lupron, Lupron Depot, Lupron Depot-3, Lupron Depot-4, Lupron Depot-Ped, Viadur.

Primary Use

This synthetic analog of a gonadotrophin-releasing hormone is used in the management of sterility, endometriosis, precocious puberty, or prostatic cancer.

Ocular Side Effects
Systemic administration – intramuscular or subcutaneous
Probable
1. Decreased vision
2. Pain
3. May aggravate or cause ocular sicca
4. Tear film
   a. Increased debris
   b. Abnormal tear meniscus – decreased, irregular
   c. Tear film break-up time – decreased
5. Eyelids
   a. Edema
   b. Injection
   c. Metaplasia meibomian gland orifices
   d. Lipid secretion abnormal

6. Visual hallucinations

Possible
1. Papilledema – pseudotumor cerebri
2. Retina
   a. Branch vein occlusions
   b. Retinal hemorrhage
3. Ptosis

Clinical Significance

Leuprorelin, like all antiandrogen drugs, has been shown to cause changes in the human meibomian gland and ocular surface. Krenzer et al showed that patients taking antiandrogen treatment compared with age-related controls had increased tear film debris, abnormal tear meniscus, irregular posterior lid margins, conjunctival tarsal injection, and orifice metaplasia of the meibomian gland with abnormal secretions.[1] They also noted increased tear film break-up times with increased light sensitivity, ocular pain, and decreased vision. This drug may cause ocular sicca with an incidence of up to 5%.[2]

The most common adverse ocular event associated with leuprorelin acetate is decreased vision.[3] In about half of the cases, this may be associated with headaches or dizziness that may occur after each injection of the drug. These symptoms occur shortly after drug administration and rarely last more than 1–2 hours. There are rare instances of decreased vision lasting 2–3 weeks. Pseudotumor cerebri has also been seen with this drug, but a direct cause-and-effect relationship has not been established. If pseudotumor cerebri occurs while the patient is receiving leuprorelin, the decision to discontinue the drug may be based on the response of the pseudotumor cerebri to therapy, the severity of the pseudotumor cerebri, and the severity of the underlying disease. Leuprorelin has been reported to be associated with thromboembolic phenomena, intraocular branch vein occlusion, or hemorrhages, but there are no firm data. Ocular pain and lid edema may be drug related because these have been seen elsewhere in the body due to this drug.

CLASS: ANTITHYROID DRUGS

Generic Names:

1. Iodide and iodine solutions and compounds; 2. radioactive iodine 125 and 131.

Proprietary Names:

1. Iodopen, Iodotope, Pima, SSKI; 2. Iodine-125, I-131.

Primary Use

Systemic

Iodide and iodine solutions and compounds are effective in the diagnosis and management of thyroid disease. They are also effective in the short-term management of respiratory tract disease and, in some instances, of fungal infections.

Ophthalmic

Topical iodide solutions are used primarily as antiseptics or chemical cautery in the treatment of herpes simplex.

Ocular Side Effects

Systemic administration – oral

Certain

1. Irritation
   a. Lacrimation
   b. Pain
   c. Burning sensation
2. Eyelids or conjunctiva
   a. Allergic reactions
   b. Hyperemia
   c. Conjunctivitis – nonspecific
   d. Edema
   e. Urticaria
   f. Nodules
3. Decreased vision

Possible (most secondary to severe allergic reactions or thyroid damage)

1. May aggravate or cause ocular sicca
2. Punctate keratitis
3. Exophthalmos
4. Hemorrhagic iritis
5. Keratoconus

Systemic administration – intravenous

Certain

1. Lacrimal system
   a. Obstruction
   b. May aggravate or cause ocular sicca
   c. Lacrimal gland dysfunction
2. Hypothyroidism – Graves' disease

Probable

1. Color vision defect – objects have green tinge

2. Visual hallucinations
3. Those mentioned for oral administration

Local ophthalmic use or exposure – topical ocular application

Certain

1. Decreased vision
2. Eyelids or conjunctiva
   a. Allergic reactions
   b. Blepharoconjunctivitis
   c. Edema
   d. Urticaria
3. Irritation
   a. Lacrimation
   b. Hyperemia
   c. Pain
   d. Edema
4. Brown corneal discoloration – transitory
5. Corneal vascularization
6. Stromal scarring
7. Delayed corneal wound healing

Possible

1. Keratitis bullosa

Clinical Significance

Iodines are used in many compounds and in many therapeutic and diagnostic procedures; therefore the information presented here is incomplete.

For oral solutions the most significant ophthalmic reaction may be the sudden onset of an acute allergic reaction affecting the eyes and periocular tissue. They may occur at small doses, with responses occurring within minutes. A delayed hypersensitivity reaction may also occur, causing iododerma with tender pustules, vesicles, and nodular eyelid lesions. This reaction may be associated with ocular irritation with epiphora, followed by ocular sicca, hemorrhagic iritis, and even vitreous opacities.

Ocular side effects due to intravenous iodides vary if used in contrast medium versus radioactive iodine for thyroid or cancer abolition. Contrast medium reactions other than allergic reactions include mild transitory ocular irritants (acute or delayed) or secondary ocular effects from Graves' disease, which are rarely a problem. Radioactive solutions may cause more permanent side effects, such as permanent lacrimal obstruction and ocular sicca. Intravenous I-131 can cause permanent obstruction of the lacrimal outflow system.[1-3] Burns et al felt that this occurred at 3.4% incidence and 4.6% documented or suspected incidences.[4] They felt that both of these percentages may be low. This may also involve salivary gland dysfunction.[5] Kloos et al pointed out that I-131 may aggravate ocular sicca.[6] When I-131 is given intravenously, this concentrates in the lacrimal sac; if concentrations are high enough, this may cause partial or complete obstruction. Radiation may also cause Graves' disease.[7,8] Radioactive plaques on the eye can cause expected destructive complications. Lee et al and Thanos et al suggested the possibility that drug-induced hypothyroidism may induce keratoconus.[9,10]

CLASS: ERECTILE DYSFUNCTION DRUGS

Generic Names:
1. Sildenafil citrate; 2. tadalafil; 3. vardenafil hydrochloride.

Proprietary Names:
1. Revatio, Viagra; 2. Adcirca, Cialis; 3. Levitra, Staxyn.

Primary Use
These phosphodiesterase-5 (PDE5) inhibitors are used for erectile dysfunction (ED). Very high dosages of these drugs are also used in the management of pulmonary hypertension.

Ocular Side Effects
Systemic administration – oral
Certain
1. Color vision defect
   a. Objects have colored tinges – usually blue or blue-green, may be pink or yellow
   b. Dark colors appear darker
   c. Increased perception of brightness
   d. Flashing lights – especially when blinking
2. Decreased vision - central haze (transitory)
3. Electroretinogram (ERG) changes
4. Conjunctival hyperemia
5. Pain
6. Photophobia
7. Subconjunctival hemorrhage
8. Blood flow – increase
   a. Choroid
   b. Retina
9. Choroidal thickness – increase

Probable
1. Nonarteritic ischemic optic neuropathy (NAION)
2. Eyelid edema

Possible
1. Central serous macular edema

Conditional/unclassified
1. Retinal vascular accidents
2. Ocular rosacea
3. Outer macular atrophy

Clinical Significance
Sildenafil has been studied far more extensively than tadalafil and vardenafil. In premarketing clinical trials, all 3 drugs have a similar incidence of visual side effects, and all were proven transitory, except possibly NAION. Sildenafil has been one of the largest-selling prescription drugs in the world. The ocular side effects most commonly associated with sildenafil are a transitory bluish tinge to objects, hypersensitivity to light, and minimal hazy vision. These reversible side effects may last from a few minutes to hours, depending on drug dosage. Visual changes are seen in approximately 3% of men taking the standard 50 mg dose and 11% of men taking 100 mg, with the incidence rising to 40% at a dose of 200 mg. At 4 times the recommended dose (200 mg) sildenafil causes minimal reversible ERG changes in b2-wave amplitude, both in phototopic and scotopic conditions, but with a less than 10% decrease in photopic implicit times in a- and b-waves. However, at normal dosage, a multicenter well-designed study showed no ERG-related findings associated with daily administration of sildenafil or tadalafil over a 6-month period.[1] Conjunctival hyperemia, ocular pain, and photophobia may occur.

Postmarketing case reports of NAION in association with PDE5 inhibitor use have raised the possibility of irreversible effects on the optic nerve. NAION is a rare event, probably caused by optic nerve hypoperfusion and infarction.[2] Individuals with a crowded optic nerve (a low cup-to-disc ratio) may be more susceptible to NAION than those with a normal cup-to-disc ratio. NAION usually presents as sudden, painless, partial unilateral vision loss, most often evident upon awakening. The degree of visual loss is variable, but usually remains static after 1–2 months. No therapy of value has been identified. Risk factors present in men receiving ED drugs are also common risk factors for NAION, including age over 50 years, diabetes, hypertension, and high lipid levels.

The US Food and Drug Administration asked manufacturers of ED drugs to address the limitations of existing data by conducting postmarketing observational phase IV studies to evaluate whether PDE5 inhibitors are associated with an increased risk of NAION. Campbell et al reported the results of the data from the Pfizer postmarketing study.[3] Data were collected on over

600 potential NAION cases from 102 ophthalmologic centers in the United States and Europe. In 81 cases, PDE5 inhibitor use had occurred within 2 months of NAION. An expert advocating committee conducted a blind review of patient records and concluded that PDE5 inhibitor use is associated with twofold increased risk of acute NAION within 5 half-lives of PDE5 inhibitor exposure. PDE5 inhibitor exposure is estimated to add 3 NAION cases per 100,000 men 50 years or older annually, giving an upper bound of 34 additional cases annually in the same population.

This large observational study is the first to provide an estimate of the risk of NAION with PDE5 inhibitors. Based on the variability in NAION severity, the risk–benefit ratio is small. Pomeranz has best summarized this complex subject with his recent publication.[4]

There are 10 published cases of macular edema and another 7 cases in the spontaneous reports.[5-10] Four of these cases have positive rechallenge of serous macular edema associated with ED drugs at normal or elevated dosages. Included are cases of chronic macular edema, which would not resolve until the drug was stopped. In total there are now some 50 cases of retinal or macular edema in the literature and spontaneous reports.[11,12] Although these data are interesting, the nature of non–drug-induced serous macular edema is recurrent and transitory. Further data are necessary; however, a few cases are suggestive, such as Aliferis et al with challenge-rechallenge data.[13] The French et al case-control study of 111 men 59 years old and younger had no increased central serous choroidopathy versus the controls.[14]

Multiple reports of retinal vascular accidents associated with the use of these drugs are given in the spontaneous reports. Because this is not an uncommon finding in elderly patients, a positive association is not possible. Murthy et al felt that tadalafil may have precipitated bilateral, concurrent central retinal artery occlusion in a patient with sickle cell disease.[15]

Gerometta et al showed a transient increase of intraocular pressure after taking sildenafil.[16] Harris et al reviewed all studies of ocular blood flow with this class of drugs.[17] Most studies have suggested an increase in choroidal blood flow with a lesser effect in the retina. Vance et al documented an increase in choroidal thickness.[18] Ioannides et al reported 10 cases of acne rosacea in patients taking these drugs.[19]

Very high dosages of this class of drugs are used in the management of pulmonary hypertension. Matieli et al reported that one-third of study patients had significant bilateral keratitis, which goes with the basic disease, but in this case-controlled study, it was aggravated by sildenafil.[20] The resistance index of the central retinal artery was diminished in the chronic users of sildenafil, which they attributed to choroidal vasodilation. Sajjad et al reported a single case involving a 32-year-old female with permanent visual loss due to bilateral outer macular atrophy.[21] She was on high-dose sildenafil for 5 years for pulmonary hypertension. This is the first report of this kind with no other cases in the spontaneous reports.

Kim et al studied the toxic retinal effects of sildenafil with full-field ERG (ffERG) and multifocal ERG.[22] They found decreased ffERG and multifocal ERG responses, especially in the macular area and with cone function. Although toxic effects were recorded, the changes were reversible, and electrophysiologic parameters were restored in 12 months. Vergis et al reported a patient with signs of retinitis pigmentosa and rapid vison loss who had been placed on high doses of tadalafil for pulmonary fibrosis.[23] There are, however, a number of studies following patients on these drugs long term or in a 3-month, double-blind, crossover study (20–80 mg tid sildenafil for pulmonary arterial hypertension versus placebo) that had complete ophthalmic examinations, including contrast sensitivity, visual fields, and color vision, and showed no permanent adverse ocular effects.[24]

Chandeclerc et al described a patient with multiple positive rechallenges of lower eyelid edema and conjunctival hyperemia, mainly in the morning, without vision loss, after taking tadalafil.[25] There are 93 cases in the spontaneous reports of eyelid edema or eye swelling.

Recommendations

1. Advise patient to stop use of all PDE5 inhibitors and to seek medical attention in the event of sudden loss of vision in 1 or both eyes. Even a transitory decrease in vision other than a mild haze should be a warning that an additional dose may cause a significant vascular ocular event.

2. Discuss with patient the possible increased risk of NAION in those who have already experienced NAION in 1 eye, with the recommendation not to take this class of drugs.

3. Most reported cases of drug-related NAION have had a small cup-to-disc ratio. It is not necessary to screen patients for this before starting these drugs.

4. Until more data are available, we do not feel informed consent is necessary.

5. In any patient on this class of drugs who develops idiopathic serous macular edema, one should be aware that if this does not resolve on its own, one may consider stopping these drugs to see if there is an association.

CLASS: ESTROGENS AND PROGESTOGENS

Generic Names:
1. Combination products of estrogens and progestogens; 2. medroxyprogesterone acetate.

Proprietary Names:
1. Allesse, Aranelle, Aviane-28, Balziva-21, Brevicon-28, Cenestin, Cyclessa, Cryselle, Delestrogen, Demulen, Desogen, Diane 35, Enjuvia, Enpresse-28, Estrostep FE, Femhrt, Gencept 10, Junel, Junel FE, Kariva, Kelnor, Lessina-28, Levora, Loestrin 21/24, Loestrin FE, Lo/orval-28, Low-ogestrel-21, Menest, Microgestrin FE, Mircette, Norethin, Norinyl, Nortdette-28, Nortrel, Nuvaring, Ogestrel, Ortho-cept, Ortho-cyclen, Ortho-Evra, Ortho-Novum, Ortho-Novum 77, Ortho-Tricyclen, Ortho-Tricyclenlo, Ovcon-35/50, Ovral birth control, Portia-28, Premarin, Previfem, Seasonale, Seasonique, Select, Sprintec, Trinorinyl-28, Triphasil, Triprevifem, Tri-Sprintec, Trivara-28, Velivet, Yasmin 28, Yaz, Zovia; 2. Amen, Depo-Provera, Depo-subQ Provera 104, Prempro/Premphase, Provera.

Primary Use
These hormonal drugs are most commonly used as oral contraceptives. They are also used in the treatment of amenorrhea, dysfunctional uterine bleeding, premenstrual tension, dysmenorrhea, and hypogonadism.

Ocular Side Effects
Systemic administration – intramuscular, intravenous, oral, subcutaneous, or vaginal
Certain
1. Decreased vision
2. Decreased contact lens tolerance
   a. Meibomian gland dysfunction
   b. May aggravate or cause ocular sicca
   c. Mucus changes
3. Color vision defect
   a. Red-green or yellow-blue defect
   b. Objects have blue tinge
   c. Colored haloes around lights – mainly blue
4. Eyelids or conjunctiva
   a. Allergic reactions
   b. Edema
   c. Hyperpigmentation
   d. Photosensitivity
   e. Urticaria
5. Cornea
   a. Steeping of curvature
   b. Fluctuation in thickness

Probable
1. Retinal vascular disorders
   a. Occlusion
   b. Thrombosis
   c. Hemorrhage (Fig. 11.1)
   d. Retinal edema
2. Decreased accommodation (diethylstilbestrol)
3. Macula
   a. Edema
   b. Thickness decreased
   c. Volume decreased
4. Cornea – copper deposit Descemet-endothelial area
5. Cataracts
6. Papilledema secondary pseudotumor cerebri

Possible
1. Retinal vascular disorders
   a. Acute macular neuroretinopathy (cofactor)
   b. Periphlebitis
2. Increased ocular mucus
3. Optic neuritis
4. Eyelids or conjunctiva
   a. Lupoid syndrome
   b. Erythema multiforme
5. Intraocular pressure in females
   a. Increase
   b. Decrease

Clinical Significance
Over 200 million women have taken this group of drugs, and still there is significant debate as to what side effects are real. This confusion is in large part due to the ever-changing formulation with newer contraceptives. A higher incidence of migraine and thrombophlebitis probably occurs in women taking oral contraceptives than in a comparable population. There is some evidence that combination oral contraceptives, which contain more progestins, have fewer side effects than those that contain mainly estrogens. There is an increased risk of venous thrombosis in patients on these medications. Risk factors include personal history of venous thrombosis, gross obesity, and abnormalities of the hemostatic mechanism.[1] Arterial thrombosis may be less likely, but aging, smoking, and hypertension may increase patient risk. Schwartz et al reported that both ischemic and hemorrhagic stroke associated with the "pill" were double over controls if the woman had a history of migraine headaches.[2] In a few cases, the courts have ruled that there is a cause-and-effect relationship between the use of oral contraceptives and retinal vascular abnormalities. In selected patients with retinal vascular abnormalities, there should probably be

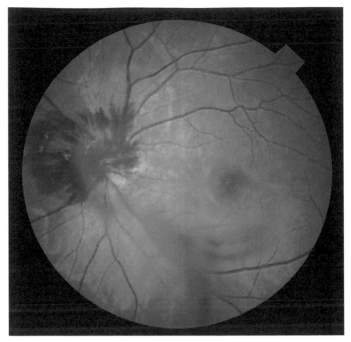

FIG. 11.1 Dense hemorrhage of the disc with vitreous hemorrhage.[29]

informed consent or even the consideration of not taking the drug. If retinal vascular abnormalities develop, the use of these drugs in that patient may need to be reevaluated. With long-term use, some data suggest there can be decreased color perception, mainly blue and yellow, and prolonged photostress recovery times. This is seldom clinically identified. If a patient has a transient ischemic attack, the oral contraceptive may need to be discontinued because the incidence of strokes is significantly increased. In the literature and spontaneous reports, there are cases that implicate these drugs in causing macular edema. A number of these patients have been rechallenged with recurrence of the edema. Rait et al stated that most patients with acute macular neuroretinopathy have been taking oral contraceptive medication in addition to other possible causative factors.[3] They postulated the "pill" as a possible cofactor. Madendag et al has shown that these drugs decrease the thickness and volume of the macula and, in some cases, also decrease the thickness of some areas of the retinal nerve fiber layer.[4] There is a suggestion that pregnancy causes progression of retinitis pigmentosa. Because these oral contraceptives cause a pseudopregnancy, there is a question of whether they may also cause progression of this retinal disease. However, there is no proof of this, and most researchers feel

these drugs are safe for the retinitis pigmentosa patient to use.

In some women, contact lens intolerance is marked. It is postulated that mucus changes, meibomian gland dysfunction, and some sicca changes may be responsible.[5-7]

Garmizo et al and Orlin et al have described patients on various estrogen-progestogens who developed bluish-green or turquoise corneal deposits in a dusting or lacy pattern.[8,9] These are worse inferiorly in the midperiphery cornea. These differ from a Kaiser-Fleischer ring by having a clear cornea between the deposit and the limbus. If the drugs are stopped, these deposits regress and disappear. In numerous studies, oral contraceptives have been associated with elevated serum copper levels.[10]

There are cases in the spontaneous reports of cataracts possibly related to the administration of oral contraceptives. Recent data by Klein et al showed no evidence to support this.[11] In fact, oral contraceptives may even have a modest protective effect on the lens. Benitez et al and Harding both support Klein's data in well-designed studies.[12,13] However, Cumming et al, in the Blue Mountain Eye Study, have supported the hypothesis that estrogen and/or progestin may be involved in cataract development.[14] The problem, in part, is the lack of an easy, accurate way to grade lenses. The Swedish Mammography Cohort study (30,861 participants) showed that women taking hormone replacement therapy for some time showed a significant positive risk of having cataract surgery versus controls.[15] They also showed that this risk was even greater if more than 1 alcoholic drink was consumed each day. There is a relationship between oral contraceptives and contact lens intolerance. Candela et al found increased tear mucus production in patients on these drugs.[16] Because there are estrogen receptors in the cornea and retina, changes can be expected. For example, Giuffre et al have shown changes in corneal thickness during menstruation.[17] Deschenes et al showed increased blood flow in the retina in females on postmenopausal hormone replacement.[18] Tomlinson et al could not confirm this.[19] Mayer found transitory decreased accommodation on diethylstilbestrol.[20] There are a number of case reports in the literature and in the spontaneous reports of retrobulbar and optic neuritis, optic nerve pathology with various visual field abnormalities, pupillary abnormalities, uveitis, transient myopia, exophthalmos, paralysis of extraocular muscles, and nystagmus. A clear cause-and-effect relationship between these events and the drug is difficult to prove. Most of these reports were from patients who were in the age range usually associated with multiple sclerosis.

Regardless, Vessey et al in 2 large UK cohort studies suggested that oral contraceptive use does not increase the risk of eye disease, with the possible exception of retinal vascular lesions.[21] However, based on the literature and spontaneous reports, our classifications are our "best guesses" at this time.

"Researchers at University of California, San Francisco, Duke University School of Medicine and the Affiliated Hospital of Nanchang University, Nanchang, China, established an increased risk of glaucoma in women who have used oral contraceptives for 3 or more years. Researchers utilized 2005–2008 data from the National Health and Nutrition Examination Survey (NHANES) which included 3,406 female participants aged 40 years or older from across the United States. It found that females who used oral contraceptives for longer than 3 years are 2.05 times more likely to also report that they have the diagnosis of glaucoma."[22]

The Pasquale et al study of 79,440 females who took oral contraceptives for more than 5 years showed a modest increased risk of primary open-angle glaucoma (POAG).[23] Hulsman et al, in a study of 3,078 females and in those who had an earlier onset of menopause,

reported that those females had a higher risk of POAG.[24] Pasquale et al, in 3,430 controls of both genders, found only in females an estrogen metabolism single nucleotide polymorphism panel that was associated with POAG.[25]

Abramov et al in a small study showed that hormone replacement therapy and lifelong estrogen and progesterone exposure does not seem to affect intraocular pressure (IOP) or cause an increased risk of IOP.[26] Tint et al reported that IOP was significantly lower in females taking hormonal therapy (HT).[27] Therefore there are data supporting HT increasing and even a decrease of IOP on HT. Further research is necessary to answer this question.

The question is, do these drugs cause papilledema secondary to pseudotumor cerebri? This is controversial, and there is a recent paper in the ophthalmology literature that states that they do not.[28]

Generic Name:
Estradiol.

Proprietary Names:
Alora, Climara, Delestrogen, Depo-Estradiol, Divigel, Elestrin, Estrace, Estraderm, Estrasorb, Estring, Estro-Gel, Evamist, FemPatch, Femring, Femtrace, Gynodiol, Gynogen LA, Imvexxy, Inofem, Menostar, Minivelle, Vagifem, Vivelle, Vivelle-Dot, Yuvafem.

Primary Use
This naturally occurring estrogen is administered in tablets, transdermal patches, and vaginal creams and is used in the management of menopause, vulval and vaginal atrophy, ovarian failure, uterine bleeding, and prevention of osteoporosis.

Ocular Side Effects
Systemic administration – oral, transdermal patch, or vaginal
Possible
1. Decreased vision
2. Decreased contact lens tolerance
3. Cornea
   a. Fluctuation of corneal curvature
   b. Increased steeping of cornea
4. Color vision defect
   a. Red-green or yellow-blue defect
   b. Objects have blue tinge
   c. Colored haloes around lights – mainly blue
5. Eyelids or conjunctiva
   a. Allergic reactions
   b. Edema

c. Hyperpigmentation
d. Photosensitivity
e. Urticaria
f. Ptosis
g. Lupoid syndrome
6. Retinal vascular disorders
    a. Occlusion
    b. Thrombosis
    c. Hemorrhage
    d. Retinal or macular edema
    e. Spasms
    f. Acute macular neuroretinopathy
    g. Periphlebitis
7. Papilledema secondary to pseudotumor cerebri

Conditional/unclassified
1. Nonarteritic ischemic optic neuropathy (NAION) – excessive dosage

Clinical Significance
This female hormone is largely responsible for the changes that take place at puberty in females and also provides their secondary sexual characteristics. These drugs are infrequently given orally because of extensive first-pass hepatic metabolism and the resulting failure to produce high enough therapeutic blood levels. However, slow, sustained release from dermal patches or creams can produce systemic effects. Most ocular side effects are the same as those listed in "Combination products of estrogens and progestogens" earlier in this section. This estrogen is commonly used in combination with levonorgestrel, a progestogen, so side effects often overlap with other contraception combination drugs. This does not allow for well-defined ocular side effects. Reports of fluctuation of corneal curvature, steepening of the cornea, and intolerance of contact lens wear have been reported.[1] Excessive dosage of this drug may cause NAION.[2]

Generic Name:
Levonorgestrel.

Proprietary Names:
EContra EZ, EContra One-Step, Fallback Solo, Kyleena, Liletta, Mirena, My Choice, My Way, Next Choice One Dose, Norplant II, Opcicon One-Step, Plan B, Plan B One-Step, React, Skyla, Take Action.

Primary Use
Synthetic progestin given as a long-term contraceptive drug.

Ocular Side Effects
Systemic administration – intrauterine or oral
Probable
1. Decreased vision

Possible
1. Papilledema secondary to pseudotumor cerebri
2. Diplopia
3. Myasthenia gravis
    a. Diplopia
    b. Ptosis
    c. Paresis of extraocular muscles
4. Ocular porphyria
5. Decreased accommodation
6. Retinal venous vascular occlusion

Clinical Significance
Levonorgestrel has been implicated in possibly causing pseudotumor cerebri.[1] Wyeth-Ayerst Laboratories, the drug manufacturer, pointed out that most patients were obese, a known risk factor for pseudotumor cerebri.[2] Also, most cases did not resolve after the implant was removed. To date there are over 300 cases of papilledema associated with this drug in the spontaneous reports; however, these data are incomplete and retrospective, and therefore it is only "possible" that there is an association. According to the package insert, patients on levonorgestrel who start to have visual symptoms should be examined by an ophthalmologist.[3]

Brittain et al reported myasthenia gravis occurring after insertion of a levonorgestrel implant and improving after its removal.[4] Levonorgestrel has been associated with acute attacks of porphyria with various ocular and acute ocular findings. These include retinal edema, cotton-wool spots, hemorrhages, and scleral ulcers. Partial third-nerve palsy, ptosis, and mydriasis may occur.

CLASS: OVULATORY DRUGS

Generic Name:
Clomifene (clomiphene) citrate.

Proprietary Names:
Clomid, Milophene, Serophene.

Primary Use
This synthetic nonsteroidal drug is effective in the treatment of anovulation.

Ocular Side Effects
Systemic administration – oral
Certain

1. Visual sensations
   a. Flashing lights
   b. Scintillating scotomas
   c. Distortion of images secondary to sensations of waves or glare
   d. Various colored lights – mainly silver
   e. Phosphene stimulation
   f. Prolongation of after image
   g. Entoptic phenomenon
2. Decreased vision
3. Mydriasis
4. Visual fields
   a. Scotomas – central, paracentral, centrocecal
   b. Constriction
5. Photophobia
6. Eyelids or conjunctiva
   a. Allergic reactions
   b. Urticaria
   c. Loss of eyelashes or eyebrows
7. Flicker sensitivity – reduced

Probable

1. Decreased tolerance to contact lenses
2. Diplopia

Possible

1. Optic neuritis
2. Uveitis
3. Central retinal vein occlusion
4. Maculopathy (Figs. 11.2 and 11.3)

Conditional/unclassified

1. Cataracts
2. Retina
   a. Phlebitis
   b. Spasms
3. Increased intraocular pressure
4. Progression keratoconus (in combination with other infertility medications)

Ocular teratogenic effects
Probable

1. Retinal aplasia
2. Cyclopia
3. Nystagmus

Clinical Significance

Clomifene appears to have a unique effect on the retina that may occur in up to 10% of patients. This consists of any or all of the following: flashing lights, glare, various colored lines (often silver), multiple images, prolonged after-images, "like looking through heat waves," objects

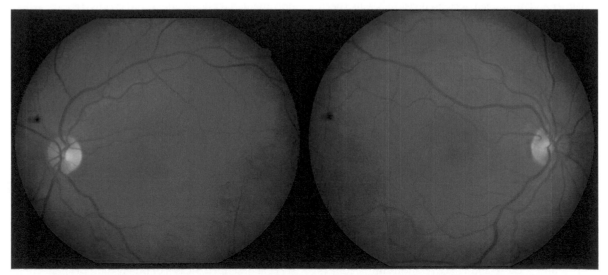

FIG. 11.2 Color fundus appearance of a patient showing oval-shaped macular atrophy in both eyes.[9]

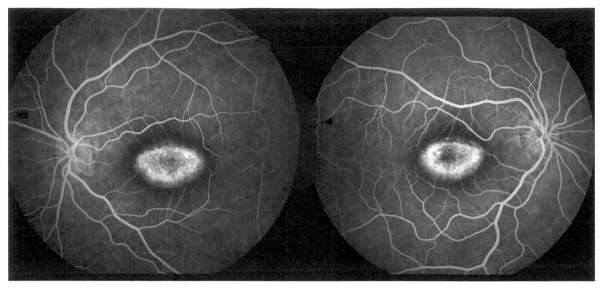

FIG. 11.3 Fluorescein angiography shows the central area of retinal pigment epithelial atrophy giving a bull's eye appearance to the macula in both eyes. There was no leakage from these areas at the later phases.[9]

have "comet" tails, phosphene stimulation, and scintillating scotomas identical to migraine. Racette et al reported that all 8 patients with ocular side effects in their study had bilateral reduction in flicker sensitivity.[1] These may occur as early as 48 hours after taking this drug and are reversible after stopping the medication. Transitory and prolonged decreased vision has also been reported. After years of prolonged use, vision loss in the 20/40–20/60 range may occur (etiology unknown), which may be slow to recover. Purvin, Choi et al, and Venkatesh et al reported cases of irreversible prolonged visual disturbances (palinopsia), as described earlier.[2–4] Cases in the spontaneous reports support this. Bilateral acute reversible loss of vision is a rare event. Mydriasis is common but of a mild degree and reversible. Of clinical significance are the unilateral or bilateral scotomas and visual field constriction seen with this drug. It is of interest that classic scintillating scotoma seems to occur secondarily to clomifene. Some of these side effects required discontinuing the medication. The causes of these are unclear, but Padron Rivas et al and several cases in the spontaneous reports suggest the possibility of an optic neuritis for some of these effects.[5] These are in females – most in the multiple sclerosis age group – and a cause-and-effect relationship is conjecture. Usually, the patient refuses to take further medication; if the drug is continued, the long-term sequelae

are unclear. Decreased contact lens wear may be due to clomifene's ability to inhibit mucus production. Monocular and binocular diplopia has been reported but is not well documented. Although the literature contains references to the cataractogenic potential of this drug, a drug-related cause has not been proven. There is 1 well-documented case in the spontaneous reports where this drug caused bilateral elevated intraocular pressure. Myers et al reported a single case of bilateral uveitis in a 30-year-old patient with polycystic ovary syndrome after starting clomifene.[6] The drug was stopped with full recovery in 3 weeks. Three months later, the drug was restarted and within 8 days bilateral uveitis returned. Lawton and Perin et al reported cases suggestive of anterior ischemic optic neuropathy on the basis that the drug may cause increased blood viscosity. Retinal vascular occlusions have been reported, but usually with complicating medical problems.[7,8] Tunc described a case of severe maculopathy (20/200) where instead of using the drug as prescribed, 100 mg per day for 5 days with a maximum of 6 cycles, the patient used the drug on her own for 3 years without follow-up.[9] It has been reported that about 1% of patients are forced to stop taking clomifene secondary to ocular side effects. Yuksel et al described 3 cases of progression of keratoconus in patients on infertility therapies that included clomifene.[10] This drug also has ocular teratogenic effects.[11]

CLASS: THYROID HORMONES

Generic Names:

1. Levothyroxine sodium; 2. liothyronine sodium; 3. thyroid.

Proprietary Names:

1. Estre, Levolet, Levo-T, Levothroid, Levoxyl, Novothyrox, Synthroid, Thyro-Tabs, Tirosint, Unithroid; 2. Cytomel, Triostat; 3. Armour Thyroid, Nature Thyroid, Nature-Throid, NP Thyroid, Westhroid, WP Thyroid.

Primary Use

These thyroid hormones are effective in the replacement therapy of thyroid deficiencies such as hypothyroidism and simple goiter.

Ocular Side Effects

Systemic administration – intravenous or oral

Certain

1. Decreased vision
2. Eyelids or conjunctiva
   a. Hyperemia
   b. Edema
3. Photophobia
4. Exophthalmos
5. Visual hallucinations

Probable

1. Papilledema secondary to pseudotumor cerebri

Possible

1. Myasthenia gravis
   a. Diplopia
   b. Ptosis
   c. Paresis of extraocular muscles
2. Open-angle glaucoma (levothyroxine)
3. Blepharospasm

Clinical Significance

Lee et al found a possible association of glaucoma and thyroid disease in the Blue Mountains Eye Study.[1] This was primarily seen in patients treated with levothyroxine. They stated, however, that further evaluation of this potential association is warranted. There are numerous articles suggesting that this group of drugs can cause pseudotumor cerebri. Prepubertal and peripubertal hypothyroid children may be the most susceptible to pseudotumor cerebri when beginning this group of drugs. Sundaram et al reported petit mal status epilepticus, with rapid rhythmic eyelid fluttering and blinking occurring in a patient approximately 1 week after starting levothyroxine therapy.[2] Lledo Carreres et al reported a case of toxic internuclear ophthalmoplegia after the use of these drugs for weight loss.[3] Visual hallucinations have appeared soon after initiation of thyroid replacement therapy in hypothyroid patients, usually in patients with an underlying psychiatric disorder. Other than the central nervous system changes, most ocular findings clear within a few months of discontinuing the medication.

REFERENCES

Drugs: Adrenal cortex injection, beclomethasone dipropionate, betamethasone dipropionate, budesonide, cortisone acetate, dexamethasone, fludrocortisone acetate, fluorometholone, fluticasone propionate, hydrocortisone, methylprednisolone, prednisolone, prednisone, rimexolone, triamcinolone acetonide

1. Garbe E, Suissa S, Lelorier J. Association of inhaled corticosteroid use with cataract extraction in elderly patients. *JAMA.* 1998;280:539–544.
2. Smeeth L, Boulis M, Hubbard R, et al. A population based case-control study of cataract and inhaled corticosteroids. *Br J Ophthalmol.* 2003;87:1247–1251.
3. Jick SS, Vasilakis-Scaramozza C, Maier WC. The risk of cataract among users of inhaled steroids. *Epidemiology.* 2001;12:229-234.
4. Wang JJ, Rochtchina E, Tan AG, et al. Use of inhaled and oral corticosteroids and the long-term risk of cataract. *Ophthalmology.* 2009;116:652–657.
5. Lipworth BJ. Systemic adverse effects of inhaled corticosteroid therapy. *Arch Intern Med.* 1999;159:941–955.
6. Çekiç O, Chang S, Tseng JJ, et al. Cataract progression after intravitreal triamcinolone injection. *Am J Ophthalmol.* 2005;139:993–998.
7. Thompson JT. Cataract formation and other complications of intravitreal triamcinolone for macular edema. *Am J Ophthalmol.* 2006;141:629–637.
8. Mitchell P, Cumming RG, Mackey DA. Inhaled corticosteroids, family history, and risk of glaucoma. *Ophthalmology.* 1999;106:2301–2306.
9. Sahni D, Darley CR, Hawk JLM. Glaucoma induced by periorbital steroid use – a rare complication. *Clin Exp Dermatol.* 2004;29:617–619.
10. Levy J, Tessler Z, Klemperer I, et al. Acute intractable glaucoma after a single low-dose sub-Tenon's corticosteroid injection for macular edema. *Can J Ophthalmol.* 2004;39:672-673.
11. Smithen LM, Ober MD, Maranan L, et al. Intravitreal triamcinolone acetonide and intraocular pressure. *Am J Ophthalmol.* 2004;138:740–743.
12. Ideta S, Noda M, Kawamura R, et al. Dehiscence of levator aponeurosis in ptosis after sub-Tenon injection of triamcinolone acetonide. *Can J Ophthalmol.* 2009;44(6):668–672.

13. Kaushik S, Gupta V, Gupta A, et al. Intractable glaucoma following intravitreal triamcinolone in central retinal vein occlusion. *Am J Ophthalmol.* 2004;137:758–760.

14. Quiram PA, Gonzales CR, Schwartz SD. Severe steroid-induced glaucoma following intravitreal injection of triamcinolone acetonide. *Am J Ophthalmol.* 2006;141:580–582.

15. Singh IP, Ahmad SI, Yeh D, et al. Early rapid rise in intraocular pressure after intravitreal triamcinolone acetonide injection. *Am J Ophthalmol.* 2004;138:286–287.

16. Leibowitz HM, Bartlett JD, Rich R, et al. Intraocular pressure-raising potential of 1.0% rimexolone in patients responding to corticosteroids. *Arch Ophthalmol.* 1996;114:933–937.

17. Bangsgaard R, Main KM, Boberg-Ans G, et al. Adrenal suppression in infants treated with topical ocular glucocorticoids. *Ophthalmology.* 2018;125:1638–1643.

18. Romano PE, Traisman HS, Green OC. Fluorinated corticosteroid toxicity in infants. *Am J Ophthalmol.* 1977;84:247–250.

19. Fukuhara D, Takiura T, Keino H, et al. Iatrogenic Cushing's syndrome due to topical ocular glucocorticoid treatment. *Pediatrics.* 2017;139(2):e20161233.

20. Rainsbury PG, Sharp J, Tappin A, et al. Ritonavir and topical ocular corticosteroid induced Cushing's syndrome in an adolescent with HIV-1 infection. *Pediatr Infect Dis J.* 2017;36(5):502–503.

21. Ustyol A, Kökali F, Duru N, et al. Cushing's syndrome caused by use of synthetic ocular steroid. *J Clin Pharm Ther.* 2017;42(6):780–782.

22. Batton DG, Roberts C, Trese M, et al. Severe retinopathy of prematurity and steroid exposure. *Pediatrics.* 1992;90(4):534–536.

23. Ehrenkranz RA. Steroids, chronic lung disease, and retinopathy of prematurity. *Pediatrics.* 1992;90(4):646–647.

24. Curragh D, McLoone E. Pseudotumor cerebri syndrome in two children on systemic steroid therapy for uveitis. *Ocul Immunol Inflamm.* 2018;26(2):295–297.

25. Liu GT, Kay MD, Bienfang DC, et al. Pseudotumor cerebri associated with corticosteroid withdrawal in inflammatory bowel disease. *Am J Ophthalmol.* 1994;117(3):352–357.

26. Romano PE. Fluorinated ocular/periocular corticosteroids have caused death as well as glaucoma in children. *Clin Experiment Ophthalmol.* 2002;31:278–279.

27. Romano PE, Traisman HS, Green OC. Fluorinated corticosteroid toxicity in infants. *Am J Ophthalmol.* 1977;84:247–250.

28. Zamir E, Read RW, Smith RE, et al. A prospective evaluation of subconjunctival injection of triamcinolone acetonide for resistant anterior scleritis. *Ophthalmology.* 2002;109:798–807.

29. Albini TA, Zami E, Read RW, et al. Evaluation of subconjunctival triamcinolone for nonnecrotizing anterior scleritis. *Ophthalmology.* 2005;112:1814–1820.

30. Abel AD, Carlson A, Bakri S, et al. Sclerosing lipogranuloma of the orbit after periocular steroid injection. *Ophthalmology.* 2003;110:1841–1845.

31. Dal Canto AJ, Downs-Kelly E, Perry JD. Ptosis and orbital fat prolapse after posterior sub-tenon's capsule triamcinolone injection. *Ophthalmology.* 2005;112:1092–1097.

32. Gallardo MJ, Johnson DA. Cutaneous hypopigmentation following a posterior sub-tenon triamcinolone injection. *Am J Ophthalmol.* 2004;137:780–799.

33. Moshfeghi DM, Lowder CY, Roth DB. Retinal and choroidal vascular occlusion after posterior sub-tenon triamcinolone injection. *Am J Ophthalmol.* 2002;134:132–134.

34. Feldman-Billard S, Du Pasquier-Frediaevsky L, Héron E. Hyperglycemia after repeated periocular dexamethasone injections in patients with diabetes. *Ophthalmology.* 2006;113:1720–1723.

35. Pendergast SD, Eliott D, Machemer R. Retinal toxic effects following inadvertent intraocular injection of Celestone Soluspan. *Arch Ophthalmol.* 1995;113(10):1230–1231.

36. Sarraf D, Vyas N, Jain A, et al. Triamcinolone-associated crystalline maculopathy. *Arch Ophthalmol.* 2010;128(6):685–690.

37. Bouzas EA, Scott MH, Mastorakos G, et al. Central serous chorioretinopathy in endogenous hypercortisolism. *Arch Ophthalmol.* 1993;111:1229–1233.

38. Haimovici R, Gragoudas ES, Duker JS, et al. Central serous chorioretinopathy associated with inhaled or intranasal corticosteroids. *Ophthalmology.* 1997;104(10):1653–1660.

39. Nicholson BP, Atchison E, Idris AA, et al. Central serous chorioretinopathy and glucocorticoids: an update on evidence for association. *Surv Ophthalmol.* 2018;63(1):1–8.

40. Iida T, Spaide RF, Negrao SG, et al. Central serous chorioretinopathy after epidural corticosteroid injection. *Am J Ophthalmol.* 2001;132:423–425.

41. Carvalho-Recchia CA, Yannuzzi LA, Negrão S, et al. Corticosteroids and central serous chorioretinopathy. *Ophthalmology.* 2002;109:1834–1837.

42. De Nijs E, Brabant P, De Laey JJ. The adverse effects of corticosteroids in central serous chorioretinopathy. *Bull Soc Belge Ophtalmol.* 2003;35:35–41.

43. Levy J, Marcus M, Belfair N, et al. Central serous chorioretinopathy in patients receiving systemic corticosteroid therapy. *Can J Ophthalmol.* 2005;40:217–221.

44. Pizzimenti JJ, Daniel KP. Central serous chorioretinopathy after epidural steroid injection. *Pharmacotherapy.* 2005;25:1141–1146.

45. Rim TH, Kim HS, Kwak JS, et al. Association of corticosteroid use with incidence of central serous chorioretinopathy in South Korea. *JAMA Ophthalmol.* 2018;136(10):1164–1169.

46. Suhler EB, Thorne JE, Mittal M, et al. Corticosteroid-related adverse events systemically increase with corticosteroid dose in noninfectious intermediate, posterior, or panuveitis. *Ophthalmology.* 2017;124(12):1799–1807.

47. VanderBeek BL, Bonaffini SG, Ma L. The association between intravitreal steroids and post-injection endophthalmitis rates. *Ophthalmology.* 2015;122(11):2311–2315.

48. Taravella MJ, Stulting RD, Mader TH, et al. Calcific band keratopathy associated with the use of topical steroid-phosphate preparations. *Arch Ophthalmol.* 1994;112:608–613.

49. Huige WM, Beekhuis WH, Rijneveld WJ, et al. Unusual deposits in the superficial corneal stroma following combined use of topical corticosteroid and beta-blocking medication. *Doc Ophthalmol.* 1991;78(3–4):169–175.

Drug: Danazol

1. Hamed LM, Glaser JS, Schatz NJ, et al. Pseudotumor cerebri induced by danazol. *Am J Ophthalmol.* 1989;107(2):105–110.
2. Loukili M, Cordonnier M, Capelluto E, et al. Pseudotumor cerebri induced by danazol. *Bull Soc Belge Ophtalmol.* 1990;239:139–144.
3. Danazol. 2018. Retrieved from http://www.pdr.net.
4. Fanous M, Hamed LM, Margo CE. Pseudotumor cerebri associated with danazol withdrawal. Letter to the editor. *JAMA.* 1991;266(9):1218–1219.
5. Sandercock PJ. Benign intracranial hypertension associated with danazol. Pseudotumor cerebri: case report. *Scottish Med J.* 1990;35:49.
6. Schmitz U, Honisch C, Zierz S. Pseudotumor cerebri and carpal tunnel syndrome associated with danazol therapy. *J Neurol.* 1991;238:355.
7. Shah A, Roberts T, McQueen IN, et al. Danazol and benign intracranial hypertension. *BMJ.* 1987;294:1323.
8. Pre-senile cataracts in association with the use of Danocrine (danazol). *PMS News Quarterly.* 1986;5.

Drug: Finasteride

1. Chatziralli IP, Peponis V, Parikakis E, et al. Risk factors for intraoperative floppy iris syndrome: a prospective study. *Eye (Lond).* 2016;30(8):1039–1044.
2. Issa SA, Dagres E. Intraoperative floppy iris syndrome and finasteride intake. *J Cataract Refect Surg.* 2007;33:2142–2143.
3. Wong AC, Mak ST. Finasteride-associated cataract and intraoperative floppy-iris syndrome. *J Cataract Refract Surg.* 2011;37(7):1351–1354.
4. Chatziralli IP, Sergentanis TN, Papazisis L, et al. Risk factors for intraoperative floppy iris syndrome: a retrospective study. *Acta Ophthalmol.* 2012;90(2):e152–e153.
5. Krenzer LK, Dana MR, Ullman MD, et al. Effect of androgen deficiency on the human meibomian gland and ocular surface. *J Clin Endocrinol Metab.* 2000;85(12):4874–4882.
6. Li K, Zhang C, Yang Z, et al. Evaluation of a novel dry eye model induced by oral administration of finasteride. *Mol Med Rep.* 2017;16(6):8763–8770.
7. Finasteride. 2018. Retrieved from http://www.pdr.net.
8. Check JH, Cohen R. Dihydrotestosterone may contribute to the development of migraine headaches. *Clin Exp Obstet Gynecol.* 2013;40(2):217–218.
9. Lombardo R, Loraschi A, Lecchini S, et al. Finasteride-associated central serous chorioretinopathy. *Drug Safety.* 2008;31(10):922.
10. Chou SY, Kao SC, Hsu WM. Propecia-associated bilateral cataract. *Clin Experiment Ophthalmol.* 2004;32(1):106–108.

Drug: Leuprolide acetate (leuprorelin acetate)

1. Krenzer LK, Dana MR, Ullman MD, et al. Effect of androgen deficiency on the human meibomian gland and ocular surface. *J Clin Endocrinol Metab.* 2000;85(12):4874–4882.
2. Leuprolide acetate. 2018. Retrieved from http://www.pdr.net.
3. Fraunfelder FT, Edwards R. Possible ocular adverse effects associated with leuprolide injections. *JAMA.* 1995;273(10):773–774.

Drugs: Iodide and iodine solutions and compounds, radioactive iodine 125 and 131

1. Yuoness S, Rachinsky I, Driedger AA, et al. Differentiated thyroid cancer with epiphora: detection of nasolacrimal duct obstruction on I-131 SPECT/CT. *Clin Nucl Med.* 2011;36(12):1149–1152.
2. Cetinkaya A, Kersten RC. Relationship between radioactive iodine therapy for thyroid carcinoma and nasolacrimal drainage system obstruction. *Ophthal Plast Reconstr Surg.* 2007;23(6):496.
3. Brockmann H, Wilhelm K, Joe A, et al. Nasolacrimal drainage obstruction after radioiodine therapy: case report and a review of the literature. *Clin Nucl Med.* 2005;30(8):543–545.
4. Burns JA, Morgenstern KE, Cahill KV, et al. Nasolacrimal obstruction secondary to I(131) therapy. *Ophthal Plast Reconstr Surg.* 2004;20(2):126–129.
5. Savage MW, Sobel RK, Hoffman HT, et al. Salivary gland dysfunction and nasolacrimal duct obstruction: stenotic changes following I-131 therapy. *Ophthalmic Plast Reconstr Surg.* 2015;31(3):e50–e52.
6. Kloos RT, Duvuuri V, Jhiang SM, et al. Nasolacrimal drainage system obstruction from radioactive iodine therapy for thyroid carcinoma. *J Clin Endocrinol Metab.* 2002;87(12):5817–5820.
7. Munigoti S, Samat A, Jones MK. Graves' disease and thyroid associated ophthalmopathy following radioiodine therapy in euthyroid multinodular goiter. *Thyroid.* 2008;18(5):585.
8. Tahrani AA, Rangan S, Moulik P. Graves' eye disease developing following radioiodine treatment for toxic nodular goiter. *Exp Clin Endocrinol Diabetes.* 2007;115(7):471–473.
9. Lee R, Hafezi F, Randleman JB. Bilateral keratoconus induced by secondary hypothyroidism after radioactive iodine therapy. *J Refract Surg.* 2018;34(5):351–353.
10. Thanos S, Oellers P, zu Hörste MM, et al. Role of thyroxine in the development of keratoconus. *Cornea.* 2016;35:1338–1346.

Drugs: Sildenafil citrate, tadalafil, vardenafil hydrochloride

1. Cordell WH, Maturi RK, Costigan TM, et al. Retinal effects of 6 months of daily use of tadalafil or sildenafil. *Arch Ophthalmol.* 2009;127(4):367–373.
2. Miller NR, Arnold AC. Current concepts in the diagnosis, pathogenesis, and management of nonarteritic anterior ischemic optic neuropathy. *Eye.* 2015;29:65–79.

3. Campbell UB, Walker AM, Gaffney M, et al. Acute non-arteritic anterior ischemic optic neuropathy and exposure to phosphodiesterase type 5 inhibitors. *J Sex Med.* 2105;12:139-151.

4. Pomeranz HD. Erectile dysfunction agents and nonarteritic anterior ischemic optic neuropathy. *Neurol Clin.* 2017;35:17–27.

5. Allibhai ZA, Gale JS, Sheidow TS. Central serous chorioretinopathy in a patient taking sildenafil citrate. *Ophthalmic Surg Las Imag.* 2004;35:165–167.

6. Gordon-Bennett P, Rimmer T. Central serous chorioretinopathy following oral tadalafil. *Eye.* 2012;26(1):168–169.

7. Park SS. Bilateral serous macular detachment in a woman on sildenafil for pulmonary hypertension. *Retin Cases Brief Rep.* 2007;1:274–276.

8. Quiram P, Dumars S, Parwar B, et al. Viagra-associated serous macular detachment. *Graefes Arch Clin Exp Ophthalmol.* 2005;243:339–344.

9. Fraunfelder FW. An overview of visual side effects associated with erectile dysfunction agents. *Am J Ophthalmol.* 2005;140:723–724.

10. Smal C, Lepiece G, Bonnet S. Central serous chorioretinopathy following the use of phosphodiesterase 5 inhibitors. *Rev Med Liege.* 2017;72(11):475–477.

11. Roy R, Panigrahi PK, Saurabh K, et al. Central serous chorioretinopathy following oral tadalafil intake. *Clin Exp Optom.* 2014;97(5):473–474.

12. Martiano D, Chevreaud O, Lam D, et al. Acute serous retinal detachment in idiopathic pulmonary arterial hypertension. *Retin Cases Brief Rep.* 2017;11(3):261–265.

13. Aliferis K, Petropoulos IK, Farpour B, et al. Should central serous chorioretinopathy be added to the list of ocular side effects of phosphodiesterase 5 inhibitors? *Ophthalmolgica.* 2012;227(2):85–89.

14. French DD, Margo CE. Central serous chorioretinopathy and phosphodiesterase-5 inhibitors. *Retina.* 2010;30:271–274.

15. Murthy RK, Perez L, Priluck JC, et al. Acute, bilateral, concurrent central retinal artery occlusion in sickle cell disease after use of tadalafil (Cialis). *JAMA Ophthalmol.* 2013;131(11):1471–1473.

16. Gerometta R, Alvarez LJ, Candia OA. Effect of sildenafil citrate on intraocular pressure and blood pressure in human volunteers. *Exp Eye Res.* 2011;93(1):103–107.

17. Harris A, Kagemann L, Ehrlich R, et al. The effect of sildenafil on ocular blood flow. *Br J Ophthalmol.* 2008;92:469–473.

18. Vance SK, Imamura Y, Freund KB. The effects of sildenafil citrate on choroidal thickness as determined by enhanced depth imaging optical coherence tomography. *Retina.* 2011;31:332–335.

19. Ioannides D, Lazaridou E, Apalla Z, et al. Phosphodiesterase-5 inhibitors and rosacea: report of 10 cases. *Br J Dermatol.* 2009;160(3):719–720.

20. Matieli L, Berezovsky A, Salomão SR, et al. Ocular toxicity assessment of chronic sildenafil therapy for pulmonary arterial hypertension. *Graefes Arch Clin Exp Ophthalmol.* 2016;254(6):1167–1174.

21. Sajjad A, Weng CY. Vison loss in a patient with primary pulmonary hypertension and long-term use of sildenafil. *Retin Cases Brief Rep.* 2017;11(4):325–328.

22. Kim HD, Chang JH, Kim YK, et al. Electrophysiologic effects of very high-dose sildenafil. *JAMA Ophthalmol.* 2017;135(2):165–167.

23. Vergis AM, Bhatt HK, Anguiano RH, et al. Blinded by science, progressive visual impairment in a patient with retinitis pigmentosa and pulmonary arterial hypertension treated with tadalafil. *Am J Respir Crit Care Med.* 2018;197. abstr A3710.

24. Wirostko BM, Tressler C, Hwang LJ, et al. Ocular safety of sildenafil citrate when administered chronically for pulmonary arterial hypertension: results from phase III, randomized, double masked, placebo controlled trial and open label extension. *BMJ.* 2012;344:e554.

25. Chandeclerc ML, Martin S, Petitpain N, et al. Tadalafil and palpebral edema. *South Med J.* 2004;97(11):1142–1143.

Drugs: Combination products of estrogens and progestogens, medroxyprogesterone acetate

1. Vandenbroucke JP, Rosing J, Bloemenkamp KWM, et al. Oral contraceptives and the risk of venous thrombosis. *N Engl J Med.* 2001;344:1527–1535.

2. Schwartz SM, Petitti DB, Siscovick DS, et al. Stroke and use of low-dose oral contraceptives in young women: a pooled analysis of two US studies. *Stroke.* 1998;29(11):2277–2284.

3. Rait JL, O'Day J. Acute macular neuroretinopathy. *Aust NZ J Ophthalmol.* 1987;15:337–340.

4. Madendag Y, Acmaz G, Atas M, et al. The effect of oral contraceptive pills on the macula, the retinal nerve fiber layer, and choroidal thickness. *Med Sci Moni.* 2017;23:5657–5661.

5. Esterified estrogens, synthetic conjugated estrogens, medroxyprogesterone acetate. 2018. Retrieved from http://www.pdr.net.

6. Asiedu K, Kyei S, Boampong F, et al. Symptomatic dry eye and its associated factors: a study of university undergraduate students in Ghana. *Eye Contact Lens.* 2017;43(4):262–266.

7. Chen SP, Massaro-Giordano G, Pistilli M, et al. Tear osmolarity and dry eye symptoms in women using oral contraception and contact lens. *Cornea.* 2013;32(4):423–428.

8. Garmizo G, Frauens BJ. Corneal copper deposition secondary to oral contraceptives. *Optom Vis Sci.* 2008;85(9):E802–E807.

9. Orlin A, Orlin SE, Makar GA, et al. Presumed corneal copper deposition and oral contraceptive use. *Cornea.* 2010;29(4):476–478.

10. Schenker JH, Jungreis E, Polishuk WZ. Oral contraceptives and serum copper concentration. *Obstet Gynecol.* 1971;37:233–237.

11. Klein BE, Klein R, Ritter LL. Is there evidence of an estrogen effect on age related lens opacities? *Arch Ophthalmol.* 1994;112:85–91.

12. Benitez Del Castillo JM, del Rio T, Garcia-Sanchez J. Effects of estrogen use on lens transmittance in postmenopausal women. *Ophthalmology*. 1997;104:970–973.

13. Harding JJ. Estrogens and cataract. *Arch Ophthalmol*. 1994;112:1511.

14. Cumming RG, Mitchell P. Hormone replacement therapy, reproductive factors, and cataract: the Blue Mountain Eye Study. *Am J Epidemiol*. 1997;145(3):242–249.

15. Lindblad BE, Kakansson N, Philipson B, et al. Hormone replacement therapy in relation to risk of cataract extraction. *Ophthalmology*. 2010;117:424–430.

16. Candela V, Castagna I. Modification of conjunctival mucus secretion by pregnancy and oral contraceptives. *Boll Oculist*. 1989;68(suppl 1):19–23.

17. Giuffre G, Di Rosa L, Fiorino F, et al. Variations in central corneal thickness during the menstrual cycle in women. *Cornea*. 2007;26(2):144–146.

18. Deschenes MC, Descovich D, Moreau M, et al. Postmenopausal hormone therapy increases retinal blood flow and protects the retinal nerve fiber layer. *Invest Ophthalmol Vis Sci*. 2010;51(5):2587–2600.

19. Tomlinson A, Pearce EI, Simmons PA, et al. Effect of oral contraceptives on tear physiology. *Ophthal Physiol Opt*. 2001;21:9–16.

20. Mayer L. Effect of diethylstilbestrol on accommodation. *Arch Ophthalmol*. 1944;32:133–134.

21. Vessey MP, Hannaford P, Mant J, et al. Oral contraception and eye disease: findings in two large cohort studies. *Br J Ophthalmol*. 1998;82:538–542.

22. American Academy of Ophthalmology. New Orleans, Louisiana: Annual Meeting; 2013:16–19.

23. Pasquale LR, Kang JH. Female reproductive factors and primary open-angle glaucoma in the nurses' health study. *Eye*. 2011;25(5):633–641.

24. Hulsman CA, Westendorp IC, Ramrattan RS, et al. Is open-angle glaucoma associated with early menopause? The Rotterdam Study. *Am J Epidemiol*. 2001;154(2):138–144.

25. Pasquale LR, Loomis SJ, Weinreb RN, et al. Estrogen pathway polymorphisms in relation to primary open angle glaucoma: an analysis accounting for gender from the United States. *Mol Vis*. 2013;19:1471–1481.

26. Abramov Y, Borik S, Yahalom C, et al. Does postmenopausal hormone replacement therapy affect intraocular pressure? *J Glauc*. 2005;14(4):271–275.

27. Tint NL, Alexander P, Tint KM, et al. Hormone therapy and intraocular pressure in nonglaucomatous eyes. *Menopause*. 2010;17(1):157–160.

28. Kilgore KP, Lee MS, Leavitt JA, et al. A population-based, case-control evaluation of the association between hormonal contraceptives and idiopathic intracranial hypertension. *Am J Ophthalmol*. 2019;197:74–79.

29. Higa A, Ayaki M, Nishihara H, et al. Vitreous haemorrhage in a 19-year-old Japanese woman using an oral contraceptive. *Acta Ophthalmol Scand*. 2004;82(2):244–246.

Drug: Estradiol

1. Estradiol. 2018. Retrieved from http://www.pdr.net.

2. Wierckx K, De Zaeytijd J, Elaut E, et al. Bilateral non-arteritic ischemic optic neuropathy in a transsexual woman using excessive estrogen dosage. *Arch Sex Behav*. 2014;43(2):407–409.

Drug: Levonorgestrel

1. Alder JB, Fraunfelder FT, Buchhalter JR. Levonorgestrel implants and intracranial hypertension. *N Engl J Med*. 1995;332(25):1720–1721.

2. Weber ME, Rofsky HE, Deitch MW. Levonorgestrel implants and intracranial hypertension. *N Engl J Med*. 1995;332(25):1721.

3. Levonorgestrel. 2018. Retrieved from http://www.pdr.net.

4. Brittain J, Lange LS. Myasthenia gravis and levonorgestrel implant. *Lancet*. 1995;346:1556.

Drug: Clomifene (clomiphene) citrate

1. Racette L, Casson PR, Claman P, et al. An investigation of the visual disturbances experienced by patients on clomiphene citrate. *Fertil Steril*. 2010;93(4):1169–1172.

2. Purvin VA. Visual disturbance secondary to clomiphene citrate. *Arch Ophthalmol*. 1995;113(4):482–484.

3. Choi SY, Jeong SH, Kim JS. Clomiphene citrate associated with palinopsia. *J Neuroophthalmol*. 2017;37(2):220–221.

4. Venkatesh R, Gujral GS, Gurav P, et al. Clomiphene citrate-induced visual hallucinations: a case report. *J Med Case Rep*. 2017;11(1):60.

5. Padron Rivas VF, Sanchez A, Lerida Arias MT, et al. Optic neuritis appearing during treatment of clomiphene (letter). *Aten Primaria*. 1994;14(7):912–913.

6. Myers TD, Fraunfelder FW. Bilateral anterior uveitis associated with clomiphene citrate. *Ocul Immunol Inflamm*. 2008;16(12):23–24.

7. Lawton AW. Optic neuropathy associated with clomiphene citrate therapy. *Fertil Steril*. 1994;61(2):390–391.

8. Perin AF, Chacko JG, Goyal S. Nonarteritic ischemic optic neuropathy associated with clomiphene citrate use. *J Neuroophthalmol*. 2017;37(1):106–107.

9. Tunc M. Maculopathy following extended useage of clomiphene citrate. *Eye (Lond)*. 2014;28(9):1144–1146.

10. Yuksel E, Yalinbas D, Aydin B, et al. Keratoconus progression induced by in vitro fertilization treatment. *J Refract Surg*. 2016;32(1):60–63.

11. Kurachi K, Aono T, Minagawa J, et al. Congenital malformations of newborn infants after clomiphene-induced ovulation. *Fertil Steril*. 1983;40(2):187–189.

Drugs: Levothyroxine sodium, liothyronine sodium, thyroid

1. Lee AJ, Rochtchina E, Wang JJ, et al. Open-angle glaucoma and systemic thyroid disease in an older population: the blue mountains eye study. *Eye*. 2004;28:600–608.

2. Sundaram MB, Hill A, Lowry N. Thyroxine-induced petit mal status epilepticus. *Neurology*. 1985;35:1792–1793.

3. Lledo Carreres M, Lajo Garrido JL, Gonzalez Rico M, et al. Toxic internuclear ophthalmoplegia related to antiobesity treatment. *Ann Pharm.* 1992;26(11):1457–1458.

FURTHER READING

Adrenal cortex injection, beclomethasone dipropionate, betamethasone dipropionate, budesonide, cortisone acetate, dexamethasone, fludrocortisone acetate, fluorometholone, fluticasone propionate, hydrocortisone, methylprednisolone, prednisolone, prednisone, rimexolone, triamcinolone acetonide

Agrawal S, Agrawal J, Agrawal TP. Conjunctival ulceration following triamcinolone injection. *Am J Ophthalmol.* 2003;136:538–540.

Bowie EM, Folk JC, Barnes CH. Corticosteroids, central serous chorioretinopathy, and neurocysticercosis. *Arch Ophthalmol.* 2004;122:281–283.

Chaine G, Haouat M, Menard-Molcard C, et al. Central serous chorioretinopathy and systemic steroid therapy. *J Fr Ophtalmol.* 2001;24:139–146.

Chen SD, Lochhead J, McDonald B, et al. Pseudohypopyon after intravitreal triamcinolone injection for the treatment of pseudophakic cystoids macular oedema. *Br J Ophthalmol.* 2004;88:843–844.

Fischer R, Henkind P, Gartner S. Microcysts of the human iris pigment epithelium. *Br J Ophthalmol.* 1979;63:750.

Fraunfelder FT, Meyer SM. Posterior subcapsular cataracts associated with nasal or inhalation corticosteroids. *Am J Ophthalmol.* 1990;109(4):489–490.

Gilles MC, Kuzniarz M, Craig J, et al. Intravitreal triamcinolone-induced elevated intraocular pressure is associated with the development of posterior subcapsular cataract. *Ophthalmology.* 2005;112:139–143.

Gupta OP, Boynton JR, Sabini P, et al. Proptosis after retrobulbar corticosteroid injections. *Ophthalmology.* 2003;110:443–447.

Gupta V, Sharma SC, Gupta A. Retinal and choroidal microvascular embolization with methylprednisolone. *Retina.* 2002;22:382–385.

Henderson RP, Lander R. Scleral discoloration associated with long-term prednisone administration. *Cutis.* 1984;34:76–77.

Jordan DR, Brownstein S, Lee-Wing MW, et al. Orbital mass following injection with depot corticosteroids. *Can J Ophthalmol.* 2001;36:153–155.

Ramanathan R, Siassi B, deLemos RA. Severe retinopathy of prematurity in extremely low birth weight infants after short-term dexamethasone therapy. *J Perinatology.* 1995;15(3):178–182.

Srinivasan S, Prasad S. Conjunctival necrosis following intravitreal injection of triamcinolone acetonide. *Cornea.* 2005;24:1027–1028.

Tognetto D, Zenoni S, Sanguinetti G, et al. Staining of the internal limiting membrane with intravitreal triamcinolone acetonide. *Retina.* 2005;25:462–467.

Yim CL, Tam M, Chan HL, et al. Association of antenatal steroid and risk of retinopathy of prematurity: a systematic review of meta-analysis. *Br J Ophthalmol.* 2018;102:1336–1341.

Finasteride

Almagro BM, Steyls MC, Navarro NL, et al. Occurrence of subacute cutaneous lupus erythematosus after treatment with systemic fluorouracil. *J Clin Oncol.* 2011;29(20):e613–e615.

Leuprolide acetate (leuprorelin acetate)

Arber N, Fadila R, Pinkhas J, et al. Pseudotumor cerebri associated with leuprorelin acetate. *Lancet.* 1990;335:668.

Boot JH. Pseudotumor cerebri as a side effect of leuprorelin acetate. *Irish J Med Sci.* 1996;165(1):60.

Federici TJ. Leuprolide acetate and central retinal vein occlusion. *Ophthalmic Surg Lasers Imaging.* 2007;38(6):497–499.

Plosker GL, Brogden RN. Leuprorelin: a review of its pharmacology and therapeutic use in prostatic cancer, endometriosis and other sex hormone-related disorders. *Drugs.* 1994;48(6):930–967.

Iodide and iodine solutions and compounds, radioactive iodine 125 and 131

Gerber M. Ocular reactions following iodide therapy. *Am J Ophthalmol.* 1957;43:879–881.

Morgenstern KE, Vadysirisack DD, Zhang Z, et al. Expression of sodium iodide symporter in the lacrimal drainage system: implication for the mechanism underlying nasolacrimal duct obstruction I(131)-treated patients. *Ophthal Plast Reconstr Surg.* 2005;21(5):337–344.

Shepler TR, Sherman SI, Faustina MM, et al. Nasolacrimal duct obstruction associated with radioactive iodine therapy for thyroid carcinoma. *Ophthal Plast Reconstr Surg.* 2003;19(6):479–481.

Sildenafil citrate, tadalafil, vardenafil hydrochloride

Bollinger K, Lee MS. Recurrent visual field defect and ischemic optic neuropathy associated with tadalafil rechallenge. *Arch Ophthalmol.* 2005;123:400–401.

Curran MP. Tadalafil: in the treatment of signs and symptoms of benign prostatic hyperplasia with or without erectile dysfunction. *Drugs Aging.* 2012;29:771–781.

Donahue SP, Taylor RJ. Pupil-sparing third nerve palsy associated with sildenafil citrate (Viagra). *Am J Ophthalmol.* 1998;126:476–477.

Egan RA, Fraunfelder FW. Viagra and anterior ischemic optic neuropathy. *Arch Ophthalmol.* 2005;123:709–710.

Egan R, Pomeranz H. Sildenafil (Viagra) associated anterior ischemic optic neuropathy. *Arch Ophthalmol.* 2000;118:291–292.

Escaravage GK, Wright JD, Givre SJ. Tadalafil associated with anterior ischemic optic neuropathy. *Arch Ophthalmol.* 2005;123:399–400.

Fraunfelder FW, Fraunfelder FT. Scientific challenges in post-marketing surveillance of ocular adverse drug reactions. *Am J Ophthalmol.* 2007;143:145–149.

Fraunfelder FT, Laties A. Visual side effects possibly associated with Viagra. *J Toxicol Cut Ocular Toxicol.* 2000;19(1):21–25.

Hayreh SS. Erectile dysfunction drugs and non-arteritic anterior ischemic optic neuropathy: is there a cause and effect relationship. *J Neuroophthalmol.* 2005;25:285–298.

Laties AM, Siegel RL. Ocular safety in patients using sildenafil citrate therapy for erectile dysfunction. *J Sex Med.* 2006;3:12–27.

Lee AG, Newman NJ. Erectile dysfunction drugs and nonarteritic anterior ischemic optic neuropathy. *Am J Ophthalmol.* 2005;140:707–708.

McGwin G, Vaphiades MS, Hall TA, et al. Non-arteritic anterior ischaemic optic neuropathy and the treatment of erectile dysfunction. *Br J Ophthalmol.* 2006;90:154–157.

Pomeranz HD, Bhavsar AR. Nonarteritic ischemic optic neuropathy developing soon after use of sildenafil (Viagra): a report of seven new cases. *J Neuroophthalmol.* 2005;25:9–13.

Pomeranz HD, Smith KH, Hart Jr WM, et al. Sildenafil-associated non-arteritic anterior ischemic optic neuropathy. *Ophthalmology.* 2002;109:584–587.

Yanoga F, Gentile RC, Chui TYP, et al. Sildenafil citrate induced retinal toxicity – electroretinogram, optical coherence tomography, and adaptive optics findings. *Retin Cases Brief Rep.* 2018;12(suppl 1):S33–S40.

Zrenner E. How should Viagra-induced vision disorders – especially retinal degeneration – be evaluated? *Klin Monatsbl Augenheilkd.* 1998;212(6):aA12–aA13.

Combination products of estrogens and progestogens, medroxyprogesterone acetate

Byrne E. Retinal migraine and the pill. *Med J Aust.* 1979;2:659–660.

Can JW. Idiopathic intracranial hypertension associated with depot medroxyprogesterone. *Eye.* 2006;20(12):1396–1397.

Chakrapani K, Balchender T, Vidyavati M, et al. Ovulation-associated uveitis. *Br J Ophthalmol.* 1982;66:320–321.

Chilvers E, Rudge P. Cerebral venous thrombosis and subarachnoid haemorrhage in users of oral contraceptives. *BMJ.* 1986;292:524.

Corbett MC, O'Brat DP, Warburton FG, et al. Biologic and environmental risk factors for regression after photorefractive keratectomy. *Ophthalmology.* 1966;103:1381–1391.

Deen BF, Shuler Jr RK, Fekrat S. Retinal venous occlusion associated with depot medroxyprogesterone acetate. *Br J Ophthalmol.* 2007;91(9):1254.

Goren SB. Retinal edema secondary to oral contraceptives: their side effects and ophthalmological manifestations. *Surv Ophthalmol.* 1969;14:90–105.

Hartge P, Tucker MA, Shields JA, et al. Case-control study of female hormones and eye melanoma. *Ophthalmology.* 1990;5(1):18.

Lalive d'Epinay SF, Trub P. Retinale vaskulare komplicationen bei oralen kontrazeptiva. *Klin Monatsbl Augenheilkd.* 1986;188:394.

Perry ND, Mallen FJ. Cilioretinal artery occlusion associated with oral contraceptives. *Am J Ophthalmol.* 1977;84:56.

Petursson GJ, Fraunfelder FT, Meyer SM. Oral contraceptives. *Ophthalmology.* 1981;88:368–371.

Rait JL, O'Day J. Acute macular neuroretinopathy. *Aust NZ J Ophthalmol.* 1987;15:337–340.

Rock T, Dinar Y, Romen M. Retinal periphlebitis after hormonal treatment. *Ann Ophthalmol.* 1989;21:75–76.

Snir M, Cohen S, Ben-Sira I, et al. Retinal manifestations of thrombotic thrombocytopenic purpura (TTP) following use of contraceptive treatment. *Ann Ophthalmol.* 1985;17:109–112.

Stowe III CC, Zakov ZN, Albert DM. Central retinal vascular occlusion associated with oral contraceptives. *Am J Ophthalmol.* 1978;86:798–801.

Tagawa H, Yoshida A, Takahashi M. A case of bilateral branch vein occlusion due to long-standing use of oral contraceptives. *Folia Ophthalmol Jpn.* 1951;32:1981.

Takahashi H, Sakai F, Sakuragi S. A case of retinal branch vein occlusion associated with oral contraceptives. *Folia Ophthalmol Jpn.* 1983;34:2670.

Thorogood M. Risk of stroke in users of oral contraceptives. *JAMA.* 1999;281(14):1255–1256.

Estradiol

Gurwood AS, Gurwood I, Gubman DT, et al. Idiosyncratic ocular symptoms associated with the estradiol transdermal estrogen replacement patch system. *Optom Vis Sci.* 1995;72(1):29–33.

See also references in the section, "Combination products of estrogens and progestogens."

Clomifene (clomiphene) citrate

Asch RH, Greenblatt RB. Update on the safety and efficacy of clomiphene citrate as a therapeutic agent. *J Reprod Med.* 1976;17:175–180.

Kistner RW. The use of clomiphene citrate in the treatment of anovulation. *Semin Drug Treatment.* 1973;3(2):159–176.

Laing IA, Steer CR, Dudgeon J, et al. Clomiphene and congenital retinopathy. *Lancet.* 1981;2:1107–1108.

Piskazeck VK, Leitsmann H. Uber die Behandlung derfunktionellen Sterilitat mit Clostylbegyt. *Zentralbl Gynaekol.* 1976;98:904.

Politou M, Gialeraki A, Merkouri E, et al. Central retinal vein occlusion secondary to clomifene treatment in a male carrier of factor V Leiden. *Genet Test Mol Biomarkers.* 2009;13(2):155–157.

Roch II LM, Gordon DL, Barr AB, et al. Visual changes associated with clomiphene citrate therapy. *Arch Ophthalmol.* 1967;77:14–17.

Rock T, Dinar Y, Romen M. Retinal periphlebitis after hormonal treatment. *Ann Ophthalmol.* 1989;21:75–76.

Van Der Merwe JV. The effect of clomiphene and conjugated oestrogens on cervical mucus. *South Afr Med J.* 1981;60(9):347–349.

Viola MI, Meyer D, Kruger T, et al. Association between clomiphene citrate and visual disturbances with special emphasis on central retinal vein occlusion: a review. *Gynecol Obstet Invest.* 2011;71(2):73–76.

Levothyroxine sodium, liothyronine sodium, thyroid

Hymes LC, Warshaw BL, Schwartz JF. Pseudotumor cerebri and thyroid replacement therapy. *N Engl J Med.* 1983;309:732.

Josephson AM, MacKensie TP. Thyroid-induced mania in hypothyroid patients. *Br J Psychiatry.* 1980;137:222–228.

Kaeser HE. Drug-induced myasthenic syndromes. *Acta Neurol Scand.* 1984;70(suppl 100):39–47.

McVie R. Pseudotumor cerebri and thyroid-replacement therapy. *N Engl J Med.* 1983;309:731.

Misra M, Khan GM, Rath S. Eltroxin induced pseudotumor cerebri? A case report. *Indian J Ophthalmol.* 1992;40(4):117.

Raghavan S, DiMartino-Nardi J, Saenger P, et al. Pseudotumor cerebri in an infant after L-thyroxine therapy for transient neonatal hypothyroidism. *J Ped.* 1997;130(3):478–480.

Van Dop C, Conte FA, Koch TK, et al. Pseudotumor cerebri associated with initiation of levothyroxine therapy for juvenile hypothyroidism. *N Engl J Med.* 1983;308:1076–1080.

CHAPTER 12

Drugs Affecting Blood Formation and Coagulability

CLASS: DRUGS USED TO TREAT DEFICIENCY ANEMIAS

Generic Name:
Cobalt.

Proprietary Name:
Generic only.

Primary Use
This drug is used in the treatment of iron-deficiency anemia.

Ocular Side Effects
Systemic administration – environmental exposure, implant, oral, or tattoo
Certain
1. Decreased vision
2. Eyelids or conjunctiva
   a. Allergic reactions
   b. Photosensitivity
   c. Urticaria
3. Uveitis (skin tattoo)
4. Optic nerve
   a. Neuropathy
   b. Atrophy
5. Retinal and choroidal pathology

Clinical Significance
Cobalt is now only occasionally used because significant systemic side effects occur and safer drugs are available. Ocular side effects have been seen with cobalt metal hip arthroplasties, environmental exposure, tattoos, and in the treatment for anemia. Only rarely are ocular side effects due to cobalt therapy seen, and decreased vision is the most common complaint. Lim et al did a review of the literature showing high serum cobalt was associated with reversible and irreversible visual loss.[1] This included optic neuropathy and atrophy, electrophysiologic evidence of retinal and retinal pigment epithelium malfunction, and fluorescein angiographic

evidence of abnormal choroidal perfusion. Rorsman et al reported 3 cases of uveitis associated with cobalt skin tattooing.[2] Each time a reaction at the tattoo site occurred, the uveitis was exacerbated. Fraunfelder et al speculated that this was a type IV hypersensitivity reaction.[3] There are well-described cases of long-term cobalt treatment causing bilateral optic atrophy or optic nerve dysfunction.[4-11] Retinal and choroidal abnormalities are also described in the literature.[4-14]

Generic Names:
1. Epoetin alfa (erythropoietin); 2. epoetin beta.

Proprietary Names:
1. Epogen, Eprex, Procrit, Retacrit; 2. NeoRecormon.

Primary Use
Recombinant human epoetin is used in the treatment of anemia in chronic renal failure in dialysis patients.

Ocular Side Effects
Systemic administration – intravenous or subcutaneous
Probable
1. Decreased vision
2. Iritis-like reaction
3. Conjunctiva – hyperemia

Possible
1. Retina
   a. Induces retinal angiogenesis
   b. Enhances retinopathy of prematurity
2. Visual hallucinations

Conditional/unclassified
1. Recurrent postoperative lens capsule opacity

Clinical Significance
Low birth weight, premature infants are at higher risk for retinitis of prematurity and may undergo treatment with epoetin to prevent anemia of prematurity. The

United Kingdom Health Regulatory Agency warns that epoetin beta possibly increases the risk of retinopathy in premature infants, particularly if born before 31 weeks gestation or in those weighing less than 1.25 kg.[1]

Manzoni et al have reported epoetin alfa as an additional independent predictor of severe threshold retinopathy of prematurity, requiring urgent ablative surgery.[2] This occurred in 31% of infants on this drug compared with 19.6% of those not receiving this drug. Kelley reported proliferation of lens capsular debris that may be due to epoetin alfa.[3] Beiran et al described 13 patients with an iritis-like reaction associated with the use of epoetin alfa.[4] They felt this may have been related to epoetin's ability to alter prostaglandin levels, which may have broken the tight junctions of the iris and ciliary epithelium. Watanabe et al reported epoetin alfa as a factor in inducing retinal angiogenesis in proliferative diabetic retinopathy.[5] Patients on hemodialysis receiving epoetin alfa may develop visual hallucinations.[6–8] Fauchere et al reported early high-dose recombinant human erythropoietin administration in very premature infants is safe with no increased mortality or major adverse side effects, including retinopathy of prematurity.[9]

Generic Names:

1. Ferrous fumarate; 2. ferrous gluconate; 3. ferrous sulfate; 4. iron dextran; 5. iron sucrose; 6. polysaccharide iron complex.

Proprietary Names:

1. Femiron, Feostat, Ferretts, Hemaspan, Hemocyte, Nephro-Fer, Vitron-C; 2. Fergon; 3. Edin-sol, Feosol, Fer-gen-sol, Fe-Iron, Feratab, Fero-Grad, Isospran, Slow-Fe; 4. Dexferrum, Infed, Proferdex; 5. Velphoro, Venofer; 6. Fe-Tinic, Ferrex, Ferrex Plus, Hytinic, Niferex, Nu-Iron, Poly-Iron.

Primary Use

These iron preparations are effective in the prophylaxis and treatment of iron-deficiency anemias.

Ocular Side Effects

Systemic administration (toxic levels) – intramuscular, intravenous, or oral
Certain
1. Decreased vision (iron dextran)
2. Yellow-brown discoloration
   a. Sclera
   b. Choroid
3. Eyelids or conjunctiva (iron dextran)
   a. Erythema
   b. Edema

   c. Urticaria
   d. Photosensitivity reactions
   e. Conjunctivitis

Probable
1. Retinal degeneration – overdosage

Possible
1. Aggravates age-related macular degeneration

Inadvertent ocular exposure
Certain
1. Irritation
   a. Hyperemia
   b. Photophobia
   c. Edema
2. Yellow-brown discoloration or deposits
   a. Eyelids
   b. Conjunctiva
   c. Cornea
   d. Sclera

Probable
1. Ulceration
   a. Eyelids
   b. Conjunctiva
   c. Cornea

Clinical Significance

Systemically administered iron preparations seldom cause ocular side effects. Adverse ocular reactions have been reported after multiple blood transfusions (over 100), with unusually large amounts of iron in the diet, or markedly prolonged iron therapy. A few cases of retinitis pigmentosa–like fundal degeneration have been reported. Hodgkins et al described a case of pigment epitheliopathy with an overlying serous retinal detachment after an infusion of iron dextran.[1] Newer iron preparations make retinal degenerations less likely. Kawada et al described photosensitivity reactions due to sodium ferrous citrate.[2] Wong et al examined the role of iron toxicity as a potential factor in age-related macular degeneration.[3] They felt that, except in overdose situations, iron was not the cause of retinal changes. However, in patients with retinal diseases, they recommended that these patients avoid taking oral iron supplements.

Direct ocular exposure to acidic ferrous salts can cause ocular irritation, but significant ocular side effects rarely occur. However, Asproudis et al described a case of self-inflicted ocular side effect in a 45-year-old female who, after grinding a ferrous sulfate tablet, placed it in the inferior fornix of her left eye and rapidly developed severe ocular siderosis with profound visual loss, corneal opacity, cataract, retinal degeneration, and ultimately phthisis bulbi.[4]

Generic Name:
Methylene blue (methylthioninium chloride).

Proprietary Names:
ProvayBlue, Urolene Blue.

Primary Use
Systemic
Methylthioninium is a weak germicidal drug used as a urinary or gastrointestinal antiseptic. It is also given intravenously in the treatment of methemoglobinemia and "cyanosis anemia" and is used as a dye to demonstrate cerebrospinal fluid fistulae or blocks.

Ophthalmic
Methylthioninium is used as a tissue marker during ocular or lacrimal surgery and has been applied to the conjunctiva to decrease glare during microsurgery.

Ocular Side Effects
Systemic administration – intrathecal, intravenous, or intraventricular (used off-label)
Certain
1. Decreased vision
2. Blue-gray discoloration
   a. Vitreous and retina
   b. Eyelids
3. Color vision defect – objects have blue tinge

Probable
1. Decreased accommodation (intravenous)
2. Mydriasis (intravenous)

Possible
1. Papilledema
2. Diplopia
3. Paresis of extraocular muscles
4. Accommodative spasm
5. Optic atrophy

Local ophthalmic use or exposure – intracameral injection (used off-label)
Certain
1. Cytotoxicity
   a. Corneal endothelium
   b. Iris

Local ophthalmic use or exposure – topical ocular application (used off-label)
Certain
1. Irritation
   a. Lacrimation
   b. Edema
   c. Burning sensation
   d. Photosensitivity
2. Blue discoloration or staining
   a. Eyelid margins
   b. Conjunctiva
   c. Corneal nerves and epithelium
3. Cornea – endothelial toxicity

Clinical Significance
Significant ocular side effects due to methylene blue have been reported only with intrathecal or intraventricular injections and with intracameral injections at high concentrations. The most common ocular side effects after intravenous administration, other than cyanopsia or blue-gray discoloration of ocular tissue, are decreased vision, mydriasis, and decreased accommodation. Porat et al have shown that this drug can be a photosensitizer, causing significant skin reactions with blue staining of tissues.[1]

Infrequent use of topical ocular application of methylene blue in low concentrations (1%) is almost free of ocular side effects. However, irritation and pain may be so severe that a topical ocular anesthetic (1-2 times) may be required for the patient's comfort. Kushner reported a case in which this drug was used to irrigate the lacrimal system in a 2-year-old child.[2] The solution broke through to the periocular tissue, causing subcutaneous necrosis and marked edema along with bluish discoloration. Edema persisted for up to 2 years, and amblyopia treatment was necessary. Staining of ocular and periocular tissue may be permanent if the dye is applied daily for years. Intracameral use appears safe if used in low concentration. Brouzas et al and Timucin et al reported that inadvertent intracameral injection of 1% methylene blue may cause extreme cytotoxicity of the corneal endothelium, taking years to recover, with iris staining.[3,4] Low concentrations may possibly aggravate already abnormal endothelium. Accidental cornea exposure to methylene blue resulted in staining of corneal nerves and reduced corneal sensitivity, which resolved within 2 weeks, in a 10-year-old child.[5]

CLASS: ANTICOAGULANTS

Generic Names:
1. Alteplase; 2. reteplase; 3. tenecteplase.

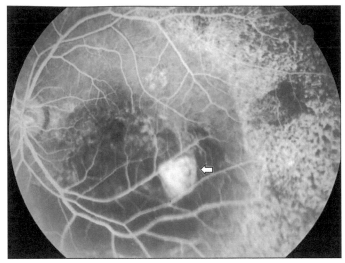

FIG. 12.1 Fluorescein angiography of diffuse granular hyperfluorescence.[13]

Proprietary Names:
1. Activase, Cathflo Activase; 2. Retavase, Rapilysin; 3. TNKase.

Primary Use
Systemic
These tissue plasminogen activators (t-PAs) are produced by recombinant DNA technology and are primarily indicated for the management of acute myocardial infarctions. Alteplase is also used in the management of acute ischemic stroke and pulmonary embolism.

Ophthalmic
Used to treat submacular hemorrhages, postvitrectomy fibrin syndrome, lysis of blood clots, and central retinal artery occlusion.

Ocular Side Effects
Systemic administration – intravenous injections
Certain
1. Hemorrhages
   a. Hyphema
   b. Retinal
   c. Orbital
   d. Choroidal
   e. Vitreous
   f. Retrobulbar
   g. Subretinal

Probable
1. Eyelids or conjunctiva
   a. Allergic reactions
   b. Edema
   c. Rashes
   d. Urticaria

Local ophthalmic use or exposure – intracameral injections
Certain
1. Hemorrhages
   a. Subconjunctival
   b. Hyphema
2. Cornea
   a. Band keratopathy
   b. Calcium phosphate precipitates
3. Retina – vitreous hemorrhage

Local ophthalmic use or exposure – intravitreal injections
Certain
1. Retina toxicity (high dosages)
   a. Diffuse pigmentary changes
   b. Exudative retinal detachment
   c. Granular hyperfluorescent lesion (fluorescein angiography) (Fig. 12.1)
2. Electroretinogram (ERG) – reduced scotopic and photopic a- and b-waves (high dose)
3. Vitreous hemorrhages

Clinical Significance

Systemically administered t-PA for various illnesses can cause bleeding anywhere within the eye or periorbital tissues. This may occur in sites of recent ocular surgery or be associated with the presence of exudative macular degeneration or retinal vascular diseases.[1-3] Visual outcomes vary from no complications to blindness or loss of the eye. Chorich et al emphasized that the onset of eye pain or vision loss after systemic t-PA should alert physicians to the possibility of an ocular or adnexal hemorrhage.[4]

Intracameral injection complications are much more frequent in single dosage over 25-μg and/or multiple t-PA intracameral injections. Hyphemas, subconjunctival hemorrhage, and vitreous hemorrhages have all been reported.[5-9] Rehfeldt et al, in their series of 185 intracameral t-PA injections, had a 5.4% incidence of hyphema and a 3.2% incidence of transient corneal edema.[10] This included 1 case of Fuch dystrophy, which had irreversible corneal endothelial decompensation. Hesse et al confirmed the temporary endothelial toxicity of t-PA.[11] Damage to the corneal endothelium allows phosphate (buffer of t-PA) and calcium from the aqueous humor to distribute within the corneal stroma. The insoluble calcium phosphate may then be precipitated within the stroma. This results in irreversible corneal opacification. Although this side effect is rare, it is easily produced in experimental animal models when the cornea endothelium is disturbed.[12]

Intravitreal injection complications increase with single dosages exceeding 50 μg and/or with repeat injections. Frequently, intravitreal t-PA is used along with pneumatic displacement, which adds a mechanical variable for possible ocular complications. Hesse et al described 4 patients given 100 μg intravitreal t-PA who developed exudative retinal detachment followed by hyperpigmentation of the retinal pigment epithelium in the area of the detachment.[12] Chen et al reported a similar case after 2 successive injections of 50 μg intravitreal t-PA 3 days apart with a minimal recovery of visual acuity.[13] Due to numerous reports of retinal toxicity in animals and humans, Chen et al advocated not using an injection over 25 μg.[13,14] Hassan et al varied this by recommending 25–100 μg, and Hesse et al felt higher dosages were indicated.[12,15] Intravitreal t-PA can cause sudden, severe vitreous hemorrhages as an immediate complication.[16]

Generic Names:

1. Apixaban; 2. dabigatran etexilate mesylate; 3. rivaroxaban.

Proprietary Names:

1. Eliquis; 2. Pradaxa; 3. Xarelto.

Primary Use

Dabigatran is a direct thrombin inhibitor, and both apixaban and rivaroxaban are specific inhibitors of factor Xa. These drugs are used in the management of atrial fibrillation, strokes, and systemic emboli.

Ocular Side Effects
Systemic administration – oral
Probable
1. Ocular bleeds from any vascular structure of ocular or periocular structures

Possible
1. Ocular myasthenia

Clinical Significance

This group of fairly new oral anticoagulants has the advantage over warfarin because they do not need coagulation monitoring or dosage adjustments due to their more predictable pharmacokinetics.[1] Statistically significant data show little difference in incidence of ocular side effects over placebos; however, subsets of patients are probably real as to a cause-and-effect relationship secondary to these drugs causing ocular bleeds. This conclusion is based on the onset occurring shortly after starting the medication, the number of bilateral ocular bleeds, the recurrent nature if staying on the medication, and the inability to control bleeding until the medication is discontinued. There are over 2000 spontaneous reports of ocular and periocular bleeds associated with the use of these drugs. Many are bilateral and a few are recurrent, with an apparent predilection for older patients. There have been reports of hyphema, subretinal, iris, and conjunctival bleeds.[2-4] Liu et al reported postoperative plastic surgery bleeds requiring procedures to protect the eye from orbital pressure increasing intraocular pressure.[5]

Shieh et al pointed out that observation and temporary cessation of the anticoagulant were sufficient in the management of these bleeding events in most patients.[4] There are cases where surgical intervention may be necessary to prevent permanent ocular damage.

Each case is individual as to how to manage and if cessation of the drug is viable. Ocular operation guidelines as to if the drug can be continued while performing surgery is also individualized, with informed consent being ideal. This whole subject may change as more data become available; however, at this point in time, major ocular complications from this class of drugs versus warfarin are as follows. Uyhazi et al, in retrospective cohort study, used a large national insurance claims database to generate 2 parallel analyses.[6] Their results suggested a decreased risk (25%) of intraocular hemorrhages associated with dabigatran and rivaroxaban compared with warfarin. They concluded that these newer anticoagulants are "at worst, equal in risk of intraocular hemorrhage and in some instances are safer than their traditional counterparts." Sun et al, using meta-analysis and randomized clinical data, also concluded that there was a 25% less incidence of ocular bleeds with these drugs versus warfarin.[7] Wormald et al evaluated these data and concluded that there is some uncertainty around relative risk estimates.[8] Therefore they felt that there are not enough data to warrant changing practice patterns.

San Norberto et al described a case of ocular myasthenia that they felt in all likelihood was caused by rivaroxaban.[9]

Generic Name:
Heparin sodium.

Proprietary Names:
Hepflush-10, Hep-Lock, Hep-Lock U/P, Monoject Prefill Advanced Heparin Lock Flush, SASH Normal Saline and Heparin.

Primary Use
This complex organic acid inhibits the blood-clotting mechanism and is used in the prophylaxis and treatment of venous thrombosis.

Ocular Side Effects
Systemic administration – intravenous or subcutaneous
Certain
1. Subconjunctival, anterior chamber, rectus muscle, or retinal hemorrhages
   a. Secondary to drug-induced anticoagulation
   b. Secondary to drug-induced anemia
2. Eyelids or conjunctiva
   a. Allergic reactions
   b. Conjunctivitis – nonspecific
   c. Edema
   d. Urticaria
   e. Necrosis

Probable
1. Lacrimation

Possible
1. Eyelids or conjunctiva – Lyell syndrome

Local ophthalmic use or exposure – subconjunctival injection
Certain
1. Subconjunctival or periocular hemorrhages

Probable
1. Subconjunctival scarring
2. Decreased intraocular pressure (minimal)

Possible
1. Exacerbation of primary disease

Clinical Significance
Ocular side effects due to systemic heparin are few and usually of little consequence. Ocular hemorrhage is the most serious adverse reaction and is probably more common in conditions with increased capillary fragility, such as diabetes.[1] Subconjunctival or periocular hemorrhage is the most common adverse reaction with subconjunctival heparin injections. It is more common after the third or fourth injection and seldom prevents continued injections of heparin. Chang et al described 2 pregnant women who developed spontaneous orbital hemorrhages after treatment with subcutaneous heparin.[2] Both women developed severe unilateral visual loss. Heparin-induced antiheparin platelet antibody leads to the thrombosis of ocular circulation.[3] Slusher et al reported hyphema in an otherwise normal eye seen 1 hour after 10,000 units of heparin were administered intravenously.[4]

Generic Name:
Streptokinase.

Proprietary Name:
Streptase.

Primary Use
This protein is used to dissolve thrombi in patients with myocardial infarction, pulmonary embolism, and other thromboembolic occlusions of veins and arteries.

Ocular Side Effects
Systemic administration – intravenous
Certain
1. Bleeding
   a. Periocular
   b. Tenon capsule
   c. Intraocular hemorrhage

    d. Hyphema
    e. Choroidal hematoma
    f. Vitreous hemorrhage
    g. Postoperative ocular bleeding
2. Anterior uveitis
3. Eyelids and orbit
    a. Urticaria
    b. Rash
    c. Edema

Conditional/unclassified
1. Central retinal artery occlusion

Clinical Significance
There are a number of reports of streptokinase causing intraocular bleeding, hyphemas, vitreous hemorrhages, or choroidal hematomas. The most serious ocular events are massive intraocular bleeds, some resulting in blindness, after intravenous streptokinase injections.[1,2] This often occurs within the first few hours after injection. This is a rare event. Cahane et al reported a total hyphema secondary to streptokinase after cataract surgery.[3] Marcus et al described a case of streptokinase-induced Tenon capsule hemorrhage after retinal detachment surgery.[4] The patient received intravenous streptokinase 2 hours after surgery when he developed a myocardial infarction. Potdar et al reported a case of unilateral central retinal artery occlusion after intravenous streptokinase, possibly due to an embolus, which caused optic atrophy and blindness.[5] There are a number of cases of primarily bilateral anterior uveitis.[6-10] Streptokinase-induced serum sickness, which Proctor et al felt occurred about 6% of the time, may occasionally exhibit a uveitis.[9] Streptokinase-induced uveitis is most likely a result of an immune complex reaction, like serum sickness, and is not due to any specific toxicity to the eye.[10] Anterior chamber injections of this drug for dissolution of fibrin exudates have had no detectable adverse intraocular effects.[11] Berger stated that there was intraocular irritation secondary to streptokinase, but it is possible that the drug used was not in as purified a form as is available now.[12] Up to one-third of patients who have received repeat injections of this drug have become hypersensitive to it. This may present with periorbital swelling and/or edema.

Generic Name:
Tranexamic acid.

Proprietary Names:
Cyklokapron, Lysteda.

Primary Use
An antifibrinolytic drug used primarily for treatment of excessive fibrinolysis. It has been used to control uterine and gastrointestinal bleeding, as well as traumatic hyphemas.

Ocular Side Effects
Systemic administration – intravenous or oral
Certain
1. Ligneous conjunctivitis
2. Color vision defect – transient
3. Decreased vision

Probable
1. Central retinal artery or venous branches
    a. Stasis
    b. Occlusion

Possible
1. Decreased corneal thickness
    a. Postintraocular surgery
    b. Bullous keratopathy

Conditional/unclassified
1. Retinal pigment epithelium disturbances

Clinical Significance
Diamond et al were the first to report ligneous conjunctivitis, including gingiva, with positive rechallenge due to tranexamic acid.[1] Hidayat et al reported 17 cases.[2] Song et al reported tranexamic acid causing ligneous conjunctivitis with positive rechallenge.[3] Scully et al showed that this drug can affect mucous membranes.[4]

Tranexamic acid use has been associated with retinal central artery and venous stasis, including occlusion.[5-7] Parsons et al described a case of branch retinal artery occlusion.[8] There are 22 additional cases in the spontaneous reports. In the *Physicians' Desk Reference*, under contraindications/precautions, the manufacturer warns that any visual changes require immediate ophthalmic evaluation.[9]

Tranexamic acid is contraindicated in patients with acquired defective color vision because this condition impedes appropriate monitoring of ocular toxicity.[9] Theil and Cravens et al have confirmed this.[10,11]

Retinal degenerations were seen in a matter of days after large dosages in animals. These changes were both central and peripheral.[10] To date this has not been seen in humans. However, Kitamura et al showed with rechallenge data that large dosages of tranexamic acid caused reversible decreased vision, probably due to malfunction of the pigment epithelium of the retina.[12] It was felt that reduction of renal function (where the drug is metabolized) was a factor. Pharmacia and UpJohn (unpublished) reported no retinal degenerative change in patients on therapeutic dosages for periods ranging from 15 months to 8 years.

Bramsen et al found that this drug decreases corneal edema in both bullous keratopathy and postintraocular surgery in humans.[13]

Generic Name:
Warfarin sodium.

Proprietary Names:
Coumadin, Jantoven.

Primary Use
This coumarin derivative is used as an anticoagulant in the prophylaxis and treatment of venous thrombosis.

Ocular Side Effects
Systemic administration – intravenous or oral
Certain
1. Bleeding
   a. Subconjunctival
   b. Hyphema
   c. Retina
   d. Vitreous
   e. Periocular
   f. Choroidal
   g. Suprachoroidal
   h. Rectus sheath
2. Eyelids or conjunctiva
   a. Allergic reactions
   b. Conjunctivitis – nonspecific
   c. Urticaria
   d. Skin necrosis

Probable
1. Lacrimation

Possible
1. Color vision defect

Ocular teratogenic effects
Possible
1. Optic atrophy
2. Cataracts
3. Microphthalmia
4. Blindness
5. Corneal opacification

Clinical Significance
Ocular side effects due to warfarin are uncommon. Massive retinal hemorrhages have been reported, especially in diseased tissue with possible capillary fragility, such as diabetic disciform degeneration of the macula.[1] However, the overall systemic bleeding rate is 1–3%.[2] Spontaneous hyphema can develop, including bilateral, which may be more common with iris fixed lenses.[3] A potentially dangerous association between the onset of a herpes zoster infection and oral anticoagulant therapy has also been found. Even so, as extensively as this drug has been used, only a few major adverse ocular side effects have been reported. Interaction of systemic doxycycline and warfarin or even topical ocular erythromycin can increase the international normalized ratio, thereby increasing the hematologic effects of warfarin.[4,5] There is some controversy as to when one might discontinue warfarin before ocular surgery to prevent an increased incidence of hemorrhaging in patients. Diabetes, hypertension, exudative age-related macular degeneration, atrial fibrillation with age-related macular degeneration, exfoliative glaucoma with vascularized posterior synechia, patients on fluconazole, and patients with other hemopoietic deficiencies have been suggested.[6-10] However, it seems that most vitreoretinal and cataract surgeons felt that the risk of stopping warfarin may outweigh the risk of ocular, intraocular, or postoperative bleeding so they do not stop the anticoagulants.[11-14] There is also a fear that stopping the anticoagulant may give a period of a transient hypercoagulable state resulting in more extensive bleeding if the drug is suddenly discontinued.[15] Caronia et al described a case of bilateral angle-closure glaucoma secondary to posterior segment intraocular hemorrhage due to anticoagulants.[16] Masri et al described acute glaucoma due to spontaneous suprachoroidal hemorrhage secondary to loss of warfarin anticoagulation control.[17] Parkin et al polled ocular plastic surgeons, and more than half have seen serious postoperative bleeding problems in patients on this drug, and about half considered stopping this drug preoperatively.[18]

Although eyelid skin necrosis is rare, if it does occur, it is typically between the third and tenth day of treatment. It is felt that this is due to a transient hypercoagulable state.[19]

There are data to suggest that this drug can cause teratogenic effects. Teratogenic effects appear to be most severe when warfarin is taken during the first trimester. Conradi-Hunermann syndrome, or chondrodysplasia punctata, and Dandy-Walker syndrome, with their associated ocular defects, have been reported in the offspring of patients receiving warfarin therapy during their pregnancies.[20]

Recommendations

1. There is controversy about how much safer, from an ocular point of view, the newer novel oral anticoagulants (apixaban, dabigatran, rivaroxaban) are compared with warfarin.[21-23] Sun et al stated a 20% reduction in bleeding ocular side effects with the novel oral anticoagulants.[21]
2. Although each case is individualized, oral versus injectable warfarin is less attractive because it requires close monitoring.

CLASS: BLOOD SUBSTITUTES

Generic Name:
Dextran.

Proprietary Names:
Gentran 40, Gentran 70, Hyskon, Macrodex, Promit, Rheomacrodex.

Primary Use
Systemic
This water-soluble glucose polymer is used for early fluid replacement and for plasma volume expansion in the adjunctive treatment of certain types of shock.

Ophthalmic
Combination dextran nanoparticles are being used in drug delivery to the eye. This drug is also used as a topical ocular demulcent.

Ocular Side Effects
Systemic administration – intravenous
Probable
1. Eyelids or conjunctiva
   a. Erythema
   b. Conjunctivitis – nonspecific
   c. Edema
   d. Urticaria
2. Irritation
   a. Lacrimation
   b. Photophobia
   c. Burning sensation
3. Keratitis

Local ophthalmic use or exposure – topical ocular application
Unconditional/unclassified
1. Corneal opacities

Clinical Significance
The most common adverse ocular reaction due to dextran is ocular irritation because this drug is secreted in the tears. An allergic keratitis, which disappeared when the drug was discontinued, has also been reported in several patients. A hypersensitivity reaction, including fever, nasal congestion, joint pain, urticaria, hypotension, and ocular irritation, can occur. This is probably due to dextran-reactivated antibodies.

Höllhumer et al described persistent epithelial opacities and corneal opacities after collagen cross-linking with substitution of dextran (T-500) with dextran sulfate in compounded topical ocular riboflavin.[1]

REFERENCES
Drug: Cobalt
1. Lim CA, Khan J, Chelva E, et al. The effect of cobalt on the human eye. *Doc Ophthalmol.* 2015;130:43–48.
2. Rorsman H, Brehmer-Andersson E, Dahlquist I, et al. Tattoo granuloma and uveitis. *Lancet.* 1969;2:27–28.
3. Fraunfelder FW, Rosenbaum JT. Drug-induced uveitis: incidence, prevention, and treatment. *Drug Saf.* 1997;17(3):197–207.
4. Licht A, Oliver M, Rachmilewitz EA. Optic atrophy following treatment with cobalt chloride in a patient with pancytopenia and hypercellular marrow. *Isr J Med Sci.* 1972;8:61–66.
5. Meecham HM, Humphrey P. Industrial exposure to cobalt causing optic atrophy and nerve deafness: a case report. *J Neurol Neurosurg Psychiat.* 1991;54:374–375.
6. Steens W, von Foerster G, Katzer A. Severe cobalt poisoning with loss of sight after ceramic-metal pairing in a hip – a case report. *Acta Orthop.* 2006;77(5):830–832.
7. Tower SS. Arthroprosthetic cobaltism: neurological and cardiac manifestations in two patients with metal-on-metal arthroplasty: a case report. *J Bone Joint Surg Am.* 2010;92(17):2847–2851.
8. Rizetti MC, Liberini P, Zarattini G, et al. Loss of sight and sound. Could it be the hip? *Lancet.* 2009;373(9668):1052.
9. Rizetti MC, Catalani S, Apostoli P, et al. Cobalt toxicity after total hip replacement: a neglected adverse effect? *Muscle Nerve.* 2011;43(1):146–147.
10. Bhardwaj N, Perez J, Peden M. Optic neuropathy from cobalt toxicity in a patient who ingested cattle magnets. *Neuroophthalmology.* 2011;35(1):24–26.
11. Apel W, Stark D, Stark A, et al. Cobalt-chromium toxic retinopathy case study. *Doc Ophthalmol.* 2013;126(1):69–78.
12. Ng SK, Ebneter A, Gilhortra JS. Hip-implant related chorio-retinal cobalt toxicity. *Indian J Ophthalmol.* 2013;61(1):35–37.
13. Apel W, Stark D, O'Hagan S. An update on cobalt-chromium toxic retinopathy. *Doc Ophthalmol.* 2013;127(2):173–175.

14. Kang JY, Lee SU, Nam KY, et al. A case of acute retinal toxicity caused by an intraocular foreign body composed of cobalt alloy. *Cutan Ocul Toxicol.* 2014;33(2):91–93.

Drugs: Epoetin alfa (erythropoietin), epoetin beta
1. Epoetin beta: increased risk of retinopathy in preterm infants cannot be excluded. *Drug Safety Update MHRA.* 2015;8(10):3.
2. Manzoni P, Maestri A, Gomirato G. Erythropoietin as a retinal angiogenic factor. *N Engl J Med.* 2005;353:782–792.
3. Kelley JS. *Recurrent Capsular Opacity and Erythropoietin.* Sea Island. GA: American Ophthalmological Society Meeting; 2002.
4. Beiran I, Krasnitz I, Mezer E, et al. Erythropoietin induced iritis-like reaction. *Eur J Ophthalmol.* 1996;6(1):14–16.
5. Watanabe D, Suzuma K, Matsui S, et al. Erythropoietin as a retinal angiogenic factor in proliferative diabetic retinopathy. *N Engl J Med.* 2005;353:782–792.
6. Stead R. Erythropoietin and visual hallucinations (reply). *N Engl J Med.* 1991;325:285.
7. Steinberg H. Erythropoietin and visual hallucinations (letter). *N Engl J Med.* 1991;325:285.
8. Steinberg H, Saravay SM, Wadhwa N, et al. Erythropoietin and visual hallucinations in patients on dialysis. *Psychosomatics.* 1996;37(6):556–563.
9. Fauchere JC, Koller BM, Tschopp A, et al. Safety of early high-dose recombinant erythropoietin for neuroprotection in very preterm infants. *J Pediatr.* 2015;167:52–57.

Drugs: Ferrous fumarate, ferrous gluconate, ferrous sulfate, iron dextran, iron sucrose, polysaccharide iron complex
1. Hodgkins PR, Morrell AJ, Luff AJ, et al. Pigment epitheliopathy with serous detachment of the retina following intravenous iron dextran. *Eye.* 1992;6(Pt 4):414–415.
2. Kawada A, Hiruma M, Noguchi H, et al. Photosensitivity due to sodium ferrous citrate. *Contact Dermatitis.* 1996;34(1):77.
3. Wong RW, Richa C, Hahn P, et al. Iron toxicity as a potential factor in AMD. *Retina.* 2007;27:997–1003.
4. Asproudis I, Zafeiropoulos P, Katsanos A, et al. Severe self-inflicted acute ocular siderosis caused by an iron tablet in the conjunctival fornix. *Acta Medica (Hradec Kralove).* 2017;60(4):160–162.

Drug: Methylene blue (methylthioninium chloride)
1. Porat R, Gilbert S, Magilner D. Methylene blue-induced phototoxicity: an unrecognized complication. *Pediatrics.* 1996;97(5):717–721.
2. Kushner BJ. Solutions can be hazardous for lacrimal system irrigation. *Arch Ophthalmol.* 1993;111:904–905.
3. Brouzas D, Droutsas S, Charakidas A. Severe toxic effect of methylene blue 1% on iris epithelium and corneal endothelium. *Cornea.* 2006;25:470–471.
4. Timucin OB, Karadaq MF, Aslanci ME, et al. Methylene blue-related corneal edema and iris discoloration. *Arq Bras Oftalmol.* 2016;79(2):121–122.
5. Peter S, Reichart E, Poyntner L, et al. Accidental staining of corneal nerves by methylene blue. *Ophthalmologe.* 2013;110(9):869–871.

Drugs: Alteplase, reteplase, tenecteplase
1. Khawly JA, Ferrone PJ, Holck DE. Choroidal hemorrhage associated with systemic tissue plasminogen activator. *Am J Ophthalmol.* 1996;121:577–578.
2. Roaf E, DaSilva C, Tsao K, et al. Orbital hemorrhage after thrombolytic therapy. *Arch Intern Med.* 1997;157:2670–2671.
3. Kaba RA, Lewis A, Bloom P, et al. Intraocular haemorrhage after thrombolysis. *Lancet.* 2005;365:330.
4. Chorich LJ, Derick RJ, Chambers RB, et al. Hemorrhagic ocular complications associated with the use of systemic thrombolytic agents. *Ophthalmology.* 1998;105:428–431.
5. Tripathi RC, Tripathi BJ, Park JK, et al. Intracameral tissue plasminogen activator for resolution of fibrin clots after glaucoma filtering procedures. *Am J Ophthalmol.* 1991;111:247–248.
6. Lundy DL, Sidoti P, Winarko T, et al. Intracameral tissue plasminogen activator after glaucoma surgery. *Ophthalmology.* 1996;103:274–282.
7. Loffler KV, Meyer JH, Wollensak G, et al. Success and complications of rTPA treatment of the anterior eye segment. *Ophthalmologe.* 1997;94:50–52.
8. Lee PF, Myers KS, Hsieh MM, et al. Treatment of failing glaucoma filtering cystic blebs with tissue plasminogen activator (t-PA). *J Ocul Pharmacol Ther.* 1995;11:227–232.
9. Kim MH, Koo TH, Sah WJ, et al. Treatment of total hyphema with relatively low dose tissue plasminogen activator. *Ophthalmic Surg Laser.* 1998;29:762–766.
10. Rehfeldt K, Hoh H. Therapeutic and prophylactic application of TPA (recombinant tissue plasminogen activator) into the anterior chamber of the eye. *Ophthalmologe.* 1999;96:587–593.
11. Hesse L, Nebelin B, Kauffmann T. Etiology of corneal opacities after plasminogen activator-induced fibrinolysis of the anterior chamber. *Ophthalmology.* 1999;96:448–452.
12. Hesse L, Schmidt J, Kroll P. Management of acute submacular hemorrhage using recombinant tissue plasminogen activator and gas. *Graefes Arch Clin Exp Ophthalmol.* 1999;237:273–277.
13. Chen S-N, Yang T-C, Cheng-Lien H, et al. Retinal toxicity of intravitreal tissue plasminogen activator: case report and literature review. *Ophthalmology.* 2003;110:704–708.
14. Hrach CJ, Johnson MW, Hassan AS, et al. Retinal toxicity of commercial intravitreal tissue plasminogen activator solution in cat eyes. *Arch Ophthalmol.* 2000;118:659–663.
15. Hassan AS, Johnson MW, Schneiderman TE, et al. Management of submacular hemorrhage with intravitreous tissue plasminogen activator injection and pneumatic displacement. *Ophthalmology.* 1999;106:1900–1907.

16. Kokame GT. Vitreous hemorrhage after intravitreal tissue plasminogen activator (t-PA) and pneumatic displacement of submacular hemorrhage. *Am J Ophthalmol.* 2000;129:546–547.

Drugs: Apixaban, dabigatran etexilate mesylate, rivaroxaban

1. Lauffenburger J, Farley J, Gehi A, et al. Factors driving anticoagulant selection in patients with atrial fibrillation in the United States. *Am J Cardiol.* 2015;115(8):1095–1101.
2. Kang TS, Lord K, Kunjukunju N. Spontaneous choroidal hemorrhage in a patient on dabigatran etexilate (Pradaxa). *Retin Cases Brief Rep.* 2014;8(3):175–177.
3. Wang K, Ehlers JP. Bilateral spontaneous hyphema, vitreous hemorrhage and choroidal detachment with concurrent dabigatran etexilate therapy. *Ophthalmic Surg Lasers Imaging Retina.* 2016;47(1):78–80.
4. Shieh WS, Sridhar J, Hong BK, et al. Ophthalmic complications associated with direct oral anticoagulant medications. *Semin Ophthalmol.* 2017;32(5):614–619.
5. Liu CY, Samimi DB, Tao JP. Hemorrhagic complications of rivaroxaban after eyelid surgery. *Ophthal Plast Reconstr Surg.* 2016;32(1):74.
6. Uyhazi KE, Miano T, Pan W, et al. Association of novel oral antithrombotics with the risk of intraocular bleeding. *JAMA Ophthalmol.* 136(2):122–130.
7. Sun MT, Wood MK, Chan WO, et al. Risk of intraocular bleeding with novel oral anticoagulants compared with warfarin. *JAMA Ophthalmol.* 2017;135(8):864–870.
8. Wormald R, Evans J. Risk of intraocular bleeding and the new anticoagulants: not such a big effect. *JAMA Ophthalmol.* 2017;135(11):1281–1282.
9. San Norberto EM, Garcia-Saiz I, Gutierrez D, et al. Ocular myasthenia induced by rivaroxaban in patient with deep vein thrombosis. *Ann Vasc Surg.* 2018;49:313e1–313e3.

Drug: Heparin sodium

1. Levartovsky S, Reisin I, Reisin I, et al. Bilateral posterior segment intraocular hemorrhage in a diabetic patient after therapy with heparin. *Isr Med Assoc J.* 2003;5:605.
2. Chang WJ, Nowinski TS, Repke CS, et al. Spontaneous orbital hemorrhage in pregnant women treated with subcutaneous heparin. *Am J Ophthalmol.* 1996;122(6):907–908.
3. Nguyen QD, Van Do D, Feke GT, et al. Heparin-induced antiheparin-platelet antibody associated with retinal venous thrombosis. *Ophthalmology.* 2003;110:600–603.
4. Slusher MM, Hamilon RW. Spontaneous hyphema during hemodialysis. *N Engl J Med.* 1975;293:561.

Drug: Streptokinase

1. Peyman M, Subrayan V. Irreversible blindness following intravenous streptokinase. *JAMA Ophthalmol.* 2013;131(10):1–2.
2. Kaba RA, Cox D, Lewis A, et al. Intraocular haemorrhage after thrombolysis. *Lancet.* 2005;365(9456):330.

3. Cahane M, Ashkenazi I, Avni I, et al. Total hyphaema following streptokinase administration eight days after cataract extraction. *Br J Ophthalmol.* 1990;74:447.
4. Marcus DM, Frederick Jr AR. Streptokinase-induced Tenon's hemorrhage after retinal detachment surgery. *Am J Ophthalmol.* 1994;118(6):815–816.
5. Potdar NA, Shinde CA, Murthy GG, et al. Unilateral central retinal artery occlusion following intravenous streptokinase. *J Postgrad Med.* 2001;47:262–263.
6. Kinshuck D. Bilateral hypopyon and streptokinase. Drug Points. *BMJ.* 1992;305(6865):1332.
7. Birnbaum Y, Barash D, Rechavia E, et al. Acute iritis and transient renal impairment following thrombolytic therapy for acute myocardial infarction (letter). *Ann Pharmacother.* 1993;27(12):1539–1540.
8. Gray MY, Lazarus JH. Iritis after treatment with streptokinase. Drug Points. *BMJ.* 1994;309:97.
9. Proctor BD, Joondeph BC. Bilateral anterior uveitis. A feature of streptokinase-induced serum sickness. *N Engl J Med.* 1994;330:576–577.
10. Fraunfelder FW, Rosenbaum JT. Drug-induced uveitis: incidence, prevention, and treatment. *Drug Saf.* 1997;17(3):197–207.
11. Cherfan GM, el Maghraby A, Tabbara KF, et al. Dissolution of intraocular fibrinous exudate by streptokinase. *Ophthalmology.* 1991;98(6):870–874.
12. Berger B. The effect of streptokinase irrigation on experimentally clotted blood in the anterior chamber of human eyes. *Acta Ophthalmol.* 1962;40:373–378.

Drug: Tranexamic acid

1. Diamond JP, Chandna A, Williams C, et al. Tranexamic acid-associated ligneous conjunctivitis with gingival and peritoneal lesions. *Br J Ophthalmol.* 1991;75(12):753–754.
2. Hidayat AA, Riddle MP. Ligneous conjunctivitis: a clinicopathologic study of 17 cases. *Ophthalmology.* 1987;94(8):949–959.
3. Song Y, Izumi N, Potts LB, et al. Tranexamic acid-induced ligneous conjunctivitis with renal failure showed reversible hypoplasminogenaemia. *BMJ Case Rep.* 2014.
4. Scully C, Gokbuget AY, Allen C, et al. Oral lesions indicative of plasminogen deficiency (hypoplasminogenemia). *Oral Surg Oral Med Oral Path Oral Radiol Endod.* 2001;91(3):334–337.
5. Snir M, Axer-Siegel R, Buckman G, et al. Central venous stasis retinopathy following the use of tranexamic acid. *Retina.* 1990;10:181–184.
6. Wijetilleka S. Central retinal artery occlusion in a 30-year-old woman taking tranexamic acid. *BMJ Case Rep.* 2017; 2017 Jul 13.
7. Dighiero P, Frau E, Bodaghi B, et al. Central retinal artery occlusion related to ingestion of tranexamic acid. *J Fr Ophtalmol.* 1996;19(12):785–786.
8. Parsons MR, Merritt DR, Ramsay RC. Retinal artery occlusion associated with tranexamic acid therapy. *Am J Ophthalmol.* 1988;105(6):688–689.

9. *Tranexamic acid.* 2018. Retrieved from http://www.pdr. net.
10. Theil PL. Ophthalmological examination of patients in long-term treatment with tranexamic acid. *Acta Ophthalmol.* 1981;59:237–241.
11. Cravens GT, Brown MJ, Brown DR, et al. Antifibrinolytic therapy use to mitigate blood loss during staged complex major spine surgery: postoperative visual color changes after tranexamic acid administration. *Anesthesiology.* 2006;105(6):1274–1276.
12. Kitamura H, Matsui I, Itoh N. Tranexamic acid-induced visual impairment in a hemodialysis patient. *Clin Exp Nephrol.* 2003;7:311–314.
13. Bramsen T, Corydon L, Ehlers N. A double-blind study of the influence of tranexamic acid on the central corneal thickness after cataract extraction. *Acta Ophthalmol.* 1978;56:121–127.

Drug: Warfarin sodium

1. Lewis H, Sloan SH, Foos RY. Massive intraocular hemorrhage associated with anticoagulation and age-related macular degeneration. *Graefes Arch Clin Exp Ophthalmol.* 1988;226:59–64.
2. Holdbrook A, Schulman S, Witt DM, et al. Evidence-based management of anticoagulant therapy: antithrombotic therapy and prevention of thrombosis, 9th ed: American College of Chest Physicians Evidence-Based Clinical Practice Guidelines. *Chest.* 2012;141(suppl 2):e152S–e184S.
3. Dharmasena A, Watts GM. Bilateral spontaneous hyphaema: case report and review of the literature. *J Thromb Thrombolysis.* 2013;36(3):343–345.
4. Hasan SA. Interaction of doxycycline and warfarin: an enhanced anticoagulant effect. *Cornea.* 2007;26(6):742–743.
5. Parker DL, Hoffmann TK, Tucker MA, et al. Elevated International Normalized Ratio associated with concurrent use of ophthalmic erythromycin and warfarin. *Am J Health Sys Pharm.* 2010;67:38–41.
6. Tilanus MA, Vaandrager W, Cuypers MH, et al. Relationship between anticoagulant medication and massive intraocular hemorrhage in age related macular degeneration. *Graefe's Arch Clin Exp Ophthalmol.* 2000;238:482–485.
7. Ung T, James M, Gray RH. Long-term warfarin associated with bilateral blindness in a patient with atrial fibrillation and macular degeneration. *Heart.* 2003;89:985.
8. Greenfield DS, Liebmann JM, Ritch R. Hyphema associated with papillary dilation in a patient with exfoliation glaucoma and warfarin therapy. *Am J Ophthalmol.* 1999;128:98–100.
9. Mootha VV, Schluter ML, Das A, et al. Intraocular hemorrhages due to warfarin-fluconazole drug interaction in a patient with presumed candida endophthalmitis. *Arch Ophthalmol.* 2002;120:94–95.
10. Younger JR, McHenry JG. Visually disabling non-traumatic orbital hemorrhage in an anticoagulated patient with factor VII deficiency. *J Neuro-Ophthalmol.* 2006;26:76–77.

11. Oh J, Smiddy WE, Kim SS. Antiplatelet and anticoagulation therapy in vitreoretinal surgery. *Am J Ophthalmol.* 2011;151(6):934–939.
12. Charles S, Rosenfeld PJ, Gayer S. Medical consequences of stopping anticoagulant therapy before intraocular surgery or intravitreal injections. *Retina.* 2007;27(7):813–815.
13. Kobayashi H. Evaluation of the need to discontinue antiplatelet and anticoagulant medications before cataract surgery. *J Cataract Refract Surg.* 2010;36(7):1115–1119.
14. Benzimra JD, Johnston RL, Jaycock P, et al. The Cataract National Dataset electronic multicentre audit of 55,567 operations: antiplatelet and anticoagulant medications. *Eye.* 2009;23(1):10–16.
15. Konstantatos A. Anticoagulation and cataract surgery: a review of the current literature. *Anaesth Intensive Care.* 2001;29:553–554.
16. Caronia RM, Sturm RT, Fastenberg DM, et al. Bilateral secondary angle-closure glaucoma as a complication of anticoagulation in a nanophthalmic patient. *Am J Ophthalmol.* 1998;126(2):307–309.
17. Masri I, Smith JM, Wride NK, et al. A rare case of acute angle closure due to spontaneous suprachoroidal haemorrhage secondary to loss of anti-coagulation control: a case report. *BMC Ophthalmol.* 2018;18(suppl 1):224.
18. Parkin B, Manner R. Aspirin and warfarin therapy in oculoplastic surgery. *Br J Ophthalmol.* 2000;84:1426–1427.
19. Rafiei N, Tabandeh H, Hirschbein M. Warfarin-induced skin necrosis of the eyelids. *Arch Ophthalmol.* 2007;125:421.
20. Kaplan LC. Congenital Dandy Walker malformation associated with first trimester warfarin: a case report and literature review. *Teratology.* 1985;32:333–337.
21. Sun MT, Wood MK, Chan W, et al. Risk of intraocular bleeding with novel oral anticoagulants compared with warfarin. *JAMA Ophthalmol.* 2017;135(8):864–870.
22. Wormald R, Evans J. Risk of intraocular bleeding and the new anticoagulants: not such a big effect. *JAMA Ophthalmol.* 2017;135(11):1281.
23. Sun MT, Wong CX. Risk of intraocular bleeding and the new anticoagulants: not such a big effect - Reply. *JAMA Ophthalmol.* 2017;135(11):1281–1282.

Drug: Dextran

1. Höllhumer R, Watson S, Beckingsale P. Persistent epithelial defects and corneal opacity after collagen cross-linking with substitution of dextran (T-500) with dextran sulfate in compounded topical riboflavin. *Cornea.* 2017;36(3):382–385.

FURTHER READING

Cobalt

Camarasa JG, Alomar A. Photosensitization to cobalt in a bricklayer. *Contact Dermatitis.* 1981;7:154–155.
Hjorth N. Contact dermatitis in children. *Acta Derm Venereal.* 1981;95(suppl):36–39.
Smith JD, Odom RB, Maibach HI. Contact urticaria from cobalt chloride. *Arch Dermatol.* 1975;111:1610–1611.

Ferrous fumarate, ferrous gluconate, ferrous sulfate, iron dextran, iron sucrose, polysaccharide iron complex

Appel I, Barishak YR. Histopathologic changes in siderosis bulbi. *Ophthalmologica*. 1978;176:205–210.

Brunette JR, Wagdi S, Lafond G. Electroretinographic alterations in retinal metallosis. *Can J Ophthalmol*. 1980;15:176–178.

Declercq SS. Desferrioxamine in ocular siderosis. *Br J Ophthalmol*. 1980;64:626–629.

Kearns M, McDonald R. Generalized siderosis from an iris foreign body. *Aust J Ophthalmol*. 1980;8:311–313.

Salminen L, Paasio P, Ekfors T. Epibulbar siderosis induced by iron tablets. *Am J Ophthalmol*. 1982;93:660–661.

Syversen K. Intramuscular iron therapy and tapetoretinal degeneration. *Acta Ophthalmol*. 1979;57:358–361.

Wolter JR. The lens as a barrier against foreign body reaction. *Ophthalmic Surg*. 1981;12:42–45.

Methylene blue (methylthioninium chloride)

Chang YS, Tseng SY, Tseng SH, et al. Comparison of eyes for cataract surgery. Part 1: cytotoxicity to corneal endothelial cells in a rabbit model. *J Cataract Refract Surg*. 2005;31:792–798.

Evans JP, Keegan HR. Danger in the use of intrathecal methylene blue. *JAMA*. 1960;174:856–859.

Lubeck MJ. Effects of drugs on ocular muscles. *Int Ophthalmol Clin*. 1971;11(2):35–62.

Morax S, Limon S, Forest A. Exogenous conjunctival pigmentation by methylene blues. *Arch Ophthalmol*. 1977;37:708A.

Norn MS. Methylene blue (methylthionine) vital staining of the cornea and conjunctiva. *Acta Ophthalmol*. 1967;45:347–358.

Pasticier-Florquin A, Boski LS, Morax S, et al. Ocular tattooing from abuse of methylene blue collyrium. *Bull Soc Ophtalmol Fr*. 1977;77:147–151.

Perry PM, Meinhard E. Necrotic subcutaneous abscesses following injections of methylene blue. *Br J Clin Pract*. 1974;8:289–291.

Raimer SS, Quevedo EM, Johnston RV. Dye rashes. *Cutis*. 1999;63(2):103–106.

Alteplase, reteplase, tenecteplase

Hesse L. Treating subretinal hemorrhage with tissue plasminogen activator. *Arch Ophthalmol*. 2002;120:102–103.

Leong JK, Ghabrial R, McCluskey PJ. Orbital haemorrhage complication following postoperative thrombolysis. *Br J Ophthalmol*. 2003;87:655–656.

Skolnick CA, Fiscella RG, Tessles HH, et al. Tissue plasminogen activator to treat impending papillary block glaucoma in patients with acute fibrinous HLA-B27 positive iridocyclitis. *Am J Ophthalmol*. 2000;129:363–366.

Smith MF, Doyle JW. Use of tissue plasminogen activator to revive blebs following intraocular surgery. *Arch Ophthalmol*. 2001;119:809–812.

Apixaban, dabigatran etexilate mesylate, rivaroxaban

Talany G, Guo M, Etminan M. Risk of intraocular hemorrhage with new oral anticoagulants. *Eye*. 2017;31(4):628–631.

Heparin sodium

Leung A. Toxic epidermal necrolysis associated with maternal use of heparin. *JAMA*. 1985;253:201.

Levine LE, Bernstein JE, Soltani K, et al. Heparin-induced cutaneous necrosis unrelated to injection sites. *Arch Dermatol*. 1983;119:400–403.

Lipson ML. Toxicity of systemic agents. *Int Ophthalmol Clin*. 1971;11(2):159–183.

Streptokinase

Beare N. "Hyperacute" unilateral anterior uveitis and secondary glaucoma following streptokinase infusion. *Eye*. 2004;18:111.

Boyer HK, Suran AA, Hogan MJ, et al. Studies on simulated vitreous hemorrhages. *Arch Ophthalmol*. 1958;59:333–336.

Oliveira DC, Coelho OR, Paraschin K, et al. Angioedema related to the use of streptokinase. *Arq Br Cardiol*. 2005;85:131–134.

Ortega-Carnicer J, Porras-Leal L, Fernandez-Ruiz A. Intraocular hemorrhage after intravenous streptokinase. *Med Clin*. 2000;115:718–719.

Steinemann T, Goins K, Smith T, et al. Acute closed-angle glaucoma complicating hemorrhagic choroidal detachment associated with parenteral thrombolytic agents. *Am J Ophthalmol*. 1988;106:752–753.

Sunderraj P. Intraocular hemorrhage associated with intravenously administered streptokinase. *Am J Ophthalmol*. 1991;112(6):734–735.

Van den Berg E, Lohmann N, Friedburg D, et al. Report of general temporary anticoagulation in the treatment of acute cerebral and retinal ischaemia. *Vasa*. 1997;26(3):222–227.

Tranexamic acid

Bramsen T, Ehlers N. Bullous keratopathy treated systemically with 4-transamino-cyclohexano-carboxylic acid. *Acta Ophthalmol*. 1977;55:665–673.

Dunn CJ, Goa KL. Tranexamic acid: a review of its use in surgery and other indications. *Drugs*. 1999;57(6):1005–1032.

Schuster V, Seregard S. Ligneous conjunctivitis. *Surv Ophthalmol*. 2003;48(4):369–388.

Warfarin sodium

Blumenkopf B, Lockhart Jr WS. Herpes zoster infection and use of oral anticoagulants. A potentially dangerous association. *JAMA*. 1983;250:936–937.

Chandra A, Barsam A, Hugkulstone C. A spontaneous suprachoroidal haemorrhage: a case report. *Cases J*. 2009;2:185.

Downie AC, Mackey DA, Vote BJ. Isolated corneal opacification and microphthalmia: a suspected warfarin embryopathy. *Clin Experiment Ophthalmol*. 2009;37(6):624–625.

Fenman SS, Bartlett RE, Roth AM, et al. Intraocular hemorrhage and blindness associated with systemic anticoagulation. *JAMA*. 1972;220:1354–1355.

Gainey SP, Robertson DM, Fay W, et al. Ocular surgery on patients receiving long-term warfarin therapy. *Am J Ophthalmol*. 1989;108:142–146.

Gordon DM, Mead J. Retinal hemorrhage with visual loss during anticoagulant therapy. *J Am Geriat Soc.* 1968;16:99–100.

Hall DL, Steen Jr WH, Drummond JW. Anticoagulants and cataract surgery. *Ann Ophthalmol.* 1980;12:759.

Harrod MJ, Sherro PS. Warfarin embryopathy in siblings. *Obstet Gynecol.* 1981;57:673–676.

Kleinebrecht J. Zur Teratogenitat von Cumarin-Derivaten. *Dtsch Med Wochenschr.* 1982;107:1929–1931.

Koehler MP, Sholiton DH. Spontaneous hyphema resulting from warfarin. *Ann Ophthalmol.* 1983;1:858–859.

Leath MC. Coumarin skin necrosis. *Texas Med.* 1983;79:62–64.

Lumme P, Laatikainen LT. Risk factors for intraoperative and early postoperative complications in extracapsular cataract surgery. *Eur J Ophthalmol.* 1994;4(3):151–158.

Marti J. Acute abdominal pain and warfarin therapy. *J Emerg Med.* 2011;41:e17–e18.

Robinson GA, Nylander A. Warfarin and cataract extraction. *Br J Ophthalmol.* 1989;73:702–703.

Schiff FS. Coumadin related spontaneous hyphemas in patients with iris fixated pseudophakos. *Ophthal Surg.* 1985;16:172–173.

Shaul WL, Hall JG. Multiple congenital anomalies associated with oral anticoagulants. *Am J Obstet Gynecol.* 1977;127:191–198.

Superstein R, Gomolin JE, Hammouda W, et al. Prevalence of ocular hemorrhage in patients receiving warfarin therapy. *Can J Ophthalmol.* 2000;35:385–389.

Taylor RH, Gibson JM. Warfarin, spontaneous hyphaemas, and intraocular lenses. *Lancet.* 1988;1:762–763.

Weir CR, Nolan DJ, Holding D, et al. Intraocular haemorrhage associated with anticoagulant therapy. *Acta Ophthalmol Scand.* 2000;78:492–493.

Dextran

Blake J, Cassidy H. Ocular hypersensitivity to dextran. *Ir J Med Sci.* 1979;148:249.

Fothergill R, Heaney GA. Reactions to dextran. *BMJ.* 1976;2:1502.

Krenzelok EP, Parker WA. Dextran 40 anaphylaxis. *Minn Med.* 1975;58:454–455.

Ledoux-Corbusier M. L'urticaire medicamenteuse. *Brux Med.* 1975;55:629.

CHAPTER 13

Homeostatic and Nutrient Drugs

CLASS: DRUGS USED TO TREAT HYPERGLYCEMIA

Generic Names:

1. Acetohexamide; 2. chlorpropamide; 3. glimepiride; 4. glipizide; 5. glyburide (glibenclamide); 6. tolazamide; 7. tolbutamide.

Proprietary Names:

1. Dymelor; 2. Diabinese; 3. Amaryl; 4. Glucotrol, Glucotrol XL; 5. Diabeta, Glycron, Gynase PresTab, Micronase 6. Tolinase; 7. Orinase, Tol-Tab.

Primary Use

These oral hypoglycemic sulfonylureas are effective in the management of selected cases of diabetes mellitus.

Ocular Side Effects

Systemic administration – oral
Certain

1. Decreased vision
2. Decreased accommodation (glyburide)
3. Eyelids or conjunctiva
   a. Allergic reactions
   b. Hyperemia
   c. Conjunctivitis – nonspecific
   d. Edema
   e. Photosensitivity
   f. Purpura
4. Color vision defect – red-green defect
5. Lens
   a. Osmotic changes
   b. Myopia
   c. Forward displacement iris-lens diaphragm

Probable

1. Decreased tear film break-up time
2. May aggravate Wernicke syndrome

Possible

1. Lens
   a. Opacities – irreversible
   b. Posterior subcapsular changes
2. Eyelids or conjunctiva – lupoid syndrome (tolazamide)

Conditional/unclassified

1. Optic nerve
   a. Vascular events
   b. Neuritis

Clinical Significance

Although there are multiple reported adverse ocular effects due to these drugs, they are difficult to evaluate. This is primarily because diabetes causes so many ocular complications that may mask or mimic adverse drug effects. Systemically, chlorpropamide has a 6% incidence of untoward reactions, whereas the incidence with acetohexamide, tolazamide, and tolbutamide is 3%.[1] First- and second-generation sulfonylureas may have more ocular side effects than more recent drugs. Tolbutamide has a 3 times higher incidence of color deficiencies than normal type 2 diabetes mellitus.[2] Chlorpropamide and tolazamide also may cause color vision defects.[3] Çakir et al have shown that tear film stability is decreased with this group of drugs.[4] However, impression cytology and Schirmer tests were unchanged compared with insulin and the control group. Isaac et al found an overall increased risk of cataracts in patients on antidiabetic drugs.[5] There are numerous reports of second-generation sulfonylureas causing lens changes.[6] Skalka et al found an increased incidence of posterior subcapsular lens changes in diabetic patients treated with oral hypoglycemic compared with diabetics controlled with diet and insulin.[7] Transient myopia and decreased accommodation have been seen in the spontaneous reports due to glyburide. Although optic nerve disease has been reported in the literature and spontaneous reports, differentiation of which changes are due to diabetes and which changes are due to a toxic drug effect is unknown.[8] Reported optic or retrobulbar neuritis with central or centrocecal scotoma has not been proven as a drug-related event.[9,10] In some cases, the optic nerve damage may be secondary to the drug-induced hypoglycemia and related vascular events. In susceptible individuals who have low thiamine reserves, hypoglycemic drugs may induce Wernicke encephalopathy, including oculomotor disturbances such as ophthalmoplegia, ptosis, and nystagmus.[11]

Generic Name:

Insulin.

Proprietary Names:

Afrezza, Apidra, Basaglar, Exubera, Humalog, Humalog Mix 50/50, Humalog Mix 75/25, Humalog Pen, Humulin 70/30, Humulin 50/50, Humulin L, Humulin N, Humulin R, Humulin U, Lantus, Lente, Levemir, Novolin 70/30, Novolin N, Novolin R, NovoLog, NovoLog Mix 70/30, Soliqua 100/33, Toujeo, Tresiba, Ultralente, Velosulin Human BR, Xultophy 100/3.6.

Primary Use

This hypoglycemic drug is effective in the management of diabetes mellitus.

Ocular Side Effects

Systemic administration – intravenous or subcutaneous

Certain

1. Decreased vision
2. Extraocular muscles
   a. Paresis
   b. Nystagmus
   c. Diplopia
3. Eyelids or conjunctiva
   a. Allergic reactions
   b. Erythema
   c. Blepharoconjunctivitis
   d. Edema
   e. Urticaria
4. Decreased tear lysozymes

Probable

1. Insulin-resistant patients
   a. Increased myopia
   b. Increased intraocular pressure

Possible

1. Immunogenic retinopathy
2. Myopia – transient
3. Acute glaucoma

Clinical Significance

The adverse ocular effects secondary to insulin are generally the result of insulin-induced hypoglycemia and not a direct toxic effect of the drug. This occurs due to an excessive dosage of insulin, omission of a meal by a patient, or increased physical activity. Ocular symptoms are primarily decreased or double vision. Although these effects are usually transitory, some cases may take many weeks to resolve. Blake et al reported

on the exceedingly rare precipitation of acute glaucoma after rapid correction of acute hyperglycemia.[1] This is probably due to intralenticular glucose-sorbitol, with a resultant swelling of the lens. It has been suggested that some diabetic retinopathy is insulin induced and immunogenic in nature.[2] Although data in primates support this, it is difficult to prove in humans. Arun et al reported that with initiation of insulin treatment in type 2 diabetes, clinically significant worsening of diabetic retinopathy over a 3-year period was uncommon in those with no retinopathy, but occurred in 31.8% of patients with retinopathy at baseline.[3] They pointed out that the risk of serious worsening of retinopathy after the start of insulin therapy in all patients with type 2 diabetes may have been previously overestimated. Gold et al pointed out cortical blindness and cerebral infarcts secondary to severe hypoglycemia.[4] Insulin may cause or aggravate lipemic retinitis in a patient with possible hyperlipoproteinemia type V. Kitzmiller et al suggested that in pregnancy, when insulin lispro therapy is given, rapid acceleration of proliferative diabetic retinopathy, without background retinopathy, may occur.[5] There are cases in the spontaneous reports of up to 3-diopter changes of myopia with overdosage of insulin. Lin et al reported 4 cases of transient hyperopia after starting insulin.[6]

In insulin-resistant patients, data suggest an increase in myopia.[7–10] This may also be a risk factor for elevated intraocular pressure.[11]

Generic Name:

Metformin hydrochloride.

Proprietary Names:

Fortamet, Glucophage, Glucophage, XR, Glumetza, Riomet.

Primary Use

A biguanide antidiabetic for the treatment of type 2 diabetes mellitus. This is the drug of choice for obese patients.

Ocular Side Effects

Systemic administration – oral

Possible

1. Decreased central corneal endothelial cell density

Conditional/unclassified

1. Protective effect of type 2 ocular complications
2. Lens – osmotic damage – transient (Fig. 13.1)
3. Eyelids or conjunctiva – erythema multiforme
4. Periorbital edema

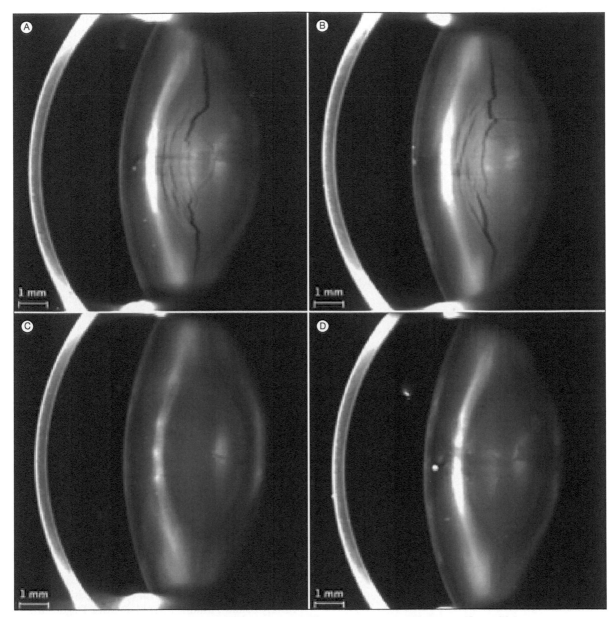

FIG. 13.1 Sugar cracks in right eye **(A)** and left eye **(B)** and spontaneous resolutions (**C** and **D**) from metformin treatment.[3])

Clinical Significance

Central corneal endothelial cell density was decreased in eye-bank eyes from patients on metformin who had glaucoma.[1] However, this was minimal and unlikely to affect the suitability of the donor corneas for transplant.

Metformin was possibly associated with a protective effect of ocular complications associated with patients who have type 2 diabetes.[2] Tangelder et al reported a single case of a unique reversible lens change called "sugar cracks."[3] These cracks were located primarily in the nucleus, running parallel to the nuclear curvature, and in a straight band nearing both ends at the equator. This occurred with decreased vision in a newly diagnosed 62-year-old diabetic 2 days after starting metformin. Two weeks later, the patient's vision was 20/80 OD and 20/33 OS. At 3 months the lens changes vanished spontaneously, and at 5 months vision was 20/20 OU. The authors felt these changes were related to a decrease in extracellular glucose and not a toxic effect of the drug.

Generic Names:
1. Pioglitazone; 2. rosiglitazone maleate.

Proprietary Names:
1. Actos; 2. Avandia.

Primary Use
Oral thiazolidinedione antidiabetic drugs, which act primarily by increasing insulin sensitivity.

Ocular Side Effects
Systemic administration – oral
Probable
1. Face
   a. Edema
   b. Periorbital edema
2. Decreased vision
3. Color vision defect
4. Decrease dark adaptation
5. Thyroid-associated orbitopathy – aggravates preexisting autoimmune thyroid disorders

Possible
1. Macular edema
2. Proptosis

Conditional/unclassified
1. Pseudotumor cerebri

Clinical Significance
Pioglitazone (bladder cancer) and rosiglitazone (cardiac effects) have caused some countries to ban these medications. Both drugs are still available in the United States, although use has significantly decreased.

There is some controversy as to if pioglitazone and rosiglitazone cause diabetic macular edema (DME), partly because macular edema may be seen in the disease for which these drugs are used. The *Physicians' Desk Reference* (PDR), under "Warnings/Precautions" for both pioglitazone and rosiglitazone, stated "macular edema reported: refer to an ophthalmologist

if visual symptoms develop"; this warning has been dropped from the current PDR; however, in rosiglitazone it does state that "[l]ong-term care facility residents receiving rosiglitazone should be monitored for visual deterioration due to new onset and/or worsening of macular edema in diabetic patients."[1] A number of studies support a cause-and-effect relationship between these drugs causing an increased incidence of macular edema, especially with pioglitazone.[2–4] In a study of 103,368 patients in the United Kingdom, both drugs equally showed higher incidences of DME than the control group at 1 and 10 years.[5] Motola et al found an incidence of 5.55% of DME on rosiglitazone.[6] Fong et al and Ryan et al found an increase of DME in this drug class's users.[2,4] The thiazolidinediones may cause systemic peripheral systemic edema in 5–7% of patients and up to 15% if pioglitazone and insulin are used in combination.[6–9] Ryan et al found that stopping the drug allowed rapid resolution of the macular edema in about 25% of patients.[6] In the other cases, the resolution was slower and may require laser treatment. The macular edema was more common in patients with peripheral edema. Ambrosius et al, in a large ACCORD eye substudy of some 9690 participants, found no association between thiazolidinedione and DME.[10] They stated that they cannot exclude a modest protective or harmful association. With these conflicting data, but thousands of cases in the literature and spontaneous reports, it is "possible," maybe even "probable," that there is an association between the use of these drugs and DME. The incidence, however, is probably small and may be primarily in patients with associated peripheral drug-induced edema.

Levin et al, Yang et al, and Clevidence et al reported proptosis due to adipogenesis properties of these drugs.[11–13] Starkey et al, Menaka et al, and Lee et al reported aggravation of preexisting thyroid eye disease.[14–16] This class of drugs probably exacerbates thyroid-associated orbitopathy in diabetic patients with a history of autoimmune thyroid diseases. Dagdelen et al described a patient with pseudotumor cerebri possibly due to rosiglitazone.[17]

Recommendations
1. If peripheral edema (primarily lower extremity) occurs, patients should be warned that if any vision changes occur, they should see an ophthalmologist to check for macular edema. Vision signs or symptoms include decreased or distorted vision, decreased dark adaptation, and/or decreased color sensation.

2. Consider recommending not using this drug if the patient has diabetic macular edema, congestive heart failure, or nephropathy.
3. Consider on a trial basis stopping the drug at the first signs of macular edema after starting the drug.

REFERENCES

Drugs: Acetohexamide, chlorpropamide, glimepiride, glipizide, glyburide (glibenclamide), tolazamide, tolbutamide

1. Acetohexamide, chlorpropamide, glimepiride, glipizide, glyburide, tolazamide, tolbutamide. 2018. Retrieved from http://www.pdr.net.
2. Tan NC, Yip WF, Kallakuri S, et al. Factors associated with impaired color vision without retinopathy amongst people with type 2 diabetes mellitus: a cross-sectional study. *BMC Endocr Disord*. 2017;17(1):29.
3. Pavan-Langston D. *Manual of Ocular Diagnosis and Therapy*. 6th ed. Philadelphia, PA: Lippincott Williams & Wilkins; 2008:464.
4. Çakir BK, Katircioğlu Y, Ünlü N, et al. Ocular surface changes in patients treated with oral antidiabetic drugs or insulin. *Eur J Ophthalmol*. 2016;26(4):303–306.
5. Isaac NE, Walker AM, Jick H, et al. Exposure to phenothiazine drugs and risk of cataract. *Arch ophthalmol*. 1991;109:256–260.
6. Hampson JP, Harvey JN. A systematic review of drug induced ocular reactions in diabetes. *Br J Ophthalmol*. 2000;84:144–149.
7. Skalka HW, Prchal JT. The effect of diabetes mellitus and diabetic therapy on cataract formation. *Ophthalmology*. 1981;88:117–125.
8. Wymore J, Carter JE. Chlorpropamide-induced optic neuropathy. *Arch Intern Med*. 1982;142:381.
9. Catros V. Bilateral axial optic neuritis in the course of treatment with D860. *Rev Otoneuropathol*. 1958;30:253–257.
10. Givner I. Centrocecal scotomas due to chlorpropamide. *Arch ophthalmol*. 1961;66:64.
11. Kwee IL, Nakada T. Wernicke's encephalopathy induced by tolazamide. *N Engl J Med*. 1983;309:599–600.

Drug: Insulin

1. Blake DR, Nathan DM. Acute angle closure glaucoma following rapid correction of hyperglycemia. *Diabetes Care*. 2003;26:3197–3198.
2. Shabo AL, Maxwell DS. Insulin-induced immunogenic retinopathy resembling the retinitis proliferans of diabetes. *Trans Am Acad Ophthalmol Otolaryngol*. 1976;81:497–508.
3. Arun CS, Pandit R, Taylor R. Long-term progression of retinopathy after initiation of insulin therapy in Type 2 diabetes: an observational study. *Diabetologia*. 2004;47:1380–1384.

4. Gold AE, Marshall SM. Cortical blindness and cerebral infarction associated with severe hypoglycemia. *Diabetes Care*. 1996;19(9):1001–1003.
5. Kitzmiller JL, Main E, Ward B, et al. Insulin lispro and the development of proliferative diabetic retinopathy during pregnancy. *Diabetes Care*. 1999;22(5):874–876.
6. Lin SF, Lin PK, Chang FL, et al. Transient hyperopia after intensive treatment of hyperglycemia in newly diagnosed diabetes. *Ophthalmologica*. 2009;233(1):68–71.
7. Galvis V, López-Jaramillo P, Tello A, et al. Is myopia another clinical manifestation of insulin resistance? *Med Hypotheses*. 2016;90:32–40.
8. Liu X, Wang P, Qu C, et al. Genetic association study between insulin pathway related genes and high myopia in a Han Chinese population. *Mol Biol Rep*. 2015;42(1):303–310.
9. Cordain L, Eaton SB, Brand Miller J, et al. An evolutionary analysis of the aetiology and pathogenesis of juvenile-onset myopia. *Acta Ophthalmol Scand*. 2002;80(2):125–135.
10. Zhuang W, Yang P, Li Z, et al. Association of insulin-like growth factor-1 polymorphisms with high myopia in the Chinese population. *Mol Vis*. 2012;18:634–644.
11. Fujiwara K, Yasuda M, Nimomiya T, et al. Insulin resistance is a risk factor for increased intraocular pressure: the Hisayama Study. *Invest Ophthalmol Vis Sci*. 2015;56(13):7983–7987.

Drug: Metformin hydrochloride

1. Chocron IM, Rai DK, Kwon JW, et al. Effect of diabetes mellitus and metformin on central corneal endothelial cell density in eye bank eyes. *Cornea*. 2018;37(8):964–966.
2. Maleškić S, Kusturica J, Gušić E, et al. Metformin use associated with protective effects for ocular complications in patients with type 2 diabetes – observational study. *Acta Med Acad*. 2017;46(2):116–123.
3. Tangelder GJ, Dubbelman M, Ringens PJ. Sudden reversible osmotic lens damage ("sugar cracks") after initiation of metformin. *N Engl J Med*. 2005;353:2621–2623.

Drugs: Pioglitazone, rosiglitazone maleate

1. Pioglitazone, rosiglitazone maleate. 2018. Retrieved from http://www.pdr.net.
2. Fong DS, Contreras R. Glitazone use associated with diabetic macular edema. *Am J Ophthalmol*. 2009;147(4):583–586.
3. Kamoi K, Takeda K, Hashimoto K, et al. Identifying risk factors for clinically significant diabetic macular edema in patients with type 2 diabetes mellitus. *Curr Diabetes Rev*. 2013;9(3):209–217.
4. Ryan EH, Han DP, Ramsay RC, et al. Diabetic macular edema associated with glitazone use. *Retina*. 2006;26:562–570.
5. Idris I, Warren G, Donnelly R. Associated between thiazolidinedione treatment and risk of macular edema among patients with Type 2 diabetes. *Arch Intern Med*. 2012;172(13):1005–1011.

6. Motola D, Piccinni C, Biagi C, et al. Cardiovascular, ocular and bone adverse reactions associated with thiazolidinediones: a disproportionality analysis of the US FDA adverse event report system database. *Drug Saf.* 2012;35(4):315–323.

7. Niemeyer NV, Janney LM. Thiazolidinedione-induced edema. *Pharmacotherapy.* 2002;22(7):924–929.

8. Avandia Package Insert (see adverse reaction section). http://us.gsk.com/products/assets/us_avandia.pdf.

9. Actos Package Insert (see adverse reaction section). http://www.fda.gov/medwatch/SAFETY/2003/03Jan_labels/Actos_PI.pdf.

10. Ambrosius WT, Danis RP, Goff DC, et al. Lack of association between thiazolidinediones and macular edema in Type 2 diabetes: the ACCORD eye substudy. *Arch ophthalmol.* 2010;128(3):312–318.

11. Levin F, Kazim M, Smith TJ, et al. Rosiglitazone-induced proptosis. *Arch ophthalmol.* 2005;123:119–121.

12. Yang CCL, Chen-Ku CH, Vagefi RM. Proptosis secondary to rosiglitazone treatment. *Int J Diabetes Metabol.* 2008;16(2):89–90.

13. Clevidence DE, Juckett MB, Lucarelli MJ. Marrow suppression with myelodysplastic features, hypoerythropoetinemia, and lipotrophic proptosis due to rosiglitazone. *Wis Med J.* 2009;108(9):462–465.

14. Starkey K, Heufelder A, Baker G, et al. Peroxisome proliferator-activated receptor-gamma in thyroid eye disease: contraindication for thiazolidinedione use? *J Clin Endocrinol Metab.* 2003;88:55–59.

15. Menaka R, Sehgal M, Lakshmi M, et al. Thiazolidinedione precipitated thyroid associated ophthalmopathy. *J Assoc Phys India.* 2010;58:243–245.

16. Lee S, Tsirbas A, Goldberg RA, et al. Thiazolidinedione induced thyroid associated orbitopathy. *BMC Ophthalmol.* 2007;7:8.

17. Dagdelen S, Gedik O. Rosiglitazone-associated pseudotumor cerebri. *Diabetologia.* 2006;49:207–208.

FURTHER READING

Acetohexamide, chlorpropamide, glimepiride, glipizide, glyburide (glibenclamide), tolazamide, tolbutamide

D'Arcy PF. Drug reactions and interactions. *Int J Pharm.* 1989;3:220–222.

Garbe E, Lelorier J, Boivin JF, et al. Risk of ocular hypertension or open angle glaucoma in elderly patients on oral glucocorticoids. *Lancet.* 1997;350:979–982.

George CW. Central scotoma due to chlorpropamide. *Arch Ophthalmol.* 1963;69:773.

Hamil MB, Suelflow JA, Smith JA. Transdermal scopolamine delivery system (Transderm-V) and acute angle closure glaucoma. *Ann Ophthalmol.* 1983;15:1011–1012.

Kanefsky TM, Medoff SJ. Stevens-Johnson syndrome and neutropenia with chlorpropamide therapy. *Arch Intern Med.* 1980;140:1543.

Kapetansky FM. Refractive changes with tolbutamide. *Ohio State Med J.* 1963;59:275–276.

Kato S, Oshika T, Numaga J, et al. Influence of rapid glycemic control on lens opacity in patients with diabetes mellitus. *Am J Ophthalmol.* 2000;130:354–355.

Kelly JT. Second generation oral hypoglycemia and lactic acidosis in a diabetic treated with chlorpropamide and phenformin. *South Med J.* 1973;66:190–192.

Lightman JM, Townsend JC, Selvin GJ. Ocular effects of second generation oral hypoglycemic agents. *J Am Optom Assoc.* 1989;60:849–853.

Paice BJ, Paterson KR, Lavson DH. Undesired effects of the sulphonylurea drugs. *Adverse Drug React Acute Poison Rev.* 1985;4:23–36.

Teller J, Rasin M, Abraham FA. Accommodation insufficiency induced by glybenclamide. *Ann Ophthalmol.* 1989;21:275–276.

Transient myopia from glibenclamide. short-sightedness with glibenclamide. *Int Pharm J.* 1989;3:221–222.

Insulin

Vermeer BJ, Polano MK. A case of xanthomatosis and hyperlipoproteinemia type V probably induced by overdosage of insulin. *Dermatologica.* 1975;151:43–50.

Metformin hydrochloride

Burger DE, Goyal S. Erythema multiforme from metformin. *Ann Pharmacother.* 2004;38:1537.

Pioglitazone, rosiglitazone maleate

Choi HK, Tan GS, Sundar G. Rosiglitazone toxicity: accidental overdose leading to macular edema. *Retin Cases Brief Rep.* 2010;4:73–77.

Colucciello M. Vision loss due to macular edema induced by rosiglitazone treatment of diabetes mellitus. *Arch Ophthalmol.* 2005;123:1273–1275.

Kendall C, Wooltorton E. Rosiglitazone (Avandia) and macular edema. *Can Med Assoc J.* 2006;174:623.

CHAPTER 14

Drugs Used to Treat Allergic and Neuromuscular Disorders

CLASS: DRUGS USED TO TREAT MYASTHENIA GRAVIS

Generic Names:
1. Edrophonium chloride; 2. pyridostigmine bromide.

Proprietary Names:
1. Enlon, Tensilon; 2. Mestinon, Regonol.

Primary Use
These drugs are effective in the treatment of myasthenia gravis. Edrophonium is primarily used as an antidote for curariform drugs and as a diagnostic test for myasthenia gravis.

Ocular Side Effects
Systemic administration – intramuscular, intravenous, or oral
Certain
1. Decreased vision
2. Miosis
3. Lacrimation
4. Paradoxical response (ptotic eye up and nonptotic eye down)

Possible
1. Oculogyric crisis (edrophonium)
2. Blepharospasm (pyridostigmine)
3. Diplopia (edrophonium)
4. Conjunctival hyperemia (edrophonium)
5. Extraocular muscles (pyridostigmine)
   a. Incyclotorsion
   b. Excyclotorsion

Clinical Significance
Ocular side effects due to these drugs are seldom of clinical significance. Most all adverse ocular reactions are reversible with discontinued drug use. Overdose may lead to a cholinergic crisis, which includes miosis, ciliary spasm, nystagmus, extraocular muscle paresis, and blepharoclonus. In rare instances, edrophonium may cause a paradoxical response when used for myasthenia gravis testing. In these cases, the ptotic eyelid goes up, while the normal eyelid goes down. Nucci et al reported an episode of oculogyric crisis within a few minutes after performing a Tensilon test (edrophonium).[1] Smith et al reported a possible case of unilateral alternating superior and inferior oblique myokymia.[2] Voon et al reported a case with rechallenge data of pyridostigmine-induced blepharospasm with cholinergic overactivity.[3]

CLASS: ANTIHISTAMINES

Generic Names:
1. Brompheniramine maleate; 2. chlorphenamine maleate (chlorpheniramine); 3. dexchlorpheniramine maleate (dexchlorpheniramine); 4. triprolidine hydrochloride.

Proprietary Names:
1. Bromfed, Dimetapp, Bromfenex, Dimetane, BPN, Lodrane; 2. Chlor-Trimeton, Piriton; 3. Mylaramine; 4. Actidil, Myidil, Actifed, Recofast Plus.

Primary Use
These alkylamine antihistamines are used in the symptomatic relief of allergic or vasomotor rhinitis, allergic conjunctivitis, and allergic skin manifestations.

Ocular Side Effects
Systemic administration – intramuscular, intravenous, oral, or subcutaneous
Certain
1. Decreased vision
2. Pupils
   a. Mydriasis – may precipitate acute glaucoma
   b. Anisocoria
3. Decreased contact lens tolerance
4. May aggravate or cause ocular sicca

Probable
1. Eyelids or conjunctiva

a. Erythema
b. Photosensitivity
c. Urticaria
d. Blepharospasm
e. Edema
2. Visual hallucinations
3. Abnormal critical flicker fusion (triprolidine)

Possible
1. Diplopia

Clinical Significance

Ocular side effects due to these antihistamines are rare and may disappear even if use of the drug is continued. These antihistamines have a weak atropine action, which accounts for the pupillary changes.[1] With chronic use, anisocoria, decreased accommodation, and decreased vision can also occur. Chlorphenamine and others in this class have been found to decrease mucus and/or tear production, which accounts for decreased contact lens tolerance and aggravation or transitory induction of ocular sicca.[2,3] Antihistamines, in large dosages or with chronic therapy, can produce facial dyskinesia, which may start with unilateral or bilateral blepharospasms.[4-6] Lack of pupillary response occurs only with chronic use or toxic states.

Generic Names:

1. Carbinoxamine maleate; 2. clemastine fumarate; 3. diphenhydramine hydrochloride; 4. doxylamine succinate.

Proprietary Names:

1. Arbinoxa, Carbihist, Carbinoxamine PD, Histex PD, Karbinal ER, Mintext PD, Palgic, RyVent; 2. Dailyhist-1, Tavist Allergy; 3. Aid to Sleep, Alka-Seltzer Plus Allergy, Aller-G-Time, Altaryl, Banophen, Benadryl, Benadryl Allergy, Benadryl Allergy Children's, Benadryl Allergy Dye Free, Benadryl Allergy Kapgel, Benadryl Allergy Ultratab, Benadryl Children's Allergy, Benadryl Children's Allergy Fastmelt, Benadryl Children's Perfect Measure, Benadryl Itch Stopping, Buckley's Bedtime, Compoz Nighttime Sleep Aid, Diphedryl, Diphen AF, Diphenhist, ElixSure Allergy, Genahist, Geri-Dryl, Hydramine, Itch Relief, Nytol, PediaCare Children's Allergy, PediaCare Nighttime Cough, PHARBEDRYL, Q-Dryl, Quenalin, Siladryl Allergy, Silphen, Simply Sleep, Sleep Tabs, Sleepinal, Sominex, Triaminic Allergy Thin Strip, Triaminic Cough and Runny Nose Strip, Tusstat, Unisom, Valu-Dryl, Vanamine PD, Vicks Qlearquil Nighttime Allergy Relief, Vicks ZzzQuil Nightime Sleep-Aid; 4. Aldex AN, Doxytex, Unisom.

Primary Use

These ethanolamine antihistamines are used in the symptomatic relief of allergic or vasomotor rhinitis, allergic conjunctivitis, and allergic skin manifestations.

Ocular Side Effects
Systemic administration – intramuscular, intravenous, oral, or topical
Certain
1. Decreased vision
2. Pupils
   a. Mydriasis – may precipitate acute glaucoma
   b. Decreased or absent reaction to light
   c. Anisocoria
3. May aggravate or cause ocular sicca
4. Decreased contact lens tolerance
5. Visual hallucinations

Probable
1. Eyelids or conjunctiva
   a. Erythema
   b. Photosensitivity
   c. Urticaria
   d. Blepharospasm
2. Decreased accommodation

Possible
1. Diplopia
2. Eyelid and periocular edema
3. Filamentary keratitis

Conditional/unclassified
1. Ocular teratogenic effects

Clinical Significance

Ocular side effects due to these antihistamines, although not uncommon, frequently disappear even if use of the drug is continued. These ethanolamines have a weak atropine action that accounts for the pupillary and ciliary body changes. The greatest concern is the precipitation of acute glaucoma, especially because most of these drugs do not require a prescription.[1] Decreased vision and changes in accommodation can occur. With long-term use, unilateral or bilateral signs have been reported, including anisocoria.[2] A decrease in mucoid and/or lacrimal secretions may account for contact lens intolerance, aggravation or induction of ocular sicca, and even filamentary keratitis.[3,4] It has been shown that these drugs, in large dosages or with chronic therapy, can produce facial dyskinesia. Many of these cases started with unilateral or bilateral blepharospasm. Lack of pupillary response, visual hallucinations, and nystagmus usually occur with chronic high-dose therapy. There are reports by both Walsh and Nigro of comas secondary to diphenhydramine ingestion in infants and teenagers where, on awakening, cortical blindness was evident.[5,6] Over time vision reverted to normal. There are cases in the spontaneous reports of possible ocular teratogenic effects secondary to diphenhydramine or doxylamine.

Generic Names:

1. Cetirizine hydrochloride; 2. desloratadine; 3. fexofenadine hydrochloride; 4. loratadine; 5. tripelennamine.

Proprietary Names:

1. All Day Allergy, All Day Allergy Children's, Pedia-Care Children's Allergy, Zyrtec, Zyrtec Children's, Zyrtec Children's Allergy, Zyrtec Children's Hives, Zyrtec Hives Relief, Zyrtec Liquid Gel, Zyrtec Pre-Filled Spoons; 2. Clarinex, Clarinex-D, Clarinex RediTab; 3. Allegra, Allegra Allergy 12 Hour, Allegra Allergy 24 Hour, Allegra Children's Allergy, Allegra Children's Allergy ODT, Allegra ODT, Allergy Relief, Children's Allergy Fexofenadine; 4. Alavert, Allergy Relief, Claritin, Claritin Chewable, Claritin-D, Claritin Liqui-Gel, Claritin RediTab, Clear-Atadine, Dimetapp Children's Non-Drowsy Allergy, QlearQuil All Day & All Night Allergy Relief, Travist ND; 5. Pyribenzamine.

Primary Use

These H_1 receptor antagonists are indicated for the treatment of allergic or vasomotor rhinitis, allergic conjunctivitis, and allergic skin manifestations of urticaria and edema.

Ocular Side Effects

Systemic administration – oral

Certain

1. Decreased vision
2. May aggravate or cause ocular sicca
3. Decreased contact lens tolerance
4. Oculogyric crisis (cetirizine)
5. Visual hallucinations

Probable

1. Eyelids or conjunctiva
   a. Erythema
   b. Photosensitivity
   c. Urticaria
   d. Blepharospasm

Possible

1. Decreased accommodation
2. Diplopia

3. Pupils
   a. Mydriasis – weak
   b. Anisocoria

Clinical Significance

Ocular side effects due to these antihistamines are uncommon and frequently disappear even if the drug is continued. These antihistamines have a weak atropine action, which accounts for pupillary changes. However, with long-term use, these effects can accumulate, so that anisocoria, decreased accommodation, or decreased vision can occur. The antimuscarine activity of H_1 antihistamines decreases basal tear production of the accessory and lacrimal glands and decreases mucin production of the conjunctival goblet cells. This accounts for decreased contact lens tolerance and aggravation or causation of ocular sicca. Ocular moisture usually returns once the drug is discontinued. These drugs all cause xerostomia, so ocular sicca is to be expected. Ousler et al showed that after 4 days of twice-a-day dosing of loratadine there were signs of ocular drying, decreased tear volume, and tear flow.[1] Nine cases of oculogyric crisis due to cetirizine therapy, with 8 occurring in the pediatric age group, were reported.[2] These drugs, in large dosages or with chronic therapy, can produce facial dyskinesia, which may start as a unilateral or bilateral blepharospasm.

Generic Name:

Cyproheptadine hydrochloride.

Proprietary Name:

Periactin.

Primary Use

This antihistamine is used in the symptomatic relief of allergic or vasomotor rhinitis, allergic conjunctivitis, and allergic skin manifestations.

Ocular Side Effects

Systemic administration – oral

Certain

1. Decreased vision
2. Mydriasis
3. Decreased contact lens tolerance
4. May aggravate or cause ocular sicca

Probable

1. Eyelids or conjunctiva
   a. Erythema
   b. Edema

c. Photosensitivity
d. Urticaria

Possible
1. Diplopia
2. Visual hallucinations

Clinical Significance

Ocular side effects due to this drug are rare and may disappear even if use of the drug is continued. This drug has atropine-like effects, such as mydriasis and decreased secretions. The package insert for cyproheptadine states that it is contraindicated in patients with narrow-angle glaucoma due to precipitation of acute glaucoma.[1] Based on spontaneous reports, this is a very rare event. Decreased lacrimal or mucoid secretion has been the cause of decreased tolerance to contact lenses and aggravation of ocular sicca.[2] Once the drug is discontinued, ocular moisture returns. This drug is known as a photosensitizer.[3]

Generic Name:
Dupilumab.

Proprietary Name:
Dupixent.

Primary Use

An interleukin-4 receptor alpha-antagonist used in the treatment of moderate to severe atopic dermatitis and as an add-on maintenance for asthma.

Ocular Side Effects
Systemic administration – subcutaneous
Certain
1. Irritation
   a. Pruritus
   b. Stinging
   c. Burning
   d. Foreign body sensation
2. Conjunctiva
   a. Conjunctivitis
      i. Toxic
      ii. Allergic
      iii. Infectious
   b. Hyperemia (Fig. 14.1)
3. Cornea
   a. Keratitis
   b. Peripheral nodules
4. Eyelids
   a. Blepharitis
   b. Edema

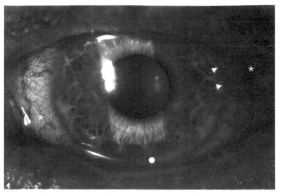

FIG. 14.1 Dupilumab-induced conjunctivitis showing conjunctival hyperemia (*white asterisks*), limbal hyperemia (*white triangles*), and tearing (*white dot*).[1]

Probable
1. Cicatricial ectropion
2. Deep corneal vascularization

Clinical Significance

Dupilumab has a high frequency of ocular side effects, some of which are serious and may be difficult to manage. The classic clinical picture is various degrees of bilateral conjunctivitis with erythema and chemosis with or without discharge. This is associated with pruritus stinging, burning, foreign body sensation, epiphora, and decreased vision. The most prominent feature is hyperemia of the limbus. In some severe cases there is nodular swelling at the limbus resembling Trantas dots, although dupilumab nodules are located a little more anterior on the limbus.[1]

According to the *Physicians' Desk Reference* (PDR), the incidence of conjunctivitis is 10–16%, blepharitis is 0–3%, keratitis is 0–4%, ocular pruritus is 1–2%, and ocular sicca is 0–2%.[2] Other clinical trials have had similar data.[3–5] Although the PDR lists incidences of ocular side effects in the range of 0–16%, if asthma patients were excluded, they may be in the 25–50% range (small series).[1,2] Ocular side effects are seen commonly in atopic dermatitis, but not in asthma or nasal polyposis trials.[6] Blood serum levels may not be elevated when side effects are most severe; therefore some of the adverse effects may be allergic, secondary infections, or immunologic effects. Wollenberg et al gave an overview of the signs and symptoms of these side effects and published the only paper that described the management of these side effects.[1] The time of onset of these side effects varied from 25–389 days.

Barnes et al reported a case of severe bilateral conjunctival hyperemia and eyelid inflammation causing a cicatricial ectropion.[6] This occurred after a 2-month period of weekly subcutaneous dupilumab injections. The ectropion worsened over a several-month period and resolved once the dupilumab injections were discontinued. Other cases, both in the literature and spontaneous reports, make this "probable."[7]

The adverse ocular side effects profile is still being developed because the drug is new and the diseases being treated may also cause the suspected drug-induced ocular side effects.

Recommendations[1]

1. Antihistamines and/or artificial tears offer little alleviation of signs or symptoms.
2. Fluorometholone 0.1% or off-label use of tacrolimus 0.03% ointment has successfully managed the ocular side effects associated with dupilumab use.

CLASS: ANTIPARKINSONISM DRUGS

Generic Names:

1. Amantadine hydrochloride; 2. memantine hydrochloride.

Proprietary Names:

1. Gocovri, Symmetrel; 2. Namenda, Namenda XR.

Primary Use

Amantadine is a N-methyl-D-aspartate (NMDA) receptor antagonist used in the treatment of Parkinson disease and tardive dyskinesia and in the prophylaxis of influenza A2 (Asian) virus infections. Memantine is closely related to amantadine and is primarily indicated in moderate to severe Alzheimer disease, vascular dementia, and symptomatic treatment of acquired pendular nystagmus.

Ocular Side Effects

Systemic administration – oral (amantadine)
Certain

1. Decreased vision
2. Visual hallucinations (also memantine)
3. Cornea (Fig. 14.2)
   a. Edema
   b. Punctate keratitis (Fig. 14.3)
   c. Subepithelial opacities
   d. Endothelium
      i. Decreased cell density
      ii. Pleomorphism
      iii. Polymegathism
      iv. Loss of endothelial cells
4. Eyelids or conjunctiva
   a. Photosensitivity
   b. Purpura
   c. Eczema
   d. Loss of eyelashes or eyebrows

Probable

1. Oculogyric crises

Possible

1. Mydriasis – may precipitate acute glaucoma
2. Cornea
   a. Abrasions
   b. Descemet's stripping endothelial keratoplasty (DSEK) failure (memantine)

Clinical Significance

Amantadine is a widely used drug in the management of many neurologic disorders, including parkinsonism. The area of ocular concern is the cornea, which may be affected in 2 ways. The first is that the drug is probably secreted in the tears and/or aqueous and appears to be toxic to the endothelium. This is a rare event and may be a hypersensitivity response occurring within a few weeks or dose dependent occurring after several years of usage. Chang et al found in 169 subjects taking amantadine orally for Parkinson disease in age-matched control groups that the endothelial cells were affected in a dose-dependent pattern.[1] There was an increased central cornea thickness, as well as a decrease in endothelial cell density compared with controls. Positive rechallenge data were reported. If recognized, this side effect is reversible; however, at some point it is irreversible.[2] French et al showed a relative risk of corneal edema on amantadine of 1.7 over a 2-year period.[3] Pathology specimens showed atrophy of the endothelium without guttata.

The second corneal pattern due to amantadine is a superficial deposit or toxic response to the corneal epithelium, possibly as a hypersensitivity event. This seems to indicate that the drug may be secreted in the tears. This presents as diffuse, white, punctate subepithelial opacities, more prominent inferonasally, occasionally associated with a superficial punctate keratitis, corneal epithelial edema, and reduced visual acuity. This usually occurs within 1–2 weeks after starting the drug and clears 2–6 days after stopping it. Amantadine was reinstituted in 2 patients, and the corneal deposits recurred.[4] Nogaki et al also noted a corneal abrasion in a patient with superficial punctate keratitis.[5]

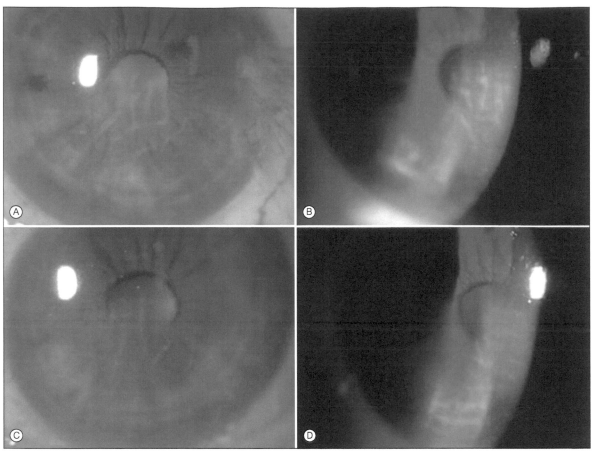

FIG. 14.2 Amantadine-induced corneal toxicity: **(A)** right cornea, **(B)** right cornea (slit lamp examination). Note the presence of corneal edema and endothelial damage, **(C)** left cornea, and **(D)** left cornea (slit lamp examination). Note corneal edema and endothelial damage.[8]

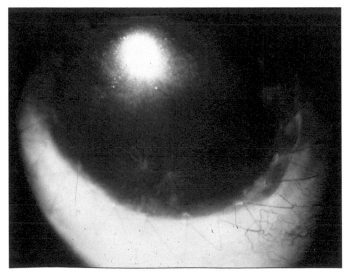

FIG. 14.3 Corneal lesions associated with superficial punctate keratitis in patient on systemic amantadine.[5]

There is only one reference to ocular toxicity associated with memantine use, a single case report with a strong suggestion of this drug causing endothelial dysfunction in an eye after Descemet's membrane endothelial keratoplasty (DMEK).[6] The DMEK was performed to improve vision after complications from Descemet's stripping automated endothelial keratoplasty (DSAEK). Three efforts to reattach the endothelium were unsuccessful until memantine was discontinued. Spontaneous reports had only 7 similar cases in a drug that reached $1.8 billion in sales in 2014, which suggests that this possible memantine-induced side effect on the corneal endothelium is weak and may be primarily in compromised cells.[7] This drug can cause visual hallucinations but few of the other ocular side effects documented with amantadine.

Generic Names:

1. Benztropine mesylate; 2. biperiden; 3. procyclidine hydrochloride; 4. trihexyphenidyl hydrochloride.

Proprietary Names:

1. Cogentin; 2. Akineton; 3. Kemadrin; 4. Artane, Trihexy-5.

Primary Use

These anticholinergic drugs are used in the management of Parkinson disease and in the control of extrapyramidal disorders due to central nervous system drugs, such as reserpine or the phenothiazines.

Ocular Side Effects

Systemic administration – intramuscular, intravenous, or oral
Certain
1. Pupils
   a. Mydriasis – may precipitate acute glaucoma
   b. Decreased reaction to light
2. Decreased vision
3. Decreased accommodation
4. Visual hallucinations
5. Decreased critical flicker fusion (procyclidine)

Probable
1. May aggravate or cause ocular sicca
2. Decreased contact lens tolerance
3. Myasthenia gravis – aggravated (trihexyphenidyl)
   a. Ptosis
   b. Diplopia
   c. Paresis of extraocular muscles

Possible
1. Oculogyric crisis

Conditional/unclassified
1. Retinal pigment changes

Clinical Significance

The degree of anticholinergic activity–induced ocular side effects varies with each drug. Adverse ocular reactions are common with benztropine, whereas they are rare with biperiden. In younger age groups decreased accommodation may cause considerable inconveniences and can be partially reversed by topical ocular application of a weak, long-acting anticholinesterase. There are cases in the literature and spontaneous reports of these drugs precipitating acute glaucoma in patients at recommended dosages. This is emphasized in the package insert.[1] These drugs, particularly trihexyphenidyl, are known to aggravate or cause ocular sicca and affect contact lens wear.[1] Visual hallucinations are primarily of people who are normal in size and color, and often they disappear if the dosage of the drug is reduced. Sharma et al showed that procyclidine reduced critical flicker fusion at therapeutic levels of 15 mg.[2] Retinal pigmentary changes have been seen in patients taking these medications, but this has not been proven as a drug-related event.

Generic Name:

Levodopa.

Proprietary Name:

Multi-ingredient preparations only.

Primary Use

This beta-adrenergic blocking drug is used in the management of Parkinson disease.

Ocular Side Effects

Systemic administration – intravenous or oral
Certain
1. Pupils
   a. Mydriasis – may precipitate acute glaucoma
   b. Miosis – delayed
2. Decreased vision
3. Diplopia
4. Blepharospasm
5. Blepharoclonus
6. Eyelids or conjunctiva
   a. Allergic reactions
   b. Edema

Probable
1. Widening of palpebral fissure
2. Extraocular muscles

a. Paresis
b. Abnormal involuntary movement
3. Oculogyric crisis

Possible
1. Horner's syndrome
2. Amblyopia
   a. Increased visual acuity
   b. Decreased binocular suppression
3. Visual hallucinations
4. Eyelids or conjunctiva – lupoid syndrome

Conditional/unclassified
1. Stimulation of malignant melanoma

Clinical Significance
Although numerous ocular side effects due to levodopa are known, they appear to be dose dependent and reversible. Rarely is the drug given alone, so to determine causation is difficult. Pupillary side effects are variable. Initially, mydriasis may occur, which has been reported to precipitate acute glaucoma.[1-3] After a few weeks of levodopa therapy, miosis is not uncommon. Eyelid responses also appear to be variable. In some patients, levodopa produces ptosis, sometimes unilateral, and blepharospasm is reported in other patients. Apraxia of lid opening has been reported due to levodopa/carbidopa, but others feel this is not caused by levodopa per se, but more likely due to a fluctuation in the brain of dopamine levels during adjustment to levodopa/carbidopa therapy.[4,5] Visual hallucinations are menacing and primarily of normal-size people and in color. These hallucinations can be stopped or decreased in frequency by reducing the drug dosage. Oculogyric crises have been precipitated by levodopa, primarily in patients with prior history of encephalitis. Gottlob et al reported that levodopa has improved contrast sensitivity, decreased the size of scotomas, and improved vision in up to 70% of amblyopic eyes.[6] This improvement is said to persist. Leguire et al reported a series of articles that suggest permanent improvement in some amblyopic eyes after administration of this drug.[7] Procianoy et al also studied the effects of levodopa in children with strabismic amblyopia.[8] Razeghinejad et al reviewed this subject and found no overall long-term benefits.[9] In a study of 16 million patients with Parkinson disease, it was found that the patients on levodopa had a decreased incidence of adult-onset macular degeneration.[10] Further studies have not yet been reported. Because levodopa is an intermediate in melanin synthesis, there is a question of whether it might induce or stimulate the growth of melanomas.[11,12] Although there are no proven data to support this, alternative forms of anti-parkinsonian therapy have been suggested for susceptible patients.

Generic Name:
Selegiline hydrochloride.

Proprietary Names:
Carbex, Eldepryl, Emsam, Zelapar.

Primary Use
This is a selective inhibitor of monoamine oxidase type B, which enhances the effects of levodopa and is used in the management of Parkinson disease.

Ocular Side Effects
Systemic administration – oral or transdermal patch
Certain
1. Decreased vision
2. Blepharospasm

Probable
1. Photophobia

Possible
1. May aggravate or cause ocular sicca
2. Chromatopsia
3. Visual hallucinations
4. Diplopia

Conditional/unclassified
1. Vortex keratopathy

Clinical Significance
This drug has had only a few ocular adverse events reported. It is a drug that increases dopaminergic activity, thereby acting as a sympathomimetic. To date, all of the side effects noted are reversible once the drug is discontinued. Buttner et al postulated a color perception problem with Parkinson disease, so the drug may not be implicated.[1] Rarely are any of these side effects a reason to discontinue the drug, except in patients with diplopia or severe blepharospasm. There is disagreement of whether or not selegiline causes visual hallucinations.[2,3] There is 1 spontaneous report of bilateral vortex keratopathy in a patient on this medication for 1 month. This cleared after the drug was discontinued. Xerostomia occurs in 4–8% of patients on this drug, and it is also mentioned as a possible cause of ocular sicca.[4] It is common that if a drug causes xerostomia, ocular sicca may also occur.

CLASS: CHOLINESTERASE REACTIVATORS

Generic Name:
Pralidoxime chloride.

Proprietary Name:
Protopam.

Primary Use
This cholinesterase reactivator is used as an antidote for poisoning due to organophosphate pesticides or other chemicals that have anticholinesterase activity. It is also of value in the control of overdosage by anticholinesterase drugs used in the treatment of myasthenia gravis.

Ocular Side Effects
Systemic administration – intramuscular, intravenous, or subcutaneous
Certain
1. Decreased vision
2. Diplopia
3. Decreased accommodation

Possible
1. May aggravate or cause ocular sicca
2. Decreased contact lens tolerance

Local ophthalmic use or exposure – subconjunctival injection
Certain
1. Irritation
   a. Hyperemia
   b. Burning sensation
2. Iritis
3. Reverses miosis
4. Reverses accommodative spasms

Possible
1. Subconjunctival hemorrhages

Clinical Significance
Pralidoxime commonly causes adverse ocular reactions after systemic administration. These effects are of rapid onset, last from a few minutes to a few hours, and are completely reversible. In 1 series, up to 60% of patients using the drug complained of misty vision, heaviness of the eye, decreased near vision, or decreased accommodation, especially after sudden head movement.[1] Ocular side effects from subconjunctival injection are also transitory and reversible. This drug may cause xerostomia and therefore may aggravate or cause ocular sicca.[2]

CLASS: MUSCLE RELAXANTS

Generic Name:
Dantrolene sodium.

Proprietary Names:
Dantrium, Revonto, Ryanodex.

Primary Use
This skeletal muscle relaxant is effective in controlling the manifestations of clinical spasticity resulting from serious chronic disorders, such as spinal cord injury, stroke, cerebral palsy, or multiple sclerosis.

Ocular Side Effects
Systemic administration – intravenous or oral
Certain
1. Decreased vision
2. Visual hallucinations

Possible
1. Eyelids or conjunctiva
   a. Photosensitivity
   b. Urticaria
2. Diplopia
3. Lacrimation
4. Pain

Clinical Significance
Ocular side effects due to dantrolene are transient and seldom of clinical significance. Decreased vision occurs in 3% of patients on this drug.[1] Diplopia and excessive lacrimation are also occasionally seen. Visual hallucinations associated with the use of this drug usually subside on drug withdrawal, but this may take several days. Low et al described eye pain once dantrolene was started.[2]

Generic Name:
Orphenadrine citrate.

Proprietary Names:
Banfelx, Norflex.

Primary Use
This antihistaminic drug is used in the treatment of skeletal muscle spasm and the associated pain of parkinsonism.

Ocular Side Effects
Systemic administration – intramuscular, intravenous, or oral
Certain
1. Decreased vision

Probable
1. Mydriasis – may precipitate acute glaucoma
2. Decreased contact lens tolerance
3. May aggravate or cause ocular sicca
4. Decreased accommodation

Possible
1. Diplopia
2. Visual hallucinations

Clinical Significance
Ocular side effects due to orphenadrine are transient and probably the result of its weak anticholinergic effect. These are seldom significant clinical problems, although rarely acute glaucoma has been precipitated secondary to drug-induced mydriasis.[1] Side effects with this drug seem to be more common in the elderly. Orphenadrine can cause ocular sicca and may interfere with contact lens wear.[1]

REFERENCES
Drugs: Edrophonium chloride, pyridostigmine bromide
1. Nucci P, Brancato R. Oculogyric crisis after the Tensilon test, Graefes. *Arch Ophthalmol Clin Exp.* 1990;228:382–385.
2. Smith TA, Cornblath WT. Alternating superior and inferior oblique myokymia. *JAMA Ophthalmol.* 2014;132(7):898–899.
3. Voon YC, Yahya WN, Hasan S, et al. Pyridostigmine-induced dystonic blepharospasm in a patient with ocular myasthenia gravis. *Mov Disord.* 2010;25(9):1299–1300.

Drugs: Brompheniramine maleate, chlorphenamine maleate (chlorpheniramine), dexchlorpheniramine maleate (dexchlorpheniramine), triprolidine hydrochloride
1. Nicholson AN, Smith PA, Spencer MB. Antihistamines and visual function: studies on dynamic acuity and the pupillary response to light. *Br J Clin Pharmacol.* 1982;14:683–690.
2. Koffler BH, Lemp MA. The effect of an antihistamine (chlorpheniramine maleate) on tear production in humans. *Ann Ophthalmol.* 1980;12:217.
3. Miller D. Role of the tear film in contact lens wear. *Int Ophthalmol Clin.* 1973;13(1):247–262.
4. Davis WA. Dyskinesia associated with chronic antihistamine use. *N Engl J Med.* 1976;294:113.
5. Granacher Jr RP. Facial dyskinesia after antihistamines. *N Engl J Med.* 1977;296:516.
6. Sovner RD. Dyskinesia associated with chronic antihistamine use. *N Engl J Med.* 1976;294:113.

Drugs: Carbinoxamine maleate, clemastine fumarate, diphenhydramine hydrochloride, doxylamine succinate
1. *Carbinoxamine maleate, clemastine fumarate, diphenhydramine hydrochloride, doxylamine succinate.* 2018. Retrieved from http://www.pdr.net.
2. Delaney Jr WV. Explained unexplained anisocoria. *JAMA.* 1980;244:1475.
3. Miller D. Role of the tear film in contact lens wear. *Int Ophthalmol Clin.* 1973;13(1):247–262.
4. Seedor JA, Lamberts D, Bergmann RB, et al. Filamentary keratitis associated with diphenhydramine hydrochloride (Benadryl). *Am J Ophthalmol.* 1986;101:376–377.
5. Walsh FB. *Clinical Neuro-Ophthalmology.* Baltimore: Williams & Wilkins; 1957.
6. Nigro SA. Toxic psychosis due to diphenhydramine hydrochloride. *JAMA.* 1968;203:301–302.

Drugs: Cetirizine hydrochloride, desloratadine, fexofenadine hydrochloride, loratadine, tripelennamine
1. Ousler III GW, Workman DA, Torkildsen GL. An open-label, investigator-masked, crossover study of the ocular drying effects of two antihistamines, topical epinastine and systemic loratadine, in adult volunteers with seasonal allergic conjunctivitis. *Clin Therap.* 2007;29(4):611–616.
2. Fraunfelder FW, Fraunfelder FT. Oculogyric crisis in patients taking cetirizine. *Am J Ophthalmol.* 2004;137:355–357.

Drug: Cyproheptadine hydrochloride
1. *Cyproheptadine hydrochloride.* 2018. Retrieved from http://www.pdr.net.
2. Miller D. Role of the tear film in contact lens wear. *Int Ophthalmol Clin.* 1973;13(1):247–262.
3. Drugs that cause photosensitivity. *Med Lett Drugs Ther.* 1986;28:51.

Drug: Dupilumab
1. Wollenberg A, Ariens L, Thurau S, et al. Conjunctivitis occurring in atopic dermatitis patients treated with dupilumab: clinical characteristics and treatment. *J Allergy Clin Immunol Pract.* 2018;6(5):1778–1780.
2. *Dupilumab.* 2018. Retrieved from http://www.pdr.net.
3. Simpson EL, Bieber T, Guttman-Yassky E, et al. Two phase 3 trials of dupilumab versus placebo in atopic dermatitis. *N Engl J Med.* 2016;375:2335–2348.
4. Blauvelt A, de Bruin-Weller M, Gooderham M, et al. Long-term management of moderate-to-severe atopic dermatitis with dupilumab and concomitant topical corticosteroids (Libery and Chronos): a 1-year, randomized, double-blinded, placebo-controlled, phase 3 trial. *Lancet.* 2017;389:2287–2303.
5. De Bruin-Weller, Thaci D, Smith CH, et al. Dupilumab with concomitant topical corticosteroids in adult patients with atopic dermatitis who are not adequately controlled

with or are intolerant to ciclosporin A, or when this treatment is medically inadvisable: a placebo-controlled, randomized phase 3 clinical trial (Liberty and Café). *Br J Dermatol.* 2018;178:1083–1101.

6. Barnes AC, Blandford AD, Perry JD. Cicatricial ectropion in a patient treated with dupilumab. *Am J Ophthalmol Case Rep.* 2017;7:120–122.
7. Levine RM, Tattersall IW, Gaudio PA, et al. Cicatrizing blepharoconjunctivitis occurring during dupilumab treatment and a proposed algorithm for its management. *JAMA Dermatol.* 2018;154(12):1485–1486.

Drugs: Amantadine hydrochloride, memantine hydrochloride

1. Chang KC, Jeong JH, Kim MK, et al. The effect of amantadine on corneal endothelium in subjects with Parkinson's disease. *Ophthalmology.* 2010;117:1214–1219.
2. Jeng BH, Galor A, Less MS, et al. Amantadine-associated corneal edema: potentially irreversible even after cessation of the medication. *Ophthalmology.* 2008;115:1540–1544.
3. French DD, Margo CE. Postmarketing surveillance of corneal edema, Fuchs dystrophy, and amantadine use in the Veterans Health Administration. *Cornea.* 2007;26:1087–1090.
4. Fraunfelder FT, Meyer SM. Amantadine and corneal deposits. *Am J Ophthalmol.* 1990;110(1):96–97.
5. Nogaki H, Morimatsu M. Superficial punctate keratitis and corneal abrasion due to amantadine hydrochloride (letter). *J Neurol.* 1993;240(6):388–389.
6. Feng MT, Price Jr FW, McKee Y, et al. Memantine-associated corneal endothelial dysfunction. *JAMA Ophthalmol.* 2015;133(10):1218–1220.
7. Memantine. In Wikipedia. Retrieved March 12, 2018, from https://en.wikipedia.org/wiki/Memantine.
8. Kubo S, Iwatake A, Ebihara N, et al. Visual impairment in Parkinson's disease treated with amantadine: case report and review of the literature. *Parkinsonism Relat Disord.* 2008;14(2):166–169.

Drugs: Benztropine mesylate, biperiden, procyclidine hydrochloride, trihexyphenidyl hydrochloride

1. *Benztropine mesylate, trihexyphenidyl hydrochloride.* 2018. Retrieved from http://www.pdr.net.
2. Sharma T, Galea A, Zachariah E, et al. Effects of 10 mg and 15 mg oral procyclidine on critical flicker fusion threshold and cardiac functioning in healthy human subjects. *J Psychopharmacol.* 2002;16:183–187.

Drug: Levodopa

1. Burdick DJ, Griffith A, Agarwal P. Mydriasis in a Parkinson's disease patient on low-dose carbidopa/levodopa. *Mov Disord.* 2013;28(3):295.
2. Burdick DJ, Griffin A, Agarwal P. Mydriasis in a Parkinson's disease patient on low-dose carbidopa/levodopa. *Mov Disord.* 2013;28(3):S218.

3. Levodopa containing products. *Risk of angle closure glaucoma. Revision of Precautions.* MHLW/PMDA; 2016.
4. Lamberti P, De Mari M, Zenzola A, et al. Frequency of apraxia of eyelid opening in the general population and in patients with extrapyramidal disorder. *Neurol Sci.* 2002;23(suppl 2):S81–S82.
5. Lee KC, Finley R, Miller B. Apraxia of lid opening: dose-dependent response to carbidopa-levodopa. *Pharmacotherapy.* 2004;24:401–403.
6. Gottlob I, Charlier J, Reinecke RD. Visual acuities and scotomas after one week levodopa administration in human amblyopia. *Invest Ophthalmol Vis Sci.* 1992;33(9):2722–2727.
7. Leguire LE, et al. Levodopa treatment for childhood amblyopia. *Invest Ophthalmol Vis Sci.* 1991;32(suppl):820.
8. Procianoy E, Fuchs FD, Procianoy L, et al. The effect of increasing doses of levodopa on children with strabismic amblyopia. *J Am Assoc Pediatr Ophthalmol Strabismus.* 1999;3(6):337–340.
9. Razeghinejad MR, Nowroozzadeh MH, Eghbal MH. Levodopa and other pharmacologic interventions in ischemic and traumatic optic neuropathies and amblyopia. *Clin Neuropharm.* 2016;39(1):40–48.
10. Brilliant MH, Vaziri K, Connor Jr TB, et al. Mining retrospective data for virtual prospective drug repurposing: l-dopa and age-related macular degeneration. *Am J Med.* 2016;129(3):292–298.
11. van Rens GN, De Jong PT, Demols EE, et al. Uveal malignant melanoma and levodopa therapy in Parkinson's disease. *Ophthalmology.* 1982;89:1464–1466.
12. Abramson DH, Rubenfield MR. Choroidal melanoma and levodopa. *JAMA.* 1984;252:1011–1012.

Drug: Selegiline hydrochloride

1. Buttner T, Kuhn W, Klotz P, et al. Disturbance of colour perception in Parkinson's disease. *J Neural Transmission Parkinsons Dis Dementia Sect.* 1993;6(1):11–15.
2. Kamakura K, Mochizuki H, Kaida K, et al. Therapeutic factors causing hallucination in Parkinson's disease patients, especially those given selegiline. *Parkinsonism Relat Disord.* 2004;10:235–242.
3. Papapetropoulos S, Argyriou AA. Administration of selegiline is not associated with visual hallucinations in advanced Parkinson's disease. *Parkinsonism Relat Disord.* 2005;11:265–266.
4. *Selegiline hydrochloride.* 2018. Retrieved from http://www.pdr.net.

Drug: Pralidoxime chloride

1. Holland P, Parkes DC. Plasma concentrations of the oxime pralidoxime mesylate (P25) after repeated oral and intramuscular administration. *Br J Ind Med.* 1976;33:43–46.
2. *Pralidoxime chloride.* 2018. Retrieved from http://www.pdr.net.

Drug: Dantrolene sodium

1. *Dantrolene sodium.* 2018. Retrieved from http://www.pdr.net.

2. Low SA, Robbins W, Tawfik VL. Complex management of a patient with refractory primary erythromelalgia lacking a SCN9A mutation. *J Pain Res.* 2017;10:973–977.

Drug: Orphenadrine citrate
1. *Orphenadrine citrate.* 2018. Retrieved from http://www.pdr.net.

FURTHER READING
Edrophonium chloride, pyridostigmine bromide
Field LM. Toxic alopecia caused by pyridostigmine bromide. *Arch Dermatol.* 1980;116:1103.

Van Dyk HJ, Florence L. The Tensilon test. A safe office procedure. *Ophthalmology.* 1980;87:210–212.

Brompheniramine maleate, chlorphenamine maleate (chlorpheniramine), dexchlorpheniramine maleate (dexchlorpheniramine), triprolidine hydrochloride
Farber AS. Ocular side effects of antihistamine-decongestant combinations. *Am J Ophthalmol.* 1982;94:565.

Halperin M, Thorig L, van Haeringen NJ. Ocular side effects of antihistamine-decongestant combinations. *Am J Ophthalmol.* 1983;95:563–564.

Schuller DE, Turkewitz D. Adverse effects of antihistamines. *Postgrad Med.* 1986;79:75–86.

Cetirizine hydrochloride, desloratadine, fexofenadine hydrochloride, loratadine, tripelennamine
Abelson MB, Allansmith MR, Friedlaender MN. Effects of topically applied ocular decongestant and antihistamine. *Am J Ophthalmol.* 1980;90:254–257.

Fraunfelder FW, Fraunfelder FT. Adverse ocular drug reactions recently identified by the national registry of drug-induced ocular side effects. *Ophthalmology.* 2004;111:1275–1279.

Grant WM, Loeb DR. Effect of locally applied antihistamine drugs on normal eyes. *Arch Ophthalmol.* 1948;39:553–554.

Hays DP, Johnson BF, Perry R. Prolonged hallucinations following a modest overdose of tripelennamine. *Clin Toxicol.* 1980;16:331–333.

Herman DC, Bartley GB. Corneal opacities secondary to topical naphazoline and antazoline (Albalon A). *Am J Ophthalmol.* 1987;103:110–111.

Amantadine hydrochloride, memantine hydrochloride
Avendano-Cantos EM, Celis-Sanchez J, Mesa-Varona D, et al. Corneal toxicity due to amantadine. *Arch Soc Esp Oftalmol.* 2012;87(9):290–293.

Beran M, Okyere B, Vova J. Amantadine induced corneal edema in a pediatric patient. *PM R.* 2017;98(10):e31–e32.

Blanchard DL. Amantadine caused corneal edema. *Cornea.* 1990;9(2):181.

Boyce TM, Cohen AW. A case of double trouble. *EyeNet.* 2013:51–53.

Drugs that. cause psychiatric symptoms. *Med Lett Drugs Ther.* 1986;28:81.

Esquenazi S. Bilateral reversible corneal edema associated with amantadine use. *J Ocul Pharmacol Therap.* 2009;25(6):567–569.

Ghaffariyeh A, Honarpisheh N. Amantadine-associated corneal edema. *Parkinsonism Relat Disord.* 2010;16:427.

Hessen MM, Vahedi S, Khoo CT, et al. Clinical and genetic investigation of amantadine-associated corneal edema. *Clin Ophthalmol.* 2018;12:1367–1371.

Hood CT, Langston RH, Schoenfield LR, et al. Amantadine-associated corneal edema treated with Descemet's stripping automated endothelial keratoplasty. *Ophthalmic Surg Lasers Imaging.* 2010;41 online:1–4.

Hughes B, Feiz V, Flynn SB, et al. Reversible amantadine-induced corneal edema in an adolescent. *Cornea.* 2004;23:823–824.

Koenig SB. Descemet stripping automated endothelial keratoplasty in the phakic eye. *Cornea.* 2010;29(5):531–533.

Naumann GO, Schlotzer-Schrehardt U. Amantadine-associated corneal edema. *Ophthalmology.* 2009;116(6):1230–1231, author reply 1231.

Pearlman JT, Kadish AH, Ramseyer JC. Vision loss associated with amantadine hydrochloride use. *JAMA.* 1977;237:1200.

Pond A, Lee MS, Hardten DR, et al. Toxic corneal oedema associated with amantadine use. *Br J Ophthalmol.* 2009;93:281.

Postma JU, Van Tilburg W. Visual hallucinations and delirium during treatment with amantadine (Symmetrel). *J Am Geriatr Soc.* 1975;23:212–215.

Selby G. Treatment of Parkinsonism. *Drugs.* 1976;11:61–70.

Soin K, Feinstein EG, Guo J. Recent-onset bilateral blurred vision. *JAMA Ophthalmol.* 2017;135(1):71–72.

Trovato E. Acute vision loss after treatment with amantadine in the setting of traumatic brain injury in a patient with history of Fuch's dystrophy: a case report. *PM R.* 2015;7(91):S96–S97.

van den Berg WH, van Ketel WG. Photosensitization by amantadine (Symmetrel). *Contact Dermatitis.* 1983;9:165.

Wilson TW, Rajput AH. Amantadine–Dyazide interaction. *Can Med Assoc J.* 1983;129:974–975.

Yang Y, Taja S, Baig K. Bilateral corneal edema associated with amantadine. *CMAJ.* 2015;187(15):1155–1158.

Benztropine mesylate, biperiden, procyclidine hydrochloride, trihexyphenidyl hydrochloride
Acute drug abuse reactions. *Med Lett Drugs Ther.* 1985;27:77.

Anticholinergic drugs are abused. *Int Drug Ther Newslett.* 1985;20:1.

Friedman Z, Neumann E. Benzhexol induced blindness in Parkinson's disease. *BMJ.* 1972;1:605.

McGucken RB, Caldwell J, Anthon B. Teenage procyclidine abuse. *Lancet.* 1985;1:1514.

Medina C, Kramer MD, Kurland AA. Biperiden in the treatment of phenothiazine-induced extrapyramidal reactions. *JAMA.* 1962;182:1127–1129.

Selby G. Treatment of Parkinsonism. *Drugs.* 1976;11:61–70.

Thaler JS. The effect of multiple psychotropic drugs on the accommodation of pre-presbyopes. *Am J Optom Physiol Optics.* 1979;56:259–261.

Thaler JS. Effects of benztropine mesylate (Cogentin) on accommodation in normal volunteers. *Am J Optom Physiol Optics.* 1982;59:918–919.

Ueno S, Takahashi M, Kajiyama K, et al. Parkinson's disease and myasthenia gravis: adverse effect of trihexyphenidyl on neuromuscular transmission. *Neurology.* 1987;37:832–833.

Levodopa

Barbeau AL. Dopa therapy in Parkinson's disease: a critical review of nine years' experience. *Can Med Assoc J.* 1969;101:791–800.

Barone DA, Martin HL. Causes of pseudotumor cerebri and papilledema. *Arch Intern Med.* 1979;139:830–831.

Casey DE. Pharmacology of blepharospasm-oromandibular dystonia. *Neurology.* 1980;30:690–695.

Cotzias GC, Papavasilliou PS, Gellene R. Modifications of Parkinsonism – chronic treatment with L-dopa. *N Engl J Med.* 1969;280:337–345.

Glantz R, Weiner WJ, Goetz CG, et al. Drug-induced asterixis in Parkinson disease. *Neurology.* 1982;32:553–555.

Goetz CG, Leurgans S, Papper EJ. et al. Prospective longitudinal assessment of hallucinations in Parkinson's disease. *Neurology.* 2001;57:2078–2082.

Leguire LE, Walson PD, Roger GL, et al. Levodopa/carbidopa for childhood amblyopia. *Invest Ophthalmol Vis Sci.* 1993;34(11):3090–3095.

Leguire LE, Walson PD, Rogers GL, et al. Levodopa/carbidopa treatment of amblyopia in older children. *J Pediatr Ophthalmol Strabismus.* 1995;32(3):143–151.

Leguire LE, Walson PD, Roger GL, et al. Longitudinal study of levodopa/carbidopa for childhood amblyopia. *J Pediatr Ophthalmol Strabismus.* 1993;30(6):354–360.

LeWitt PA. Conjugate eye deviations as dyskinesias induced by levodopa in Parkinson's disease. *Mov Disord.* 1998;13(4):731–734.

Linazasoro F, Van Blercom N, Lasa A. Levodopa-induced ocular dyskinesias in Parkinson's disease. *Mov Disord.* 2002;17:186–220.

Martin WE. Adverse reactions during treatment of Parkinson's disease with levodopa. *JAMA.* 1971;216:1979–1983.

Shimizu N, Cohen B, Bala SP, et al. Ocular dyskinesias in patients with Parkinson's disease treated with levodopa. *Ann Neurol.* 1977;1:167–171.

Pralidoxime chloride

Bryon HM, Posner H. Clinical evaluation of Protopam. *Am J Ophthalmol.* 1964;57:409–418.

Dekking HM. Stopping the action of strong miotics. *Ophthalmologica.* 1964;148:428–430.

Jager BV, Stagg GN. Toxicity of diacetyl monoxime and of pyridine-2-aldoxime methiodide in man. *Bull Johns Hopkins Hosp.* 1958;102:203–211.

Taylor WJ, Llewellyn-Thomas E, Sellers EA, et al. Effects of a combination of atropine, metaraminol and pyridine aldoxime methanesulfonate (AMP therapy) on normal human subjects. *Can Med Assoc J.* 1965;93:957–961.

Dantrolene sodium

Andrews LG, Muzumdar AS, Pinkerton AC. Hallucinations associated with dantrolene sodium therapy. *Can Med Assoc J.* 1975;112:148.

Pembroke AC, Saxena SR, Kataria M, et al. Acne induced by dantrolene. *Br J Dermatol.* 1981;104:465–468.

Silverman HI, Harvie RJ. Adverse effects of commonly used systemic drugs on the human eye –Part III. *Am J Optom Physiol Optics.* 1975;52:275–287.

Orphenadrine citrate

Bennett NB, Kohn J. Case report: orphenadrine overdose. Cerebral manifestations treated with physostigmine. *Anaesth Intens Care.* 1976;4:67.

Davidson SI. Reports of ocular adverse reactions. *Trans Ophthalmol Soc UK.* 1973;93:495–510.

Furlanut M, Bettio D, Bertin I, et al. Orphenadrine serum levels in a poisoned patient. *Hum Toxicol.* 1985;4:331–333.

Heinonen J, Heikkilä J, Mattila MJ, et al. Orphenadrine poisoning. A case report supplemented with animal experiments. *Arch Toxicol.* 1968;23:264.

Selby G. Treatment of Parkinsonism. *Drugs.* 1976;11:61–70.

Stoddart JC, Parkin JM, Wytne NA. Orphenadrine poisoning: a case report. *Br J Anaesth.* 1968;40:786.

CHAPTER 15

Oncolytic Drugs

CLASS: ANTINEOPLASTIC DRUGS

Generic Name:
Alemtuzumab.

Proprietary Names:
Campath, Campath-1H, Lemtrada, MabCampath.

Primary Use
A monoclonal antibody used in the management of some leukemias, in multiple sclerosis, and as an anti-rejection drug.

Ocular Side Effects
Systemic administration – intravenous
Certain
1. Graves' ophthalmopathy
2. Hypothyroidism

Probable
1. Increased risk of
   a. Cytomegalovirus retinitis (Fig. 15.1)
   b. Intraocular aspergillosis
   c. Herpes simplex and zoster
   d. Fungal infection
   e. Tuberculosis

Clinical Significance
Alemtuzumab causes infusion-related reactions such as autoimmune disorders, especially Graves' oph-thalmopathy, and may allow secondary pathogens to invade the eye.

Graves' disease likely occurs as the lymphocytes start to recover and there is a loss of self-tolerance during lym-phocytic proliferation. This appears to be more com-mon in those with a family history of thyroid disease or in smokers.[1,2] In multiple sclerosis patients, Graves' ophthalmopathy seems to occur most frequently 12-36 months after starting therapy.[3-7] The incidence may be as high as 22%, with 23% reverting spontaneously to a euthyroid state.[7] This may occur after more than 1 course of treatment with alemtuzumab.

Song et al described 4 cases of cytomegalovirus (CMV) retinitis after the use of an alemtuzumab-conditioning regimen in patients with acute leukemia.[8] Tang et al and Derzko-Dzulynsky et al have also reported CMV retinitis after this same drug protocol in patients with low-grade lymphoma.[9,10] Alemtuzumab has been shown to cause a high incidence of CMV reactivation systemically.[11,12] With decreased immunologic response secondary to this drug, other second pathogens may invade the eye.[13]

Generic Names:
1. Atezolizumab; 2. ipilimumab; 3. nivolumab; 4. pembrolizumab.

Proprietary Names:
1. Tecentriq; 2. Yervoy; 3. Opdivo; 4. Keytruda.

Primary Use
Monoclonal antibodies used to treat malignant mela-noma and various cancers.

Ocular Side Effects
Systemic administration – intravenous
Certain
1. Decreased vision
2. Blindness

Probable
1. Uveitis (must be differentiated from inflammation – secondary to tumor necrosis)
   a. Anterior
   b. Posterior
   c. Panuveitis
2. May aggravate or cause ocular sicca
3. Myasthenia-like syndrome
   a. Ptosis
   b. Paresis of extraocular muscles
   c. Diplopia
   d. Myositis of ocular and periocular muscles
4. Orbit
   a. Mimic thyroid-associated orbitopathy
   b. Inflammation
   c. Edema
   d. Proptosis
5. Extraocular muscles and orbicularis oculi
   a. Myositis

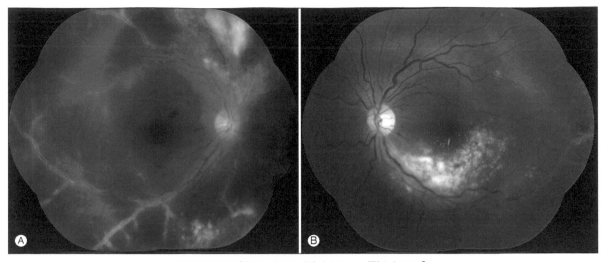

FIG. 15.1 CMV retinitis: **(A)** right eye, **(B)** left eye.[8]

b. Various degrees of paresis
  c. Diplopia
6. Conjunctiva and cornea
  a. Keratitis
  b. Ulceration
  c. Edema
7. Eyelids
  a. Edema
  b. Ptosis
  c. Blepharitis
8. Uveal effusions
9. Retina and choroid
  a. Choroiditis
    i. Serous retinal detachments
    ii. Whitest deposits
  b. Pigment clumping
    i. Window defect
  c. Vasculitis
  d. Macular edema
  e. Vascular occlusions
  f. Choroidal folds

Possible

1. Optic nerve
  a. Neuritis
  b. Edema
2. Vogt-Koyangi-Harada (VKH) disease
  a. Uveitis
  b. Vitiligo
  c. Poliosis
  d. Retinal changes

Conditional/unclassified

1. Corneal erosion
2. Episcleritis
3. Nerve paresis

Clinical Significance

These checkpoint inhibitors primarily affect the immune system for therapeutics, as well as causing their ocular side effects. The ocular side effects profile is made up of limited data from single case reports and small case series. Most reports are with ipilimumab, which was one of the first approved and which also seems to have a more generalized effect on the immune system. This class of drugs can cause significant and irreversible ocular side effects via multiple mechanisms, including immune-mediated reactions, direct toxic drug effects, the drugs and their metabolites via the tears, or secondary effects from drug-induced tumor necrosis. These side effects may be dose, time, and location dependent. Although ocular side effects are uncommon, they may be blinding and affect all ocular or periocular tissues.

Uveitis is probably the most well-documented significant ocular side effect. There are over 35 publications often reporting multiple cases of probable immunologically induced anterior, posterior, or panuveitis.[1–6] In addition, there are over 200 spontaneous reports of these drugs causing uveitis. The severity is usually dependent on when discovered, but cases of permanent blindness have been reported. Onset typically occurs after 2-3 injections of the drug. The uveitis occurs if the treatment is for an intraocular or extra-ocular melanoma. The uveitis may be unilateral or bilateral. Any and all parts of the eye may be affected causing macular edema, optic nerve inflammation, and choroidal inflammation with resultant serous retinal detachments. Steroids often control this uveitis.

Pham et al pointed out that severe ocular or periocular inflammation can occur by an aggressive intraocular tumor outgrowing its blood supply precipitated by this class of drugs, which may increase tumor necrosis with a resultant severe intraocular reaction.[7]

This group of drugs may mimic thyroid-associated orbitopathy. Patients may have unilateral, but most often bilateral, pain, swelling of upper and lower eyelids, proptosis, diplopia, chemosis, and erythema of the conjunctiva. There are various degrees of limitation, including total, of the extraocular muscles. Corneal exposure with keratitis and ulceration may be seen. This usually occurs after 2 or more courses of intravenous therapy. There have been 10 cases reported in the literature and over 20 spontaneous reports of these drugs causing a thyroid-mimicking effect.[5,8-12] Imaging tests may be nearly identical to thyroid eye disease with marked thickening of any and all extraocular muscles. Treatment is with steroids but may take months to resolve.

There have been case reports of ocular sicca caused by these drugs, as well as numerous spontaneous reports.[13,14] It has been postulated that this occurs as an immunologic-mediated response. There have been rare reports of keratitis, corneal erosion, and perforation.

Retinal and choroidal adverse events are rare. Inflammation of the choroid causing macular edema and/or serous retinal detachments was reported, and numerous spontaneous reports make this a possible side effect.[1,2,6,15-19] Roberts et al described multiple chorioretinal scars, pigment clumping, and window defects.[17] Modjtahedi et al reported a possible association between ipilimumab and the formation of bilateral choroidal neovascularization membranes.[20]

Optic nerve changes possibly occurring secondarily to severe uveitis may cause edema, optic neuritis, papillitis, or neuropathy.[21-23] There are numerous spontaneous reports of Optic nerve inflammation associated with severe uveitis.

This new group of drugs may possibly cause or simulate VKH disease. VKH is a syndrome characterized by inflammation involving the eye, skin, hair, meninges of the central nervous system (CNS), and the inner ear. Eye findings include uveitis, poliosis, vitiligo, and chorioretinal pathology. There are 5 reports of VKH along with 14 cases from spontaneous reports (nivolumab 9, ipilimumab 6, and pembrolizumab 4).[19,24-27] The *Physicians' Desk Reference* (PDR) mentions VKH as an adverse drug effect.[28] There are a few reports of just poliosis or vitiligo.[29]

There are 6 reported cases of myasthenia with ocular findings, including ptosis, diplopia, extraocular muscle weakness, and orbicularis oculi muscle weakness.[30-33] There are over 130 spontaneous reports of ptosis, diplopia, or diagnosis of ocular or systemic myasthenia. Some cases are probably not myasthenia, but possibly a direct immunologic response causing myositis of any or all of the extraocular muscles and eyelid.[9,34]

Diamantopoulos et al reported a unique case of ptosis after a single injection of pembrolizumab. Systemic findings include various neuromyopathies.[35] Ruff et al described bilateral phrenic nerve paralysis during treatment with ipilimumab, and Hsiao et al described corneal epithelial sloughing after administration of pembrolizumab.[36,37] Both were on the basis of an immune-mediated response.

Uveal effusions have been reported in the literature and spontaneous reports with atezolizumab, nivolumab, and pembrolizumab.[19,38] Dalvin et al recently did a review of systemic and ocular side effects.[39] They noted that ocular side effects were most prominent with generalized systemic adverse drug effects.

Generic Names:
1. Binimetinib; 2. cobimetinib; 3. trametinib.

Proprietary Names:
1. Generic only; 2. Cotellic; 3. Mekinist.

Primary Use
Trametinib is the only mitogen-activated extracellular kinase (MEK) drug approved by the US Food and Drug Administration (FDA) used to treat *BRAF*-mutated melanoma. Cobimetinib is used in combination with vemurafenib for the management of advanced melanoma with *BRAF* V600E or V600K mutations. Binimetinib is prescribed for various types of cancer.

Ocular Side Effects
Systemic administration – oral
Certain
1. Decreased vision
   a. Altered color perception
   b. Shadows
   c. Metamorphopsia
   d. Glare

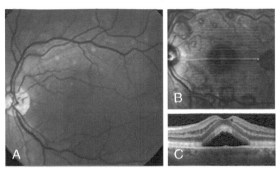

FIG. 15.2 Multimodal imaging illustrating the clinical course of serous retinopathy associated with binimetinib treatment. Multifocal, variably sized serous neuroretinal detachments on red-free fundus photography **(A)** and infrared reflectance (IRR) imaging **(B)** in a 64-year-old patient with metastatic cutaneous melanoma (CM) treated with binimetinib. Bilateral mild intraretinal fluid accumulation and a dome-shaped serous neuroretinal detachment with subretinal fluid (SRF) accumulation were seen on optical coherence tomography (OCT) **(C)**. The intraretinal fluid appeared 20 days after the start of binimetinib and disappeared in 12 days. The binimetinib dose was tapered 7 days after appearance of the intraretinal fluid. Resolution of the intraretinal fluid occurred faster than the resolution of the subfoveal SRF, which was still present at ophthalmologic follow-up 11 weeks later.[2]

2. Retina
    a. Serous retinal detachment (single or multifocal) (Fig. 15.2)
    b. Macular edema
       i. Cystoid
       ii. Subfoveal
3. Photosensitivity
4. Eyelid and periorbital edema

Possible
1. Uveitis
2. Retina
    a. Detachment (if ocular melanoma present)
    b. Intraretinal cysts
    c. Bleeds
    d. Vascular abnormalities
3. May aggravate or cause ocular sicca

Clinical Significance

MEK inhibitors, a targeted therapy, cause ocular side effects that are generally symmetrical and time and dose dependent. Many new MEK inhibitors are in clinical trials, and they all seem to have similar side effects, including decreased vision, serous retinal detachment, photophobia, and periorbital edema. Some MEK inhibitors are used in combination with other anticancer drugs, so their ocular side effects profile may be varied or enhanced.

Visual changes, even with MEK retinopathy, vary widely but most are mild, transitory, self-limiting, and do not interfere with quality of life. MEK retinopathy, unique to this class of drugs, may occur within days of the first dose or up to 15 months after starting therapy. The clinical picture most often presents with a choroiditis causing a serous retinal detachment, which may be single or progress to a multifocal pattern. These may resolve, even on medication. The macula may be involved and progress to cystoid macular edema. Pigment epithelial detachments occur and may resolve on their own.

Eyelid and periorbital edema may occur, but rarely cause significant problems, although diplopia may occur.

Although trametinib is the only FDA-approved drug, many are in clinical trials, and a few are available on an orphan drug basis. Binimetinib is still an investigational drug, but it may well be the most studied for delineating MEK inhibitor–associated retinopathy (MEKAR).[1–4] This side effect appears to be unique and apparently occurs with all MEK inhibitors at an incidence of over 90% in most studies. The clinical findings are dramatic and seem well out of proportion of the symptomatology. Onset of this entity may occur within days or as long as 15 months after starting therapy. The condition is always bilateral, so if not, consider other conditions. The basic lesion is central serous retinopathy. Macular involvement is common, and focal lesions often extend into the midperiphery, primarily around the vascular arcades. Lesions may darken or become yellowish with age. Francis et al has outlined the difference between MEKAR and classic central serous retinopathy as shown by pattern, location, and manner of fluid location.[4] MEKAR is a distinct entity. It is time dependent and is reversible even if the drug is continued. There have been rare reports of vision not fully returning to normal and other ocular abnormalities, drug or nondrug related, so communication between the oncologist and ophthalmologist may be necessary.

Although uveitis has been reported in the literature as well as in spontaneous reports, it seems to primarily occur when dabrafenib is added to trametinib.[5-7] The uveitis is usually bilateral, and it can be a panuveitis and may be severe.

Ocular sicca has been reported with trametinib and in spontaneous reports.[8] Because most antimetabolites are secreted in the tears, irritation or inflammatory sicca complaints would be expected.

Generic Names:
1. Bleomycin sulfate; 2. dactinomycin; 3. daunorubicin hydrochloride; 4. doxorubicin hydrochloride.

Proprietary Names:
1. Blenoxane; 2. Cosmegen; 3. Cerubidine, Daunoxome; 4. Adriamycin, Adriamycin PFS, Doxil, Rubex.

Primary Use
These antibiotics are used in a variety of malignant conditions.

Ocular Side Effects
Systemic administration – intramuscular, intrapleural, intravenous, or subcutaneous
Certain
1. Decreased vision – transitory
2. Eyelids or conjunctiva
   a. Conjunctivitis
   b. Edema
   c. Erythema
3. Epiphora

Probable
1. Pseudotumor cerebri (dactinomycin)

Possible
1. May aggravate herpes infections
2. Ocular teratogenic effects

Inadvertent ocular exposure
Certain
1. Keratoconjunctivitis
2. Chemosis
3. Subepithelial dot infiltrates
4. Transitory anterior uveitis

Clinical Significance
All of these drugs are antimetabolites and, when given systemically, may be concentrated in the tears and cause irritation of the conjunctiva, cornea, and lid margin. This usually occurs within a few days after drug exposure and may return to normal a few days after the drug is stopped and, in some cases, even if the drug is continued. Conjunctivitis and decreased vision are the most frequent drug-induced side effects. Daunorubicin causes mild to moderate visual disturbances in 3%, severe in 2%, and conjunctivitis and eye pain in <5%.[1,2] Blum stated that up to 25% of patients on doxorubicin may have increased lacrimation.[3] The cause may be secondary to ocular irritation. Dactinomycin is the only drug in this group that is probably causing pseudotumor cerebri.[4] Young et al described transient cortical blindness due to bleomycin.[5] These drugs may be cofactors in cataractogenesis. In most instances, this group of drugs is only given systemically for cancer therapy, and their systemic side effects are often so severe that ocular side effects may be insignificant to the overall clinical disability.

Inadvertent topical ocular exposure causes transitory ocular effects. Keratoconjunctivitis, with or without punctate subepithelial dot infiltrates, may occur. These effects resolve after a few days without sequelae. McLoon et al reported muscle loss secondary to direct injection of doxorubicin in the management of blepharospasm.[6]

Generic Name:
Bortezomib.

Proprietary Name:
Velcade.

Primary Use
A first-generation orphan-drug proteasome inhibitor used intravenously and subcutaneously for multiple myeloma and multiple lymphomas.

Ocular Side Effects
Systemic administration – intravenous or subcutaneous
Certain
1. Decreased vision
2. Irritation
3. Conjunctivitis

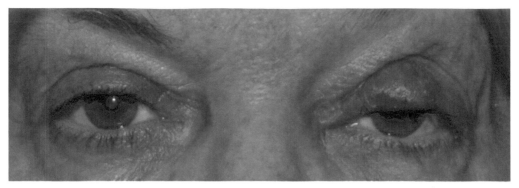

FIG. 15.3 Large left upper eyelid chalazion associated with bortezomib.[1]

Probable

1. Eyelids or conjunctiva
   a. Meibomitis
   b. Chalazion (Fig. 15.3)
   c. Blepharitis
2. Oculomotor nerve palsy

Possible

1. Diplopia

Clinical Significance

This drug is primarily given intravenously. There are few significant rare ocular side effects. However, its association with multiple giant (involving half of the eyelid) chalazions is fairly unique.[1] In a review of 24 cases, chalazions occurred as early as 3 months after the start of bortezomib.[2] These lesions often required multiple therapies and surgeries, and a number of patients had to stop the drug due to this side effect. There were many cases of positive dechallenge and rechallenge. Withdrawal of bortezomib usually leads to resolution or in some cases marked improvement of the chalazion. Min et al proposed that bortezomib may enhance the release of proinflammatory cytokines, increasing an inflammatory response.[3]

Toema et al reported a case of unilateral, partially reversible oculomotor palsy with positive rechallenge data.[4] There are 37 spontaneous reports of diplopia or ptosis associated with bortezomib use.

Chacko et al recently described 2 cases of optic atrophy associated with bortezomib use.[5] In both patients the neuropathy stabilized once the drug was discontinued.

Generic Names:

1. Bromocriptine mesylate; 2. cabergoline.

Proprietary Names:

1. Cycloset, Parlodel; 2. Dostinex.

Primary Use

Dopaminergic agonist primarily used to treat macroprolactinoma pituitary tumors.

Ocular Side Effects

Systemic administration – oral

Probable

1. Bilateral hemianopsia
2. Visual hallucinations

Possible

1. Acute glaucoma
   a. Uveal effusions
   b. High myopia

Conditional/unclassified

1. Central retinal vein occlusion

Clinical Significance

There are numerous reports of a unique ophthalmic finding due to these drugs.[1-7] Patients with a pituitary tumor, primarily a prolactinoma, present with bilateral hemianopsia. They are treated with 1 of the drugs listed, and their visual field markedly improves or goes away. While on therapy, 3–9 months later the bilateral hemianopsia returns, in spite of significant or total regression of the tumor. Although the exact mechanism is open to debate, many have felt that this is due to secondary chiasmal herniation. Others suggest compromised chiasmal vascular blood supply, direct toxicity of the drug, vasospasm-induced ischemia, or reversible perivascular fibrosis. Raverot et al felt that this was an underrecognized phenomena and suggested long-term follow-up of these patients, especially by an ophthalmologist.[2]

Razmjoo et al reported a case of bilateral acute glaucoma associated with cabergoline.[8] This occurred 5 hours after a single 0.5-mg oral tablet. The cause of the acute glaucoma was bilateral effusion of the ciliary body with anterior rotation of the iris–ciliary body. This was associated with 8–9 diopters of myopia, which resolved to normal after 80 days. There are 3 cases of acute glaucoma and 6 cases of glaucoma in the spontaneous reports. No data are available, however, to determine whether these were also associated with ciliary body effusions.

Nagaki et al reported a case of central retina vein occlusion (CRVO) in a 34-year-old female after starting bromocriptine.[9] She had no risk factors for CRVO, and they postulated an unknown paradoxical response to bromocriptine that caused vasoconstriction.

Generic Name:
Busulfan.

Proprietary Names:
Busulfex, Myleran.

Primary Use
This alkylating drug, which is now an orphan drug, is used in the palliative treatment of chronic granulocytic leukemia and other blood dyscrasias.

Ocular Side Effects
Systemic administration – intravenous or oral
Certain
1. Decreased vision
2. Visual hallucinations

Probable
1. May aggravate or cause ocular sicca

Possible
1. Cataracts
   a. Posterior subcapsular
   b. Punctate cortical opacities

Conditional/unclassified
1. Myasthenia gravis
   a. Diplopia
   b. Ptosis
   c. Paresis of extraocular muscles

Ocular teratogenic effects
Possible
1. Retinal degeneration
2. Microphthalmia

Clinical Significance
In general, the ocular side effects associated with busulfan are reversible and seldom of major clinical significance.[1] They include decreased vision, visual hallucinations, and ocular sicca. The incidence of xerostomia is 0–26% in patients taking this drug, which speaks for a probability of the drug also aggravating or causing ocular sicca; the incidence of ocular sicca is 0–1%.[2]

The area of controversy, with no clear conclusion, is busulfan's role in the causation of lens changes, especially in children. The drug manufacturer looked at the clinical data of a 5-year cumulative incidence of extensive chronic graft versus host disease, as well as a 7-year study in acute myeloid leukemia, and concluded that the incidence of lens cataracts was insignificant.[2] Others feel that this drug causes posterior subcapsular lens opacities after 4–5 years of therapy or a cumulative amount of 2000 mg of the drug.[3] These lens changes are often associated with scattered punctate cortical opacities and/or a polychromatic sheen to the posterior capsule of the lens. The incidence and severity increase with duration and total dosage. Although many consider cataract formation rare, Shi-Xia et al, using meta-analysis in a long-term study, found an incidence of 12.7%.[4] Holmström et al, in their series of children who received total-body radiation and busulfan, found that the incidence of cataracts increased along with the cataractogenic additive cofactor effects of corticosteroids and other cytostatic drugs.[5] They stressed early diagnosis by observing lens changes to prevent the development of amblyopia. Kaida et al described a 42-year-old patient on a very high dosage of busulfan who showed signs of posterior subcapsular lens changes after 4 days.[6] Al-Tweigeri et al suggested that the mechanism of busulfan-induced cataracts is related to decreased DNA synthesis in the lens epithelium.[7] The basis for concluding that this drug is cataractogenic is primarily 4 papers in the literature that involved patients with serious diseases who were on multiple medications, especially steroids, and often total-body radiation.[3-6] Both are major cofactors in causing lens changes. Also, the primary description of busulfan lens changes is posterior subcapsular sheen or opacities, both of which are classic for steroid-induced lens changes. We classify busulfan as a "possible" cataractogenic drug and possible cofactor. Regardless, at worst, busulfan is a weak cataractogenic drug.

This drug may cause teratogenic effects, such as microphthalmia or retinal degeneration.[2]

Generic Name:
Capecitabine.

Proprietary Name:
Xeloda.

Primary Use
This antimetabolite is an orally administered fluoropyrimidine carbamate used for the treatment of metastatic breast and colorectal cancers.

Ocular Side Effects
Systemic administration – oral
Certain
1. Ocular irritation
2. Epiphora
3. Cornea
   a. Superficial punctate keratitis
   b. Keratoconjunctivitis
   c. Keratitis
4. Photophobia
5. Conjunctiva
   a. Chemosis
   b. Erythema
   c. Conjunctivitis
6. Decreased vision

Probable
1. May aggravate or cause ocular sicca
2. Superficial corneal deposits (Fig. 15.4)
3. Stenosis of lacrimal drainage system

Conditional/unclassified
1. Purtscher-like retinopathy
2. Cranial nerve palsy
3. Ocular teratogenic effects

Clinical Significance
Capecitabine, acting as a prodrug, is converted to fluorouracil (5FU) through which it acts.[1] However, the ocular side effects of capecitabine are significantly milder than those of 5FU. For example, 5FU has an incidence rate of 5–14% for canalicular

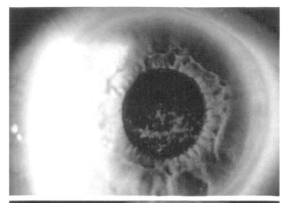
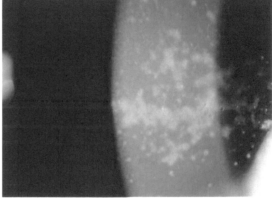
FIG. 15.4 Slit lamp photographs of corneal deposits.[5]

stenosis, whereas it rarely occurs with capecitabine.[2] The most common ocular side effects due to capecitabine are ocular irritation (5–15%), epiphora (12%), decreased vision (5%), and conjunctivitis or keratoconjunctivitis (0–5%).[2] There is an incidence rate of 6% of xerostomia; therefore ocular sicca may be part of the ocular irritation signs and symptoms.[2]

Tsoucalas et al reported 2 cases of lacrimal drainage system stenosis due to capecitabine, and Noguchi et al reported a case of lacrimal duct obstruction caused by capecitabine.[3,4] There are 38 cases in the spontaneous reports of lacrimal outflow problems. Because capecitabine is a prodrug for 5FU, which does cause lacrimal outflow problems, a rare "probable" association seems plausible.

Waikhom et al reported 2 cases of bilateral superficial white corneal deposits in a whorl pattern.[5] Both cases were in ocular sicca patients with incapacitating visual and ocular symptoms. In 1 case there were 2 positive rechallenges with complete clearing in between. These signs and symptoms may take 4–6 weeks to develop and take an equal amount of time to resolve. Although reversible when the drug is discontinued, they may lessen if the dosage is decreased. These corneal findings may include corneal neovascularization, and inflammatory infiltrates in the anterior corneal stroma have been seen in capecitabine-exposed dogs.[6]

Purtscher-like retinopathy was associated with 1000 mg capecitabine twice daily.[7] The patient developed bilateral scattered cotton-wool spots and intraretinal hemorrhages.

Dasgupta et al reported a case of cranial nerve palsy possibly due to capecitabine therapy.[8]

Congenital abnormalities may occur if capecitabine is taken during pregnancy.[2]

Generic Name:
Carboplatin.

Proprietary Name:
Paraplatin.

Primary Use
Systemic
A platinum coordination compound used intravenously primarily in ovarian cancer, non–small cell lung cancers, and various other cancers.

Ophthalmic
Intra-arterial injections are used in the management of ocular retinal blastomas.

Ocular Side Effects
Local ophthalmic use or exposure – orbital or subconjunctival injection
Certain
1. Decreased vision
2. Blindness
3. Edema, necrosis, and scarring
   a. Conjunctiva
   b. Ocular muscles
   c. Orbit
4. Proptosis
5. Optic nerve
   a. Edema
   b. Ischemic necrosis
   c. Atrophy

Systemic administration – intravenous
Possible
1. Decreased vision

2. Color vision defect
3. Conjunctivitis
4. Pain (transient)

Systemic administration – intracarotid or ophthalmic artery injection
Certain
1. Decreased vision
2. Blindness
3. Acute glaucoma
4. Uveal effusion
5. Orbital inflammation
6. Proptosis
7. Uveitis
8. Retinal detachment
9. Chorioretinal atrophy
10. Optic atrophy

Clinical Significance
Carboplatin is 45 times less toxic than cisplatin.[1] It is most often given in combination with other anticancer drugs, especially paclitaxel, and therefore it is difficult to define "certain" ocular side effects. Ocular side effects due to carboplatin are heavily dependent on the site of injection, dosage, and duration of treatment. In general, ocular side effects due to carboplatin are uncommon and reversible. The exceptions include subconjunctival, periocular, and subtenon injections for adjunctive therapy for retinoblastoma. Irreversible changes include fat necrosis with fibrosis, ocular muscle restriction, and ischemic necrosis with atrophy of the optic nerve.[2–4]

A single case of unilateral uveal effusion and angle-closure glaucoma resulted within 7 hours of an intracarotid injection of carboplatin with etoposide phosphate.[5] After 4 days the patient had orbital inflammation, count-fingers vision, and proptosis. Uveitis occurred 2 weeks later. After 2 months vision returned to 20/70 and near-normal motility. A similar case of severe ocular and orbital toxicity was reported by Watanabe et al.[6]

Zegans et al presented a histopathologic study of a patient receiving intra-arterial carboplatin for glioblastoma multiforme.[7] Five months later the patient developed retinal pigment epithelial (RPE) clumping in a bull's-eye pattern with normal vision. At autopsy there was significant loss of retinal receptors in the macula with RPE hypertrophy and hyperplasia.

Generic Name:
Carmustine.

Proprietary Names:
BiCNU, Gliadel.

Primary Use

This nitrosourea is used in the treatment of brain tumors and various malignant neoplasms.

Ocular Side Effects

Systemic administration – intravenous

Certain

1. Decreased vision
2. Eyelids and conjunctiva
   a. Allergic reactions
   b. Hyperemia (Fig. 15.5A)
   c. Blepharoconjunctivitis
   d. Chemosis
3. Irritation
   a. Lacrimation
   b. Photophobia
   c. Burning sensation
4. Visual hallucinations

Probable

1. Orbit
   a. Vasodilatation
   b. Proptosis
   c. Pain
   d. Edema
2. May aggravate or cause
   a. Herpes infections
   b. Ocular sicca

Possible

1. Cornea
   a. Edema
   b. Opacities (see Fig. 15.5B)

Conditional/unclassified

1. Optic nerve
   a. Neuritis
   b. Atrophy
2. Arteriovenous shunting

Systemic administration – intracarotid

Certain

1. Decreased vision
2. Orbit
   a. Vasodilation
   b. Proptosis
   c. Pain
   d. Edema
3. Eyelids and conjunctiva
   a. Hyperemia
   b. Blepharoconjunctivitis
   c. Chemosis
4. Irritation
   a. Lacrimation
   b. Photophobia
   c. Burning sensation
5. Optic nerve
   a. Neuritis
   b. Atrophy
6. Retinal vascular disorders
   a. Occlusion
   b. Thrombosis

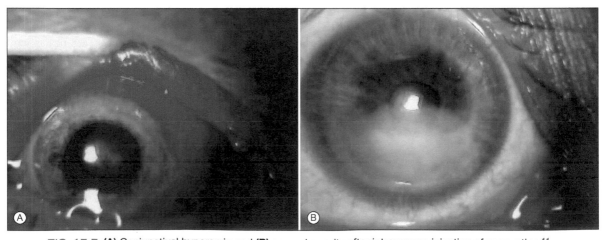

FIG. 15.5 **(A)** Conjunctival hyperemia and **(B)** corneal opacity after intravenous injection of carmustine.[11]

c. Hemorrhages
d. Exudates
7. Cornea
  a. Edema
  b. Opacities
8. Extraocular muscle
  a. Fibrosis of recti muscles
  b. Internal ophthalmoplegia
9. Electroretinogram (ERG) abnormalities
10. Vitreous opacities

Probable
1. May aggravate or cause
  a. Herpes infections
  b. Ocular sicca

Possible
1. Arteriovenous shunting

Systemic administration – implanted wafers
Certain
1. Any and all of those noted earlier
2. Pseudotumor cerebri

Clinical Significance
Ocular side effects associated with carmustine use are related to dose, injection site, frequency of injections, and speed of infusion. Many side effects are delayed, possibly implying long-lasting active metabolites. Ocular side effects from high-dose intravenous carmustine are primarily conjunctival hyperemia and nonspecific decreased vision. The incidence of ocular pain and diplopia is around 1% and 5% for hallucinations.[1] Color vision may be affected, primarily blue and yellow. This drug, like most all antimetabolites, is secreted in the tears and therefore the irritative signs and symptoms of the ocular anterior segment. These mostly resolve within a few days after discontinuing the drug.

The ocular side effects due to intracarotid carmustine and implanted carmustine wafers are more severe. Ocular side effects of intracarotid injections can be limited by the intracarotid catheter placement. Applying pressure on the eye with a Honan balloon during the infusion may decrease the amount of drug getting to the eye.[2] If these measures are not done, up to 70% of patient eyes will have significant ocular side effects from intracarotid infusions within 2–14 weeks.[2] Even with proper placement of the catheter, various degrees of decreased vision, retrobulbar pain, conjunctival hyperemia, corneal edema and opacities, secondary glaucoma, internal ophthalmoplegia, vitreous opacities, various orbital vascular pathologies, optic

neuropathy, bleeding, retinal arterial narrowing, nerve-fiber layer infarcts, and intraretinal hemorrhages can occur.[3-6] Various degrees of recovery occur after therapy is stopped. Carmustine wafer implants may have a 4–9% incidence of pseudotumor cerebri.[1] This may require implant removal.

This drug is often used in combination with various other antimetabolites. Due to this drug's ability to penetrate the blood–retina barrier, increased neuroretinal toxicity may occur. It can also cause ischemic changes with vascular narrowing.[7] Various reports have shown a variety of the same ocular side effects as those associated with carmustine, including blindness.[8-10]

Generic Names:
1. Cetuximab; 2. erlotinib; 3. gefitinib; 4. osimertinib; 5. panitumumab.

Proprietary Names:
1. Erbitux; 2. Tarceva; 3. Iressa; 4. Tagrisso; 5. Vectibix.

Primary Use
These epidermal growth factor receptor (EGFR) antagonists are used in the treatment of various cancers.

Ocular Side Effects
Systemic administration – intravenous or oral
Certain
1. Conjunctivitis
  a. Photophobia
  b. Pain
2. Eyelids
  a. Squamous blepharitis
  b. Meibomitis
  c. Telangiectasias
  d. Hyperpigmentation
3. Eyelashes and eyebrows (Fig. 15.6) (no reports with osimertinib)
  a. Elongated
  b. Increased rigidity
  c. Tortuous
  d. Darkening of lashes
  e. Decrease in number
  f. Misdirected
4. Tear film dysfunction
  a. May aggravate or cause ocular sicca
  b. Decreased tear film break-up time
5. Periocular
  a. Acneiform skin change
  b. Erythema
  c. Edema

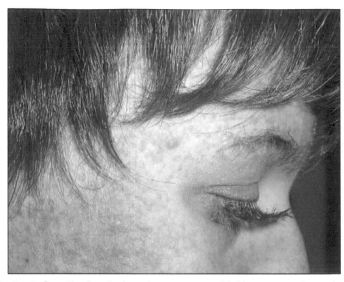

FIG. 15.6 Growth of eyelashes after treatment with irinotecan and cetuximab.[6]

6. Cornea (Fig. 15.7)
   a. Erosions
   b. Delayed wound healing
   c. Superficial punctate keratitis

Possible
1. Cornea
   a. Persistent epithelial defects
   b. Perforation
2. Ectropion
3. Uveitis (erlotinib)

Conditional/unclassified
1. Vortex keratopathy (osimertinib)
2. Cataracts (erlotinib, osimertinib)

Clinical Significance
The most common side effects of this class of drugs are skin changes, which occur in 60–80% of patients,[1] whereas ocular side effects are uncommon. The exact mechanism as to how ocular side effects occur secondary to EGFR inhibitors is unknown. EGFR sites are present in the basal epithelial cells of the conjunctiva, limbus, and cornea. EGFRs are most prominent in the basal layers of the epidermis, outer root sheath of hair follicles, capillary systems, and sebaceous glands.

The different EGFR inhibitors appear to have a similar ocular side effect pattern, may differ in time of onset and frequency, and are fully reversible with discontinuation of the drug. The unique eyelash changes are not found with osimertinib. The most common ocular side effects are conjunctivitis, blepharitis, meibomitis, and ocular sicca with presenting symptoms of photophobia, pruritus, foreign body sensation, and eye pain. These effects are probably secondary to the direct toxic effects on EGFR sites in periocular skin, hair follicles, and/or mucosal epithelium; it is unproven that the drug or its metabolites are secreted in the tears. These could also be the most likely cause of ocular tear film dysfunction. The most striking side effect, and the latest to occur (usually after 2–3 months of treatment), is trichomegaly of the eyelashes and eyebrows.

It appears the more profound the generalized skin changes are near the eyes, the more marked the ocular side effects. In high-dose human studies, spontaneous corneal erosions occurred with delayed would healing probably secondary to a direct drug effect.[2] Some of these effects may be secondary to misdirected eyelashes.[3] However, Saint-Jean et al have reported cases of corneal melting, persistent corneal defects, and corneal perforation, which they felt was a direct drug effect.[4] These findings were also seen with panitumumab and erlotinib. Most ocular side effects were reversible, which usually resolved within a few days, and trichomegaly within 6–8 weeks.

Chia et al reported a case of bilateral vortex keratopathy with corneal deposits at the level of the epithelium in a whorl-like pattern.[5]

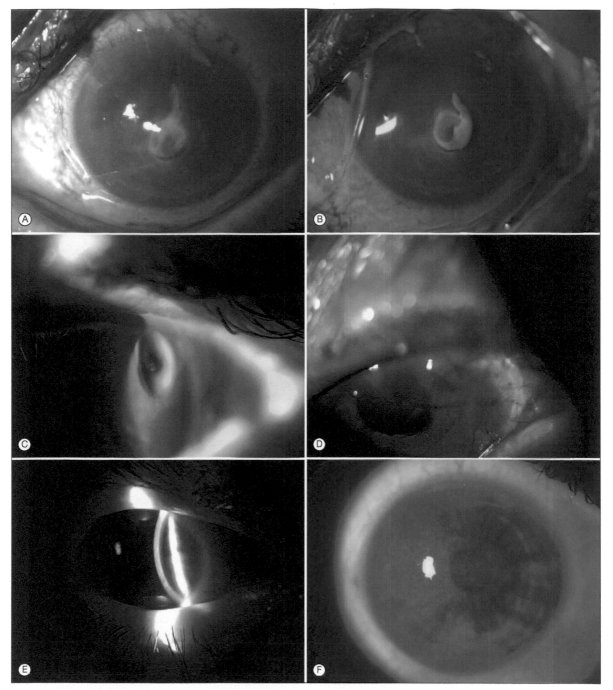

FIG. 15.7 Various corneal changes associated with EGFR: **(A)** noninfiltrated severe central corneal stromal thinning with iris incarceration, **(B)** diffuse punctate fluorescein staining and aqueous leakage, **(C)** noninfiltrated perforated peripheral corneal ulcer with iris incarceration, **(D)** peripheral lamellar keratoplasty, **(E)** severe superficial punctate keratitis, and **(F)** diffuse punctate fluorescein staining.[4]

Generic Name:
Cisplatin (cisplatinum).

Proprietary Names:
Platinol, Platinol-AQ.

Primary Use
This platinum-containing antineoplastic drug is used for the treatment of metastatic testicular or ovarian tumors, advanced bladder carcinoma, and a wide variety of other neoplasms.

Ocular Side Effects
Systemic administration – intravenous
Certain
1. Decreased vision
2. Color blindness – blue-yellow axis
3. Abnormal electroretinogram (ERG), electrooculogram (EOG), or visual evoked potential (VEP)
4. Loss of contrast sensitivity
5. Macular pigment changes – mild
6. Eyelids or conjunctiva
   a. Erythema
   b. Conjunctivitis – nonspecific
   c. Edema
   d. Urticaria
   e. Loss of eyelashes or eyebrows
7. Orbital pain

Probable
1. Optic nerve
   a. Edema
   b. Neuritis
   c. Retrobulbar neuritis
2. Cortical blindness
3. Visual fields
   a. Central visual constricted
   b. Hemianopsia
4. May aggravate herpes infections

Possible
1. Myasthenic neuromuscular blocking effect
   a. Diplopia
   b. Ptosis
   c. Paresis of extraocular muscles
2. Oculogyric crises
3. Nystagmus

Systemic administration – intracarotid injection
Certain
1. Ipsilateral vision loss
2. Ipsilateral orbital pain
3. Periorbital erythema and edema
4. Cavernous sinus-like syndrome
5. Blindness
6. ERG – abnormal
7. Optic nerve degeneration
8. Retina (Fig. 15.8)
   a. Pigmentary maculopathy
   b. Cotton-wool spots
   c. Intraretinal hemorrhage
   d. Neovascularization

Possible
1. Nystagmus

Clinical Significance
Cisplatin (cisplatinum) is given by intravenous or intracarotid arterial injection, often with other chemotherapeutic drugs, which makes it difficult to define this drug's ocular toxicity.

Intravenous cisplatin ocular side effects differ significantly from intracarotid injections. With intravenous injections, the more significant ocular side effects are neuroretinal with decreased vision, color vision defects, and ERG changes. Changes in the optic nerve include edema, neuritis, and retrobulbar neuritis. These side effects are dose dependent and, unless given over only 2-3 courses, are seldom significant in dosages of 60–100 mg/m^2.[1,2] Ozols et al felt advancing age and being female to be risk factors for increased ocular toxicity.[3] In patients taking dosages above 200 mg/m^2 divided into 5 daily dosages, decreased vision occurred in 62% of patients, decreased color vision (blue-yellow axis) in 23%, and 84% of patients had some cone dysfunction demonstrated by color vision testing or ERG.[4] Both Caruso et al and Wilding et al showed mild, irregular macular pigmentary changes in many patients, with decreased vision rarely worse than 20/25.[4,5] Decreased vision returns to normal after discontinuing the drug, but persistent color defects may continue for up to 16 months. There are also numerous single case reports of optic neuritis, retrobulbar neuritis, and disc edema.[6] It is felt that this drug can cause reversible segmented nerve demyelination, similar to heavy-metal CNS toxicity. High-dose cisplatin (85–200 mg/m^2), alone or with other antimetabolites, has been associated with reversible cortical blindness. Prim et al reported nystagmus secondary to cisplatin-induced vestibular pathology.[7] Metastases, infarcts, infections, and bleeding may mimic drug toxicity.

Dulz et al reported clinical, but irreversible, reduction of the nerve-fiber layer in 11 or 14 patients (75%)

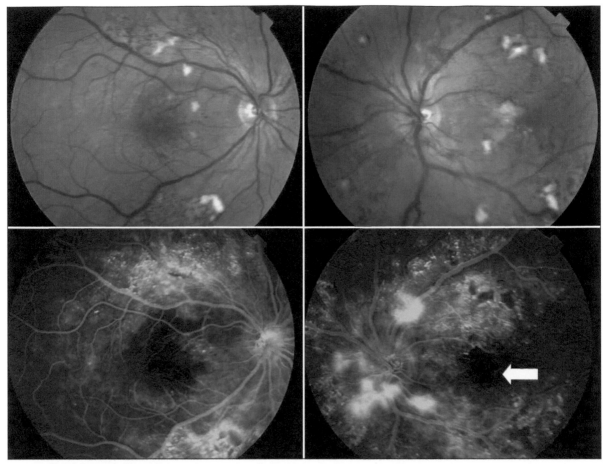

FIG. 15.8 Color photographs and fluorescein angiogram of retinal ischemia with *arrow* pointing to macular ischemia.[11]

examined after cisplatin therapy.[8] Mild changes in cone a- and b-wave latency were also observed. Although these changes occurred, they were mild, and the authors concluded that this should "never preclude or delay curative intended platinum-based chemotherapy."

The side effects from intra-arterial injection differ in part because many of the effects are due to the high drug concentration in the eye, resulting in direct drug retinal toxicity.[9-11] Retinal pathology, besides pigmentary disturbances, also includes ischemic changes such as cotton-wool spots, intraretinal hemorrhages, and neovascularization. These are clearly dose related and include ipsilateral visual loss in 15–60% of patients. Some patients also received carmustine, which may also be toxic to ocular pigment epithelium.[12] Miller et al described a patient who, after the second intracarotid injection of cisplatin and carmustine, developed ophthalmoplegia and only light perception within a few days.[13] To limit these side effects, the intra-arterial catheter can be advanced beyond the ophthalmic artery; however, this appears to increase the risk of cerebral toxicity. Margo et al described a patient who had infusion of intra-arterial cisplatin distal to the ophthalmic artery and in a matter of days had unilateral massive orbital edema, uveal effusion, exudative retinal detachment, ophthalmoplegia, nonreactive pupil, and irreversible loss of vision.[14] Wu et al reported a case of extreme facial periorbital edema, proptosis, and chemosis.[15] This was followed by permanent unilateral loss of vision (light perception) and complete ophthalmoplegia with retinal changes. They felt this was due to a combination of chemotherapeutic drugs, including cisplatin.

Barr-Hamilton et al reported increased ototoxicity secondary to cisplatin in patients with darker irises.[16] The melanin content of the inner ear is related to eye color. Melanin accumulates cisplatin, which is toxic to the vestibular area, and hence a possible cause of nystagmus.

Generic Name:
Crizotinib.

Proprietary Name:
Xalkori.

Primary Use
Oral inhibitor of receptor tyrosine kinases used in the management of metastatic non–small cell lung cancer.

Ocular Side Effects
Systemic administration – oral
Certain
1. Decreased vision
2. Photopsia
3. Photophobia
4. Diplopia
5. Floaters – increased

Possible
1. Optic nerve
   a. Optic neuritis
   b. Optic atrophy
2. Light-dark accommodation abnormalities

Clinical Significance
Visual disturbances occur in 62% of recipients enrolled in phase I and II clinical trials.[1-3] However, in further phase II trials, most all visual disturbances were short-term in duration and had minimal impact on patient activities. Regardless, the *Physicians' Desk Reference* (PDR) warns that optic neuritis may occur after crizotinib exposure.[4] There are 6 spontaneous reports of significant optic nerve toxicity and 1 report in the literature.[5] Although optic nerve pathology is a rare event, it has been reported to start as early as 2 weeks after drug exposure. Chun et al had a case of possible drug-induced optic neuritis, which had a positive rechallenge.[5] Shaw et al described an abnormal light-dark accommodation phenomenon.[6]

Recommendations[4]
1. Full ophthalmic work-up, including retinal and disc photography, visual fields, and optic coher-

ence tomography (OCT). This should be performed at the first signs of unexplained visual loss.
2. Discontinue crizotinib in patients with new onset of severe visual loss.
3. There are insufficient data on when or if to restart the drug.
4. Patients on this drug should use caution when driving or operating machinery when experiencing visual disorders.

Generic Name:
Cyclophosphamide.

Proprietary Names:
Cytoxan, Lyophilized Cytoxan, Neosar.

Primary Use
This alkylating drug is used in the treatment of various malignant diseases, including lymphoma, myeloma, and a variety of solid tumors.

Ocular Side Effects
Systemic administration – intravenous or oral
Certain (high dosages)
1. Decreased vision
2. Irritation
   a. Lacrimation
   b. Hyperemia
   c. Photophobia
   d. Burning sensation
3. Eyelids and conjunctiva
   a. Allergic reactions
   b. Hyperemia
   c. Blepharoconjunctivitis
   d. Edema
4. May aggravate or cause ocular sicca
5. Visual hallucinations
6. Pupils – pinpoint
7. Loss of eyelashes and eyebrows

Possible
1. Accommodative spasm
2. Myopia – transient
3. May aggravate
   a. CMV retinitis
   b. Cataract formation
4. Graft versus host disease

Conditional/unclassified
1. Congenital ocular abnormalities
2. Conjunctival lymphoma

Clinical Significance

This anticancer drug is generally used in combination with others, which makes it difficult to specify the ocular side effects. At normal dosages, the incidence of ocular side effects is fairly rare. In high dosages, especially when given intravenously, transitory decreased vision may occur within minutes to 24 hours.[1] This resolves within 1–14 days. Blepharoconjunctivitis or conjunctivitis may occur secondary to the antimetabolite effects or toxic effects of the drug in the tears.[2] Pinpoint pupils are probably secondary to the parasympathomimetic effects of this drug, which may rarely include accommodative spasms and transient myopia.[3] Other adverse ocular effects may be graft versus host disease, Stevens-Johnson syndrome, and possibly enhancement of lens changes.[4] Agrawal et al reported on 4 patients on long-term cyclophosphamide for collagen vascular disease who developed CMV retinitis.[5] Cyclophosphamide's main systemic toxicity is bone marrow depression, so subconjunctival and retinal hemorrhages can occur. London et al reported a nodular lymphocytic conjunctival infiltrate, which developed after 6 months of cyclophosphamide therapy.[6]

With the growing trend among women to postpone pregnancy, there are increasing chances to develop breast cancer; therefore prenatal exposure to chemotherapy may occur. Cyclophosphamide has been implicated in causing congenital ocular abnormalities.[7]

Generic Name:
Cytarabine (cytosine arabinoside).

Proprietary Names:
Cytosar-U, Depocyt, Ara-C.

Primary Use
This antimetabolite is effective in the management of acute granulocytic leukemia, polycythemia vera, and malignant neoplasms.

Ocular Side Effects
Systemic administration – intrathecal, intravenous, or subcutaneous
Certain
1. Decreased vision
2. Cornea
   a. Punctate keratitis
   b. Subepithelial granular deposits
   c. Refractive microcysts (Fig. 15.9)
   d. Stromal edema
   e. Stria in Descemet's membrane
3. Irritation
   a. Lacrimation
   b. Hyperemia
   c. Photophobia
   d. Pain
   e. Burning sensation
4. Eyelids or conjunctiva
   a. Allergic reactions
   b. Erythema
   c. Conjunctivitis – hemorrhagic
   d. Hyperpigmentation
   e. Urticaria
   f. Purpura
   g. Edema
5. Extraocular muscles – intrathecal
   a. Paresis
   b. Diplopia
   c. Nystagmus

Probable
1. Uveitis

Possible
1. Pseudotumor cerebri
2. Papilledema
3. Corneal endothelial cell damage

Clinical Significance
The frequency of the ocular toxicity due to cytarabine is both time and dose dependent. The most common ocular side effects are decreased vision and keratoconjunctivitis. The keratitis may occur in 100% of patients on high dosages, regardless of the method of administration. Barletta et al reported corneal and conjunctival changes even on low-dose systemic cytosine arabinoside.[1] Cytarabine-induced ocular toxicity usually occurs after 5–7 days of therapy and is associated with pain, lacrimation, foreign body sensation, and decreased vision. Clinically, one may see central punctate corneal opacities, subepithelial granular deposits, refractile microcysts, superficial punctate keratitis, and, rarely, mild corneal edema with stria in Descemet's membrane. Symptoms improve after a few days off the drug, vision improves in 1–2 weeks, and the corneal opacities within 4 weeks. The cause of these adverse effects may primarily be due to the nonselective inhibition of DNA synthesis by this drug. This explains the 5- to 7-day delay in onset of corneal changes (i.e. the length of time it takes the basal cells of the corneal epithelium to reach the surface). Cytarabine can be found in the tears from systemic administration, which can account for immediate ocular and periocular symptoms. Weak topical ocular steroids and frequent

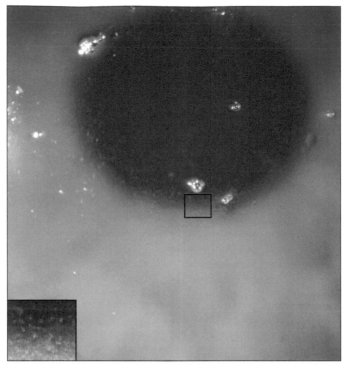

FIG. 15.9 Corneal cyst from systemic cytarabine.[16]

preservative-free artificial tears often improve these ocular symptoms. Krema et al described a case of bilateral cytarabine toxicity to the corneal endothelium.[2] There are several cases of anterior uveitis in the literature, and there are a few in spontaneous reports.[3-7] These were mainly on higher dosages.

Adverse effects associated with high-dose intravenous regimens may also include cerebral or cerebellar dysfunction, which is usually reversible. Ocular manifestations of this CNS toxicity may include lateral gaze nystagmus, diplopia, and lateral rectus palsy.[8] Neurotoxicity after intrathecal injection and intravenous cytarabine has been associated with pseudotumor cerebri, optic atrophy, and blindness.[9-11] Lopez et al, Sommers et al, Tziotzios et al, and Wiznia et al pointed to an additive effect of cytarabine and low-dosage radiation on occlusive microvascular retinopathy in patients with leukemia.[8,12-15]

There are 10 cases from the spontaneous reports of papilledema occurring within 3-11 weeks after starting the drug. Where data were available, this resolved once the drug was discontinued.

Topical ocular cytarabine caused significant corneal toxicity, and therefore was replaced by equally effective and less toxic antiviral drugs.

Generic Names:
1. Dabrafenib; 2. vemurafenib.

Proprietary Names:
1. Tafinlar; 2. Zelboraf.

Primary Use
BRAF kinase inhibitors used alone or in combination in the management of unresectable or metastatic melanoma.

Ocular Side Effects
Systemic administration – oral
Certain
1. Decreased vision
2. Uveitis
3. Photophobia

Possible
1. Panuveitis – severe
2. Macular edema
3. Palsy (vemurafenib)
   a. Extraocular muscles
   b. Facial

4. Eyelid neoplasms (vemurafenib)
5. Conjunctivitis

Conditional/unclassified
1. Scleritis
2. Episcleritis
3. VKH disease (vemurafenib)

Clinical Significance

Choe et al and Guedj et al have the largest published series of vemurafenib-associated uveitis.[1,2] They reported that 22% of patients on varying dosages had ocular side effects, which were usually mild in nature; uveitis occurred in 4%, and conjunctivitis occurred in 2.8% of patients. Uveitis may be a potentially significant side effect. Onset may occur within a few days or as late as 1.5 years after starting therapy. In most cases the uveitis is bilateral, responsive to topical ocular steroid therapy, and seldom required stopping the anticancer therapy. There are numerous cases in the literature and spontaneous reports with positive dechallenge and rechallenge data; therefore this is a "certain" association of a drug-related event. There are reports and some well-documented spontaneous reports where, within weeks to months of starting vemurafenib, an acute panuveitis with severe visual loss, with or without scleritis, occurred.[2,3] Outcomes were variable, some with long-lasting sequelae.

Klein et al and Shailesh et al reported facial and extraocular muscle palsy, but there is little data from spontaneous reports to support a relationship.[4,5]

It is well known that these drugs can cause skin neoplasms. Yin et al reported 3 cases of keratinocytic neoplasms, including 1 invasive squamous cell carcinoma of the eyelid.[6] There are 4 spontaneous reports of VKH disease occurring after the start of vemurafenib.

Generic Names:
1. Dasatinib; 2. imatinib mesylate; 3. nilotinib.

Proprietary Names:
1. Sprycel; 2. Gleevec; 3. Tasigna.

Primary Use

These selective inhibitors of the *BCR-ABL* and platelet-derived growth factor receptor (PDGFR) tyrosine kinase are used in targeted therapy for the management of myelogenous leukemia and gastrointestinal stromal tumors.

Ocular Side Effects
Systemic administration – oral
Certain
1. Decreased vision
2. Edema
   a. Orbital (Fig. 15.10)
   b. Eyelid
   c. Conjunctiva
3. Conjunctivitis
4. May aggravate or cause ocular sicca

Probable
1. Epiphora
2. Eyelids and conjunctiva
   a. Hypopigmentation
   b. Purpura

Possible
1. Optic nerve
   a. Neuritis
   b. Pseudotumor cerebri
   c. Vascular events
2. Retina
   a. Macular bleeds
   b. Edema
   c. Cystoid macular edema
3. Ocular bleeding – postsurgery

Conditional/unclassified
1. Madarosis

Clinical Significance

These drugs have markedly prolonged the life of patients with certain leukemias. This confuses the profile of possible drug-induced ocular side effects because they could be due to the basic disease or the drug. Therefore more adverse effects are listed as "possible" until more data are available to sort this out. For example, Breccia et al reported a number of cases of glaucoma in their series, some secondary to ocular bleeds or other predisposing factors.[1] Various bleeds and vascular effects may be disease related.

These antimetabolites cause various degrees of systemic edema. Periorbital is one of the more common sites of edema, and the swelling may be so severe that it causes visual obstruction that requires surgical debulking or topical steroids.[2,3] In the spontaneous reporting systems, the top 3 ocular side effects for these 3 drugs were periorbital edema, eyelid edema, and eye swelling; imatinib had 1,184 cases. Fraunfelder et al

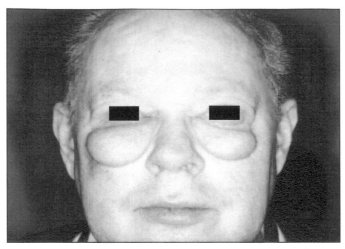

FIG. 15.10 Periorbital edema after imatinib treatment.[3]

and Demetri et al reported 70–74% of patients taking the standard dose of imatinib (400 mg/day) showed orbital edema, making this the most common ocular side effect due to this drug.[4,5] This reaction is dose dependent, and the mean onset is 68 days. Edema is mild to moderate in most patients and may occur within a few weeks of starting therapy. Orbital edema is twice as common as peripheral edema.[4] Conjunctival chalasis may occlude the punctum, or severe orbital edema may interfere with the lacrimal pump.[4] Esmaeli et al, Fraunfelder et al, Govind Babu et al, Masood et al, Radaelli et al, and 29 cases in the spontaneous reporting systems suggest a higher incidence of cystoids macular edema often in post–cataract surgery patients on these drugs.[2-4,6–8]

Decreased vision is probably multifactorial, with an onset occurring shortly after drug exposure, and appears to be most common with dasatinib. The *Physicians' Desk Reference* (PDR) states that this can occur in up to 10% of cases; with nilotinib and imatinib, it is only 0.1–1.0%.[9] Irritation and ocular sicca have a 1–10% incidence.[9] This may result in epiphora as a primary complaint in some patients, especially in those taking imatinib.[2]

Optic neuritis has been reported.[1,6] Monge et al reported a case of unilateral optic neuritis possibly secondary to dasatinib.[10] The drug was stopped with full recovery. Nilotinib was started, which possibly caused a mild and transient recurrence of the optic neuritis. Nilotinib was continued without progression. The PDR reports the incidence of optic neuritis as 0.1%.[9]

Optic disc edema secondary to this class of drugs has been reported by DeLuca et al, Kwon et al, Napolitano et al, Mbekeani et al, and in 64 spontaneous case reports.[11-14] Many of the papilledema cases are probably secondary to pseudotumor cerebri. This group of patients have disease-related increases in vascular and hematologic events, as well as retinal and macular changes, which cannot be distinguished from drug events.

Kusumi et al reported a case of retinal macular edema (between the pigment epithelium and the neurosensory retina), causing a significant decrease in vision, occurring within 2 months of starting imatinib and completely resolving within 2 weeks of stopping this drug.[15] Imatinib may block the PDGF receptors in the retina, allowing edema to occur. Georgalas et al reported bilateral macular edema, and there are many cases in the spontaneous reports as well.[16] Bajel et al reported bilateral retinal edema and hemorrhages in a patient with chronic myeloid leukemia.[17]

Naithani attributes dasatinib in causing madarosis.[18]

Recommendations

1. Orbital edema can be managed conservatively by either observation alone or, in more symptomatic patients, with low-dose diuretics in short pulses. Surgical excision of periocular soft tissue may, in rare instances, be necessary to improve visual function.
2. Epiphora is not improved by probing or irrigating the nasal lacrimal system. Topical steroids or, rarely, conjunctivochalasis surgery may be considered.

3. The physician may want to discuss with preoperative cataract patients the possibility of postoperative cystoid maculopathy and/or increased ocular bleeding.

Generic Names:

1. Docetaxel; 2. nab-paclitaxel; 3. paclitaxel.

Proprietary Names:

1. Docefrez, Taxotere; 2. Abraxane; 3. Onxol, Taxol.

Primary Use

These antimicrobial drugs are used alone and in combination with other anticancer drugs in various stages of cancer therapy, but most often in advanced cases.

Ocular Side Effects

Systemic administration – intraarterial, intravenous, or oral

Certain

1. Decreased vision
2. Irritation (primarily docetaxel)
   a. Lacrimation
   b. Photophobia
   c. Pain
3. Cystoid macular edema
4. Eyelids and conjunctiva (primarily docetaxel)
   a. Occlusion of lacrimal canaliculi and punctum – various degrees
   b. Blepharoconjunctivitis
   c. Erosive conjunctivitis
5. Photopsia (paclitaxel)
6. Scintillating scotoma (paclitaxel)

Probable

1. Optic neuropathy (docetaxel)
   a. Color vision defect
   b. Decreased visual field
   c. Scotoma
   d. Optic nerve edema
   e. Optic disc microhemorrhages

Possible

1. Cicatricial entropion (docetaxel)
2. Crystalline keratopathy (docetaxel) (immune suppressed)

Conditional/unlikely

1. Glaucoma
2. Optic neuropathy (paclitaxel)

Clinical Significance

Initially many felt that the ocular side effects profile of these 3 drugs differed; however, with time, the profiles have become more similar. Nab-paclitaxel is an orphan drug with improved therapeutic outcomes, although probable increased side effects. Overall, significant ocular side effects are rare, but if not recognized can cause irreversible reactions. Adverse reactions are more common in those above age 65.

Docetaxel has been shown to be secreted in the tears, which is possibly also true for paclitaxel, but less so. Their anterior side effects profiles are similar.[1] Stenosis of the punctum and/or canaliculus occurs in up to 77% of patients on weekly docetaxel injections.[2] Esmaeli et al felt that stenosis was probably based on total dose.[3] If the drug is given every 3 weeks rather than weekly, both conjunctivitis and effects on the lacrimal outflow system are decreased. Esmaeli et al pointed out that early diagnosis of drug-related stenosis may prevent irreversible occlusion.[4] This has been confirmed by others.[5,6] Epiphora is usually well tolerated with adjustment of dosage and frequency; artificial tears and/or topical steroids usually suffices.

Docetaxel, paclitaxel to a mild degree, or their metabolites, which are likely secreted in the tears, may irritate the cornea, conjunctiva, and eyelids. Erosive conjunctivitis has been reported and resolved when the docetaxel was discontinued.[5] Cetinkaya et al described cicatricial entropion after docetaxel therapy.[7] Gupta et al described meibomian gland inflammation, meibomian orifice blockage, and chalazion induced by docetaxel.[8] Infectious crystalline keratopathy in an immune-suppressed patient on docetaxel has been reported.[9]

Intra-arterial or intravenous paclitaxel causes scintillating scotoma in 20% of patients, usually starting toward the end of the infusion and lasting 15 minutes to 3 hours.[10] This is usually mild, nonvision threatening, and reversible. Photopsia often occurs.[11] This is associated with visual evoked potential (VEP) changes suggestive of changes in the optic nerve pathway.[12]

Well-documented bilateral cystoid macular edema (CME) without evidence of leakage has been seen with all 3 of these drugs.[13–17] To date there are 24 cases in the literature and 187 cases in the spontaneous reports of CME associated with the taxanes, 95% of which were associated with docetaxel. The edema is mild to moderate and resolves with drug withdrawal.[14,16] Continued therapy may result in permanent damage. OCT scans have shown that CME associated with these drugs causes an impaired filling of the choriocapillaris, and if the drug is stopped the CME resolves over a 6-month period.[18]

Valeshabad et al reported a case of docetaxel and gemcitabine possibly causing uveal effusion and outer retinal disruption.[19]

There are reports of docetaxel causing optic nerve pathology, including neuritis and neuropathy.[20-22] Bakbak et al have shown that paclitaxel decreases the thickness of the peripapillary retinal nerve-fiber layer.[23] There are 14 cases of docetaxel-associated optic neuritis in the spontaneous reports.

Recommendations

1. It is probably best not to use these drugs in patients who have a history of CME.
2. If CME occurs, stop the drug, if possible, and switch to a nontaxane anticancer drug.
3. Consider treating CME with topical acetazolamide.[24]
4. Because these drugs are irritating to the eye, immediate lavage is required if inadvertent ocular exposure occurs.
5. Many suggest closer ophthalmic monitoring of patients on taxanes for epiphora, CME, and toxic neuropathies.

Generic Name:
Etoposide.

Proprietary Names:
Eposin, Etopophos, Toposar, Vepesid.

Primary Use
This antineoplastic drug is used for various systemic malignancies and irreversibly inhibits CMV replication.

Ocular Side Effects
Systemic administration – intracarotid, intravenous, or oral
Certain
1. Decreased vision
2. Loss of eyelashes or eyebrows
3. Ocular bleeding
4. Yellow pigmentation
   a. Eyelids
   b. Sclera
5. Secondary infections

Possible
1. Uveal effusion
2. Orbital inflammation
3. Proptosis (Fig. 15.11)

4. Anterior uveitis
5. Macular pigmentary changes
6. Cortical blindness – transient
7. Optic neuritis

Clinical Significance
Etoposide is seldom used alone. It is primarily used with carboplatin. Decreased vision may occur, but it is uncommon. Once the drug is discontinued, vision returns to its prior level.[1] As with most antimetabolites, ocular bleeds may occur due to low platelet counts, icterus secondary to liver damage, and with decreased body resistances, secondary pathogens may occur. Loss of eyelashes or eyebrows usually starts gradually over a 2- to 3-week period once treatment begins, but it is rare. These grow back once treatment is stopped; however, it may take several months and the hair may be softer and curlier, and there may be some change in color.[1] Optic neuritis has also been seen.[2]

The acute possible ocular-orbital inflammatory response is based on 1 well-documented case.[3] These are primarily in patients who are given carboplatin and etoposide via intracarotid injections. Many antineoplastic drugs given via the intracarotid route have also caused drug-induced acute orbital and ocular inflammation syndromes.

Generic Name:
Fludarabine phosphate.

Proprietary Name:
Fludara.

Primary Use
A nucleoside analog used primarily in chronic leukemias and to achieve immunosuppression for stem-cell transplants.

Ocular Side Effects
Systemic administration – intravenous or oral
Certain
1. Vision loss
   a. Decreased vision
   b. Blindness
2. Optic nerve
   a. Neuritis
   b. Atrophy
3. Uveitis
   a. Anterior
   b. Posterior
4. Atrophy
   a. Occipital lobes

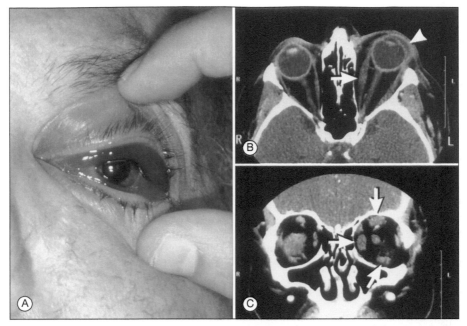

FIG. 15.11 **(A)** Four days after intracarotid etoposide phosphate and carboplatin, the left eye is proptotic by 8 mm, the eyelids are swollen and erythematous, and the ptotic eyelid is elevated digitally. Superior subconjunctival hemorrhage and inferior chemosis are apparent. **(B)** The orbital computed axial tomogram with contrast taken 4 days after intracarotid etoposide phosphate and carboplatin. Axial view shows proptosis with straightening of the optic nerve and tenting of the posterior pole. The left medial rectus muscle is enlarged (*arrow*), and a subconjunctival hemorrhage is apparent (*arrowhead*). **(C)** Coronal view discloses enlarged left superior, medial, and inferior recti (*arrows*).[3]

b. Parietal lobes

5. Activation of pathogens

Clinical Significance

Ocular toxicity due to fludarabine, although infrequent, may include rapid irreversible loss of vision. Although this is largely dose dependent, even at normal dosages, rare, severe, rapid ocular events may occur. The most significant side effect of this drug is neurotoxicity, and visual side effects may be the first to present. If the drug is immediately stopped, some visual recovery may occur. Otherwise, the visual side effect is usually irreversible. Ocular toxicity includes inflammation and atrophy of the optic nerve and inner retina, loss of white matter, and gliosis of the occipital and parietal lobes causing various degrees of blindness. Because this drug also suppresses the immune and hematologic systems, secondary opportunistic pathogens may affect the eye, causing inflammation in any part of the eye.[1] The most complete review of the ocular side effects due to fludarabine was done by Ding et al.[2] In a large study at higher dosages with 5-year follow-up, Sorenson et al showed incidences of subtotal blindness at 1% and blindness at 0.3%.[3] Other data showed visual impairment with early onset at a varying incidence of 3–15%.[4]

Topical ocular exposure of this drug is highly toxic and requires immediate lavage.

Generic Name:

Fluorouracil (5FU).

Proprietary Names:

Adrucil, Carac, Efudex, Fluoroplex, Tolak.

Primary Use
Systemic

This fluorinated pyrimidine antimetabolite is used in the management of carcinoma of the colon, rectum, breast, stomach, and pancreas. Fluorouracil is also used topically for actinic keratoses and intradermally for skin cancer.

Ophthalmic

Fluorouracil is used subconjunctivally to enhance glaucoma filtration surgery. Topical ocular fluorouracil is used for carcinoma in situ and squamous cell carcinoma.

Ocular Side Effects

Systemic administration – intravenous or topical
Certain

1. Irritation
   a. Lacrimation
   b. Photosensitivity
   c. Pain
2. Decreased vision
3. Eyelids or conjunctiva
   a. Conjunctivitis
   b. Occlusion of lacrimal canaliculi or punctum
   c. Blepharoconjunctivitis
   d. Erythema
   e. Edema
   f. Keratinization lid margin
   g. Dermatitis
4. Cornea
   a. Superficial punctate keratitis
   b. Epithelial erosion
   c. Opacity
5. Circumlimbal edema
6. Epiphora

Possible

1. Nystagmus (coarse)
2. Decreased convergence or divergence
3. Diplopia
4. Blepharospasm
5. May aggravate herpes infections
6. Decreased accommodation
7. Optic neuritis

Local ophthalmic use or exposure – subconjunctival injection or topical ocular application
Certain

1. Irritation
   a. Lacrimation
   b. Pain
   c. Edema
   d. Burning sensation
2. Conjunctiva
   a. Edema
   b. Hyperpigmentation
   c. Keratinization
   d. Cicatricial changes
   e. Delayed wound healing

3. Periorbital edema
4. Cornea
   a. Superficial punctate keratitis
   b. Ulceration
   c. Scarring – stromal
   d. Keratinized plaques
   e. Delayed wound healing
   f. Striate melanokeratosis
   g. Endothelial damage
   h. Limbal stem-cell deficiency
   i. Crystalline keratopathy (Fig. 15.12)
   j. Pannus
5. Filtering blebs
   a. Delayed leaks
   b. Giant blebs
   c. Thin walled
   d. Infections
   e. Cystic blebs
   f. Ectasia
6. Anterior uveitis
7. Hypotonous maculopathy

Local ophthalmic use or exposure – eyelid injection
Certain

1. Eyelid
   a. Edema
   b. Erythema
   c. Cicatricial reaction
   d. Ectropion
   e. Hyperpigmentation
   f. Allergic or toxic reaction
2. Conjunctival
   a. Chemosis
   b. Erythema
   c. Cicatricial reaction

Possible

1. Loss of eyelashes or eyebrows
2. Crystalline keratopathy
3. Lid necrosis if followed by cryotherapy

Clinical Significance

Fluorouracil (5FU) has been used for over 4 decades and is one of the more commonly used cytotoxic drugs in the palliative treatment of solid tumors. Because its therapeutic dose is often close to its toxic level, 25–35% of patients on systemic therapy have side effects. However, ocular side effects at suggested dosages are rare. Reviews of the ocular side effects from systemic 5FU have been done by Eiseman et al and Singh et al.[1,2] Adverse ocular effects can be divided into those

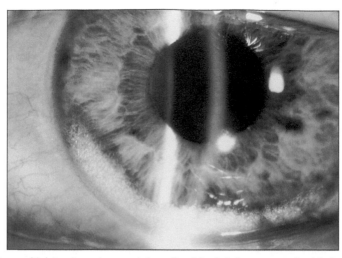

FIG. 15.12 Left eye with intrastromal corneal deposits at the inferior corneoscleral limbus secondary to subconjunctival injection of 5FU.[14]

occurring in the first 3 months of therapy and those occurring with chronic therapy. The most common early adverse ocular effects, besides decreased vision, are low-grade blepharitis and conjunctival irritation, with symptoms well out of proportion to the clinical findings. These reactions usually peak in the second and third weeks of therapy and, in rare instances, are severe enough to cause discontinuation of treatment. The reason for discomfort is multifactorial, including 5FU or its antimetabolite secreted in the tears, decrease in basal cell secretion, and excessive lacrimation. Eiseman et al found epiphora to be the most common adverse ocular event, with the highest incidence among African Americans.[1] With long-term therapy, up to one-third of patients may have a cicatricial reaction occurring in the conjunctiva, punctum, canaliculi, or lacrimal sac. If recognized early, this may be reversed, but if unrecognized, the scarring is irreversible with resulting epiphora.[3,4] There are a number of reports of irreversible punctual, canalicular, or lacrimal sac stenosis, as well as cicatricial changes in the fornices.[5-7] Agarwal et al reported severe squamous metaplasia in the lacrimal canaliculi.[8] Toxic effects to the cornea can occur for the same reasons as noted earlier. Fortunately, other than corneal sloughs, this uniformly resolves within a few weeks of the drug being discontinued. Corneal opacities can occur. Neurotoxicity, which possibly affects the brainstem and causes oculomotor disturbance, has been reported. This may include various ocular motor defects, including blepharospasm, nystagmus, and diplopia.[6] Delval et al reported a case of bilateral anterior optic neuropathy in a patient with dihydropyrimidine dehydrogenase deficiency.[9] Bixenman et al reported diplopia heralding the onset of further cerebral dysfunction.[10] Sato et al reported that injections of 5FU in the superficial temporal artery caused complete bilateral visual loss.[11] There are cases of possible optic nerve toxicity secondary to 5FU in the literature and spontaneous reports.

Direct injection of 5FU into the eyelids for the treatment of basal cell carcinoma can cause cicatricial ectropion and hyperpigmentation. This drug should be used with caution in patients with preexistent corneal pathology and in diabetics. There is a case of lid necrosis in the spontaneous reports of a patient receiving cryotherapy for trichiasis when the patient was also on 5FU.

5FU has gained increasing popularity in the management of difficult glaucoma patients requiring filtration surgery. Initially, significant ocular side effects occurred but with the method of application and the ideal concentration of the drug being determined, this has decreased. 5FU is most commonly given as a subconjunctival injection, which enhances bleb formation. However, adverse ocular effects, most reversible, occur in up to 50% of cases. The most common is superficial keratitis, which may rarely become ulcerated. Hayashi et al reported a permanent corneal opacity requiring a lamellar keratoplasty when this drug was used after a trabeculectomy.[12] Patitsas et al reported an infectious and Rothman et al a noninfectious reversible crystalline keratopathy secondary to subconjunctival 5FU injections in postoperative filtering surgery.[13,14] Stank et al and Peterson et al reported striate melanokeratosis after trabeculectomy with 5FU.[15,16] Libre reported a profound transient cataract secondary to subconjunctival 5FU in after-filtering surgery.[17] Pires et al reported a late complication of limbal stem-cell deficiency in 2 patients after 5FU subconjunctival injections.[18] These required stem-cell transplantations to correct. Other defects include conjunctival wound leaks, excessive filtration with shallow-to-flat anterior chambers, and conjunctival or corneal keratinization. Ticho et al reviewed long-term complications and incidences with 8.6% mild iridocyclitis, 3.8% endophthalmitis, 2.9% hypotony, and 1.9% transient leaking blebs.[19] Stamper et al reported on hypotonous maculopathy, and Oppenheim et al suggested that some of these may be due to drug-induced ciliary body shutdown.[20,21] Hickey-Dwyer et al felt that 5FU subconjunctival injections should be used with great care in diabetic patients due to potential corneal complications and may be contraindicated in corneas with band keratopathy.[22]

Topical ocular 5FU has had some popularity in the management of conjunctival and corneal neoplasia.[23] Ocular irritation and other side effects are directly related to concentration, dose, and length of treatment. All the signs of severe ocular toxicity of the anterior segment may be seen, including corneal erosions, opacities (permanent), pannus, and scleral melts.

Recommendations

1. Ocular symptoms may be decreased by preservative-free topical ocular artificial tears or mild steroids during peak serum levels of 5FU.
2. If patients are given the drug intravenously, ocular ice packs should be applied for 30 minutes in total, starting 5 minutes before the injection. This significantly decreases ocular symptoms.[24]
3. If chronic therapy is necessary, a prophylactic silastic intubation of the lacrimal system is advised.[8,25]
4. If topic ocular 5FU is used, consider using punctual plugs.
5. Pires et al found amniotic membrane transplants or conjunctival limbal autografts to be of value for limbal cell deficiency induced by 5FU post–glaucoma surgeries.[18]
6. Use with caution in diabetic patients.

Generic Name:

Gemcitabine.

Proprietary Name:

Gemzar.

Primary Use

A deoxycytidine antimetabolite related to cytarabine. This drug is used in the management of pancreatic, lung, breast, bladder, kidney, ovarian, and head and neck cancers.

Ocular Side Effects

Systemic administration – intravenous
Possible

1. Decreased vision
2. Retina
   a. Preretinal hemorrhages
   b. Cotton-wool spots
   c. Yellowish plaques
   d. Venous beading
   e. Capillary nonprofusion
   f. Macular exudates
   g. Subretinal fluid
   h. Intraretinal cysts
   i. Hard exudates
   j. Capillary leakage

Clinical Significance

This drug is primarily used in severe cancers with a high mortality rate. It is often used with other anticancer drugs; therefore a visual side effect profile is difficult to establish. Even so, and based on only a small number of cases, a possible pattern may occur. This is based on 5 single case reports in the literature and 11 additional cases of various forms of acute retinopathies found in spontaneous reporting systems.[1-6] The pattern starts between 1 and 6 cycles (with a 6-week clear-out between cycles) of intravenous gemcitabine, often with another anticancer drug (docetaxel, oxaliplatin, or cisplatin) with a progressive decrease in vision with significant posterior pole retinopathy over 1–6 weeks. On fluorescein angiography and OCT there is a diffuse ischemic retinal vasculopathy, possibly in large part due to endothelial cell dysfunction. This includes preretinal hemorrhages, cotton-wool spots, hard exudates, areas of capillary nonprofusion, subretinal fluid, intraretinal cysts, and capillary leakage. If the drug is stopped, some improvement occurs, but not always. There are 2 cases of positive rechallenge. It is common for most of these hematologic effects to also occur systemically. Valeshabad et al reported a case of the pattern noted earlier associated with choroidal effusion; however, they felt the effusions were secondary to the concomitant use of docetaxel.[4]

Generic Name:

Imiquimod.

Proprietary Names:
Aldara Cream, Zyclara.

Primary Use
Topical cream used in the management of actinic keratosis, as well as basal and squamous cell carcinomas.

Ocular Side Effects
Local ophthalmic use or exposure – topical ocular application or periocular application with intentional and unintentional ocular exposure
Certain
1. Decreased vision
2. Irritation
   a. Pain
   b. Pruritus
   c. Burning
   d. Epiphora
3. Conjunctiva
   a. Erythema
   b. Edema
   c. Ulceration
   d. Chemosis
4. Cornea
   a. Ulceration
   b. Superficial punctate keratitis
5. Eyelids and periocular
   a. Edema
   b. Irritation
   c. Pigmentation
      i. Increased
      ii. Decreased

Probable
1. Cicatricial ectropion

Conditional/unclassified
1. Retinal vein occlusion
2. Anterior uveitis

Clinical Significance
Although the manufacturer does not recommend it and the FDA has not approved it, there are dozens of articles regarding the use of imiquimod in periocular and conjunctival treatment.[1-16] If the patient is closely monitored, then the ocular side effects are manageable and resolve with a month of cessation of treatment. This may require lubrication, topical antibiotics, decreased dosage, and periods without treatment to allow tissue to recover. There have been reports of cicatricial ectropion, retinal vein occlusion, and even loss of the eye.[17] Hong et al reported a case of retinal vein occlusion after using imiquimod cream.[18] They postulated that it may have been due to retinal vasculitis or local pressure effect due to swelling, leading to impaired drainage of the retinal veins. The authors were not aware of any other cases of this.

Generic Name:
Interferon (alpha, beta, gamma, or PEG).

Proprietary Names:
Actimmune, Alferon N, Avonex, Betaseron, Extavia, Infergen, Intron A, Pegasys, PegIntron, Rebif, Roferon-A, Sylatron.

Primary Use
These proteins and glycoproteins have antiviral, antiproliferative, and immunomodulatory activity. They are therefore used in a variety of diseases, including chronic viral infections, chronic blood diseases, and various malignancies.

Ocular Side Effects
Systemic administration – intramuscular, intravenous, or subcutaneous
Certain (primarily interferon alpha-2b)
1. Decreased vision
2. Pain
3. Diplopia
4. Eyelids or conjunctiva
   a. Conjunctivitis – nonspecific
   b. Subconjunctival hemorrhage
   c. Increased eyelash growth
5. Retina – choroid
   a. Hemorrhages
   b. Cotton-wool spots (Fig. 15.13)
   c. Microaneurysm
   d. Vascular tortuosity
   e. Vascular occlusion
   f. Vascular dilation
   g. Macular edema
6. Abnormal visual evoked potential (VEP)
7. Visual hallucinations
8. Photophobia

Probable
1. Myasthenia gravis
   a. Diplopia
   b. Ptosis
   c. Paresis of extraocular muscles
2. Graves' ophthalmopathy
3. Cornea
   a. Squamous metaplasia

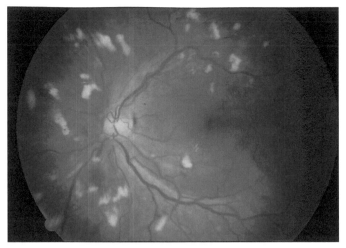

FIG. 15.13 Multiple cotton-wool spots and hemorrhage in patient taking systemic interferon.[2]

b. Epithelial cysts
4. Orbital myositis
5. Causes ocular sarcoid

Possible
1. May aggravate herpes infections
2. Nonarteritic anterior ischemic optic neuropathy (NAION)
3. May aggravate or cause ocular sicca
4. Optic neuritis

Conditional/unclassified
1. Papilledema
2. Uveitis
3. Nystagmus
4. Conjunctiva – reactive lymphoid hyperplasia
5. VKH-like disease

Clinical Significance
There are well over 8000 cases in the spontaneous reports of the interferons and possible adverse ocular side effects. The best studied with the most serious adverse ocular side effects is interferon alpha-2b. Interferon alpha-2b, as per the package insert, requires an ophthalmic exam before beginning therapy with periodic follow-up.[1] The second most common is interferon beta-1a with similar, but milder, adverse ocular side effects. Of greatest clinical interest is the adverse effects that interferon alpha-2b has on the retina. These ocular side effects characteristically occur between 2 weeks and 3 months after drug exposure.

These changes may spontaneously regress while on the drug or when it is stopped. They are more commonly seen with diabetics, hypertensive patients, and at higher dosages. Ocular side effects may occur within 15 minutes after first exposure or not for many months. Decreased vision may be transitory and may occur after each drug exposure. The primary complication is retinal ischemic changes, both in large vessels and capillaries, as shown by fluorescein angiography. Retinal capillary nonperfusion and/or cotton-wool spots due to vascular occlusion can occur, but usually good central vision remains.[2] There are a number of reports of branch arterial or venous obstruction. Only a small percentage of patients have permanent changes. Why these retinal changes occur is open to debate. Anything from deposition of immune complexes, to leukocyte infiltrates, to anemia, to exacerbation of autoimmune disease has been postulated. The drug or underlying disease causes various blood dyscrasias as well as anemia, and this may also be the cause of the adverse event. Retinopathy is seen with both interferon alpha-2b and beta-1a. Visual changes may include bright afterimages that are reversible. Ocular or orbital pain can occur, which can be intense. The drug can cause conjunctivitis, subconjunctival hemorrhages, or corneal changes, probably because the drug may be secreted in the tears.[3] Deng-Huang et al reported impairment of tears as well as squamous metaplastic changes on the ocular surface in patients with chronic hepatitis C receiving long-term interferon and ribavirin.[4] Although these changes were reversible, abnormal tear function and metaplasia persisted for up to 6 months after the drugs were discontinued. There are reports of eyelash growth, which required up to twice-weekly trimming.[5] Myasthenia and Graves' disease can be related to drug-associated development of autoimmune-induced pathology. Thyroid dysfunction is seen in up to 40% of patients on interferon alpha-2a with resultant Graves' ophthalmopathy occurring.[6] Because the drug can cause immune suppression, activation of various virus- or immune-mediated disease can occur. Sene et al, along with many others, reported cases of uveitis and VKH disease.[7] Orbital myositis, diplopia, and diplopia secondary to Graves' ophthalmopathy have also been reported.[8,9] Cases in the spontaneous reports support a "possible" association. Damasceno et al pointed out recurrence of uveitis after taking this drug.[10] Uveitis secondary to sarcoid and reactive lymphoid hyperplasia has also been reported.[11,12]

There are over 360 cases in the spontaneous reports of the interferons causing optic nerve side effects. Fraunfelder et al reviewed 36 cases of anterior ischemic optic neuropathy (AION) in patients on interferon alpha therapy.[13] The median duration of therapy to onset to AION was 4.5 months, with 50% having some form of permanent visual loss. In this series, there were 3 positive rechallenge cases. There are a number of optic neuritis cases reported in the literature and in the spontaneous reports, but as with AION, many patients on these drugs have diseases with a higher incidence of neurologic disorders to begin with, so it is difficult to determine drug-related events.[14,15]

Interferon beta-1a has been associated with ocular sicca (1–3%), and interferon alpha-2b has been associated with xerostomia (1–28%).[1] If a drug causes xerostomia, there is a possibility that ocular sicca may also occur. There are over 350 cases in the spontaneous reports of these drugs being associated with ocular sicca.

Recommendations

1. The manufacturer suggested retinal examination before starting interferon; if any retinal ischemic changes are seen, the drug should probably not be used.[1]
2. The manufacturer also suggested following the patient for retinal problems on a monthly basis.[1]
3. Assessing the risk factors, i.e. high dosage, diabetics, hypertension, and a patient's underlying disease, will help the clinician to decide how best to monitor these patients.
4. If optic neuropathy is suspected, rapid cessation of interferon therapy may portend a better prognosis because permanent visual loss is possible if this adverse effect goes unrecognized.[13]

Generic Name:
Lenalidomide.

Proprietary Name:
Revlimid.

Primary Use

Immunomodulator, angiogenesis inhibitor, and thalidomide analog used in the management of transfusion-dependent anemia, multiple myeloma, stem-cell transplantation, mantle cell lymphoma, and amyloidosis.

Ocular Side Effects
Systemic administration – oral
Certain
1. Decreased vision

Probable
1. Mimic thyroid-associated orbitopathy
   a. Ptosis
   b. Proptosis
   c. Eyelid retraction
   d. Enlargement extraocular muscles

Possible
1. May aggravate or cause ocular sicca

Conditional/unclassified
1. Cataracts

Clinical Significance

Decreased vision occurs shortly after taking lenalidomide but returns to normal without stopping treatment. Its incidence is 17%.[1] This drug appears to dysregulate the thyroid with various progressions or regressions of the gland. Iams et al reported a 5–10% incidence of hypothyroidism.[2] Figaro et al reported thyroid abnormalities in 6% of their series of 170 patients; 6 patients became hypothyroid and 4 became hyperthyroid based on thyroid-stimulating hormone measurements.[3] Stein et al reported an acute case of thyroiditis within 5 days after starting the drug.[4] Samara et al documented a case in which a patient initially became hyperthyroid followed by hypothyroidism.[5] There are a number of proposed mechanisms.[6]

An area of most interest is the incidence of cataracts at 17%.[1] The are 659 spontaneous reports of cataracts in patients taking this drug. This drug is often used in the treatment of multiple myeloma in which concomitant oral steroids are commonly used. In those spontaneous reports, 533 of the patients were on either dexamethasone or prednisone. Therefore this drug probably does not cause cataracts, but rather the associated oral steroid is likely the cause. We can find no description of the reported lens changes, but suspect that most are posterior subcapsular. We cannot rule out this drug as being a cofactor in causing lens changes.

Lim et al reported a suspected case of CMV retinitis after starting lenalidomide.[7] They postulated that the drug penetrated the blood–retinal barrier, allowing reactivation of the CMV in the retina.

Recommendations[6]
1. Monitor patients on lenalidomide for thyroid changes while on the medication.
2. Watch for thyroid disease, even years later while off lenalidomide.
3. Lid retraction is often the sign of thyroid abnormalities.

Generic Name:
Melphalan.

Proprietary Names:
Alkeran, Evomela.

Primary Uses
Systemic
A nitrogen mustard analog used orally and intravenously for various cancers.

Ophthalmic
Used in ophthalmology, intracamerally and intra-arterially, in the management of retinal blastomas on an orphan-drug basis.

Ocular Side Effects
Local ophthalmic use or exposure – intravitreal injection
Certain
1. Irritation at injection site
2. Eyelids or conjunctiva
   a. Blebs – at injection site
   b. Edema
   c. Ptosis
3. Iris
   a. Depigmentation
   b. Thinning
   c. Synechiae
   d. Recession
   e. Atrophy
4. Uveitis
5. Cornea
   a. Edema
   b. Fold in Descemet's membrane

6. Sclera
   a. Thinning
   b. Atrophy
   c. Scleritis
7. Retina
   a. Electroretinogram (ERG) changes – decreased
   b. Vascular
      i. Bleeding
      ii. Edema
      iii. Sheathing
      iv. Sclerosis
      v. Fibrosis
      vi. Salt-and-pepper retinopathy
      vii. Diffuse atrophy
      viii. Drug accumulates in pigment epithelium
      ix. Occlusion
8. Orbit
   a. Fat atrophy
   b. Decreased perfusion
   c. Edema
9. Cataracts
10. Impaired ocular growth
11. Phthisis bulbi
12. Optic atrophy

Local ophthalmic use or exposure – intra-arterial injection
Certain
1. Same as intravitreal injection – may be more extensive
2. Intravascular birefringent foreign bodies
3. Periocular blanching erythematous edematous patches
4. Ocular nerve palsy – older catheterization technique

Clinical Significance
Although it is not uncommon for melphalan to be used with other drugs, especially topotecan, it is frequently used alone, and therefore an accurate profile of adverse ocular side effects can be outlined. This drug's toxic ocular profile is less than what is presented here because the refined technique of selective catheterization of the ophthalmic artery allows for safer drug delivery.

Intravitreal injection is the most common method of administration. This may cause posterior and anterior ocular toxicity most prevalent in the meridian of the injection, where the drug is at its highest concentration. In the largest series to date, salt-and-pepper retinopathy occurred in 43–50% of patients and was significantly associated with a pronounced degradation of ERG responses.[1-4] At the irritation site, both pigment and conjunctival blebs are common. Blebs and irritation are transitory, and it has been postulated that they are the result of patency of a potential trans-scleral fistula.[2] Scleral thinning in this area may occur to the degree that the underlying uvea may be seen. Iris recession may occur with retinal necrosis and hypotony.[2]

The most serious side effects are the drug's direct toxic effect on the vascularity of the retina and choroid. Although many of the anterior segment side effects are reversible, those of the posterior segment are not. These changes have been felt to be possibly due to the toxic effects on the endothelium. The severity of the retinal and choroidal vascular toxicity is dependent on dosage, method of administration, concomitant arterial melphalan injections (within a week), and addition of other anticancer drugs.[3] Melphalan also appears to be more toxic in heavily pigmented eyes.

Lens changes can occur for multiple reasons, including drug toxicity, uveitis, and vascular shutdown.

Intra-arterial injections can cause all of the noted side effects, although they are often more severe. Marr et al discuss ciliary madarosis and skin changes after intraarterial chemotherapy.[5] In their series, 16% of patients developed blanching, erythematous, and edematous periocular skin changes. These all resolved within 3 months after the drug was discontinued. Muen et al and others have reported intra-arterial melphalan causing isolated infarcts of the third nerve, causing palsy and/or ptosis.[6] Steinle et al pointed out that direct drug toxicity, pH of infusate, mechanical stress, and/or particle size all trigger endothelial cell inflammation.[7] Using histopathologic analysis, Eagle et al and Munier et al found that possible intravascular emboli can cause a granulomatous-like inflammatory response, which can lead to total vascular occlusion.[8,9]

Generic Name:
Methotrexate.

Proprietary Names:
Otrexup, Rasuvo, Rheumatrex, Trexall, Xatmep.

Primary Use
Systemic
This folic acid antagonist is effective in the systemic treatment of certain neoplastic diseases and immune system suppressants, as with rheumatoid arthritis, psoriasis, and uveitis.

Ophthalmic
Intravitreal methotrexate is used in the management of intraocular lymphomas, both primary CNS lymphomas and non-Hodgkin lymphomas. It is also used in the management of uveitis and advanced diabetic retinopathy.

Ocular Side Effects
Systemic administration – intramuscular, intrathecal, intravenous, oral, or subcutaneous
Certain
1. Eyelids or conjunctiva
   a. Allergic reactions
   b. Erythema
   c. Blepharoconjunctivitis
   d. Seborrheic blepharitis
   e. Depigmentation
   f. Hyperpigmentation
   g. Urticaria
   h. Loss of eyelashes or eyebrows
2. Decreased vision
3. Irritation
   a. Lacrimation
   b. Hyperemia
   c. Photophobia
   d. Pain
   e. Burning sensation
4. Periorbital edema
5. Keratitis (Fig. 15.14)
6. Retinal pigmentary changes (intrathecal or carotid artery infusion)

Possible
1. May aggravate or cause ocular sicca
2. Paresis of extraocular muscles (intrathecal or carotid artery infusion with mannitol)
3. Optic nerve (intrathecal or carotid artery infusion)
   a. Neuritis
   b. Atrophy
4. May aggravate
   a. Herpes infections
   b. Molluscum contagiosum
5. Eyelids or conjunctiva
   a. Erythema multiforme
   b. Lyell syndrome

Local ophthalmic use or exposure – intravitreal injection
Certain
1. Conjunctival hyperemia
2. Corneal epitheliopathy
   a. Punctate keratopathy
   b. Severe epitheliopathy
3. Intravitreal hemorrhage

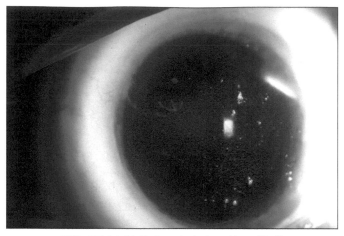

FIG. 15.14 Methotrexate-induced keratitis.[15]

Probable
1. Cataract
2. Posterior capsule fibrosis – pseudophakia

Possible
1. Loss of vision
2. Maculopathy
3. Band keratopathy
4. Toxic anterior segment syndrome

Clinical Significance
Ocular side effects such as periorbital edema, blepharitis, conjunctival hyperemia, increased lacrimation, or photophobia may occur in about 25% of patients on methotrexate.[1] Despite minimal drug-related blepharoconjunctivitis, some patients have marked subjective complaints. The drug is secreted in the tears, probably causes a direct irritation, and interferes with the metabolism of the meibomian glands as well as the corneal and conjunctival epithelium. Lacrimation is increased initially and is probably secondary to ocular irritation, but some have reported a decrease in lacrimation, with the drug possibly damaging the lacrimal gland or basic secretors. Peak methotrexate drug levels were measured in tears and found to be equivalent to plasma levels 48 hours after therapy in both symptomatic and asymptomatic patients.

O'Neill et al reported a small-vessel vasculitis in the skin after low-dose methotrexate.[2] Cursiefen et al reported methotrexate-induced immunosuppression that may be associated with the onset of multiple bilateral eyelid molluscum contagiosum lesions.[3,4] This drug is a probable cause of lymphomas, including intraocular lymphoma, orbital lymphoma, and ocular intravascular lymphoma.[5–7]

Methotrexate-induced retinal or optic nerve pathology is not clear-cut. Oral methotrexate, given on a weekly basis for 8.5 years to a 13-year-old patient, had shown partially reversible decreased vision and abnormal electroretinogram (ERG) findings 3 years after stopping the drug. Balachandran et al reported bilateral optic neuropathy in a 53-year-old female on methotrexate 15 mg/week.[8] The authors felt that the long-term drug interfered with folate metabolism. Folate deficiency is associated with optic neuropathy. Millay et al reported that RPE changes developed ipsilateral to carotid arterial infusion of mannitol and methotrexate in patients with intracranial malignant neoplasms.[9] A mannitol-induced "opening" of the blood–retina barrier may have potentiated these changes. Intrathecal or intracarotid injections of methotrexate suggest the potential for optic nerve toxicity. There are only a few case reports of neurotoxicity, and many are complicated by the co-administration of other anticancer drugs and/or radiation. Clare et al reported a case of possible low-dose methotrexate causing irreversible optic neuropathy.[10] Balachandran et al reported a case of possible methotrexate-induced central scotoma, reduction in vision, and optic atrophy.[8] Boogerd et al described a case with histology of intrathecal methotrexate and cytarabine showing major CNS and optic nerve damage.[11] Epstein et al described a case of seesaw nystagmus after intrathecal methotrexate and other complicating factors.[12] In children with acute leukemia, intrathecal methotrexate in conjunction with radiation therapy has been associated with reports of optic nerve atrophy at radiotherapy doses below those usually associated with such toxicity.

Many variables of intravitreal methotrexate toxicity include trauma of injection, frequency of injections, or associated silicone injection clouds. Hardwig et al described the side effects of intravitreal methotrexate in eyes containing silicone.[13] These eyes usually have much more extensive pathology to begin with, so the side effects may be more extensive due in part to the underlying pathology. Most all intravitreal injections of methotrexate cause conjunctival hyperemia and some degree of epitheliopathy.[13] These are relatively mild and temporary, although some cases of epitheliopathy may be severe. Gorovoy et al reported cases of severe corneal changes after intravitreal injections.[14] They have theorized that methotrexate disturbs the mitotically active limbal progenitor cells and corneal epithelial cells resulting in significant corneal pathology. Depending on dosage and frequency, cataract formation can occur. In pseudophakic eyes, this drug probably also causes some posterior lens fibrosis.

Generic Name:
Mitoxantrone hydrochloride.

Proprietary Name:
Novantrone.

Primary Use
This is a synthetic anthracycline derivative used for its antineoplastic properties to treat acute leukemias and various malignant neoplasms of the breast and ovary.

Ocular Side Effects
Systemic administration – intravenous
Certain
1. Decreased vision
2. Sclera
   a. Blue pigmentation
   b. Blue-green pigmentation
3. Eyelids and conjunctiva
   a. Edema
   b. Blue or blue-green pigmentation
   c. Conjunctivitis

Possible
1. Alopecia primarily in areas of white hair

Clinical Significance
As with most antineoplastic drugs, this drug is probably secreted via the lacrimal gland, causing color changes in the conjunctiva, eyelid, and sclera.[1,2] The drug, either mechanically or chemically, is the probable reason for conjunctivitis. The conjunctivitis is self-limiting and resolves once therapy is stopped. The incidence of conjunctivitis is up to 5%.[3] Pigmentation of the sclera and eyelids is transitory and secondary to the deposition of the dark-blue drug. All ocular side effects are transitory and of no major clinical significance.

Generic Name:
Nilutamide.

Proprietary Name:
Nilandron.

Primary Use
This antiandrogen is used in the treatment of prostatic cancer and as a feminizing hormone.

Ocular Side Effects
Systemic administration – oral
Certain
1. Decreased vision – transitory
2. Photostress – slow recovery
3. Decreased dark adaptation – transitory
4. Chromatopsia – transitory

Possible
1. May aggravate or cause ocular sicca
2. Diplopia
3. Decreased accommodation

Clinical Significance
Some of the most common adverse drug-related effects of nilutamide are visual. Multiple well-controlled clinical trials state that, after roughly 2 weeks, anywhere from 12–65% of patients receiving this drug experienced delayed adaptation to darkness after exposure to bright illumination (sun, television, or bright light).[1-3] In general, photostress recovery time values were from 9–25 minutes, where the normal upper limit was 1.3 minutes. This delayed adaptation to dark was reversed on discontinuation of therapy, dosage reduction, and spontaneously in some patients despite continuation of therapy. Dukman et al noted that the "transient visual disturbance" that occurred at entrance into a dark area was seldom troublesome and only mild in nature.[4] Dole, however, felt that this adverse event was a reason to discontinue the medication.[5] Patients may take up to a year before recovery is complete after the drug is discontinued. Theoretically, this may be due to a delayed regeneration of the visual pigments. Anatomically, no cause of retinal changes, clinical or histologic, can be found. In a randomized double-blind study, Namer et al showed a 3% incidence of

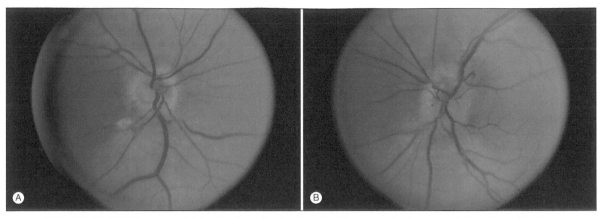

FIG. 15.15 **(A)** Edematous right optic disc after treatment with oprelvekin. On presentation, the patient was noted to have disc edema with exudates inferotemporal to the nerve. **(B)** Edematous left optic disc after treatment with oprelvekin. The left disc was also noted to be edematous during the initial examination.[3]

chromatopsia, a 1% incidence of diplopia, and a 1% incidence of abnormal accommodation, whereas the placebo group showed none of these adverse events.[6] Because there is a 2% incidence of xerostomia, ocular sicca may occur or be aggravated.[7] There is 1 case in the spontaneous reports of bilateral magenta anterior subcapsular cataracts in a patient after 7 years of nilutamide therapy.

Generic Name:
Oprelvekin.

Proprietary Name:
Neumega.

Primary Use
A recombinant form of interleukin engineered by combining the antibody with a toxin. It is primarily used to treat chemotherapy-related thrombocytopenia and Wiskott-Aldrich syndrome.

Ocular Adverse Effects
Systemic administration – subcutaneous
Certain
1. Decreased vision – mild
2. Conjunctiva – hyperemia
3. Optic discs (Fig. 15.15)
   a. Papilledema
   b. Peripapular exudates
4. Periorbital edema
5. Subconjunctival hemorrhages

Clinical Significance
This drug is rarely given in isolation; therefore adverse events are difficult to evaluate. In the manufacturer's clinical trials, 13% of patients had conjunctival injections compared with 2% in the placebo group, edema anywhere in the body was 41% on the drug versus 10% in the control group, and bilateral disc edema occurred in 1% of adults and 16% of children.[1] In a letter to health care professionals, 25% of pediatric patients on 100 µg/kg/day developed papilledema.[2] None of the 9 patients at 75 µg developed this complication. Peterson et al reported a well-documented case of oprelvekin-associated bilateral optic disc edema in a 38-year-old male, which resolved when the drug was discontinued.[3] There are 14 cases of disc edema in the spontaneous reports, some with peripapular exudates. One case had a positive rechallenge. Most of the disc edema improved markedly when the drug was discontinued. To date, all ocular signs and symptoms from this drug are reversible on stopping the drug.

Recommendation
As per the manufacturer, use this drug with caution if the patient has preexisting papilledema, known increased intracranial pressure, or tumors involving the CNS.[1]

Generic Name:
Oxaliplatin.

Proprietary Name:
Eloxatin.

Primary Use
Intravenous anticancer drug used to treat multiple types of cancers. It is often used in combination with other anticancer drugs to treat advanced cancers.

Ocular Side Effects
Systemic administration – intravenous
Certain
1. Decreased vision
2. Ptosis
3. Conjunctivitis
4. Pain
5. Lacrimation

Probable
1. Visual field defects
2. Cortical blindness
3. Abducens nerve palsy (diplopia)

Possible
1. Optic neuritis
2. Color vision defect
3. Pseudotumor cerebri

Conditional/unclassified
1. Retinitis pigmentosa – progression

Clinical Significance
Possible ocular side effects appear to be infrequent and reversible. Acute side effects (occurring within the first or second dose) include decreased vision, ptosis, increased lacrimation, ocular pain, and visual field defects. Delayed reactions include conjunctivitis, optic-nerve changes, and pseudotumor cerebri.

The most complete data as to incidence are from Japan, which reported a possible ocular side effects incidence of 18%, which included ptosis, 9%; decreased vision, 6%; and visual field defects, 4%.[1] The *Physicians' Desk Reference* (PDR) states an incidence of conjunctivitis from 2–8% and increased lacrimation from 1–9%.[2]

Neurotoxicity may be the most significant side effect. This may be seen in both acute and delayed phases. The acute-phase ocular side effects are often associated with a systemic hyperexcitability state caused by oxaliplatin. This is manifested as bilateral ptosis, which may occur as early as the first infusion.[3,4] This typically resolves in 6–24 hours without sequelae. Some of these cases have been precipitated by cold temperatures, too rapid an infusion, or increased drug dosage. Another neurotoxic effect brought on by similar circumstances as ptosis, is bilateral transient abducens nerve palsy. This may occur during or shortly after infusion and may last 15–120+ minutes. All cases have been fully reversible. As with ptosis, the incidence rate decreases with a warmer environment, slower infusion, or decreased dosage.[5,6] There have been 47 cases of ptosis and 56 cases of eye movement disorders or diplopia from spontaneous reporting agencies. There has been a case of positive rechallenge with both of these side effects.

Other examples of neurotoxicity include transient visual field defects, cortical blindness, optic neuritis, and color vision defects.[1,7-9] Mesquida et al reported a case of mild residual visual field defects and an abnormal electrooculogram 8 months after stopping the drug.[9]

Pseudotumor cerebri with papilledema has been reported in association with this drug.[7,10]

There are 2 cases in the spontaneous reports and 1 in the literature that suggest worsening of retinitis pigmentosa after oxaliplatin exposure.[11]

Generic Names:
1. Pazopanib; 2. sorafenib; 3. sunitinib.

Proprietary Names:
1. Votrient; 2. Nexavar; 3. Sutent.

Primary Use
Anticancer drugs that are multitargeted, multi–protein kinase inhibitors that block angiogenesis and signals that cause cancer cells to grow.

Ocular Side Effects
Systemic administration – oral
Certain
1. Decreased vision
2. Eyelids
   a. Edema
   b. Erythema
   c. Blepharitis
3. Conjunctiva
   a. Chemosis
   b. Erythema
4. Periocular edema
5. May aggravate or cause ocular sicca
6. Irritation
   a. Photophobia
   b. Epiphora
   c. Discharge
7. Keratitis

Possible

1. Retinal detachment – serous
2. Bleeding
   a. Conjunctiva
   b. Intravitreal
   c. Retina
3. Poliosis

Conditional/unclassified

1. Retina
   a. Detachment - rhegmatogenous
   b. Arterial or venous occlusions
2. Macular edema
3. Uveitis
4. Optic nerve disorders
5. Extraocular muscle disorders, including ptosis

Clinical Significance

The European Medicines Agency (EMA) and Japanese Pharmaceuticals and Medical Devices Agency (PMDA) have required the pazopanib package inserts to include the possibility of this drug causing retinal tears and retinal detachments.[1,2] The requirements do not differentiate between rhegmatogenous and nonrhegmatogenous retinal detachments. There have been 74 cases of retinal detachments reported in the spontaneous reporting systems (FDA, World Health Organization [WHO], EMA, and PMDA).[3] Unfortunately, few of these differentiate between rhegmatogenous and nonrhegmatogenous. Additionally, there are 2 single-case reports of rhegmatogenous retinal detachments in the literature.[4,5] To date, no oral medication has been proven to cause rhegmatogenous retinal detachments, although oral fluoroquinolones have been implicated by Etminan et al.[6] Wegner reported a single case of serous retinal detachment (nonrhegmatogenous) with triple positive rechallenge.[7] There are 2 positive rechallenge cases from the spontaneous reports, making this a "possible" drug-related side effect.

This class of drugs (sunitinib) is now being used experimentally with success in metastatic ocular melanomas.[8]

As with most systemic anticancer drugs, anterior segment ocular signs and symptoms may occur. These adverse anterior ocular side effects are most likely multifactorial, including the drug or its metabolites being secreted in the tears, toxicity to the lacrimal gland, etc. Decreased vision is the most commonly reported adverse ocular event. Followed equally are ocular or periocular edema and anterior segment toxicity. Although edema is a known systemic side effect of these drugs, ocular and periocular edema may be secondary to drug-tear-related exposure.

Reports of extraocular muscle and ptosis disorders are difficult to evaluate because metastatic disease may be involved. Thirty-eight spontaneous reports of poliosis are a substantial number. This side effect has been described as secondary to various benign and malignant growths to both oral and topical medications. Bleeding and vascular events are also known systemic side effects of oral anti–vascular endothelial growth factor (VEGF) drugs. Insufficient data are available to evaluate the spontaneous reports of optic nerve pathology, uveitis, and macular edema.[3]

Recommendations

1. Patients started on this class of drugs should be told the signs and symptoms of retinal tears and detachments. They should be instructed to seek immediate ophthalmic consultation if these signs or symptoms occur.
2. If a serous retinal detachment is found, the drug may not necessarily need to be discontinued. Some of these drugs are given in a cyclic manner, and the serous detachment often resolves during the usual 2 weeks without the drug in the prescribing cycle (pazopanib, sunitinib).
3. The next generation of oral anti-VEGF drugs should have a similar ocular side effect panel as presented here. We do not know which retinal side effects are real, but they need close observation. This requires better differentiation of retinal findings (type of retinal detachments).

Generic Name:

Pemetrexed disodium.

Proprietary Name:

Alimta.

Primary Use

Pyrimidine-based antifolate used in the treatment of mesothelioma and non–small cell cancers.

Ocular Side Effects

Systemic administration – intravenous

Certain

1. Edema
   a. Eyelid (Fig. 15.16)
   b. Periorbital
   c. Orbital

Probable

1. Conjunctivitis
2. Lacrimation

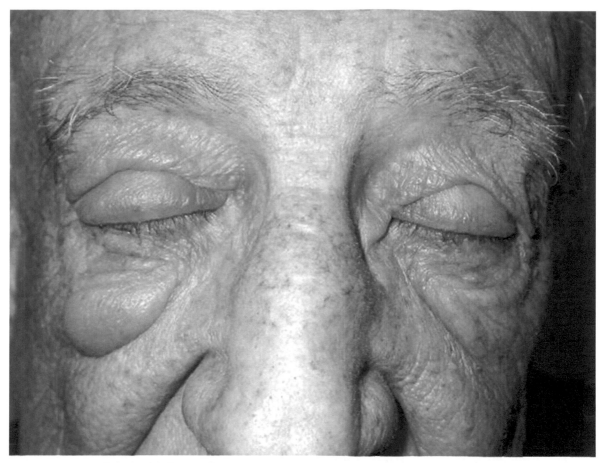

FIG. 15.16 Edema of the lower eyelids 10 days after the first dose of pemetrexed.[4]

Clinical Significance

This drug is fairly unique in causing significant eyelid edema after only a few daily intravenous injections of a 21-day therapy cycle and occurring as late as during the 16th cycle. The incidence is estimated at around 2.3%.[1,2] Approximately half of the cases are bilateral. There are multiple reports of positive rechallenge. In some cases, swelling of the feet also occurs. The vast majority of this edema resolves on its own once the medication is discontinued. However, there is 1 case reported by Mangla et al and 4 cases in the spontaneous reports where the edema did not resolve.[3] Surgery may be necessary. Although the pathogenesis of this swelling is unknown, the drug does cause capillary protein leakage resulting in soft tissue and nonmalignant effusions. The anatomy of the periocular area, especially with age and loss of elasticity of the tissue, is an ideal location to allow edema to cause significant anatomic changes.

Conjunctivitis is uncommon and rarely seen after a few cycles of therapy. Epiphora is also rare and usually occurs shortly after starting therapy.

Generic Name:

Raloxifene hydrochloride.

Proprietary Name:

Evista.

Primary Use

Used in postmenopausal women in the treatment and prevention of osteoporosis. Also, a prophylaxis for postmenopausal women with osteoporosis for invasive breast cancer or for those at high risk for developing this cancer.

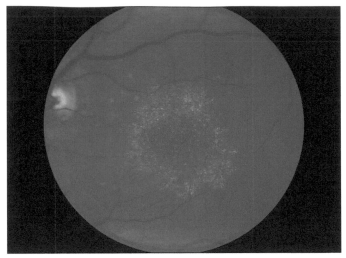

FIG. 15.17 Tamoxifen retinopathy with intraretinal white deposits.[24]

Ocular Side Effects
Systemic administration – oral
Probable
1. Cataracts
2. Conjunctivitis - nonspecific

Possible
1. Retina
   a. Venous thrombosis
   b. Vein occlusion

Clinical Significance
Vogel et al, in a large prospective, double-blind, randomized clinical trial (STAR P-2), showed a statistically significant incidence of cataracts for both tamoxifen and raloxifene.[1] However, the data showed a 21% lower rate of cataract development and an 18% lower rate of cataract surgery in patients on raloxifene compared with patients on tamoxifen. They also reported a possible slight increase in nonspecific conjunctivitis and venous thromboembolism during the first 4 months of therapy.

In the *Physicians' Desk Reference* (PDR) there is a black box warning of increased risk of deep venous thrombosis and pulmonary embolism.[2] There are 5 cases of possible vascular retinopathy associated with this drug.[3] There are over 150 cases of retinal vascular events in the spontaneous reports.

Siesky et al studied 24 postmenopausal women in a cross-sectional study with 12 receiving placebo and 12 receiving raloxifene daily for 3 months.[4] They found no impact on intraocular pressure, ocular blood flow, visual acuity, or contrast sensitivity.

Generic Name:
Tamoxifen citrate.

Proprietary Names:
Nolvadex, Soltamox.

Primary Use
Tamoxifen is a first-generation selective estrogen receptor inhibitor in the palliative treatment of breast carcinoma, ovarian cancer, pancreatic cancer, and malignant melanoma. It is also used as an adjuvant therapy for early and late-stage breast cancer.

Ocular Side Effects
Systemic administration – oral
Certain
1. Decreased vision
2. Corneal opacities
   a. Whorl-like, subepithelial
   b. Calcium
   c. Map dot
3. Retina or macula (Fig. 15.17 and Fig. 15.18)
   a. Superficial yellow-white refractile opacities – inner retinal layers
   b. Punctate gray lesions – outer retinal layers and pigment epithelium
   c. Edema
   d. Degeneration

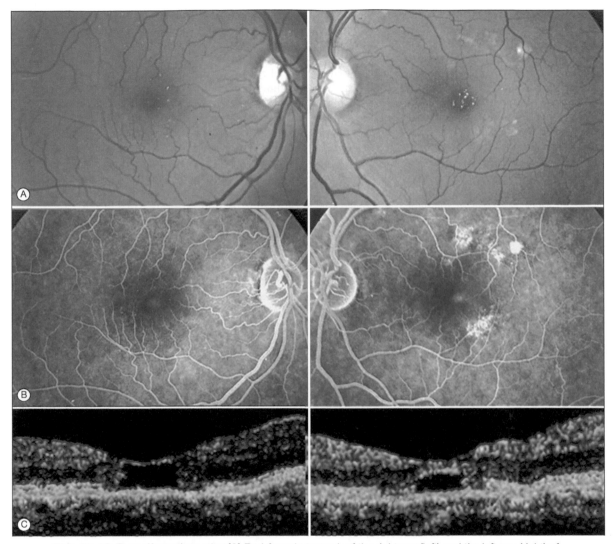

FIG. 15.18 Tamoxifen retinopathy. **(A)** Red-free photograph of the right eye (left) and the left eye (right) of a 64-year-old woman showing tamoxifen retinopathy with tiny refractile crystalline deposits in the macula. **(B)** Fluorescein angiography shows foveolar hyperfluorescence. Several patchy areas of hyperfluorescence are also present around the macula. **(C)** A horizontal OCT scan showed a foveolar cystoid space, combined with focal disruption of the photoreceptor line. Macular thickness was measured with calipers at 175 μm at the center.[15]

e. Pigmentary changes
f. Hemorrhages
4. Posterior subcapsular cataracts
5. Color vision defect

Probable

1. Visual fields
   a. Constriction
   b. Paracentral scotoma

Possible

1. Macular hole

Clinical Significance

Tamoxifen has 30-plus years of clinical use, and there is an extensive, ever-changing adverse ocular profile for it. Gallicchio et al reported an incidence of 13% of tamoxifen users having an adverse ocular side effect.[1] They have shown that women who complain of visual side effects have high serum blood levels of tamoxifen and its metabolite, N-desmethyltamoxifen, compared with those without visual complaints. Gorin et al reported the largest series of more detailed ocular-studied patients.[2,3] Although it is clear that tamoxifen can affect vision and the eye, serious side effects are rare and primarily at high doses. Serious effects are seldom seen at total dosages of less than 10 g. However, in highly susceptive individuals, at only a few grams, ocular side effects have been seen. More extensive retinal and corneal findings were evident when the drug was given at daily doses of up to 180 mg per day (standard dosage is 20 mg per day or less). At lower dosages, the severity, incidence, and reversibility of ocular complications are significantly lower. In a prospective study by Pavlidis et al at higher tamoxifen doses, 6.3% of patients developed keratopathy or retinopathy.[4] However, most incidence levels in the literature are in the 1–2% range. Tamoxifen is secreted in the tears, which may cause reduced vision, photophobia, and ocular irritation. Corneal deposits are seldom of major clinical significance and are typically white, whorl-like, subepithelial corneal deposits. These deposits are similar to other amphiphilic-like compounds, such as chloroquine and amiodarone, and they are reversible; however, Andreanos et al reported a case in which there was still no clearing 4 years after the initial drug withdrawal.[5] Hollander et al felt these are usually dose related.[6] On rare occasions, hypercalcemia developed with associated tamoxifen corneal changes.

Gorin et al were the first to do a long-term, follow-up study that included a tamoxifen exposed and unexposed group.[2,3] This study included a standardized clinical examination of the lens. They found a markedly elevated risk for posterior subcapsular cataracts. Fisher et al reported an increased risk of cataract surgery for women on tamoxifen versus women on placebo.[7] Paganini-Hill et al found a 70% increase in cataracts for long-term users of tamoxifen compared with those never exposed to this drug.[8] Bradbury et al, in a large matched case-controlled study done by family practitioners, found no increased risk of cataracts, but no systematic ophthalmic examinations were performed.[9] Gorin et al were also the first to describe subclinical color discrimination in women on long-term tamoxifen.[2,3] Eisner et al studied these phenomena using various sophisticated electrophysiologic techniques, showing changes in both the peripheral and central retina.[10–12] To date, these changes are reversible and subclinical.

Typical tamoxifen retinopathy (i.e. striking white-to-yellow refractile bodies perimacular and temporal to the macula) most commonly occurs after 1+ years of therapy with at least 100+ g of the drug.[13] Bourla et al reported that at higher dosages peripheral crystalline retinopathy may occur.[14] There are a number of cases in the spontaneous reporting systems and in the literature of minimal retinal pigmentary changes without visual loss, occurring after a few months with only a few grams of tamoxifen. Retinal deposits may be associated with cystoid macular edema, punctate macular RPE changes, parafoveal hemorrhages, and peripheral reticular pigment changes. These deposits are refractile bodies located in the inner retina and histologically may be the products of axonal degeneration. Gualino et al suggested that tamoxifen maculopathy may include the cystoid space different from macular edema.[15] The lesions do not appear to regress if the drug is discontinued. Doshi et al suggested "crystalline retinopathy represents an earlier manifestation of Müller cell damage while cavitation represents a later stage of atrophy in which both crystals and Müller cell architecture have degenerated."[16] Gorin et al, using a single-masked treatment and placebo cohort study, showed a low risk for tamoxifen-related retinal toxicity.[3] Loss of visual acuity in this chronic form of maculopathy is often progressive, dose dependent, and irreversible unless the cystoid macular edema or hemorrhage is the cause of the visual loss. Retinopathy due to tamoxifen can be seen without refractile bodies being present. Park et al pointed out microcystic maculopathy due to tamoxifen can be diagnosed by Fourier-domain OCT in normal-appearing fundi, which may, in some cases, explain visual loss.[17] Cronin et al and Hu et al suggested a link, although a rare finding, between tamoxifen use and the development of macular holes.[18,19] There are 7 possible cases of macular holes associated with tamoxifen usage in the spontaneous reporting systems. Kalina et al pointed out that idiopathic juxtafoveal retinal telangiectasias can also be confused with tamoxifen retinopathy.[20] Gorin et al showed that tamoxifen is associated with thromboembolic events in large vessels, but they found little evidence for this occurring in small vessels as in the eye.[2] The incidence of retinal occlusive disease due to tamoxifen in their study was consistent with chance.

What effect tamoxifen has on the optic nerve is uncertain. In the literature and in the spontaneous reporting systems, there are reports of unilateral and bilateral optic neuritis or neuropathy. It is uncertain if these are drug-related events. There are cases of optic-nerve pallor and atrophy.[21] Eisner et al have documented some subclinical swelling of the optic nerve in women with small optic cups, possibly secondary to the action of this drug on estrogen receptors.[12] There is no evidence of any clinical effect in the optic nerve due to tamoxifen from this edema.

Recommendations

There are many who believe that low-dose tamoxifen (less than 10 g cumulative) causes few to no significant ocular side effects. They recommend not seeing an ophthalmologist until visual symptoms occur. At that point, even with retinal crystals, see the patient every 3 months and stay in close contact with the oncologist.[22] Gianni et al, through the American Cancer Society, do not recommend stated times for ocular examinations.[23] Rather, they recommend the patient be told the ocular signs and symptoms due to tamoxifen, "so that they may seek prompt ophthalmic evaluation for ocular complaints."

Guidelines for management (modified after Gorin et al)[2,3] include the following:

1. If requested, do a baseline examination within the first year of starting tamoxifen. This should include slit lamp biomicroscopy of the anterior and posterior segments. Baseline color vision testing should be done. Warn the patient to contact you at the first sign of any change in vision. Unexplained visual loss may require temporary cessation of therapy to evaluate cause and reversibility.
2. In keeping with the American Academy of Ophthalmology's current recommendations, in normal adults, do a complete eye examination at least every 2 years. More frequent examinations are recommended if ocular symptoms occur.
3. The discovery of a limited number of intraretinal crystals in the absence of macular edema or visual impairment does not seem to warrant discontinuation of the drug.
4. Significant color loss may be a valid reason to consider discontinuing the drug. Gorin et al recommend considering stopping the drug for 3 months (in patients on prophylactic therapy) and retesting.[2,3] If the color vision returns to normal, restart the drug and retest in 3 months. If at any time there is no rebound from stopping the drug or continued progression, then one may need to consult the oncologist and reevaluate the risk–benefit ratio.
5. The presence of posterior subcapsular cataracts is not an indication to stop the drug because the con-

dition usually progresses even if the drug is discontinued.
6. The presence of age-related maculopathy is not a contraindication to the use of tamoxifen. However, informed consent may be advisable in our litigious society.
7. Consultation with the oncologist is recommended if significant ocular findings occur.

Generic Name:
Thiotepa.

Proprietary Name:
Tepadina.

Primary Use
Systemic
This ethylenimine derivative is used in the management of carcinomas of the breast and ovary, lymphomas, Hodgkin disease, and various sarcomas.

Ophthalmic
This topical drug is used to inhibit pterygium recurrence and possibly to prevent corneal neovascularization after chemical injuries.

Ocular Side Effects
Systemic administration – intramuscular or intravenous
Certain
1. Decreased vision
2. Eyelids or conjunctiva
   a. Erythema
   b. Edema
   c. Urticaria
   d. Periorbital depigmentation

Possible
1. Loss of eyelashes or eyebrows
2. Hyperpigmentation
3. Ocular teratogenic effects

Local ophthalmic use or exposure – topical ocular application
Certain
1. Irritation
2. Eyelids or conjunctiva
   a. Edema
   b. Conjunctivitis – nonspecific
   c. Allergic reactions
   d. Depigmentation
   e. Poliosis

3. Cornea
   a. Edema
   b. Keratitis
   c. Delayed healing
   d. Ulceration
4. Occlusion of lacrimal punctum

Clinical Significance

Systemic thiotepa rarely has ocular side effects. The most common are decreased vision and eyelid or orbital edema, all of which are reversible. Periorbital pigmentation can occur.[1] Grant et al reported a single case of acute bilateral plastic uveitis.[2] There are no other cases of this in the spontaneous reports.

Topical ocular thiotepa may be contraindicated in dark-skinned individuals because permanent depigmentation of the eyelid or eyelashes can occur. Depigmentation may occur within a few weeks or at various times up to 6 years after exposure.[3-5] The depigmentation effect seems to be enhanced by excessive sunlight exposure and in rare cases can be permanent, especially in heavily pigmented skin.[6] Irritative reactions are common and dependent on dosage. Allergic reactions are rare.[7] Use of thiotepa for many months in dosages 4-6 times daily has caused keratitis. There are reports in the literature and in the spontaneous reports of punctal occlusion due to topical ocular use of this drug. Thiotepa probably retards wound healing and possibly retards corneal blood vessel ingrowth. It has been implicated in either causing or enhancing preexisting corneal ulceration.

Thiotepa can enter the bloodstream through the mucous membrane. Because the drug is potentially mutagenic and teratogenic, topical ocular application is contraindicated in pregnancy. The drug also has been shown to be carcinogenic.

Smith et al reviewed the limited ocular side effects data on intravitreal injection of thiotepa for retinoblastomas.[8]

Generic Name:

Trastuzumab.

Proprietary Name:

Herceptin.

Primary Use

Monoclonal antibody used primarily in adjuvant breast cancer, metastatic breast cancer, and metastatic gastric cancer. Off-label use with other anticancer drugs for breast and gastric cancers.

Ocular Side Effects

Systemic administration – intravenous

Probable

1. Decreased vision

Possible

1. Lacrimation
2. May aggravate or cause ocular sicca
3. Cornea
   a. Superficial punctate keratitis
   b. Ulceration
   c. Epithelial microcysts

Conditional/unclassified

1. Macular ischemia
2. Madarosis
3. Conjunctivitis

Clinical Significance

Trastuzumab should not be confused with trastuzumab emtansine, a completely different drug whose only ocular side effects may be conjunctivitis and possible limbal lesions.

Trastuzumab is difficult to pinpoint as to its ocular side effects because they are uncommon and seldom of major clinical significance. It is also often used in combination with other anticancer drugs. There are, however, many positive rechallenge cases, primarily with corneal pathology, which, in most all cases, clears after stopping the drug. Eaton et al gave an overview of this class of drugs, which may affect the ocular surface, causing transitory decreased vision, ocular sicca, and corneal epithelial microcysts.[1] Orlandi et al presented a case of persistent, bilateral corneal ulceration with infiltrates resistant to antibiotics and steroids.[2] The spontaneous reporting systems have 3 similar cases. Trastuzumab causes xerostomia, so it is likely to cause ocular sicca, with the early sign of this disease being increased lacrimation. Increased lacrimation may also be due to the drug or its metabolites being secreted in the tears, causing irritation.

There is 1 case of bilateral macular ischemia attributed to trastuzumab.[3] There are no spontaneous reports to support this.

Generic Name:

Vinblastine sulfate.

Proprietary Name:

Velban.

Primary Use

Primarily used for inoperable malignant neoplasms of the breast, the female genital tract, the lungs, the testis, and the gastrointestinal tract.

Ocular Side Effects

Systemic administration – intravenous

Probable

1. Photosensitivity

Possible

1. Nystagmus
2. May aggravate or cause ocular sicca

Inadvertent ocular exposure

Probable

1. Irritation
   a. Lacrimation
   b. Hyperemia
   c. Photophobia
   d. Edema
2. Cornea
   a. Keratitis
   b. Superficial gray opacities
   c. Edema
   d. Ulceration
   e. Subepithelial scarring
3. Blepharospasm
4. Decreased vision
5. May aggravate or cause ocular sicca

Possible

1. Nystagmus
2. Diplopia
3. Ptosis

Clinical Significance

Intravenous vinblastine only rarely may cause "possible" ocular side effects. Photosensitivity or phototoxic reactions to the skin are the most likely.[1] Nystagmus and, rarely, diplopia have been mentioned as unproven adverse ocular side effects; however, because significant vestibular toxicity can occur from this drug, these may possibly be drug related.[2] The drug or its metabolites are probably secreted in the tears; therefore sicca symptoms may be aggravated.

The accidental splashing of vinblastine, which causes characteristic keratopathy, is the main ophthalmic interest with this drug. This includes microcystic edema, superficial punctate keratitis, and corneal erosion with or without low-grade anterior uveitis. Corneal epithelial damage is usually apparent within the first few days along with decreased vision. The keratitis resolves within weeks to months.[3,4] Some cases develop ocular sicca, some show opacities in the area of Bowman's layer, and some have become permanent. Ocular sicca may be caused by severe initial inflammation or vinblastine-induced neuropathy.[3]

Generic Name:

Vincristine sulfate.

Proprietary Names:

Oncovin, Vincasar PFS.

Primary Use

Primarily used in the treatment of Hodgkin disease, lymphosarcoma, reticulum cell sarcoma, rhabdomyosarcoma, neuroblastoma, and Wilms tumor.

Ocular Side Effects

Systemic administration – intravenous

Certain

1. Extraocular muscles
   a. Ptosis (Fig. 15.19)
   b. Paresis or paralysis
   c. Diplopia
   d. Nystagmus
   e. Lagophthalmos
2. Decreased corneal reflexes
3. Visual hallucinations

Probable

1. Optic nerve
   a. Retrobulbar or optic neuritis
   b. Atrophy
2. Visual fields
   a. Scotomas – central or centrocecal
   b. Constriction
   c. Hemianopsia
3. Cortical blindness
4. Nystagmus

Possible

1. Loss of eyelashes or eyebrows
2. Decreased accommodation
3. Color vision defect – red-green defect
4. Decreased dark adaptation
5. Ocular signs of gout

Clinical Significance

Vincristine neurotoxicity is dose related; if recognized, at least 80% of the drug-induced side effects are reversible. The reversibility is variable even at a reduced

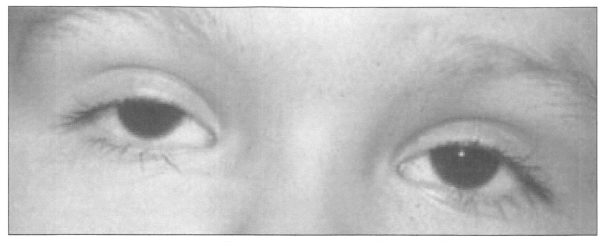

FIG. 15.19 Bilateral ptosis after treatment with vincristine.[5]

dosage. The most common ocular side effect involves the cranial nerves and may be manifested by ptosis, extraocular muscle palsies, internuclear ophthalmoplegia, corneal anesthesia, and lagophthalmos occurring in one form or another in up to 50% of the cases.[1-3] These findings may occur acutely or gradually. Ptosis may be the only presenting sign of neurotoxicity, and it may be unilateral or bilateral.[4] Müller et al reported the benefits of pyridoxine and pyridostigmine therapy to improve vincristine-induced ptosis.[5] Optic neuropathy has been reported with vincristine, which can improve in some cases if the drug is discontinued.[6,7] There are numerous additional cases of possible vincristine-associated optic atrophy and resultant blindness.[1,5,8-11] Most patients were also on other anticancer drugs. An additional 35 cases of optic neuropathy with visual loss are in the spontaneous reports. These cases often involved additional anticancer drugs. Optic neuropathy may not be dose related, and recovery is variable. Optic nerve toxicity is rare and may be an idiopathic response to the drug. Its onset is usually slow and progressive, but Teichmann et al reports a case of acute onset.[10] Retinal damage can occur based on autopsy findings.[6,12] Transient cortical blindness has also been reported, with recovery in 1-14 days.[13,14] The latter case showed transient neuroradiologic lesions in the occipital cortex. The ocular signs of gout that may occur include conjunctival hyperemia, uveitis, scleritis, and corneal deposits or ulcerations. Ripps et al extensively studied a patient who developed night blindness after vincristine therapy.[15] They felt that this drug interferes with the transmission between the photoreceptors and their second-order neurons.

REFERENCES
Drug: Alemtuzumab
1. Dick AD, Meyer P, James T, et al. Campath-1H therapy in refractive ocular inflammatory disease. *Br J Ophthalmol.* 2000;84:107–109.
2. Coles AJ, Wing M, Smith S, et al. Pulsed monoclonal antibody treatment and autoimmune thyroid disease in multiple sclerosis. *Lancet.* 1999;345:1691–1695.
3. Coles AJ, Twyman CL, Arnold DL, et al. Alemtuzumab for patients with relapsing multiple sclerosis after disease-modifying therapy: a randomized controlled phase 3 trial. *Lancet.* 2012;380(9856):1829–1839.
4. Gilbert D, Vladic A, Brinar V, et al. Alemtuzumab-related thyroid dysfunction in a phase 2 trial of patients with relapsing-remitting multiple sclerosis. *J Clin Endocrinol Metab.* 2014;99:80–89.
5. Trinh T, Haridas AS, Sullivan TJ. Ocular findings in alemtuzumab (Campath 1-H)-induced thyroid eye disease. *Ophthal Plast Reconstr Surg.* 2016;32(6): 3128–e129.
6. Willis MD, Pickersgill TP, Robertson NP, et al. Alemtuzumab-induced remission of multiple sclerosis-associated uveitis. *Int Ophthalmol.* 2017;37(5):1229–1233.
7. Weetman AP. Graves' disease following immune reconstitution or immunomodulatory treatment: should we manage it any differently? *Clin Endocrinol.* 2014;80:629–632.
8. Song WK, Min YH, Kim YR, et al. Cytomegalovirus retinitis after hematopoietic stem cell transplantation with alemtuzumab. *Ophthalmology.* 2008;115:1766–1770.
9. Tang SC, Hewitt K, Reis MD, et al. Immunosuppressive toxicity of CAMPATH1H monoclonal antibody in the treatment of patients with recurrent low grade lymphoma. *Leuk Lymphoma.* 1996;24:93–101.
10. Derzko-Dzulynsky LA, Berger AR, Berinstein NL. Cytomegalovirus retinitis and low-grade non-Hodgkin's lym-

phoma: case report and review of the literature. *Am J Hematol.* 1998;57:228–232.

11. Borthakur G, Lin E, Faderl S, et al. Low serum albumin level is associated with cytomegalovirus reactivation in patients with chronic lymphoproliferative diseased treated with alemtuzumab (Camphath-1H)-based therapies. *Cancer.* 2007;110:2478–2483.

12. Chakrabart S, Mackinnon S, Chopra R, et al. High incidence of cytomegalovirus infection after nonmyeloablative stem cell transplantation: potential role of Campath-1H in delaying immune reconstitution. *Blood.* 2002;99:4357–4363.

13. Alemtuzumab. 2018. Retrieved from http://www.pdr.net.

Drugs: Atezolizumab, ipilimumab, nivolumab, pembrolizumab

1. Mantopoulos D, Kendra KL, Letson AD, et al. Bilateral choroidopathy and serous retinal detachments during ipilimumab treatment for cutaneous melanoma. *JAMA Ophthalmol.* 2015;133(8):965–967.

2. Diem S, Keller F, Ruesch R, et al. Pembrolizumab-triggered uveitis: an additional surrogate marker for responders in melanoma immunotherapy. *J Immunother.* 2016;39(9):379–382.

3. Fierz FC, Meier F, Chaloupka K, et al. Intraocular inflammation associated with new therapies for cutaneous melanoma: case series and review. *Klin Monbl Augenheilkd.* 2016;233(4):540–544.

4. Hahn L. Bilateral neuroretinitis and anterior uveitis following ipilimumab treatment for metastatic melanoma. *J Ophthalmic Inflamm Infect.* 2016;6(1):14.

5. Papavasileiou E, Prasad S, Freitag SK, et al. Ipilimumab-induced ocular and orbital inflammation: a case series and review of the literature. *Ocul Immunol Inflamm.* 2016;24(2):140–146.

6. Zimmer L, Goldinger SM, Hofmann L, et al. Neurological, respiratory, musculoskeletal, cardiac and ocular side-effects of anti-PD-1 therapy. *Eur J Cancer.* 2016;60:210–225.

7. Pham CM, Kalyam K, Smith BT, et al. Acute angle closure precipitated by hemorrhage and necrosis of a large uveal melanoma in the setting of systemic immunomodulatory therapy. *Ocul Oncol Pathol.* 2017;3(4):254–258.

8. Min L, Vaidaya A, Becker C. Thyroid autoimmunity and ophthalmopathy related to melanoma biologic therapy. *Eur J Endocrinol.* 2011;164(2):303–307.

9. Lecouflet M, Verschoore M, Giard C, et al. Orbital myositis associated with ipilimumab. *Ann Dermatol Venereol.* 2013;140(6-7):448–451.

10. McElnea E, Ni Mhealoid A, Moran S, et al. Thyroid-like ophthalmopathy in a euthyroid patient receiving ipilimumab. *Orbit.* 2014;33(6):424–427.

11. Henderson AD, Thomas DA. A case report of orbital inflammatory syndrome secondary to ipilimumab. *Ophthal Plast Reconstr Surg.* 2015;31(3):e68–e70.

12. Sheldon CA, Kharlip J, Tamhankar MA. Inflammatory orbitopathy associated with ipilimumab. *Ophthal Plast Reconstr Surg.* 2017;33(3S):S155–S158.

13. Nguyen AT, Elia M, Materin MA, et al. Cyclosporine for dry eye associated with nivolumab: a case progressing to corneal perforation. *Cornea.* 2016;35:399–401.

14. Dein E, Sharfman W, Kim J, et al. Two cases of sinusitis induced by immune checkpoint inhibition. *J Immunother.* 2017;40(8):312–314.

15. Crews J, Agarwal A, Jack L, et al. Ipilimumab-associated retinopathy. *Ophthalmic Surg Lasers Imaging Retina.* 2015;46(6):658–660.

16. Hanna KS. A rare case of pembrolizumab-induced uveitis in a patient with metastatic melanoma. *Pharmacotherapy.* 2016;36(11):e183–e188.

17. Roberts P, Fishman GA, Joshi K, et al. Chorioretinal lesions in a case of melanoma-associated retinopathy treated with pembrolizumab. *JAMA Ophthalmol.* 2016;134(10):1184–1188.

18. Theillac C, Straub M, Breton AL, et al. Bilateral uveitis and macular edema induced by nivolumab: a case report. *BMC Ophthalmol.* 2017;17(1):227.

19. Conrady CD, Larochelle M, Pecen P, et al. Checkpoint inhibitor-induced uveitis: a case series. *Graefes Arch Clin Exp Ophthalmol.* 2018;256(1):187–191.

20. Modjtahedi BS, Maibach H, Park S. Multifocal bilateral choroidal neovascularization in a patient on ipilimumab for metastatic melanoma. *Cutan Ocul Toxicol.* 2013;32(4):341–343.

21. Yeh OL, Francis CE. Ipilimumab-associated bilateral optic neuropathy. *J Neuroophthalmol.* 2015;35(2):144–147.

22. Abu Samra K, Valdes-Navarro M, Lee S, et al. A case of bilateral uveitis and papillitis in a patient treated with pembrolizumab. *Eur J Ophthalmol.* 2016;26(3):e46–e48.

23. Boisseau W, Touat M, Berzero G, et al. Safety of treatment with nivolumab after ipilimumab-related meningoradiculitis and bilateral optic neuropathy. *Eur J Cancer.* 2017;83:28–31.

24. Crosson JN, Laird PW, Debiec M, et al. Vogt-Koyanagi-Harada-like syndrome after CTLA-4 inhibition with ipilimumab for metastatic melanoma. *J Immunother.* 2015;38(2):80–84.

25. Arai T, Harada K, Usui Y, et al. Case of acute uveitis and Vogt-Koyanagi-Harada syndrome-like eruptions induced by nivolumab in a melanoma patient. *J Dermatol.* 2017;44(8):975–976.

26. Bricout M, Petre A, Amini-Adle M, et al. Vogt-Koyanagi-Harada-like syndrome complicating pembrolizumab treatment for metastatic melanoma. *J Immunother.* 2017;40(2):77–82.

27. Matsuo T, Yamasaki O. Vogt-Koyanagi-Harada disease-like posterior uveitis in the course of nivolumab (anti-PD-1 antibody), interposed by vemurafenib (BRAF inhibitor), for metastatic cutaneous malignant melanoma. *Clin Case Rep.* 2017;5(5):694–700.

28. Ipilimumab, nivolumab, pembrolizumab, atezolizumab. 2019. Retrieved from http://www.pdr.net.

29. Wolner ZJ, Marghoob AAK, Pulitzer MP, et al. A case report of disappearing pigmented skin lesions associated with pembrolizumab treatment for metastatic melanoma. *Br J Dermatol.* 2018;178(1):265–269.

30. Johnson DB, Saranga-Perry V, Lavin PJ, et al. Myasthenia gravis induced by ipilimumab in patients with metastatic melanoma. *J Clin Oncol.* 2015;33(33):e122–e124.

31. Montes V, Sousa S, Pita F, et al. Myasthenia gravis induced by ipilimumab in a patient with advanced melanoma. *Eur J Neuro.* 2016;23(suppl 2):548.

32. Nguyen BH, Kuo J, Budiman A, et al. Two cases of clinical myasthenia gravis associated with pembrolizumab use in responding melanoma patients. *Melanoma Res.* 2017;27(2):152–154.

33. Earl DE, Loochtan AI, Bedlack RS. Refractory myasthenia gravis exacerbation triggered by pembrolizumab. *Muscle Nerve.* 2018;57(4):E120–E121.

34. Pushkarevskaya A, Neuberger U, Dimitrakopoulou-Strauss A, et al. Severe ocular myositis after ipilimumab treatment for melanoma: a report of 2 cases. *J Immunother.* 2017;40(7):282–285.

35. Diamantopoulos PT, Tsatsou K, Benopoulou O, et al. Inflammatory myopathy and axonal neuropathy in a patient with melanoma following pembrolizumab treatment. *J Immunother.* 2017;40(6):221–223.

36. Ruff MW, Mauermann ML. The Mayo Clinic experience with the neurological complications of the CTLA-4 inhibitor ipilimumab. *Neurologist.* 2018;23(3):98–99.

37. Pembrolizumab Hsiao. induced acute corneal toxicity after allogeneic stem cell transplantation. *Clin Exp Ophthalmol.* 2018;46(6):698–700.

38. Tsui E, Madu A, Belinsky I, et al. Combination ipilimumab and nivolumab for metastatic melanoma associated with ciliochoroidal effusion and exudative retinal detachment. *JAMA Ophthalmol.* 2017;135:1455–1457.

39. Dalvin LA, Shields CL, Orloff M, et al. Checkpoint inhibitor immune therapy: systemic indications and ophthalmic side effects. *Retina.* 2018;38:1063–1078.

Drugs: Binimetinib, cobimetinib, trametinib

1. Urner-Bloch U, Urner M, Stieger P, et al. Transient MEK inhibitor-associated retinopathy in metastatic melanoma. *Ann Oncol.* 2014;25(7):1437–1441.

2. van Dikj EH, van Herpen CM, Marinkovic M, et al. Serous retinopathy associated with mitogen-activated protein kinase inhibition (binimetinib) for metastatic cutaneous and uveal melanoma. *Ophthalmology.* 2015;122(9):1907–1916.

3. Weber ML, Liang MC, Flaherty KT, et al. Subretinal fluid associated with MEK inhibitor use in the treatment of systemic cancer. *JAMA Ophthalmol.* 2016;134(8):855–862.

4. Francis JH, Habib LA, Abramson DH, et al. Clinical and morphologic characteristics of MEK inhibitor-associated retinopathy. *Ophthalmology.* 2017;124(12):1788–1798.

5. Joshi L, Karydis A, Gemenetzi M, et al. Uveitis as a result of MAP kinase pathway inhibition. *Case Rep Ophthalmol.* 2013;4(3):279–282.

6. Draganova D, Kerger J, Caspers L, et al. Severe bilateral panuveitis during melanoma treatment by dabrafenib and trametinib. *J Ophthalmic Inflamm Infect.* 2015;5(6):17.

7. Sarny S, Neumayer M, Kofler J, et al. Ocular toxicity due to trametinib and dabrafenib. *BMC Ophthalmol.* 2017;17(1):146.

8. Lyons YA, Frumovitz M, Soliman PT. Response to MEK inhibitor in small cell neuroendocrine carcinoma of the cervix with a KRAS mutation. *Gynecol Oncol Rep.* 2014;10:28–29.

Drugs: Bleomycin sulfate, dactinomycin, daunorubicin hydrochloride, doxorubicin hydrochloride

1. Curran CF, Luce JK. Ocular adverse reactions associated with Adriamycin (doxorubicin). *Am J Ophthalmol.* 1989;108(6):709–711.

2. Wickremasinghe S, Dansingani KK, Tranos P, et al. Ocular presentations of breast cancer. *Acta Ophthalmol Scand.* 2007;85(2):133–142.

3. Blum R. An overview of studies with adriamycin in the United States. *Cancer Chemother Rep.* 1975;6:247–251.

4. Bleomycin sulfate, dactinomycin, daunorubicin hydrochloride, doxorubicin hydrochloride. 2018. Retrieved from http://www.pdr.net.

5. Young DC, Mitchell A, Kessler J, et al. Cortical blindness and seizures possibly related to cisplatin, vinblastine, and bleomycin treatment of ovarian dysgerminoma. *J Am Osteopath Assoc.* 1993;93:502–504.

6. McLoon LK, Wirtschafter J. Doxorubicin chemomyectomy: injection of monkey orbicularis oculi results in selective muscle injury. *Inv Ophthalmol Vis Sci.* 1988;29(12):1854–1859.

Drug: Bortezomib

1. Grob SR, Jakobiec FA, Rashid A, et al. Chalazia associated with bortezomib therapy for multiple myeloma. *Ophthalmology.* 2014;121(9):1845–1847.

2. Fraunfelder FW, Yang HK. Association between bortezomib therapy and eyelid chalazia. *JAMA Ophthalmol.* 2016;134(1):88–90.

3. Min CK, Lee S, Kim YJ, et al. Cutaneous leucoclastic vasculitis (LV) following bortezomib therapy in a myeloma patient; association with pro-inflammatory cytokines. *Eur J Haematol.* 2006;76:265–268.

4. Toema B, El-Sweilmeen H, Helmy T. Oculomotor nerve palsy associated with bortezomib in a patient with multiple myeloma: a case report. *J Med Case Rep.* 2010;4:342.

5. Chacko JG, Behbehani R, Hundley KN, et al. Bortezomib-associated optic atrophy in two patients with multiple myeloma. *J Neuro-Ophthalmol.* 2018;38:473–475.

Drugs: Bromocriptine mesylate, cabergoline

1. Taxel P, Waitzman DM, Harrington Jr JF, et al. Chiasmal herniation as a complication of bromocriptine therapy. *J Neuroophthalmol.* 1996;16(4):252–257.

2. Raverot G, Jacob M, Jouanneau E, et al. Secondary deterioration of visual field during cabergoline treatment for macroprolactinoma. *Clin Endocrinol.* 2009;70(4):588–592.

3. Jones SE, James RA, Hall K, et al. Optic chiasmal herniation, an under recognized complication of dopamine agonist therapy for macroprolactinoma. *Clin Endocrinol.* 2000;53:529–534.
4. Chuman H, Cornblath WT, Trobe JD, et al. Delayed visual loss following pergolide treatment of a prolactinoma. *J Neuroophthalmol.* 2002;22(2):102–106.
5. Zhang N, Guo L, Ge J, et al. Endoscopic transsphenoidal treatment of a prolactinoma patient with brain and optic chiasmal herniations. *J Craniofacial Surg.* 2014;25(3):e271–e272.
6. Alvarez Berastegui GR, Raza SM, Anand VK, et al. Endonasal endoscopic transsphenoidal chiasmapexy using a clival cranial base cranioplasty for visual loss from massive empty sella following macroprolactinoma treatment with bromocriptine: case report. *J Neurosurg.* 2016;124(4):1025–1031.
7. Papanastasiou L, Fountoulakis S, Pappa T, et al. Brain and optic chiasmal herniation following cabergoline treatment for a giant prolactinoma: wait or intervene? *Hormones.* 2014;13(2):290–295.
8. Razmjoo H, Rezaei L, Dehghani A, et al. Bilateral angle-closure glaucoma in a young female receiving cabergoline: a case report. *Case Rep Ophthalmol.* 2011;2:30–33.
9. Nagaki Y, Hayasaka S, Hiraki S, et al. Central retinal vein occlusion in a woman receiving bromocriptine. *Ophthalmologica.* 1997;211(6):397–398.

Drug: Busulfan
1. Sidi Y, Douer D, Pinkhas J. Sicca syndrome in a patient with toxic reaction to busulfan. *JAMA.* 1977;238:1951.
2. Busulfan. 2018. Retrieved from http://www.pdr.net.
3. Honda A, Dake Y, Amemiya T. Cataracts in a patient treated with busulfan (Mablin powder) for eight years. *Nippon Ganka Gakkai Zasshi Acta Societatis.* 1993;97(1):1242–1245.
4. Shi-Xia X, Xian-Hua T, Hai-Qin X, et al. Total body irradiation plus cyclophosphamide versus busulphan with cyclophosphamide as conditioning regimen for patients with leukemia undergoing allogeneic stem cell transplantation: a meta-analysis. *Leuk Lymphoma.* 2010;51(1):50–60.
5. Holmström G, Borgström B, Calissendorff B. Cataract in children after bone marrow transplantation: relation to conditioning regimen. *Acta Ophthalmol Scand.* 2002;80:211–215.
6. Kaida T, Ogawa T, Amemiya T. Cataract induced by short term administration of large doses of busulfan: a case report. *Ophthalmologica.* 1999;213:397–399.
7. Al-Tweigeri T, Nabholtz JM, Mackey JR. Ocular toxicity and cancer chemotherapy. *Cancer.* 1996;78:1359–1373.

Drug: Capecitabine
1. Capecitabine. The American Society of Health-System Pharmacists. 15 April 2016.
2. Capecitabine. 2018. Retrieved from http://www.pdr.net.

3. Tsoucalas GI, Tzovaras AA, Ntokou AP, et al. Dacryoscintigraphy for the detection of ocular drainage system stenosis induced by docetaxel and fluorouracil. *Hell J Nucl Med.* 2012;15(2):159–161.
4. Noguchi Y, Mitani T, Kawara H, et al. A case of lacrimal duct obstruction caused by capecitabine. *Gan To Kagaku Ryoho.* 2015;42(1):123–125.
5. Waikhom B, Fraunfelder FT, Henner WD. Severe ocular irritation and corneal deposits associated with capecitabine use. *N Engl J Med.* 2000;343:1428.
6. Zarfoss M, Bentley E, Milovancev M, et al. Histopathologic evidence of capecitabine corneal toxicity in dogs. *Vet Pathol.* 2007;44(5):700–702.
7. Shah RJ, Choudhry N, Leiderman YI. Purtscher-like retinopathy in association with metastatic pancreatic adenocarcinoma and capecitabine therapy. *Retin Cases Brief Rep.* 2013;7(3):196–197.
8. Dasgupta S, Adilieje C, Bhattacharya A. et al. Capecitabine and sixth cranial nerve palsy. *J Cancer Res Ther.* 2010;6(1):80–81.

Drug: Carboplatin
1. Carboplatin. 2018. Retrieved from http://www.pdr.net.
2. Mulvihill A, Budning A, Jay V, et al. Ocular motility changes after subtenon carboplatin chemotherapy for retinoblastoma. *Arch Ophthalmol.* 2003;121:1120–1124.
3. Schmack I, Hubbard B, Kang SJ, et al. Ischemic necrosis and atrophy of the optic nerve after periocular carboplatin injection for intraocular retinoblastoma. *Am J Ophthalmol.* 2006;142(2):310–315.
4. Kim JW, Yau JW, Moshfeghi D, et al. Orbital fibrosis and intraocular recurrence of retinoblastoma following periocular carboplatin. *J Pediatr Ophthalmol Strabismus.* 2011;48:e1–e4.
5. Lauer AK, Wobig JL, Shults WT, et al. Severe ocular and orbital toxicity after intracarotid etoposide phosphate and carboplatin therapy. *Am J Ophthalmol.* 1999;127(2):230–233.
6. Watanabe W, Kuwabara R, Nakahara T, et al. Severe ocular and orbital toxicity after intracarotid injection of carboplatin for recurrent glioblastomas. *Graefes Arch Clin Exp Ophthalmol.* 2002;240:1033–1035
7. Zegans M, Gonzalez-Fernandez F, Newman S. Carboplatin retinal toxicity. *ARVO Invest Ophthalmol Vis Sci Annual Meeting Abstract.* 1997;906(27):1448.

Drug: Carmustine
1. Carmustine. 2018. Retrieved from http://www.pdr.net.
2. Imperia PS, Lazarus HM, Lass JH. Ocular complications of systemic cancer chemotherapy. *Surv Ophthalmol.* 1989;34(3):209–230.
3. Greenberg HS, Ensminger WD, Chandler WF, et al. Intra-arterial BCNU chemotherapy for treatment of malignant gliomas of the central nervous system. *J Neurosurg.* 1984;61:423–429.

4. Grimson BS, Mahaley MS, Dubey HD, et al. Ophthalmic and central nervous system complications following intracarotid BCNU (Carmustine). *J Clin Neuroophthalmol.* 1981;1:261–264.

5. Al-Tweigeri T, Nubholtz TM, Mackey JR. Ocular toxicity and cancer chemotherapy. *Cancer.* 1996;78:1359–1373.

6. Walsh TJ, Clark AW, Parhad IM, et al. Neurotoxic effects of cisplatin therapy. *Arch Neurol.* 1982;39:719–720.

7. Wang MY, Arnold AC, Vinters HV, et al. Bilateral blindness and lumbosacral myelopathy associated with high dose carmustine and cisplatin therapy. *Am J Ophthalmol.* 2000;120:297–368.

8. Singleton BJ, Bienfang DC, Albert DM, et al. Ocular toxicity associated with high dose carmustine. *Arch Ophthalmol.* 1982;100:1766–1772.

9. Miller DF, Bay JW, Lederman RJ, et al. Ocular and orbital toxicity following intracarotid injection of BCNU (Carmustine) and cisplatinum for malignant gliomas. *Ophthalmology.* 1985;92:402–406.

10. Johnson DW, Cagnoni PJ, Schossau TM, et al. Optic disc and retinal microvasculopathy after high-dose chemotherapy and autologous hematopoietic progenitor cell support. *Bone Marrow Transplant.* 1999;24:785–792.

11. Schmid KE, Kornek GV, Scheithauer W, et al. Update on ocular complication of systemic cancer chemotherapy. *Surv Ophthalmol.* 2006;51:19–40.

Drugs: Cetuximab, erlotinib, gefitinib, osimertinib, panitumumab

1. Agero AC, Dusza SW, Benvenuto-Andrade C, et al. Dermatologic side effects associated with the epidermal growth factor inhibitors. *J Am Acad Dermatol.* 2006;55(4):657–670.

2. Johnson KS, Levin F, Chu DS. Persistent corneal epithelial defect associated with erlotinib treatment. *Cornea.* 2009;28(6):706–707.

3. Plotkin SR, Halpin C, McKenna MJ, et al. Erlotinib for progressive vestibular schwannoma in neurofibromatosis 2 patients. *Otol Neurotol.* 2010;31(7):1135–1143.

4. Saint-Jean A, Sainz de la Maza M, Morral M, et al. Ocular adverse events of systemic inhibitors of the epidermal growth factor receptor: report of 5 cases. *Ophthalmology.* 2012;119:1798–1802.

5. Chia PL, John T. Vortex keratopathy presumed secondary to AZD9291. *J Thorac Oncol.* 2015;10(12):1807–1808.

6. Dueland S, Sauer T, Lund-Johansen F, et al. Epidermal growth factor receptor inhibition induces trichomegaly. *Acta Oncol.* 2003;42:345–346.

Drug: Cisplatin (cisplatinum)

1. Einhorn LH, Donahue J. Cis-diamminedichloroplatinum, vinblastine and bleomycin combination chemotherapy in disseminated testicular cancer. *Ann Intern Med.* 1977;87:293–298.

2. Young RC, VonHoff DD, Gormley P, et al. Cis-diamminedichloroplatinum (II) for the treatment of advanced ovarian cancer. *Cancer Treat Rep.* 1979;63:1539–1544.

3. Ozols RF, Deisseroth AB, Javadpour N, et al. Treatment of poor prognosis nonseminomatous testicular cancer with a 'high dose' platinum combination chemotherapy regimen. *Cancer.* 1983;51:1803–1807.

4. Wilding G, Caruso R, Lawrence TS, et al. Retinal toxicity after high-dose cisplatin therapy. *J Clin Oncol.* 1985;3:1683–1689.

5. Caruso R, Wilding G, Ballintine E, et al. Cis-platinum retinopathy. *Invest Ophthalmol Vis Sci.* 1985;26:34.

6. Katz BJ, Ward JH, Digre KB, et al. Persistent severe visual and electroretinographic abnormalities after intravenous cisplatin therapy. *J Neuroophthalmol.* 2003;23:132–135.

7. Prim MP, de Diego JI, de Sarria MJ, et al. Vestibular and oculomotor changes in subjects with Cisplatin. *Acta Otorrinolaringol Esp.* 2001;52:370–397.

8. Dulz S, Asselborn NH, Dieckmann KP, et al. Retinal toxicity after cisplatin-based chemotherapy in patients with germ cell cancer. *J Cancer Res Clin Oncol.* 2017;143:1319–1325.

9. Khawly JA, Rubin P, Petros W, et al. Retinopathy and optic neuropathy in bone marrow transplantation for breast cancer. *Ophthalmology.* 1996;103(1):87–95.

10. Gonzalez F, Menedez D, Gomez-Ulla F. Monocular visual in a patient undergoing cisplatin Chemotherapy. *Int Ophthalmol.* 2001;24:301–304.

11. Kwan AS, Sahu A, Palexes G. Retinal ischemia with neovascularization in cisplatin related retinal toxicity. *Am J Ophthalmol.* 2006;141:196–197.

12. Kupersmith MJ, Seiple WH, Holopigian K, et al. Maculopathy caused by intra-arterially administered cisplatin and intravenously administered carmustine. *Am J Ophthalmol.* 1992;113(4):435–438.

13. Miller DF, Bay JW, Lederman RJ, et al. Ocular and orbital toxicity following intracarotid injection of BCNU (carmustine) and cisplatinum for malignant gliomas. *Ophthalmology.* 1985;92:402–406.

14. Margo CE, Murtagh FR. Ocular and orbital toxicity after intracarotid cisplatin therapy. *Am J Ophthalmol.* 1993;116(4):508–509.

15. Wu H, Lee A, Lehane D, et al. Ocular and orbital complications of intraarterial cisplatin: a case report. *J Neuroophthalmol.* 1997;17(3):195–198.

16. Barr-Hamilton RM, Matheson LM, Keay DG. Ototoxicity of cisplatinum and its relationship to eye color. *J Laryngol Otol.* 1991;105(1):7–11.

Drug: Crizotinib

1. Pfizer Inc. Xalkori oral capsules (crizotinib). US prescribing information [online]. Available from URL: http://labeling.pfizer.com. (Accessed 2011 Sep 27).

2. Camidge DR, Bang Y, Kwak EL, et al. Progression-free survival (PFS) from a phase I study of crizotinib (PF-02341066) in patients with ALK-positive non-small cell lung cancer (NSCLC) [abstract no. 2501]. *J Clin Oncol.* 2011;29 Suppl. Plus oral presentation at the 47th Meeting

of the American Society of Clinical Oncology. Chicago, IL; 2011 Jul 3–7.

3. Kim DW, Blackhall F, Soria JC, et al. A global phase 2 study including efficacy, safety, and patient-reported outcomes with crizotinib in patients with ALK-positive non-small cell lung cancer [abstract no. 9084 plus oral presentation]. Stockholm: European Multidisciplinary Cancer Congress; 2011: 23–27.

4. Crizotinib. 2018. Retrieved from http://www.pdr.net.

5. Chun SG, Iyengar P, Gerber DE, et al. Optic neuropathy and blindness associated with crizotinib for non-small-cell lung cancer with EML4-ALK translocation. *J Clin Oncol.* 2015;33(5):e25–e26.

6. Shaw AT, Yeap BY, Solomon BJ, et al. Effect of crizotinib on overall survival in patients with advanced non-small-cell lung cancer harbouring ALK gene rearrangement: a retrospective analysis. *Lancet Oncol.* 2011;12(11):1004–1012.

Drug: Cyclophosphamide

1. Kende G, Sirkin S, Thomas PR, et al. Blurring of vision – a previously undescribed complication of cyclophosphamide therapy. *Cancer.* 1979;44:69–71.

2. Johnson DR, Burns RP. Blepharoconjunctivitis associated with cancer therapy. *Trans Pac Coast Oto-Ophthalmol.* 1965;46:43–49.

3. Arranz JA, Jiménez R, Alvarez-Mon M, et al. Cyclophosphamide-induced myopia. *Ann Intern Med.* 1992;116:92–93.

4. Porter R, Crombie AL. Cataracts after renal transplantation. *BMJ.* 1972;3:766.

5. Agrawal A, Dick AD, Olson JA. Visual symptoms in patients on cyclophosphamide may herald sight threatening disease. *Br J Ophthalmol.* 2003;87:122–123.

6. London NJ, Siverio Jr C, Cunningham Jr ET. Conjunctival lymphoma following treatment with cyclophosphamide. *Eye.* 2010;24(7):1294–1295.

7. Rengasamy P. Congenital malformations attributed to prenatal exposure to cyclophosphamide. *Anticancer Agents Med Chem.* 2017;17(9):1211–1227.

Drug: Cytarabine (cytosine arabinoside)

1. Barletta JP, Fanous MM, Margo CE. Corneal and conjunctival toxicity with low-dose cytosine arabinoside. *Am J Ophthalmol.* 1992;113(5):587–588.

2. Krema H, Santiago RA, Schuh A. Cytarabine toxicity of the corneal endothelium. *Ann Hematol.* 2013;92:559–560.

3. Fintelmann RE, Qian Y, Skalet A, et al. Anterior uveitis associated with high-dose cytosine arabinoside. *Ocul Immunol Inflamm.* 2010;18(6):485–487.

4. Moberg J, Carlsson M, Holm C, et al. Severe anterior uveitis as a complication of high-dose cytosine-arabinoside. *Acta Ophthalmol.* 2009;87(8):922–923.

5. Planer D, Cukirman T, Liebster D, et al. Anterior uveitis as a complication of treatment with high dose cytosine-arabinoside. *Am H Hematol.* 2004;76:304–306.

6. Cho AR, Yoon YH, Kim JG, et al. Uveoretinal adverse effects presented during systemic anticancer chemotherapy: a 10-year single center experience. *J Korean Med Sci.* 2018;33(7):e55.

7. Grewal DS, Holland PM, Frankfurt O, et al. Asymmetric anterior uveitis as a delayed complication of treatment with systemic high-dose cytosine-arabinoside: a case report and literature review. *Ocul Immunol Inflamm.* 2014;22(4):322–325.

8. Sommer C, Lackner H, Benesch M, et al. Neuroophthalmological side effects following intrathecal administration of liposomal cytarabine for central nervous system prophylaxis in three adolescents with acute myeloid leukaemia. *Ann Hematol.* 2008;87:887–890.

9. Lunskens S, Lammertijn L, Deeren D, et al. Intracranial hypertension following intrathecal administration of liposomal cytarabine. *J Neurol.* 2011;258(1):162–163.

10. Hoffman DL, Howard JR, Sarma R, et al. Encephalopathy, myelopathy, optic neuropathy, and anosmia associated with intravenous cytosine arabinoside. *Clin Neuropharmacol.* 1993;16(3):258–262.

11. Schwartz J, Alster Y, Ben-Tal O, et al. Visual loss following high-dose cytosine arabinoside (ara-c). *Eur J Hematol.* 2000;64:208–209.

12. Lopez JA, Agarwal RP. Acute cerebellar toxicity after high-dose cytarabine associated with CNS accumulation of its metabolite, uracil arabinoside. *Cancer Treat Rep.* 1984;68:1309–1310.

13. Lopez PF, Sternberg P, Dabbs CK, et al. Bone marrow transplant retinopathy. *Am J Ophthalmol.* 1991;112(6):635–646.

14. Tziotzios C, Follows G, Sarkies N, et al. Bilateral irreversible blindness in leukaemic meningitis: cause or cure? *Ann Hematol.* 2011;90(12):1487–1488.

15. Wiznia RT, Rose A, Levy AL. Occlusive microvascular retinopathy with optic disc and retinal neovascularization in acute lymphocytic leukemia. *Retina.* 1994;14(3):253–255.

16. Krachmer JH, Palay DA. *Cornea Atlas.* 2nd ed. London: Mosby Elsevier; 2006.

Drugs: Dabrafenib, vemurafenib

1. Choe CH, McArthur GA, Caro I, et al. Ocular toxicity in BRAF mutant cutaneous melanoma patients treated with vemurafenib. *Am J Ophthalmol.* 2014;158(4):831–837.

2. Guedj M, Queant A, Funck-Brentano E, et al. Uveitis in patients with late-stage cutaneous melanoma treated with vemurafenib. *JAMA Ophthalmol.* 2014;132(12):1421–1425.

3. Wolf SE, Meenken C, Moll AC, et al. Severe pan-uveitis in a patient treated with vemurafenib for metastatic melanoma. *BMC Cancer.* 2013;13:561.

4. Klein O, Ribas A, Chmielowski B, et al. Facial palsy as a side effect of vemurafenib treatment in patients with metastatic melanoma. *J Clin Oncol.* 2013;31(12):e215–e217.

5. Shailesh FN, Singh M, Tiwari U, et al. Vemurafenib-induced bilateral facial palsy. *J Postgrad Med.* 2014;60(2):187–188.

6. Yin VT, Wiraszka TA, Tetzlaff M, et al. Cutaneous eyelid neoplasms as a toxicity of vemurafenib therapy. *Ophthal Plast Reconstr Surg.* 2015;31(4):e112–e115.

Drugs: Dasatinib, imatinib mesylate, nilotinib

1. Breccia M, Gentilini F, Cannella L, et al. Ocular side effects in chronic myeloid leukemia patients treated with imatinib. *Leuk Res.* 2007;32(7):1022–1025.
2. Esmaeli B, Diba R, Ahmadi MA. et al. Periorbital oedema and epiphora as ocular side effects of imatinib mesylate (Gleevec). *Eye.* 2004;18:760–762.
3. Esmaeli B, Prieto VG, Butler CE, et al. Severe periorbital edema secondary to STI571 (Gleevec). *Cancer.* 2002;95:881–887.
4. Fraunfelder FW, Solomon J, Druker BJ, et al. Ocular side effects associated with imatinib mesylategleevec), 2003 mesylate (gleevec). *J Ocul Pharmacol Ther.* 2003;19:371–375.
5. Demetri G, vonMehren M, Blank CD, et al. Efficacy and safety of imatinib mesylate in advanced gastrointestinal stromal tumors. *N Engl J Med.* 2002;347:472–480.
6. Govind Babu K, Attili VS, Bapsy PP, et al. Imatinib-induced optic neuritis in a patient of chronic myeloid leukemia. *Int Ophthalmol.* 2007;27(1):43–44.
7. Masood I, Negi A, Dua HS. Imatinib as a cause of cystoids macular edema following uneventful phacoemulsification surgery. *J Cataract Refract Surg.* 2005;31(12):2427–2428.
8. Radaelli F, Vener C, Ripamonti F, et al. Conjunctival hemorrhagic events associated with imatinib mesylate. *Int J Hematol.* 2007;86(5):390–393.
9. Dasatinib, imatinib, nilotinib. 2018. Retrieved from http://www.pdr.net.
10. Monge KS, Galvez-Ruiz A, Alvarez-Carron A, et al. Optic neuropathy secondary to dasatinib in the treatment of a chronic myeloid leukemia case. *Saudi J Ophthalmol.* 2015;29(3):227–231.
11. DeLuca C, Shenouda-Awad N, Haskes C, et al. Imatinib mesylate (Gleevec) induced unilateral optic disc edema. *Optom Vis Sci.* 2012;89(10):e16–e22.
12. Kwon SI, Lee DH, Kim YJ. Optic disc edema as a possible complication of imatinib mesylate (Gleevec). *Jpn J Ophthalmol.* 2008;52(4):331–333.
13. Napolitano M, Santoro M, Mancuso S, et al. Late onset of unilateral optic disk edema secondary to treatment with imatinib mesylate. *Clin Case Rep.* 2017;5(10):1573–1575.
14. Mbekeani JN, Abdel Fattah M, Al Nounou RM, et al. Chronic myelogenous leukemia relapse presenting with central nervous system blast crisis and bilateral optic nerve infiltration. *J Neuroophthalmol.* 2016;36(1):73–77.
15. Kusumi E, Arakawa A, Kami M, et al. Visual disturbance due to retinal edema as a complication of imatinib. *Leukemia.* 2004;18:1138–1139.
16. Georgalas I, Pavesio C, Ezra E. Bilateral cystoids macular edema in a patient with chronic myeloid leukaemia under treatment with imatinib mesylate: report of an unusual side effect. *Graefes Arch Clin Exp Ophthalmol.* 2007;245(10):1585–1586.
17. Bajel A, Bassili S, Seymour JF. Safe treatment of a patient with CML using dasatinib after prior retinal oedema due to imatinib. *Leuk Res.* 2008;32(11):1789–1790.
18. Naithani R. Dasatinib-induced loss of eyebrows. *Br J Haematol.* 2017;179(3):362.

Drugs: Docetaxel, nab-paclitaxel, paclitaxel

1. Esmaeli B, Ahmadi A, Rivera E, et al. Docetaxel secretion in tears. *Arch Ophthalmol.* 2002;120:1180–1182.
2. Burstein HJ, Manola J, Younger J, et al. Docetaxel administered on a weekly basis for metastatic breast cancer. *J Clin Oncol.* 2000;18:1212–1219.
3. Esmaeli B, Hortobagyi GN, Esteva FJ, et al. Canalicular stenosis secondary to weekly versus every-3-weeks docetaxel in patients with metastatic breast cancer. *Ophthalmology.* 2002;109(6):1188–1191.
4. Esmaeli B, Hidaji L, Adinin RB, et al. Blockage of the lacrimal drainage apparatus as a side effect of docetaxel therapy. *Cancer.* 2003;98:504–507.
5. Skolnick CA, Doughman DJ. Erosive conjunctivitis and punctal stenosis secondary to docetaxel (Taxotere). *Eye Contact Lens.* 2003;29(2):134–135.
6. Chan A, Su C, de Boer RH, et al. Prevalence of excessive tearing in women with early breast cancer receiving adjuvant docetaxel-based chemotherapy. *J Clin Oncol.* 2013;31(17):2123–2127.
7. Cetinkaya A, Hudak D, Kulwin D. Cicatricial entropion following docetaxel (Taxotere) therapy. *Ophthal Plast Reconstr Surg.* 2011;27(5):e113–e116.
8. Gupta S, Silliman CG, Trump DL. Docetaxel-induced meibomian duct inflammation and blockage leading to chalazion formation. *Prostate Cancer Prostatic Dis.* 2007;10(4):396–397.
9. Sridhar MS, Laibson PR, Rapuano CJ, et al. Infectious crystalline keratopathy in an immunosuppressed patient. *CLAO J.* 2001;27(2):108–110.
10. Capri G, Munzone E, Tarenzi E, et al. Optic nerve disturbances: new form of paclitaxel neurotoxicity. *J Natl Cancer Inst.* 1994;86:1099–1101.
11. Seidman AD, Barrett S, Canezo S. Photopsia during 3-hour paclitaxel administration at doses > or = 250 mg/m². *J Clin Oncol.* 1994;12(8):1741–1742.
12. Scaioli V, Caraceni A, Martini C, et al. Electrophysiologic evaluation of visual pathways in paclitaxel-treated patients. *J Neurooncol.* 2006;77(1):79–87.
13. Georgakopoulos CD, Makri OE, Vasilakis P, et al. Angiography silent cystoids macular oedema secondary to paclitaxel therapy. *Clin Exp Optom.* 2012;95(2):233–236.
14. Joshi MM, Garretson BR. Paclitaxel maculopathy. *Arch Ophthalmol.* 2007;125(5):709–710.
15. Murphy CG, Walsh JB, Hudis CA, et al. Cystoid macular edema secondary to nab-paclitaxel therapy. *J Clin Oncol.* 2010;28(33):e684–e687.
16. Teitelbaum BA, Tresley DJ. Cystic maculopathy with normal capillary permeability secondary to docetaxel. *Optom Vis Sci.* 2003;80(4):277–279.
17. Telander DG, Sarraf D. Cystoid macular edema with docetaxel chemotherapy and the fluid retention syndrome. *Semin Ophthalmol.* 2007;22(3):151–153.

18. Shih CH, Lee YC. Impaired retinal pigment epithelium in paclitaxel-induced macular edema. *Medicine (Baltimore).* 2018;97(26):e11229.

19. Valeshabad AK, Mieler WF, Setlur V, et al. Posterior segment toxicity after gemcitabine and docetaxel chemotherapy. *Optom Vis Sci.* 2015;92(5):e110–e113.

20. Docetaxel. 2018. Retrieved from http://www.pdr.net.

21. Moloney TP, Xu W, Rallah-Baker K, et al. Toxic optic neuropathy in the setting of docetaxel chemotherapy. *BMC Ophthalmol.* 2014;14:18.

22. Naidu Sugnanam KK, Turner NH, O'Hagan S. Docetaxel-related toxic optic neuropathy in management of prostate adenocarcinoma. *Clin Genitourin Cancer.* 2017;15(1):e115–e118.

23. Bakbak B, Gedik S, Koktekir BE, et al. Assessment of ocular neurotoxicity in patients treated with systemic cancer chemotherapeutics. *Cutan Ocul Toxicol.* 2014;33(1): 7–10.

24. Dwivedi R, Tiroumal S. Possible efficacy of topical dorzolamide in the treatment of paclitaxel-related cystoid macular edema. *Retin Cases Brief Rep.* 2018;12(1):75–79.

Drug: Etoposide

1. Etoposide. 2018. Retrieved from http://www.cancerresearchuk.org.

2. Etoposide. 2018. Retrieved from http://www.pdr.net.

3. Lauer AK, Wobig JL, Shults WT, et al. Severe ocular and orbital toxicity after intracarotid etoposide phosphate and carboplatin therapy. *Am J Ophthalmol.* 1999;127(2):230–233.

Drug: Fludarabine phosphate

1. Chee YL, Culligan DJ, Olson JA, et al. Sight-threatening varicella zoster virus infection after fludarabine treatment. *Br J Haematol.* 2000;11:874–875.

2. Ding X, Herzlich AA, Bishop R, et al. Ocular toxicity of fludarabine: a purine analog. *Expert Rev Ophthalmol.* 2008;3(1):97–109.

3. Sorensen JM, Vena DA, Fallavollita A, et al. Treatment of refractory chronic lymphocytic leukemia with fludarabine phosphate via the group C protocol mechanism of the National Cancer Institute: five-year follow-up report. *J Clin Oncol.* 1997;15(2):458–465.

4. Fludarabine phosphate. 2018. Retrieved from http://www.pdr.net.

Drug: Fluorouracil (5FU)

1. Eiseman AS, Flanagan JC, Brooks AB, et al. Ocular surface, ocular adnexal, and lacrimal complications associated with the use of systemic 5-fluorouracil. *Ophthal Plast Reconstr Surg.* 2003;19:216–224.

2. Singh P, Singh A. Ocular adverse effects of anti-cancer chemotherapy. *J Cancer Ther Res.* 2012;1:1–5.

3. Mansur C, Pfeiffer ML, Esmaeli B. Evaluation and management of chemotherapy-induced epiphora, punctal and canalicular stenosis, and nasolacrimal duct obstruction. *Ophthal Plast Reconstr Surg.* 2017;33:9–12.

4. Hassan A, Hurwitz JJ, Burkes RL. Epiphora in patients receiving systemic 5-fluorouracil therapy. *Can J Ophthalmol.* 1998;33:14–19.

5. Brink HM, Beex LV. Punctal canalicular stenosis associated with systemic fluorouracil therapy. *Doc Ophthalmol.* 1995;90:1–6.

6. Prasad S, Kamath GG, Phillips RP. Lacrimal canalicular stenosis associated with systemic 5-fluorouracil therapy. *Acta Ophthalmol.* 2000;78:110–113.

7. Stevens A, Spooner D. Lacrimal duct stenosis and other ocular toxicity associated with adjuvant cyclophosphamide, methotrexate and 5-fluorouracil combination chemotherapy for early stage breast cancer. *Clin Oncol.* 2001;13:438–440.

8. Agarwal MR, Esmaeli B, Burnstine MA. Squamous metaplasia of the canaliculi associated with 5-fluorouracil: a clinicopathologic case report. *Ophthalmology.* 2002;109:2359–2361.

9. Delval L, Klastersky J. Optic neuropathy in cancer patients. Report of a case possibly related to 5-fluorouracil toxicity and review of the literature. *J Neurooncol.* 2002;60:165–169.

10. Bixenman WW, Nicholls JV, Warwick OH. Oculomotor disturbances associated with 5-fluorouracil chemotherapy. *Am J Ophthalmol.* 1968;83:604–608.

11. Sato K, Watanabe J, Nakayama T, et al. Clinical investigation of corneal damage induced by 5-fluorouracil. *Folia Ophthalmol.* 1988;39(1):1754–1760.

12. Hayashi M, Ibaraki N, Tsuru T. Lamellar keratoplasty after trabeculectomy with 5-fluorouracil. *Am J Ophthalmol.* 1994;117(2):268–269.

13. Patitsas C, Rockwood EJ, Meisler DM, et al. Infectious crystalline keratopathy occurring in an eye subsequent to glaucoma filtering surgery with postoperative subconjunctival 5-fluorouracil. *Ophthalmic Surg.* 1991;22(7):412–413.

14. Rothman RF, Liebmann JM, Ritch R. Noninfectious crystalline keratopathy after postoperative subconjunctival 5-fluorouracil. *Am J Ophthalmol.* 1999;128(2):236–237.

15. Stank TM, Krupin T, Feitl ME. Subconjunctival 5-fluorouracil-induced transient striate melanokeratosis. *Arch Ophthalmol.* 1990;108:1210.

16. Peterson MR, Skuta GL, Phelan MJ, et al. Striate melanokeratosis following trabeculectomy with 5-fluorouracil. *Arch Ophthalmol.* 1990;108:1216–1217.

17. Libre PE. Transient, profound cataract associated with intracameral 5-fluorouracil. *Am J Ophthalmol.* 2003;135:101–102.

18. Pires RT, Chokshi A, Tseng SC. Amniotic membrane transplantation or conjunctival limbal autograft for limbal stem cell deficiency induced by 5-fluorouracil in glaucoma surgeries. *Cornea.* 2000;19:284–287.

19. Ticho U, Ophir A. Late complications after glaucoma filtering surgery with adjunctive 5-fluorouracil. *Am J Ophthalmol.* 1993;115:506–510.

20. Stamper RL, McMenemy MG, Lieberman MF. Hypotonous maculopathy after trabeculectomy with subconjunctival 5-fluorouracil. *Am J Ophthalmol.* 1992;114(5):544–553.

21. Oppenheim B, Ortiz JM. Hypotonous maculopathy after trabeculectomy with subconjunctival 5-fluorouracil. *Am J Ophthalmol.* 1993;115(4):546–547.

22. Hickey-Dwyer M, Wishart PK. Serious corneal complication of 5-fluorouracil. *Br J Ophthalmol.* 1993;77:250–251.

23. Yeatts RP, Engelbrecht NE, Curry CD, et al. 5-fluorouracil for the treatment of intraepithelial neoplasia of the conjunctiva and cornea. *Ophthalmology.* 2000;107:2190–2195.

24. Loprinzi CL, Wender DB, Veeder MH, et al. Inhibition of 5-fluorouracil-induced ocular irritation by ocular ice packs. *Cancer.* 1994;74:945–948.

25. Imperia PS, Lazarus HM, Lass JH. Ocular complications of systemic cancer chemotherapy. *Surv Ophthalmol.* 1989;34:209–230.

Drug: Gemcitabine

1. Banach MJ, Williams GA, Oak R. Purtscher retinopathy and necrotizing vasculitis with gemcitabine therapy. *Arch Ophthalmol.* 2000;118(5):726–727.

2. Tran THC, Desauw C, Rose C. Gemcitabine-induced retinopathy in a diabetic patient. *Acta Ophthalmol.* 2009;87(1):114–115.

3. Sheyman AT, Wald KJ, Pahk PJ, et al. Gemcitabine associated retinopathy and nephropathy. *Retin Cases Brief Rep.* 2014;8(2):107–109.

4. Valeshabad AK, Mieler WF, Setlur V, et al. Posterior segment toxicity after gemcitabine and docetaxel chemotherapy. *Optom Vis Sci.* 2015;92(5):110–113.

5. Jhaj G, Jhaj R, Shrier EM. Gemcitabine-induced retinopathy. *Retina.* 2017;37(11):e130–e131.

6. Kovach JL. Gemcitabine-induced retinopathy. *Retin Cases Brief Rep.* 2018;12(3):240–241.

Drug: Imiquimod

1. Cannon PS, O'Donnell B, Huilgo SC, et al. The ophthalmic side-effects of imiquimod therapy in the management of periocular skin lesions. *Br J Ophthalmol.* 2011;95(12):1682–1685.

2. Murchison AP, Washington CV, Soloman AR, et al. Ocular effects of imiquimod with treatment of eyelid melanoma in situ. *Dermatol Surg.* 2007;33(9):1136–1138.

3. Ross AH, Kennedy CT, Collins C, et al. The use of imiquimod in the treatment of periocular tumours. *Orbit.* 2010;29(2):83–87.

4. Attili SK, Ibbotson SH, Fleming C. Role of non-surgical therapies in the management of periocular basal cell carcinoma and squamous intra-epidermal carcinoma: a case series and review of the literature. *Photodermatol Photoimmunol Photomed.* 2012;28:68–79.

5. Brannan PA, Anderson HK, Kersten RC, et al. Bowen disease of the eyelid successfully treated with imiquimod. *Ophthal Plast Reconstr Surg.* 2005;21:321–322.

6. Carneiro RC, de Macedo EM, Matayoshi S. Imiquimod 5% cream for the treatment of periocular Basal cell carcinoma. *Ophthal Plast Reconstr Surg.* 2010;26:100–102.

7. Demirci H, Shields CL, Bianciotto CG, et al. Topical imiquimod for periocular lentigo maligna. *Ophthalmology.* 2010;117:2424–2429.

8. Garcia-Martin E, Idoipe M, Gil LM, et al. Efficacy and tolerability of imiquimod 5% cream to treat periocular basal cell carcinomas. *J Ocul Pharmacol Ther.* 2010;26:373–379.

9. O'Neill J, Ayers D, Kenealy J. Periocular lentigo maligna treated with imiquimod. *J Dermatolog Treat.* 2011;22:109–112.

10. Blasi MA, Giammaria D, Balestrazzi E. Immunotherapy with imiquimod 5% cream for eyelid nodular basal cell carcinoma. *Am J Ophthalmol.* 2005;140:1136–1139.

11. Karabulut GO, Kaynak P, Ozturker C, et al. Imiquimod 5% cream for the treatment of large nodular basal cell carcinoma at the medial canthal area. *Indian J Ophthalmol.* 2017;65(1):48–51.

12. Choontanom R, Thanos S, Busse H, Stupp T. Treatment of basal cell carcinoma of the eyelids with 5% topical imiquimod: a 3-year follow-up study. *Graefes Arch Clin Exp Ophthalmol.* 2007;245:1217–1220.

13. Bath-Hextall F, Bong J, Perkins W, Williams H. Interventions for basal cell carcinoma of the skin: systematic review. *BMJ.* 2004;329:705.

14. Tsang HH, Huynh NT, Hollenbach E. Topical therapy with imiquimod for eyelid lesion. *Clin Exp Ophthalmol.* 2006;34:179–181.

15. Rowlands MA, Giacometti JN, Servat J, et al. Topical imiquimod in the treatment of conjunctival actinic keratosis. *Ophthal Plast Reconstr Surg.* 2017;33(1):e21–e23.

16. Costales-Alvarez C, Alvarez-Coronado M, Rozas-Reyes P, et al. Topical imiquimod 5% as an alternative therapy in periocular basal cell carcinoma in two patients with surgical complication. *Arch Soc Esp Oftalmol.* 2017;92(2):93–96.

17. Cannon PS, O'Donnell B, Huilgol SC, et al. The ophthalmic side-effects of imiquimod therapy in the management of periocular skin lesions. *Br J Ophthal.* 2011;95:1682–1685.

18. Hong E, Cooper A. Incipient retinal vein occlusion following immunotherapy of periorbital basal cell carcinoma. *Aust J Dermatol.* 2012;53(2):139–140.

Drug: Interferon (alpha, beta, gamma, or PEG)

1. Interferon alfa-2b, interferon beta-1a. 2018. Retrieved from http://www.pdr.net.

2. Esmaeli B, Koller C, Papadopoulos N. et al. Interferon-induced retinopathy in asymptomatic cancer patients. *Ophthalmology.* 2001;108:858–860.

3. Fracht HU, Harvey TJ, Bennett TJ. Transient corneal microcysts associated with interferon therapy. *Cornea.* 2005;24:480–481.

4. Deng-Huang S, Ying-Chun C, Shu-Lang L. et al. Lanreotide treatment in a patient with interferon-associated Graves' ophthalmopathy. *Graefes Arch Clin Exp Ophthalmol.* 2005;243:269–272.

5. Foon KA, Dougher G. Increased growth of eyelashes in a patient given leukocyte A interferon. *N Engl J Med.* 1984;111:1259.

6. Ghembaza MEA, Lounici A. Safety of interferon alpha-2a in patients with severe ophthalmic Behcet's disease: response to Bielefeld et al's letter. *Ocul Immunol Inflamm.* 2018;26(5):793–794.

7. Sene D, Touitou V, Bodaghi B, et al. Intraocular complications of IFN-alpha and ribavirin therapy in patients with chronic viral hepatitis C. *World J Gastroenterol.* 2007;13(22):3137–3140.

8. Rajak S, Sullivan T, Dinesh S. Orbital myositis: a rare effect of interferon alpha 2b treatment. *Ophthal Plast Reconstr Surg.* 2015;31(1):75.

9. Fukumoto Y, Shigemitsu T, Kajii N, et al. Abducent nerve paralysis during interferon alpha-2a therapy in a case of chronic active hepatitis C. *Intern Med.* 1994;33(10):637–640.

10. Damasceno EF, Damasceno NA. Anterior uveitis after treatment of hepatitis C with alpha interferon: the recurrence of a previous inflammatory process due to presumed ocular toxocariasis. *Ocul Immunol Inflamm.* 2012;20(1):53–55.

11. Nigam N, Hedaya J, Freeman WR. Interferon induced sarcoid uveitis with papillitis and macular edema. *Retin Cases Brief Rep.* 2009;3(1):102–104.

12. Lee GA, Hess L, Glasson WJ, et al. Topical interferon alpha-2b induced reactive lymphoid hyperplasia masquerading as orbital extension of ocular surface squamous neoplasia. *Cornea.* 2018;37(6):796–798.

13. Fraunfelder FW, Fraunfelder FT. Interferon alfa-associated anterior ischemic optic neuropathy. *Ophthalmology.* 2011;118:408–411.

14. Matsuo T, Takabatake R. Multiple sclerosis-like disease secondary to alpha interferon. *Ocul Immunol Inflamm.* 2002;10(4):299–304.

15. Fuzzard DR, Mack HG, Symons RC. Bilateral retrobulbar optic neuropathy in the setting of interferon alpha-2a therapy. *Case Rep Ophthalmol.* 2014;5(2):270–276.

Drug: Lenalidomide

1. Lenalidomide. 2018. Retrieved from http://www.pdr.net.

2. Iams WT, Hames ML, Tsai JP, et al. Increased serum tumor necrosis factor α levels in patients with lenalidomide-induced hypothyroidism. *Exp Hematol.* 2015;43(2):74–78.

3. Figaro MK, Clayton Jr W, Usoh C, et al. Thyroid abnormalities in patients treated with lenalidomide for hematological malignancies: results of a retrospective case review. *Am J Hematol.* 2011;86(6):467–470.

4. Stein EM, Rivera C. Transient thyroiditis after treatment with lenalidomide in a patient with metastatic renal cell carcinoma. *Thyroid.* 2007;17(7):681–683.

5. Samara WA, Harary S, Burks ML, et al. Recurrent painless thyroiditis with sequential thyrotoxicosis and hypothyroidism after 2 courses of lenalidomide. *AACE Clin Case Rep.* 2016;2(3):e228–e232.

6. Slean GR, Silkiss RZ. Lenalidomide-associated thyroid-related eyelid retraction. *Ophthal Plast Reconstr Surg.* 2018;34(2):e46–e48.

7. Lim HY. Cytomegalovirus retinitis after treatment with lenalidomide in multiple myeloma. *Retin Cases Brief Rep.* 2013;7(2):172–175.

Drug: Melphalan

1. Francis JH, Schaiquevich P, Buitrago E, et al. Local and systemic toxicity of intravitreal melphalan for vitreous seeding in retinoblastoma. *Ophthalmology.* 2014;121(9):1810–1817.

2. Francis JH, Marr BP, Brodie SE, et al. Anterior ocular toxicity of intravitreous melphalan for retinoblastoma. *JAMA Ophthalmol.* 2015;133(12):1459–1463.

3. Francis JH, Brodie SE, Marr BP, et al. Efficacy and toxicity of intravitreous chemotherapy for retinoblastoma: four-year experience. *Ophthalmology.* 2017;124(4):488–495.

4. Munier FL, Gaillard M-C, Balmer A, et al. Intravitreal chemotherapy for vitreous disease in retinoblastoma revisited: from prohibition to conditional indications. *Br J Ophthalmol.* 2012;96(8):1078–1083.

5. Marr B, Gobin PY, Dunkel IJ, et al. Spontaneously resolving periocular erythema and ciliary madarosis following intra-arterial chemotherapy for retinoblastoma. *Middle East Afr J Ophthalmol.* 2010;17(3):207–209.

6. Muen WJ, Kingston JE, Robertson F, et al. Efficacy and complications of super-selective intra-ophthalmic artery melphalan for the treatment of refractory retinoblastoma. *Ophthalmology.* 2012;119(3):611–616.

7. Steinle JJ, Zhang Q, Thompson KE, et al. Intra-ophthalmic artery chemotherapy triggers vascular toxicity through endothelial cell inflammation and leukostasis. *Invest Ophthalmol Vis Sci.* 2012;53(4):2439–3445.

8. Eagle Jr RC, Shields CL, Bianciotto C, et al. Histopathologic observations after intra-arterial chemotherapy for retinoblastoma. *Arch Ophthalmol.* 2011;129(11):1416–1421.

9. Munier FL, Beck-Popovic M, Balmer A, et al. Occurrence of sectoral choroidal occlusive vasculopathy and retinal arteriolar embolization after superselective ophthalmic artery chemotherapy for advance intraocular retinoblastoma. *Retina.* 2011;31(3):566–573.

Drug: Methotrexate

1. Fraunfelder FT. Interim report: National Registry of Drug-Induced Ocular Side Effects. *Ophthalmology.* 1980;87:87–90.

2. O'Neill T, Simpson J, Smyth SJ, et al. Porphyria cutanea tarda associated with methotrexate therapy. *Br J Rheumatol.* 1993;32:411–412.

3. Cursiefen C, Holbach LM. Molluscum contagiosum in immunosuppression with methotrexate: multiple warts with central depressions of the eyelids. *Linische Monatsblatter fur Augenheilkunde.* 1998;212(2):123–124.

4. Cursiefen C, Grunke M, Dechant C, et al. Multiple bilateral eyelid molluscum contagiosum lesions associated with TNF α-antibody and methotrexate therapy. *Am J Ophthalmol.* 2012;134:270–271.

5. Rizkalla K, Rodrigues S, Proulx A, et al. Primary intraocular lymphoma arising during methotrexate treatment of temporal arteritis. *Can J Ophthalmol.* 2005;40:585–592.

6. Kobayashi Y, Kimura K, Fujitsu Y, et al. Methotrexate-associated orbital lymphoproliferative disorder in a patient with rheumatoid arthritis: a case report. *Jpn J Ophthalmol.* 2016;60(3):212–218.

7. Winegarner A, Hashida N, Koh S, et al. Hemorrhagic hypopyon as presenting feature of intravascular lymphoma: a case report. *BMC Ophthalmol.* 2017;17(1):195.

8. Balachandran C, McCluskey PJ, Champion GD, et al. Methotrexate-induced optic neuropathy. *Clin Exp Ophthalmol.* 2002;30:440–441.

9. Millay RH, Klein ML, Shults WT, et al. Maculopathy associated with combination chemotherapy and osmotic opening of the blood–brain barrier. *Am J Ophthalmol.* 1986;102:626–632.

10. Clare G, Colley S, Kennett R, et al. Reversible optic neuropathy associated with low-dose methotrexate therapy. *J Neuroophthalmol.* 2005;25:109–112.

11. Boogerd W, Moffie D, Smets LA. Early blindness and coma during intrathecal chemotherapy for meningeal carcinomatosis. *Cancer.* 1990;65:452–457.

12. Epstein JA, Moster ML, Spiritos M. Seesaw nystagmus following whole brain irradiation and intrathecal methotrexate. *J Neuroophthalmol.* 2001;21:264–265.

13. Hardwig PW, Jose SP, Bakri SJ. The safety of intraocular methotrexate in silicone-filled eyes. *Retina.* 2008;28(8):1082–1086.

14. Gorovoy I, Prechanond T, Abia M, et al. Toxic corneal epitheliopathy after intravitreal methotrexate and its treatment with oral folic acid. *Cornea.* 2013;32(8):1171–1173.

15. Fraunfelder FT. Methotrexate-induced keratitis [photograph]. Portland, OR: Casey Eye Institute, Oregon Health & Science University; ©1990. 1 photograph: color.

Drug: Mitoxantrone hydrochloride

1. Kumar K, Kochipillai V. Mitoxantrone induced hyperpigmentation. *N Z Med J.* 1990;103:55.

2. Leyden MJ, Sullivan JR, Cheng ZM, et al. Unusual side effect of mitoxantrone. *Med J Aust.* 1983;2(10):514.

3. Mitoxantrone. 2018. Retrieved from http://www.pdr.net.

Drug: Nilutamide

1. Brisset JM, Bertagna C, Proulx L. Ocular toxicity of Anandron. *Br J Ophthalmol.* 1987;71:639–640.

2. Dukman GA, Klotz LH, Diokno AC, et al. Clinical experiences of visual disturbances with nilutamide (comment). *Ann Pharmacother.* 1997;31:1550–1551.

3. Harnois C, Malenfant M, Dupont A, et al. Ocular toxicity of Anandron I patients treated for prostatic cancer. *Br J Ophthalmol.* 1986;70:471–473.

4. Dukman GA, Klotz LH, Diokno AC, et al. Clinical experiences of visual disturbances with nilutamide (comment). *Ann Pharmacother.* 1997;31(12):1550–1552.

5. Dole EJ. Comment. Clinical experiences of visual disturbances with nilutamide (author's reply). *Ann Pharmacother.* 1997;31:1551–1552.

6. Namer M, Toubol J, Caty A, et al. A randomized double-blind study evaluating Anandron associated with orchiectomy in stage D prostate cancer. *J Steroid Biochem Molec Biol.* 1990;37(6):909–915.

7. Nilutamide. 2018. Retrieved from http://www.pdr.net.

Drug: Oprelvekin

1. Oprelvekin. 2018. Retrieved from http://www.pdr.net.

2. Data on file (Protocol C9504-14, Final Clinical Study Report 1998). Genetics Institute, Inc.

3. Peterson DC, Inwards DJ, Younge BR. Oprelvekin-associated bilateral optic disc edema. *Am J Ophthalmol.* 2005;139:367–368.

Drug: Oxaliplatin

1. Noguchi Y, Kawashima Y, Kawara H, et al. A retrospective analysis of eye disorders due to oxaliplatin. *Gan To Kagaku Ryoho.* 2015;42(11):1401–1405.

2. Oxaliplatin. 2018. Retrieved from http://www.pdr.net.

3. Lau SC, Shibata SI. Blepharoptosis following oxaliplatin administration. *J Oncol Pharm Pract.* 2009;15(4):255–257.

4. La Verde N, Garassino MC, Spinelli G, et al. Reversible palpebral ptosis following oxaliplatin infusion. *Dig Liver Dis.* 2007;39(11):1041.

5. Winquist E, Vincent M, Stadler W. Acute bilateral abducens paralysis due to oxaliplatin. *J Natl Cancer Inst.* 2003;95(6):488–489.

6. Tan MH, Chay WY, Ng JH, et al. Transient bilateral abducens neuropathy with post-tetanic facilitation and acute hypokalemia associated with oxaliplatin: a case report. *J Med Case Rep.* 2010;4:36.

7. O'Dea D, Handy CM, Wexler A. Ocular changes with oxaliplatin. *Clin J Oncol Nurs.* 2006;10(2):227–229.

8. Saif MW. Management of a patient with metastatic colorectal cancer and liver metastases. *Case Rep Oncol Med Mar.* 2014;2014:790192.

9. Mesquida M, Sanchez-Dalmau B, Ortiz-Perez S, et al. Oxaliplatin-related ocular toxicity. *Case Rep Oncol.* 2010;3(3):423–427.

10. Painhas T, Amorim M, Soares R, et al. Idiopathic intracranial hypertension and oxaliplatin: a causal association. *Cutan Ocul Toxicol.* 2015;34(3):237–241.

11. Garcia Villanueva C. Accelerated retinitis pigmentosa progression following folfox chemotherapy for advanced colorectal cancer. *Ophthalmic Res.* 2011;46(4):239.

Drugs: Pazopanib, sorafenib, sunitinib

1. Pazopanib. Retinal detachment. *Rev Prescrire.* 2014;34(373):827.

2. Revision of Precautions. MHLW/PMDA. 24 March 2015 (www.pmda.go.jp/english/).

3. Fraunfelder FT, Fraunfelder FW. Oral anti-vascular endothelial growth factor drugs and ocular adverse events. *J Ocul Pharmacol Ther.* 2018;34(6):432–435.

4. Gaertner KM, Caldwell SH, Rahma OE. A case of retinal tear associated with use of sorafenib. *Front Oncol.* 2014;4(196):1–2.

5. Hasan R. A retinal tear induced by pazopanib therapy: a case report. *The Medicine Forum.* 2015;16(13):1–3.

6. Etminan M, Forooghian F, Brophy JM, et al. Oral fluoroquinolones and the risk of retinal detachment. *JAMA.* 2012;307(13):1414–1419.

7. Wegner A, Khoramnia R. Neurosensory retinal detachment due to sunitinib treatment. *Eye.* 2011;25(11):1517–1518.

8. Valsecchi ME, Orloff M, Sato R, et al. Adjuvant sunitinib in high-risk patients with uveal melanoma: comparison with institutional controls. *Ophthalmology.* 2017;125(2):210–217.

Drug: Pemetrexed disodium

1. Schallier D, Decoster L, Fontaine C, et al. Pemetrexed-induced eyelid edema: incidence and clinical manifestations. *Anticancer Res.* 2010;30(12):5185–5188.

2. Eguia B, Ruppert AM, Fillon J, et al. Skin toxicities compromised prolonged pemetrexed treatment. *J Thorac Oncol.* 2011;6(12):2083–2089.

3. Mangla N, Carlson A, Wakil A, et al. Pemetrexed-associated eyelid edema: effective treatment by excision of lymphedematous eyelid tissue. *Ophthal Plast Reconstr Surg.* 2015;31(6):e155–e157.

4. Guhl G, Diaz-Lay B, Sanchez-Perez J, et al. Pemetrexed-induced edema of the eyelid. *Lung Cancer.* 2010;69(2):249–250.

Drug: Raloxifene hydrochloride

1. Vogel VG, Costantino JP, Wickerman DL, et al. Effects of tamoxifen vs raloxifene on the risk of developing invasive breast cancer and other disease outcomes. *JAMA.* 2006;295:2727–2741.

2. Raloxifene hydrochloride. 2018. Retrieved from http://www.pdr.net.

3. Bourgeois N, Chavant F, Lafay-Chebassier C, et al. Drugs and retinal disorders: a case/non-case study in the French pharmacovigilance database. *Therapie.* 2016;71(4):365–374.

4. Siesky B, Harris A, Kheradiya N, et al. The effects of raloxifene hydrochloride on ocular hemodynamics and visual function. *Int Ophthalmol.* 2009;29(4):225–230.

Drug: Tamoxifen citrate

1. Gallicchio L, Lord G, Tkaczuk K, et al. Association of tamoxifen (TAM) and TAM metabolite concentrations with self-reported side effects of TAM in women with breast cancer. *Breast Cancer Res Treat.* 2004;85:89–97.

2. Gorin MB, Costantino JP, Kulacoglu DN, et al. Is tamoxifen a risk factor for retinal vaso-occlusive disease? *Retina.* 2005;25:523–526.

3. Gorin MB, Day R, Costantino JP, et al. Long-term tamoxifen citrate use and potential ocular toxicity. *Am J Ophthalmol.* 1998;125:493–501.

4. Pavlidis NA, Petris C, Briassoulis E, et al. Clear evidence that long-term, low-dose tamoxifen treatment can induce ocular toxicity. A prospective study of 63 patients. *Cancer.* 1992;69(12):2961–2964.

5. Andreanos K, Oikonomakis K, Droutsas K, et al. Refractory tamoxifen-induced keratopathy despite drug withdrawal. *Cornea.* 2017;36(3):377–378.

6. Hollander DA, Aldave AJ. Drug-induced corneal complications. *Curr Opin Ophthalmol.* 2004;15:541–548.

7. Fisher B, Costantino JP, Wickerham L, et al. Tamoxifen for prevention of breast cancer: report of the national surgical adjuvant breast and bowel project P-1 study. *J Natl Cancer Inst.* 1998;90:1371–1388.

8. Paganini-Hill A, Clark LJ. Eye problems in breast cancer patients treated with tamoxifen. *Breast Cancer Res Treat.* 2000;60:167–172.

9. Bradbury BD, Lash TL, Kaye JA, et al. Tamoxifen and cataracts: a null association. *Breast Cancer Res Treat.* 2004;87:189–196.

10. Eisner A, Austin DF, Samples JR. Short wavelength automated perimetry and tamoxifen use. *Br J Ophthalmology.* 2004;88:125–130.

11. Eisner A, Incognito LJ. The color appearance of stimuli detected via short-wavelength-sensitive cones for breast cancer survivors using tamoxifen. *Vis Res.* 2006;46:1816–1822.

12. Eisner A, O'Malley JP, Incognito LJ, et al. Small optic cup sizes among women using tamoxifen: assessment with scanning laser ophthalmoscopy. *Curr Eye Res.* 2006;31:367–379.

13. Kaiser-Kupfer MI, Kupfer C, Rodrigues MM. Tamoxifen retinopathy: a clinicopathologic report. *Ophthalmology.* 1981;88:89–93.

14. Bourla DH, Sarraf D, Schwartz SD. Peripheral retinopathy and maculopathy in high-dose tamoxifen therapy. *Am J Ophthalmol.* 2007;144(1):126–128.

15. Gualino V, Cohen SY, Dalyfer M-N, et al. Optical coherence tomography findings in tamoxifen retinopathy. *Am J Ophthalmol.* 2005;140(4):757–758.

16. Doshi RR, Fortun JA, Kim BT, et al. Pseudocystic foveal cavitation in tamoxifen retinopathy. *Am J Ophthalmol.* 2014;157(6):1291–1298.

17. Park SS, Zawadzki RJ, Truong S, et al. Microcystoid maculopathy associated with tamoxifen use diagnosed by high-resolution Fourier-domain optical coherence tomography. *Retin Cases Brief Rep.* 2009;3(1):33–35.

18. Cronin BG, Lekich CK, Bourke RD. Tamoxifen therapy conveys increased risk of developing a macular hole. *Intern Ophthalmol.* 2005;26:101–105.

19. Hu Y, Liu N, Chen Y. The optical imaging and clinical features of tamoxifen associated macular hole: a case report and review of the literatures. *Photodiagnosis Photodyn Ther.* 2017;17:35–38.

20. Kalina RE, Wells CG. Screening for ocular toxicity in asymptomatic patients treated with Tamoxifen. *Am J Ophthalmol.* 1995;119:112–113.

21. Zvornicanin J. Tamoxifen associated bilateral optic neuropathy. *Acta Neurol Belg.* 2015;115(2):173–175.

22. Heier JS, Dragoo RA, Enzenauer RW, et al. Screening for ocular toxicity in asymptomatic patients treated with tamoxifen. *Am J Ophthalmol.* 1994;117:772–775.
23. Gianni L, Panzini I, Li S, et al. Ocular toxicity during adjuvant chemoendocrine therapy for early breast cancer. *Cancer.* 2006;106:505–513.
24. Spalton DJ, Hitchings RA, Hunter PA. *Atlas of Clinical Ophthalmology.* 3rd ed. London: Mosby Elsevier; 2005.

Drug: Thiotepa

1. Horn TD, Beveridge RA, Egorin MJ, et al. Observations and proposed mechanism of N, N', N″ – triethylenethiophosphoramide (thiotepa)-induced hyperpigmentation. *Arch Dermatol.* 1989;125:524–527.
2. Grant WM, Schuman JS. *Toxicology of the Eye.* 4th ed. Springfield, IL: Charles C Thomas; 1993:1412–1414.
3. Berkow JW, Gill JP, Wise JB. Depigmentation of eyelids after topically administered thiotepa. *Arch Ophthalmol.* 1969;82:415–420.
4. Howitt D, Karp EJ. Side effects of topical thiotepa. *Am J Ophthalmol.* 1969;68:473–474.
5. Hornblass A, Adler RI, Vukcevich WM, et al. A delayed side effect of topical thiotepa. *Ann Ophthalmol.* 1974;6:1155–1157.
6. Asregadoo ER. Surgery, thiotepa, and corticosteroid in the treatment of pterygium. *Am J Ophthalmol.* 1972;74:960–963.
7. Weiss RB, Bruno S. Hypersensitivity reactions to cancer chemotherapeutic agents. *Ann Intern Med.* 1981;94:66–72.
8. Smith SJ, Smith BD, Mohney BG. Ocular side effects following intravitreal injection therapy for retinoblastoma: a systematic review. *Br J Ophthalmol.* 2014;98:292–297.

Drug: Trastuzumab

1. Eaton JS, Miller PE, Mannis MJ, et al. Ocular adverse events associated with antibody-drug conjugates in human clinical trials. *J Ocul Pharmacol Ther.* 2015;31(10):589–604.
2. Orlandi A, Fasciani R, Cassano A, et al. Trastuzumab-induced corneal ulceration: successful no-drug treatment of a "blind" side effect in a case report. *BMC Cancer.* 2015;15:973.
3. Saleh M, Bourcier T, Noel G, et al. Bilateral macular ischemia and severe visual loss following trastuzumab therapy. *Acta Oncol.* 2011;50(3):477–478.

Drug: Vinblastine sulfate

1. Breza TS, Halprin KM, Taylor R. Photosensitivity reaction to vinblastine. *Arch Dermatol.* 1975;111:1168–1170.
2. Vinblastine sulfate. 2019. Retrieved from http://www.pdr.net.
3. Chowers I, Frucht-Pery J, Siganos CS, et al. Vinblastine toxicity to the ocular surface. *Anticancer Drugs.* 1996;7(7):805–808.
4. McLendon BF, Bron AJ. Corneal toxicity from vinblastine solution. *Br J Ophthalmol.* 1978;62:97–99.

Drug: Vincristine sulfate

1. Albert DM, Wong V, Henderson ES. Ocular complications of vincristine therapy. *Arch Ophthalmol.* 1967;78:709–713.
2. Lash SC, Williams CP, Marsh CS, et al. Acute sixth-nerve palsy after vincristine therapy. *J AAPOS.* 2004;8:67–68.
3. Schmid KE, Kornek GV, Scheithauer W, et al. Update on ocular complications of systemic cancer chemotherapy. *Surv Ophthalmol.* 2006;51:19–40.
4. Batta B, Trechot F, Cloche V, et al. Vincristine-induced unilateral ptosis: case report and review of the literature. *J Fr Ophthalmol.* 2013;36(8):683–686.
5. Müller L, Kramm C, Tenenbaum T. Treatment of vincristine-induced bilateral ptosis with pyridoxine and pyridostigmine. *Pediatr Blood Cancer.* 2004;42:287–288.
6. Sanderson PA, Kuwabara T, Cogan DG. Optic neuropathy presumably caused by vincristine therapy. *Am J Ophthalmol.* 1976;81:146–150.
7. Norton SW, Stockman III JA. Unilateral optic neuropathy following vincristine chemotherapy. *J Pediatr Ophthalmol Strabismus.* 1979;16:190–193.
8. Awidi AS. Blindness and vincristine. *Ann Intern Med.* 1980;93:781.
9. Shurin SB, Rekate HL, Annable W. Optic atrophy induced by vincristine. *Pediatrics.* 1982;70:288–291.
10. Teichmann KD, Dabbagh N. Severe visual loss after a single dose of vincristine in a patient with spinal cord astrocytoma. *J Ocular Pharmacol.* 1989;4:149–151.
11. Weisfeld-Adams JD, Dutton GN, Murphy DM. Vincristine sulfate as a possible cause of optic neuropathy. *Pediatr Blood Cancer.* 2007;48(2):238–240.
12. Munier F, Uffer S, Herbort CP, et al. Loss of ganglion cells in the retina secondary to vincristine therapy. *Klin Monatsbl Augenheilkd.* 1992;200(5):550–554.
13. Byrd RL, Rohrbaugh TM, Raney Jr RB, et al. Transient cortical blindness secondary to vincristine therapy in childhood malignancies. *Cancer.* 1981;47:37–40.
14. Schouten D, de Fraff SSN, Verrips A. Transient cortical blindness following vincristine therapy. *Med Pediatr Oncol.* 2003;41:470.
15. Ripps H, Carr RE, Siegel IM, et al. Functional abnormalities in vincristine-induced night blindness. *Invest Ophthalmol Vis Sci.* 1984;25:787–794.

FURTHER READING

Alemtuzumab

Anoop P, Stanford M, Saso R, et al. Ocular and cerebral aspergillosis in a non-neutropenic patient following alemtuzumab and methyl prednisolone treatment for chronic lymphocytic leukaemia. *J Infect Chemother.* 2010;16(2):150–151.

Atezolizumab, ipilimumab, nivolumab, pembrolizumab

Acaba-Berrocal LA, Lucio-Alvarez JA, Mashayekhi A, et al. Birdshot-like chorioretinopathy associated with pembrolizumab treatment. *JAMA Ophthalmol.* 2018;136(10):1205–1207.

Hassanzadeh B, Desanto J, Kattah JC. Ipilimumab-induced adenohypophysitis and orbital apex syndrome: importance of early diagnosis and management. *Neuro-Ophthalmology.* 2018;42(3):176–181.

Binimetinib, cobimetinib, trametinib

Duncan KE, Chang LY, Patronas M. MEK inhibitors: a new class of chemotherapeutic agents with ocular toxicity. *Eye.* 2015;29(8):1003–1012.

Giuffre C, Miserocchi E, Modorati G, et al. Central serous chorioretinopathy-like mimicking multifocal vitelliform macular dystrophy: an ocular side effect of mitogen/extracellular signal-regulated kinase inhibitors. *Retin Cases Brief Rep.* 2018;12(3):172–176.

Stjepanovic N, Velazquez-Martin JP, Bedard PL. Ocular toxicities of MEK inhibitors and other targeted therapies. *Ann Oncol.* 2016;27(6):998–1005.

Bleomycin sulfate, dactinomycin, daunorubicin hydrochloride, doxorubicin hydrochloride

Kirschen McLoon L, Wirtschafter JD, Cameron JD. Muscle loss from doxorubicin injections into the eyelids of a patient with blepharospasm. *Am J Ophthalmol.* 1993;116(5):646–648.

Knowles RS, Virden JE. Handling of injectable antineoplastic agents. *BMJ.* 1980;2:589–591.

Bortezomib

Veys MC, Delforge M, Mombaerts I. Treatment with doxycycline for severe bortezomib-associated blepharitis. *Clin Lymphoma Myeloma Leuk.* 2016;16(7):e109–e112.

Yun C, Mukhi N, Kremer V, et al. Chalazia development in multiple myeloma: a new complication associated with bortezomib therapy. *Hematol Rep.* 2015;7(2):5729.

Busulfan

Dahlgren S, Holm G, Svanborg N, et al. Clinical and morphological side effects of busulfan (Myleran) treatment. *Acta Med Scand.* 1972;192:129–135.

Grimes P, von Sallmann L, Frichette A. Influence of Myleran on cell proliferation in the lens epithelium. *Invest Ophthalmol.* 1965;3:566–576.

Imperia PS, Lazarus HM, Lass JH. Ocular complication of systemic cancer chemotherapy. *Surv Ophthalmol.* 1989;34:209–230.

Podos SM, Canellos GP. Lens changes in chronic granulocytic leukemia. *Am J Ophthalmol.* 1969;68:500–504.

Ravindranathan MP, Paul VJ, Kuriakose ET. Cataract after busulphan treatment. *BMJ.* 1972;1:218–219.

Schmid KE, Kornek GV, Scheithauer W, et al. Update on ocular complications of systemic cancer chemotherapy. *Surv Ophthalmol.* 2006;51:19–40.

Smalley RV, Wall RL. Two cases of busulfan toxicity. *Ann Intern Med.* 1966;64:154–164.

Soysal T, Bavunoglu I, Baslar Z, et al. Cataract after prolonged busulphan therapy. *Acta Haematol.* 1993;90:213.

Carboplatin

Shah PK, Kalpana N, Narendran V, et al. Severe aseptic orbital cellulitis with subtenon carboplatin for intraocu-lar retinoblastoma. *Indian J Ophthalmol.* 2011;59(1):49–51.

Carmustine

Chrousos GA, Oldfield EH, Doppman JL, et al. Prevention of ocular toxicity of carmustine (BCNU) with supraophthalmic intracarotid infusion. *Ophthalmology.* 1986;93:1471–1475.

Elsås T, Watne K, Fostad K, et al. Ocular complications after intracarotid BCNU for intracranial tumors. *Acta Ophthalmol.* 1989;67:83–86.

Greenberg HS, Ensminger WD, Chandler WF, et al. Intra-arterial BCNU chemotherapy for treatment of malignant gliomas of the central nervous system. *J Neurosurg.* 1984;61:423–429.

Pickrell L, Purvin V. Ischemic optic neuropathy secondary to intracarotid infusion of BCNU. *J Clin Neuro-Ophthalmol.* 1987;7:87–91.

Cetuximab, erlotinib, gefitinib, osimertinib, panitumumab

Basti S. Ocular toxicities of epidermal growth factor receptor inhibitors and their management. *Cancer Nurs.* 2007;30(4S):S10–S16.

Borkar DS, Lacouture ME, Basti S. Spectrum of ocular toxicities from epidermal growth factor receptor inhibitors and their intermediate-term follow-up: a five-year review. *Support Care Cancer.* 2013;21(4):1167–1174.

Burtness B, Anadkat M, Basti S, et al. NCCN task force report: management of dermatologic and other toxicities associated with EGFR inhibition in patients with cancer. *J Natl Compr Canc Netw.* 2009;7(suppl 1):S5–S21.

Fabbrocini G, Panariello L, Cacciapuoti S, et al. Trichomegaly of the eyelashes during therapy with epidermal growth factor receptor inhibitors: report of 3 cases. *Dermatitis.* 2012;23(5):237–238.

Fraunfelder FT, Fraunfelder FW. Trichomegaly and other external eye side effects associated with epidermal growth factor. *Cut Ocul Toxicol.* 2012;31(3):195–197.

Guarnieri A, Alfonso-Bartolozzi B, Ciufo G, et al. Plasma rich in growth factors for the treatment of rapidly progressing refractory corneal melting due to erlotinib in nonsmall cell lung cancer. *Medicine (Baltimore).* 2017;96(22):e7000.

Ho WL, Wong H, Yau T. The ophthalmological complications of targeted agents in cancer therapy: what do we need to know as ophthalmologists. *Acta Ophthalmol.* 2013;91(7):604–609.

Hollhumer R, et al. Corneal edema with a systemic epidermal growth factor receptor inhibitor. *Can J Ophthalmol.* 2017;52(3):e96–e97.

Kau H-C, Tsai C-C. Erlotinib-related keratopathy in a patient underwent laser in situ Keratomileusis. *Cutan Ocul Toxicol.* 2016;35(3):257–259.

Kumar I, Ali K, Usman-Saeed M, et al. Follow-up of erlotinib related uveitis. *BMJ Case Reports.* 2012.

Lane K, Goldstein SM. Erlotinib-associated trichomegaly. *Ophthal Plast Reconstr Surg.* 2007;23(1):65–66.

Lim LT, Blum RA, Cheng CP, et al. Bilateral anterior uveitis secondary to erlotinib. *Eur J Clin Pharmacol.* 2010;66(12):1277–1278.

Liu Y. A survey on the ADRs of cetuximab in hospitalized patients of our hospital in 2012. *Chin J New Drugs.* 2013;22(20):2445-2448.

Morishige N, Hatabe N, Morita Y, et al. Spontaneous healing of corneal perforation after temporary discontinuation of erlotinib treatment. *Case Rep Ophthalmol.* 2014;5(1):6-10.

Saif MW, Gnanaraj J. Erlotinib-induced trichomegaly in a male patient with pancreatic cancer. *Cutan Ocul Toxicol.* 2010;29(1):62-66.

Salman A, Cerman E, Seckin D, et al. Erlotinib induced ectropion following papulopustular rash. *J Dermatol Case Rep.* 2015;9(2):46-48.

Sun P, Long J, Chen P, et al. Rapid onset of conjunctivitis associated with overdosing of erlotinib. *J Clin Pharm Ther.* 2018;43(2):296-298.

Zhang G, Basti S, Jampol LM. Acquired trichomegaly and symptomatic external ocular changes in patients receiving epidermal growth factor receptor inhibitors: case reports and a review of the literature. *Cornea.* 2007;26(7):858-860.

Zhu H, Zhu Z, Huang W, et al. Common and uncommon adverse cutaneous reactions to erlotinib: a study of 20 Chinese patients with cancer. *Cutan Ocul Toxicol.* 2018;37(1):96-99.

Cisplatin (cisplatinum)

Bachmeyer C, Decroix Y, Medioni J, et al. Hypomagnesemic and hypocalcemic coma, convulsions, and ocular motility disorders after chemotherapy with platinum compounds. *Revue de Medecine Interne.* 1996;17(6):467-469.

Caraceni A, Martini C, Spatti G, et al. Recovering optic neuritis during systemic cisplatin and carboplatin chemotherapy. *Acta Neurol Scand.* 1997;96(4):260-261.

Chalam KV, Tsao K, Malkani S, et al. Cisplatin causes neuroretinal toxicity. *J Toxicol Cut Ocular Toxicol.* 1999;18:270.

Cohen RJ, Cuneo RA, Cruciger MP, et al. Transient left homonymous hemianopsia and encephalopathy following treatment of testicular carcinoma with cisplatinum, vinblastine, and bleomycin. *J Clin Oncol.* 1983;1:392-393.

Diamond SB, Rudolph SH, Lubicz SS, et al. Cerebral blindness in association with cis-platinum chemotherapy for advanced carcinoma of the fallopian tube. *Obstet Gynecol.* 1982;59:84S-86S.

Feun LG, Wallace S, Stewart DJ, et al. Intracarotid infusion of cisdiamminedichloroplatinum in the treatment of recurrent malignant brain tumors. *Cancer.* 1984;54:794-799.

Hilliard LM, Berkow RL, Watterson J, et al. Retinal toxicity associated with cisplatin and etoposide in pediatric patients. *Med Pediatr Oncol.* 1997;28:310-313.

Pollera CF, Cognetli F, Nardi M, et al. Sudden death after acute dystonic reaction to high-dose metoclopramide. *Lancet.* 1984;2:460-461.

Shimamur Y, Chikama M, Tanimoto T, et al. Optic nerve degeneration caused by supraophthalmic carotid artery infusion with cisplatin and ACNU. *J Neuro-Surg.* 990;72:285-288.

Solak Y, Dikbas O, Altundag K, et al. Myasthenic crisis following cisplatin chemotherapy in a patient with malignant thymoma. *J Exp Clin Cancer Res.* 2004;23:343-344.

Swan I, Gatehouse S. Cisplatinum ototoxicity and eye colour. *J Laryngol Otol.* 1992;105(1):294.

Tang RA, et al. Ocular toxicity and cisplatin. *Invest Ophthalmol Vis Sci.* 1983;24(suppl):284.

Walsh TJ, Clark AW, Parhad IM, et al. Neurotoxic effects of cisplatin therapy. *Arch Neurol.* 1982;39:719-720.

Crizotinib

Curran MP. Crizotinib in local advanced or metastatic non-small cell lung cancer. *Drugs.* 2012;72(1):99-107.

Ho WL, Wong H, Yau T. The ophthalmological complications of targeted agents in cancer therapy: what do we need to know as ophthalmologists. *Acta Ophthalmol.* 2013;91(7):604-609.

Cyclophosphamide

Fraunfelder FT, Meyer SM. Ocular toxicity of antineoplastic agents. *Ophthalmology.* 1983;90:1-3.

Jack MK, Hicks JD. Ocular complications in high dose chemo-radiotherapy and marrow transplantation. *Ann Ophthalmol.* 1981;13:709-711.

Cytarabine (cytosine arabinoside)

Doan T, Lacayo N, Fisher PG. et al. Dorsolateral midbrain MRI abnormalities and ocular motor deficits following cytarabine-based chemotherapy for acute myelogenous leukemia. *J Neuroophthalmol.* 2011;31(1):52-53.

Gressel MG, Tomsak RL. Keratitis from high dose intravenous cytarabine. *Lancet.* 1982;2:273.

Hopen G, Mondino BJ, Johnson BL, et al. Corneal toxicity with systemic cytarabine. *Am J Ophthalmol.* 1981;91:500-504.

Hwang TL, Yung WK, Estey EH, et al. Central nervous system toxicity with high-dose Ara-C. *Neurology.* 1985;35:1475-1479.

Lass JH, Lazarus HM, Reed MD, et al. Topical corticosteroid therapy for corneal toxicity from systemically administered cytarabine. *Am J Ophthalmol.* 1982;94:617-621.

Lochhead J, Salmon JF, Bron AJ. Cytarabine-induced corneal toxicity. *Eye.* 2003;17:677-678.

Mori T, Kato J, Yamane A, et al. Prevention of cytarabine-induced kerato-conjunctivitis by eye rinse in patients receiving high-dose cytarabine and total body irradiation as a conditioning for hematopoietic stem cell transplantation. *Intern J Hematol.* 2011;94(3):261-265.

Ritch PS, Hansen RM, Heuer DK. Ocular toxicity from high-dose cytosine arabinoside. *Cancer.* 1983;51:430-432.

Dabrafenib, vemurafenib

Fonollosa A, Mesquida M. Adan A Uveitic macular oedema after treatment with vemurafenib. *Acta Ophthalmol.* 2015;93(8):e686-e687.

Dasatinib, imatinib mesylate, nilotinib

Anzalone CL, Cohen PR, Kurzrock R, et al. Imatinib-induced postoperative periorbital purpura: GASP (Gleevec-Associated Surgical Purpura) in a woman with imatinib-treated chronic myelogenous leukemia. *Dermatol Online.* 2014;20(1):21242.

Caccavale A, Ferrari D, Girmenia G, et al. Optic nerve head leakage in chronic myeloid leukemia treated with imatinib mesylate: successful therapy with antiangiotensin converting enzyme. *Blood.* 2002;100:329–330.

do Carmo LL, Mendonca LG, Yung AA. Imatinib-related conjunctival pigmentation. *Ophthalmology.* 2018;125(7):1002.

Dogan SS, Esmaeli B. Ocular side effects associated with imatinib mesylate and perifosine for gastrointestinal stromal tumor. *Hematol Oncol Clin N Am.* 2009;23:109–114.

Grossman WJ, Wilson DB. Hypopigmentation from imatinib mesylate (gleevec). *J Pediatr Hematol Oncol.* 2004;26:214.

Mistry S, Sudharshan S, Ganesean S, et al. Vogt-Koyanagi-Harada disease like presentation in patients with chronic myeloid leukemia. *Am J Ophthalmol Case Rep.* 2018;10:221–225.

Tsao AS, Kantarjian H, Cortes J, et al. Imatinib mesylate causes hypopigmentation of the skin. *Cancer.* 2003;98:2483–2487.

Valeyrie L, Basuji-Garin S, Revuz J, et al. Adverse cutaneous reactions to imatinib (STI571) in Philadelphia chromosome-positive leukemias: a prospective study of 54 patients. *J Am Acad Dermatol.* 2003;48:201–206.

Docetaxel, nab-paclitaxel, paclitaxel

Chang SY, Tsai SH, Chen LJ, et al. Paclitaxel-induced cystoid macular edema. *Acta Ophthalmol.* 2018;96(5):e649–e650.

Fabre-Guillevin E, Tchen N, Anibali-Charpiat M-F, et al. Taxane-induced glaucoma. *Lancet.* 1999;354(9185):1181–1182.

Ito S, Okuda M. A case of cystic maculopathy during paclitaxel therapy. *Nihon Ganka Gakkai Zasshi.* 2010;114(1):23–27.

Kintzel PE, Michaud LB, Lange MK. Docetaxel-associated epiphora. *Pharmacotherapy.* 2006;26(6):853–867.

Li J, Tripathi RC, Tripathi BJ. Drug-induced ocular disorders. *Drug Safety.* 2008;31(2):127–141.

Mansur C, Pfeiffer ML, Esmaeli B. Evaluation and management of chemotherapy-induced epiphora, punctal and canalicular stenosis, and nasolacrimal duct obstruction. *Ophthal Plast Reconstr Surg.* 2017;33(1):9–12.

Smith SV, Benz MS, Brown DM. Cystoid macular edema secondary to albumin-bound paclitaxel therapy. *Arch Ophthalmol.* 2008;126(11):1605–1606.

Tan WW, Walsh T. Ocular toxicity secondary to paclitaxel in two lung cancer patients. *Med Pediatr Oncol.* 1998;31(3):177.

Etoposide

Hilliard LM, Berkow RL, Watterson J, et al. Retinal toxicity associated with cisplatin and etoposide in pediatric patients. *Med Pediatr Oncol.* 1997;28:310–313.

Luke C, Bartz-Schmidt KU, Walter P, et al. Effects of etoposide (VP 16) on vertebrate retinal function. *J Toxicol Cut Ocular Toxicol.* 1999;18(1):23–32.

Peyman GA, Greenberg D, Fishman GA. Evaluation of toxicity of intravitreal antineoplastic drugs. *Ophthalmic Surg.* 1984;15:411–413.

Fludarabine phosphate

Bishop RJ, Ding X, Heller III CK, et al. Rapid vision loss associated with fludarabine administration. *Retina.* 2010;30:1272–1277.

Chun HG, Leyland-Jones BR, Caryk SM, et al. Central nervous systemic toxicity of fludarabine phosphate. *Cancer Treat Rep.* 1986;70:1225–1228.

Spriggs DR, Stpa E, Mayer RJ, et al. Fludarabine phosphate infusions for the treatment of acute leukemia: phase I and neuropathological study. *Cancer Res.* 1986;46:5953–5958.

Verma A, Llanes N, Rose D, et al. Cortical blindness following fludarabine therapy: a case report and review of literature. *Neurology.* 2008;70(suppl 1):261.

Warrell Jr RP, Berman E. Phase I and II study of fludarabine phosphate in leukemia: therapeutic efficacy with delayed central nervous system toxicity. *J Clin Oncol.* 1986;4:74–79.

Fluorouracil (5FU)

Adams JW, Bofenkamp TM, Kobrin J, et al. Recurrent acute toxic optic neuropathy secondary to 5-FU. *Cancer Treat Rep.* 1984;68:565–566.

Alward WLM, Farrell T, Hayreh S, et al. Fluorouracil filtering surgery study one-year follow-up. *Am J Ophthalmol.* 1989;108(6):625–635.

Baldassare RD, Brunette I, Desjardine DC, et al. Corneal ectasia secondary to excessive ocular massage following trabeculectomy with 5-fluorouracil. *Can J Ophthalmol.* 1996;31(5):252–254.

Baskin Y, Amirfallah A, Unal OU, et al. Dihydropyrimidine dehydrogenase 85T>C mutation is associated with ocular toxicity of 5-fluorouracil: a case report. *Am J Ther.* 2015;22(2):e36–e39.

Caravella Jr LP, Burns JA, Zangmeister M. Punctal-canalicular stenosis related to systemic fluorouracil therapy. *Arch Ophthalmol.* 1981;99:284–286.

Forbes JE, Brazier DJ, Spittle M. 5-Fluorouracil and ocular toxicity. *Br J Ophthalmol.* 1993;77(7):465–466.

Galentine P, Sloas H, Hargett N, et al. Bilateral cicatricial ectropion following topical administration of 5-fluorouracil. *Ann Ophthalmol.* 1981;13:575–577.

Hurwitz BS. Cicatricial ectropion: a complication of systemic fluorouracil. *Arch Ophthalmol.* 1993;111:1608–1609.

Jansman FG, Sleijfer DT, de Graaf JC, et al. Management of chemotherapy-induced adverse effects in the treatment of colorectal cancer. *Drug Saf.* 2001;24:353–367.

Khaw PT, Sherwood MB, MacKay SL, et al. Five-minute treatments with fluorouracil, floxuridine, and mitomycin have long-term effects on human Tenon's capsule fibroblasts. *Arch Ophthalmol.* 1992;110:1150–1154.

Knapp A, Heuer DK, Stern GA. et al. Serious corneal complications of glaucoma filtering surgery with postoperative 5-fluorouracil. *Am J Ophthalmol.* 1987;103:183–187.

Lemp MA. Striate melanokeratosis. *Arch Ophthalmol.* 1991;109(7):917.

Mannis MJ, Sweet EH, Lewis RA. The effect of fluorouracil on the corneal endothelium. *Arch Ophthalmol.* 1988;106:816–817.

Ophir A, Ticho U. Subconjunctival 5-fluorouracil and herpes simplex keratitis. *Ophthalmic Surg.* 1991;22(2):109–110.

Schmid KE, Kornek GV, Scheithauer W, et al. Update on ocular complications of systemic cancer chemotherapy. *Surv Ophthalmol.* 2006;51:19–40.

Solomon LM. Plastic eyeglass frames and topical fluorouracil therapy. *JAMA.* 1985;253:3166.

Imiquimod
O'Neill J, Ayers D, Kenealy J. Periocular lentigo maligna treated with imiquimod. *J Dermatolog Treat.* 2011;22(2):109–112.

Interferon (alpha, beta, gamma, or PEG)
Borgia G, Reynaud L, Gentile I, et al. Myasthenia gravis during low-dose IFN-α therapy for chronic hepatitis C. *J Interferon Cytokine Res.* 2001;21:469–470.

Cuthbertson FM, Davies M, McKibbin M. Is screening for interferon retinopathy in hepatitis C justified? *Br J Ophthalmol.* 2004;88:1518–1520.

Färkkilä M, Iivanainen M, Roine R, et al. Neurotoxic and other side effects of high-dose interferon in amyotrophic lateral sclerosis. *Acta Neurol Scand.* 1984;70:42–46.

Gupta R, Singh S, Tang R, et al. Anterior ischemic optic neuropathy caused by interferon alpha therapy. *Am J Med.* 2002;112:683–684.

Hayasaka S, Nagaki YU, Matsumoto M, et al. Interferon associated retinopathy. *Br J Ophthalmol.* 1998;82:323–325.

Hejny C, Sternber P, Lawson DH, et al. Retinopathy associated with high dose interferon alfa-2b therapy. *Am J Ophthalmol.* 2001;131:782–787.

Huang F, Shih M, Tseng S, et al. Tear function changes during interferon and ribavirin treatment in patients with chronic hepatitis C. *Cornea.* 2005;24:561–566.

Isler M, Akhan G, Bardak Y, et al. Dry cough and optic neuritis: two rare complications of interferon treatment in chronic viral hepatitis. *Am J Gastroenterol.* 2001;96:1302–1303.

Rohatiner AZ, Prior PF, Burton AC, et al. Central nervous system toxicity of interferon. *Br J Cancer.* 1983;47:419–422.

Rubio JE, Charles S. Interferon-associated combined branch retinal artery and central retinal vein obstruction. *Retina.* 2003;23:546–548.

Scott GM, Secher DS, Flowers D, et al. Toxicity of interferon. *BMJ.* 1981;282(25):1345–1348.

Tokai R, Ikeda T, Miyaura T. et al. Interferon-associated retinopathy and cystoid macular edema. *Arch Ophthalmol.* 2001;119:1077–1079.

Vardizer Y, Linhart Y, Loewenstein A, et al. Interferon-α-associated bilateral simultaneous ischemic optic neuropathy. *J Neuroophthalmol.* 2003;23:256–259.

Lenalidomide
Min L, Vaidya A, Becker C. Thyroid autoimmunity and ophthalmopathy related to melanoma biological therapy. *Eur J Endocrinol.* 2011;164(2):303–307.

Melphalan
Chao A-N, Kao L-Y, Liu L, et al. Diffuse chorioretinal atrophy after a single standard low-dose intravitreal melphalan injection in a child with retinoblastoma: a case report. *BMC Ophthalmol.* 2016;16:27.

Lambert NG, Winegar BA, Feola GP, et al. Ocular dysmotility after intra-arterial chemotherapy for retinoblastoma. *J AAPOS.* 2015;19(6):574–577.

Monroy JE, Orbach DB, VanderVeen D, et al. Complications of intra-arterial chemotherapy for retinoblastoma. *Semin Ophthalmol.* 2014;29(5-6):429–433.

Schaiquevich P, Fabius AW, Francis JH, et al. Ocular pharmacology of chemotherapy for retinoblastoma. *Retina.* 2017;37(1):1–10.

Methotrexate
Chaput F. Intraocular T-cell lymphoma: clinical presentation, diagnosis, treatment, and outcome. *Ocul Immunol Inflamm.* 2017;25(5):639–648.

Doroshow JH, Locker GY, Gaasterland DE, et al. Ocular irritation from high-dose methotrexate therapy: pharmacokinetics of drugs in the tear film. *Cancer.* 1981;48:2158–2162.

Fishman ML, Beati SC, Cogan DC. Optic atrophy following prophylactic chemotherapy and cranial radiation for acute lymphocytic leukemia. *Am J Ophthalmol.* 1976;82:571–576.

Frenkel S, Hendler K, Siegal T, et al. Intravitreal methotrexate for treating vitreoretinal lymphoma: 10 years of experience. *Br J Ophthalmol.* 2008;92:383–388.

Galor A, Jabs DA, Leder HA, et al. Comparison of antimetabolite drugs as corticosteroid-sparing therapy for noninfectious ocular inflammation. *Ophthalmology.* 2008;115(10):1826–1832.

Hussain MI. Ocular irritation from low-dose methotrexate therapy. *Cancer.* 1982;50:605.

Imperia PS, Lazarus HM, Lass JH. Ocular complications of systemic cancer chemotherapy. *Surv Ophthalmol.* 1989;34(3):209–230.

Johansson BA. Visual field defects during low-dose methotrexate therapy. *Doc Ophthalmol.* 1992;79(1):91–94.

Knowles RS, Virder JE. Handling of injectable antineoplastic agents. *BMJ.* 1980;281:589–591.

Lepore FE, Nissenblatt MJ. Bilateral internuclear ophthalmoplegia after intrathecal chemotherapy and cranial irradiation. *Am J Ophthalmol.* 1980;92:851–853.

Margileth DA, Poplack DG, Pizzo PA, et al. Blindness during remission in two patients with acute lymphoblastic leukemia. A possible complication of multimodality therapy. *Cancer.* 1977;39:58–61.

Nelson RW, Frank JT. Intrathecal methotrexate-induced neurotoxicities. *Am J Hosp Pharm.* 1981;38:65–68.

Ohguro N, Hashida N, Tano Y. Effect of intravitreous rituximab injections in patients with recurrent ocular lesions associated with central nervous system lymphoma. *Arch Ophthalmol.* 2008;126(7):1002–1003.

Oster MW. Ocular side effects of cancer chemotherapy. In: Perry MC, Yarbro JW, eds. *Toxicity of Chemotherapy.* New York: Grune & Stratton; 1984:181–197.

Ponjavic V, Gränse L, Stigma EB, et al. Reduced full-field electroretinogram (ERG) in a patient treated with methotrexate. *Acta Ophthalmol Scand.* 2004;82:96–99.

Nilutamide

Harris MG, Coleman SG, Faulds D, et al. Nilutamide: a review of its pharmacodynamic and pharmacokinetic properties, and therapeutic efficacy in prostate cancer. *Drugs Aging.* 1993;3(1):9–25.

Kuhn JM, Billebaud T, Navratil H, et al. Prevention of the transient adverse effects of a gonadotropin releasing hormone analogue (buserelin) in metastatic prostatic carcinoma by administration of an antiandrogen (nilutamide). *N Engl J Med.* 1989;321:413–418.

Migliari R, Scarpa RM, Campus G, et al. Evaluation of efficacy and tolerability of nilutamide and buserelin in the treatment of advanced prostate cancer. *Arch It Urol.* 1991;63:147–153.

Oxaliplatin

Leonard G, Wright M, Quinn M, et al. Survey of oxaliplatin-associated neurotoxicity using an interview-based questionnaire in patients with metastatic colorectal cancer. *BMC Cancer.* 2005;5:116–125.

Pemetrexed disodium

Martins-Filho PR, Kameo SY, Mascarenhas-Oliveira AC, et al. Pemetrexed-induced eyelid edema in lung cancer. *J Craniofac Surg.* 2013;24(4):e401–e403.

Shih C, Chen VJ, Gossett LS, et al. LY231514, a pyrrole[2,3-d] pyrimidine-based antifolate that inhibits multiple folate-requiring enzymes. *Cancer Res.* 1997;57:1116–1123.

Tamoxifen citrate

Ah-Song R, Sasco AJ. Tamoxifen and ocular toxicity. *Rev Cancer Detect Prevent.* 1997;21:522–531.

Alwitry A, Gardner I. Tamoxifen maculopathy. *Arch Ophthalmol.* 2002;120:1402.

Ashford AR, Donev I, Tiwari RP, et al. Reversible ocular toxicity related to tamoxifen therapy. *Cancer.* 1988;61:33–35.

Chang T, Gonder JR, Ventresca MR. Case report: Low-dose tamoxifen retinopathy. *Can J Ophthalmol.* 1992;27:148–149.

Colley SM, Elston JS. Tamoxifen optic neuropathy. *Clin Exp Ophthalmol.* 2004;32(1):105–106.

Griffiths MF. Tamoxifen retinopathy at low dosage. *Am J Ophthalmol.* 1987;104:185–186.

Imperia PS, Lazarus HM, Lass JH. Ocular complications of systemic cancer chemotherapy. *Surv Ophthalmol.* 1989;34(3):209–230.

McKeown CA, Swartz M, Blom J, et al. Tamoxifen retinopathy. *Br J Ophthalmol.* 1981;65:177–179.

Nayfield SG, Gorin MB. Tamoxifen associated eye disease: a review. *J Clin Oncol.* 1996;14:1018–1026.

Pugesgaard T, von Eyben F. Bilateral optic neuritis evolved during tamoxifen treatment. *Cancer.* 1986;58:383–386.

Robinson E, Kimmick GG, Muss HB. Tamoxifen in postmenopausal women, a safety perspective. *Review.* 1996;8:329–337.

Sadowski B, Kriegbaum C, Apfelstedt-Sylla E. Tamoxifen side effects, age related macular degeneration (AMD) or cancer associated retinopathy (CAR)? *Eur J Ophthalmol.* 2001;11:309–312.

Tamoxifen and venous thromboembolism. *WHO ADR Newslett.* 1999;2:3.

Tang R, Shields J, Schiffman J, et al. Retinal changes associated with tamoxifen treatment for breast cancer. *Rev Eye.* 1997;11:295–297.

Tsai D-C, Chen S-J, Chiou S-H, et al. Should we discontinue tamoxifen in a patient with vision-threatening ocular toxicity related to low-dose tamoxifen therapy? *Eye.* 2003;17:276–278.

Vinding T, Nielsen NV. Retinopathy caused by treatment with tamoxifen in low dosage. *Acta Ophthalmol.* 1983;61:45–50.

Vogel VG, Costantino JP, Wickerman DL, et al. Effects of tamoxifen vs raloxifene on the risk of developing invasive breast cancer and other disease outcomes. *JAMA.* 2006;295:2727–2741.

Zinchuk O, Watanabe M, Hayashi N, et al. A case of tamoxifen keratopathy. *Arch Ophthalmol.* 2006;124:1046–1048.

Thiotepa

Cooper JC. Pterygium. prevention of recurrence by excision and postoperative thiotepa. *Eye Ear Nose Throat Monthly.* 1966;45:59–61.

Greenspan EM, Jafrrey I, Bruckner H. Thiotepa, cutaneous reactions, and efficacy. *JAMA.* 1977;237:2288.

Harben DJ, Cooper PH, Rodman OG. Thiotepa-induced leukoderma. *Arch Dermatol.* 1979;115:973–974.

Olander K, Haik KG, Haik GM. Management of pterygia. Should thiotepa be used? *Ann Ophthalmol.* 1978;10:853–862.

Trastuzumab

Beeram M, Krop IE, Burris HA, et al. A phase 1 study of weekly dosing of trastuzumab emtansine (T-DM1) in patients with advanced human epidermal growth factor 2-positive breast cancer. *Cancer.* 2012;118(23):5733–5740.

Burriss 3rd HA, Rugo HS, Vukelja SJ, et al. Phase II study of the antibody drug conjugate trastuzumab-DM1 for the treatment of human epidermal growth factor receptor 2 (HER2) – positive breast cancer after prior HER2-directed therapy. *J Clin Oncol.* 2011;29(4):398–405.

Kreps EO, Derveaux T, Denys H. Corneal changes in trastuzumab emtansine treatment. *Clin Breast Cancer.* 2018;18(4):e427–e429.

Krop IE, Beeram M, Modi S, et al. Phase I study of trastuzumab-DM1, an HER2 antibody-drug conjugate, given every 3 weeks to patients with HER2-positive metastatic breast cancer. *J Clin Oncol.* 2010;28(16):2698–2704.

Vinblastine sulfate

Cohen RJ, Cuneo RA, Cruciger MP, et al. Transient left homonymous hemianopsia and encephalopathy following treatment of testicular carcinoma with cisplatinum, vinblastine, and bleomycin. *J Clin Oncol.* 1983;1:392–393.

Vincristine sulfate

Elomaa I, Pajunen M, Virkkunen P. Raynaud's phenomenon progressing to gangrene after vincristine and bleomycin therapy. *Acta Med Scand.* 1984;216:323–326.

Holland JF, Scharlau C, Gailani S, et al. Vincristine treatment of advanced cancer: a cooperative study of 392 cases. *Cancer Res.* 1973;33:1258–1264.

Imperia PS, Lazarus HM, Lass JH. Ocular complications of systemic cancer chemotherapy. *Surv Ophthalmol.* 1989;34(3):209–230.

Kaplan RS, Wiernik PH. Neurotoxicity of antineoplastic drugs. *Semin Oncol.* 1982;9:103–130.

Margileth DA, Polplack DG, Tizzo PA, et al. Blindness during remission in two patients with acute lymphoblastic leukemia: a possible complication of multimodality therapy. *Cancer.* 1977;39:5–61.

Toker E, Yenice O, Ogut MS. Isolated abducens nerve palsy induced by vincristine therapy. *J AAPOS.* 2004;8:69–71.

CHAPTER 16

Heavy Metal Antagonists and Miscellaneous Drugs

CLASS: DRUGS USED TO TREAT ALCOHOLISM

Generic Name:
Disulfiram.

Proprietary Name:
Antabuse.

Primary Use
This thiuram derivative is used as an aid in the management of chronic alcoholism.

Ocular Side Effects
Systemic administration – oral
Certain
1. Decreased vision
2. Optic nerve
   a. Hyperemia
   b. Edema
   c. Neuritis
   d. Retrobulbar neuritis
   e. Pallor
3. Scotomas – central or centrocecal
4. Color vision defect – red-green defect

Probable
1. Eyelids or conjunctiva
   a. Allergic reactions
   b. Erythema
   c. Urticaria
2. Visual hallucinations

Possible
1. Extraocular muscles – paresis or paralysis

Clinical Significance
Disulfiram has been in use for over 60 years as a "psychological threat" to treat alcoholism because of the severity of the disulfiram–ethanol interaction. On rare occasions marked decreased vision may occur. Retrobulbar and optic neuritis have been documented by numerous authors.[1-8] Optic nerve disease may occur as early as a few weeks or as late as 18 months after starting the drug.[5-8] Improvement of optic or retrobulbar neuritis may occur within 7 weeks to 3 months after stopping the drug.[8] In general, the vision loss secondary to retrobulbar or optic neuritis occurs 1–5 months after disulfiram is discontinued. These ocular side effects may be more common at higher dosages, in the elderly, or in patients with impaired hepatic function. Peripheral neuropathy due to disulfiram occurs in 1 in 15,000 patients; therefore optic nerve disorders are plausible.[9] Most patients have a comorbid alcohol and nicotine abuse, which complicates determining if all of the neurologic effects are due to disulfiram. However, there are enough cases of drug withdrawal with complete remission and cases of positive rechallenge after relapse to support a "certain" association. Other ocular side effects are reversible and seldom of importance. In the spontaneous reports, there is a case of sisters on disulfiram who experienced transient repeating episodes of vertical diplopia. They were not related to time, day, or activity and lasted only a matter of minutes, then spontaneously resolved. Acheson et al reported a case of decreased and delayed visual evoked potential in a patient with bilateral optic neuropathy with full recovery after 8 months off disulfiram.[10]

CLASS: CALCIUM-REGULATING DRUGS

Generic Names:
1. Alendronate sodium; 2. etidronate disodium; 3. ibandronate sodium; 4. pamidronate disodium; 5. risedronate sodium; 6. zoledronic acid.

Proprietary Names:
1. Binosto, Fosamax; 2. Didronel; 3. Boniva; 4. Aredia; 5. Actonel, Atelvia; 6. Reclast, Zometa.

Primary Use
These bisphosphonate calcium-regulating drugs are used primarily in the management of hypercalcemia of malignancy, metastasis bone pain, osteoporosis, and Paget disease of bone.

Ocular Side Effects
Systemic administration – intravenous or oral
Certain
1. Decreased vision
2. Conjunctiva – transitory
   a. Lacrimation
   b. Hyperemia
   c. Pain
   d. Burning sensation
   e. Gritty sensation
   f. Irritation
   g. Edema
3. Photophobia
4. Uveitis – anterior or posterior
5. Eyelids
   a. Edema
   b. Inflammation
   c. Blepharitis
6. Scleritis
7. Episcleritis
8. Visual hallucinations

Probable
1. Orbit
   a. Inflammation
   b. Edema
2. Color vision defect

Possible
1. Optic neuritis

Conditional/unclassified
1. Conjunctival squamous metaplasia (risedronate)

Clinical Significance
The adverse ocular side effects listed may be caused by the bisphosphonate, but not by all bisphosphonates. There are hundreds of published case reports and thousands of cases in the spontaneous reports concerning possible adverse ocular side effects from this class of drugs. Especially with intravenous bisphosphates, there is well-documented dechallenge and rechallenge data. Anterior ocular external reactions, including conjunctivitis and eyelid edema, may occur after each intravenous infusion. Visual side effect incidences seldom exceed 1% for oral bisphosphonates; however, with intravenous use, especially in the elderly and with long-term use, the incidence may increase.[1]

Nonspecific conjunctivitis usually occurs within 6–48 hours after drug exposure. This conjunctivitis is transitory and seldom requires treatment. The cause for the nonspecific conjunctivitis is also unknown, but the pattern suggests that the drug or its metabolites are secreted into the tears by the lacrimal gland and then cause transitory irritation to the mucous membranes. Rare cases of anterior or posterior uveitis may occur unilaterally or bilaterally within 24–48 hours after drug exposure.[2] Patel et al, in a prospective randomized control trial, found a 1.1% incidence of anterior uveitis confirmed by an ophthalmologist after intravenous zoledronate versus controls.[3] The mean onset was 3 days, and about 60% were unilateral with all gradations of severity. Rechallenge with intravenous zoledronate was not contraindicated, as the ocular side effects may not recur; however, close ophthalmic follow-up was recommended. Episcleritis or scleritis can occur as early as 1–6 days after exposure.[2] The onset is more rapid and intense with intravenous medication. Fraunfelder et al reported 17 cases of unilateral scleritis and 1 case of bilateral scleritis after intravenous pamidronate, with the first positive rechallenge data for any drug causing scleritis.[4,5] The cause of the uveitis, scleritis, and episcleritis is conjecture, but because this is a high-molecular-weight drug, the potential for an immune complex formation has been suggested. If patients develop a uveitis, episcleritis, or scleritis, one needs to monitor these patients more closely and, in some cases, discontinue the drug. Etminan et al, in a retrospective cohort study, found first-time users of bisphosphonates, who saw an ophthalmologist, may be at a higher risk for scleritis or uveitis compared with nonusers.[6] Based on this data and the strong rechallenge data with the need to stop the drug to have scleritis resolve, we feel that uveitis and scleritis due to these drugs, although rare events, are "certain."

It is probable that all of the bisphosphonates have the potential to cause orbital inflammation. This is primarily true of zoledronate, but also alendronate and pamidronate. There are 35 cases documented in the literature and 600+ undocumented cases in the spontaneous reports.[7-10] Although this side effect is primarily seen when the drug is given intravenously, it may occasionally be seen when given orally. With intravenous bisphosphonates, the onset of orbital inflammation may be preceded by a prodromal illness of fever, myalgias, and arthralgias in 30% of the cases.[7] This typically occurs 2–6 days after infusion along with anterior uveitis in 29%. Most cases are bilateral and may be associated with conjunctival chemosis, hyperemia, and subconjunctival hemorrhage.[7] There is obvious periorbital and eyelid edema, which is often associated with proptosis, ocular mobility defects, diplopia, and pain. Meaney et al reported a case with positive rechallenge of a possible early-phase orbital inflammation with bilateral chemosis, lid edema, erythema, and vertical diplopia 2 hours after intravenous pamidronate.[8]

There are little rechallenge data for orbital inflammation. There are some suggestions that some serious bisphosphonate side effects may not occur on rechallenge, and in many cases the drug can be restarted without any fear of recurrence; however, close monitoring is required.[9] There may or may not be cross sensitivity between drugs; however, informed consent is essential. The diagnosis in absence of biopsy is clinical radiology, computed tomography (CT), or magnetic resonance imaging (MRI). Regardless, the close temporal association between exposure to the drug, pattern of onset, CT or MRI findings, side effect, response, sequelae, and the plausible inflammatory pathogenesis supports a connection.[10]

Des Grottes et al described a patient with porphyria who developed reversible retrobulbar neuritis after intravenous pamidronate.[11] Ghose et al also reported a case with orbital pain, proptosis, ptosis, chemosis, and partial 3rd and 4th nerve palsies.[12] The patient had a negative neurologic work-up, and all findings resolved after a course of oral steroids. Stach et al reported a case of possible optic neuritis due to alendronate.[13]

There are a few published case reports of optic neuritis – it is possibly more common with pamidronic acid and zoledronic acid.[14–16] Also, based on 2 cases in the spontaneous reports, xanthopsia occurred with positive rechallenge within 2 hours of drug exposure.

Mammo et al reported that continued users of long-term oral bisphosphonates are at a higher risk of developing wet age-related macular degeneration.[17] Grzybowski et al and Mammo et al have discussed that the changes are small.[18,19]

Bursztyn et al reported a case of severe visual loss after intravenous zoledronic acid in a patient with 15 years of quiescence chloroquine maculopathy.[20]

Unusual cases associated with this class of drugs include risedronate-associated squamous metaplasia of the conjunctiva.[21]

Recommendations

1. Any patients on this group of drugs who report any persistent change in vision or ocular pain should see an ophthalmologist.
2. Nonspecific conjunctivitis seldom requires treatment and usually decreases in intensity with repeat exposure to the drug. Use of preservative-free artificial tears may give temporary relief.

3. One needs to be aware that multiple ocular side effects may occur in the same patients, so a complete dilated ophthalmic examination is necessary. In some instances, the drug may need to be discontinued for severe uveitis to resolve; but for the most part, anterior uveitis can be controlled with topical steroids.
4. In our experience, for the scleritis to resolve, even with the patient on full medical therapy, the bisphosphonate must be discontinued.
5. Orbital inflammation requires intravenous steroids to control. Signs and symptoms usually completely resolve.

CLASS: CHELATING DRUGS

Generic Name:
Deferasirox.

Proprietary Names:
Exjade, Jadenu.

Primary Use
Tridentate iron chelator used in patients needing frequent blood transfusions and in patients with non–transfusion-dependent thalassemia syndromes.

Ocular Side Effects
Systemic administration – oral
Possible
1. Decreased vision
2. Retinopathy
3. Maculopathy

Conditional/unclassified
1. Optic neuritis
2. Cataracts

Clinical Significance
Deferasirox is given orally once per day, whereas deferoxamine, the leading chelating drug for these diseases, is given intravenously, intramuscularly, or subcutaneously. Deferoxamine is classified by the World Health Organization as one of the safest and most effective drugs; therefore patients are often started on deferoxamine and if visual side effects occur or progress, then they may be switched to deferasirox. However, there are 3 cases in the literature where starting deferasirox after stopping deferoxamine caused either progression of prior deferoxamine maculopathy or new visual symptoms.[1–3] After stopping deferasirox the visual acuity in all 3 reports reverted to its prior baseline.

There are 37 spontaneous case reports of retinal problems associated with deferasirox use. Bui et al described increased macular thickness and decreased dark adaptation in a patient with prior deferoxamine-associated pseudovitelliform maculopathy when deferasirox was started.[3] Pan et al described optic coherence tomography revealing thinning of the outer retinal layers with disruption of the inner and outer segment junction in the perifoveal region.[1] Walia et al described mild funduscopic changed with marked electrophysical abnormalities; however, no pattern was found.[2]

Sanford et al reported episcleritis associated with this drug.[4] We found no other reports in the literature and only 1 case in the spontaneous reports.

Generic Name:
Deferoxamine mesylate (desferrioxamine).

Proprietary Name:
Desferal.

Primary Use
Systemic
This chelating drug is used in the treatment of iron-storage diseases and acute iron poisoning.

Ophthalmic
This topical drug is used in the treatment of ocular siderosis and hematogenous pigmentation of the cornea.

Ocular Side Effects
Systemic administration – intramuscular, intravenous, or subcutaneous
Certain
1. Decreased vision
2. Night blindness
3. Color vision defect
4. Decreased dark adaptation
5. Retina
   a. Pigment epithelium (Fig. 16.1)
      i. Opacification
      ii. Loss of transparency
      iii. Molting
6. Macula
   a. Decreased foveal reflex
   b. Cystoid macular edema
   c. Vitelliform maculopathy
   d. Bull's-eye maculopathy
7. Optic nerve
   a. Disc edema
   b. Pallor
   c. Atrophy
8. Abnormal – electroretinogram (ERG), multifocal ERG, electrooculogram (EOG), or visual evoked potential (VEP)
9. Visual field defects
   a. Scotoma – central, centrocecal, and ring
   b. Constriction
10. Eyelids and conjunctiva
   a. Allergic reactions
   b. Urticaria
   c. Edema

Possible
1. Cataracts
2. Optic neuritis

Local ophthalmic use or exposure – topical ocular application
Certain
1. Eyelids or conjunctiva
   a. Allergic reactions
   b. Hyperemia

Clinical Significance
Deferoxamine has been used clinically for 40+ years, and with refinement of the product, it is being used for more diseases. One must keep in mind the clinical features of the disease being treated to not confuse the disease and the drug's possible side effects. Ocular toxicity usually occurs with long-term therapy, although acute toxicity may occur with rechallenge exposure, in dialysis patients, or in end-stage renal disease.[1-7] The acute reactions are no different from those found in patients on long-term deferoxamine therapy and may be irreversible, even with only a single dose.[1,8] Although ocular toxicity is rare, it varies from minimal reversible changes in approximately two-thirds of cases to irreversible changes, including blindness, in approximately one-third of cases. With current preparations, the one-third figure is probably high. Acute adverse ocular effects are seen most frequently in high dosages, whereas low-dose chronic exposure over a 20-year period may show no retinal toxicity.[9]

No clear-cut relationship between drug dosage and retinopathy has been established for deferoxamine. The earliest signs of retinal toxicity include blurred or decreased night vision. Retinal pigment epithelial mottling changes are seen only after the onset of color abnormalities or after nyctalopia occurs. Haimovici et al reported that the earliest fundus findings are subtle opacifications or loss of transparency of the outer retina and retinal pigment epithelium.[10] Fluorescein angiography in the earliest stage of toxicity is variable.

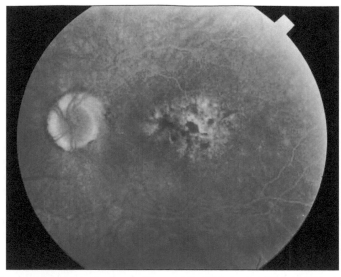

FIG. 16.1 Late fluorescein angiogram showing foveal retinal pigment epithelial (RPE) pigment clumping after deferoxamine treatment.[10]

During the transition stage, there is often block fluorescence and then late fluorescence in the late stage. This occurs before retinal pigment epithelium molting. If vitelliform maculopathy develops, permanent visual loss may occur.[3,11] Gonzales et al pointed out that persistent hyperfluorescence within the macula may represent a poor prognostic finding due to irreversible retinal pigment epithelium damage.[11] This molting is primarily foveal, but with time it may extend to the paramacular, papillomacular, and peripapillary areas. Electrophysiologic studies suggest widespread retinal involvement, not just focal areas, as seen on funduscopic examination.[10] Electrophysiologic testing is important in diagnosis, management, and predicting progression.[12,13] Spectral domain–optical coherence tomography is a noninvasive tool for detection and long-term follow-up.[14,15]

Toxic cerebral and optic neuropathies with central or centrocecal scotomas and peripheral constriction of visual fields have also been reported in patients receiving deferoxamine.[4,16,17] Various symmetrical and asymmetrical disc changes have been described, including edema and atrophy. Although these events may well be drug related, there are a few with no clear pattern or mechanism. This drug can cause cataracts in animals, but there are only a few reports in humans.[18-20] Popescu et al suggested that deferoxamine may even be protective against cataracts.[21] To date, there is no strong evidence that this drug is cataractogenic in humans; however, postmarketing data, especially in geriatric patients on long-term therapy, shows that cataracts can occur on deferoxamine therapy.[22] It is unknown if this is due to the drug, age factors, the disease, or a combination of all of these. The exact mechanism of deferoxamine toxicity to the eye is unknown and varies, in part, according to the condition that is being treated. However, in some cases, it is probably due to the drug's capacity to chelate the essential trace elements required for normal enzymatic activity and cellular function.

Recommendations

There are no universally accepted ophthalmic guidelines for following patients on deferoxamine. It is clear that with low and even standard dosages, very few ocular side effects are seen. However, in patients receiving intravenous medication; patients receiving higher-than-standard dosages; patients who are diabetic; and patients with rheumatoid arthritis, metabolic encephalopathy, low ferritin concentration, or renal failure, the following should be considered:

1. Baseline ocular examination, including dilated funduscopy, color vision testing, visual fields testing, dark adaptometry, and angiography. An electrophysiologic study is ideal and, if possible, include multifocal ERG in high-risk patients.[23]

2. If intravenous deferoxamine is necessary, the patient should undergo an ophthalmic examination with

visualization of the fundus, and frequent serum ferritin levels (<0.025) may be taken.[24]

3. Baath et al, in a review of a large pediatric hospital, found it was not cost-effective to do regular annual screenings if the drug was given subcutaneously or at standard dosages.[25] They felt that this was not true for patients on higher dosages or intravenous therapy.

4. Patients should be told to see an ophthalmologist at the first signs of a change in vision, color perception, or night vision.

5. Late hyperfluorescence on fluorescein angiography seems to be a reliable indicator of active retinopathy. Retinal pigment epithelium molting does not resolve with stopping deferoxamine. Electrophysiologic tests are confirmatory and may show more widespread dysfunction than seen by fundoscopy alone.[10]

6. At the first signs of toxicity to the retina, the risk–benefit ratio needs to be called to the attention of the treating physician.

7. As Arora et al pointed out, even using these guidelines and stopping the drug early, some patients will develop significant visual loss.[26]

8. Pinna et al suggested oral zinc sulfate for presumed optic neuropathy and hearing loss.[17]

Generic Name:
Methoxsalen (8-methoxypsoralen).

Proprietary Names:
8-MOP, Oxsoralen, Oxsoralen-Ultra, Uvadex.

Primary Use
This psoralen is used in the treatment of psoriasis. It is also used in the management of various skin cancers.

Ocular Side Effects
Systemic administration – cutaneous, extracorporeal, or oral
Certain
1. Eyelids
   a. Hyperpigmentation
   b. Erythema
   c. Phytodermatitis
2. Conjunctival hyperemia
3. Keratitis
4. Photophobia
5. Decreased electrophysiologic tests

Probable
1. Eyelids and periocular skin – increased incidence of malignancies

Possible
1. Eyelids – hypertrichosis
2. Lacrimation decreased
3. Cataracts

Conditional/unclassified
1. Pigmentary glaucoma

Clinical Significance
This medication is given orally as a photosensitizing drug before ultraviolet A therapy (PUVA) for treatment of various skin disorders. Wraparound ultraviolet (UV)–protecting sunglasses are given to the patient during and for at least 12 hours after treatment. To date, this regimen has had little to no ocular side effects other than a photosensitizing effect on the periocular skin. Most ocular adverse effects are transitory and reversible and have been due to inadvertent light exposure or not wearing protective lenses. Other than the typical photosensitivity reaction of the anterior segment (conjunctival hyperemia, keratitis, photophobia), occasionally a patient may also complain of sicca-like symptoms for 48–72 hours after therapy. In a study of 82 patients who refused goggles and posttreatment UV-blocking lenses over a 2- to 4-year period, about one-quarter had transitory conjunctival hyperemia and decreased lacrimation.[1] Souêtre et al reported increased sensitivity of the retina to visible light.[2] Reported visual field changes are transitory and probably functional rather than drug related.[3] There are a few cases in the spontaneous reports of pigmentary glaucoma after PUVA therapy, but this is not a proven drug-related event. Because this therapy causes proliferation of pigment epithelial cells, this association may not be coincidental. The increased incidence of skin cancers is probable.[4,5]

The area of greatest controversy is whether PUVA therapy causes cataracts. It has been shown in animals without UV ocular protection that systemic psoralens can cause anterior inferior cortical cataracts. Lerman et al detected methoxsalen in the lens for at least 12 hours after oral administration.[6] Lerman et al and Woo et al stated that this drug is photo bound in the lens and may be cumulative with additional therapy.[6,7] Van Deenen et al reported transitory punctiform opacities in the nucleus and cortex of patients undergoing PUVA treatment.[8] There have been numerous reports both supporting and denying lens changes in patients with proper eye protection after long-term PUVA therapy. Glew et al wrote a comprehensive review of a series of patients undergoing PUVA therapy followed up for 14 years.[9] With proper UV-blocking lenses, they found no evidence of a higher incidence of lens changes, even with long-term therapy, versus that expected with normal aging change. Stern et al reported the results of 1235 patients enrolled in a PUVA follow-up study with an average follow-up of 10 years.[10,11] Although they showed an increase in posterior subcapsular cataracts and a 4 times higher incidence of cataract extraction in the PUVA cohorts, the authors concluded that these differences may be attributable to variations in the lens abnormalities, nonuniform examination techniques, or exposure to other drugs. A review of the literature, US Food and Drug Administration (FDA) data, and more than 40 cases in the spontaneous reports of lens changes associated with psoralen use seems to support the following conclusions. Usually, a drug causes a certain type of cataract. To date, no characteristic pattern of lens abnormalities in humans has been associated with psoralen use. Few, if any, lens changes occur with proper UV-blocking lenses. Theoretically, PUVA therapy without UV-blocking lenses could cause cataracts in humans, but a definite cause-and-effect relationship has not been proven. However, the *Physicians' Desk Reference* (PDR) states that cataracts may occur after methoxsalen therapy.[12] Maitray et al reported the only case of macular toxicity arising from methoxsalen use.[13] The 41-year-old male had been on this drug for 15 years. Over 3 years he developed metamorphopsia with yellowish-white deposits in both macula and blunted foveal reflexes. With progressive changes, after 1 year the drug was discontinued. Minimal change on electrophysiologic tests were seen. There are 3 questionable cases in the spontaneous reports of retinal changes. Shoeibi et al reported significant acute electrophysiologic changes associated with methoxypsoralen and UVA, which were prevented if UV-blocking lenses were used.[14]

Recommendations[12]

1. Patients receiving oral methoxsalen should have an ophthalmic examination before starting therapy and then yearly thereafter.
2. This drug is contraindicated in aphakic patients.

Generic Name:
Penicillamine.

Proprietary Names:
Cuprimine, D-PENAMINE, Depen.

Primary Use

This amino acid derivative of penicillin is a potent chelating drug effective in the management of Wilson disease; cystinuria; and copper, iron, lead, or mercury poisonings. It is also a second-line drug in the management of rheumatoid arthritis.

Ocular Side Effects
Systemic administration – oral
Certain
1. Myasthenia gravis
   a. Diplopia
   b. Ptosis
   c. Paresis of extraocular muscles

Possible
1. Eyelids or conjunctiva
   a. Blepharoconjunctivitis
   b. Urticaria
   c. Pemphigoid lesion with symblepharon
   d. Trichomegaly
   e. Yellowing and wrinkling of eyelids
   f. Chalazion
2. Color vision defect – red-green defect
3. Extraocular muscles
   a. Decreased convergence
   b. Nystagmus
   c. Internuclear ophthalmoplegia
4. Irritation
   a. Lacrimation
   b. Hyperemia
   c. Photophobia
   d. Edema
5. Retina
   a. Pigmentary changes
   b. Hemorrhages
   c. Serous detachment
6. Retrobulbar or optic neuritis
7. Visual fields
   a. Scotomas – centrocecal
   b. Constriction
8. Eyelids or conjunctiva
   a. Lupoid syndrome
   b. Lyell syndrome

Clinical Significance

Adverse ocular reactions to penicillamine are rare. Myasthenia gravis is a well-documented complication from long-term penicillamine therapy.[1] Ptosis, diplopia, or extraocular muscle paresis may be the first signs of this drug-related event. The onset usually occurs within 6–7 months, but in some cases, it may take years to manifest.[2] These side effects usually resolve spontaneously once the drug is stopped, but some patients require anticholinesterase therapy. This adverse drug event may be more common in the immunosuppressed or in those with a genetic predisposition to developing myasthenia.

The drug appears to affect the nervous system, so neuro-ophthalmic complications seem plausible. Damaske et al, Klingele et al, and the *Physicians' Desk Reference* (PDR) suggested that retrobulbar or optic neuritis may be associated with the use of penicillamine.[3-5] The unmarked DL and L forms of penicillamine probably cause optic nerve changes. Pless et al reported chronic internuclear ophthalmoplegia secondary to D-penicillamine–associated cerebral vasculitis.[6] There are cases in the literature that suggest this drug can cause an ocular pemphigoid clinical picture.[7,8] Penicillamine has been implicated in delayed corneal wound healing, decreased proliferation of connective tissue, and corneal superficial punctate keratitis. Penicillamine-induced zinc deficiency may be the cause of keratitis, blepharitis, and loss of eyelashes, but this is unproven. Retinal pigment epithelial defects, serous detachments of the macula, and subretinal or choroidal hemorrhages have also been reported with this drug.[9,10]

CLASS: DIAGNOSTIC AIDS

Generic Name:
Amidotrizoate (diatrizoate meglumine and/or sodium).

Proprietary Names:
Cystografin, Gastrografin, Hypaque, Hypaque-76, MD-76R, MD-Gastroview, Reno-30, Reno-60, Renocal-76, Reno-Dip, Renografin 60, Renografin 76, Urografin.

Primary Use
This organic iodide is used in excretion urography, angiography, joint and computer tomography, and peripheral arteriography.

Ocular Side Effects
Systemic administration – catheter, intravenous, oral, or rectal
Certain
1. Decreased vision
2. Eyelids or conjunctiva
   a. Allergic reactions
   b. Hyperemia
   c. Conjunctivitis – follicular
   d. Edema
   e. Urticaria
3. Irritation
   a. Lacrimation
   b. Photophobia
   c. Pain
   d. Burning sensation
4. Corneal infiltrates
5. Cortical blindness

Possible
1. Visual fields
   a. Scotomas – paracentral
   b. Hemianopsia
2. Retinal vascular disorders
   a. Hemorrhages
   b. Thrombosis
   c. Occlusion
3. Acute macular neuroretinopathy
4. Oculogyric crisis

Clinical Significance
Rare ocular complications associated with radiopaque contrast media arteriography have been well documented. In the spontaneous reports, over half were transitory orbital edema. Most complications usually result from either the toxic irritative or hypersensitivity responses on blood vessels or emboli. A number of hypersensitivity responses have occurred with amidotrizoate, especially perilimbal corneal infiltrates.[1] These are not unlike those seen with staphylococcal hypersensitivity reactions. These may or may not be associated with ocular pain, hyperemia, and chemosis. These infiltrates clear on application of topical ocular steroids without complication. There are cases in the spontaneous reports where amidotrizoate has layered out in the anterior chamber, like a hypopyon, in postoperative cataract surgery patients. No complications from this have been reported. In the absence of pathologic confirmation, retinal or cerebral emboli with resultant secondary complications have been variously interpreted as cholesterol crystals, fat, air, dislodged atheromatous plaques, and the injected contrast media. These have caused various degrees of retinal, choroidal, or optic nerve infarcts with permanent loss of vision. Lantos described 4 cases of acute cortical blindness after the use of amidotrizoate, including hemianopic or complete visual loss.[2] These cases reverted to normal in hours or days. Guzak et al and Priluck et al described cases of acute macular neuroretinopathy after intravenous diatrizoate.[3,4] Findings included swollen macules and subtle opacification of the parafoveal retina. Deep retinal lesions developed later. There were 6 cases in the spontaneous reports of oculogyric crisis.

Generic Name:
Iodipamide meglumine (adipiodone).

Proprietary Name:
Cholografin.

Primary Use
This radiographic contrast medium is used for intravenous cholecystography and cholangiography.

Ocular Side Effects
Systemic administration – intravenous
Certain
1. Eyelids or conjunctiva
    a. Allergic reactions
    b. Erythema
    c. Edema
2. Transient cortical blindness
3. Corneal infiltrates
4. Periorbital edema

Possible
1. Lateral rectus palsy

Clinical Significance
There are multiple case reports of transient cortical blindness (TCB) reported in the literature.[1-10] This is seen most often after vascular intervention after contrast-enhanced coronary, cerebral, and other arterial perfusion studies.

TCB is a bilateral amblyopia or amaurosis with normal fundi, normal papillary reflex, and unaltered extraocular movements. This occurs within minutes up to 12 hours after injection of the contrast medium. Most often it resolves within 2–7 days, but may take 3 weeks.[3] This may be associated with headache, mental changes, hallucinations, memory loss, and blindness denial. TCB can also be associated with hemiparesis, dysplasia, and seizures.[2] Light and motion perception are the first to recover, followed by form and color vision. In a few patients, some residual effects to the visual system may remain, primarily in their visual field.[11]

Although the precise mechanism of the toxic effect is unknown and many explanations have been given, more recent publications favor factors resulting in an osmotic disruption of the blood–brain barrier that seem selective for the occipital cortex. Yeh et al published a table of conditions that can cause leptomeningeal breakdown of the blood–brain barrier, including iodipamide.[10] Junck et al and Lantos felt that this was a direct toxic effect of iodipamide.[6,12] Petrus et al and Wang et al reported cases of TCB after inadvertent arterial entry during venous catheterization.[11,13] Neetans et al reported a patient who developed corneal infiltrates after intravenous iodipamide.[14] The corneal

lesion disappeared with topical ocular corticosteroid treatment. This is a classic finding in most intravenous contrast agents. Bell et al reported a case of transient lateral rectus palsy, which is not unlike those reported with other intravenous contrast media.[15] Although it appears to be a direct toxic event of the contrast agent, the role the procedure plays is unknown. As with other contrast media, transitory periorbital edema is not uncommon.

Generic Names:
1. Iomeprol; 2. iopamidol; 3. iopromide.

Proprietary Names:
1. Imeron; 2. Iopamiro, Isovue, Iopamiron, Niopam; 3. Ultravist.

Primary Use
Intravascularly injected iodinated, nonionic radiographic contrast agents used in showing vasculature in almost all areas of the body.

Ocular Side Effects
Systemic administration – intravascular
Certain
1. Eyelids or conjunctiva
    a. Pruritus
    b. Lacrimation
    c. Chemosis
2. Periorbital edema
3. Extraocular muscles
    a. Paresis
    b. Diplopia

Possible
1. Uveitis
2. Oculogyric crisis
3. Vision loss
    a. Decreased vision
    b. Cortical blindness
    c. Transient visual loss

Clinical Significance
Significant adverse ocular events are rare and usually transient and completely reversible. Allergic ocular reactions occur within a few minutes after injection and present as ocular pruritus lacrimation, and edema. Allergic individuals have twice the adverse reaction as those in the normal population. Another acute pattern is 6th-nerve paresis occurring within a few hours or as late as 12 days later after otherwise uneventful myelograms.[1] These are usually transient with full recovery; however, some have

taken 6 months to recover.[2] Bell et al reported the incidence of this occurring after a myelogram with iopamidol was 1 in 500.[3] Welzl-Hinterkörner et al reported a case of unilateral recurrent uveitis, vitritis, and retinal bleeds, which occurred every 3 months after intravenous iopamidol injections.[4] These ocular side effects resolved within a week after topical ocular steroids.

There are over 30 cases in the literature and spontaneous reports of iopromide- or iopamidol-induced TCB.[5-10] The age range was 17–72 years. In all instances, where data were available, these occurred within minutes to hours after the contrast media was injected. Most all patients' vision returned to normal within 24–72 hours. In 3 instances there was no apparent recovery. The overall incidence rate of TCB occurring in clinical trials was 1.1% with iopromide.[11]

Generic Name:
Iotalamic acid (iothalamic acid, iothalamate sodium, or meglumine iothalamate).

Proprietary Names:
Conray, Conray-30, Conray-43, Cysto-Conray, Glofil-125.

Primary Use
This radiopaque contrast medium is used for excretion urography, contrast enhancement of computed tomography (CT) of the brain, aortography, selective renal arteriography, angiocardiography, and selective coronary arteriography.

Ocular Side Effects
Systemic administration – intravenous or intravesical
Certain
1. Decreased vision
2. Eyelids or conjunctiva
   a. Allergic reactions
   b. Erythema
   c. Conjunctivitis – nonspecific
   d. Edema
3. Irritation
   a. Lacrimation
   b. Photophobia
4. Cortical blindness
5. Cornea – superficial, cloudy peripheral infiltrates

Possible
1. Myasthenia gravis
   a. Diplopia
   b. Ptosis
   c. Paresis of extraocular muscles

d. Divergent strabismus
2. Scotomas – paracentral
3. Retina or macular
   a. Edema
   b. Wedge-shaped lesions
4. Increased intraocular pressure (transitory)

Clinical Significance
Potential rare complications of cerebral angiography may include temporary disturbances in vision and neuromuscular disorders. Visual field losses are usually transient, although permanent changes have been reported after intravenous iothalamate. Guzak et al reported 2 cases of acute macular neuroretinopathy associated with scotoma, metamorphopsia, macular swelling, and typical wedge-shaped retinal lesions.[1] Neetens et al reported a rapid onset of anaphylactic corneal perilimbal superficial marginal infiltrates, which cleared in a few days on topical ocular steroid application.[2] These are also seen with other iodine-containing contrast agents. Smith et al reported a 20–45% decrease in intraocular pressure after intravenous iothalamate sodium.[3] The peak effect is at 30 minutes and returns to baseline in 120 minutes. Lantos reported 4 cases of cortical blindness secondary to this agent, all recovering within 1 month.[4] He postulated that the cause of the clinical manifestations of cortical blindness could be the drug passing through the blood–brain barrier along with toxic effects of the contrast agent on neural elements. Canal et al reported a myasthenic crisis precipitated by an iothalamic acid injection.[5]

CLASS: IMMUNOSUPPRESSANTS

Generic Name:
Azathioprine.

Proprietary Names:
Azasan, Imuran.

Primary Use
This imidazolyl derivative of mercaptopurine is used as an adjunct to help prevent rejection in homograft transplantation and to treat various autoimmune diseases.

Ocular Side Effects
Systemic administration – intravenous or oral
Probable
1. Decreased resistance to infection
2. Delayed corneal wound healing
3. Photosensitivity reactions

Possible

1. Subconjunctival or retinal hemorrhages secondary to drug-induced dyscrasias
2. Loss of eyelashes or eyebrows

Conditional/unclassified

1. Fine macular pigmentation

Ocular teratogenic effects
Possible

1. Cataracts

Clinical Significance

Ocular side effects are uncommon and are reversible on withdrawing the drug. There are reports of activation of ocular viral disease, such as cytomegalic inclusion disease, vaccinia, and bacterial and herpes zoster.[1-5] There is evidence that this drug impedes corneal wound healing.[6,7] This drug has been implicated in numerous blood dyscrasias. Sudhir et al reported bilateral macular hemorrhages due to azathioprine-induced aplastic anemia.[8] Miserocchi et al reported blood dyscrasias in patients treated with this drug for ocular cicatricial pemphigoid.[9] Apaydin et al, along with 2 cases in the spontaneous reports, show an increase in macular pigment while on azathioprine.[10] Patients were on multiple other drugs, and an association could not be made without more cases being reported. Lareb reported 10 cases of various photosensitivity reactions to this drug.[11]

Generic Name:

Cyclosporine (ciclosporin or cyclosporin).

Proprietary Names:

Cequa, Gengraf, Neoral, Restasis, Sandimmune.

Primary Use

Systemic

This immunosuppressive drug is used for prevention of kidney, liver, or heart allografts. Disorders of the skin, blood, gastrointestinal tract, liver, neurologic system, and kidney, as well as collagen vascular diseases, have been treated with this drug.

Ophthalmic

Topical ocular use in the management of uveitis, Behçet syndrome, corneal disease, scleritis, and severe conjunctivitis.

Ocular Side Effects

Systemic administration – intravenous or oral
Certain

1. Decreased vision
2. Conjunctiva
   a. Hyperemia
   b. Conjunctivitis
3. Eyelids
   a. Blepharitis
   b. Edema
4. Irritation
   a. Pain
   b. Discharge
   c. Pruritus
   d. Foreign body sensation
5. Optic nerve (primarily bone marrow transplants)
   a. Edema
   b. Neuropathy
6. Retinal and optic nerve ischemia (with total body radiation)
   a. Cotton-wool spots
   b. Hemorrhages
   c. Lipid deposits
7. Posterior leukoencephalopathy
8. Visual hallucinations
9. Cortical blindness

Probable

1. Extraocular muscles
   a. 6th-nerve palsy
   b. Ocular flutter
   c. External ophthalmoplegia
   d. Nystagmus

Possible

1. Pseudotumor cerebri
2. Increased lymphoproliferative disease

Local ophthalmic use or exposure – topical ocular application
Certain

1. Irritation
   a. Burning sensation
   b. Pain
   c. Pruritus
   d. Discharge
      i. Clear fluid
      ii. Yellow fluid
2. Increased corneal sensitivity

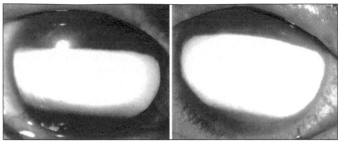

FIG. 16.2 Dense white deposits after topical ocular cyclosporine treatment.[22]

Possible
1. Cornea
    a. Superficial punctate keratitis
    b. Superficial deposits (Fig. 16.2)
2. Eyelids and conjunctiva
    a. Edema
    b. Hyperemia
    c. Neoplasia

Conditional/unclassified
1. Anterior subcapsular cataract (with prednisolone)
2. Superficial ocular neoplasia
3. Trichomegaly

Clinical Significance
This drug is used systemically for medical conditions of some complexity where multiple medications and procedures (i.e. bone marrow transplants, total-body radiation) are complicating factors in determining specific drug side effects. However, with the drug now in clinical use for over 30 years, drug-induced ocular side effects are fairly well understood. The drug or its metabolites are probably secreted in the tears, causing symptoms in 1–6% of patients, including pain, foreign body sensation, epiphora, pruritus and ocular irritation.[1] They are reversible when the drug is continued and may get better with time without decreasing the dosage.

Bone marrow transplantation patients seem to have unique ocular toxicity due to cyclosporine and associated drugs. Avery et al described 8 cases of optic disc edema that resolved after discontinuing or decreasing the cyclosporine dosage.[2] Optic disc edema is not uncommon in some bone marrow transplant series.[3] Optic disc edema due to cyclosporine may be a direct toxic effect of the drug on the optic nerve or papilledema secondary to pseudotumor cerebri. Bernauer et al described retinal and optic nerve ischemia in 13 patients, including bilateral disc edema, cotton-wool spots, retinal hemorrhages, and lipid deposits.[4] This occurred within the first 6 months of cyclosporine therapy after bone marrow transplantation and was reversible in 9 of the 13 cases after the drug was discontinued. The authors concluded that this adverse event was due to a combined effect of cyclosporine along with total-body radiation. Other ocular side effects may include cortical blindness, papilledema, and pseudotumor cerebri. This drug rarely affects the optic nerve in renal transplant patients.[5] There have been a few reports of pseudotumor cerebri with this drug, but a clear-cut cause-and-effect relationship has not been proven.[6,7] There are 4 cases of unilateral or bilateral 6th-nerve palsy with or without ptosis in patients on both cyclosporine and ganciclovir.[8,9] Magnetic resonance imaging (MRI) showed this was due to abnormalities in the region of the 6th-nerve nucleus rather than a localized ocular neuromuscular event. The palsies reverted to normal in a matter of days once cyclosporine was stopped. The MRI findings also resolved. Ocular flutter in bone marrow transplant patients taking cyclosporine has been described by Apsner et al.[10] Porges et al reported a case of cyclosporine-induced optic neuropathy, ophthalmoplegia, and nystagmus in a patient with Crohn's disease.[11] Palmer et al showed that in renal allograft patients, systemic cyclosporine increased tear flow even when no lacrimal autoimmune disease exists.[12]

Cyclosporine can cause posterior leukoencephalopathy, which includes various degrees of visual loss, encephalopathy, white matter changes, and seizures. These changes usually return to near normal after stopping cyclosporine. There are at least 40 well-documented cases of this syndrome, primarily in bone marrow or liver transplant cases, but also in patients with leukemia or aplastic anemia. Visual abnormalities have a variable presentation, but most commonly occur within the first 2 months after starting cyclosporine.

The retinal examination is negative, although Estel et al described yellow retinal exudates.[13] When this syndrome is discovered, one must reduce dosage or discontinue the drug. Recovery of vision is often directly proportional to the severity of the syndrome.[14] Although complete recovery is common, there are cases of permanent blindness.[13,15]

There have been reports with positive rechallenge of cortical blindness caused by cyclosporine after lung transplantation.[16] With systemic administration, severe ocular pain may occur for unexplained reasons with or without evidence of an ocular abnormality. This may occur while taking the drug or when the drug is discontinued. Various irritative reactions may occur around the eye, but these are seldom of major clinical significance. Visual hallucinations may be so severe that they require cyclosporine to be discontinued. Cho et al reported 4 cases of posttransplant lymphoproliferative disorders, including uveitis and iris nodules.[17] They attributed this to a cyclosporin side effect. Oktay Kacmaz et al, in a large series, showed increased ocular and systemic side effect rates associated with cyclosporine use in patients over 55 years old.[18]

Topical ocular cyclosporine has recently had a significant increase in commercial interest, with newer vehicles and forms of this drug being developed. Therefore the ocular side effects profile of this drug is in flux.

Commercial topical ocular cyclosporine (0.05%) may, in up to 17% of patients, cause some burning or stinging on application. Occasionally patients may develop lid irritation, superficial punctate keratitis, and erythema of the lids and/or conjunctiva. Sall et al reported few ocular side effects other than burning and stinging.[19] Peyman et al, in laser-assisted in situ keratomileusis (LASIK) patients, and Toker et al, in dry eye patients, showed increased corneal sensitivity after topical cyclosporine.[20,21] Kachi et al reported a patient developing corneal deposits bilaterally within 5 days of starting topical ocular cyclosporine (2%) 3 times daily.[22] This was associated with severe disturbances of the corneal epithelium and decreased tear production. After 12 months without the drug, no improvement in the density of the opacities was seen, other than some peripheral clearing. Barber et al found no associated systemic side effects when using a 0.1% ophthalmic emulsion for up to 3 years.[23]

Topical ocular immunosuppression may carry an increased risk of malignant tumors. Touzeau et al, Macarez et al, and the spontaneous reports have a few reports of conjunctival intraepithelial neoplasia and/or squamous cell carcinoma of the conjunctiva or limbus.[24,25] Flynn et al reported benign papillomatous lesions of the conjunctiva.[26] Mohammadpour et al described a 25-year-old patient with bilateral anterior subcapsular cataracts after 3 years of prednisolone, cyclosporine, and mycophenolate mofetil after a second kidney transplant.[27] Histology showed anterior subcapsular fibrosis. Siak et al described reactivation of cytomegalovirus uveitis after topical ocular cyclosporine.[28]

Generic Name:
Tacrolimus (FK506 or fujimycin).

Proprietary Names:
Astagraf XL, Envarsus, Hecoria, Prograf, Protopic.

Primary Use
Systemic
This potent immunosuppressant is used in the prophylaxis treatment of organ rejection.

Ophthalmic
Used off-label for graft rejection and other conditions helped by immunosuppression.

Ocular Side Effects
Systemic administration – intravenous or oral
Certain
1. Decreased vision
2. Visual hallucinations
3. Eyelids or conjunctiva
   a. Photosensitivity
   b. Increased susceptibility to bacterial, viral, or fungal infections

Probable
1. Cortical blindness – posterior reversible leukoencephalopathy syndrome
2. Optic nerve
   a. Neuropathy
   b. Neuritis
3. Abnormal visual evoked potential (VEP)

Possible
1. Increase incidence of malignancies, lymphoma, intraepithelial neoplasia, and various viruses
2. Oculogyric crisis
3. Myasthenia gravis

Conditional/unclassified
1. Downward gaze deviation
2. Internuclear ophthalmoplegia
3. Retinal vasculitis – vessel occlusion

Local ophthalmic use of exposure – ointment 0.1–0.3%
Certain
1. Decreased vision
2. Irritation
   a. Burning
   b. Pruritus
   c. Erythema

Conditional/unclassified
1. Mucosal pigmentary changes
2. Hypertrichosis
3. Reactivation of herpes simplex
4. Aqueous tear deficiency

Clinical Significance

Ocular side effects due to this drug are uncommon. The most common central nervous system toxicity probably due to tacrolimus is posterior reversible leukoencephalopathy syndrome. This typically presents with bilateral white matter lesions in the parieto-occipital lobes with significant visual consequences.[1-3] Once the drug is stopped, vision usually improves within 1–2 weeks. Devine et al reported 3 cases of cortical blindness that followed a pattern similar to ciclosporin-induced cortical blindness, early in the course of therapy.[2] No direct correlation to blood levels of the drug and continued improvement while still on the drug were seen. MRI findings appeared to lag behind the clinical improvements. There are 7 cases of cortical blindness attributed to this drug in the spontaneous reports.

Rasool et al recently did a review of their 3 cases and 9 cases in the literature of probable tacrolimus-induced optic neuropathy.[4-13] This entity may start with minimal or severe changes in visual acuity, often unilateral, with most progressing to bilateral involvement. Optic nerve appearance is variable from normal to disc edema with or without peripapillary hemorrhages. Length of drug exposure is from 2 months to 2 years. There is no correlation between optic nerve toxicity and concomitant immunosuppressants. There may be some evidence of a genetic predisposition.[4] Spontaneous reports concerning this drug and the optic nerve include 39 cases of optic neuropathy, 18 cases of papilledema, 14 cases of optic atrophy, and 6 cases of ischemic optic neuropathy. Cases were reversible 1 month after discontinuing treatment, deterioration continued even when the drug was stopped, and cases occurred at the normal or low therapeutic dose range.[5-15] There are isolated reports of downward gaze deviation in tacrolimus-induced mutism, reversible bilateral internuclear

ophthalmoplegia, and decreased vision with MRI cerebral abnormalities.[16-18] Lauzurica et al reported severe bilateral noninfectious corneal ulcers after oral tacrolimus.[19] Yamazoe et al reported activation in corneal grafts of herpes simplex and cytomegalovirus endotheliitis.[20] Plosker et al pointed out, as with most immunosuppressive therapy, an increased rate of malignancy can happen, especially lymphomas.[21] Pournaras et al reported conjunctival intraepithelial neoplasm after tacrolimus therapy.[22]

Topical ocular 1–3% tacrolimus ointment is well tolerated and seldom requires discontinuation of the drug due to ocular side effects. The drug-induced irritation that occurs often decreases in intensity, even if drug use is continued.[23,24] Freeman et al and Russell treated 20 patients with atopic eyelid disease using 0.1% tacrolimus ointment.[25,26] They found that 60–80% reported burning and 25–50% reported itching on application of the ointment, but neither reaction was severe enough to stop using the drug. Kang et al, in treating dermatitis in children, found up to an 11% increase in skin changes after topical tacrolimus, including herpes simplex, varicella, and eczema herpeticum.[27] Russell felt there was a higher incidence of recurrence of herpes after this drug is applied to or around the eye.[26] Shen et al reported hyperpigmentation of the oral mucosa after topical tacrolimus.[28] Caelles et al reported a case, and there are an additional 5 cases in the spontaneous reports, of hypertrichosis in the area where tacrolimus ointment was applied.[29] There are reports that find no significant adverse ocular events due to tacrolimus ointment applied to the eyelids.[30] The FDA has terminated topical ocular application of this drug in solution form for ocular sicca.

CLASS: RETINOIDS

Generic Names:
1. Acitretin; 2. isotretinoin.

Proprietary Names:
1. Neotigason, Soriatane; 2. Absorica, Accutane, Amnesteem, Claravis, Sotret.

Primary Use
These retinoids are used in the treatment of psoriasis, cystic acne, and various other disorders of the skin.

Ocular Side Effects
Systemic administration – oral
Certain
1. Eyelids or conjunctiva

a. Blepharoconjunctivitis
b. Erythema
c. Edema
d. Conjunctivitis – nonspecific
    i. Alterations in both exposed and nonexposed epithelium
    ii. Renders epithelium to become nonsecretory
e. Photosensitivity
f. Pruritus
2. Decreased vision
3. Meibomian glands
    a. Meibomitis
    b. Increased viscosity of secretion
    c. Atrophy
    d. Associated increased staphylococcus
4. Lacrimation – variable
5. Tears
    a. Decreased osmolarity
    b. Decreased tear film break-up times
    c. Drug found in tears
    d. May aggravate or cause ocular sicca – evaporative form
6. Cornea
    a. Superficial opacities – fine, rough
    b. Superficial punctate keratitis
    c. Ulceration
    d. Thinning
7. Decreased dark adaptation
    a. Night blindness
    b. Permanent night blindness
8. Myopia – transitory
9. Abnormal electroretinogram (ERG) (scopic)
10. Decreased contact lens tolerance
11. Papilledema secondary to pseudotumor cerebri

Probable
1. Color vision defect

Possible
1. Optic neuritis
2. Giant cobblestone-like conjunctival papillae
3. 6th-nerve palsy
4. Peripapillary choroidal layer – increased thickness

Ocular teratogenic effects
Certain
1. Microphthalmia
2. Optic nerve hypoplasia
3. Orbital hypertelorism
4. Cortical blindness
5. Epicanthus folds

Possible
1. Cataracts
2. Keratoconus

Clinical Significance

Isotretinoin is the most used and best studied of these retinoids. The ocular side effects profile for these 2 drugs is probably identical. Acitretin is a more potent teratogen, which limits its use.

Ocular side effects associated with isotretinoin use are dose related, and probably the most frequent adverse drug reactions are blepharoconjunctivitis, subjective complaints of dry eyes, and transient decreased vision.[1] Acute refractive changes, especially myopic shifts, are transitory and well documented. The drug is secreted in the tears via the lacrimal gland, which may be the cause of an irritative or drug-induced conjunctivitis. Bozkurt et al and Mathers et al believe if given in low doses and not in multiple cycles, the sicca is reversible, but in rare instances it may be permanent.[2–4] Some of these signs and symptoms are secondary to isotretinoin's direct effect of decreasing meibomian gland function with resultant increased tear evaporation and tear osmolarity. Isotretinoin may cause keratoconjunctivitis sicca.[4] This again confirms that drugs that cause oral dryness have the potential to cause ocular sicca as well.[5] Aragona et al discussed the problems of ocular-surface disease in patients on isotretinoin and its management.[6] Karalezli et al and de Queiroga et al, using conjunctival impression cytology, pointed out that many patients on oral isotretinoin have an alteration in exposed and nonexposed conjunctiva.[7,8] Miles et al pointed out the problems of doing laser-assisted in situ keratomileusis (LASIK) in patients on isotretinoin and recommend not using this drug for 6 months postsurgery.[9] The fine, rounded, subepithelial opacities found in the central and peripheral corneas of patients treated with this medication rarely interfere with vision. They may be of variable sizes, white to gray in color, and disappear within 2–10 months after discontinuation of the drug. This probably occurs partially by changes in tear film along with the drug being secreted in the tears. These factors also affect patients who wear contact lenses. Some recommend not fitting patients with lenses while on the drug. Approximately 20% of previously successful wearers may need to discontinue their contact lens use, decrease their wearing time, or use additional preservative-free lubricating eye drops while on isotretinoin.

There are well-documented cases of decreased ability to see at night in patients after taking isotretinoin.[4] This may occur as early as after a few weeks or after prolonged drug exposure. This may be irreversible. Retinal dysfunction is probably due to the competition for binding sites between retinoic acid and retinol (vitamin A). The risk of a photosensitizing drug, such as isotretinoin, enhancing the effects of light on the macula and retina is unclear. Although there are spontaneous reports of retinal pigmentary changes, these are few in number and may be unrelated.

Fraunfelder et al reported on 179 cases of pseudotumor cerebri in patients on isotretinoin.[10] The mean onset was 2.3 months after starting the drug. Six patients in this series had positive rechallenge. Isotretinoin is a synthetic derivative of vitamin A, a well-known cause of pseudotumor cerebri. It is felt that this class of drugs alters the lipid concentration of the arachnoid villi, thereby impeding absorption of cerebrospinal fluid.[11]

The role of isotretinoin as a cataractogenic drug is not yet defined. Although there are several spontaneous reports of cataracts as well as a publication, there is little data to prove that isotretinoin is a cataractogenic drug.[12] This drug has been in widespread use for more than 2 decades, and very few cataracts are reported. This suggests that this drug is, at worst, a very weak cataractogenic drug. Drug exposure is often short-term (i.e. a number of months), indicating the reports are chance events or consist of a subset of individuals whose lenses are highly sensitive to the drug. Regardless, there is no clear-cut pattern to the cataracts. There are a few spontaneous reports of patients in high-light environments who have taken multiple cycles of isotretinoin developing multiple small, cortical punctate opacities of various sizes.

Optic neuritis, unilateral and bilateral, has been seen shortly after starting isotretinoin. Most of these patients are in the multiple sclerosis age group; therefore it is difficult to be confident as to a cause-and-effect relationship. To our knowledge, no case has been rechallenged. However, there are cases that suggest a possible relationship; therefore the manufacturer recommends stopping the drug if this occurs. Aydogan et al, using neurologic and neurophysiologic testing, felt that cortical sensory and retinal function were affected by this drug.[13]

Although keratoconus has been reported with isotretinoin usage, the drug is used in atopic individuals. Keratoconus is seen in 4–6% of atopic individuals. We doubt keratoconus is caused by this drug.

Yavuz et al, using optic coherence tomography, reported an increased peripapillary choroidal thickness in the superior temporal and temporal areas of the retina in patients taking isotretinoin.[14]

Offspring of mothers exposed to these drugs during pregnancy may have various congenital abnormalities involving the eyes.[15]

Acitretin has very few published or spontaneous reports of visual side effects, in large part due to its limited use. In premarketing studies, the ocular side effect profile is basically the same as with isotretinoin, with superficial anterior segment signs and symptoms most prominent. The most significant ocular side effects may be night blindness (1–10%), pseudotumor cerebri (incidence unknown), and the fear of congenital abnormalities.[16] The fear of congenital abnormalities is so great that patients on these drugs should not conceive until off the medication for 3 years.

Recommendations

1. If the patient is below the age of 40 and has not had an eye examination for a few years or is above the age of 40 and has not had one within 2 years, it may be prudent to have a baseline dilated ocular examination before starting this class of drugs.
2. Explain the risk–benefit ratio to patients with:
   a. Retinitis pigmentosa (theoretical)
   b. Severe or chronic blepharoconjunctivitis
   c. Significant tear film abnormalities
3. In selected patients with anterior segment pathology, consider ultraviolet (UV)–blocking lenses because these drugs are photosensitizers.
4. Some feel one should consider discontinuing or delaying fitting of contact lenses while on this drug and discontinue the drug during and 6 months postoperatively to LASIK surgery.
5. Patients on long-term isotretinoin should have an annual eye examination.
6. Suggest that patients see you if any significant ocular signs or symptoms occur.
7. Question all patients concerning night blindness, ocular sicca, and decreased color vision. If they persist for a number of weeks, consider closer monitoring and further testing and possibly stopping the drug. If the patient wants to continue the medication, informed consent should be considered.
8. Consider discontinuing these drugs if any of the following occurs until a cause is determined:
   a. Pseudotumor cerebri
   b. Optic neuritis
   c. Persistent night blindness
   d. Color vision defect

Generic Name:

Tretinoin (retinoic acid, vitamin A acid, or all-trans retinoic acid).

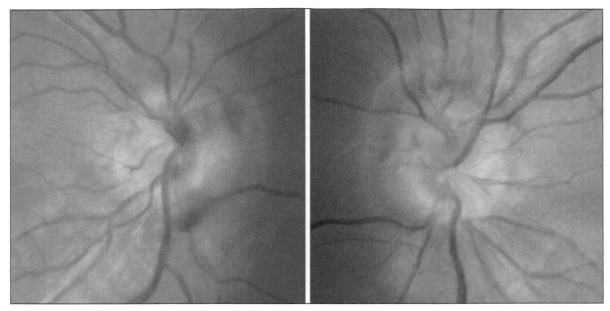

FIG. 16.3 Fundus photo showing optic disc edema and hemorrhage after tretinoin treatment.[5]

Proprietary Names:
Altinac, Altreno, Atralin, Avita, Refissa, Renova, Retin-A, Retin-A Micro, Tretin-X, Vesanoid.

Primary Use
Systemic
Used in the treatment of various leukemias, various forms of acne vulgaris, and aging changes.

Ophthalmic
Primarily used as a topical ocular medication for ocular sicca.

Ocular Side Effects
Systemic administration – oral or topical
Certain
1. Eyelids or conjunctiva
   a. Blepharoconjunctivitis
   b. Erythema
   c. Edema
   d. Conjunctivitis
   e. Photosensitivity
   f. Keratoconjunctivitis
2. Papilledema secondary to pseudotumor cerebri – optic nerve edema (Fig. 16.3)
   a. Visual field defect
   b. Decreased vision
3. Visual hallucinations

Possible
1. Hypercalcemia – ocular surface

Local ophthalmic use or exposure – periocular or topical ocular application
Certain
1. Cornea
   a. Vascularization
   b. Scarring
   c. Opacities in band or ring pattern
   d. Enhanced epithelial healing
   e. Keratitis
2. May aggravate or cause ocular sicca
   a. Decreased meibomian gland function
   b. Increased tear evaporation
3. Eyelids or conjunctiva
   a. Irritation
   b. Edema
   c. Hypopigmentation
   d. Hyperpigmentation
   e. Contact allergy
   f. Erythema
   g. Peeling
   h. Photosensitivity
   i. Blister formation

Clinical Significance

The oral use of this drug has increased; however, ocular side effects are rare. In high doses the drug is probably secreted in the tears because eyelid and conjunctival findings are similar to topical ocular use of this drug. The most severe ocular side effect is pseudotumor cerebri with resultant optic nerve edema. There are numerous reports of pseudotumor cerebri due to tretinoin.[1-6] Vanier et al pointed out that various drugs, including fluconazole, may interfere with the metabolism of tretinoin, causing increases in plasma levels and resulting in an increased incidence of pseudotumor cerebri.[7] The duration and dosage of tretinoin use and the correlation of the onset of pseudotumor cerebri are variable because of individual variation in the pharmacokinetics of this drug.[8] Increased mucosal and skin dryness is not uncommon with tretinoin use. Hypercalcemia may cause increased corneal deposits.

Topical ocular tretinoin preparations are undergoing changes to make it less toxic. The amount of ocular irritation is directly proportional to the concentration of the drug and the frequency of application. These products have few side effects if used at lower concentrations and less frequency. In low dosages, the primary ocular side effects are transient hyperemia, irritation, and burning. All other ocular side effects rarely occur except in higher concentrations with 5 or more applications per day. Avisar et al noted that with the use of topical ocular tretinoin in sicca patients, calcium-like deposits can appear in the epithelium of the cornea.[9] These calcium deposits disappeared over a 2-month period if the drug was stopped; however, a few were permanent. Samarawickrama et al have reviewed the current thinking on the topical ocular use of retinoic acid on the ocular surface, which included the drug's negative effect on the meibomian glands causing ocular sicca and its beneficial effect on the conjunctival and corneal tissue.[10]

Recommendations

1. Topical tretinoin is flammable – do not use near heat, open flame, or while smoking.[12]
2. Therapeutic concentrations of topical tretinoin creams, gels, lotions, and liquids are too high for ocular use. Significant irritation will occur.
3. Topical ocular retinoic acid is contraindicated in meibomian gland disease because it may cause ocular sicca.[11]
4. May alter polymers of soft contact lenses.

CLASS: SOLVENTS

Generic Name:
Dimethyl sulfoxide (DMSO).

Proprietary Name:
Rimso-50.

Primary Use
This is a solvent for various drug deliveries. It is also used in the treatment of musculoskeletal pain, interstitial cystitis, and elevated intracranial pressure and as an anti-inflammatory drug.

Ocular Side Effects
Systemic administration – intravesical or topical
Certain
1. Potentiates the adverse effects of any drug with which it is combined
2. Color vision defect (transitory)
3. Photophobia
4. Eyelids or conjunctiva
   a. Allergic reactions
   b. Erythema
   c. Urticaria
5. Lens – change in nuclear refractive index (chronic use)

Local ophthalmic use or exposure – topical ocular application
Certain
1. Irritation
   a. Hyperemia
   b. Burning sensation
2. Eyelids
   a. Erythema
   b. Photosensitivity
3. Lens – change in nuclear refractive index (chronic use)

Clinical Significance
Dimethyl sulfoxide (DMSO) may enhance ocular side effects when combined with other drugs by increasing the speed and volume of tissue penetration. Changes in lens refractive errors have been detected in animals and in humans after systemic DMSO. We have followed over 100 patients on large doses of DMSO daily for up to 25 years. In fact, the founder of DMSO took a few ounces of oral DMSO daily for 30+ years. There was no evidence of any pattern of lens opacity, but there was a marked, clear delineation of the lens nucleus from the cortex

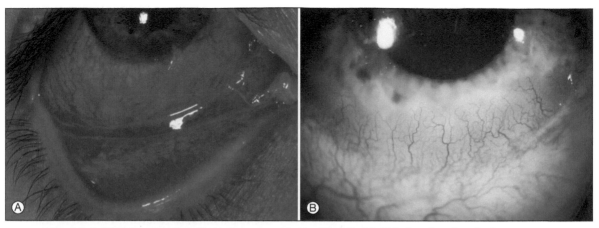

FIG. 16.4 **(A)** Delayed methyl ethyl ketone peroxide keratitis with third failed graft and marked vascularization with conjunctival and corneal hyperesthesia 26 years after injury. **(B)** Typical exacerbations with bulbar, palpebral, conjunctival, and limbus areas injected markedly 11 years after a single ocular exposure to methyl ethyl ketone peroxide.[1]

with a change in the refractive index. In our opinion, even with prolonged administration of large amounts of DMSO, no cases of lens opacities have been proven due to systemic, topical, or local ophthalmic administration. Using the Scheimpflug camera to follow patients on high-dosage DMSO for many years, we could not show any lens opacities due to DMSO in humans (unpublished). There was a change in the refractive index. Rowley et al reported a 58-year-old female who developed bilateral fine brown/red pigment deposits in the anterior and posterior lens cortex after 1 year.[1] Vision was unaffected for 2 years. However, a small decrease in vision occurred in 1 eye, and she elected to stop her DMSO for bladder instillation for interstitial cystitis. A 6-month follow-up showed no lens changes. Metelitsyna reported that in rabbits, DMSO does potentiate lens changes in combination with polychromatic light.[2] Although color vision defects have been reported, they are only of a transient nature. Topical ocular DMSO used in high concentrations for its anti-inflammatory properties (i.e. uveitis) commonly causes ocular irritation. This is uncommon, however, with newer, more refined preparations.

Generic Name:

Methyl ethyl ketone peroxide (MEKP).

Proprietary Names:

Butanox, Chaloxyd, Esperfoam, FR 222, Hi-Point, Kayamek, Lucidol, Lupersol, Permek, Quickset, Sprayset MEKP, Superox, Trigonox M.

Primary Use

Used as a curing agent for thermosetting polyester resins and a cross-linking agent and catalyst in the production of other polymers. It is a lipophilic peroxide used in the automobile, airline, boating, fabric, and paint industries. It is a catalyst for most polyester resins.

Ocular Side Effects

Inadvertent ocular exposure

Certain

1. Pain
2. Lacrimation
3. Photophobia
4. Eyelids – erythema
5. Conjunctiva – bulbar and palpebral
   a. Hyperemia
   b. Chemosis
6. Vision loss
   a. All grades
   b. Total blindness
7. Cornea (Fig. 16.4)
   a. Demyelination of nerves
   b. Edema – superficial to full thickness
   c. Epithelial erosions
   d. Endothelial cell death
   e. Pannus
   f. Interstitial keratitis
   g. Abnormal tear film break-up time
   h. Thinning
   i. Necrosis

8. Anterior uveitis
9. Increased intraocular pressure
10. Phthisis

Clinical Significance

Clinically, the main factor as to severity and prognosis of methyl ethyl ketone peroxide (MEKP) ocular injury is the speed of getting the eye irrigated (especially with a local anesthetic so that adequate irrigation can occur). This needs to be performed in a manner of seconds rather than minutes. No severe cases, even with marked exposure, have been reported where immediate irrigation occurred.

Mild exposure occurs with hand-to-eye contact with MEKP, vapor exposure, minimal inadvertent contact with MEKP solutions, or with immediate irrigation. Even with mild exposure, lid erythema resolved in 3–7 days and conjunctiva hyperemia without corneal findings after a few weeks. However, symptoms of ocular discomfort may persist for many months.

Moderate-to-extensive exposure is due to a rupture of a container by dropping or an object falling on the container, explosion of a canister or tubing containing MEKP, or confusing a bottle with MEKP and an eye dropper, resulting in directly dropping MEKP onto the eye. The classic syndrome of moderate exposure is recurring corneal and conjunctival abnormalities, which are triggered by external ocular stimulus (wind, dust, and light). This pattern of multiple recurrences, lasting for 6 months, is the sign of a moderate injury. If signs and symptoms are severe or last for more than 6 months, there is usually progression or persistence of corneal edema, pannus, or interstitial keratitis; the prognosis is poor. A cyclic course of recurrences may extend over a 20-year-plus period. In cases when irrigation was delayed for over 1 hour, the eye sustained complete corneal endothelial cell death, chronic corneal edema, and possible phthisis.[1]

The long-term course of MEKP ocular injury mimics nitrogen mustard gas injury in many ways, with a slow progression of multiple exacerbations and remission over decades. It differs in lack of eyelid changes, conjunctival ischemia, scleral disease, tortuous corneal blood vessels, and corneal lipoidal-cholesterol deposit degeneration. MEKP may act by causing molecular alteration of tissue macromolecules such as DNA. This creates an autoimmune response primarily in the limbus and cornea. Surprisingly, the rest of the eye and eyelid are generally not affected in the long term, unless damaged at the time of the original exposure.

Recommendations

1. Main effort should be on prevention with:
   a. Safety goggles
   b. Local anesthetic drops available – pain from the chemical is so severe one cannot adequately perform immediate irrigation without an anesthetic. Make sure to single- and double-evert lids while using copious amounts of saline irrigation.
2. Use of topical ocular steroids over the first few weeks should be avoided. Treat frequently with preservative-free lubricants, reduction of external stimulant (light and/or fumes), protection of the eyes with goggles or patching, and use of as few irritating topical ocular medications as possible. Avoid preservatives in all topical ocular medications.
3. Cases with delayed irrigation are universally the most difficult to treat. There is no effective treatment for serious MEKP injury. The primary goal is to attempt to decrease or impede corneal neovascularization to maintain the immune privilege. The use of topical ocular steroids, limiting external stimuli, oral or injectable vitamin E (alpha-tocopherol), or topical ocular sulfhydryl agents (N-acetylcysteine) should be considered after the first month.[2-5] We have found liquid nitrogen application to the limbus impedes and destroys limbal blood vessels as shown by regrafts of corneal transplants, which have a high success rate.[1] This may be considered in severe cases, although no one has treated any MEKP injuries in this way. Once extensive corneal pannus or interstitial keratitis occurs, the prognosis is universally poor.

CLASS: VACCINES

Generic Name:
Bacillus Calmette-Guérin (BCG) vaccine.

Proprietary Names:
Pacis, TheraCys, TICE.

Primary Use
BCG vaccine is used for active immunization against tuberculosis and in the treatment of various malignant diseases. Intravesical BCG has gained popularity as an adjunctive immunotherapy for superficial carcinomas of the urinary bladder.

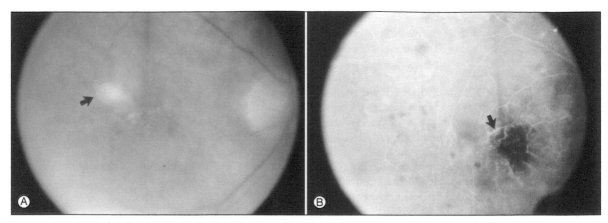

FIG. 16.5 **(A)** Chorioretinal infiltrate in the macular of the right eye at presentation (*arrow*). Vitreous haze and scattered midperipheral infiltrates are also present in the right eye. **(B)** Fundus fluorescein angiography of the right eye at presentation shows a focal vasculitis surrounding the infiltrate (*arrow*).[11]

Ocular Side Effects

Systemic administration – intradermal, intravesical, or percutaneous

Certain

1. Decreased vision
2. Uveitis
3. Conjunctivitis – nonspecific

Probable

1. Reiter syndrome

Possible

1. Eyelids or conjunctiva
   a. Urticaria
   b. Purpura
   c. Lupoid syndrome
   d. Erythema multiforme
   e. Eczema
2. Optic neuritis
3. Retinopathy
   a. Focal areas of depigmentation
   b. Choroiditis
   c. Attenuated vascular tree
4. Endophthalmitis (Fig. 16.5)
5. Vitritis
6. Subconjunctival or retinal hemorrhages secondary to drug-induced anemia

Inadvertent ocular exposure

Certain

1. Follicular conjunctivitis

Clinical Significance

Ocular complications after the BCG vaccine are rare, but acute ocular inflammatory or hypersensitivity reactions within the eye, along with a concurrent systemic inflammatory response, have been reported.[1–6] Whereas most patients are HLA-B27 positive, Wertheim et al reported bilateral anterior uveitis presumed secondary to BCG that was HLA-B27 negative.[6] In general, the uveitis is bilateral and anterior, but may also be a panuveitis.[7] Some authors have postulated that uveitis may be more likely if an individual has a positive antinuclear antibody (ANA).[8] These reactions may occur with or without associated systemic findings, such as arthritis, during the first course or after multiple courses of BCG therapy. The uveitis may be granulomatous but is more often nongranulomatous. Clavel et al reported 26 cases of reactive arthritis secondary to intravesicular BCG.[5] About 8% of these had an associated uveitis, and all patients were HLA-B27 positive. Proof of a cause-and-effect relationship is difficult to determine, but the number of reported cases and their similar patterns make an association almost certain. Donaldson et al reported 2 melanoma patients treated with BCG vaccine that developed uveitis associated with vitiligo.[9] Price reported a patient who, after a second course of BCG therapy for bladder cancer, had his first episode of peripheral arthritis and bilateral iritis with secondary glaucoma.[2] Cases in the spontaneous reports and in the literature suggest that in some patients, conjunctivitis may occur, often lasting throughout the injection series. The conjunctivitis is nonspecific, but appears to have more chemosis than normally seen. This can be controlled with topical ocular steroids. Hegde et al, as well as Hogarth et al, reported bilateral panuveitis with optic neuritis after BCG vaccination.[7,10] Han et al reported a single case of endophthalmitis due to *Mycobacterium bovis,* possibly secondary to BCG therapy.[11] It occurred 14 months after the patient's last treatment (BCG contains live attenuated mycobacteria).

BCG's effect on the retina is not as well established. Cases resembling cancer-associated retinopathy (CAR) without a serum reaction to the CAR autoantigen have been reported.[12] This includes areas of pigmentary disturbances, usually focal, and choroiditis often with narrowed arterioles. There are 2 similar cases in the spontaneous reports. Hodish et al reported retinitis syndrome after intravesical BCG.[13] There are multiple reports of panuveitis and additional reports of endophthalmitis due to treatment with BCG for bladder cancer.[14-19]

Pollard et al described a case of inadvertent direct ocular exposure to BCG vaccine causing follicular conjunctivitis, which was controlled by topical ocular steroids.[20]

Generic Names:

1. Diphtheria (D) vaccine (receiving a tetanus toxoid booster); 2. diphtheria and tetanus (DT) vaccine; 3. diphtheria, tetanus, and pertussis (DTaP) vaccine.

Proprietary Names:

1. Menactra, Menveo; 2. Decavac, Tenivac; 3. Adacel, Boostrix, Daptacel, Infranix, Pediarix, Pentacel, Tripedia.

Primary Use

These combinations of diphtheria and tetanus toxoids with pertussis vaccine are the recommended preparations for routine primary immunizations and recall injections in children younger than 7 years of age.

Ocular Side Effects
Systemic administration – intramuscular
Possible
1. Eyelids or conjunctiva
   a. Allergic reactions
   b. Erythema
   c. Conjunctivitis – nonspecific (DPT)
   d. Edema
   e. Urticaria
   f. Eczema (DT)
   g. Erythema multiforme
   h. Periorbital edema

Conditional/unclassified
1. Optic neuritis
2. Extraocular muscles
   a. Paresis or paralysis (D)
   b. Ptosis (DPT)
3. Pupils
   a. Mydriasis (D)
   b. Decreased reaction to light (D)
4. Subconjunctival or retinal hemorrhages secondary to drug-induced anemia (DPT)
5. Corneal graft rejection (tetanus toxoid booster)
6. Papilledema secondary to pseudotumor cerebri (DPT)
7. Visual field defects (DT)
8. Guillain-Barré syndrome
9. Retinal vasculitis

Clinical Significance

For the many millions exposed to these vaccines, there are comparatively few ocular complications. The most common ocular side effect in the spontaneous reports is periorbital edema. Rarely, a partial paralysis of accommodation may occur. This may be unilateral or bilateral and take a few weeks to develop and a few weeks to resolve. The pupils are usually normal or slightly dilated with a normal papillary response to light.[1] Generalized urticarial reactions have been reported to occur immediately or several hours after injection. Allergic reactions may be due to preservatives or contaminants of the antigens, but are rarely seen. Conjunctivitis has been seen after DTaP injections, but it is transitory and inconsequential. Neurologic complications, including papilledema, optic neuritis, and decreased vision, have been reported as transient adverse effects, sometimes accompanying encephalitis.[2-4] Cabrera-Maqueda et al reported 2 pregnant women who developed optic neuritis within 3 weeks of vaccination.[5] There was complete recovery in both case reports. There are cases of transitory strabismus after DTaP injections in the spontaneous reports, but a cause-and-effect relationship is hard to establish. Steinemann et al reported a 33-year-old woman with a graft rejection requiring a repeat graft after receiving a tetanus toxoid booster.[6]

Generic Name:
Hepatitis A vaccine.

Proprietary Names:
Havrix, Twinrix (include hepatitis B vaccine), Vaqta.

Primary Use
Active immunization against disease caused by hepatitis A virus in persons older than 1 year.

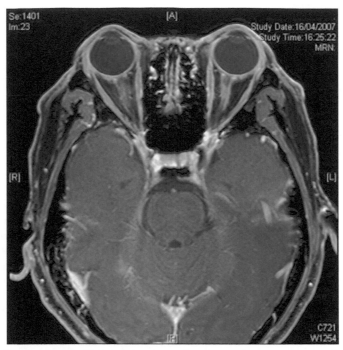

FIG. 16.6 MRI of brain using gadolinium; T1-weighted image showing enhancement of the intraconal segment of the left optic nerve, sparing the prechiasmal portion.[1]

Ocular Side Effects
Systemic administration – intramuscular
Possible
1. Conjunctivitis
2. Diplopia
3. Eyelid and periorbital edema
4. Multiple evanescent white dot syndrome
5. Retrobulbar optic neuritis
6. Uveitis

Clinical Significance
Ocular side effects from hepatitis A virus are very rare, and most reports lack dechallenge and rechallenge data. From the literature, there is the possibility that retrobulbar optic neuritis could occur after vaccination. Huang et al reported a case of a man with HIV who received a hepatitis A vaccination and 6 days later developed visual loss and light sensitivity.[1] Then 12 days later, an afferent pupillary defect developed in his left eye. He improved dramatically after 3 days of methylprednisolone treatment. Voigt et al described a patient who developed irreversible loss of vision in the left eye.[2] This was in a 21-year-old, otherwise healthy woman who was receiving the hepatitis A vaccination in preparation for travel to Africa. This occurred 2 weeks after the vaccination. Both of these case reports had magnetic resonance images (MRIs), which demonstrated enhancement of the intraconal segment of the optic nerve (Fig. 16.6).[1] O'Dowd et al described a 57-year-old man who developed bilateral optic neuritis and irreversible loss of vision 2 weeks after vaccination with hepatitis A vaccine.[3]

Generic Name:
Hepatitis B vaccine.

Proprietary Names:
Comvax (includes Haemophilus B conjugate vaccine), Engerix-B, HepaGam B, Heplisav-B, HyperHEP B S/D, Nabi-HB, Recombivax HB, Twinrix (includes hepatitis A vaccine).

Primary Use
Active immunization against disease caused by all hepatitis B virus subtypes.

Ocular Side Effects
Systemic administration – intramuscular
Possible
1. Conjunctivitis
2. Diplopia

3. Eyelid and periorbital edema
4. Gaze palsy (mononeuritis)
5. Optic neuritis
6. Uveitis

Clinical Significance

The most common ocular side effects, although rare, are conjunctivitis, periorbital and eyelid edema, gaze palsy with diplopia and transitory strabismus, uveitis, and rare cases of optic neuritis. The most serious of these with potential for permanent visual loss is optic neuritis. There are 2 cases of optic neuritis after hepatitis B vaccination in the literature.[1,2] Erguven et al discussed a case of a 9-year-old girl who developed vision loss and pain in the left eye 1 week after receiving the hepatitis B vaccine.[1] The clinical condition improved after systemic corticosteroid treatment. A case report from Voigt et al described an otherwise healthy, 21-year-old woman receiving hepatitis B vaccination in preparation for a trip to Africa.[2] She developed permanent irreversible vision loss 2 weeks after vaccination, with an MRI demonstrating retrobulbar optic neuritis. This case was confounded by the fact that she also received hepatitis A vaccine. A relatively large case series by Fraunfelder et al described 32 case reports of uveitis due to hepatitis B vaccination.[3] The mean time to development of uveitis was 3 days, and the condition resolved with topical ocular steroid treatment. Grewal et al reported a gaze palsy from a mononeuritis of the 6th cranial nerve in a 4-day-old infant who received the vaccine at birth, which resolved completely in a few days and did not recur on subsequent vaccinations.[4]

Generic Names:

1. Herpes zoster (shingles) vaccine; 2. measles, mumps, rubella, and varicella virus vaccine live; 3. varicella (chickenpox) vaccine.

Proprietary Names:

1. Shingrix, Zostavax; 2. Proquad; 3. Varilrix, Varivax, Varivax II.

Primary Use

These vaccines are used to provide active immunity to chickenpox and herpes zoster infection.

Ocular Side Effects

Systemic administration – intramuscular or subcutaneous
Possible

1. Acute posterior multifocal placoid pigment epitheliopathy
2. Exacerbation of zoster keratitis

3. Eyelids or conjunctiva
   a. Allergic reactions
   b. Eyelid edema
   c. Periorbital edema
4. Gaze palsy
5. Keratouveitis
6. Ocular hypertension
7. Optic neuritis
8. Retinal necrosis
9. Sclerokeratitis
10. Uveitis (Fig. 16.7)

Clinical Significance

Vaccination with varicella virus vaccine induces a cell-mediated immune response against varicella-zoster virus infection. The vaccine is indicated for children older than 1 year and in adults for prevention of shingles and zoster infection. There are multiple cases in the spontaneous reports of ocular side effects, with the majority being case reports of eyelid and periorbital edema, conjunctivitis, gaze palsy, and rare cases of uveitis and vitritis. There is a case report of anterior uveitis from Esmaeli-Gutstein et al.[1] From this case report, it appears a facial rash occurred 2 days after vaccination with unilateral uveitis 7 days after vaccination. The condition improved within 7 days with topical ocular steroids and oral acyclovir 800 mg 5 times daily. Of particular concern are case reports of acute retinal necrosis (ARN) after zoster vaccination first reported by Charkoudian et al and Gonzales et al.[2,3] They described patients aged 20, 77, and 80; the ARN was noted at 1 month, 1 week, and 2 months, respectively, after vaccination with Zostavax. There are case reports of bilateral ARN in an immunocompetent subject and bilateral ARN in a patient with HIV.[4,5] By polymerase chain reaction, the vitreous aspirate and core vitrectomy specimens can be positive for DNA from the Oka strain of varicella-zoster virus, the viral strain used in both Varivax and Zostavax. Although ocular side effects from zoster vaccine are probably exceedingly rare, clinicians should be aware of the possibility of uveitis, ARN, gaze palsies, and periorbital and eyelid edema. There is strong evidence that stromal keratitis can arise in rare patients who have received the varicella-zoster virus vaccine in any form. The zoster keratitis can occur even if there is no history of corneal disease. Subjects at particularly high risk are those who have had zoster keratitis in the past and then receive the varicella virus vaccine. Because the vaccine is a live virus, there appears to be a reactivation of the inflammatory response in patients who have had stromal keratitis due to zoster in the past. Liu et al have shown no increase in complications using live virus vaccines.[6] Clinicians may need to consider discouraging

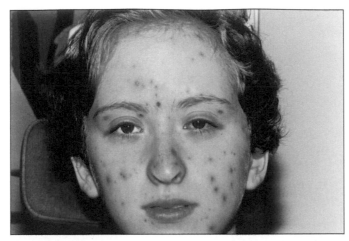

FIG. 16.7 The patient with a generalized vesicular rash involving the face and periocular soft tissues associated with ciliary injection of the left eye.1

vaccination with this vaccine if zoster keratitis has been diagnosed in the patient's ocular history.[7-9]

Generic Name:
Human papillomavirus (HPV) vaccine.

Proprietary Name:
Gardasil 9.

Primary Use
Recombinant vaccine used in the prophylaxis of preventing inoculation with HPV.

Ocular Side Effects
Systemic administration – intramuscular
Possible
1. Decreased vision
2. Photophobia
3. Eyelids or conjunctiva
   a. Edema
   b. Hypersensitivity reactions
4. Periorbital edema
5. Uveitis
6. Extraocular muscles
   a. Palsy
   b. Ptosis

Clinical Significance
No ocular side effects have been proven. Those reported to spontaneous reporting systems are generally mild, reversible, and rare. The type of papilloma vaccine has varied with time; therefore data presented here is suspect. Regardless, some of the time, temporal relationships make the clinician suspect a possible association in certain individuals.

The most commonly reported visual side effect is a reversible decreased vision occurring shortly after the intramuscular injection. Hypersensitivity reactions have been reported, varying in onset from 5–540 minutes after injection.[1] Ocular findings included edema and pruritus. This was with HPV vaccine recombinant quadrivalent. Chen et al reported acute panuveitis within 4 days of receiving the 3rd dose of HPV vaccine recombinant quadrivalent.[2] Sawai et al reported 2 cases of tubulointerstitial nephritis with uveitis: one 4 days before and one 14 days before the 3rd dose of the HPV vaccine.[3] Holt et al reviewed 24 possible unproven cases of uveitis in women ages 12–26 years who developed uveitis 0–476 days after exposure to the HPV vaccine.[4] Some cases included papillitis, retinitis, and papilledema. Ogino et al reported multiple evanescent white dot retinal symptoms with possible progressive visual field loss.[5] Dansingani et al reported a 20-year-old female who developed panuveitis with exudative retinal detachments 3 weeks after her second injection of the vaccine.[6] Khalifa et al reported bilateral choroiditis in a 17-year-old female.[7] Dimario et al reported a 16-year-old patient who developed bilateral visual field loss 10 days after receiving the vaccine.[8] These cases do not prove causation, but a temporal relationship may be a rare event.

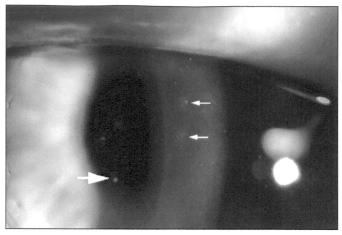

FIG. 16.8 Small *arrows* showing infiltrates and large *arrow* showing keratic precipitate of graft rejection.[27]

Generic Name:
Influenza virus vaccine.

Proprietary Names:
Afluria, Agriflu, Fluad, Fluarix, Fluarix Quadrivalent, Flublok, Flublok Quadrivalent, Flucelvax Quadrivalent, Flulaval, Flulval Quadrivalent, FluMist Quadrivalent, Fluvirin, Fluzone, Fluzone High-Dose, Fluzone Intradermal, Fluzone Intradermal Quadrivalent, Fluzone Quadrivalent, H1N1.

Primary Use
Influenza virus vaccines are used to provide active immunity to influenza virus strains.

Ocular Side Effects
Systemic administration – intramuscular or intranasal
Certain
1. Oculorespiratory syndrome
   a. Conjunctivitis
   b. Eyelid edema
   c. Photophobia
   d. Decreased vision
   e. Conjunctival discharge
   f. Pain

Probable
1. Corneal graft rejection (Fig. 16.8)

Possible
1. Decreased vision

2. Eyelids or conjunctiva
   a. Allergic reactions
   b. Erythema
   c. Blepharoconjunctivitis
   d. Urticaria
   e. Purpura
   f. Edema
3. Optic nerve
   a. Neuritis
   b. Neuropathy
   c. Ischemic optic neuropathy
   d. Edema
4. Extraocular muscles – paresis or paralysis
5. Bell palsy
6. Color vision defect – red-green defect
7. Retinal vasculitis
8. Acute posterior multifocal placoid pigment epitheliopathy
9. Multiple evanescent white dot syndrome
10. Uveitis
11. Central serous chorioretinopathy

Conditional/unclassified
1. Episcleritis
2. Scleritis
3. Orbital myositis
4. Sjögren syndrome

Clinical Significance
Earlier influenza vaccines were from swine, but these have discontinued due to an increased incidence of neurologic complications, including optic neuritis,

optic atrophy, and blindness.[1,2] Poser reported isolated trochlear and 59 facial nerve palsies also using swine vaccine.[3] There is a case report of 6th-nerve palsy in the literature.[4] Manufacturers use various virus strains that may produce different ocular effects. The best-studied adverse ocular side effect is an influenza vaccine–induced oculorespiratory syndrome, which consists of cough, wheeze, chest tightness, difficulty breathing, and/or sore throat. The ocular manifestation is bilateral conjunctivitis, which can occur within hours of inoculation. This may or may not include facial edema. Fredette et al noted photophobia, blurred vision, lid edema, ocular pain, and conjunctival concentrates as part of the syndrome.[5] Onset varies between 2 and 24 hours after exposure and resolves within 48 hours. Up to 16% of women between the ages of 50 and 59 had this syndrome, making them the highest-risk group.[6] De Serres et al have shown that an earlier onset of this syndrome (less than 2 hours) is more likely in younger patients who have more coughs and sore throats, and a later onset (after 2 hours) is more likely in the older population, which has more ocular symptoms.[7] The frequency of this syndrome substantially decreased with each annual injection over a 4-year, follow-up series.[8] Although the data cited are mainly from a specific manufacturer, this vaccine was minimally retrogenic; therefore this syndrome can be associated with influenza vaccines in general.[9,10] Hull et al reported a case of bilateral optic neuritis developing within 2 weeks of being vaccinated by the newer influenza vaccination.[11] This happened on 2 separate occasions, 1 year apart. Ray et al and Laffon-Pioger et al reported similar cases without rechallenge data.[12,13] There have been various reports of unilateral and bilateral optic neuritis after vaccination with good recovery, with or without treatment.[14–19] Kawasaki et al reported bilateral ischemic optic neuropathy with 2 cases of permanent visual loss.[20] The authors speculated that an immune complex–mediated vasculopathy after vaccination can cause anterior ischemic optic neuropathy. There are other reports of optic neuropathy in the literature, including a case of nonarteritic ischemic optic neuropathy.[21,22] Knopf reported a case of complicated cataract surgery with secondary uveitis that had complete recovery.[23] Four months later, after a flu vaccination, the patient had a recurrence of her uveitis with decreased vision and cystoid macular edema. Two case reports of serous retinal detachment and uveitis were reported by Tao et al with resolution 1 month after vaccination.[24] When a rare case of extraocular muscle abnormalities or uveitis occurs, this is usually within 2–14 days after inoculation. These may last from a few days to a few weeks.

Patients with corneal grafts who are vaccinated are probably at higher risk for a graft rejection. Most patients who react usually only have mild graft reactions that can be controlled with topical ocular steroids. However, severe reactions requiring regrafts have occurred. Steinemann et al, Solomon et al, and Wertheim et al have all reported cases of graft rejection, and there are cases in the spontaneous reports.[25–27] Thurairajan et al reported a case of bilateral orbital myositis and posterior scleritis after influenza vaccination.[28] The authors found no other cause for this and felt these ocular side effects, including an associated acute symmetrical polyarthropathy, were due to the vaccine. Mutsch et al reported 46 cases of Bell palsy with an influenza vaccine that was only used in Switzerland.[29] There are cases of episcleritis after inoculation in the spontaneous reports.

Generic Names:

1. Measles, mumps and rubella virus vaccine live; 2. measles, mumps, rubella, and varicella virus vaccine live; 3. measles virus vaccine live; 4. mumps virus vaccine live; 5. rubella and mumps virus vaccine live; 6. rubella virus vaccine live.

Proprietary Names:

1. MMR II; 2. Proquad; 3. Attunvax; 4. Mumpsvax; 5. Biavax II; 6. Meruvax II.

Primary Use

These vaccines are used to provide active immunity to measles, mumps, and rubella.

Ocular Side Effects
Systemic administration – subcutaneous
Possible

1. Optic nerve – optic or retrobulbar neuritis (measles, rubella)
2. Eyelids or conjunctiva
   a. Allergic reactions
   b. Hyperemia
   c. Erythema
   d. Conjunctivitis – nonspecific
   e. Ptosis (measles)
   f. Edema
   g. Urticaria
   h. Purpura
   i. Eczema
3. Pseudotumor cerebri
4. Pain

Conditional/unclassified
1. Decreased vision
2. Extraocular muscles
   a. Paresis or paralysis
   b. Strabismus
3. Scotomas – centrocecal
4. Retinopathy (rubella)
5. Uveitis

Inadvertent ocular exposure
Certain
1. Keratitis (measles)
2. Conjunctival edema (measles)

Conditional/unclassified
1. Ocular teratogenic effects (rubella)

Clinical Significance
Millions of people have been exposed to these vaccines, and there are only a few scattered reports of significant ocular side effects. The most noteworthy ocular side effect reported is optic or retrobulbar neuritis. Onset varies, with Arshi et al reporting occurrence within a few hours, Kline et al reporting onset within 1 week, and Stevenson et al and Kazarian et al reporting onset within 2–3 weeks.[1-4] All cases were bilateral, and 4 of the 6 had good visual outcomes within days to a few weeks. From the spontaneous reports there are 5 additional reports of optic neuritis, each with an incidence of 1 in 1,600,000 in the United Kingdom. Most authors felt there was a cause-and-effect relationship between the reports of optic neuritis and the measles vaccination, perhaps due to the demyelinating effect. Regardless, causation has not been proven. In time, some of these patients may develop multiple sclerosis. There are 2 cases of 3rd nerve palsy reported by Manzotti et al and Chan et al.[5,6] The risk of neurologic complications after natural rubella infections is greater than after rubella vaccines.[7] Islam et al reported 2 cases of patients developing anterior uveitis at 4 weeks and at 6 weeks after measles, mumps, and rubella vaccinations.[8] Months of conventional therapy were required for management. There are many reports of uveitis in the spontaneous reports and in the literature.[9,10] Maspero et al reported, via a patient survey, a 6% incidence of conjunctivitis after measles vaccine.[11] This is transitory and of no clinical consequence. Marshall et al reported diffuse retinopathy after rubella vaccination in children, but there are no such reports in the spontaneous reports.[12]

Cases of direct ocular exposure to live measles virus vaccine that resulted in keratoconjunctivitis, which resolved within 2 weeks, are in the spontaneous reports.

Generic Names:
1. Rabies immune globulin; 2. rabies vaccine.

Proprietary Names:
1. BayRab, HyperRAB, HyperRAB S/D, Imogam, KEDRAB; 2. Imovax, RabAvert.

Primary Use
Rabies immune globulin is used to provide passive immunity to rabies for postexposure prophylaxis of individuals exposed to the disease or virus. Rabies vaccine is used to promote active immunity to rabies in individuals exposed to the disease or virus.

Ocular Side Effects
Systemic administration – intramuscular
Certain
1. Eyelids or conjunctiva
   a. Allergic reactions
   b. Erythema
   c. Edema
   d. Urticaria

Possible
1. Optic nerve
   a. Optic neuritis
   b. Retrobulbar neuritis
2. Diplopia
3. Multiple evanescent white dot syndrome (MEWDS)
4. Photophobia
5. Scotomas – centrocecal
6. Decreased vision

Conditional/unclassified
1. Neuroretinitis
   a. Optic disc edema
   b. Macular edema
   c. Hard exudates

Clinical Significance
Neurologic adverse reactions were much more common with the earlier preparations of rabies vaccine made from infected rabbit brain tissue than from later-generation vaccines. There are reports of optic neuritis.[1-6] Optic neuritis usually occurs from a few weeks to 3 months after vaccination and is often part of acute disseminated encephalomyelitis.[7] There are cases where the optic neuritis was the only neurologic finding.[8,9] Mostly, patients can recover good vision, but some permanent damage to the retinal fibers may occur.[8] Although neurologic complications due to rabies vaccinations are rare, encephalitis, myelitis, and encephalomyelitis are well

documented. This includes varying degrees of paralysis, including the oculomotor nerve.[10] Chayakul et al, along with cases in the spontaneous reports, reported paralysis of the ocular motor nerve.[3] This is usually associated with a vaccine-induced encephalomyelitis.

Yang et al reported a case report of MEWDS 7 days after rabies vaccination.[11] There was complete recovery upon examination 3 years later. Saxena et al reported bilateral neuroretinitis using chick embryo cell antirabies vaccine.[12] The neuroretinitis was an acute swelling of both optic discs associated with hard exudates and macular edema.

Generic Name:
Smallpox (vaccinia) vaccine.

Proprietary Names:
ACAM2000, Dryvax.

Primary Use
Used as a vaccination against the vaccinia virus.

Ocular Side Effects
Systemic administration – percutaneous
Certain
1. Eyelids and conjunctiva
   a. Blepharoconjunctivitis
   b. Vesicles
   c. Pustules
   d. Profound edema
   e. Periorbital erythema (Fig. 16.9)
   f. Preauricular and submandibular lymphadenopathy
   g. Scarring
   h. Madarosis
   i. Conjunctivitis
      i. Papillary reaction
      ii. Serous and mucopurulent discharge
      iii. Ulceration
      iv. Symblepharon
   j. Punctal stenosis
2. Cornea
   a. Superficial punctate keratitis
   b. Interstitial and stromal keratitis
   c. Disciform keratitis
   d. Necrosis
   e. Perforation
   f. Subepithelial opacities
   g. Ring infiltrates
3. Iritis
4. Photophobia

Conditional/unclassified
1. Retina

   a. Cotton-wool spots
   b. Branch arteriolar occlusions
   c. Vasculitis
2. Optic nerve
   a. Neuropathy
   b. Neuritis

Clinical Significance
In the 1980s, the World Health Organization declared smallpox eradicated, but countries not abiding by the promise to destroy the virus have now perpetuated a fear that smallpox may become a biologic weapon.

This has required mass vaccination in the US military. It is estimated that 10–20 per 1 million smallpox immunizations develop ocular complications. The worst complications are in those who are immunocompromised, i.e. patients who are allergic to any components of the vaccine or who have coronary artery disease.[1] Ocular complications primarily occur in the very young (age 1–4 years) and occur from autoinoculation from the vaccination site to the eyelid or eye. The most common finding is blepharoconjunctivitis, which occurs between 5 and 11 days after vaccination.[2] Only rarely does this go on to cornea involvement, often with significant scarring of the lids and conjunctiva. Uveitis has only been reported with severe corneal involvement.[3] Surprisingly, those with the most severely involved corneal disease rarely have significant visual defects after 5 years.[2]

There are reports of retinal complications primarily as multiple branch retinal artery occlusions.[4,5] Smallpox and vaccinia have been implicated in encephalopathy and other neurologic disorders. Mathur et al reported a case of bilateral optic nerve inflammation.[6] In 2003, 2 patients developed ocular vaccinia after coming into contact with subjects who had a recent smallpox vaccination.[7]

Generic Names:
1. Tetanus immune globulin; 2. tetanus toxoid.

Proprietary Names:
1. BayTET, HyperTET S/D; 2. Acthib, Te Anatxal.

Primary Use
Tetanus immune globulin is used prophylactically for wound management in patients not completely immunized. Tetanus toxoid is used for active immunization against tetanus.

Ocular Side Effects
Systemic administration – intramuscular
Possible
1. Eyelids or conjunctiva

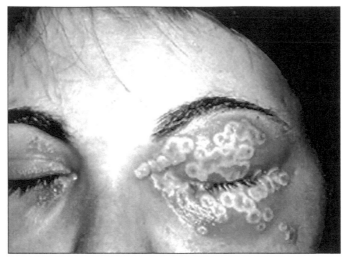

FIG. 16.9 Periorbital edema and erythema after smallpox immunization.[2]

a. Allergic reactions
b. Erythema
c. Conjunctivitis – nonspecific
d. Edema
e. Urticaria
f. Purpura
2. Corneal graft rejection
3. Photophobia

Conditional/unclassified
1. Decreased accommodation
2. Horizontal nystagmus
3. Visual hallucinations
4. Decreased pupillary response to light
5. Optic neuritis

Clinical Significance
Except for local reactions, such as erythema or urticaria, adverse ocular reactions after tetanus immunization are exceedingly rare. Steinmann et al reported a 33-year-old woman who developed a severe graft rejection within 4 days after receiving a tetanus toxoid booster.[1] This required a repeat graft. She received an influenza immunization 2 years later, 6 months after her repeat graft, and she again had a mild graft rejection. A similar case with a corneal graft reaction after a tetanus immunization is in the spontaneous reports. Neurologic complications probably occur at a rate of 0.4 per 1 million.[2] Nystagmus and accommodative paresis have been reported in the spontaneous reports as adverse ocular symptoms after tetanus vaccine. Optic neuritis and myelitis were reported in an 11-year-old child after a tetanus booster.[3] A 39-year-old male developed 3rd nerve palsy after a tetanus shot, and it resolved in 7 days.[4]

Generic Name:
Yellow fever vaccine.

Proprietary Names:
STAMARIL, YF-Vax.

Primary Use
Used to prevent yellow fever infection.

Ocular Side Effects
Systemic administration – subcutaneous
Possible
1. Multiple evanescent white dot syndrome (MEWDS)
2. Uveitis
   a. Anterior
   b. Intermediate

Clinical Significance
Biancardi et al describe 2 patients, a 35-year-old and a 21-year-old, who received the yellow fever vaccine 10 days and 2 weeks prior, respectively.[1] They developed an anterior and an intermediate uveitis, which resolved completely with conservative treatment. In addition, there is a single case report of MEWDS, which occurred 1 week after vaccination.[2] This resolved completely within 6 weeks after vaccination.

REFERENCES

Drug: Disulfiram

1. Chick J. Safety issues concerning the use of disulfiram in treating alcohol dependence. *Drug Saf.* 1999;20:427–435.
2. Orakzai A, Guerin M, Beatty S. Disulfiram-induced transient optic and peripheral neuropathy: a case report. *Ir J Med Sci.* 2007;176(4):319–321.
3. Bessero AC, Daeppen JB, Borruat FX. Optic neuropathy while taking disulfiram. *J Fr Ophtalmol.* 2006;29:924–928.
4. Trelohan A, Milea D. Reversible optic neuropathy related to disulfiram. *J Fr Ophtalmol.* 2011;34(6):382(e1–e3).
5. Appelmans M. Discussion following paper of Humblet M. *Bull Soc Belge Ophtalmol.* 1953;104:301.
6. Woillez M, Asseman R, Blerbacque A. Nevrite toxique medicamenteuse au cours de la desintoxication ethylique. *Bull Soc Ophtalmol Fr.* 1962;75:350–357.
7. Humblet M. Nevrite retrobulbaire chronique par Antabuse. *Bull Soc Belge Ophtalmol.* 1953;104:297–301.
8. Perdriel G, Chevaleraud J. A propos d'un nouveau cas de nevrite optique due au disulfirame. *Bull Soc Ophtalmol Fr.* 1966;66:159–165.
9. Bevilacqua JA, Diaz M, Diaz V, et al. Disulfiram neuropathy. Report of 3 cases. *Rev Med Chil.* 2002;130:1037–1042.
10. Acheson JF, Howard RS. Reversible optic neuropathy associated with disulfiram. A clinical and electrophysiological report. *J Neuroophthalmol.* 1988;8:175–177.

Drugs: Alendronate sodium, etidronate disodium, ibandronate sodium, pamidronate disodium, risedronate sodium, zoledronic acid

1. Alendronate sodium, etidronate disodium, pamidronate disodium, risedronate sodium, ibandronate sodium, zoledronic acid. 2019. Retrieved from http://www.pdr.net.
2. Haverbeke G, Pertile G, Claes C, et al. Posterior uveitis: an under recognized adverse effect of pamidronate: 2 case reports. *Bull Soc Belge Ophtalmol.* 2003;290:71–76.
3. Patel DV, Bolland M, Nisa Z, et al. Incidence of ocular side effects with intravenous zoledronate: secondary analysis of a randomized controlled trial. *Osteoporos Int.* 2015;26:499–503.
4. Fraunfelder FW, Fraunfelder FT. Bisphosphonates and ocular inflammation. *N Engl J Med.* 2003;348:1187–1188.
5. Fraunfelder FW, Fraunfelder FT, Jensvold B. Scleritis and other ocular side effects associated with pamidronate disodium. *Am J Ophthalmol.* 2003;135:219–222.
6. Etminan M, Forooghian F, Maberley D. Inflammatory ocular adverse events with the use of oral bisphosphonates: a retrospective cohort study. *CMAJ.* 2012;184(8):E431–E434.
7. Umunakwe OC, Herren D, Kim SJ, et al. Diffuse ocular and orbital inflammation after zoledronate infusion – case report and review of the literature. *Digit J Ophthalmol.* 2017;23(4):18–21.
8. Meaney TPJ, Musadiq M, Corridan PGJ. Diplopia following intravenous administration of pamidronate. *Eye.* 2004;18:103–104.
9. Patel DV, Horne A, Mihov B, et al. The effects of re-challenge in patients with a history of acute anterior uveitis following intravenous zoledronate. *Calcif Tissue Int.* 2015;97(1):58–61.
10. Pirbhai A, Rajak SN, Goold LA, et al. Bisphosphonate-induced orbital inflammation: a case series and review. *Orbit.* 2015;34(6):331–335.
11. Des Grottes JM, Schrooyen M, Dumon JC, et al. Retrobulbar optic neuritis after pamidronate administration in a patient with a history of cutaneous porphyria. *Clin Rheum.* 1997;16(1):93–95.
12. Ghose K, Waterworth R, Trolove P, et al. Uveitis associated with pamidronate. *Aust N Z J Med.* 1994;24:320.
13. Stach R, Tarr K. Drug-induced optic neuritis and uveitis secondary to bisphosphonates. *N Z Med J.* 2006;119:74–76.
14. Brulinksi P, Nikapota AD. Zolendronic acid-induced retrobulbar optic neuritis: a case report. *Clin Oncol (R Coll Radiol).* 2013;25(5):328–329.
15. Lavado FM, Prieto MP, Osorio MRR, et al. Bilateral retrobulbar optic neuropathy as the only sign of zoledronic acid toxicity. *J Clin Neurosci.* 2017;44:243–245.
16. Boyd I. Pamidronic acid and optic neuritis. *WHO Pharmaceuticals Newsletter.* 2014;5:18–20.
17. Mammo Z, Guo M, Maberley D, et al. Oral bisphosphonates and risk of wet age-related macular degeneration. *Am J Ophthalmol.* 2016;168:62–67.
18. Grzybowski A, Iribarren R, Iribarren G, et al. Oral bisphosphonates and risk of wet age-related macular degeneration. *Am J Ophthalmol.* 2017;176:255.
19. Mammo Z, Guo M, Maberley D, et al. Reply: oral bisphosphonates and risk of wet age-related macular degeneration. *Am J Ophthalmol.* 2017;176:255–256.
20. Bursztyn LL, Masri M, Sheidow TG. Severe visual loss secondary to retinal toxicity after intravenous use of bisphosphonate in an eye with known chloroquine maculopathy. *Retin Cases Brief Rep.* 2014;8(4):322–325.
21. Geneva II, Eagle RC, Barker-Griffith A, et al. Squamous metaplasia of the conjunctiva: a previously unrecognized adverse effect of risedronate sodium. *JAMA Ophthalmol.* 2013;131(2):249–251.

Drug: Deferasirox

1. Pan Y, Keane PA, Sadun AA, et al. Optic coherence tomography findings in deferasirox-related maculopathy. *Retin Cases Brief Rep.* 2010;4(3):229–232.
2. Walia HS, Yan J. Reversible retinopathy associated with oral deferasirox therapy. *BMJ Case Rep.* 2013.
3. Bui KM, Sadda SR, Salehi-Had H. Pseudovitelliform maculopathy associated with deferoxamine toxicity: multimodal imaging and electrophysiology of a rare entity. *Digit J Ophthalmol.* 2017;23(1):11–15.
4. Sanford D, Hsia CC. A case of transfusion independence in a patient with myelodysplastic syndrome using deferasirox, sustained for two years after stopping therapy. *Curr Oncol.* 2015;22(2):e128–e132.

Drug: Deferoxamine mesylate (desferrioxamine)

1. Bene C, Manzler A, Bene D, et al. Irreversible ocular toxicity from single "challenge" dose of deferoxamine. *Clin Nephrol.* 1989;31(1):45–48.
2. Yaqoob M, Prabhu P, Ahmad R. Comment on "Irreversible ocular toxicity from single challenge dose of desferrioxamine" by Bene C, et al. *Clin Nephrol.* 1991;36(3):155.
3. Mehta AM, Engstrom RE, Kreiger AE. Deferoxamine-associated retinopathy after subcutaneous injection. *Am J Ophthalmol.* 1994;118(2):260–262.
4. Blake DR, Winyard P, Lunec J, et al. Cerebral and ocular toxicity induced by desferrioxamine. *Q J Med.* 1985;56:345–355.
5. Davies SC, Marcus RE, Hungerford JL, et al. Ocular toxicity of high-dose intravenous desferrioxamine. *Lancet.* 1983;2:181–184.
6. Rubinstein M, Dupont P, Doppee JP, et al. Ocular toxicity of desferrioxamine. *Lancet.* 1985;1:817–818.
7. Cases A, Kelly J, Sabater J, et al. Acute visual and auditory neurotoxicity in patients with end-stage renal disease receiving desferrioxamine. *Clin Nephrol.* 1988;29(4):176–178.
8. Pengloan J, Dantal J, Rossazza C, et al. Ocular toxicity after a single intravenous dose of desferrioxamine. *Nephron.* 1990;56:19–23.
9. Elison JR, Liss JA, Lee TC, et al. Effects of Long-Term Deferoxamine on Retinal Function. *Scientific Poster 184.* American Academy of Ophthalmology Meeting; 2005.
10. Haimovici R, D'Amico DJ, Gragoudas ES, et al. The expanded clinical spectrum of deferoxamine retinopathy. *Ophthalmology.* 2002;109:164–171.
11. Gonzales CR, Lin AP, Engstrom RE, et al. Bilateral vitelliform maculopathy and deferoxamine toxicity. *Retina.* 2004;24:464–467.
12. Viola F, Barteselli G, Dell'Arti L, et al. Multimodal imaging in deferoxamine retinopathy. *Retina.* 2014;34:1428–1438.
13. Georgakopoulos CD, Tsapardoni F, Kostopoulou EV, et al. Pattern dystrophies in patients treated with deferoxamine: report of two cases and review of the literature. *BMC Ophthalmol.* 2018;18:246.
14. Wu CH, Yang CP, Lai CC, et al. Deferoxamine retinopathy: spectral domain-optical coherence tomography findings. *BMC Ophthalmol.* 2014;14:88.
15. Van Bol L, Alami A, Benghiat FS, et al. Spectral domain optical coherence tomography findings in early deferoxamine maculopathy: report of two cases. *Retin Cases Brief Rep.* 2014;8(2):97–102.
16. Lakhanpal V, Schocket SS, Jiji R. Deferoxamine (Desferal)-induced toxic retinal pigmentary degeneration and presumed optic neuropathy. *Ophthalmology.* 1984;91:443–451.
17. Pinna A, Corda L, Carta F. Rapid recovery with oral zinc sulphate in deferoxamine-induced presumed optic neuropathy and hearing loss. *J Neuroophthalmol.* 2001;21:32–33.
18. Jacobs J, Greene H, Grendel BR. Acute iron intoxication. *N Engl J Med.* 1965;273:1124–1127.
19. Ciba Pharmaceutical Company. Official literature on new drugs: deferoxamine mesylate. *Clin Pharmacol Ther.* 1969;10:595–596.
20. Bloomfield SE, Markenson AL, Miller DR, et al. Lens opacities in thalassemia. *J Pediatr Ophthalmol Strabismus.* 1978;15:154–156.
21. Popescu C, Siganos D, Zanakis E, et al. The mechanism of cataract formation in persons with beta-thalassemia. *Oftalmologia.* 1998;45(4):10–13.
22. Deferoxamine Mesylate. 2019. Retrieved from http://www.pdr.net.
23. Kertes PJ, Lee TKM, Couplan SG. The utility of multifocal electroretinography in monitoring drug toxicity: deferoxamine retinopathy. *Can J Ophthalmol.* 2004;39:656–661.
24. Lai TY, Lee GK, Chan W-M, et al. Rapid development of severe toxic retinopathy associated with continuous intravenous deferoxamine infusion. *Br J Ophthalmol.* 2006;90:243–244.
25. Baath JS, Lam W-C, Kirby M, et al. Deferoxamine-related ocular toxicity: incidence and outcome in a pediatric population. *Retina.* 2008;28:894–899.
26. Arora A, Wren S, Evans KG. Desferrioxamine related maculopathy: a case report. *Am J Hematol.* 2004;76:386–388.

Drug: Methoxsalen (8-methoxypsoralen)

1. Calzavara-Pinton PG, Carlino A, Manfred E, et al. Ocular side effects of PUVA-treated patients refusing eye sun protection. *Acta Derm Venereol (Stockh).* 1994;186:164–165.
2. Souêtre E, De Galeani B, Gastaud P, et al. 5-Methoxypsoralen increases the sensitivity of the retina to light in humans. *Eur J Clin Pharmacol.* 1989;36:59–61.
3. Fenton DA, Wilkinson JD. Dose-related visual-field defects in patients receiving PUVA therapy. *Lancet.* 1983;1:1106.
4. Forman AB, Roenigk Jr HH, Caro WA, et al. Long-term follow-up of skin cancer in the PUVA-48 cooperative study. *Arch Dermatol.* 1989;125:515–519.
5. Lever LR, Farr PM. Skin cancers or premalignant lesions occur in half of high-dose PUVA patients. *Br J Dermatol.* 1994;131:215–219.
6. Lerman S, Megaw J, Willis I. Potential ocular complications from PUVA therapy and their prevention. *J Invest Dermatol.* 1980;74:197–199.
7. Woo TY, Wong RC, Wong JM, et al. Lenticular psoralen photoproducts and cataracts of a PUVA treated psoriatic patient. *Arch Dermatol.* 1985;121:1307–1308.
8. Van Deenen WL, Lamers WP. PUVA therapy and the lens reconsidered. *Doc Ophthalmol.* 1988;70:179–184.
9. Glew WB, Nigra TP. PUVA and the eye. In: Elizabeth AA, ed. *Photochemotherapy in Dermatology.* Stanford, CA: IG-AKU-SHOIN Medical Publishers; 1992:241–253.
10. Stern RS. Photochemotherapy follow-up study: ocular lens findings in patients treated with PUVA. *Am J Ophthalmol.* 1995;119(2):252–253.
11. Stern RS, Parrish JA, Fitzpatrick TB. Ocular findings in patients treated with PUVA. *J Invest Dermatol.* 1985;85:269–273.

12. Methoxsalen. 2019. Retrieved from http://www.pdr.net.
13. Maitray A, Rishi P. Methoxsalen-induced macular toxicity. *Ind J Ophthalmol*. 2017;65(11):1243–1245.
14. Shoeibi N, Taheri A, Nikandish M, et al. Effect of oral photochemotherapy (8-methoxypsoralen + UVA) on the electrophysiologic function of retina. *Cutan Ocul Toxicol*. 2016;35(2):104–109.

Drug: Penicillamine

1. Delamere JP, Jobson S, Mackintosh LP, et al. Penicillamine-induced myasthenia in rheumatoid arthritis: its clinical and genetic features. *Ann Rheum Dis*. 1983;42:500–504.
2. Katz LJ, Lesser RL, Merikangas JR, et al. Ocular myasthenia gravis after D-penicillamine administration. *Br J Ophthalmol*. 1989;73:1015–1018.
3. Damaske E, Althoff W. Optic neuritis in a child with Wilson's disease. *Klin Monatsbl Augenheilkd*. 1972;160:168–175.
4. Klingele TG, Burde RM. Optic neuropathy associated with penicillamine therapy in a patient with rheumatoid arthritis. *J Clin Neuro-Ophthalmol*. 1984;4:75–78.
5. Penicillamine. 2019. Retrieved from http://www.pdr.net.
6. Pless M, Sandson T. Chronic internuclear ophthalmoplegia. A manifestation of D-penicillamine cerebral vasculitis. *J Neuro-Ophthalmol*. 1997;17(1):44–46.
7. Peyrí J, Servitje O, Ribera M, et al. Cicatricial pemphigoid in a patient with rheumatoid arthritis treated with D-penicillamine. *J Am Acad Dermatol*. 1986;14:681.
8. Marti-Huguet T, Quintana M, Cabiro I. Cicatricial pemphigoid associated with D-penicillamine treatment. *Arch Ophthalmol*. 1989;107:115.
9. Bigger JF. Retinal hemorrhages during penicillamine therapy of cystinuria. *Am J Ophthalmol*. 1968;66:954–955.
10. Klepach GL, Way SH. Bilateral serous retinal detachment with thrombocytopenia during penicillamine therapy. *Ann Ophthalmol*. 1981;13:201–203.

Drug: Amidotrizoate (diatrizoate meglumine and/or sodium)

1. Baum JL, Bierstock SR. Peripheral corneal infiltrates following intravenous injection of diatrizoate meglumine. *Am J Ophthalmol*. 1978;85:613–614.
2. Lantos G. Cortical blindness due to osmotic disruption of the blood-brain barrier by angiographic contrast material: CT and MRI studies. *Neurology*. 1989;39:567–571.
3. Guzak SV, Kalina RE, Chenoweth RG. Acute macular neuroretinopathy following adverse reaction to intravenous contrast media. *Retina*. 1983;3:312–317.
4. Priluck IA, Buettner H, Robertson DM. Acute macular neuroretinopathy. *Am J Ophthalmol*. 1978;86:775–778.

Drug: Iodipamide meglumine (adipiodone)

1. Alsarraf R, Carey J, Sires BS, et al. Angiography contrast-induced transient cortical blindness. *Am J Otolaryngol*. 1999;20:130–132.
2. Boyes LA, Tew K. Cortical blindness after subclavian arteriography. *Australas Radiol*. 2000;44(3):315–317.

3. Demirtas M, Birand A, Usal A, et al. Transient cortical blindness after second coronary angiography: is immunological mechanism possible? *Cathet Cardiovasc Diagn*. 1994;31(2):161.
4. Hinchey J, Sweeney PJ. Transient cortical blindness after coronary angiography. *Lancet*. 1998;351:1513–1514.
5. Kwok BW, Lim TT. Cortical blindness following coronary angiography. *Singapore Med J*. 2000;41(12):604–605.
6. Lantos G. Cortical blindness due to osmotic disruption of the blood-brain barrier by angiographic contrast material: CT and MRI studies. *Neurology*. 1989;39(4):567–571.
7. Mentzel H-J, Blume J, Malich A, et al. Cortical blindness after contrast-enhanced CT: complication in a patient with diabetes insipidus. *Am J Neuroradiol*. 2003;24:1114–1116.
8. Shyn PB, Bell KA. Transient cortical blindness following cerebral angiography. *J La State Med Soc*. 1989;141:35–37.
9. Till V, Koprivsek K, Stojanovic S, et al. Transient cortical blindness following vertebral angiography in a young adult with cerebellar haemangioblastoma. *Pediatr Radiol*. 2009;39(11):1223–1226.
10. Yeh S, Bazzaz S, Foroozan R. Transient cortical blindness with leptomeningeal enhancement after attempted peripherally inserted central venous catheter placement. *Arch Ophthalmol*. 2005;123:700–702.
11. Petrus LV, Lois JF, Lo WW. Iatrogenically induced cortical blindness associated with leptomeningeal enhancement. *Am J Neuroradiol*. 1998;19:1522–1524.
12. Junck L, Marshall WH. Neurotoxicity of radiological contrast agents. *Ann Neurol*. 1983;13:469–484.
13. Wang RC, Katz SE, Lubow M. Visual loss and central venous catheterization: cortical blindness and hemianopsia after inadvertent subclavian artery entry. *J Neuroophthalmol*. 2000;20:32–34.
14. Neetans A, Buroenich H. Anaphylactic marginal keratitis. *Bull Soc Belge Ophthalmol*. 1979;186:69–72.
15. Bell JA, Dowd TC, McIlwaine GG, et al. Postmyelographic abducent nerve palsy in association with the contrast agent iopamidol. *J Clin Neuro-Ophthalmol*. 1990;10(2):115–117.

Drugs: Iomeprol, iopamidol, iopromide

1. Bell JA, Dowd TC, McIllwaine GG, et al. Postmyelographic abducent nerve palsy in association with the contrast agent iopamidol. *J Clin Neuroophthalmol*. 1990;10(2):115–117.
2. Bell JA, McIllwaine CG. Postmyelographic lateral rectus palsy associated with iopamidol. *BMJ*. 1990;300(6735):1343–1344.
3. Bell JA, McIllwaine GG, O'Neill D. Iatrogenic lateral rectus palsies: a series of five postmyelographic cases. *J Neuroophthalmol*. 1994;14(4):205–209.
4. Welzl-Hinterkörner E, Haefner M, Mengiardi B. Unilateral uveitis induced by a nonionic iodinated contrast agent. *Am J Ophthalmol*. 2003;136(5):958–960.
5. Fischer-Williams M, Gottschalk PG, Browell JN. Transient cortical-blindness: an unusual complication of coronary angiography. *Neurology*. 1970;20(4):353–355.

6. Boyes LA, Tew K. Cortical blindness after subclavian arteriography. *Australas Radiol.* 2000;44(3):315–317.
7. Mentzel HJ, Blume J, Malich A, et al. Cortical blindness after contrast-enhanced CT: complication in a patient with diabetes insipidus. *Am J Neuroradiol.* 2003;24(6):1114–1116.
8. Till V. Transient cortical blindness following vertebral angiography in a young adult with cerebellar haemangiobloastoma. *Pediatr Radiol.* 2009;39(11):1223–1226.
9. Akhtar N. Transient cortical blindness after coronary angiography: a case report and literature review. *J Pak Med Assoc.* 2011;61(3):295–297.
10. Pasha K. Transient loss of vision after coronary angiogram – case report. *Mymensingh Med J.* 2015;24(3):615–618.
11. Iopromide. 2018. Retrieved from http://www.pdr.net.

Drug: Iotalamic acid (iothalamic acid, iothalamate sodium, or meglumine iothalamate)

1. Guzak SV, Kalina RE, Chenoweth RG. Acute macular neuroretinopathy following adverse reaction to intravenous contrast media. *Retina.* 1983;3:312–317.
2. Neetens A, Buroenich H. Anaphylactic marginal keratitis. *Bull Soc Belge Ophthalmol.* 1979;186:69–72.
3. Smith RE, Carlson DW. Intravenous pyelography contrast media acutely lowers intraocular pressure. *Invest Ophthalmol Vis Sci.* 1994;35(4):1387.
4. Lantos G. Cortical blindness due to osmotic disruption of the blood-brain barrier by angiographic contrast material. CT and MRI studies. *Neurology.* 1989;39:567–571.
5. Canal N, Francesci M. Myasthenic crisis precipitated by iothalamic acid. *Lancet.* 1983;1:1288.

Drug: Azathioprine

1. Scott WJ, Giangiacoma J, Hodges KE, et al. Accelerated cytomegalovirus retinitis secondary to immunosuppressive therapy. *Arch Ophthalmol.* 2004;104(1117–1118):1124.
2. Squirrell DM, Bhatta S, Mudhar HS, et al. Hypersensitive iridocyclitis associated with delayed onset biopsy proven cytomegalovirus retinitis. *Indian J Ophthalmol.* 2014;62(5):656–658.
3. Thomas MH. Azathioprine and severe vaccinia. *Arthritis Rheum.* 1976;19:270.
4. Speerstra F, Boerbooms AM, van de Putte LB, et al. Side-effects of azathioprine treatment in rheumatoid arthritis: analysis of 10 years of experience. *Ann Rheum Dis.* 1982;41(suppl):37–39.
5. Lawson DH, Lovatt GE, Gurton CS, et al. Adverse effects of azathioprine. *Adverse Drug React Acute Poison Rev.* 1984;3:161–171.
6. Elliott JH, Leibowitz HM. The influence of immunosuppressive agents upon corneal wound healing. *Arch Ophthalmol.* 1966;76:334–337.
7. Francois J, Feher J. The effect of azathioprine and chlorpromazine on corneal regeneration. *Exp Eye Res.* 1972;14:69–72.
8. Sudhir RR, Rao SK, Shanmugam MP, et al. Bilateral macular hemorrhage caused by azathioprine-induced aplastic anemia in a corneal graft recipient. *Cornea.* 2002;21:712–714.
9. Miserocchi E, Baltatzis S, Roque MR, et al. The effect of treatment and its related side effects in patients with severe ocular cicatricial pemphigoid. *Ophthalmology.* 2002;109:111–118.
10. Apaydin C, Gur B, Yakupoglu G, et al. Ocular and visual side effects of systemic cyclosporine. *Ann Ophthalmol.* 1992;24(12):465–469.
11. Azathioprine and photosensitivity reactions. 2008. Retrieved from http://www.lareb.nl.

Drug: Cyclosporine (ciclosporin or cyclosporin)

1. Cyclosporine. 2019. Retrieved from http://www.pdr.net.
2. Avery R, Jabs DA, Wingard JR, et al. Optic disc edema after bone marrow transplantation. *Ophthalmology.* 1991;98:1294–1301.
3. Walter SH, Bertz H, Gerling J. Bilateral neuropathy after bone marrow transplantation and cyclosporine A therapy. *Graefe's Arch Clin Exp Ophthalmol.* 2000;238:472–476.
4. Bernauer W, Gratwohl A, Keller A, et al. Microvasculopathy in the ocular fundus after bone marrow transplantation. *Ann Int Med.* 1991;115(12):925–930.
5. Rodriguez E, Delucchi A, Cano F. Neurotoxicity caused by cyclosporine A in renal transplantation in children. *Rev Med Child.* 1992;120:300–303.
6. Cruz OA, Fogg SG, Roper-Hall G. Pseudotumor cerebri associated with cyclosporine use. *Am J Ophthalmol.* 1996;122(3):436–437.
7. Büschen R, Vij O, Hudde T, et al. Pseudotumor cerebri following cyclosporine A treatment in a boy with tubulointerstitial nephritis associated with uveitis. *Pediatr Nephrol.* 2004;19:558–560.
8. Openshaw H, Slatkin NE, Smith E. Eye movement disorders in bone marrow transplant patients on cyclosporin and ganciclovir. *Bone Marrow Transplant.* 1997;19(5):503–505.
9. Openshaw H. Eye movement abnormality associated with ciclosporin. *J Neurol Neurosurg Psychiatry.* 2001;70:809.
10. Apsner R, Schulenburg A, Steinhoff N, et al. Cyclosporin A induced ocular flutter after marrow transplantation. *Bone Marrow Transplant.* 1997;20(3):255–256.
11. Porges Y, Blumen S, Fireman Z, et al. Cyclosporine-induced optic neuropathy, ophthalmoplegia, and nystagmus in a patient with Crohn's disease. *Am J Ophthalmol.* 1998;126(4):607–608.
12. Palmer SL, Bowen II A, Green K. Tear flow in cyclosporine recipients. *Ophthalmology.* 1995;102(1):118–121.
13. Estel RM, Gupta N, Garvin PJ. Permanent blindness after cyclosporine neurotoxicity in a kidney-pancreas transplant recipient. *Clin Neuropharmacol.* 1996;19:259–266.
14. DeGroen PC, Aksamit AJ, Rakela J, et al. Central nervous system toxicity after liver transplantation: the role of cyclosporine and cholesterol. *N Engl J Med.* 1987;317:861–866.

15. Casanova B, Prieto M, Deya E. Persistent cortical blindness after cyclosporine leukoencephalopathy. *Liver Transplant Surg.* 1997;3:638–640.
16. Knower MT, Pethke SD, Valentine VG. Reversible cortical blindness after lung transplantation. *South Med J.* 2003;96:606–612.
17. Cho AS, Holland GN, Glasgow BJ, et al. Ocular involvement in patients with posttransplant lymphoproliferative disorder. *Arch Ophthalmol.* 2001;119:183–189.
18. Oktay Kacmaz R, Kempen JH, Newcomb C, et al. Cyclosporine for ocular inflammatory diseases. *Ophthalmology.* 2010;117:576–584.
19. Sall K, Stevenson OD, Mundorf TK, et al. Two multicenter, randomized studies of the efficacy and safety of cyclosporine ophthalmic emulsion in moderate to severe dry eye disease. *Ophthalmology.* 2000;107:631–639.
20. Peyman GA, Sanders DR, Batlle JF, et al. Cyclosporine 0.05% ophthalmic preparation to aid recovery from loss of corneal sensitivity after LASIK. *J Refract Surg.* 2008;24:337–343.
21. Toker E, Asfuroglu E. Corneal and conjunctival sensitivity in patients with dry eye: the effect of topical cyclosporine therapy. *Cornea.* 2010;29(2):133–140.
22. Kachi S, Hirano K, Takesue Y, et al. Unusual corneal deposit after the topical use of cyclosporine as eyedrops. *Am J Ophthalmol.* 2000;130:667–669.
23. Barber LD, Pflugfelder SC, Tauber J, et al. Phase III safety evaluation of cyclosporine 0.1% ophthalmic emulsion administered twice daily to dry eye disease patients for up to 3 years. *Ophthalmology.* 2005;112:790–794.
24. Touzeau O, Borderie VM, Laroche L. Carcinoma of the corneoscleral limbus in a patient treated with cyclosporine after heart transplantation. *N Engl J Med.* 1999;341(5):374–375.
25. Macarez R, Bossis S, Robinet A, et al. Conjunctival epithelial neoplasias in organ transplant patients receiving cyclosporine therapy. *Cornea.* 1999;18(4):495–497.
26. Flynn TH, Manzouri B, Tuft SJ. Ocular surface squamous neoplasia in an immunosuppressed patient with atopic keratoconjunctivitis. *Int Ophthalmol.* 2012;32(5):471–473.
27. Mohammadpour M, Hashemi H, Jabbarvand M, et al. Clinicopathologic report of anterior subcapsular cataracts after combined administration of corticosteroids and cyclosporine following renal transplantation. *JCRS Online Case Rep.* 2013;1(2):e37–e40.
28. Siak J, Chee SP. Cytomegalovirus anterior uveitis following topical cyclosporine A. *Ocul Immunol Inflamm.* 2018;26(1):90–93.

Drug: Tacrolimus (FK506 or fujimycin)

1. Shutter LA, Green JP, Newman NJ, et al. Cortical blindness and white matter lesions in a patient receiving FK506 after liver transplantation. *Neurology.* 1993;43:2417–2418.
2. Devine SM, Newman NJ, Siegel JL, et al. Tacrolimus (FK506)-induced cerebral blindness following bone marrow transplantation. *Bone Marrow Transplant.* 1996;18:569–572.
3. Steg RE, Kessinger A, Wszolek ZK. Cortical blindness and seizures in a patient receiving FK506 after bone marrow transplantation. *Bone Marrow Transplant.* 1999;23:956–962.
4. Rasool N, Boudreault K, Lessell S, et al. Tacrolimus optic neuropathy. *J Neuroophthalmol.* 2018;38(2):160–166.
5. Brazis PW, Spivey JR, Bolling JP, et al. A case of bilateral optic neuropathy in a patient on tacrolimus (FK506) therapy after liver transplantation. *Am J Ophthalmol.* 2000;129:536–538.
6. Venneti S, Moss HE, Levin MH, et al. Asymmetric bilateral demyelinating optic neuropathy from tacrolimus toxicity. *J Neurol Sci.* 2011;301(1–2):112–115.
7. Lake DB, Poole TRG. Tacrolimus. *Br J Ophthalmol.* 2003;87:121–122.
8. Ascaso FJ, Mateo J, Huerva A, et al. Unilateral tacrolimus-associated optic neuropathy after liver transplantation. *Cutan Ocul Toxicol.* 2012;31(2):167–170.
9. Akers G, Carnero G, Govindasamy R, et al. *Tacrolimus (FK506) Toxicity Presenting as Unilateral Optic Papillitis.* Nashville, TN: Poster Presented At: National Kidney Foundation; 2009.
10. Shao X, He Z, Tang L, et al. Tacrolimus-associated ischemic optic neuropathy and posterior reversible encephalopathy syndrome after small bowel transplantation. *Transplantation.* 2012;94:e58–e60.
11. Yun J, Park KA, Oh SY. Bilateral ischemic optic neuropathy in a patient using tacrolimus (FK506) after liver transplantation. *Transplantation.* 2010;89(12):1541–1542.
12. Kessler L, Lucescu C, Pinget M. Tacrolimus-associated optic neuropathy after pancreatic islet transplantation using a sirolimus/tacrolimus immunosuppressive regimen. *Transplantation.* 2005;81:636–637.
13. Gupta M, Bansal R, Beke N, et al. Tacrolimus-induced unilateral ischaemic optic neuropathy in a non-transplant patient. *BMJ Case Rep.* 2012.
14. Mezza E, et al. Calcineurin Inhibitors (CNI) Related Optic Neuropathy After Kidney Transplantation (KT): Results of Conversion to an m-TOR Regimen in Three Cases. *14th Congress of the European Society for Organ Transplantation* (abstr P-377). 2009.
15. Bartolome I, Lopez Sangros I, Marco Monzon S, et al. Bilateral tacrolimus-associated optic neuropathy after kidney transplant. *Acta Ophthalmol.* 2017;95(suppl 259):no pagination.
16. Sokol DK, Molleston JP, Filo RS, et al. Tacrolimus (FK560)-induced mutism after liver transplant. *Pediatr Neurol.* 2003;28:156–158.
17. Lai MM, Kerrison JB, Miller NR. Reversible bilateral internuclear ophthalmoplegia associated with FK506. *J Neurol Neurosurg Psychiatr.* 2004;75:776–778.
18. Bova D, Shownkeen H, Goldberg K, et al. Delayed transient neurologic toxicity due to tacrolimus: CT and MRI. *Neuroradiology.* 2000;42:666–668.
19. Lauzurica R, Loscos J, Diaz-Couchod P, et al. Tacrolimus-associated severe bilateral corneal ulcer after renal transplantation. *Trans.* 2002;73:1006–1007.

20. Yamazoe K, Yamazoe K, Yamaguchi T, et al. Efficacy and safety of systemic tacrolimus in high-risk penetrating keratoplasty after graft failure with systemic cyclosporine. *Cornea*. 2014;33(11):1157–1163.
21. Plosker GL, Foster RH. Tacrolimus: a further update of its pharmacology and therapeutic use in the management of organ transplantation. *Drugs*. 2000;59:323–389.
22. Pournaras J-AC, Chamot L, Uffer S, et al. Conjunctival intraepithelial neoplasia in a patient treated with tacrolimus after liver transplantation. *Cornea*. 2007;26(10):1261–1262.
23. Marquezan MC, Nascimento H, Vieira LA, et al. Effect of topical tacrolimus in the treatment of Thygeson's superficial punctate keratitis. *Am J Ophthalmol*. 2015;160(4):663–668.
24. Al-Amri AM. Long-term follow-up of tacrolimus ointment for treatment of atopic keratoconjunctivitis. *Am J Ophthalmol*. 2014;157(2):280–286.
25. Freeman AK, Serle J, VanVeldhuisen P, et al. Tacrolimus ointment in the treatment of eyelid dermatitis. *Cutis*. 2004;73:225–227.
26. Russell JJ. Topical tacrolimus. a new therapy for atopic dermatitis. *Am Fam Physician*. 2002;66:1899–1902.
27. Kang S, Luck AW, Pariser D, et al. Long-term safety and efficacy of tacrolimus ointment for the treatment of atopic dermatitis in children. *J Am Acad Dermatol*. 2001;44(suppl 1):S58–S64.
28. Shen JT, Pedvis-Leftick A. Mucosal staining after using topical tacrolimus to treat erosive oral lichen planus. *J Am Acad Dermatol*. 2004;50:326.
29. Caelles IP, Pinto PH, Casado ELD, et al. Focal hypertrichosis during topical tacrolimus therapy for childhood vitiligo. *Pediatr Dermatol*. 2005;22:86–87.
30. Rikker SM, Holland GN, Drayton GE, et al. Topical tacrolimus treatment of atopic eyelid disease. *Am J Ophthalmol*. 2003;135:297–302.

Drugs: Acitretin, isotretinoin

1. Cumurcu T, Sezer E, Kilic R, et al. Comparison of dose-related ocular side effects during systemic isotretinoin administration. *Eur J Ophthalmol*. 2009;19(2):196–200.
2. Bozkurt B, Irkec MT, Atakan N, et al. Lacrimal function and ocular complications in patients treated with systemic isotretinoin. *Eur J Ophthalmol*. 2002;12:173–176.
3. Mathers WD, Shields WJ, Schdev MS, et al. Meibomian gland morphology and tear osmolarity: changes with Accutane therapy. *Cornea*. 1991;10(4):286–290.
4. Fraunfelder FT, Fraunfelder FW, Edwards R. Ocular side effects possible associated with isotretinoin usage. *Am J Ophthalmol*. 2001;132:299–305.
5. Bots CP, van Nieuw-Amerongen A, Brand HS. Enduring oral dryness after acne treatment. *Ned Tijdschr Tandheelkd*. 2003;110:295–297.
6. Aragona P, Cannavó SP, Borgia F, et al. Utility of studying the ocular surface in patients with acne vulgaris treated with oral isotretinoin: a randomized controlled trial. *Br J Dermatol*. 2005;152:576–578.
7. Karalezli A, Borazan M, Altinors DD, et al. Conjunctival impression cytology, ocular surface, and tear-film changes in patients treated with systemic isotretinoin. *Cornea*. 2009;28(1):46–50.
8. De Queiroga IB, Vieira LA, de Nadai Barros J, et al. Conjunctival impression cytology changes induced by oral isotretinoin. *Cornea*. 2009;28(9):1009–1013.
9. Miles S, McGlathery W, Abernathie B. The importance of screening for laser-assisted in situ keratomileusis operation (LASIK) before prescribing isotretinoin. *J Am Acad Dermatol*. 2006;54:180–181.
10. Fraunfelder FW, Fraunfelder FT, Corbett JJ. Isotretinoin-associated intracranial hypertension. *Ophthalmology*. 2004;111:1248–1250.
11. Roytman M, Frumkin A, Bohn TG. Pseudotumor cerebri caused by isotretinoin. *Cutis*. 1988;42:399–400.
12. Herman DC, Dyer JA. Anterior subcapsular cataracts as a possible adverse ocular reaction to isotretinoin. *Am J Ophthalmol*. 1987;103:236–237.
13. Aydogan K, Turan OF, Onart S, et al. Neurological and neurophysiological effects of oral isotretinoin: a prospective investigation using auditory and visual evoked potentials. *Eur J Derm*. 2008;18(6):642–646.
14. Yavuz C, Ozcimen M. An evaluation of peripapillary choroidal thickness in patients receiving systemic isotretinoin treatment. *Cutan Ocul Toxicol*. 2019;38(1):25–28.
15. Guirgis MF, Wong AMF, Tychsen L, et al. Congenital restrictive external ophthalmoplegia and gustatory epiphora associated with fetal isotretinoin toxicity. *Arch Ophthalmol*. 2002;120:1094–1095.
16. Acitretin. 2018. Retrieved from http://www.pdr.net.

Drug: Tretinoin (retinoic acid, vitamin A acid, or all-trans retinoic acid)

1. Colucciello M. Pseudotumor cerebri induced by all-trans retinoic acid treatment of acute promyelocytic leukemia. *Arch Ophthalmol*. 2003;121:1064–1065.
2. Guirgis MF, Leuder GT. Intracranial hypertension secondary to all-trans retinoic acid treatment for leukemia: diagnosis and management. *JAAPOS*. 2003;7:432–434.
3. Schroeter T, Lanvers C, Herding H, et al. Pseudotumor cerebri induced by all-trans-retinoic acid in a child treated for acute promyelocytic leukemia. *Med Pediatr Oncol*. 2000;34:284–286.
4. Tiamkao S, Sirijirachai C. Pseudotumor cerebri caused by all-trans-retinoic acid: a case report. *J Med Assoc Thai*. 2000;83:1420–1423.
5. Yeh YC, Tang HF, Fang IM. Pseudotumor cerebri caused by all-trans-retinoic acid treatment for acute promyelocytic leukemia. *Jpn J Ophthalmol*. 2006;50:295–296.
6. Teichmann LL. Idiopathic intracranial hypertension resulting from ATRA therapy in acute promyelocytic leukemia: an important adverse effect. *Oncol Res Treat*. 2016;39(suppl 3):193.
7. Vanier KL, Mattiussi AJ, Johnston DL. Interaction of all-trans-retinoic acid with fluconazole in acute promyelocytic leukemia. *J Pediatr Hematol Oncol*. 2003;25:403–404.

8. Lanvers C, Wagner A, Dubber A, et al. Pharmacokinetics and metabolism of low-dose ATRA in children – first observations. In: Hiddemann W, et al, eds. *Acute Leukemias VII*. Berlin: Springer-Verlag; 1998:565–569.

9. Avisar R, Deutsch D, Savir H. Corneal calcification in dry eye disorders associated with retinoic acid therapy. *Am J Ophthalmol*. 1988;106:753–755.

10. Samarawickrama C, Chew S, Watson S. Retinoic acid and the ocular surface. *Surv Ophthalmol*. 2015;60:183–195.

11. Tretinoin. 2019. Retrieved from http://www.pdr.net.

Drug: Dimethyl sulfoxide (DMSO)

1. Rowley S, Baer R. Lens deposits associated with RIMSO-50 (dimethylsulphoxide). *Eye*. 2001;15:332–333.

2. Metelitsyna IP. Potentiation of the cataractogenic effect of light by dimethylsulfoxide and adrenaline. *Ukr Biokhim Zh*. 2001;73:114–119.

Drug: Methyl ethyl ketone peroxide (MEKP)

1. Fraunfelder FT, Coster DJ, Drew R, et al. Ocular injury induced by methyl ethyl ketone peroxide. *Am J Ophthalmol*. 1990;110:635–640.

2. Ando M, Tappel AL. Effect of dietary vitamin E on methyl ethyl ketone peroxide damage to microsomal cytochrome P-450 peroxidase. *Chem Biol Interact*. 1985;55:317–326.

3. Floyd EP, Stokinger HE. Toxicity studies of certain organic peroxides and hydroperoxides. *Am Ind Hyg Assoc J*. 1958;19:205–212.

4. Litov RE, Mathews LC, Tappel AL. Vitamin E protection against in vivo lipid peroxidation initiated in rats by methyl ethyl ketone peroxide as monitored by pentane. *Toxicol Appl Pharmacol*. 1981;59:96–106.

5. Slansky HH, Berman MB, Dohlman CH, et al. Cysteine and acetylcysteine in the prevention of corneal ulcerations. *Ann Ophthalmol*. 1970;2:488.

Drug: Bacillus Calmette-Guérin (BCG) vaccine

1. Lamm DL, Stodgdill VD, Stodgill B, et al. Complications of bacillus Calmette-Guérin immunotherapy in 1278 patients with bladder cancer. *J Urol*. 1986;135(2):272–274.

2. Price GE. Arthritis and iritis after BCG therapy for bladder cancer. *J Rheum*. 1994;21(3):564–565.

3. Missioux D, Hermabessier J, Sauvezie B. Arthritis and iritis after bacillus Calmette-Guérin therapy. *J Rheumatol*. 1995;22:2010.

4. Chevrel G, Zech C, Miossec P. Severe uveitis followed by reactive arthritis after bacillus Calmette-Guérin therapy. *J Rheumatol*. 1999;26:1011.

5. Clavel G, Grados F, Cayrolle G, et al. Polyarthritis following intravesical BCG immunotherapy. *Rev Rheum Engl Ed*. 1999;66:115–118.

6. Wertheim M, Astbury N. Bilateral uveitis after intravesical BCG immunotherapy for bladder carcinoma. *Br J Ophthalmol*. 2002;86:706.

7. Hegde V, Dean F. Bilateral panuveitis and optic neuritis following bacillus Calmette-Guérin (BCG) vaccination. *Acta Paediatr*. 2005;94:635–636.

8. Parafita-Fernandez A, Parafita MA. Bilateral iritis after vaccine for bladder cancer. *Optom Vis Sci*. 2015;92(10):e368–e370.

9. Donaldson RC, Canaan Jr SA, McLean RB, et al. Uveitis and vitiligo associated with BCG treatment for malignant melanoma. *Surgery*. 1974;76:771–778.

10. Hogarth MB, Thomas S, Seifert MH, et al. Reiter's syndrome following intravesical BCG immunotherapy. *Postgrad Med J*. 2000;76:791–793.

11. Han DP, Simons KB, Tarkanian CN, et al. Endophthalmitis from mycobacterium bovis-bacille Calmette-Guérin after intravesicular bacilli Calmette-Guérin injections for bladder cancer. *Am J Ophthalmol*. 1999;128:648–650.

12. Sharon S, Thirkill CE, Grigg JR. Autoimmune retinopathy associated with intravesical BCG therapy. *Br J Ophthalmol*. 2005;89:927–928.

13. Hodish I, Ezra D, Gur H, et al. Reiter's syndrome after intravesical bacillus Calmette-Guérin therapy for bladder cancer. *Isr Med Assoc J*. 2000;2:240–241.

14. Garip A, Diedrichs-Mohring M, Thurau SR, et al. Uveitis in a patient treated with Bacilli-Calmette-Guérin: possible antigenic mimicry of mycobacterial and retinal antigens. *Ophthalmology*. 2009;116:2457–2462.

15. Gerbrandy SJ, Schreuders LC, de Smet MD. Mycobacterium bovis endophthalmitis from BCG immunotherapy for bladder cancer. *Ocul Immunol Inflamm*. 2008;16(3):95–97.

16. Imperia PS, Lazarus HM, Lass JH. Ocular complications of systemic cancer chemotherapy. *Surv Ophthalmol*. 1989;34(3):209–230.

17. Loukil I, Ammari L, Hachicha F. Unilateral panuveitis following intravesical therapy with bacilli of Calmette et Guérin. *Bull Soc Belge Ophtalmol*. 2012;320:23–28.

18. Takeuchi A, Taguchi M, Satoh Y, et al. Bilateral orbital inflammation following intravesical bacille Calmette-Guérin immunotherapy for bladder cancer. *Jpn J Ophthalmol*. 2012;56(2):187–189.

19. Uppal GS, Shan AN, Tossounis CM, et al. Bilateral panuveitis following intravesical BCG immunotherapy for bladder cancer. *Ocul Immunol Inflamm*. 2010;18(4):292–296.

20. Pollard AJ, George RH. Ocular contamination with BCG vaccine (letter). *Arch Dis Child*. 1994;70(1):71.

Drugs: Diphtheria (D) vaccine (receiving a tetanus toxoid booster), diphtheria and tetanus (DT) vaccine, diphtheria, tetanus, and pertussis (DTaP) vaccine

1. Lewin L, Guillery H. *Die Wirkungen Von Arzneimitteln Und Giften Auf Das Auge*. 2nd ed. Berline: August Hirschwald; 1913.

2. McReynolds WU, Havener WH, Petrohelos MA. Bilateral optic neuritis following smallpox vaccination and diphtheria-tetanus toxoid. *Am J Dis Child*. 1953;86:601–603.

3. Hamed LM, Silbiger J, Guy J, et al. Parainfectious optic neuritis and encephalomyelitis. a report of two cases with thalamic involvement. *J Clin Neuro-Ophthalmol*. 1993;13(1):18–23.

4. Burkhard C, Choi M, Wilhelm H. Optic neuritis as a complication in preventive tetanus-diphtheria-poliomyelitis vaccination: a case report. *Klin Monatsbl Augenheilkd.* 2001;218:51–54.

5. Cabrera-Maqueda JM, Hernandez-Clares R, Baidez-Guerrero AE, et al. Optic neuritis in pregnancy after Tdap vaccination: report of two cases. *Clin Neurol Neurosurg.* 2017;160:116–118.

6. Steinemann TL, Koffler BH, Jennings CD. Corneal allograft rejection following immunization. *Am J Ophthalmol.* 1988;106:575–578.

Drug: Hepatitis A vaccine

1. Huang EH, Lim SA, Lim PL, et al. Retrobulbar optic neuritis after hepatitis a vaccination in a HIV-infected patient. *Eye.* 2009;23(12):2267–2271.

2. Voigt U, Baum U, Behrendt W, et al. Neuritis of the optic nerve after vaccinations against hepatitis A, hepatitis B and yellow fever. *Klin Monbl Augenheilkd.* 2001;218(10):688–690.

3. O'Dowd S, Bafig R, Ryan A, et al. Severe bilateral optic neuritis post hepatitis A virus (HAV) and typhoid fever vaccination. *J Neurol Sci.* 2015;357(1-2):300–301.

Drug: Hepatitis B vaccine

1. Erguven M, Guven S, Akyuz U, et al. Optic neuritis following hepatitis B vaccination in a 9-year-old girl. *J Chin Med Assoc.* 2009;72(11):594–597.

2. Voigt U, Baum U, Behrendt W, et al. Neuritis of the optic nerve after vaccinations against hepatitis A, hepatitis B and yellow fever. *Klin Monbl Augenheilkd.* 2001;218(10):688–690.

3. Fraunfelder FW, Suhler EB, Fraunfelder FT. Hepatitis B vaccine and uveitis: an emerging hypothesis suggested by review of 32 case reports. *Cutan Ocul Toxicol.* 2010;29(1):26–29.

4. Grewal DS, Zeid JL. Isolated abducens nerve palsy following neonatal hepatitis B vaccination. *J AAPOS.* 2014;18(1):75–76.

Drugs: Herpes zoster (shingles) vaccine, measles, mumps, rubella, and varicella virus vaccine live, varicella (chickenpox) vaccine

1. Esmaeli-Gutstein B, Winkelman JZ. Uveitis associated with varicella virus vaccine. *Am J Ophthalmol.* 1999;127(6):733–734.

2. Charkoudian LD, Kaiser GM, Steinmetz RL, et al. Acute retinal necrosis after herpes zoster vaccination. *Arch Ophthalmol.* 2011;129(11):1495–1497.

3. Gonzales JA, Levison AL, Stewart JM, et al. Retinal necrosis following varicella-zoster vaccination. *Arch Ophthalmol.* 2012;130(10):1355–1356.

4. Host B. Zostavax vaccine triggering bilateral acute retinal necrosis due to wild-type varicella zoster virus. *Clin Exp Ophthalmol.* 2017;45(suppl 1):147.

5. Navalkele BD, Henig O, Fairfax M, et al. First case of vaccine-strain varicella infection as manifestation of HIV in

healthcare worker: a case report and review of the literature. *J Hosp Infect.* 2017;97(4):384–388.

6. Liu RT, Yeung SN, Carleton B, et al. Risk of anterior segment complications associated with the live herpes zoster vaccine: evidence from a health-claim database. *Cornea.* 2018;37(8):952–956.

7. Grillo AP, Fraunfelder FW. Keratitis in association with herpes zoster and varicella vaccines. *Drugs Today (Barc).* 2017;53(7):393–397.

8. Krall P, Kubal A. Herpes zoster stromal keratitis after varicella vaccine booster in a pediatric patient. *Cornea.* 2014;33(9):988–989.

9. Jastrzebski A, Brownstein S, Ziai S, et al. Reactivation of herpes zoster keratitis with corneal perforation after zoster vaccination. *Cornea.* 2017;36(6):740–742.

Drug: Human papillomavirus (HPV) vaccine

1. Crawford NW, Hodgson K, Gold M, et al. Adverse events following HPV immunization in Australia: Establishment of a clinical network. *Hum Vaccin Immunother.* 2016;12(10):2662–2665.

2. Chen Y-H, Chang Y-H, Lee Y-C. Panuveitis following administration of quadrivalent human papillomavirus vaccine. *Tzu Chi Med J.* 2014;26(1):44–46.

3. Sawai T, Shimizu M, Sakai T, et al. Tubulointerstitial nephritis and uveitis syndrome associated with human papillomavirus vaccine. *J Pediatr Ophthalmol Strabismus.* 2016;53(3):190–191.

4. Holt HD. Human papilloma virus vaccine associated with uveitis. *Curr Drug Saf.* 2014;9(1):65–68.

5. Ogino K, Kishi S, Yoshimura N. Multiple evanescent white dot syndrome after human papillomavirus vaccination. *Case Rep Ophthalmol.* 2014;5(1):38–43.

6. Dansingani KK, Suzuki M, Naysan J, et al. Panuveitis with exudative retinal detachments after vaccination against human papilloma virus. *Ophthalmic Surg Lasers Imaging Retina.* 2015;46(9):967–970.

7. Khalifa YM, Monahan PM, Acharya NR. Ampiginous choroiditis following quadrivalent human papilloma virus vaccine. *Br J Ophthalmol.* 2010;94(1):137–139.

8. Dimario Jr FJ, Hajjar M, Ciesielski T. A 16-year old girl with bilateral visual loss and left hemiparesis following an immunization against human papilloma virus. *J Child Neurol.* 2010;25(3):321–327.

Drug: Influenza virus vaccine

1. Cangemi FE, Bergen RL. Optic atrophy following swine flu vaccination. *Am Ophthalmol.* 1980;12:857.

2. Macoul KL. Bilateral optic nerve atrophy and blindness following swine influenza vaccination. *Ann Ophthalmol.* 1982;14:398–399.

3. Poser CM. Neurological complications of swine influenza vaccination. *Acta Neurol Scand.* 1982;66:413–431.

4. Leiderman YI, Lessell S, Cestari DM. Recurrent isolated sixth nervy palsy after consecutive annual influenza vaccinations in a child. *J AAPOS.* 2009;13(3):317–318.

5. Fredette MJ, De Serres G, Malenfant M. Ophthalmological and biological features of the oculorespiratory syndrome after influenza vaccination. *Clin Infect Dis*. 2003;37:1136–1138.

6. Skowronski DM, Strauss B, Kendall P, et al. Low risk of recurrence of oculorespiratory syndrome following influenza revaccination. *CMAJ*. 2002;167:853–858.

7. De Serres G, Grenier JL, Toth E, et al. The clinical spectrum of the oculo-respiratory syndrome after influenza vaccination. *Vaccine*. 2003;21:2354–2361.

8. De Serres G, Toth E, Ménard S, et al. Oculo-respiratory syndrome after influenza vaccination: trends over four influenza seasons. *Vaccine*. 2005;23:3726–3732.

9. De Serres G, Boulianne N, Duval B, et al. Oculo-respiratory syndrome following influenza vaccination: evidence for occurrence with more than one influenza vaccine. *Vaccine*. 2003;21:2346–2353.

10. Scheifele DW, Duval B, Russell ML, et al. Ocular and respiratory symptoms attributable to inactivated split influenza vaccine: evidence from a controlled trial involving adults. *Clin Infect Dis*. 2003;36:850–857.

11. Hull TP, Bates JH. Optic neuritis after influenza vaccination. *Am J Ophthalmol*. 1997;124(5):703–704.

12. Ray CL, Dreizin IJ. Bilateral optic neuropathy associated with influenza vaccination. *J Neuro-Ophthalmol*. 1996;16(3):182–184.

13. Laffon-Pioger M, Rocher F, Cohen M, et al. Bilateral optic neuropathy with loss of vision after an influenza vaccination in a patient suffering from mixed connective tissue disease. *Rev Neurol*. 2010;166(12):1024–1027.

14. Crawford C, Grazko MB, Raymond 4th WR, et al. Reversible blindness in bilateral optic neuritis associated with nasal flu vaccine. *Binocul Vis Strabolog Q Simms Romano*. 2012;27(3):171–173.

15. Rubinov A, Beiran I, Krasnitz I, et al. Bilateral optic neuritis after inactivated influenza vaccination. *Isr Med Assoc J*. 2012;14(11):705–707.

16. Jun B, Fraunfelder RW. Atypical optic neuritis after inactivated influenza vaccination. *Neuroophthalmology*. 2017;42(2):105–108.

17. Jöhr N, Tschopp M, Hollbach N, et al. Optic neuritis after influenza vaccination in a patient after stem cell transplantation. *Klin Monbl Augenheilkd*. 2015;232(4):484–486.

18. Crawford CM, Grazko MB, Raymond 4th WR, et al. Retrobulbar optic neuritis and live attenuated influenza vaccine. *J Pediatr Ophthalmol Strabismus*. 2013;50(1):61.

19. Influenza HA vaccine: risk of optic neuritis. *WHO Pharmaceuticals Newsletter*. 2015;4:8–9.

20. Kawasaki A, Purvin VA, Tang R. Bilateral anterior ischemic optic neuropathy following influenza vaccination. *J Neuro-Ophthalmol*. 1998;18(1):56–59.

21. Manasseh G, Donovan D, Shao EH, et al. Bilateral sequential non-arteritic ischaemic optic neuropathy following repeat influenza vaccination. *Case Rep Ophthalmol*. 2014;5(2):267–269.

22. Papke D, McNussen PJ, Rasheed M, et al. A case of unilateral optic neuropathy following influenza vaccination. *Semin Ophthalmol*. 2017;32(4):517–523.

23. Knopf HL. Recurrent uveitis after influenza vaccination. *Ann Ophthalmol*. 1991;23(6):213–214.

24. Tao Y, Chang LB, Zhao M, et al. Two cases of exudative retinal detachment and uveitis following H1N1 influenza vaccination. *Chin Med J*. 2011;124(22):3838–3840.

25. Steinemann TL, Koffler BH, Jennings CD. Corneal allograft rejection following immunization. *Am J Ophthalmol*. 1988;106:575–578.

26. Solomon A, Frucht-Pery J. Bilateral simultaneous corneal graft rejection after influenza vaccination. *Am J Ophthalmol*. 1996;121(6):708–709.

27. Wertheim MS, Keel M, Cook SD, et al. Corneal transplant rejection following influenza vaccination. *Br J Ophthalmol*. 2006;90:925–926.

28. Thurairajan G, Hope-Ross MW, Situnayake RD, et al. Polyarthropathy, orbital myositis and posterior scleritis: an unusual adverse reaction to influenza vaccine. *Br J Rheum*. 1997;36:120–123.

29. Mutsch M, Zhou W, Rhodes P, et al. Use of the inactivated intranasal influenza vaccine and the risk of Bell's palsy in Switzerland. *N Engl J Med*. 2004;350:896–903.

Drugs: Measles, mumps and rubella virus vaccine live, measles, mumps, rubella, and varicella virus vaccine live, measles virus vaccine live, mumps virus vaccine live, rubella and mumps virus vaccine live, rubella virus vaccine live

1. Arshi S, Sadeghi-Bazargani H, Ojaghi H, et al. The first rapid onset optic neuritis after measles-rubella vaccination: case report. *Vaccine*. 2004;22:3240–3242.

2. Kline L, Margulie SL. Optic neuritis and myelitis following rubella vaccination. *Arch Neurol*. 1982;39:443–444.

3. Stevenson VL, Acheson JF, Ball J, et al. Optic neuritis following measles/rubella vaccination in two 13-year-old children. *Br J Ophthalmol*. 1996;80(12):1110–1111.

4. Kazarian EL, Gager WE. Optic neuritis complicating measles, mumps, and rubella vaccination. *Arch Neurol*. 1982;39:443.

5. Manzotti F, Menozzi C, Porta MR, et al. Partial third nerve palsy after measles mumps rubella vaccination. *Ital J Pediatr*. 2010;36:59.

6. Chan CC, Sogg RL, Steinman L. Isolated oculomotor palsy after measles immunization. 0 1980;89:446–448.

7. Krugman S. Present status of measles and rubella immunization in the United States: a medical progress report. *Pediatrics*. 1977;90:1–12.

8. Islam SMM, El-Sheikh HF, Tabbara KF. Anterior uveitis following combined vaccination for measles mumps and rubella (MMR): a report of two cases. *Acta Ophthalmol Scand*. 2000;78:590–592.

9. Ferrini W, Aubert V, Balmer A, et al. Anterior uveitis and cataract after rubella vaccination: a case report of a 12-month-old girl. *Pediatrics*. 2013;132(4):e1035–e1038.

10. ten Berge JC, van Daele PL, Rothova A. Rubella virus-associated anterior uveitis in a vaccinated patient: a case report. *Ocul Immunol Inflamm*. 2016;24(1):113–114.
11. Maspero A, Sesana B, Ferrante P. Adverse reactions to measles vaccine. *Boll 1st Sieroter Milan*. 1984;63(2):125–129.
12. Marshall GS, Wright PF, Fenichel GM, et al. Diffuse retinopathy following mumps and rubella vaccination. *Pediatrics*. 1985;76:989–991.

Drugs: Rabies immune globulin, rabies vaccine

1. Cormack HS, Anderson LAP. Bilateral papillitis following antirabic inoculation: recovery. *Br J Ophthalmol*. 1934;18:167–168.
2. Srisupan V, Konyama K. Bilateral retrobulbar optic neuritis following antirabies vaccination. *Siriraj Hosp Gaz*. 1971;23:403.
3. Chayakul V, Ishikawa S, Chotibut S, et al. Convergence insufficiency and optic neuritis due to antirabies inoculation – a case study. *Jpn J Ophthalmol*. 1975;19:307–314.
4. Francois J, Van Lantschoot G. Optic neuritis and atrophy due to drugs. *T Geneesk*. 1976;32:151.
5. Van de Geijn E, Tukkie E, Van Philips L, et al. Bilateral optic neuritis with branch retinal artery occlusion associated with vaccination. *Doc Ophthalmol*. 1994;86:403–408.
6. Dadeya S, Guliani BP, Gupta VS, et al. Retrobulbar neuritis following rabies vaccination. *Trop Doct*. 2004;34:174–175.
7. Brain WR. *Diseases of the Nervous System*. 6th ed. New York: Oxford University Press; 1962.
8. Consul BN, Purohit GK, Chhabra HN. Antirabic vaccine optic neuritis. *Indian J Med Sci*. 1968;22:630–632.
9. Stratton KR, Howe CJ, Johnston Jr RB, eds. Adverse Events Associated with Childhood Vaccines: Evidence Bearing on Causality. Vaccine Safety Committee. *Division of Health Promotion and Disease Prevention Institute of Medicine*. Washington, DC: National Academy Press; 1994.
10. Walsh FB. *Clinical Neuro-Ophthalmology*. 2nd ed. Baltimore: Williams and Wilkins; 1957:477.
11. Yang JS, Chen CL, Hu YZ, et al. Multiple evanescent white dot syndrome following rabies vaccination: a case report. *BMC Ophthalmol*. 2018;18(1):312.
12. Saxena R, Sethi HS, Rai HK, et al. Bilateral neuro-retinitis following chick embryo cell anti-rabies vaccination: a case report. *BMC Ophthalmol*. 2005;5:20.

Drug: Smallpox (vaccinia) vaccine

1. Maki DG, Wis M. National preparedness for biological warfare and bioterrorism. *Arch Ophthalmol*. 2003;121:710–711.
2. Pepose JS, Marcolis TP, LaRussa P, et al. Ocular complications of smallpox vaccination. *Am J Ophthalmol*. 2003;136:343–352.
3. Lee SF, Butler R, Chansue E, et al. Vaccinia keratouveitis manifesting as a masquerade syndrome. *Am J Ophthalmol*. 1994;117:480–487.
4. Redslob E. Cecite foudroyanted chez un efant en bas age après vaccination antivariolique. *Bull Men Soc Franc Ophtalmol*. 1935;48:126–139.
5. Landa G, Marcovich A, Leiba H, et al. Multiple branch retinal arteriolar occlusions associated with smallpox vaccination. *J Infect*. 2006;52:e7–e9.
6. Mathur SP, Makhija JM, Mehta MC. Papillitis with myelitis after revaccination. *Indian J Med Sci*. 1967;21:469–471.
7. US Centers for Disease Control and Prevention. Smallpox vaccine adverse events among civilians – United States. *Arch Dermatol*. 2003;13:683–684.

Drugs: Tetanus immune globulin, tetanus toxoid

1. Steinmann TL, Koffler BH, Jennings CD. Corneal allograft rejection following immunization. *Am J Ophthalmol*. 1988;106:575–578.
2. Immunization practices advisory committee. centers for disease control: diphtheria tetanus and pertussis: guidelines for vaccine prophylaxis and other preventive measures. *Ann Intern Med*. 1981;95:723–728.
3. Topaloglu H, Berker M, Kansu T, et al. Optic neuritis and myelitis after booster tetanus toxoid vaccination. *Lancet*. 1992;339:178–179.
4. Mohammad J, Kefah AH, Abdel AH. Oculomotor neuropathy following tetanus toxoid injection. *Neurol India*. 2008;56(2):214–216.

Drug: Yellow fever vaccine

1. Biancardi AL, Moraes HV. Anterior and intermediate uveitis following yellow fever vaccination with fractional dose: case reports. *Ocul Immunol Inflamm*. 2018:1–3.
2. Stangos A, Zaninetti M, Petropoulos I, et al. Multiple evanescent white dot syndrome following simultaneous hepatitis-A and yellow fever vaccination. *Ocul Immunol Inflamm*. 2006;14(5):301–304.

FURTHER READING

Disulfiram

Geffray L, Dao T, Cevallos R, et al. Retrobulbar optic neuritis caused by disulfiram. *Revue de Medecine Interne*. 1995;16(12):973.

Graveleau J, Ecoffet M, Villard A. Les neuropathies peripheriques dues au disulfirame. *Nouv Presse Med*. 1980;9:2905–2907.

Hautala N, Nevalainen J, Mustonen E, et al. Disulfiram-induced bilateral optic disc oedema with disc-related visual field loss and sparing central vision. *Neuro-Ophthalmo*. 2009;33(1–2):47–51.

Kulkarni RR, Pradeep AV, Bairy BK. Disulfiram induced combined irreversible anterior ischemic optic neuropathy and reversible peripheral neuropathy: a prospective case report and review of the literature. *J Neuropsychiatry Clin Neurosci*. 2013;25(4):339–342.

Mokri B, Ohnishi A, Dyck PJ. Disulfiram neuropathy. *Neurology*. 1981;31:730–735.

Morcamp D, Boudin G, Mizon JP. Complications neurologiques inhabituelles du disulfirame. *Nouv Presse Med*. 1981;10:338–339.

Trélohan A, Milea D. Reversible optic neuropathy related to disulfiram. *J Fr Ophtalmol*. 2011;34(6):382(e1–e3).

Alendronate sodium, etidronate disodium, ibandronate sodium, pamidronate disodium, risedronate sodium, zoledronic acid

Adverse Drug Reactions Advisory Committee. Bisphosphonates and ocular inflammation. *Aust Adv Drug React Bull*. 2004;23:7–8.

Coleman CI, Perkerson KA, Lewis A. Alendronate-induced hallucinations and visual disturbance. *Pharmacotherapy*. 2004;24:799–802.

Colucci A, Modorati G, Miserocchi E, et al. Anterior uveitis complicating zolendronic acid infusion. *Ocul Immunol Inflamm*. 2009;17(4):267–268.

Dasanu CA, Alexandrescu DT. Acute retinal epithelial detachment secondary to pamidronate administration. *J Oncol Pharm Pract*. 2009;15(2):119–121.

De S, Meyer P, Crisp AJ. Pamidronate and uveitis (letter to the editor). *Br J Rheumatol*. 1995;34(5):479.

French DD, Margo CE. Postmarketing surveillance rates of uveitis and scleritis with bisphosphonates among a national veteran cohort. *Retina*. 2008;28(6):889–893.

Hemmati I, Wade J, Kelsall J. Risedronate-associated scleritis: a case report and review of the literature. *Clin Rheumatol*. 2012;31:1403–1405.

Kaur H, Uy C, Kelly J, et al. Orbital inflammatory disease in a patient treated with zoledronate. *Endocr Pract*. 2011;17(4):e101–e103.

Lespagnard S, Bonnet S, Betz P. Clinical case of the month. Bilateral optic neuropathy secondary to bisphosphonate therapy. *Rev Med Liege*. 2010;65(7–8):434–436.

Leung S, Ashar BH, Miller RG. Bisphosphonates-associated scleritis: a case report and review. *South Med J*. 2005;98:733–735.

Macarol V, Fraunfelder FT. Disodium pamidronate and adverse ocular drug reactions. *Am J Ophthalmol*. 1994;118:220–224.

Mbekeani JN, Slamovits TL, Schwartz BH, et al. Ocular inflammation associated with alendronate therapy. *Arch Ophthalmol*. 1999;117:837–838.

MHRA. Final Report on TGN1412 Clinical Trial. *Media release* 2006. Retrieved from http://www.mhra.gov.uk.

Morton AR, et al. Disodium pamidronate (APD) for the management of single-dose versus daily infusions and of infusion duration. In: *Disodium Pamidronate (APD) in the Treatment of Malignancy-Related Disorders*. Toronto: Hans Huber Publishers; 1989:85–100.

O'Donnell NP, Rao GP, Aguis-Fernandez A. Paget's disease: ocular complications of disodium pamidronate treatment. *Br J Clin Pract*. 1995;49(5):272–273.

Ortiz-Perez S, Fernandez E, Molina JJ, et al. Two cases of drug-induced orbital inflammatory disease. *Orbit*. 2011;30(1):37–39.

Patel DV, Horne A, House M, et al. The incidence of acute anterior uveitis after intravenous zoledronate. *Ophthalmology*. 2013;120:773–776.

Peterson JD, Bedrossian Jr EH. Bisphosphonate-associated orbital inflammation – a case report and review. *Orbit*. 2012;31(2):119–123.

Richards JC, Wiffen SJ. Corneal graft rejection precipitated by uveitis secondary to alendronate sodium therapy. *Cornea*. 2006;25(9):1100–1101.

Ryan PJ, Sampath R. Idiopathic orbital inflammation following intravenous pamidronate. *Rheumatol*. 2001;40:956–957.

Siris ES. Bisphosphonates and iritis. *Lancet*. 1993;342:436–437.

Stewart GO, Stuckey BG, Ward LC, et al. Iritis following intravenous pamidronate. *Aust N Z J Med*. 1996;26(3):414–415.

Subramanian PS, Kerrison JB, Calvert PC, et al. Orbital inflammatory disease after pamidronate treatment for metastatic prostate cancer. *Arch Ophthalmol*. 2003;121:1335–1336.

Vinas G, Olive A, Holgado S, et al. Episcleritis secondary to risedronate. *Med Clin*. 2002;118:598–599.

Yeo J, Jafer AK. Zolendronate associated inflammatory orbital disease. *N Z Med J*. 2010;123(1323):50–52.

Deferoxamine mesylate (desferrioxamine)

Albalate M, Velasco L, Ortiz A, et al. High risk of retinal damage by desferrioxamine in dialysis patients [letter]. *Nephron*. 1996;73(4):726–727.

Arden GB, Wonke B. Desferrioxamine (DFX) and ocular toxicity. *Invest Ophthalmol Vis Sci*. 1984;25(suppl):336.

Bansal V, Elgarbly I, Ghanchi FD, et al. Bull's eye maculopathy with deferoxamine. *Eur J Haematol*. 2003;70:420–421.

Bentur Y, McGuigan M, Koren G. Deferoxamine (desferrioxamine) new toxicities for an old drug. *Drug Safety*. 1991;6(1):37–46.

Borgna-Pignatti C, de Stefano P, Broglia AM. Visual loss in patient on high dose subcutaneous desferrioxamine. *Lancet*. 1984;1:681.

Haimovici R. The Deferoxamine Retinopathy Study Group: the expanded clinical spectrum of desferrioxamine retinopathy. *IOVS*. 1998;39(4):S1133.

Marciani MG, Stefani N, Stefanini F, et al. Visual function during long-term desferrioxamine treatment [letter]. *Lancet*. 1993;341(8843):491.

Olivieri NF, Buncic JR, Chew E, et al. Visual and auditory neurotoxicity in patients receiving subcutaneous deferoxamine infusions. *N Engl J Med*. 1986;314:869–873.

Orton RB, de Veber LL, Sulh HM. Ocular and auditory toxicity of long-term, high-dose subcutaneous deferoxamine therapy. *Can J Ophthalmol*. 1985;20:153–156.

Porter JB. A risk–benefit assessment of iron chelation therapy. *Drug Safety*. 1997;17:407–421.

Simon P, Ang KS, Meyrier A, et al. Desferrioxamine, ocular toxicity, and trace metals. *Lancet*. 1983;2:512–513.

Methoxsalen (8-methoxypsoralen)

Archier E, Devaux S, Castela E, et al. Ocular damage in patients with psoriasis treated by psoralen UV-A therapy or narrow band UVB therapy: a systemic literature review. *J Eur Acad Dermatol Venereol.* 2012;26(suppl 3):32–35.

Bartley GB. Ocular lens findings in patients treated with PUVA. *Am J Ophthalmol.* 1995;119(2):252–253.

Farber EM, Abel EA, Cox AJ. Long-term risks of psoralens and UV-A therapy for psoriasis. *Arch Dermatol.* 1983;119:426–431.

Lafond G, Roy PE, Grenier R. Lens opacities appearing during therapy with methoxsalen and long-wavelength ultraviolet radiation. *Can J Ophthalmol.* 1984;19:173–175.

Penicillamine

Atcheson SG, Ward JR. Ptosis and weakness after start of D-penicillamine therapy. *Ann Intern Med.* 1978;89:939–940.

Dingle J, Havener WH. Ophthalmoscopic changes in a patient with Wilson's disease during long-term penicillamine therapy. *Ann Ophthalmol.* 1978;10:1227–1230.

Fenton DA. Hypertrichosis. *Semin Dermatol.* 1985;4:58.

George J, Spokes E. Myasthenic pseudo-internuclear ophthalmoplegia due to penicillamine. *J Neurol Neurosurg Psychiatry.* 1984;47:1044.

Haviv YS, Safadi R. Rapid progression of scleroderma possibly associated with penicillamine therapy. *Clin Drug Invest.* 1998;15(1):61–63.

Kimbrough RL, Mewis I, Stewart RH. D-penicillamine and the ocular myasthenic syndrome. *Ann Ophthalmol.* 1981;13:1171–1172.

Loffredo A, Sammartino A, Cecio A, et al. Hepatolenticular degeneration. *Acta Ophthalmol.* 1983;61:943–946.

Moore AP, Williams AC, Hillenbrand P. Penicillamine induced myasthenia reactivated by gold. *BMJ.* 1984;288:192–193.

Amidotrizoate (diatrizoate meglumine and/or sodium)

Haney WP, Preston RE. Ocular complications of carotid arteriography in carotid occlusive disease. *Arch Ophthalmol.* 1962;67:127–137.

Junck L, Marshall WH. Neurotoxicity of radiological contrast agents. *Ann Neurol.* 1983;13:469–484.

McMahon KA, Frewin DB, Easterbrook EG, et al. Adverse reactions to drugs: A 12-month hospital survey. *Aust N Z J Med.* 1977;7:382–385.

Iodipamide meglumine (adipiodone)

McMahon KA, Frewin DB, Easterbrook EG, et al. Adverse reactions to drugs: a 12-month hospital survey. *Aust N Z J Med.* 1977;7:382–385.

Iotalamic acid (iothalamic acid, iothalamate sodium, or meglumine iothalamate)

Junck L, Marshall WH. Neurotoxicity of radiological contrast agents. *Ann Neurol.* 1983;13:469–484.

Azathioprine

Knowles RS, Virden JE. Handling of injectable antineoplastic agents. *BMJ.* 1980;2:589–591.

Schneider F. Progressive multifocal leukoencephalopathy as a cause of neurologic symptoms in sharp syndrome. *Zeitschrft Fur Rheumatologie.* 1991;50(4):222–224.

Tuchmann-Duplessis H, Mercier-Parot L. Dissociation of antitumor and teratogenic properties of a purine antimetabolite, azathioprine. *C R Soc Biol.* 1965;159:2290–2294.

Cyclosporine (ciclosporin or cyclosporin)

Ahern MJ, Harrison W, Hollingsworth P, et al. A randomized double-blind trial of cyclosporin and azathioprine in refractory rheumatoid arthritis. *Aust N Z J Med.* 1991;21:844–849.

Akagi T, Manabe S, Ishigooka H. A case of cyclosporine-induced optic neuropathy with a normal therapeutic level of cyclosporine. *Jpn J Ophthalmol.* 2010;54(1):102–104.

Dawson DG, Trobe JD. Blindness after liver transplant. *Surv Ophthalmol.* 2002;47:387–391.

Filipec M, Phan TM, Zhao TZ, et al. Topical cyclosporine A and corneal wound healing. *Cornea.* 1992;11:546–552.

Ghalie R, Fitzsimmons WE, Bennett D, et al. Cortical blindness: a rare complication of cyclosporine therapy. *Bone Marrow Transplant.* 1990;6:147–149.

González-Vincent M, Díaz MA, Madero L. "Pseudotumor cerebri" following allogeneic bone marrow transplantation (BMT). *Ann Hematol.* 2001;80:236–237.

Katirji MB. Visual hallucinations and cyclosporine. *Transplantation.* 1987;43:768–769.

Laibovitz RA, Solch S, Andriano K, et al. Pilot trial of cyclosporine 1% ophthalmic ointment in the treatment of keratoconjunctivitis sicca. *Cornea.* 1993;12:315–323.

Marchiori PE, Mies S, Scaff M. Cyclosporine A-induced ocular opsoclonus and reversible leukoencephalopathy after orthotopic liver transplantation. *Clin Neuropharmacol.* 2004;27:195–197.

Meyers-Elliott RH, Chitjian PA, Billups CB. Effects of cyclosporine A on clinical and immunological parameters in herpes simplex keratitis. *Invest Ophthalmol Vis Sci.* 1987;28:1170–1180.

Noll RB, Kulkarni R. Complex visual hallucinations and cyclosporine. *Arch Neurol.* 1984;41:329–330.

Obermoser G, Weber F, Sepp N. Discoid lupus erythematosus in a patient receiving cyclosporine for liver transplantation. *Acta Derm Venereol.* 2001;81:319.

Palmer SL, Bowen II A, Green K. Longitudinal tear study after cyclosporine in kidney transplant recipients. *Ophthalmology.* 1996;103(4):670–673.

Rubin AM, Kang H. Cerebral blindness and encephalopathy with cyclosporin A toxicity. *Neurology.* 1987;37:1072–1076.

Stevenson D, Tauber J, Reis BL, et al. Efficacy and safety of cyclosporine A ophthalmic emulsion in the treatment of moderate-to-severe dry eye disease. *Ophthalmology.* 2000;107:967–974.

Stucrenschneider BJ, Meiler WF. Ocular findings following bone marrow transplantation. *Ophthalmology.* 1992;92(suppl):152.

Tang-Liu DD, Acheampong A. Ocular pharmacokinetics and safety of ciclosporin, a novel topical treatment for dry eye. *Clin Pharmacokinet.* 2005;44:247–261.

Uoshima N, Karasuno T, Yagi T, et al. Late onset cyclosporine-induced cerebral blindness with abnormal SPECT imagings in a patient undergoing unrelated bone marrow transplantation. *Bone Marrow Transplant*. 2000;26:105–108.

Wilson SE, de Groen PC, Aksamit AJ, et al. Cyclosporin A-induced reversible cortical blindness. *J Clin Neuro-Ophthalmol*. 1988;8:215–220.

Tacrolimus (FK506 or fujimycin)

Donnadieu B, Amouyal F, Hoffart L, et al. Central retinal vein occlusion-associated tacrolimus after liver transplantation. *Transplantation*. 2014;98(12):e94–e95.

Joseph MA, Kaufman HE, Insler M. Topical tacrolimus ointment for treatment of refractory anterior segment inflammatory disorders. *Cornea*. 2005;24:417–420.

Nakamura M, Fuchinouc S, Sato S, et al. Clinical and radiological features of two cases of tacrolimus-related posterior leukoencephalopathy in living related liver transplantation. *Transplant Proc*. 1998;30:1477–1478.

Oliverio PJ, Lucas R, Mitchell SA, et al. Reversible tacrolimus-induced neurotoxicity isolated to the brain stem. *Am J Neuroradiol*. 2000;21:1251–1254.

Uygun V, Daloğlu H, Öztürkmen SI, et al. Extracorporeal photopheresis did not prevent the development of an autoimmune disease: myasthenia gravis. *Transfusion*. 2016;56(12):3081–3085.

Acitretin, isotretinoin

Alam MS, Agarwal S. Presumed isotretinoin-induced extraocular myopathy. *J Pharmacol Pharmacother*. 2016;7(4):187–189.

Arnault J-P, Petitpain N, Granel-Brocard F, et al. Acitretin and sixth nerve palsy. *J Eur Acad Dermatol Venereol*. 2007;21(9):1258–1259.

Barbero P, Lotersztein V, Bronberg R, et al. Acitretin embryopathy: a case report. *Birth Defects Res A Clin Mol Teratol*. 2004;70(10):831–833.

Bastos PR, Avelleira JCR, Cruz MA, et al. Granulation tissue in palpebral conjunctivae associated with acitretin therapy. *J Am Acad Dermatol*. 2008;58(suppl 2):S41–S42.

Bergler-Czop B, Bilewicz-Stebel M, Stankowska A, et al. Side effects of retinoid therapy on the quality of vision. *Acta Pharm*. 2016;66(4):471–478.

Brown RD, Grattan CEH. Visual toxicity of synthetic retinoids. *Br J Ophthalmol*. 1989;73:286–288.

Chua WC, Martin PA, Kourt G. Watery eye: a new side-effect of isotretinoin therapy. *Eye*. 2001;15:115–116.

Ellies P, Dighiero P, Legeais JM, et al. Persistent corneal opacity after oral isotretinoin therapy for acne. *Cornea*. 2000;19:238–239.

Farhidnia N, Memarian A. Congenital anomalies following use of isotretinoin: emphasis on its legal aspects. *Med Leg J*. 2017;85(1):33–34.

Faustino JF, Ribeiro-Silva A, Dalto RF, et al. Vitamin A and the eye: an old tale for modern times. *Arg Bras Oftalmol*. 2016;79(1):56–61.

Fraunfelder FW. Ocular side effects associated with isotretinoin. *Drugs Today*. 2004;40:23–27.

Gold JA, Shupack JL, Nemec MA. Ocular side effects of the retinoids. *Int J Dermatol*. 1989;28:218–225.

Gürel G, Sahin S, Cölgecen E. Pityriasis rosea-like eruption induced by isotretinoin. *Cutan Ocul Toxicol*. 2018;37(1):100–102.

Hazen PG, Carney JM, Langston RH, et al. Corneal effect of isotretinoin: possible exacerbation of corneal neovascularization in a patient with the keratitis, ichthyosis, deafness ("KID") syndrome. *J Am Acad Dermatol*. 1986;14:141–142.

Horlings RK. A "chicken skin" due to blood disorders: MGUS-associated lichen myxedematosus. *Ned Tijdschr Geneeskd*. 2017;27(2):81–84.

Johnson M. Recurrent corneal erosion syndrome associated with oral isotretinoin: a cautionary tale. *Clin Exp Dermatol*. 2016;41(5):564.

Kiratli H, Diketas Ö. Bilateral lacrimal gland enlargement associated with isotretinoin treatment. *Ophthal Plast Reconstr Surg*. 2013;29(6):e156–e157.

Lammer EJ, Chen DT, Hoar RM. Retinoic acid embryopathy. *N Engl J Med*. 1985;313(14):837–841.

Larsen FG, Andersen SR, Weismann K, et al. Keratoconus as a possible side-effect of acitretin (neotigason) therapy. *Acta Cerm Venereol*. 1993;73(2):156.

Li Y-Y, Song Y-L, Zhang B-L, et al. Treatment of multiple Bowen's disease with squamous cell and basal cell carcinomas with oral acitretin combined with excision. *Dermatol Sinica*. 2014;32(3):189–190.

Madke B, Prasad K, Kar S. Isotretinoin-induced night blindness. *Indian J Dermatol*. 2015;60(4):424.

Moy A, McNamara NA, Lin MC. Effects of isotretinoin on meibomian glands. *Optom Vis Sci*. 2015;92(9):925–930.

Ozlu E, Karadag AS, Akdeniz N, et al. Acitretin-induced alopecia areata: a case report. *Cutan Ocul Toxicol*. 2015;34(3):248–250.

Palestine AJ. Transient acute myopia resulting from isotretinoin (Accutane) therapy. *Ann Ophthalmol*. 1984;16:661.

Pan Y, Zhao H, Chen A, et al. A Mal De Meleda patient with severe flexion contractures of hands and feet: a case report in West China. *Medicine (Baltimore)*. 2017;96(36):e7972.

Park YM, Lee TE. Isotretinoin-induced angle closure and myopic shift. *J Glaucoma*. 2017;26(11):e252–e254.

Polat M, Kükner S. The effect of oral isotretinoin on visual contrast sensitivity and amount of lacrimation in patients with acne vulgaris. *Cutan Ocul Toxicol*. 2017;36(1):35–38.

Rismondo V, Ubels JL. Isotretinoin in lacrimal gland fluid and tears. *Arch Ophthalmol*. 1987;105:416–420.

Rosen E, Raz J, Segev F. Giant cobblestone-like papillae during isotretinoin therapy. *Ocul Immunol Inflamm*. 2009;17(5):312–313.

Saray Y, Seckin D. Angioedema and urticaria due to isotretinoin therapy. *J Eur Acad Dermatol Venereol*. 2006;20:118–120.

Sarkar S, Das K, Roychoudhury S, et al. Pseudotumor cerebri in a child treated with acitretin: a rare occurrence. *Indian J Pharmacol*. 2013;45(1):89–90.

Weleber RG, Denman ST, Hanifin JM, et al. Abnormal retinal function associated with isotretinoin therapy for acne. *Arch Ophthalmol.* 1986;104:831–837.

Yap J. Cystoid macular edema associated with acitretin. *Digit J Ophthalmol.* 2013;19(4):56–58.

Yilmaz Ugur, Kücük E, Cagdas K, et al. Comparison of autologous serum versus preservative free artificial tear in patients with dry eyes due to systemic isotretinoin therapy. *Curr Eye Res.* 2017;42(6):827–831.

Yuksel N, Ozer MD, Akcay E, et al. Reduced central corneal thickness in patients with isotretinoin treatment. *Cutan Ocul Toxicol.* 2015;34(4):318–321.

Tretinoin (retinoic acid, vitamin A acid, or all-trans retinoic acid)

Frankel SR, Eardley A, Heller G, et al. All-trans-retinoic acid for acute promyelocytic leukemia: results of the New York study. *Ann Intern Med.* 1994;120:278–286.

Gillis JC, Goa KL. Tretinoin: a review of its pharmacodynamic and pharmacokinetic properties and use in the management of acute promyelocytic leukaemia. *Drugs.* 1995;50(5):897–923.

Smolin G, Okumoto M. Vitamin A acid and corneal epithelial wound healing. *Ann Ophthalmol.* 1981;13:563–566.

Smolin G, Okumoto M, Friedlaender M. Tretinoin and corneal epithelial wound healing. *Arch Ophthalmol.* 1979;97:545–546.

Somsak T, Sirijirachai C. Pseudotumor cerebri caused by all-trans-retinoic acid: a case report. *J Med Assoc Thai.* 2000;83:1420–1423.

Soong HK, Martin NF, Wagoner MD, et al. Topical retinoid therapy for squamous metaplasia of various ocular surface disorders. A multicenter, placebo-controlled double-masked study. *Ophthalmology.* 1988;95(10):1442–1446.

Stonecipher KG, Jensen HG, Rowsey JJ, et al. Topical application of all-trans-retinoic acid, a look at the cornea and limbus. *Graefes Arch Clin Exp Ophthalmol.* 1988;226:371–376.

Wright P. Topical retinoic acid therapy for disorders of the outer eye. *Trans Ophthalmol Soc UK.* 1985;104:869–874.

Dimethyl sulfoxide (DMSO)

Dimethyl sulfoxide (DMSO). *Med Lett Drugs Ther.* 1980;22:94.

Garcia CA. Ocular toxicology of dimethyl sulfoxide and effects on retinitis pigmentosa. *Ann NY Acad Sci.* 1983;411:48–51.

Hanna C, Fraunfelder FT, Meyer SM. Effects of dimethylsulfoxide on ocular inflammation. *Ann Ophthalmol.* 1977;9:61–65.

Kluxen G, Schultz U. Comparison of human nuclear cataracts with cataracts induced in rabbits by dimethylsulfoxide. *Lens Res.* 1986;3:161.

Rubin LF. Toxicologic update of dimethyl sulfoxide. *Ann NY Acad Sci.* 1983;411:6–10.

Use of DMSO for unapproved indications. *FDA Drug Bull.* 1980;10:20.

Yellowless P, Greenfield C, McIntyre N. Dimethylsulphoxide-induced toxicity. *Lancet.* 1980;2:1004–1006.

Methyl ethyl ketone peroxide (MEKP)

Chaudiere J, Clement M, Gerard D, et al. Brain alterations induced by vitamin E deficiency and intoxication with methyl ethyl ketone peroxide. *Neurotoxicology.* 1988;2:173–179.

Summerfield FW, Tappel AL. Vitamin E protects against methyl ethyl ketone peroxide-induced peroxidative damage to rat brain DNA. *Mutat Res.* 1984;126:113–120.

Bacillus Calmette-Guérin (BCG) vaccine

Bouchard R, Bogert M, Tinthoin JF. Eczematides post-BCG. *Bull Soc Fr Dermatol Syph.* 1965;72:126.

Dogliotti M. Erythema multiforme – an unusual reaction to BCG vaccination. *S Afr Med J.* 1980;57:332–334.

Krebs W, Schumann M. Allgenerkrankkung nach BCG-Impfung. *Monatsschr Tuberk-Bekampf.* 1971;14:80.

Llorenc V, Mesquida M, Molins B, et al. Bacillus Calmette-Guerin infection and cytotoxicity in the retinal pigment epithelium. *Ocul Immunol Inflamm.* 2018;26(5):786–792.

Nakagawa T, Shigehara K, Naito R, et al. Reiter's syndrome following intravesical Bacillus Calmette-Guerin therapy for bladder carcinoma: a report of five cases. *Int Cancer Conf J.* 2018;7(4):148–151.

Spratt A, Key T, Vivian AJ. Chronic anterior uveitis following bacilli Calmette-Guérin vaccination: molecular mimicry in action? *J Pediatr Ophthalmol Strabismus.* 2008;45(4):252–253.

Valenzuela-Suarez H, Javier GG, Dominguez-Gordillo L, et al. A 74-year-old male with bilateral conjunctival hyperemia, pollakiuria, dysuria, burning pain in the urinary meatus, lower back pain and reactive arthritis secondary to BCG vaccine application. *Gac Med Mex.* 2008;144(4):345–347.

Vogt D. Tuberkuloseschutz-Impfung. Die Komplikationen der BCG-Impfung. In: Herrlich A, ed. *Handbuch der Schutzimpfungen.* Berlin: Springer-Verlag; 1965:345.

Diphtheria (D) vaccine (receiving a tetanus toxoid booster), diphtheria and tetanus (DT) vaccine, diphtheria, tetanus, and pertussis (DTaP) vaccine

Dolinova L. Bilateral uveoretinoneuritis after vaccination with DTaP (diphtheria, tetanus, and pertussis vaccine). *Cs Oftal.* 1974;30:114–116.

Frederiksen MS, Brenoe E, Trier J. Erythema multiforme following vaccination with pediatric vaccines. *Scand J Infect Dis.* 2004;36:154–155.

Kongbunkiat K, Kasemsap N, Tiamkao S, et al. Clinical manifestations and outcomes of Guillain-Barre syndrome after diphtheria and tetanus vaccine (DT) during a diphtheria outbreak in Thailand: a case series. *Neurology Asia.* 2014;19(2):149–155.

O'Brien P, Wong RW. Optic neuritis following diphtheria, tetanus, pertussis, and inactivated poliovirus combined vaccination: a case report. *J Med Case Rep.* 2018;12(1):356.

Pembroke AC, Marten RH. Unusual cutaneous reactions following diphtheria and tetanus immunization. *Clin Exp Dermatol.* 1979;4:345–348.

Hepatitis A vaccine

Benage M, Fraunfelder FW. Vaccine-associated uveitis. *Missouri Med.* 2016;113(1):48–49.

Stangos A, Zaninetti M, Petropoulos I, et al. Multiple evanescent white dot syndrome following simultaneous hepatitis-A and yellow fever vaccination. *Ocul Immunol Inflamm.* 2006;14(5):301–304.

Hepatitis B vaccine

Benage M, Fraunfelder FW. Vaccine-associated uveitis. *Missouri Med.* 2016;113(1):48–49.

Fried M, Conen D, Conzelmann M, et al. Uveitis after hepatitis B vaccination. *Lancet.* 1987;2(8559):631–632.

Herpes zoster (shingles) vaccine, measles, mumps, rubella, and varicella virus vaccine live, varicella (chickenpox) vaccine

Fine HF, Kim E, Flynn TE, et al. Acute posterior multifocal placoid pigment epitheliopathy following varicella vaccination. *Br J Ophthalmol.* 2010;94(3):282–283. 363.

Han SB, Hwang JM, Kim JS, et al. Optic neuritis following varicella zoster vaccination: report of two cases. *Vaccine.* 2014;32(39):4881–4884.

Khalifa YM, Jacoby RM, Margolis TP. Exacerbation of zoster interstitial keratitis after zoster vaccination in an adult. *Arch Ophthalmol.* 2010;128(8):1079–1080.

Lin P, Yoon MK, Chiu CS. Herpes zoster keratouveitis and inflammatory ocular hypertension 8 years after varicella vaccination. *Ocul Immunol Inflamm.* 2009;17(1):33–35.

Naseri A, Good WV, Cunningham ET, et al. Herpes zoster virus sclerokeratitis and anterior uveitis in a child following varicella vaccination. *Am J Ophthalmol.* 2003;135(3):415–417.

Influenza virus vaccine

Belliveau MJ, Kratky V, Evans GA, et al. Acute orbital inflammation syndrome following H1N1 immunization. *Can J Ophthalmol.* 2011;46(6):552–553.

Ghosh C. Periorbital and orbital cellulites after H. influenza b vaccination. *Ophthalmology.* 2001;108:1514–1515.

Goyal S, Nazarian SM, Thayi DR, et al. Multiple evanescent white dot syndrome following recent influenza vaccination. *Can J Ophthalmol.* 2013;48(5):e115–e116.

Hamilton A, Massera R, Maloof A. Stromal rejection in a deep anterior lamellar keratoplasty following influenza vaccination. *Clin Exp Ophthalmol.* 2015;43(9):838–839.

Kim M. Vogt-Koyanagi-Harada syndrome following influenza vaccination. *Indian J Ophthalmol.* 2016;64(1):98.

Kwok T, Al-Bermani A. Two rare cases of retinal vasculitis following vaccination. *Scott Med J.* 2013;58(2):e10–e12.

Liu JC, Nesper PL, Fawzi AA, et al. Acute macular neuroretinopathy associated with influenza vaccination with decreased flow at the deep capillary plexus on OCT angiography. *Am J Ophthalmol Case Rep.* 2018;10:96–100.

Manusow JS, Rai A, Yeh S, et al. Two cases of panuveitis with orbital inflammatory syndrome after influenza vaccination.

Can J Ophthalmol. 2015;50(5):e71–e74.

Skowronski DM, Bjornson G, Husain E, et al. Oculo-respiratory syndrome after influenza immunization in children. *Pediatr Infect Dis J.* 2005;24:63–69.

Skowronski DM, De Serres G, Hebert J, et al. Skin testing to evaluate oculo-respiratory syndrome (ORS) associated with influenza vaccination during the 2000–2001 season. *Vaccine.* 2002;20:2713–2719.

Skowronski DM, Lu H, Warrington R, et al. Does antigen-specific cytokine response correlate with the experience of oculorespiratory syndrome after influenza vaccine? *J Infect Dis.* 2003;187:495–499.

Skowronski DM, Strauss B, De Serres G, et al. Oculo-respiratory syndrome: a new influenza vaccine-associated adverse event? *Clin Infect Dis.* 2003;36:705–713.

Toussirot E, Bossert M, Herbein G, et al. Comments on the article by Tabache F et al. Acute poly arthritis after influenza A H1N1 immunization. Joint Bone Spine 2011: Primary Sjögren's syndrome occurring after influenza H1N1 vaccine administration. *Joint Bone Spine.* 2012;79(1):107.

Tzoukeva and et al, 2010 Tzoukeva A, et al. Optic neuropathy after influenza vaccination in a patient with rheumatoid arthritis. *14th Congress of the European Federation of Neurological Societies.* 2010;abstr P2574.

Williams GW, Evans S, Yeo D, et al. Retinal vasculitis secondary to administration of influenza vaccine. *BMJ Case Rep.* 2015;2015 Aug 27.

Measles, mumps and rubella virus vaccine live, measles, mumps, rubella, and varicella virus vaccine live, measles virus vaccine live, mumps virus vaccine live, rubella and mumps virus vaccine live, rubella virus vaccine live

Behan PO. Diffuse myelitis associated with rubella vaccination. *BMJ.* 1977;1:166.

Gowda VK, Reddy B, Reddy H, et al. Idiopathic intracranial hypertension following measles vaccine. *J Ped Neurol.* 2014;12(1):55–58.

Hassin H. Ophthalmoplegic migraine wrongly attributed to measles immunization. *Am J Ophthalmol.* 1987;104:192–193.

Herman JJ, Radin R, Schneiderman R. Allergic reactions to measles (rubeola) vaccine in patients hypersensitive to egg protein. *J Pediatr.* 1983;102:196–199.

Miller CL. Surveillance after measles vaccination in children. *Practitioner.* 1982;226:535–537.

Morton-Kute L. Rubella vaccine and facial paresthesias. *Ann Intern Med.* 1985;102:563.

Preblud SR, Stetler HC, Frank Jr JA, et al. Fetal risk associated with rubella vaccine. *JAMA.* 1981;246:1413–1417.

Riikonen R. The role of infection and vaccination in the genesis of optic neuritis and multiple sclerosis in children. *Acta Neurol Scand.* 1989;80:425–431.

Rios L, Martin I, Mercadal M. Unilateral vi cranial nerve palsy after vaccination. *An Pediatr (Barc).* 2014;81(6):e44–e45.

Thomas E, Champagne S. A case of mumps meningitis: a complication of a vaccine? *CMAJ.* 1988;138:135.

Uysal P. Anaphylaxis developing after measles vaccine in an infant with cow's milk allergy. *Asim Allergi Immunoloji.* 2018;16(3):171–174.

World Health Organization. Adverse reactions to measles-rubella vaccine. *WHO ADR Newslett.* 1995;4:10.

Rabies immune globulin, rabies vaccine

Cremieux G, Dor JF, Mongin M. Paralysies faciales peripheriques et polyradiculoneurites post-vaccino-rabiques. *Acta Neurol Belge.* 1978;78:279.

Gupta V, Bandyopadhyay S, Bapuraj JR, et al. Bilateral optic neuritis complicating rabies vaccination. *Retina.* 2004;24:179–181.

Van der Meyden CH, Van den Ende J, Uys M. Neurological complications of rabies vaccines. *S Afr Med J.* 1978;53:478.

Smallpox (vaccinia) vaccine

Fillmore GL, Ward TP, Bower KS, et al. Ocular complications in the Department of Defense Smallpox Vaccination Program. *Ophthalmology.* 2004;111:2086–2093.

Francois J, Molder ED, Gildemyn H. Ocular vaccinia. *Acta Ophthalmol.* 1967;45:25–31.

Hu G, Wang MJ, Miller MJ, et al. Ocular vaccinia following exposure to a smallpox vaccine. *Am J Ophthalmol.* 2004;137:554–556.

McMahon AW, Bryant-Genevier MC, et al. Photophobia following smallpox vaccination. *Vaccine.* 2005;23:1097–1098.

Perera C. Vaccinial disciform keratitis. *Arch Ophthalmol.* 1940;24:352–356.

Rennie A, Cant JS, Foulds WS, et al. Ocular vaccinia. *Lancet.* 1974;3:273–275.

Ruben F, Lane J. Ocular vaccinia: epidemiologic analysis of 348 cases. *Arch Ophthalmol.* 1970;84:45–48.

Semba RD. The ocular complications of smallpox and smallpox immunization. *Arch Ophthalmol.* 2003;121:715–719.

Tetanus immune globulin, tetanus toxoid

Chopra A, Drage LA, Hanson EM, et al. Stevens-Johnson syndrome after immunization with smallpox, anthrax and tetanus vaccines. *Mayo Clin Proc.* 2004;79:1193–1196.

Harrer VG, Melnizky U, Wendt H. Akkommodationsparese und schlucklahmung nach tetanus-toxoid-auffrischungsimpfung. *Wien Med Wochenschr.* 1971;15:296.

Jacobs RL, Lowe RS, Lanier BQ. Adverse reactions to tetanus toxoid. *JAMA.* 1982;247:40–42.

McReynolds WU, Havener WH, Petrohelos MA. Bilateral optic neuritis following smallpox vaccination and diphtheria-tetanus toxoid. *Am J Dis Child.* 1953;86:601–603.

Quast U, Hennessen W, Widmark RM. Mono- and polyneuritis after tetanus vaccination (1970–1977). *Dev Biol Stand.* 1979;43:25–32.

Schlenska GK. Unusual neurological complications following tetanus toxoid administration. *J Neurol.* 1977;215:299–302.

Yellow fever vaccine

Moysidis SN, Koulisis N, Patel VR, et al. The second blind spot: small retinal vessel vasculopathy after vaccination against Neisseria meningitidis and yellow fever. *Retin Cases Brief Rep.* 2017;11(suppl 1):S18–S23.

CHAPTER 17

Drugs Used in the Management of Human Immunodeficiency Virus/ Acquired Immunodeficiency Syndrome

CLASS: ANTIRETROVIRAL DRUGS

Generic Names:

1. Abacavir; 2. didanosine; 3. emtricitabine; 4. lamivudine; 5. stavudine; 6. zidovudine.

Proprietary Names:

1. Ziagen; 2. Videx, Videx EC; 3. Emtriva; 4. Epivir, Epivir HBV; 5. Zerit; 6. Retrovir.

Primary Use

These nucleoside/nucleotide reverse transcriptase inhibitors (NRTIs) are most often used in combination with other anti–acquired immunodeficiency syndrome (AIDS) drugs.

Ocular Side Effects

Systemic administration – oral (primarily didanosine and zidovudine)

Probable

1. Lipodystrophy
   a. Increased superior lid sulcus
   b. Ptosis
2. Mitochondrial myopathy syndrome
   a. Ptosis
   b. Extraocular muscle weakness
      i. Diplopia
      ii. Gaze paresis
3. Chronic progressive external ophthalmoplegia
   a. Ptosis
   b. Diplopia
   c. Orbicularis
   d. Ophthalmoplegia
   e. Cannot elevate eyebrows
4. Immune recovery syndrome (only in cytomegalovirus [CMV] retinitis patients)
   a. Uveitis
   b. Vitritis
   c. Macular edema
5. Retina (didanosine)
   a. Retinal pigment epithelium (RPE) mottling
   b. RPE atrophy

   c. Abnormality of neurosensory retina
   d. Loss of choriocapillaris

Possible

1. Macular edema (zidovudine)
2. Hyperpigmentation (zidovudine)
   a. Eyelids
   b. Conjunctiva
3. Hypertrichosis (zidovudine)
4. Photosensitivity (zidovudine)
5. Color vision defect (zidovudine)
6. Optic neuritis (didanosine)
7. Night blindness (didanosine)

Clinical Significance

AIDS patients normally have associated ocular diseases, which include noninfectious retinal vasculopathy, ocular infections (herpes zoster, herpes simplex, and molluscum contagiosum), retinitis due to CMV, ocular tuberculosis, syphilis, toxoplasmosis, and metastatic fungi. Neuro-ophthalmic complications due to these conditions, as well as progressive multifocal leukoencephalopathy, can occur. Ocular neoplasms such as Kaposi sarcoma and conjunctival squamous cell carcinoma can also occur. These diseases, plus the drugs used to treat them, can interact and mimic side effects that may unjustly place blame on antiretroviral therapy (ART) drugs.

Based on our review of the literature, *Physicians' Desk Reference* (PDR), and a host of spontaneous reports, we have found that most of the available ART drugs have very few important ocular side effects, and they are all rare. Most clinically important ocular side effects are from the original NRTIs, which are didanosine and zidovudine and, less so, stavudine. Newer NRTIs have fewer and seldomly significant ocular side effects. However, these older drugs are still in use, and decades of daily therapy, even with the newer drugs, has the potential to cause visual side effects. This outline is not without a significant margin of error, but it is our best interpretation of this complex, ever-changing field.

A known effect of some ART drugs is lipoatrophy. This affects the orbit with resultant increased superior lid sulcus and ptosis.

Although the mechanisms of most ocular side effects are not known, there are data to support mitochondrial toxicity with didanosine and zidovudine. This may manifest itself by causing weakness of the levator extraocular muscles, including progressive external ophthalmoplegia. The direct effect of these drugs on the mitochondria may be weak; however, the prolonged daily exposure may allow these side effects to occur. These effects are more common in older patients, those on higher dosages, and those with advanced human immunodeficiency virus (HIV) disease.

Chronic progressive external ophthalmoplegia (CPEO) has been reported in association with long-term ART therapy.[1,2] CPEO is the most frequent manifestation of mitochondrial myopathies. The first signs are ptosis, but with time the orbicularis muscle and extraocular muscles are affected. Ophthalmoplegia is most marked horizontally with downward gaze. This is usually slowly progressive over a 5- to 15-year period.[3]

Didanosine is somewhat unique in that significant neurosensory retinal problems may occur without visual fundoscopic changes. Whitcup et al described retinal lesions that first appeared as patches of RPE mottling and atrophy in the midperiphery of the fundi in children taking didanosine.[4,5] In time, these lesions became more circumscribed and developed a border of RPE hypertrophy. Cobo et al described similar changes in adults.[6] Electrophysiologic and ophthalmologic findings suggest diffuse dysfunction of the RPE. Histologic findings confirm multiple areas of RPE loss. Electron microscopic findings show normal mitochondria, but with membranous lamellar inclusions and cytoplasmic bodies in the RPE. If didanosine therapy continues, progression may occur, although there may be some improvement if the drug is stopped. Night blindness and electrooculogram (EOG) changes appear to be reversible once the drug is discontinued. Although the midperiphery is the area first involved, lesions may encroach on the posterior pole if the drug is continued at high dosage. To date, central visual acuity has been preserved. Didanosine's toxic effects on the retina appear related both to peak dosage and accumulated dosage. Haug et al reviewed 19 cases of chorioretinal degeneration secondary to didanosine.[7] Three cases clearly showed progression despite stopping the drug, and 4 were in children. To date, there are 40+ cases in the spontaneous reports. Patients taking this drug should be monitored for the development and progression of retinal lesions. Cobo et al contend that retinal toxicity to this drug is under-recognized.[6] The PDR has previously recommended periodic ocular examinations seeking retinal or optic-nerve changes.[8]

Immune recovery syndrome consists of uveitis, vitritis, and macular edema that develop after significant immune recovery after ART. This condition only occurs in patients with CMV retinitis.[9,10]

There have been a few reports of macular edema associated with zidovudine use in the literature and in the spontaneous reports.[9,11] It is difficult to prove a cause-and-effect relationship; however, Lalonde et al supported an association with positive dechallenge and rechallenge data.[12] Klutman et al reported that zidovudine could cause hypertrichosis.[13] Geier et al reported cases of tritan color vision defects secondary to zidovudine.[14] Merenich et al reported hyperpigmentation (similar to adrenal insufficiency) of the eyelids and conjunctiva, especially in already heavily pigmented individuals, which they felt was due to zidovudine.[15]

Optic neuritis has been mentioned as a possible adverse event secondary to didanosine.[16] There have been a few cases of night blindness in the spontaneous reports, but these patients were taking many drugs, some of which may cause this as well.

Recommendations
1. Patients on didanosine should be questioned as to visual symptoms, including specific questions regarding night vision, scotoma, and constriction of visual fields.
2. If any of these problems occur, visual field and/or electrophysiologic studies (i.e. EOGs) should be considered.
3. Because many patients are unaware of visual changes, consider a visual field test in patients who have been on didanosine for over 2 years.
4. Didanosine may need to be discontinued in some patients based on retinal changes.

Generic Name:
Foscarnet sodium.

Proprietary Name:
Foscavir.

Primary Use
Systemic
Pyrophosphate analog used in the treatment of mucocutaneous herpes simplex.

Ophthalmic

Used in the management of cytomegalovirus (CMV) and acute retinal necrosis.

Ocular Side Effects

Systemic administration – intravenous
Probable
1. Periocular edema
2. Conjunctivitis
3. Pain

Possible
1. May aggravate or cause ocular sicca

Local ophthalmic use or exposure – intravitreal injection
Probable
1. Foscarnet crystalline formation

Clinical Significance

As with other drugs in this class, periorbital edema may occur. This may be due to water retention. According to the *Physicians' Desk Reference* (PDR), conjunctivitis (delayed), ocular pain (early), and xerostomia (early) occur with an incidence of 1–5%.[1] Ocular pain and delayed conjunctivitis may be related to the drug or its metabolites being secreted in the tears. Xerostomia is often a strong indicator that ocular sicca may occur or be aggravated.

Intravitreal foscarnet injections are used to avoid serious systemic toxicity to this drug. The safety of even high-dose intravitreal foscarnet is well established, and adverse effects, including retinal detachment, vitreous hemorrhage, endophthalmitis, and cataract, are due to the injection technique and most likely not the drug.[2-4] Martinez-Castillo et al reported a single case of a 42-year-old patient receiving 11 intravitreal injections of foscarnet who developed crystalline deposits of the drug on the retina, the internal limiting membrane, and detached posterior hyaloids.[4] The authors postulated that a possible change in the pH of the vitreous after that many injections may have precipitated the crystallization of the drug. Injections were not stopped because there was no apparent local toxicity.

Generic Name:
Ritonavir.

Proprietary Name:
Norvir.

Primary Use

Antiviral protease inhibitor used in the treatment of AIDS.

Ocular Side Effects

Systemic administration – oral
Certain
1. Decreased vision
2. Eyelid edema

Probable
1. Retinal pigment epitheliopathy
   a. Mottling
   b. Atrophy
2. Macula
   a. Foveal distortion
   b. Edema
   c. Cystoid edema
   d. Bull's-eye maculopathy
3. Retina
   a. Thinning
   b. Crystals
   c. Telangiectasias
   d. Hyperautofluorescence
4. Visual field
   a. Scotoma – central, paracentral
   b. Peripheral loss
5. Choroid
   a. Choroiditis
   b. Thinning
6. Lipodystrophy
   a. Deepening superior lid sulcus
   b. Ptosis
7. Autoimmune reconstitution syndrome
   a. Iritis
   b. Uveitis
   c. Vitritis
   d. Choroiditis
8. Myopathy
   a. Extraocular muscles
   b. Diplopia
   c. Ptosis

Possible
1. Decreased night vision
2. Graves' ophthalmopathy
3. Blepharitis
4. Conjunctivitis

Clinical Significance

Decreased vision is the most common and earliest adverse ocular side effect associated with ritonavir use.

The incidence is 6.4%.[1] Myopathy is a delayed effect (months to years) occurring at a rate of 3.8%.[1] Also occurring as a late effect (months to years) is lipodystrophy, which may affect the orbital fat causing an increased superior lid sulcus and/or ptosis.[1]

Of greatest clinical interest is what effect this drug may have on the retina and choroid. The problems in identifying drug toxicity include the number of drugs often taken at the same time, the severity of the human immunodeficiency virus (HIV) infection with its associated ocular complications, and the small numbers of cases that are actually reported. This is complicated by the same inconsistencies in the overall reported pattern of retinal findings. Regardless, there are enough data to make it a strong possibility. This effect is time and dose related, and may be on an individual basis in terms of susceptibility.[2] Another drug in this purine analogue class, didanosine, also causes retinal toxicity as a rare event.[3] In addition, ritonavir has been shown to cause retinal toxicity in exposed animals.[4] With so few cases, most with similar patterns, we may be seeing various stages of the spectrum of toxicity.

Cases of retinal toxicity have occurred as early as 19 months and as late as 8 years after starting the drug. The first symptom is usually slowly progressive visual loss and, in 2 cases, decreased night vision. All cases have been bilateral except the cases reported by Tu et al.[5] Their case, after 6 years on ritonavir, developed sudden mild liver problems with vision in 1 eye decreasing from 20/20 to 20/400 over a 2-week period. The drug was discontinued, and after 2 weeks vision returned to 20/25. In most all other cases, even with stopping the drug, there was mild to significant progression of retinal pathology. Early detection and stopping the drug possibly have the best prognosis for some recovery. The typical pattern of retinal and choroidal pathology was in the initial report of 3 cases by Roe et al.[6] This consisted of retinal pigment epitheliopathy, para foveal telangiectasias, and intraretinal crystal deposits.

Temporal optic nerve atrophy was only seen in 1 case.[7] There were cases that also had some features of retinitis pigmentosa.[8,9] Papavasileiou and a few spontaneous reports pointed out that night blindness can occur as an early sign of retinal toxicity.[8] Bull's-eye maculopathy has been reported.[7] Electrophysiologic tests include:

- Fluorescein angiography – window defects and parafoveal telangiectasias[6,10]
- Multifocal electroretinogram (ERG) – shows little response rings first, second, and third[2]
- Optic coherence tomography (OCT) – shows thickening of the macula, inner foveal cysts[6]

- Spectral domain OCT – confirms choroidal thinning[8]
- Autofluorescence – increase in central macula with loss of autofluorescence in area of RPE disturbance[2,8]

A risk factor may be liver damage.[6] Even with mild liver damage, serum blood levels of ritonavir may cause 3 times the normal therapeutic dosage.[5] Immune reconstitution syndrome (IRS) refers to the initial phase of HIV treatment in patients whose immune system responds to the antiviral treatment, but they may develop an inflammatory reaction to indolent or residual opportunistic infections. Some of the opportunistic infections occur in the eye, such as CMV and tuberculosis. IRS may also cause Graves' disease and polymyositis. The time to onset is variable and may occur months after treatment has been started.[1] Faure et al feel that the retinal side effects due to this drug are underreported.[2]

REFERENCES

Drugs: Abacavir, didanosine, emtricitabine, lamivudine, stavudine, zidovudine

1. Chen T, Pu C, Shi Q, et al. Chronic progressive external ophthalmoplegia with inflammatory myopathy. *Int J Clin Exp Pathol.* 2014;7(12):8887–8892.
2. Jones AM, Starte J, Dunn H, et al. Surgical technique for pulled in two syndrome: three cases with chronic progressive external ophthalmoplegia. *J Pediatr Ophthalmol Strabismus.* 2017;54:e83–e87.
3. Riordan-Eva P, Whitcher JP. *Vaughan and Asbury's General Ophthalmology.* 17th ed. USA: McGraw Hill; 2008:293.
4. Whitcup SM, Butler KM, Caruso R, et al. Retinal toxicity in human immunodeficiency virus infected children treated with 2',3'-dideoxyinosine. *Am J Ophthalmol.* 1992;113:1–7.
5. Whitcup SM, Dastgheib K, Nussenblatt RB, et al. A clinicopathologic report of the retinal lesions associated with didanosine. *Arch Ophthalmol.* 1994;112:1594–1598.
6. Cobo J, Ruiz MF, Figueroa MS, et al. Retinal toxicity associated with didanosine in HIV-infected adults. *AIDS.* 1996;10:1297–1300.
7. Haug SJ, Wong RW, Day S, et al. Didanosine retinal toxicity. *Retina.* 2016;36(Suppl 1):S159–S167.
8. Physicians' Didanosine. *Desk Reference.* 67th ed. Montvale, NJ: Thomson PDR; 2013.
9. Jabs DA, Van Natta ML, Holbrook JT, et al. Longitudinal study of the ocular complications of AIDS: 2. Ocular examination of results at enrollment. *Ophthalmology.* 2007;114(4):787–793.
10. Leeamornsiri S, Choopong P, Tesavibul N. Frosted branch angiitis as a result of immune recovery uveitis in a patient with cytomegalovirus retinitis. *J Ophthalmic Inflamm Infect.* 2013;3(1):52.

11. Jabs DA, Van Natta ML, Thorne JE, et al. Course of cytomegalovirus retinitis in the era of highly active antiretroviral therapy: 1. Retinitis progression. *Ophthalmology.* 2004;111(12):2224–2231.

12. Lalonde RG, Deschênes JG, Seamone C. Zidovudine-induced macular edema. *Ann Int Med.* 1991;114(4):297–298.

13. Klutman NE, Hinthorn DR. Excessive growth of eyelashes in a patient with AIDS being treated with zidovudine. *N Engl J Med.* 1991;324(26):1896.

14. Geier SA, Held M, Bogner J, et al. Impairment of tritan colour vision after initiation of treatment with zidovudine in patients with HIV disease or AIDS. *Br J Ophthalmol.* 1993;77:315–316.

15. Merenich JA, Hannon RN, Gentry RH, et al. Azidothymidine-induced hyperpigmentation mimicking primary adrenal insufficiency. *Am J Med.* 1989;86:469–470.

16. Didanosine. Retrieved from http://www.pdr.net; 2019.

Drug: Foscarnet sodium

1. *Foscarnet sodium.* ; 2019. Retrieved from http://www.pdr.net.

2. Diaz-Llopis M, Espana E, Munoz G, et al. High dose intravitreal foscarnet in the treatment of cytomegalovirus retinitis in AIDS. *Br J Ophthalmol.* 1994;78:120–124.

3. Wong R, Pavesio CE, Laidlaw AH, et al. Acute retinal necrosis: the effects of intravitreal foscarnet and virus type on outcome. *Ophthalmology.* 2010;117:556–560.

4. Martinez-Castillo S, Marin-Lambies C, Gallego-Pinazo R, et al. Crystallization after intravitreous foscarnet injections. *Arch Ophthalmol.* 2012;130(5):658–659.

Drug: Ritonavir

1. Ritonavir. Retrieved from http://www.pdr.net; 2019.

2. Faure C, Paques M, Audo I. Electrophysiological features and multimodal imaging in ritonavir-related maculopathy. *Doc Ophthalmol.* 2017;135(3):241–248.

3. Whitcup SM, Butler KM, Caruso R, et al. Retinal toxicity in human immunodeficiency virus-infected children treated with 2′,3′-dideoxyinosine. *Am J Ophthalmol.* 1992;113:1–7.

4. European Medicines Agency. Scientific Discussion for the Approval of Novir. Retrieved from http://www.ema.europa.eu.

5. Tu Y, Poblete RJ, Freilich BD, et al. Retinal toxicity with ritonavir. *Int J Ophthalmol.* 2016;9(4):640–642.

6. Roe RH, Jumper JM, Gualino V, et al. Retinal pigment epitheliopathy, macular telangiectasis, and intraretinal crystal deposits in HIV-positive patients receiving ritonavir. *Retina.* 2011;31:559–565.

7. Non L, Jeroudi A, Smith BT, et al. Bull's eye maculopathy in an HIV-positive patient taking ritonavir. *Antivir Ther.* 2016;21(4):365–367.

8. Papavasileiou E, Younis S, Zygoura V, et al. Ritonavir-associated toxicity mimicking retinitis pigmentosa in an HIV-infected patient on highly active antiretroviral therapy. *Retin Cases Brief Rep.* 2017;11(4):306–309.

9. Muccioli C, Gonzalez-Fernandez D, Alfonso V, et al. Didanosine-associated toxicity mimicking retinitis pigmentosa in a HIV infected patient. *JSM Ophthalmol.* 2013;2:1011.

10. Biancardi AL, Curi AL. Retinal toxicity related to long-term use of ritonavir. *Retina.* 2016;36(1):229–231.

FURTHER READING
Abacavir, didanosine, emtricitabine, lamivudine, stavudine, zidovudine

Chapman KO, Lelli G. Blepharoptosis and HAART related mitochondrial myopathy. *Orbit.* 2014;33(6):459–461.

Dinges WL, Witherspoon R, Itani KM. et al. Blepharoptosis and external ophthalmoplegia associated with long-term antiretroviral therapy. *Clin Infect Dis.* 2008;47:845–852.

Fernando AI, Anderston OA, Holder GE, et al. Didanosine-induced retinopathy in adults can be reversible. *Eye.* 2006;20(12):1435–1437.

Kumarasamy N, Venkatesh KK, Devaleenol B, et al. Regression of Kaposi's sarcoma lesions following highly active antiretroviral therapy in an HIV-infected patient. *Int J STD AIDS.* 2008;19(11):786–788.

Pfeffer G, Mezei M, Li CX, et al. Mitochondrial toxicity in HIV patients treated with antiretrovirals manifesting as a syndrome resembling chronic progressive external ophthalmoplegia. *10th International Workshop on Adverse Drug Reactions and Lipodystrophy in HIV.* 2008;A71 abstr:66.

Silkiss RZ, Lee H, Gills Ray VL. Highly active antiretroviral therapy-associated ptosis in patients with human immunodeficiency virus. *Arch Ophthalmol.* 2009;127:345–346.

Spear JB, Kessler HA, Nusinoff Lehrman S, et al. Zidovudine overdose. First report of ataxia and nystagmus: case report. *Ann Int Med.* 1988;109:76–77.

Steinfeld SD, Demols P, Van Vooren JP. et al. Zidovudine in primary Sjögren's syndrome. *Rheumatol.* 1999;38(9):814–817.

Strominger MB, Sachs R, Engel HM. Macular edema from zidovudine? *Ann Int Med.* 1991;115(1):67.

Ritonavir

Leiner S. Re: retinal pigment epitheliopathy, macular telangiectasis, and intraretinal crystal deposits in HIV-positive patients receiving ritonavir. *Retina.* 2012;32(2):411.

CHAPTER 18

Drugs Used in Ophthalmology

CLASS: DRUGS USED TO TREAT AGE-RELATED MACULAR DEGENERATION

Generic Names:
1. Aflibercept; 2. bevacizumab; 3. pegaptanib sodium; 4. ranibizumab.

Proprietary Names:
1. Eylea; 2. Avastin; 3. Macugen; 4. Lucentis.

Primary Use
These intravitreal drugs are intended to treat the "wet" form of age-related macular degeneration (AMD). Their use has expanded to include macular edema following retinal vein occlusion, diabetic macular edema, and diabetic retinopathy in patients with diabetic macular edema.

Ocular Side Effects
Local ophthalmic use or exposure – intravitreal injection
Certain
1. Visual disturbance – transitory
   a. Decreased vision
   b. Photopsia
2. Irritation – transitory
   a. Discharge
   b. Pain
   c. Discomfort
   d. Inflammation
3. Increased intraocular pressure (IOP)
   a. Acute, transitory
   b. Long-term decrease
   c. Subset long-term increase (except aflibercept)
4. Vitreous (injection trauma)
   a. Floaters
   b. Opacities
   c. Detachment
5. Cataract
6. Conjunctival hemorrhage

Probable
1. Retinal pigment epithelium (RPE)
   a. Atrophy
   b. Tear

Possible
1. Ocular inflammation
   a. Sterile endophthalmitis
   b. Uveitis
2. Increased IOP – sustained
3. Retina
   a. Pigment epithelial tear (Fig. 18.1)
   b. Edema
   c. Detachment
4. Macular holes
5. Fetal abnormalities

Clinical Significance
These drugs have been in widespread clinical use for well over a decade and have had a good safety record. Many of the reported adverse events may be due to the trauma of the injection procedure and not the drug itself. There is little data to support any significant differences in the side effect profiles of each of these drugs. Initial concerns of systemic adverse events were similar to controls.[1,2] According to a product update from Regeneron Pharmaceuticals, there is a potential risk of systemic arterial thromboembolic events after intravitreal aflibercept injections for all types of intracameral injections of 6.4% (37 out of 578) compared with 4.2% (12 out of 287) in the control group.[3] A recent report by the American Academy of Ophthalmology assessed intravitreal injections of anti–vascular endothelial growth factor (VEGF) therapies over a 2-year period and found them safe and effective for neovascular AMD, but longer-term follow-up is needed.[4]

Retinal and retinal pigment epithelial detachments or tears have been reported. There are multiple variables, including anatomic considerations and long-term effects of contraction of neovascularization. There are no conclusive data that the drug itself, via a toxic mechanism, is the cause. However, Chang et al felt that in some instances these events are anti-VEGF related.[5] Hata et al described retinal pigment atrophy in 36.6% of eyes during the first year of anti-VEGF therapy.[6] The presence of refractile drusen at baseline was a significant risk factor in predicting this atrophy to occur. The number of injections did not seem to be associated with macular atrophy.[7] Kabanarou et al, in a retrospective

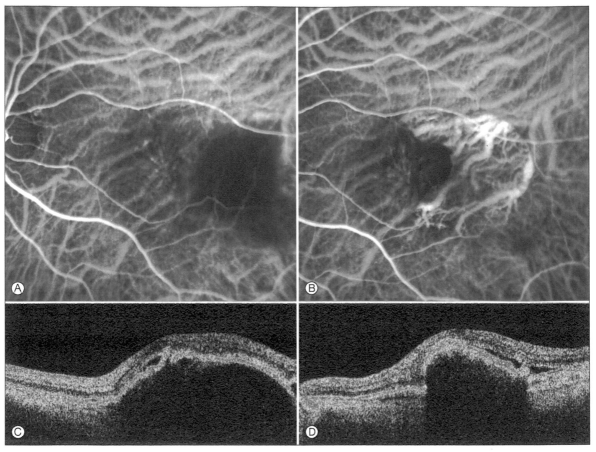

FIG. 18.1 Before and after treatment with intravitreal ranibizumab. **(A)** Before treatment with intravitreal ranibizumab. Indocyanine green angiography shows hyperfluorescence resulting from choroidal neovascularization. **(B)** One month after injection of intravitreal ranibizumab. The indocyanine green angiogram shows a well-demarcated area of hyperfluorescence in the temporal macula corresponding to the RPE tear. **(C)** Optical coherence tomogram (OCT) before injection showing a serous pigment epithelial detachment with overlying subretinal fluid. **(D)** OCT after the second injection of ranibizumab showing a retinal pigment epithelium tear.[4]

case series, described 4 cases of full-thickness macular hole associated with these drugs.[8]

Intraocular bleeding may be caused by the injection, a secondary underlying disease, or the drug itself. Data are inconclusive as to cause and effect. Ocular inflammation, including iritis, iridocyclitis, uveitis, and vitritis, have been reported. In 2 detailed prospective side effect studies, on the first postoperative day, a statistically significant increased flare was found and a statistically significant decreased flare at 1 week.[9,10] There are a few reports of recurrent ocular inflammation after injections.[11] Of most concern to the ophthalmologist is a sterile endophthalmitis after intravitreal injection of 1 of these drugs. This is

described as an acute intraocular inflammation without pain, conjunctival injection, or hypopyon. The incidence may be in the range of 0.37–0.47%; however, Vander-Beek et al found no association.[12–14] The incidence is so small that it is difficult to determine cause and effect. Still, possibly with the small subset, classic presentation, and occurrence within 1–3 days postinjection, a cause-and-effect relationship is likely. This, however, may just be due to the trauma of the injection, bubbles in the syringe, protein denaturation, or impurities. To date, there is no firm conclusion as to cause.

Cataract may occur secondary to trauma in about 0.07%.[15] Changes due to the drug were 2 times controls,

12.5% versus 6.3%.[16] Studies over 2 years did not seem to increase cataract progression, even with an increased number of intravitreal injections. The incidence of cataract extraction within 2 years of the start of therapy was 2.6%.[17]

A sudden raise in IOP after any intravitreal injection is well known because of the injection volume. These elevated pressures are uncommon and transient. They rarely necessitate stopping therapy. The area of controversy is if sustained elevation of IOP occurs.[18] Although most reports in the literature are small series or case reports, large clinical trials and controlled studies do not support a cause-and-effect relationship of intravitreal anti-VEGF drugs causing glaucoma long-term. Regardless, many believe a relationship exists, and further studies are necessary. There are many theories as to why it occurs, as it is probably a multifactorial process.[18,19] Some data support that ranibizumab may be more likely than aflibercept or bevacizumab to cause this.[19,20] There is enough suspicion that this sustained elevation is real, and therefore careful monitoring of IOP is required once one is started on this type of treatment. The American Academy of Ophthalmology Intelligent Research in Sight (IRIS) Registry evaluated 524,485 patients who received 2,419,931 anti-VEGF injections.[21] Their analysis showed a statistically significant decrease in IOP over time. A subset of patients (2.6%) experienced a sustained, clinically significant IOP rise compared with 1.5% in the fellow untreated eye. This increase was not found with aflibercept.

Based on data from the Diabetic Retinopathy Clinical Research Network, persistent diabetic macular edema was more likely with bevacizumab than with aflibercept or ranibizumab.[22]

Lass et al have shown that intravitreal aflibercept injections every 8 weeks for unilateral neovascular AMD over a 1-year period had no endothelial corneal changes compared with the fellow control eye.[23]

Systemic side effects are debatable; however, 2 well-documented cases of hypersensitivity reactions have been reported, 1 of oral angioedema and generalized urticaria 35 minutes after intravitreal injection of pegaptanib, which required hospitalization.[24] The other case, generalized urticaria, occurred within 12 hours after each of 4 intravitreal injections of pegaptanib.

There have been numerous reports of serious and nonserious systemic hematologic events in patients taking these drugs; however, it is difficult to prove a cause-and-effect relationship because the group of patients receiving these drugs is already at a higher risk for thromboembolic and hematologic events.[25] Regardless, some systemic side effects may occur.

Polizzi et al reviewed the safety of these drugs in pregnancy and concluded that there are potential risks to the fetus and that each case is individualized as to whether to treat.[26]

Generic Name:
Verteporfin.

Proprietary Name:
Visudyne.

Primary Use

Used during photodynamic therapy in the treatment of choroidal neovascularization. It is photoactivated in the eye by a low-power laser and generates oxygen radicals that damage neovascular endothelial cells and cause thrombus formation, resulting in choroidal vascular occlusion. A half dose (off-label use) is used in refractory macular edema.

Ocular Side Effects
Systemic administration – intravenous
Certain
1. Eyelids or conjunctiva
   a. Blepharitis
   b. Conjunctivitis
   c. Conjunctival injection
   d. Photosensitivity
   e. Allergic hypersensitivity reaction
2. Irritation
   a. May aggravate or cause ocular sicca
   b. Pruritus
3. Retina
   a. Subretinal hemorrhage
   b. Detachment (exudative) (Fig. 18.2)
   c. Retinal or choroidal vessel nonperfusion
   d. Pigment epithelial detachment
   e. Pigment epithelial tears
   f. Pigment epithelial changes
4. Vitreous hemorrhage
5. Decreased vision
6. Visual field defects
7. Choroidal hypoperfusion and infarcts

Probable
1. Abnormal electroretinogram (ERG)
2. Visual hallucinations
3. Lacrimation disorder

Possible
1. Diplopia
2. Cataracts

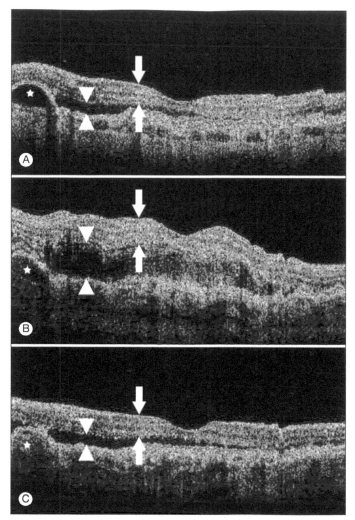

FIG. 18.2 Optical coherence tomography (OCT) examination before and after photodynamic therapy in occult choroidal neovascularization due to age-related macular degeneration (scan length = 6 mm). **(A)** Before PDT, cross-sectional OCT image showing a hyporeflective area in the subneuroretinal space due to fluid accumulation (*arrowheads*). The foveal architecture appears normal; retinal elevation = 280 μm; retinal thickness is indicated by *arrows*. A focal pigment epithelial detachment is present at the left border of the scan (width = 805 μm, indicated by star). **(B)** Two days after PDT, cross-sectional OCT image demonstrates a significant enlargement of the hyporeflective area, representing the amount of fluid accumulation (increased retinal elevation of >600 μm). Although the thickness of the neurosensory retina increased moderately (*arrows*), no change of the intraretinal structure and the foveal depression became obvious. The size of the focal pigment epithelial detachment remained unchanged (*asterisk*). **(C)** Seven days after PDT, the subretinal fluid absorbed almost completely, resulting in a reduced retinal elevation of 275 μm, appearing similar to the pretreatment OCT. Whereas the width of the focal pigment epithelial detachment seems unchanged, the height is reduced in size *(star)*.[11]

3. Increased retinal neovascularization
4. Ischemic optic neuropathy – if lasering too close to the optic nerve

Systemic administration – intravenous (half dosage)
Certain
1. Decreased vision – blurred, transient
2. Photosensitivity – transient

Probable
1. Acute exudative maculopathy

Conditional/unclassified
1. Polypoidal choroidal vasculopathy

Systemic Side Effects
Systemic administration – intravenous
Certain
1. Headaches
2. Back pain – especially during or around time of infusion
3. Joint pain
4. Muscle weakness

Possible
1. Malaise
2. Nausea
3. Constipation
4. Flu-like symptoms (chills, fever, body aches, sore throat)

Clinical Significance
Many of the adverse ocular events listed here are due to the intended mechanism of action of the drug and not necessarily due to the inherent toxicity of verteporfin. Some feel photosensitivity is the most common side effect from photodynamic therapy (PDT) with verteporfin. Photosensitivity reactions to the eye, eyelid, and periocular skin usually occur in the form of an irritation after exposure to sunlight, even 5 days after injection, if patients are exposed to bright lights. Other reported ocular side effects due to verteporfin PDT include blurred or decreased vision, inflammatory response, edema, and ocular pain, all at incidences of 10–30%.[1] Delayed responses include ocular bleeds, scotomas, cataracts, and conjunctivitis.[1] Rapid or early side effects, including ocular sicca, increased lacrimation, blepharitis, ocular pruritus and diplopia, occur at an incidence of 1–10%.[1] Severe vision decreases, the equivalent of 4 lines or more, within 7 days after treatment have been reported in 1–5% of patients.[1] Partial recovery of vision was observed in some patients. Retinal detachment occurred in 0–1%.[1]

Alteration of RPE has been reported by several investigators.[2-4] These changes are felt to be, in part, due to destruction of the choroidal choriocapillaris, which causes RPE alteration.[3] Variation of this same process of PDT accounts for various bleeding complications, detachments, exudative reactions, tears, and infarcts.[5-18]

Half-dosage PDT for central serous retinopathy has caused a transient increase in intraretinal edema in 5 patients.[19] Additional cases, which named this response acute exudative maculopathy, all resolved with time.[20,21]

There were no systemic side effects in a placebo-controlled trial with half-dosage for central serous retinopathy,[22] although there is a host of literature (see Further Reading) and spontaneous reports that dispute this. The events may be so rare that it is possible that the placebo trial does not have the power to detect them.

Neovascularization is a reason for PDT treatment with verteporfin, although there may be increased neovascularization after PDT therapy for choroidal hemangioma or for central serous retinopathy.[23,24] Because PDT with verteporfin can cause total occlusion of blood vessels, various effects can occur; e.g. if therapy is too close to the optic disc, ischemic optic neuropathy can occur.[25]

A host of systemic side effects may occur secondary to infusion of verteporfin. Few are serious – they are mainly aggravating. The most common is back pain during or after infusion. Headaches and joint pain may be the next most common.[26] In placebo-controlled studies, systemic adverse effects were transient, and mild or moderate back pain occurred at an incidence of 2.4% versus 0% with placebo.[27] Fossarello et al described a case of acute respiratory distress 8 minutes after verteporfin was intravenously injected.[28] They pointed out the need for the same emergency resources to be available as with fluorescein angiography.

CLASS: DRUGS USED TO TREAT ALLERGIES

Generic Name:
Emedastine difumarate.

Proprietary Name:
Emadine.

Primary Use
Relatively selective H_1 receptor antagonist used as a topical ocular drug for the treatment of allergic conjunctivitis.

Ocular Side Effects
Local ophthalmic use or exposure – topical ocular application
Certain
1. Decreased vision
2. Irritation
   a. Burning and stinging
   b. Foreign body sensation
   c. Epiphora
   d. Discomfort
   e. Photophobia
3. Cornea
   a. Infiltrates
   b. Superficial punctate keratitis
4. Conjunctival hyperemia

Probable
1. Pruritus
2. May aggravate or cause ocular sicca

Systemic Side Effects
Local ophthalmic use or exposure – topical ocular application
Certain
1. Headaches
2. Drowsiness

Probable
1. Bad taste

Possible
1. Abnormal dreams
2. Asthenia
3. Dermatitis
4. Rhinitis
5. Sinusitis

Clinical Significance
This topical ocular antihistamine is one of the stronger antihistamines available, but it is still relatively free of significant side effects. The manufacturer states that many of the reported side effects may be secondary to the underlying disease or the preservative. The most common ocular side effect is decreased vision. The incidence of anterior segment irritation varies from 0–5%.[1] This side effect, plus most of the others, may be the same as the signs and symptoms of the allergic reaction for which the drug is being used. Corneal infiltrates are seldom of any consequence. The most common systemic side effects are headache and drowsiness. The reported incidence of headache is 11%.[1] Occasionally patients have a significant impairment of the ability to

drive due to the sedating effect of emedastine.[2] Some patients complain of unusual dreams or nightmares. Other systemic side effects appear fairly insignificant, and all are reversible.

Recommendation[1]
This product contains benzalkonium chloride, so patients should remove contact lenses before administering emedastine and wait 15 minutes before reinsertion.

Generic Name:
Loteprednol etabonate.

Proprietary Names:
Alrex, Lotemax.

Primary Use
Ophthalmic corticosteroid used for allergic conjunctivitis and various ocular irritations.

Ocular Side Effects
Local ophthalmic use or exposure – topical ocular application
Certain
1. Decreased vision
2. Photophobia
3. Epiphora
4. Foreign body sensation
5. Pruritus
6. Hyperemia
7. Eyelid or conjunctiva edema
8. May aggravate or cause ocular sicca
9. Keratitis
10. Intraocular pressure elevation

Probable
1. Cataract – posterior subcapsular (many years of exposure)

Possible
1. Uveitis

Clinical Significance
Loteprednol is a unique steroid preparation that has anti-inflammatory properties with less intraocular pressure elevation and cataract potential.[1,2] This drug, even if given orally, has not been detected in the bloodstream, so drug interactions are unlikely.

Ocular side effects are common and seldom of major clinical importance. Topical ocular application causes photophobia, visual impairment, epiphora, foreign body sensation, hyperemia, pruritus and edema in 5–15% of patients.[3] These only occasionally require discontinuation of the drug. These side effects may be secondary to benzalkonium chloride, which is the preservative used with this drug. There are case reports where, in hyperemic eyes, within a few days intraocular pressure elevated to 50 mmHg in both eyes.[4] This drug may aggravate existing glaucoma.[5] Spontaneous case reports support causation of both of these side effects. These, however, are very rare events if the drug is used for less than 10 days.

After many years of exposure, cataracts are "probable" because they are posterior subcapsular, as with other steroids.[3] Rare reports of uveitis, as with other topical steroids, have occurred. Even though this drug has not been found in the bloodstream, there are spontaneous case reports of systemic side effects with positive rechallenge. This could be real or psychological. Reported side effects include dizziness, diarrhea, and vomiting. Pharyngitis may occur due to exposure to the drug and its preservative via the nasal lacrimal system.

Recommendations

1. This product contains benzalkonium chloride, so the patient should remove contact lenses before administering loteprednol and wait 15 minutes before reinsertion.[3]
2. If used over 10 days, intraocular pressure should be monitored in patients with open-angle glaucoma. Long-term use also requires monitoring of intraocular pressure.
3. Use with caution in patients with corneal abrasions.
4. Side effects are more frequent in hyperemic eyes.
5. Be aware of fungal, herpes, mycobacterial, varicella, or viral infection with loteprednol exposure.

Generic Name:
Olopatadine hydrochloride.

Proprietary Names:
Pataday, Patanol, Pazeo.

Primary Use
Topical ocular histamine H_1 receptor antagonist, with a mast cell stabilizing effect, used in the management of ocular allergies.

Ocular Side Effects
Local ophthalmic use or exposure – topical ocular application
Certain
1. Cornea and conjunctiva
   a. Foreign body sensation – stinging

   b. Hyperemia
   c. Keratitis
   d. Hyperemia
   e. Conjunctivitis
2. Eyelids
   a. Edema
   b. Blepharitis
   c. Pruritus
3. Decreased vision

Possible
1. May aggravate or cause ocular sicca

Conditional/unclassified
1. Increased intraocular pressure after deep anterior lamella keratoplasty

Systemic Side Effects
Local ophthalmic use or exposure – topical ocular application
Certain
1. Headache

Probable
1. Nausea
2. Taste perversion

Possible
1. Cold syndrome
2. Pharyngitis
3. Rhinitis
4. Sinusitis

Clinical Significance
This antihistamine and mast cell stabilizer is unique due to its longer duration of action, lower probability of ocular irritation, and approved use in children 2 years of age and older. Ocular side effects are minimal and reversible. As with any eye drop, if the preservative is benzalkonium chloride, ocular irritation is a given. Whether the effect is from the preservative or the drug is speculative. The incidences of these irritative effects vary from 0–5%.[1] All irritative ocular side effects are acute; however, keratitis, conjunctivitis, and hyperemia are delayed. Decreased vision occurred in 0–5% and was transient.[1,2] Patients with deep anterior lamellar keratoplasty who were on preoperative olopatadine had increased postoperative intraocular pressure versus controls.[3] The authors concluded that these patients most likely had an allergic eye disease and had corticosteroids as part of their management. Headaches are reported at an incidence of 7%.[1] Less than 5% of

patients may experience burning or stinging, cold syndrome, ocular sicca, foreign body sensation, hyperemia, nausea, taste perversion, and upper respiratory inflammatory symptoms. Studies by the manufacturer showed no effect on tear film stability.[4]

Recommendation[1]

This product contains benzalkonium chloride, so the patient should remove contact lenses before administering olopatadine and wait 15 minutes before reinsertion.

CLASS: DRUGS USED TO TREAT GLAUCOMA

Generic Name:
Apraclonidine hydrochloride.

Proprietary Name:
Iopidine.

Primary Use
This topical ocular alpha-adrenergic antagonist is used primarily in the short-term control of elevated ocular pressure. It is also used for acute pressure change after laser or surgical procedures.

Ocular Side Effects
Local ophthalmic use or exposure – topical ocular exposure (short exposure, only a few dosages)
Certain
1. Ocular hyperemia
2. Upper eyelid elevation
3. Conjunctival blanching
4. Pupil
   a. Miosis – early
   b. Mydriasis
5. Pruritus

Local ophthalmic use or exposure – topical ocular exposure (long-term therapy, not recommended by manufacturer)
Certain
1. Loss of vision
2. Tachyphylaxis
3. Eyelids and conjunctiva
   a. Pruritus
   b. Conjunctivitis – follicular (Fig. 18.3)
   c. Hyperemia
   d. Contact dermatitis
   e. Blepharitis
   f. Conjunctival blanching
   g. Discharge
4. Upper eyelid elevation
5. Mydriasis
6. Photophobia
7. Cornea
   a. Keratitis
   b. Erosions
   c. Foreign body sensation

Possible
1. May aggravate or cause ocular sicca
2. Uveitis

Systemic
Certain
1. Xerostomia and rhinitis sicca
2. Taste abnormalities

Possible
1. Headaches
2. Fatigue
3. Gastrointestinal symptoms
   a. Nausea
   b. Abdominal pain
   c. Diarrhea
4. Cardiovascular episodes
   a. Bradycardia
   b. Palpitations
   c. Orthostatic episodes

Clinical Significance
With short-term use, apraclonidine has a less than 2% adverse event rate, with few adverse events becoming clinically significant.[1] In long-term use, tachyphylaxis occurs in 48% of patients within 3 months. Araujo et al best summarized long-term apraclonidine use in a series of patients who were followed for 35 weeks.[2] Of those patients, 39% had side effects occurring as early as after the first drop to as late as the thirty-fifth week. Around 23% of the patients had to stop the drug secondary to adverse drug reactions. The most common side effect was decreased vision. In most cases this was a one-line loss on the Snellen chart and was transient. However, a few patients lost 2–4 lines, and in 2 cases the vision did not return. Allergic reactions were the second-most-common side effect and the primary reason for stopping the drug. Once the drug was stopped, the allergic reaction usually resolved within 5 days. Robin et al noted, in their series, that 50% had lid retraction, between 20% and 50% had a drug-induced allergic reaction, and 45% had a small amount

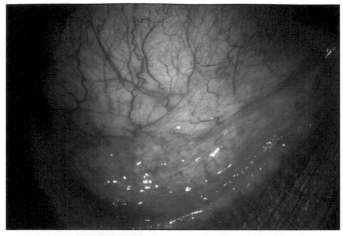

FIG. 18.3 Follicular conjunctivitis involving the palpebral conjunctiva of the lower eyelid.[9]

(0.4 mm) of mydriasis.[3] Cambron et al studied normal volunteers using infrared pupillography and showed that with 1 drop of 1% apraclonidine, a relative miosis occurred, peaking at 30–60 minutes.[4] Others have found that mydriasis tends to occur later.[3,5,6] Apraclonidine is a strong vasoconstrictor, and conjunctival blanching occurred in 85% of patients.[3] There are a few cases in the spontaneous reports of anterior granulomatous uveitis that promptly resolved when the drug was stopped. A cause-and-effect relationship has not been established, although this may be secondary to an anterior segment ischemic response. Some of these side effects may be due to or aggravated by the preservative benzalkonium chloride.

Systemic adverse drug-related events may occur, although they are rare. The sensation of dry mouth and nose is not unexpected because this group of drugs was initially intended as nasal decongestants. The drug reaches the nasal pharynx through the lacrimal outflow system to cause this effect. Occasionally patients complain of an abnormal taste. Lethargy has been reported in children and pulmonary edema in a 6-year-old child after 1 topical ocular application of apraclonidine.[7,8] This drug has minimal effects on the respiratory, cardiovascular, and gastrointestinal systems.

Recommendation[1]

This product contains benzalkonium chloride, so the patient should remove contact lenses before administering apraclonidine and wait 15 minutes before reinsertion.

Generic Names:

1. Betaxolol hydrochloride; 2. levobunolol hydrochloride; 3. timolol maleate.

Proprietary Names:

1. Betoptic, Betoptic S, Kerlone; 2. Ak-Beta, Betagan; 3. Betimol, Blocadren, Istalol, Timoptic, Timoptic Ocudose, Timoptic Ocumeter, Timoptic-XE.

Primary Use
Systemic

Timolol is effective in the management of hypertension and myocardial infarction.

Ophthalmic

These beta-adrenergic blockers are used in the treatment of glaucoma.

Ocular Side Effects
Systemic administration – oral (timolol)
Probable

1. Decreased vision
2. Eyelids or conjunctiva
   a. Allergic reactions
   b. Hyperpigmentation
3. Myasthenia gravis
   a. Diplopia
   b. Ptosis
   c. Paresis of extraocular muscles
4. Visual hallucinations
5. Decreased intraocular pressure

Possible
1. Loss of eyelashes or eyebrows
2. May aggravate or cause ocular sicca

Local ophthalmic use or exposure – topical ocular application
Certain
1. Decreased vision
2. Irritation
   a. Hyperemia
   b. Foreign body sensation
   c. Pain
   d. Burning sensation
   e. Pruritus
3. Cornea
   a. Superficial punctate keratitis
   b. Anesthesia
   c. Slows epithelial wound healing
   d. Decreased tear film break-up time
4. Eyelids
   a. Allergic reactions
   b. Contact dermatitis
5. Conjunctiva – chronic use
   a. Symblepharon
   b. Squamous metaplasia
   c. Increased subepithelial collagen density
   d. Subepithelial degenerative changes
   e. Decreased number of secretory epithelial cells
   f. Decreased desmogenous and zonula occludens on conjunctival surface cells
6. Myasthenia gravis
   a. Ptosis
   b. Diplopia
   c. Paresis of extraocular muscles
7. Nasolacrimal system obstruction (most common with combination eye drops)
8. Visual hallucinations
9. Myopia

Possible
1. Eyelids or conjunctiva
   a. Edema
   b. Loss of eyelashes or eyebrows
2. Uveitis
3. Recurrent choroidal detachments
4. Iris depigmentation
5. Cystoid macular edema

Systemic Side Effects
Local ophthalmic use or exposure – topical ocular application
Certain
1. Asthma
2. Bradycardia
3. Dyspnea
4. Cardiac arrhythmia
5. Aggravation of chronic obstructive pulmonary disease
6. Bronchospasms
7. Syncope
8. Apnea – children
9. Rebound increased blood pressure on beta blocker withdrawal
10. Increase in high-density lipoprotein
11. Respiratory failure
12. Palpitation
13. Myasthenia-like syndrome

Probable
1. Hypotension
2. Dizziness
3. Hypoglycemia

Possible
1. Headache
2. Asthenia
3. Cerebral vascular accident
4. Nausea
5. Nightmares
6. Raynaud syndrome
7. Arthralgia
8. Alopecia (Fig. 18.4)
9. Confusion
10. Psoriasis
11. Cardiac arrest
12. Cerebral ischemia
13. Hyperkalemia
14. Impotence
15. Nail pigmentation

Clinical Significance
The potential side effects from the various beta blockers are all based on timolol, either the oral formulation or eye drops. The other beta blockers should have similar side effect profiles. The more selective beta blockers, such as betaxolol, in all probability have fewer side effects, especially on the respiratory system. Regardless, any of the beta blockers seem to have the potential for causing many of the side effects listed. The most common topical ocular timolol side effect is blurred vision, with an incidence of 33%; followed by ocular irritation, at 12.5%; and conjunctivitis, ocular pruritus discharge, foreign body sensation, pain, and lacrimation, all occurring in the 1–5% incidence range.[1] The topical ocular administration of timolol usually has its peak systemic blood level between 30 and 90 minutes after application, which can reach systemic therapeutic blood levels.

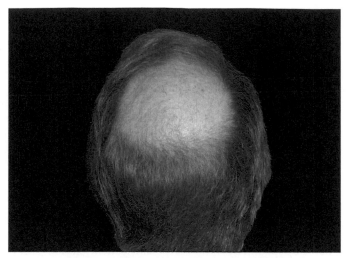

FIG. 18.4 Hair loss from topical ocular timolol.[30]

The adverse effects from this drug may occur shortly after application, or may not occur for many weeks, months, or even years on therapy. It should be noted that all adverse reactions reported due to systemic beta blockers have been seen possibly secondary to topical ocular beta blockers. Examples include fingernail and toenail pigmentation, myasthenia gravis, neuroblocking effects, psoriasis, and impotency.[2-4] The local ocular effects from ophthalmic use are only occasionally of major consequence causing discontinuation of the drug. Newer formulations and vehicles have decreased some of the initial burning associated with some of these drugs. However, if the clinician notices superficial punctate keratitis or erosions, the probability is that the patient is getting an effect from the medication, including benzalkonium chloride. Long-term ocular medications, either due to the drug or its preservative, can cause pemphigoid-like symblepharon, especially in the inferior cul-de-sac, as well as damage to the meibomian gland.[5,6] Many believe that beta blockers can enhance sicca (possibly after long-term use by affecting the microvilli), decrease tear film break-up time, and decrease goblet cell density.[7] Hong et al showed, as with all chronic topical ocular glaucoma medications, that significant squamous metaplasia occurs with long-term use.[8] This may be due to the preservative as well. An overview of antiglaucoma medications and their side effects is given by Servat et al.[9] The suspicion that timolol decreases tear production is real, but in most cases, it is of a mild nature. Seider et al reported nasal lacrimal duct obstruction due to chronic topical glaucoma medication.[10] The role of the preservative could not be separated from the drug. Combination antiglaucoma medications were the most common cause.

The area in which the beta blockers cause the greatest concern is their systemic side effects from topical ocular application. The most severe side effects affect the cardiovascular system and the respiratory system. Cardiovascular side effects include bradycardia, which can be an indication for stopping the drug. However, for diabetic patients who depend on an increased heart rate (i.e. hypoglycemic attack) as an indication for insulin use, this is of importance because the beta blocker may mask the increase in heart rate. It is also of importance in exertion because some patients are unable to increase their heart rate. Additional problems include arrhythmia, syncope, congestive heart failure, and a possible increase in cerebral vascular accidents, especially in patients with carotid insufficiency with drug-induced decreased blood pressure or pulse rate. In very rare instances, this may be associated with a fatality. Lee et al, in reviewing data from the Blue Mountain Eye Study, suggested a higher cardiovascular mortality in glaucoma patients taking topical ocular timolol.[11] Lama's editorial on this article concurs, but he felt further studies were necessary.[12] Müskens et al could not find an association between topical ocular beta blockers and excessive mortality.[13] Because the nonselective beta blockers decrease heart rate in a different location than the calcium channel blockers, there have been reports of sudden death in patients who are taking both drugs. The combination of these drugs playing a role is only theoretical. The adverse respiratory effects are the most perplexing. It has been well documented that these drugs have caused bronchospasm and status asthmaticus, with death reported shortly after the use of topical ocular beta blockers. There are many cases in spontaneous reports of status asthmaticus, including death. In approximately two-thirds of patients with a significant bronchospastic attack, there has been a previous history of asthma. This group of drugs may especially cause problems in patients with chronic obstructive lung disease. Patients recognize that they can breathe more easily after discontinuing these drugs, especially with the nonselective beta blockers. Approximately one-third of patients who develop bronchospasm recognize the problem with the beta blockers within the first week, and one-quarter within the first day. It seems that patients with chronic pulmonary disease who are taking these drugs may suffer a decrease in their forced expiratory volume as measurable by spirometry.

There have been reports of apnea in infants who received topical ocular timolol.[14–16] The central nervous system may also be affected.[17] Systemic beta blockers can cause depression in some patients, and in the younger age group there have been reports of an increased incidence of suicide attempts.[18–20] Kaiserman et al, however, could not find an association in 274,000 patients.[21] The elderly suffer increased emotional liability, vivid dreams, and increased anxiety, which may improve after discontinuation of the medication.[22] Recently, Hackethal reported 4 cases of topical ocular timolol causing visual hallucinations with positive rechallenge in an elderly white woman.[23] Nanda et al reported an additional case.[24] There have been numerous reports of sexual dysfunction in both men and women while taking timolol.[4] Skin changes from timolol are rare. However, there are well-documented reports of psoriasis, various rashes, increased pigmentation of fingernails and toenails, and male-pattern baldness in men and women.[2,25–27] This baldness is interesting because it usually does not occur until at least 4 months after the medication is started, although it may take many years for this to occur. Once it is recognized and the drug discontinued, it usually takes 4–8 months for recovery. Myasthenia has been associated with beta blockers, as has Raynaud phenomena, arthralgias, and 1 well-documented case with rechallenge of recurrent hyperkalemia.[28] Only with timolol are there data as to interactions between topical ocular medication and oral medication. Timolol and quinine enhance bradycardia. Timolol and halothane also enhance bradycardia and hypotension. Madadi et al showed topical ocular timolol in lactating mothers' milk, however not in high enough concentrations to likely cause systemic effects in healthy, breast-fed infants.[29]

Recommendations

To decrease systemic effects:

1. Have the patient only use 1 drop.
2. Close the lids for 3–5 minutes. You can also lay the head on the side away from the inner canthus with lids closed. Gravity will decrease the amount of drug reaching the lacrimal outflow system with resultant nasal mucosal absorption of the drug.
3. Before and immediately after opening the eyelids, use a tissue to absorb as much of the tears as possible to decrease the amount of medication reaching the puncta.
4. Applying pressure over the lacrimal sac during the period of lid closure and while removing excess medication is ideal, but difficult for many patients.
5. This product contains benzalkonium chloride, so the patient should remove contact lenses before administering the drug and wait 15 minutes before reinsertion.[1]

Generic Names:

1. Bimatoprost; 2. latanoprost; 3. tafluprost; 4. travoprost.

Proprietary Names:

1. Latisse, Lumigan; 2. Xalatan; 3. Zioptan; 4. Travatan.

Primary Use

Indicated for the reduction of intraocular pressure in ocular hypertensives and various forms of glaucoma.

Ocular Side Effects

Local ophthalmic use or exposure – topical ocular application

Certain

1. Decreased vision – transitory
2. Irritation
   a. Burning
   b. Stinging
   c. Foreign body sensation
   d. Pruritus
   e. Pain
   f. Photophobia
3. Conjunctiva
   a. Hyperemia
   b. Pigmentation
4. Eyelashes
   a. Increased pigmentation
   b. Increased curling
   c. Increased growth – length and thickness
   d. Increased number
   e. Poliosis

5. Iris
  a. Increased darkening
  b. Cysts
6. Eyelids
  a. Deepening lid sulcus
  b. Dermatochalasis
    i. Decreased
    ii. Increased – rare
  c. Eyelid pigmentation
    i. Increased
    ii. Decreased – rare
  d. Edema
  e. Erythema
  f. Ptosis
  g. Allergic reactions
  h. Contact dermatitis
  i. Lower lid retraction
  j. Punctal stenosis or occlusion – may be due to the preservative
7. Orbit – fat atrophy
8. Cornea
  a. Reduced central thickness
  b. Superficial punctate keratitis
9. May aggravate or cause ocular sicca
10. Photosensitivity
11. Cystoid macular edema

Probable
1. Uvea
  a. Iritis
  b. Uveitis

Possible
1. Bilateral optic disc edema
2. Myopia
3. Acute glaucoma
4. Cornea
  a. Edema (travoprost)
  b. Neovascularization

Conditional/unclassified
1. Choroidal detachment
2. Activation of herpes simplex
3. Meibomian gland dysfunction
4. Cataracts

Systemic Side Effects
Local ophthalmic use or exposure – topical ocular application
Probable
1. Flu-like symptoms
  a. Abdominal cramps
  b. Malaise
  c. Upper respiratory tract–like infection
2. Facial burning
3. Facial rash
4. Headache

Possible
1. Dyspnea
2. Aggravates asthma
3. Sweating
4. Muscle, joint, and back pain – aggravation of arthritis
5. Angina
6. Migraine

Clinical Significance

Topical ocular prostaglandin analogs (PGAs) are similar to the topical ocular beta-adrenergic blockers, in that many ocular and systemic side effects were not appreciated until after the drugs were marketed. It has taken many years to get a fairly accurate side effect profile. Most data available are with latanoprost because it was first introduced in the mid-1990s. However, it appears that there may be very few and no major differences in the side effect profile for this group of drugs. Because benzalkonium chloride is the preservative in all of these drugs except tafluprost, some of the listed side effects may be due to the preservative.

The most common adverse ocular events, occurring in 5–15% of subjects, are decreased vision, burning, stinging, conjunctival hyperemia, foreign body sensation, pruritus, increased pigmentation of the iris, and punctate epithelial keratopathy. Conjunctival hyperemia appears to occur more commonly with travoprost and bimatoprost. Ocular sicca, excessive tearing, eye pain, lid crusting, lid discomfort/pain, lid edema, lid erythema, or photophobia are seen in 1–4% of patients.

Johnstone pointed out the rapidity of onset of eyelash changes.[1] For example, curling can occur in less than 5 days, with increased growth and number occurring less than 3 weeks after starting the drug. Incidence is between 45% and 57% after 1 year.[1,2] The length of lashes increases an average of between 13% and 19% and in extreme cases may touch the patient's spectacles. Poliosis may occur. Uva et al, in a case of unilateral congenital glaucoma in an infant, reported that latanoprost caused the usual iris and eyelash changes.[3] These changes, however, regressed off the drug over a 3-year period.

Iris pigmentation is most evident in patients with mixed-color irises and may be permanent. The darkening occurs around the pupil initially and spreads with time peripherally. Uniformly blue or brown irises do not undergo darkening. Dark irises in Japan, Taiwan, and parts of Europe may not have increased pigmentation. Huang et al reported a higher incidence of iris hyperpigmentation in Chinese with homochromatic brown eyes than in Caucasians.[4] Albert et al noted that the incidence of iris color changes may occur in more than 50% of patients.[5] Length of time on the drug and age (over 75 years old) are risk factors for this effect. There may be a race or genetic component because it appears that there is an increase in melanin content in melanosomes, but there does not appear to be a predisposition toward malignant transformation. Alm et al, after a review of the literature, concluded that there was no substantial evidence that this group of drugs provoked precancerous events, iris inflammation, or secondary glaucoma.[6] Esteve et al, however, reported 3 cases of melanomas after taking latanoprost eye drops.[7] One was on a lower eyelid, another choroidal, and 1 on the ear lobe. We have heard of no other cases.

There has been a large number of case reports of possible iris cysts associated with PGA therapy. This was first reported by Krohn et al.[8] In almost all cases, the cysts decreased in size or within a matter of weeks disappeared after the drug was discontinued. Most did not recur if the drug was restarted. This has occurred in unilateral and in bilateral treated eyes.[9] Not all concur that this is a cause-and-effect relationship. However, Krohn et al have more recently reported iris cysts with positive rechallenge with bimatoprost therapy.[8]

The role of PGA in causation of uveitis, macular edema, or cystoid macular edema (CME) is open to debate. Miyake et al have shown latanoprost using the laser flare cell meter to cause disruption of the blood–aqueous barrier and to show an increased incidence of angiographic CME after cataract surgery.[10] Furuichi et al, using ocular coherence tomography, found no change in retinal thickness after taking latanoprost, but eyes with prior uveitis or intraocular surgery (potential risk factors) were excluded.[11] There are a number of cases in the literature and in spontaneous reports of uveitis, macular edema, or CME associated with the use of PGA. Most all are in patients with risk factors; however, there are a few well-documented positive dechallenge and rechallenge cases. In all likelihood there is an association, but it's probably weak. The risk factors appear to be aphakia; pseudophakia with ruptured posterior capsule during surgery; and history of uveitis, retinal inflammatory, or vascular disease.

Eyelids may have color changes, usually a darkening in color, but there are cases of lightening in color, some in a spotty pattern. There are also cases of depigmentation.[12] Doshi et al reported on 37 Caucasian subjects

who developed periocular skin hyperpigmentation that was cosmetically noticeable after 3–6 months of topical ocular Bimatoprost.[13] This may even occur in ocular skin grafts.[14] Priluck et al, in their series of skin hyperpigmentation after direct application of PGA to the eyelid, found that pigmentation may occur between 3 and 8 weeks.[15] If, however, given to the conjunctival cul-de-sac, it takes 3–6 months. Others report a range of 50–618 days.[1] They point out that pigmentation may extend away from the direct area of drug contact. These types of pigmentation are reversible when the PGA is discontinued.

Shah et al, in a cross-sectional survey, studied topical ocular prostaglandin use and ocular adnexal changes and reported involution of dermatochalasis of the upper eyelid, inferior eyelid extraconal orbital fat herniation, upper eyelid ptosis, and lower eyelid retraction.[16] Deeping of the upper eyelid sulci and loss of inferior eyelid periorbital fat were confirmed.[17–20]

Mocan et al has linked long-term therapy with this group of drugs to meibomian gland dysfunction.[21] Chronic benzalkonium chloride use may also cause this.

Abedi et al reported an unusual case of clearly audible clicking sounds from both eyelids associated with each blink after 7 years of topical ocular travoprost use.[22]

There is disagreement if PGA can reactivate herpes simplex virus-1 (HSV-1). Kaufman et al first showed that latanoprost could worsen HSV-1 in rabbits.[23,24] Also, in rabbits, Gordon et al reported that latanoprost does not appear to promote HSV-1 ocular shredding.[25] There are 11 cases in the literature and 31 cases of HSV and 9 cases of herpes zoster in the spontaneous reports of activation of cornea or periocular skin herpes activation. Cases were unilateral and bilateral after start of PGA in patients with a positive history of prior ocular herpes. Bean et al evaluated 411 patients with ocular HSV and could not correlate any particular antiglaucoma therapy with increased HSV compared with the general population.[26] Based on case reports and laboratory data, although HSV on its own is a recurring disease, the authors feel it is prudent to inquire on HSV and maybe zoster history when starting these medications; if there is a positive history, consider alternatives to PGA.

Gutierrez-Ortiz et al has shown a decrease in anterior chamber depth after 1 month of treatment with latanoprost.[27] Yalvac et al has reported 2 cases of acute narrow-angle glaucoma associated with the use of a PGA.[28]

The most common systemic side effect is an upper respiratory tract infection flu-like syndrome, which occurs in 4% of patients. Chest pain/angina pectoris, muscle/joint/back pain, and rash/allergic skin reactions occur at a rate of 1–2%.[29] Although it is not proven that this drug can exacerbate arthritis symptoms, positive rechallenge cases in spontaneous reports suggest that some patients are convinced and refuse to continue this drug. Facial burning and facial rashes occur but are rare. An unproven association includes darkening of scalp hair and, in elderly males, increased difficulty urinating. Because prostaglandins cause smooth muscle constriction, this possible PGA side effect cannot be ruled out. Increased headaches and increased dreaming or nightmares have also been reported. There are no data to support that this drug causes postmenopausal bleeding, although there are a small number of spontaneous reports of this nature. Goodwin et al reported an accidental travoprost overdose, which was associated with severe menstrual bleeding.[30] Fahim et al reported heightened cough sensitivity after latanoprost use.[31]

Recommendations

1. Forewarn patients of probable permanent color changes of iris; however, eyelid or eyelash pigmentation changes regress, and most all return to normal. Especially warn patients who only take the PGA unilaterally.
2. Use with caution in patients with aphakia, pseudophakia, torn posterior capsules, or any other risk factors for macular edema.
3. Use with care in patients who have a past history of uveitis or macular edema. Do not use in patients who currently have uveitis.
4. Use with caution in patients with a prior history of ocular or periocular herpes simplex.
5. May affect the Clinical Activity Score for Graves' ophthalmopathy, as the drug, not the disease, may cause signs of erythema, pain, edema, and impaired ocular function.[32] This then increases and misrepresents more active Graves' disease.
6. This product contains benzalkonium chloride, so the patient should remove contact lenses before administering bimatoprost, latanoprost, tafluprost, or travoprost and wait 15 minutes before reinsertion.[29]
7. Use is contraindicated in closed-angle, inflammatory, or neovascular glaucoma.
8. The PGA has been isolated from the mother's milk after topical ocular application.
9. The safety profile in pediatric patients appears to be acceptable on long-term treatment.[33]

Generic Name:
Brimonidine tartrate.

Proprietary Names:
Alphagan, Alphagan P, Mirvaso.

Primary Use
This relatively selective alpha-2 adrenergic agonist is an effective intraocular pressure–lowering drug for open-angle glaucoma and ocular hypertension.

Ocular Side Effects
Local ophthalmic use or exposure – topical ocular application
Certain
1. Irritation
   a. Allergic reactions (Fig. 18.5A)
   b. Hyperemia
   c. Pain
   d. Pruritus
   e. Foreign body sensation
   f. Pain
2. Conjunctiva
   a. Blanching
   b. Hyperemia
   c. Edema
   d. Follicles (Fig. 18.5B)
   e. Hemorrhage
   f. Discharge
3. Eyelids
   a. Blepharitis
   b. Hyperemia
   c. Edema
4. Decreased vision
5. Cornea
   a. Staining
   b. Superficial punctate keratitis
   c. Increased thickness
6. May aggravate or cause ocular sicca
7. Miosis
8. Anterior uveitis
   a. Cells and flare
   b. Granulomatous
   c. Stellate keratic precipitates

Probable
1. Charles Bonnet syndrome (CBS)
   a. Visual loss
   b. Visual hallucinations

Possible
1. Tachyphylaxis – may lose pressure-lowering effect
2. Ectropion
3. Pressure elevation
4. Cornea
   a. Infiltrates

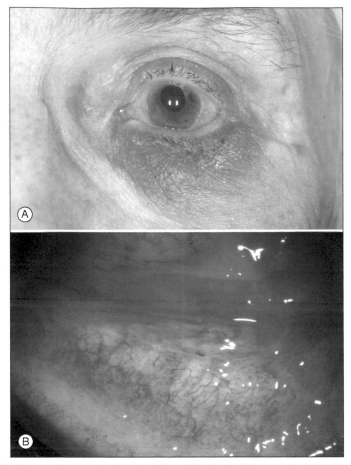

FIG. 18.5 **(A)** Allergic reaction to topical ocular brimonidine in the left eye only. **(B)** Follicular conjunctivitis from topical ocular brimonidine.[29]

b. Opacities
c. Neovascularization

Systemic Side Effects
Local ophthalmic use or exposure – topical ocular application
Certain
1. Headaches
2. Rhinitis sicca
3. Xerostomia
4. Drowsiness, fatigue, or somnolence
5. Reduction in systolic blood pressure
6. Upper respiratory symptoms
7. Dizziness
8. Gastrointestinal disorders
9. Abnormal taste
10. Infants
    a. Bradycardia
    b. Hypotension
    c. Hypothermia
    d. Hypotonia
11. Contact dermatitis
12. Loss of laser-assisted in situ keratomileusis (LASIK) flap adherence
13. Flu-like syndrome

Probable
1. Syncope
2. Muscle pain

Possible

1. Infants – apnea

Clinical Significance

Brimonidine tartrate with benzalkonium chloride (BAK) as a preservative has more ocular side effects than preparations preserved with Purite. Side effects increase with increased concentrations of the drug. With BAK and 0.2% concentration, adverse ocular side effects occur at an incidence between 10% and 30% and in descending order of incidence include ocular hyperemia, burning, stinging, blurred vision, foreign body sensation, conjunctival follicles, ocular allergies, ocular pruritus and ocular sicca.[1] Those at 3–9% incidence in descending order include corneal staining/erosion, blepharitis, ocular irritation, conjunctival blanching, and decreased vision.[1] Those side effects occurring at an incidence of less than 3% include conjunctival hemorrhage and ocular discharge.[1] Postmarketing ocular side effects with an unknown incidence include iritis, miosis, eyelid erythema, pruritus and vasodilation.[1]

Brimonidine tartrate may need to be discontinued in 5–10% of patients due to ocular or systemic side effects. The most common reason for discontinuing this drug is allergic reactions, which present as ocular hyperemia, pain, pruritus, foreign body sensation with a follicular conjunctival response, and eyelid swelling. In postmarketing follow-up, the unexpected finding has been granulomatous uveitis usually due to long-term brimonidine therapy.[2-10] There has been some concern about the role of BAK in causing uveitis; however, McKnight et al reported 5 cases of granulomatous uveitis where the preservative was polyquaternium-1.[6] In the majority of cases, the patients were above age 75 and had used brimonidine for over 11 months. Byles et al reported 4 cases of positive rechallenge within 3 weeks of restarting brimonidine.

In addition to the corneal changes listed, corneal infiltrates and opacities may occur rarely.[11,12] There are a number of reports of this drug causing miosis.[13,14] In fact, McDonald et al found it useful postoperatively in refractive patients who reported night vision problems.[15] This was confirmed by Edwards et al.[16] Grueb et al reported reversible increase of central corneal thickness.[17] Walter et al reported preoperative brimonidine had an adverse effect on flap adherence on LASIK patients.[18] Hedge et al report that brimonidine, as with many chronic topical ocular medications, may induce ectropion.[19] This study was done with BAK as the preservative.

Problems that may require discontinuing the drug include headache, fatigue, and somnolence. This drug rarely affects the respiratory or cardiovascular system.

Patients may have rhinitis sicca or xerostomia.[1] This is not surprising, because this group of drugs was initially developed as nasal decongestants. This is probably due to a direct drug effect via the nasal lacrimal system on the nasal pharynx.

Topical ocular brimonidine may cause bradycardia, hypotension, hypothermia, hypotonia, and apnea in neonates and infants. There are now multiple reports in the literature and spontaneous reports of central nervous system depression, hypotension, bradycardia, hypersomnolence, and even coma secondary to brimonidine eye drops in infants.[20-23] Fortunately, the side effects resolve upon discontinuation of the medication and supportive care.

CBS has been attributed to topical ocular brimonidine use.[24-27] This syndrome, probably induced by brimonidine use, consists of bilateral visual loss with persistent or repetitive formed visual hallucinations not routinely accompanied by other psychiatric symptoms. Onset of CBS is from 5 days to 2.5 months after starting brimonidine. Most have full recovery within days after the drug is discontinued or improve markedly.

Recommendations – modified after McKnight et al[6]

1. If the intraocular pressure is elevated, a trial of brimonidine withdrawal should precede a decision to embark on potentially unnecessary surgery.
2. Withdrawal of brimonidine may obviate the need for unnecessary topical steroid treatment.
3. Withdrawal of brimonidine should be considered before embarking on extensive investigation of uveitis.
4. In the presence of ocular surface signs of brimonidine allergy, clinicians should actively look for signs of uveitis.
5. This drug is contraindicated in patients taking monoamine oxidase (MAO) inhibitors.[1]
6. Use with caution in patients with severe cardiovascular diseases.[1]
7. Use with caution in patients with hepatic or renal disease.[1]
8. Use with caution in patients with depression, cerebral or coronary insufficiency, Raynaud phenomenon, orthostatic hypotension, or thromboangiitis obliterans.[1]
9. This product contains benzalkonium chloride, so the patient should remove contact lenses before administering brimonidineand wait 15 minutes before reinsertion.[1]
10. Topical ocular irritation from this drug interferes in the grading of Graves' disease.[28]

Generic Names:

1. Brinzolamide; 2. dorzolamide hydrochloride.

Proprietary Names:

1. Azopt; 2. Trusopt.

Primary Use

These topical ocular carbonic anhydrase inhibitors are effective in suppressing aqueous humor production in the management of elevated intraocular pressure.

Ocular Side Effects

Local ophthalmic use or exposure – topical ocular application

Certain

1. Irritation
   a. Burning
   b. Stinging
   c. Epiphora
   d. Pruritus
   e. Allergic reaction
   f. Photophobia
   g. Foreign body sensation
2. Decreased vision
3. Conjunctiva
   a. Follicular reaction
   b. Conjunctivitis
4. Eyelids
   a. Irritation
   b. Allergic reaction
   c. Blepharitis
   d. Edema
5. Cornea
   a. Superficial punctate keratitis (Fig. 18.6)
   b. Erosions

Probable

1. Hypotony – ciliochoroidal detachment

Possible

1. Iritis
2. Cornea

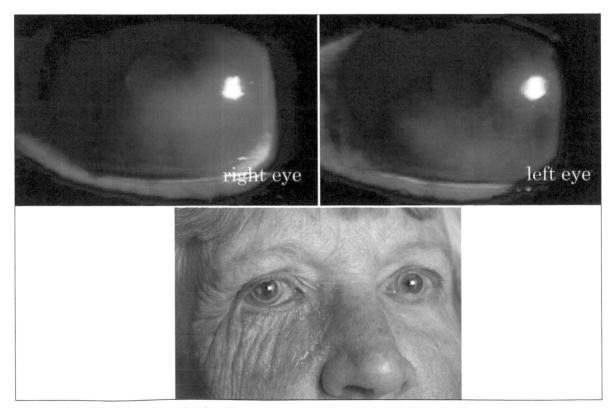

FIG. 18.6 Superficial punctate keratitis with late staining centered on the inferior cornea after treatment with topical ocular brinzolamide.[6]

a. Endothelial decompensation
b. Edema
3. May aggravate or cause ocular sicca
4. Choroidal detachment
5. Symblepharon – long-term administration
6. Myopia

Systemic Side Effects
Local ophthalmic use or exposure – topical ocular application
Certain
1. Drug in contact with nasal and oral mucosa
   a. Taste disturbance
   b. Numbness
   c. Edema
   d. Increased salivation
   e. Nasal congestion
   f. Epistaxis
   g. Dysphonia
   h. Loss of appetite
2. Gastrointestinal disturbances
   a. Gastrointestinal upsets (abdominal cramping)
   b. Nausea
   c. Heartburn
3. Central nervous system effects
   a. Headaches
   b. Asthenia/fatigue
   c. Insomnia
   d. Depression
   e. Paresthesia

Possible
1. Nephrolithiasis

Clinical Significance
It is difficult to separate some of the side effects of the drug from the side effects of the preservative, benzalkonium chloride. Still, most all topical ocular side effects are transitory and of minimal clinical importance, except for possible corneal edema. Konowal et al have shown a subset of patients (usually having had previous ocular surgery, often with borderline endothelial function and disturbed corneal epithelium) who, after starting a topical ocular carbonic anhydrase inhibitor (CAI), developed irreversible corneal decompensation.[1] There are pharmacologic and toxicologic data to support a cause-and-effect relationship. These drugs can also cause superficial punctate keratitis and corneal erosions; however, these are seldom indications to stop the drug. On occasion, the transitory stinging is severe enough that the patient refuses the medication. These effects are, in part, probably secondary to the relatively low pH of the ocular solution. In rare instances, a low-grade iritis is possibly caused by these drugs. As with any topical medication, the intended drug effect may not occur (i.e. pressure lowering). However, in individuals hypersensitive to these drugs, ocular hypotony may occur.

The most common nonocular side effect in this class (up to one-third of patients) is the bitter metallic-like taste, which may increase salivation. In others, it may be associated with tongue or perioral numbness and edema. The second-most-common side effects are gastrointestinal complaints, which have occurred in as many as 10% of patients in some series. This may be one of the primary reasons that patients discontinue the drug. The central nervous system effects are much less common, but striking in some patients (i.e. headaches). Dermatologic conditions may be drug related and may cross-react with other sulfa medications. There are no proven or suspected blood dyscrasias in the literature or spontaneous reports associated with the topical CAIs. There are numerous spontaneous reports of dyspnea, but there is not a positive cause-and-effect relationship. Seizures, as with oral CAI, have also been reported, but not proven, with topical ocular CAIs. Carlsen et al suggested an association with nephrolithiasis and stated, "perhaps alternative topical glaucoma medication should be considered in patients with a history of renal calculi."[2] This is also an unproven association.

Recommendations
1. We do not feel that informed consent is necessary for systemic side effects because these effects appear to be rare and most all are reversible.
2. If bitter taste is a major problem, consider some form of punctal occlusion.
3. It may be contraindicated to use oral and systemic CAI concomitantly.
4. It may be safe to use topical CAI in patients who report sulfa allergies.[3]
5. Use with caution in patients with renal calculi, severe kidney disease, or liver disease.
6. Topical ocular irritation from these drugs may interfere in the grading of Graves' disease.[4]
7. This product contains benzalkonium chloride, so the patient should remove contact lenses before administering brinzolamide or dorzolamide and wait 15 minutes before reinsertion.[5]

Generic Name:
Carteolol hydrochloride.

Proprietary Name:
Ocupress.

Primary Use
A nonselective beta blocker that is used in the management of glaucoma.

Ocular Side Effects
Local ophthalmic use or exposure – topical ocular application
Certain
1. Decreased intraocular pressure
2. Irritation
   a. Pain
   b. Burning sensation
   c. Epiphora
   d. Hyperemia
   e. Photophobia
3. Decreased vision
4. Eyelids or conjunctiva
   a. Allergic reactions
   b. Contact dermatitis
   c. Erythema blepharoconjunctivitis
   d. Chemosis
5. Corneal punctate staining
6. Ptosis

Systemic Side Effects
Local ophthalmic use or exposure – topical ocular application
Certain
1. Pulmonary
   a. Asthma
   b. Aggravates chronic obstructive pulmonary disease
   c. Bronchospasms
   d. Respiratory failure
   e. Dyspnea
2. Cardiovascular
   a. Bradycardia
   b. Cardiac arrhythmia
   c. Hypotension
3. Depression
4. Headache
5. Asthenia
6. Dizziness
7. Syncope

Probable
1. Rhinitis
2. Confusion
3. Taste perversion

Possible
1. Congestive heart failure
2. Cerebral vascular accident
3. Skin disease

Clinical Significance
In general, carteolol's ocular and systemic side effects are similar to timolol. Most ocular side effects decrease with time. Ocular pain may be a significant side effect, but rarely an indication for discontinuing the drug. To date, the local anesthetic effect of this drug has not been reported in humans. Transient ocular irritation, however, may occur in about 25% of patients.[1] Baudouin et al have shown that using a preservative-free solution enhances the stability of the tear film.[2]

It is apparent from controlled trials that there seem to be fewer systemic side effects with this drug than with timolol. Although this drug can reduce the mean heart rate and possibly the mean blood pressure, these have been insignificant clinically.[3,4] There have been cases in the literature and spontaneous reports of asthma, heart failure, headaches, asthenopia, and dizziness, but these are in a much smaller proportion than seen with other nonselective beta blockers. There are spontaneous reports, with both dechallenge and rechallenge data, of a bleeding diathesis with nose bleeds and easy bruisability while taking this drug. This has not been reported with the other beta blockers. Stewart et al have shown that topical ocular carteolol does not affect serum lipid levels.[5] This is in contrast to timolol maleate, which adversely affects the high-density lipoprotein (HDL) and total cholesterol/high-density lipoprotein (TC/HDL) ratio in females age 60 and older (see timolol).

Recommendation[1]
This product contains benzalkonium chloride, so the patient should remove contact lenses before administering carteolol and wait 15 minutes before reinsertion.

Generic Name:
Metipranolol.

Proprietary Name:
Optipranolol.

Primary Use
This noncardioselective beta blocker is used to reduce intraocular pressure associated with glaucoma.

Ocular Side Effects
Local ophthalmic use or exposure – topical ocular application
Certain
1. Decreased intraocular pressure
2. Irritation
   a. Hyperemia
   b. Photophobia
   c. Pain
   d. Burning sensation
3. Anterior uveitis
   a. Granulomatous
   b. Nongranulomatous
4. Eyelids or conjunctiva
   a. Allergic reactions
   b. Erythema
   c. Blepharoconjunctivitis
5. Decreased contact lens tolerance
   a. Corneal erosion
   b. Inability to wear

Probable
1. Punctate keratitis
2. Decreased tear film break-up time
3. Corneal anesthesia

Possible
1. Conjunctival keratinization

Systemic Side Effects
Similar to timolol.

Clinical Significance
This nonselective beta blocker has a lower cost, lower concentration of preservatives, fewer central nervous system (CNS) side effects, and, possibly, less corneal anesthesia than seen with other beta blockers. This drug has the potential to cause any of the systemic side effects seen with other nonselective beta blockers (see timolol). All nonselective beta blockers have been reported to cause anterior uveitis in rare instances. When metipranolol was initially released at a 0.6% dose, the incidence of uveitis was excessive. This dosage was removed from the market in 1990. The incidence at 0.3% dosage was 0.38% and 0.49%.[1,2] Onset varies from 7–31 months with cells and flare, rarely with granulomatous keratic precipitates and posterior synechiae. With discontinuing metipranolol and adding topical corticosteroids, resolution of inflammation usually occurs after 3–5 weeks.[1-6] Beck et al found no cases of uveitis in retrospective studies of 1928 patients on 0.3% metipranolol or in 3903 patients on other topical ocular beta blockers.[3] There are cases of positive rechallenge, and there is an increased incidence with higher drug concentrations.[3,4] De Groot et al described 3 cases of contact allergies secondary to this drug.[7] Wolf et al showed that both systemic and topical ocular metipranolol lead to increased retinal blood flow velocity.[8]

The drug plus an irritating preservative, benzalkonium chloride, may cause anterior segment irritation, which may cause discontinuation of metipranolol.[9] Seldom are any changes irreversible.

Recommendation[9]
This product contains benzalkonium chloride, so the patient should remove contact lenses before administering metipranolol and wait 15 minutes before reinsertion.

Generic Name:
Netarsudil.

Proprietary Name:
Rhopressa.

Primary Use
Used for ocular pressure control in open-angle glaucoma and ocular hypertension.

Ocular Side Effects
Local ophthalmic use or exposure – topical ocular application
Certain
1. Conjunctiva
   a. Hyperemia
   b. Hemorrhage
   c. Edema
2. Cornea
   a. Deposits
   b. Verticillata
   c. Punctate keratitis
3. Decreased vision
4. Lacrimation
5. Irritation
   a. Pruritus
   b. Pain
   c. Foreign body sensation
6. Eyelids
   a. Erythema
   b. Edema

Systemic Side Effects
Local ophthalmic use or exposure – topical ocular application
Possible
1. Upper respiratory tract inflammation
2. Headaches
3. Dermatitis
4. Respiratory, thoracic, and mediastinal disorders
5. Lowered blood pressure

Clinical Significance
This is the first in the series of rho-kinase inhibitors and the first new class of drugs used to treat intraocular pressure in over a decade. This is a once-daily medication, probably because it is quite effective at the recommended dosage and when used twice daily patients had a rejection rate of 10–12%.[1]

Hyperemia is the most common side effect, with an incidence rate of up to 53%.[2] This is most prominent at the instillation site and resolves typically within hours. This reaction usually becomes less with time so that at 6 weeks the incidence rate drops to around 14%. If the medication is taken at bedtime, little, if any, cosmetic issues should occur.[3] The redness is almost always rated as mild. Cornea verticillata, pain at the instillation site, and conjunctival hemorrhage are seen at a 20% incidence. To date, corneal verticillata appear to be fully reversible and cause no visual acuity change. The onset is variable from 1–3 months.

Subconjunctival hemorrhages are usually small, unilateral, near the limbus, and typically last 1– 3 weeks. Instillation site erythema, corneal staining, decreased vision, increased lacrimation, lid erythema, and reduced visual acuity are reported at a 5–10% rate.[1]

Arnold et al pointed out that this drug has the potential to reduce the intraocular pressure–lowering effect of timolol maleate presumably because of increased systemic elimination of timolol through the conjunctival vasculature.[4] This could possibly increase the systemic side effects of timolol.

Systemic side effects secondary to these eye drops are seldom a reason to stop the medication. This class of drugs lowers blood pressure and vascular resistance and thus has potential consequences.[5]

CLASS: ANTI-INFECTIVES

Generic Name:
Vancomycin.

Proprietary Names:
First-Vancomycin, FIRVANQ, Vancocin.

Primary Use
US Food and Drug Administration (FDA)–unapproved intracameral injection as a prophylaxis for intraocular infections after cataract surgery.

Ocular Side Effects
Local ophthalmic use or administration – intracameral injection
Probable
1. Hemorrhagic occlusive retinal vasculitis (HORV) (Fig. 18.7)
   a. Decreased vision
   b. Retina
      i. Hemorrhages
      ii. Vasculitis
      iii. Peripheral ischemia
   c. Macula
      i. Whitening
      ii. Edema
      iii. Cystic changes
2. Uveitis
3. Corneal edema

Clinical Significance
Intracameral injections of vancomycin alone or in combination with other drugs is unapproved by the FDA.[1] Nicholson et al were the first to report HORV.[2] There have been several other reports since.[3-9] The most complete review with recommendations as to management is by Witkin et al, who in a retrospective case series, tabulated data from the American Society of Cataract and Refractive Surgery and the American Society of Retinal Specialists.[10] All of their cases had intracameral vancomycin at the time of cataract surgery. There were 36 eyes of 23 patients diagnosed with HORV, which they found to be a rare event but potentially blinding. Significant ocular pain is often the presenting symptom. Their data suggested this to be a delayed hypersensitivity reaction rather than a toxic reaction to vancomycin. This is based on HORV always appearing in the second eye if both eyes had undergone cataract surgery using intracameral vancomycin, even if the second surgery was performed months to years later. HORV is often associated with a mild anterior-chamber reaction and vitritis. Todorich et al suggested that the pathophysiology is complex: "it is grounded in a necrotizing retinal vasculopathy

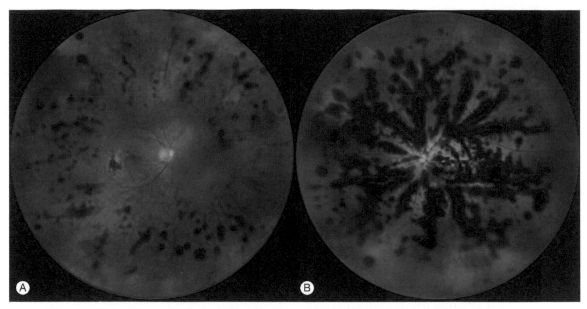

FIG. 18.7 Bilateral hemorrhagic occlusive retinal vasculitis in a 55-year-old man after cataract surgery with intracameral vancomycin 18 days (**A** [right eye]) and 11 days (**B** [left eye]) before presentation.[10]

in the absence of retinal vasculitis, chronic nongranu-lomatous choroiditis, and an unusual glomeruloid proliferation of endothelial cells in the choroid and elsewhere in the eye."[11]

CLASS: ANTIVIRAL DRUGS

Generic Name:
Acyclovir (aciclovir).

Proprietary Names:
Sitavig, Zovirax.

Primary Use
This purine nucleoside antiviral medication is used in the treatment of herpes simplex, zoster, and varicella disease.

Ocular Side Effects
Systemic administration – intravenous or oral
Certain
1. Visual hallucinations

Probable
1. Periocular edema
2. Decreased vision – transitory
3. May aggravate or cause ocular sicca

Possible
1. Eyelids
   a. Edema
   b. Erythema
   c. Urticaria
2. Phospholipidosis
   a. Corneal epithelial vacuoles
   b. Conjunctival hyperemia

Local ophthalmic use or exposure – topical ocular application
Certain
1. Irritation
   a. Lacrimation
   b. Hyperemia
   c. Pain
   d. Edema
   e. Burning sensation
   f. May aggravate or cause ocular sicca
2. Superficial punctate keratitis
3. Eyelids or conjunctiva
   a. Allergic reaction
   b. Blepharitis
   c. Conjunctivitis – follicular

Possible
1. Narrowing or occlusion of lacrimal puncta

Clinical Significance

Oral acyclovir has very few ocular side effects. The most common is probably periocular edema with or without perioral numbness. Because the drug can cause severe angioedema, it is likely that it can also cause periorbital edema.[1] Almost half of the spontaneous reports associated with acyclovir are periorbital edema. Because the drug is secreted in human tears, ocular sicca can be aggravated. Visual hallucinations have been reported secondary to systemic acyclovir therapy.[1] This drug is a known neurotoxic drug. Chevret et al reported random eye movement and loss of eye contact in a 6-month-old infant who was given acyclovir after liver transplant to prevent herpes simplex infection.[2]

Topical ophthalmic acyclovir is occasionally prescribed for herpes keratitis; it is being replaced, in part, by ganciclovir. It is generally well tolerated. A mild transient burning or a stinging sensation has been reported immediately after application of the drug. Punctate epithelial staining of the inferior bulbar conjunctiva and limbus is reversible with discontinuation of the drug. Punctal stenosis or occlusion, follicular conjunctivitis, contact blepharoconjunctivitis, palpebral allergy, or other signs of hypersensitivity have also occurred occasionally.[3-6]

Acyclovir does not appear to interfere significantly with the healing of stromal wounds. Colin et al felt that healing rates were better with ganciclovir than with acyclovir gel, but these data were not statistically significant.[3] Ohashi reviewed herpes simplex keratitis treated with topical ocular acyclovir.[5] He suggested that a more persistent superficial punctate keratitis can occur with emergence of an acyclovir-resistant strain of the virus and an increase in progressive corneal endotheliitis. Wilhelmus et al felt that drug-induced phospholipidosis is a cause of punctate epitheliopathy seen in AIDS patients, but it is not clear if this is due to acyclovir and/or ganciclovir given systemically.[7]

Generic Name:
Cidofovir.

Proprietary Name:
Vistide.

Primary Use

A nucleotide analog used in the treatment of cytomegalovirus retinitis in patients with AIDS.

Ocular Side Effects

Local ophthalmic use or exposure – intravitreal injection OR systemic administration – intravenous
Certain
1. Anterior uveitis (Fig. 18.8)
2. Intraocular pressure
    a. Decreased
    b. Hypotony

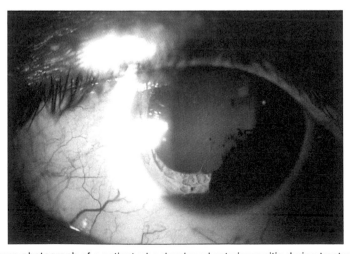

FIG. 18.8 Slit-lamp photograph of a patient who developed anterior uveitis during treatment with cidofovir showing ciliary flush and posterior synechiae.[7]

3. Decreased vision
4. Vitritis (intravitreal injections)
5. Visual hallucinations

Clinical Significance

Ocular side effects occur from either intravenous administration or intravitreal injection.[1] The 2 main ocular side effects are anterior uveitis and hypotonia. Although the drug may need to be discontinued due to severe uveitis with synechiae and cataracts, this is unusual. Iritis or uveitis occurs at an incidence of 3–4% and chronic hypotony at 3% with intravitreal injections.[1-3] It is not unusual to lose more than 2 lines on the Snellen chart, but patients often recover most of this vision loss. It is unclear how much loss is drug related versus the cytomegalovirus disease. In most cases the iritis is controlled with lower dosages of topical ocular steroids and cycloplegics.[4,5] Although retinal detachments have been reported, it is unclear whether this is drug related or associated with the intraocular injection. Chavez de la Paz et al felt concomitant use of probenecid would decrease the incidence and severity of iritis.[4] Pretreatment with topical ocular steroids was ineffective in decreasing the severity or incidence of the iritis. Davis et al pointed out that reduction of the dosage was effective in decreasing the severity of the ocular adverse reaction; however, if severe inflammation or hypotony persists, other medication should be considered.[6] They also pointed out that it was unclear whether the drug and its ocular side effects are cumulative, although they have 1 case that suggests this. They reported 3 cases of positive rechallenge.

Hypotony occurs at an incidence of 4% and chronic hypotony at 3% after intravitreal injections.[1-3] Iritis and uveitis are associated in all severe hypotony cases.[7] Ocular hypotony may be irreversible, even with appropriate management. Once chronic hypotony occurs, it is not uncommon that poor vision results.[7-11] It is felt that the physiopathology of this complication is a direct toxicity of cidofovir on the ciliary body.[2,3,11] Orssaud described a Urrets–Zavalia-like syndrome with rigid and widely dilated pupils, posterior synechia, and iris atrophy.[9] Their case, however, had severe hypotony rather than increased intraocular pressure, which they felt was due to intravenous cidofovir.

Topical ocular application of cidofovir 1% eye drops has been attempted without success due to local toxicity.[12]

Generic Names:

1. Idoxuridine (IDU); 2. trifluridine (F3T, trifluorothymidine); 3. vidarabine (ara-A).

Proprietary Names:

1. Dendrid, Herplex; 2. Viroptic; 3. VIRA-A.

Primary Use

These antivirals are used in the treatment of herpes simplex keratitis and vaccinia virus infections of the eye.

Ocular Side Effects

Local ophthalmic use or exposure – topical ocular application
Certain

1. Irritation
   a. Lacrimation
   b. Hyperemia
   c. Photophobia
   d. Pain
   e. Edema
2. Cornea
   a. Superficial punctate keratitis
   b. Edema
   c. Filaments
   d. Delayed wound healing
   e. Erosions or indolent ulceration
   f. Stromal opacities
   g. Superficial vascularization (late)
3. Eyelids or conjunctiva
   a. Allergic reactions
   b. Hyperemia
   c. Blepharitis
   d. Conjunctivitis – follicular
   e. Edema
   f. Pemphigoid-like lesion with symblepharon
   g. Perilimbal filaments
   h. Conjunctival punctate staining
   i. Conjunctival scarring
   j. Conjunctival squamous metaplasia (Fig. 18.9)
4. Lacrimal system
   a. Canaliculitis
   b. Stenosis
   c. Occlusion
5. Ptosis

Probable

1. Cornea – epithelial dysplasia (chronic therapy)

Possible

1. Eyelids or conjunctiva – ischemia (trifluridine)

Clinical Significance

The ocular side effects mentioned are a wide spectrum of early and long-term use (much longer than the 21 days recommended by the manufacturers).[1] The most severe

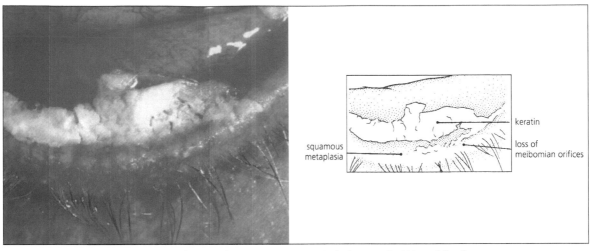

FIG. 18.9 Conjunctiva squamous metaplasia from topical idoxuridine.[5]

are primarily seen with idoxuridine (IDU), which is more toxic and less effective than trifluridine. The appearance of corneal clouding may occur early, with stippling and small punctate defects in the corneal epithelium occurring later. These corneal changes can be painful, even in partially anesthetic corneas. Late ocular side effects secondary to these drugs are confusing, in large part due to the normal sequelae of the disease and already compromised tissue being exposed frequently to the toxicity of the drug and its preservative. However, a late clinically important side effect is when the epithelial viral disease is in check but the antiviral medication plus the preservatives will not allow the epithelium to heal. Topical rose bengal stain of the epithelial edges will be ragged (fiord pattern), meaning the virus is still active, while a smooth, often slightly elevated edge means the viral process is inactive. Although most of the ocular side effects listed are reversible once the drug is stopped, some are quite indolent or irreversible. Ptosis, either from habit, chronic edema, or possibly drug enhancement, may never completely recover. Occlusion of the lacrimal outflow system may be permanent. Some of the stromal scarring may be enhanced by the delay in wound healing by these drugs.[2] Ischemic changes have been reported in the conjunctiva and anterior segment, possibly secondary to trifluridine.[2,3] These changes were described as irreversible, including iris atrophy. Jayamanne et al described a case of reversible anterior ischemia possibly due to trifluridine.[4] There is evidence of cross-reactivity with the other pyrimidine analogs, not only ocular but cutaneous as well.

Although several instances of premalignant changes have occurred after application of topical antivirals, the causal relationship has not been proven. It is best not to use these drugs during pregnancy. Although they have teratogenic effects in animals in high dosages, at the dosages used in ophthalmology, with manual punctual occlusion, they may be safe. However, every effort should be made not to use them during pregnancy; if they are so used, a signed informed consent may be prudent. The drugs should be safe in nursing mothers, because the dosages are low; however, again, it is prudent not to use these drugs, even though they are probably safe.[1]

CLASS: CARBONIC ANHYDRASE INHIBITORS

Generic Names:
1. Acetazolamide; 2. methazolamide.

Proprietary Names:
1. Diamox, Diamox Sequels; 2. Neptazane.

Primary Use
These enzyme inhibitors are effective in the treatment of glaucoma. Acetazolamide is also effective in edema due to congestive heart failure, drug-induced edema, and centrencephalic epilepsies.

Ocular Side Effects
Systemic administration – intravenous or oral
Certain
1. Decreased vision
2. Myopia

3. Uveal effusion syndrome
   a. Acute glaucoma – often bilateral
   b. Uveal effusion
   c. Iritis
   d. Lens
      i. Hydration
      ii. Forward displacement
      iii. Cataract – glaucoma type
4. Eyelids or conjunctiva
   a. Allergic reactions
   b. Erythema
   c. Photosensitivity
   d. Urticaria
   e. Purpura
5. Color vision defect – objects have yellow tinge (methazolamide)

Probable

1. Loss of eyelashes or eyebrows
2. Ocular signs of gout
3. Palinopsia

Possible

1. Electroretinogram (ERG) changes
2. Eyelids or conjunctiva
   a. Erythema multiforme
   b. Stevens-Johnson syndrome (Fig. 18.10)
   c. Lyell syndrome

Systemic Side Effects
Systemic administration – intravenous or oral
Certain

1. Malaise syndrome
   a. Acidosis
   b. Asthenia
   c. Anorexia
   d. Weight loss
   e. Depression
   f. Somnolence
   g. Confusion
   h. Impotence
2. Paresthesia
3. Taste disorders
4. Gastrointestinal disorder
   a. Nausea
   b. Vomiting
   c. Gastrointestinal irritation
5. Renal disorder (usually in persons with preexisting renal disease)
   a. Urolithiasis
   b. Polyuria
   c. Hematuria

d. Glycosuria
e. Calculi
f. Tubular acidosis
6. Respiratory problems
   a. Acidosis
   b. Aggravation of severe chronic lung disease
7. Increased aspirin-induced central nervous system (CNS) toxicity
8. Blood dyscrasia
   a. Aplastic anemia
   b. Pancytopenia
   c. Thrombocytopenia
   d. Agranulocytosis
   e. Hypochromic anemia
   f. Eosinophilia
9. Gout
   a. Increased serum uric acid
   b. Gouty arthritis
10. Ammonia intoxication

Probable

1. Osteomalacia – primarily with Dilantin use
2. Teratogenicity – contraindicated in pregnancy (in animal studies)

Possible

1. Anaphylactic shock or death
2. Hypophosphatemia

Clinical Significance

Ocular side effects secondary to carbonic anhydrase inhibitors (CAIs) are transient and usually insignificant. Acute reversible myopia, ranging from 1–8 diopters, may occur within hours to days after starting the drug. This can occur especially in the last months of pregnancy when the drug is given for water retention without toxemia. Although the side effects listed earlier are primarily for acetazolamide, most are also seen with methazolamide. Of greatest clinical significance, and probably an underrecognized syndrome associated with these drugs, is bilateral acute secondary angle-closure glaucoma.[1-6] This is associated with acute ocular pain, headache, nausea and vomiting, pupillary changes, hyperemia, corneal edema, cataract, retinal vascular accidents, visual field defects, and blindness (if not recognized early). This is also associated with uveal effusion causing a forward rotation of the ciliary process resulting in angle closure. Lenticular swelling with forward rotation of the iris lens diaphragm may cause increased curvature of the lens surface resulting in myopia. Szawarski et al felt that myopia may be seen in mountain climbers taking this drug for mountain

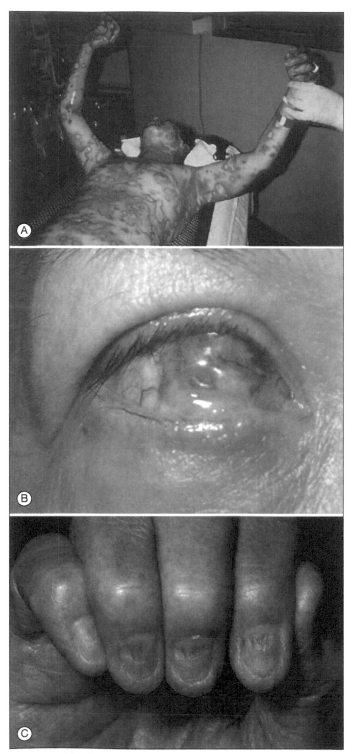

FIG. 18.10 **(A)** Painful, bullous, denuded skin lesions cover the patient's entire body. **(B)** Right eye after corneal perforation and several surgeries, including multiple penetrating keratoplasties and both mucosal and conjunctival grafts. **(C)** Right and left hands demonstrate permanent loss of fingernails.[15]

sickness.[7] Firth et al reported corneal edema also in mountain climbers.[8] Mancino et al and Parthasarathi et al also reported choroidal effusions after taking CAIs.[1,2] Apushkin et al reported a rebound effect of cystoids macular edema after continued use of CAI in 3 of 6 patients with retinitis pigmentosa.[9] Other ocular side effects are usually of minimal importance and do not appear to be dose related.

Systemic side effects from oral or intravenous CAIs are common. Patients may be unaware of how poorly they tolerate these drugs until they are discontinued. The quality of life in some patients is profoundly affected. One of the most bothersome side effects is the overall malaise and weakness that these drugs may cause. This syndrome may include marked changes in perception of taste, anorexia, generalized malaise, severe depression, decreased libido, and impotence. This overall syndrome is the primary cause of patients discontinuing the drug.[10,11] Paresthesia is one of the most common initial side effects, with numbness and tingling around the mouth, face, and extremities. This side effect may improve with time. Gastrointestinal disturbances are common and characterized by generalized stomach and gastrointestinal irritation. Delayed-release forms of this medicine have improved this side effect. Acetazolamide has been implicated in causing kidney stones, but this is uncommon and usually occurs in the first 18 months of therapy.[12,13] Uric acid retention with elevation of serum uric acid, occasionally with gouty arthritis, can be seen secondary to oral CAI.[10]

Numerous skin problems have been reported. Most are those typically seen with sulfa drugs and are usually transitory if the medication is stopped.[14] However, reports by Flach et al pointed out a possible increased incidence of Stevens-Johnson syndrome in Japanese Americans exposed to CAIs.[15] In patients with severe chronic obstructive lung disease, CAIs may cause significant CO_2 retention with respiratory acidosis and respiratory failure.[10] In the elderly, the severely diabetic, and those with severe renal disease, metabolic acidosis may also occur. This may be enhanced in patients simultaneously receiving medication that causes hypokalemia.[10] The need to watch for potassium depletion is well recognized. Tabbara et al recently reported that CAIs, when used in a uveitis patient on cyclosporine, may have a marked elevation in blood levels of cyclosporine.[16]

In severe liver disease, including cirrhosis, CAIs are contraindicated because ammonia intoxication can result. In patients on high oral dosages of salicylates, CAIs may increase salicylate concentration in the CNS, causing salicylate toxicity, including convulsions.[10]

As with all pure-sulfa preparations, drug-induced blood dyscrasias can occur. However, few sulfas are used for as long a period as those for glaucoma patients. Keisu et al reported that exposure to acetazolamide has an aplastic anemia incidence 25 times higher in males and 10 times higher in females than the control group.[17] They calculated 1 case of aplastic anemia for 18,000 patient-years of exposure, which is significantly higher than with oral chloramphenicol. There are almost 400 cases of possible CAI-related blood dyscrasias in the spontaneous reports, between 35% and 45% display aplastic anemia, with the remainder consisting of leukopenia, agranulocytosis, pancytopenia, thrombocytopenia, hypochromic anemia, or eosinophilia.

Recommendations

There are no spontaneous reports of blood dyscrasia from oral CAI exposure with less than 2 weeks of therapy. We consider short-term CAI therapy to be safe. Our current recommendations for following patients on oral CAIs include:

1. Before starting a possible longer-term use of these drugs, obtain a complete blood count, which should be repeated every 2 months during the first 6 months, and then every 6–12 months.
2. Have the patient call you if any of the following develop:
   persistent sore throat
   pallor
   fever
   fatigue
   easy bruising
   jaundice
   nosebleeds
   red blotches
3. A drop in any level of formed blood element calls for stopping the drug and seeking hematologic consultation. The majority of the ophthalmic community has not accepted these recommendations, nor require informed consent; therefore this may not be considered at this point in time to be the standard of ophthalmic practice.

CLASS: DECONGESTANTS

Generic Names:

1. Naphazoline hydrochloride; 2. tetryzoline hydrochloride (tetrahydrozoline).

Proprietary Names:

1. AK-Con, Albalon, All Clear, All Clear AR, Clear Eyes, Nafazair, Napha Forte, Naphcon Forte, Ocu-Zoline, Vasocon; 2. Tyzine, Visine.

Primary Use

These sympathomimetic amines are effective in the symptomatic relief of ophthalmic congestion of allergic or inflammatory origin.

Ocular Side Effects

Local ophthalmic use or exposure – topical ocular application
Certain
1. Conjunctival vasoconstriction
2. Irritation
   a. Lacrimation
   b. Reactive hyperemia
   c. Pain
   d. Burning sensation
3. Mydriasis – may precipitate angle-closure glaucoma
4. Decreased vision
5. Punctate keratitis
6. Allergic reactions
   a. Conjunctivitis
   b. Blepharoconjunctivitis
7. Decreased contact lens tolerance

Possible
1. Increased width of palpebral fissures
2. Occlusion of puncta and/or lacrimal outflow system (extended use)
3. Conjunctival synechia (extended use)

Systemic Side Effects

Local ophthalmic use or exposure – topical ocular application (primarily overdose situations)
Probable
1. Headache
2. Hypertension
3. Nervousness
4. Nausea
5. Dizziness
6. Asthenia
7. Somnolence

Possible
1. Stroke
2. Cardiac arrhythmia
3. Hyperglycemia
4. Hypothermia

Clinical Significance

Because these drugs do not require a prescription, abuse is the main reason for significant side effects. Both drugs have been used in intended or unintended harm via eye drops or oral ingestion.[1,2] Otherwise, ocular side effects are per short-term use and are exceedingly rare. Of greatest concern is that the drugs can induce transient mydriasis and this can precipitate narrow-angle glaucoma.[3–6] These drugs cause vasoconstriction of the conjunctival blood vessels, which may exacerbate the effects of glaucoma.[7] Many of the irritative effects, even at the manufacturer's recommended dosages, are due to the preservative, benzalkonium chloride.

Some individuals get addicted to keeping their eyes white with these decongestants, resulting in significant ocular side effects. Kisilevsky et al described a woman taking tetryzoline for 25 years with resultant conjunctival corkscrew blood vessels and dilated tortuous retinal arteries and veins.[8] Soparkar et al did a landmark study of these over-the-counter vasoconstrictors, used from 8 hours to 20 years.[9] Clinical patterns included conjunctival hyperemia, follicular conjunctivitis, and eczematoid blepharoconjunctivitis. They reported that the length of time off medication before these adverse effects resolved ranged from 1–24 weeks with a mean of 4 weeks. On rare occasions the side effect may not resolve if the drug was used for many years. Prolonged use may cause the lack of vasostructure effect to occur. This may result in a rebound hyperemia. Mendonca et al described the use of naphazoline to temporarily correct upper lid ptosis.[10]

Systemic side effects are primarily in children with overdose exposure.[2,11,12]

Recommendations[7]

1. This product contains benzalkonium chloride, so the patient should remove contact lenses before administering these drugs and wait 15 minutes before reinsertion.
2. Caution glaucoma patients to not use these drugs for prolonged periods.
3. Use with caution in patients with cardiac disease, hypertension, hyperthyroidism, and diabetes.
4. Not known if any effect on fetus during pregnancy.
5. Not known if secreted in mothers' milk.

CLASS: MIOTICS

Generic Name:
Acetylcholine chloride.

Proprietary Name:
Miochol-E.

Primary Use

This intraocular quaternary ammonium parasympathomimetic drug is used to produce prompt, short-term miosis.

Ocular Side Effects
Local ophthalmic use or exposure – intracameral or subconjunctival injection
Certain
1. Paradoxical mydriasis – rare
2. Cornea
   a. Clouding
   b. Edema
   c. Decompensation
3. May worsen uveitis – especially in children

Possible
1. Decreased intraocular pressure
2. Conjunctival hyperemia
3. Accommodative spasm
4. Decreased anterior-chamber depth
5. Lacrimation
6. Blepharoclonus

Conditional/unclassified
1. Cataract – transient

Systemic Side Effects
Local ophthalmic use or exposure – intracameral or subconjunctival injection
Probable
1. Bradycardia
2. Hypotension
3. Vasodilation
4. Dyspnea
5. Perspiration

Clinical Significance
The primary concern and most common side effect, occurring in less than 1% of patients, is corneal edema with clouding and, in extreme cases, corneal decompensation.[1,2] This problem has improved since initial reports with the addition of an improved buffering system.[3,4] The manufacturer cautions that this drug should be avoided in patients with acute iritis or inflammation of the anterior segment because it may worsen these conditions.[2] The safety and efficiency of this drug have not been established in adolescents and younger.[2] Transient lens changes have been reported, probably on an osmotic basis, and are not a toxic effect of the drug.[5,6]

Systemic side effects from intraocular injections, although rare, may occur.[7–9] These effects occur in less than 0.1%.[3] Some may be life threatening.

Generic Name:
Echothiophate iodide (ecothiophate).

Proprietary Name:
Phospholine Iodide.

Primary Use
This topical anticholinesterase is used in the management of open-angle glaucoma, in conditions in which movement or constriction of the pupil is desired, and in accommodative esotropia.

Ocular Side Effects
Local ophthalmic use or exposure – topical ocular application
Certain
1. Miosis
2. Decreased vision
3. Accommodative spasm
4. Irritation
   a. Lacrimation
   b. Hyperemia
   c. Photophobia
   d. Pain
   e. Edema
   f. Burning sensation
5. Eyelids or conjunctiva
   a. Allergic reactions
   b. Conjunctivitis – follicular
   c. Chemosis
6. Myopia
7. Iris or ciliary body cysts – especially in children
8. Intraocular pressure
   a. Increased – initial
   b. Decreased
9. Iritis
   a. Occasional fine keratic precipitates
   b. Activation of latent iritis or uveitis
   c. Formation of anterior or posterior synechiae
10. Decreased scleral rigidity
11. Occlusion of lacrimal canaliculi
12. Decreased anterior chamber depth
13. Retinal detachment
14. Myasthenia gravis - aggravated
15. Pemphigoid-like lesion – symblepharon

Probable
1. Cataracts – anterior or posterior subcapsular
2. Decreased size of filtering bleb

Possible
1. Blepharoclonus
2. Hyphema – during surgery
3. Vitreous hemorrhages
4. Cystoid macular edema

Systemic Side Effects
Local ophthalmic use or exposure – topical ocular application
Probable
1. Gastrointestinal disorders
   a. Nausea
   b. Vomiting
   c. Abdominal pain
   d. Diarrhea
2. Urinary incontinence
3. Increased saliva
4. Dyspnea
5. Bradycardia
6. Cardiac arrhythmia
7. Perspiration
8. Asthenia

Clinical Significance
Visual complaints, with or without accommodative spasm, are the most frequent adverse ocular reactions. Drug-induced lens changes are primarily seen in the older age group. In shallow anterior-chamber angles, this drug is contraindicated because it may precipitate angle-closure glaucoma. This is probably due to peripheral vascular congestion of the iris and a possible forward shift of the iris–lens diaphragm, which may further aggravate an already compromised angle. Whereas irritative conjunctival changes are common with long-term use, allergic reactions are rare.[1-4].

This strong miotic, primarily in aphakic eyes with diseased retinas, may cause retinal detachments by exerting traction on the peripheral retina.[5] Halperin et al reported a case of cystoid macular edema after echothiophate iodide.[6] Cases of irreversible miosis due to long-term therapy have been reported in spontaneous reports. A slowly progressive echothiophate-related cicatricial process of the conjunctiva may be clinically indistinguishable from ocular cicatricial pemphigoid.[7-9] Patients receiving topical ocular anticholinesterases and those being treated for myasthenia may have increased systemic and ocular side effect risks if exposed to organic phosphorus insecticides.[10] Mezer et al described a case of hyperthyroidism and hypothyroidism induced by ecothiopate iodide eye drops.[11] They felt that the thyroid dysfunction was secondary to excessive iodide intake found in the eye drops.

Systemic side effects from this drug are well documented.[1,12]

Recommendations[1]
1. Use with caution with preexisting retinal disease and in aphakia.

2. Contraindicated in cases of iritis.
3. This product contains benzalkonium chloride, so the patient should remove contact lenses before administering echothiophate and wait 15 minutes before reinsertion.
4. Use methods such as lacrimal sac pressure to minimize systemic absorption when applying echothiophate eye drops in a mother who is breast-feeding to protect the infant from echothiophate exposure.
5. Use with caution with cardiac disease, asthma, bradycardia, hypotension, gastrointestinal obstruction, Parkinson disease, peptic ulcer disease, seizure disorder, and urinary obstruction.
6. In some patients, limit night driving or operating machinery.
7. May cause paradoxical increase in ocular pressure in infants, children, and adolescents with primary congenital glaucoma, anterior segment dysgenesis, or uveitis when echothiophate is used to control ocular pressure.
8. If given before ocular surgery, echothiophate has a higher incidence of hyphemia occurring.

Generic Name:
Pilocarpine hydrochloride.

Proprietary Names:
Adsorbocarpine, Akarpine, Isopto Carpine, Pilocar, Pilopine HS, Salagen.

Primary Use
This topical ocular parasympathomimetic drug is used in the management of glaucoma and in conditions in which constriction of the pupil is desired.

Ocular Side Effects
Local ophthalmic use or exposure – topical ocular application
Certain
1. Pupils
   a. Miosis
   b. Mydriasis – rare
2. Decreased vision (light hunger)
3. Paralysis or spasm of accommodation
4. Intraocular pressure
   a. Increased – initial
   b. Decreased
5. Anterior chamber
   a. Decreased depth
   b. Increased angle width in narrow angles
6. Eyelids or conjunctiva
   a. Allergic reactions

b. Hyperemia
c. Conjunctivitis – follicular
d. Muscle spasms
7. Irritation
  a. Lacrimation
  b. Burning sensation
8. Myopia – transient
9. Retina
  a. Bleeds (vitreous hemorrhage)
  b. Detachment
10. Cornea
  a. Punctate keratitis
  b. Edema
  c. Epithelial microcysts
  d. Atypical band keratopathy (preservative)
11. Decreased dark adaptation
12. Iris cysts
13. Increased axial lens diameter
14. Decreased scleral rigidity
15. Malignant glaucoma
16. Meibomian gland dysfunction

Probable

1. Eyelids or conjunctiva
  a. Pseudomembrane
  b. Cicatricial shortening of fornices
  c. Conjunctival dysplasia or epithelial proliferation (Fig. 18.11)
  d. Conjunctival hemorrhage

2. Cornea – dysplasia or epithelial proliferation
3. Blepharoclonus
4. Cataracts
5. Iritis
6. Punctal or canalicular stenosis
7. Enlarged Schlemm's canal

Possible

1. Retina – macular hole
2. Color vision defect
3. May aggravate or cause ocular sicca

Systemic Side Effects
Local ophthalmic use or exposure – topical ocular application
Probable

1. Headache, brow ache
2. Perspiration
3. Gastrointestinal disorder
  a. Nausea
  b. Vomiting
  c. Diarrhea
  d. Spasms
4. Saliva increased
5. Tremor
6. Bradycardia
7. Hypotension
8. Bronchospasm
9. Pulmonary edema

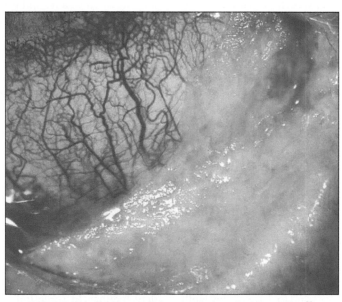

FIG. 18.11 Dyskeratosis from topical ocular pilocarpine.[22]

10. Mental status changes
    a. Confusion
    b. Short-term memory loss
    c. Depression
    d. Aggravation of Alzheimer syndrome
    e. Aggravation of Parkinson syndrome
11. Rhinorrhea
12. Epistaxis
13. Voice changes, including hoarseness

Possible
1. Tenesmus

Clinical Significance

The use of pilocarpine has been reduced significantly. It is, however, still in use for diagnostic testing of a dilated pupil, reversal of pupillary dilation, and therapeutic miosis. Side effects from pilocarpine can be divided into those that are primarily seen within minutes to hours and those that may take weeks, months, or years to develop. The most frequent immediate effects are those that affect the pupil, including miosis that causes "light hunger," effects on accommodation, transient myopia, and periocular muscle spasms. Acute toxic or allergic reactions of the anterior segment are infrequent. The most bothersome effects are superficial punctate keratitis and, rarely, corneal edema. Cases of edema are primarily seen with a defective corneal epithelium, possibly allowing a direct drug or preservative effect on the corneal endothelium.[1-4]

The most serious side effects, however, are retinal detachment and malignant glaucoma. Retinal detachments or macular holes may be aggravated by drug-induced accommodation with forward displacement of the posterior lens surface and elongation of the eye.[5-7] Walker et al reported a case of macular changes after a single application of pilocarpine.[8] This causes a more anterior position of the vitreous face and body. This forward movement may cause traction in areas where the vitreous is attached to the retina. A partial macular hole (Stage 1-A) that resolved on discontinuation of the miotic has also been reported.[7] Animal data show that a miotic can cause a pull on the peripheral retina by constriction of the ciliary body. Either of these mechanisms (i.e. forward vitreous displacement or accommodation in already diseased retinas) may precipitate a retinal hole or tear in an already compromised area of the retina.[9] Vitreous hemorrhages have been reported secondary to this process involving a retinal vessel. Pilocarpine's abilities to increase the anteroposterior diameter of the lens and to decrease the depth of the anterior chamber may also play prominent roles

in some forms of malignant glaucoma. Massry et al and spontaneous reports suggest that pilocarpine does diminish corneal allograft immune privilege and enhances graft rejection.[10] Kobayashi et al have shown that pilocarpine increases angular width in angle-closure eyes, and this is the reason that it is of value in the management of angle-closure glaucoma.[11] Nuzzi et al described decreased tear secretion compared with controls after topical ocular pilocarpine.[3] Fraunfelder et al reported bizarre behavior after topical ocular pilocarpine was administered in elderly patients.[12] This is possibly due to miosis causing "light hunger," thereby causing a decrease in sensory input that may be enough to cause confusion in some patients. Reyes et al believe that this is most common in subclinical Alzheimer syndrome patients.[13] They postulated that this may be a direct effect of pilocarpine on the central nervous system and noted an increase of symptomatology in patients with Parkinson disease after taking topical ocular pilocarpine. Fox et al and Tsao et al support that anticholinergics impair cognition in older adults.[14,15]

Ocular changes secondary to the long-term use of pilocarpine may be divided into those specifically due to the drug itself or those due to various combinations of the drug, preservatives, or vehicles. These side effects are due to repeated exposure over a period of months to many years. This includes conjunctival, corneal, and lacrimal outflow system changes. Epithelial microcysts similar in appearance to Cogan microcystic dystrophy can be seen after long-term pilocarpine therapy, but they are often smaller and usually clear.[16] Corneal and conjunctival dysplasia or hyperplasia occurs most often on the inferior nasal limbus. Chronic topical ocular drug exposure has been implicated in changes in the conjunctiva and Tenon capsule to the extent that they may adversely influence the success of filtration procedures for glaucoma.[17] These effects in the conjunctiva and trabecular meshwork are mainly due to benzalkonium chloride, but chronic exposure to the drug itself can also play a minor role.[1,3] Pilocarpine and/or the preservative can also cause cicatricial shortening in the fornices, lacrimal outflow system, and even pseudo-ocular pemphigoid.[18-20]

The most frequent finding in the spontaneous reporting systems includes literally hundreds of reports of pilocarpine, of various concentrations, having no effect on intraocular pressure. Iritis has been reported secondary to pilocarpine use. Human data support the fact that pilocarpine increases the blood–aqueous barrier's permeability to plasma protein in a dose-dependent manner. In some individuals this will give cells and flare on slit-lamp examination.[4]

Mothers on topical ocular pilocarpine giving birth may have infants with signs mimicking neonatal meningitis – hyperthermia, restlessness, convulsions, and diaphoresis. Pediatricians should be made aware of this syndrome so unnecessary tests and manipulations are avoided. It is not known whether pilocarpine is excreted in human milk, but caution should be advised when miotics are administered to nursing mothers.[4,21]

Recommendations[4]
1. Use with caution with preexisting retinal disease.
2. May be contraindicated in cases of iritis.
3. This product contains benzalkonium chloride, so the patient should remove contact lenses before administering pilocarpine and wait 15 minutes before reinsertion.
4. Use methods such as lacrimal sac pressure, lid closure, and removal of excess medication with a tissue to minimize systemic absorption when applying pilocarpine eye drops in a mother who is breast-feeding to protect the infant from pilocarpine exposure.
5. Use with caution in biliary tract disease, cholelithiasis, cardiac disease, and nephrolithiasis.
6. In some patients, limit night driving or operating machinery.
7. May cause paradoxical increase in ocular pressure in infants, children, and adolescents with primary congenital glaucoma, anterior segment dysgenesis, or uveitis when pilocarpine is used to control ocular pressure.

CLASS: MYDRIATICS AND CYCLOPLEGICS

Generic Names:
1. Cyclopentolate hydrochloride; 2. tropicamide.

Proprietary Names:
1. AK-Pentolate, Cyclogyl, Cylate, Ocu-Pentolate, Pentolair; 2. Mydral, Mydriacyl, Ocu-Tropic, Ophthalmic-myd, Tropicacyl.

Primary Use
These topical ocular short-acting anticholinergic mydriatic and cycloplegic drugs are used in refractions and fundus examinations.

Ocular Side Effects
Local ophthalmic use or exposure – topical ocular application
Certain
1. Decreased vision
2. Mydriasis – may precipitate angle-closure glaucoma

3. Irritation
   a. Hyperemia
   b. Photophobia
   c. Pain
   d. Burning sensation
4. Decreased accommodation
5. Increased intraocular pressure
6. Eyelids or conjunctiva
   a. Allergic reactions
   b. Blepharoconjunctivitis
   c. Urticaria
7. Keratitis
8. Amblyopia (patients 3 months of age or younger)

Systemic Side Effects
Local ophthalmic use or exposure – topical ocular application
Certain
1. Central nervous system (CNS) effects
   a. Personality disorders
   b. Psychosis
   c. Ataxia
   d. Speech disorder
   e. Agitation
   f. Visual hallucinations
   g. Confusion
   h. Convulsion
   i. Emotional changes
   j. Loss of equilibrium
   k. Seizures
2. Tachycardia
3. Fever
4. Vasodilation
5. Urinary retention
6. Nausea
7. Xerostomia
8. Paresthesia
9. Generalized urticaria
10. Myasthenia-like syndrome
11. Weakness

Probable
1. Gastrointestinal disorder
2. Paralytic ileus

Possible
1. Anaphylaxis
2. Peripheral numbness and paresis

Clinical Significance
Significant ocular side effects due to these drugs are quite rare. Topical ocular cyclopentolate and tropicamide can

elevate intraocular pressure in open-angle glaucoma and can precipitate angle-closure glaucoma, as with any mydriatics.[1] Cycloplegics have been shown to decrease the coefficient of outflow. Some have suggested that the use of these drugs may cause an instability of vitreous face, which could aggravate cystoid macular edema. Mori et al showed that tropicamide reduces aqueous barrier permeability.[2] McCormack showed reduced mydriasis from both of these drugs with repeat dosage and recommended that they not be used the day before surgery if the goal is to achieve maximum dilation at surgery.[3] Topical ocular cyclopentolate and/or tropicamide have been used for mood elevation. Individuals have noted an increase in pleasure; a decrease in depression; and an increase in energy, relaxation, and getting along with the group. There are numerous reports of addiction.[4-10]

Systemic adverse reactions from these drugs can occur, especially in premature children. Disorientation, somnolence, hyperactivity, vasomotor collapse, tachycardia, and even death have been reported. Kellner et al have the most complete review of cyclopentolate-induced acute psychosis with onset between 20 and 60 minutes after ocular exposure.[11] This is followed by disorientation, dysarthria, ataxia, various types of hallucinations, and retrograde amnesia. Recovery is between 30 minutes and 7 hours. There are cases in the literature and in the spontaneous reports of dilation (due to decrease in sensory input) aggravating patients who are elderly or those with Alzheimer disease.[12-14] Hermansen et al and Isenberg et al warned against the use of 0.5% cyclopentolate in preterm infants because there appears to be a risk of developing necrotizing enterocolitis.[15,16] They performed studies that showed that 0.25% cyclopentolate has no effect on gastric functions; however, case reports from Sarici et al and Lim et al described bowel obstruction in neonates using cyclopentolate.[17,18] There are numerous cases in the spontaneous reports of necrotizing enterocolitis occurring after a single dose of topical ocular cyclopentolate, especially within the first 2 months of life. Newman et al reported a case of generalized urticaria secondary to topical ocular cyclopentolate.[19] Meyer et al reported a case with rechallenge of a myasthenia-like syndrome induced by 1.0% tropicamide.[20] Tayman et al reported a case of anaphylaxis in a 4-year-old child possibly due to cyclopentolate.[21]

Generic Name:

Hydroxyamphetamine hydrobromide (hydroxyamfetamine).

Proprietary Names:

Paredrine, Paremyd (with tropicamide).

Primary Use

This topical sympathomimetic amine is used as a mydriatic to dilate the pupil and as a diagnostic test for Horner's syndrome. Also used in combination with other mydriatics for a more rapid miosis (compared with other mydriatics) after a dilated retinal examination.

Ocular Side Effects

Local ophthalmic use or exposure – topical ocular application

Certain

1. Mydriasis – may precipitate angle-closure glaucoma
2. Decreased vision – transitory
3. Irritation
   a. Lacrimation
   b. Photophobia
   c. Pain
4. Palpebral fissure – increase in vertical width
5. Paradoxical pressure elevation in open-angle glaucoma
6. Eyelids or conjunctiva – allergic reactions
7. Paralysis of accommodation – minimal
8. Anisocoria (Horner's syndrome)

Probable

1. Color vision defect – objects have a blue tinge

Clinical Significance

In the United States, Paredrine is not commercially available and is made by some pharmacies in a 1% solution for neuro-ophthalmic testing. Paremyd is available commercially as a combination mydriatic. Other than precipitating angle-closure glaucoma, ocular side effects from topical ocular administration of hydroxyamphetamine are insignificant and reversible.[1-3] An increase in vertical palpebral fissure width reaching a maximum within 30 minutes after topical ocular application is common. This is secondary to stimulation of Müeller's muscle.[4] Some feel this may be the safest mydriatic to use with a shallow anterior chamber because it is slow acting and probably more easily counteracted by miotics. Administration of 1% hydroxyamphetamine eye drops causes a more pronounced mydriasis in patients with Down syndrome.[5] A letter to ophthalmologists from the manufacturer described 3 cases of significant cardiac events following the use of a topical ocular hydroxyamphetamine/tropicamide ophthalmic solution (1%/0.25%).[6]

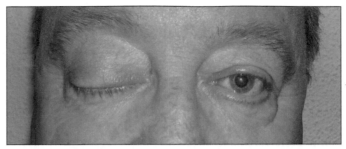

FIG. 18.12 Botulinum toxin-induced ptosis in the treatment of corneal pathology.[16]

CLASS: NEUROTOXINS

Generic Names:

1. Botulinum toxin A (abobotulinumtoxinA, incobotulinumtoxinA, onabotulinumtoxinA); 2. botulinum toxin B (rimabotulinumtoxinB).

Proprietary Names:

1. Botox, Botox Cosmetic, Dysport, Xeomin; 2. Myobloc.

Primary Use

These neurotoxins are used primarily to treat blepharospasm, hemifacial spasms, and Meige syndrome. They have also been used in selected strabismus and various neuromuscular disorders of the head and neck. Retrobulbar injections for acquired nystagmus have been advocated.

Ocular Side Effects

Local ophthalmic use or exposure – periocular injection
Certain

1. Ptosis
   a. Eyelids (Fig. 18.12)
   b. Eyebrows
2. Decreased vision
3. Extraocular muscles
   a. Paresis (in muscles other than those intended)
   b. Diplopia
   c. Hyperdeviation
4. Eyelids
   a. Lagophthalmos
   b. Edema
   c. Pruritus
   d. Paralytic ectropion
   e. Paralytic entropion
   f. Allergic reaction
5. Keratitis – exposure

6. Facial weakness or numbness
7. Epiphora (associated with dry eye reflex tearing)

Probable
1. Photophobia
2. Tear film
   a. Increased tear film break-up time
   b. Decreased Schirmer's test

Possible
1. Eyelids
   a. Permanent cutaneous depigmentation
   b. Erythema multiforme
2. Pupil
   a. Mydriasis
   b. Acute glaucoma
   c. Inverse Argyll Robertson pupil
3. Myasthenia gravis - aggravated
   a. Ptosis
   b. Diplopia
   c. Paresis of extraocular muscles

Local ophthalmic use or exposure – retrobulbar injection
Certain
1. Diplopia
2. Ptosis
3. Ophthalmoplegia
4. Filamentary keratitis (associated with ocular sicca)

Systemic Side Effects

Local ophthalmic use or exposure – periocular injection
Probable
1. Immediate hypersensitivity reaction
2. Weakness
   a. Generalized
   b. Neck

3. Fatigue
4. Flu-like syndrome
5. Dyspnea
6. Urinary incontinence
7. Dysphagia
8. Hoarseness

Clinical Significance

The listed side effects are primarily for botulinum toxin A (BTX-A) because it is more commonly used and is more toxic to the ocular system. The side effects vary with the injection technique, pathology treated, level of injection, volume, and experience of the physician. Ocular side effects are transitory and are usually gone from with a few hours, but may take up to 2–6 weeks. The most frequently encountered side effect is ptosis with or without lagophthalmos and decreased blink rate. Sicca is the second-most commonly seen adverse effect. Although there are numerous reports, pro and con, on BTX-A and botulinum toxin B (BTX-B) causing ocular sicca and changes in tear film break-up times and decreased Schirmer's tests, these are mainly insignificant.[1] The incidence of ptosis varies from 0–21% and dry eyes varies from 0–6%.[2] Ptosis, or "heavy" eyelid events, occur within 2 weeks after injection and last at least 2 weeks.[3] In a major review of 8,787 patients for facial aesthetics, the incidences after BTX-A injections were 2.5% for ptosis and 3.1% for brow ptosis.[4] Nonallergic eyelid edema occurs in 1.4% of patients, mainly Asians.[5] The next most common side effect is diplopia, which occurs in up to 3% in some series.[6] The inferior oblique is the most commonly involved extraocular muscle, which occurs in about 2%. This side effect is surprisingly well tolerated by most patients. Keratitis caused by exposure and evaporation occurred in 0–3%.[2] There have been reports of injection around eyelids for blepharospasm in which mydriasis and tonic pupil occurred.[7] Mydriasis due to these drugs may cause secondary acute glaucoma.[8] Keech et al reported possible enhancement of anterior segment ischemia after vertical muscle transposition after botulinum injection.[9] Sanders et al reported a case of the toxin causing transitory paresis of an arm after periocular injection.[10] Roehm et al treated 26 African Americans without any alteration of skin pigmentation, although Friedland et al reported 3 Caucasian patients with permanent periocular cutaneous depigmentation.[11,12] Nussgens et al compared the incidence of side effects of Dysport with Botox.[13] Statistically significant data showed fewer cases of ptosis with Botox (1.4% versus 6.6%) and fewer side effects with Botox (17.0% versus 24.1%). Reports of herpes simplex or zoster occurred after injection of botulinum toxic.[14,15]

Although rare, systemic side effects can occur. A black box warning in the *Physicians' Desk Reference* (PDR) outlines these side effects, which include an immediate hypersensitivity reaction, generalized weakness, fatigue, flu-like syndrome, dyspnea, urinary incontinence, difficulty swallowing, and death.[2]

CLASS: OPHTHALMIC DYES

Generic Name:
Fluorescein sodium.

Proprietary Names:
AK-Fluor, Fluorescite, Fluor-I-Strip, Ful-Glo.

Primary Use
Intravenous fluorescein is used to study various ocular and systemic vascular perfusions. Topical ocular fluorescein is used as a diagnostic test.

Ocular Side Effects
Systemic administration – intravenous
Certain
1. Stains ocular fluids and tissues yellow-green
2. Eyelids or conjunctiva
   a. Allergic reactions
   b. Hyperemia
   c. Yellow-orange discoloration
   d. Edema
   e. Urticaria
   f. Eczema
3. Decreased vision – transient
4. Photosensitivity

Local ophthalmic use or exposure – fluorescein strips
Certain
1. Ocular fluids and tissues stained yellow-green
2. Eyelids or conjunctiva
   a. Yellow-orange discoloration
   b. Chemosis
3. Tears and/or contact lenses stained yellow-green
4. Phototoxicity
5. Irritation

Possible
1. Phototoxic response in diseased macula

Conditional/unclassified
1. Iritis (radial keratotomy)

Systemic Side Effects
Systemic administration – intravenous
Certain
1. Nausea
2. Vomiting
3. Urine discoloration
4. Headache
5. Dizziness
6. Fever
7. Syncope
8. Hypotension
9. Dyspnea
10. Shock
11. Thrombophlebitis – injection site
12. Skin necrosis – injection site
13. Cardiac arrest
14. Myocardial infarction
15. Anaphylaxis
16. Generalized seizure
17. Phototoxic reactions

Systemic administration – intrathecal
Probable
1. Lower extremity weakness
2. Numbness
3. Generalized seizures
4. Opisthotonos
5. Cranial nerve paralysis
6. Lower extremity paralysis

Possible
1. Status epilepticus

Clinical Significance
Hundreds of thousands of intravenous fluorescein angiographies are done annually. Although widely perceived as a safe drug, significant adverse events rarely occur. The most common systemic reactions are nausea and vomiting, which occur between 3% and 9% of the time, and pruritus and urticaria from a type 1 reaction approximately 0.5–1.5% of the time.[1] Bregu et al showed a significantly higher incidence of nausea when fluorescein was injected over 10 seconds compared with 2 seconds.[2] The most serious and occasionally fatal reactions include laryngeal edema or anaphylactic reactions.[3-6] Bearelly et al and Butrus et al reported cases of elevated levels of beta-tryptase in serum, which indicated a systemic reaction to fluorescein that was mast-cell dependent.[3,4] This test can be done several hours after the reaction to confirm an anaphylactic reaction. Danis et al reported 3 patients who experienced marked cutaneous erythema, edema, and pain in the sun-exposed areas 1 hour after sunlight exposure after an ocular fluorescein angiogram.[7] Fluorescein is a photosensitive agent, and patients have complained that their vision became worse after an ocular fluorescein angiogram. Although possible, this is hard to prove because these may be in diseased maculae. However, as it occurred shortly after exposure, there is a possibility that there is a relationship. Johnson et al reported a delayed allergic reaction that resulted in a rash, chills, and fever 2 hours after an intravenous injection.[8] Hara et al reported 1787 patients who had oral fluorescein for ocular angiography and stated that the side effects were significantly less than with intravenous injections.[9] Local reactions from infiltration of fluorescein in the area of the injection site range from pain and tenderness to tissue necrosis.[10]

Ocular side effects due to topical ocular fluorescein are rare and transient. Brodsky et al reported that microperforations occurred after radial keratotomy incisions; topical ocular fluorescein entered the eye and may have caused acute iritis with an inflammatory membrane.[11] Corneal transplant surgeons use topical ocular fluorescein to test wound integrity and have not reported this problem. Solutions of fluorescein can become contaminated with *Pseudomonas* because fluorescein inactivates the preservatives found in most ophthalmic solutions. Valvano et al reported a case of periorbital urticaria after topical ocular fluorescein.[12]

Generic Name:
Indocyanine green (ICG).

Proprietary Name:
IC Green.

Primary Use
Staining posterior segment structures and intravenous for angiography.

Ocular Side Effects
Local ophthalmic use or exposure – intraocular injection
Certain
1. Visual field defect
2. Retinal pigment epithelium toxicity
3. Nerve-fiber layer toxicity

Systemic administration – intravenous
Possible
1. Reduced efficacy of infrared laser treatment
2. Enhanced photothermal effect with infrared laser treatment

Systemic Side Effects
Local ophthalmic use or exposure – intraocular injection
Certain
1. Nausea and vomiting
2. Urticaria
3. Vasovagal episodes
4. Cardiorespiratory arrest
5. Hypotension
6. Urge to defecate
7. Anaphylactic shock

Clinical Significance
Intraocular injections of ICG use in enhancing the visualization of diaphanous collagenous tissue has a narrow safety profile; however, newer preparations have made this dye safer along with refinement of surgical techniques. There have been reports of ICG causing permanent central scotoma after ICG-assisted macular hole surgery.[1-4] ICG is toxic to retinal pigment epithelial cells in vitro.[5] Ho et al found it was nontoxic to the retinal pigment epithelium for up to 5 minutes of exposure.[6,7] Gale et al showed that ICG dye demonstrated more toxicity than trypan blue to the human retinal pigment epithelium in cell cultures.[5] Gulkilik et al reported a unique case of a 60-year-old woman with bilateral internal limiting membrane peels for macular holes.[6] For staining, brilliant blue was used for 1 eye and ICG for the other. After 6 months the eye exposed to ICG had retinal pigment damage with outer segment–inner segment damage under the fovea. Disc atrophy, retinal toxicity, and ocular hypotony have been observed. To prevent toxicity, residual ICG and ICG-stained internal limiting membrane must be removed as completely as possible.

Intravenous ICG dye has been used for more than 35 years in other areas of medicine and has some popularity in ophthalmology. In the main, trypan blue has replaced ICG for intravitreal surgery; however, some clinicians have increased their use of ICG for retinal choroidal angiography. The side effects of intravenous ICG are less frequent than with fluorescein. Mild adverse reactions to fluorescein were 1–10%, and mild adverse reactions to ICG dye were approximately 0.15%. The rate of moderate reactions to fluorescein was 1.6% compared with 0.2% for ICG. Severe reactions were 0.05% with ICG, which was similar to that with fluorescein.[9] ICG dye may absorb infrared laser light and could produce a photothermal effect, leading to unwanted damage to the inner retinal layers during retinal laser surgery.

ICG dye is an established iodine allergen, is metabolized in the liver, and will cross the placental barrier;

therefore its use is contraindicated in patients with iodine allergies, those who are pregnant, or those who have liver or kidney disease. Patients with uremia have a higher incidence of significant adverse systemic reactions to ICG than normal. The reason for this is unknown, but may be due to an allergic hypersensitivity reaction. Deaths have been reported with this agent, and are probably due to an anaphylactic reaction and cardiorespiratory arrest.[10-13] There may be an increased incidence of reactions with repeat administration, but this has not been proven.

Generic Names:
1. Lissamine green; 2. rose bengal.

Proprietary Names:
1. Greenglo; 2. Rosettes.

Primary Use
These dyes are used for surface ocular diagnostic tests.

Ocular Side Effects
Local ophthalmic use or exposure – topical ocular application
Certain
1. Staining
   a. Mucus
   b. Devitalized epithelium
   c. Epithelium not adequately covered by periocular tear film
   d. Connective tissue
2. Irritation
   a. Pain
   b. Burning sensation
3. Eyelids or conjunctivitis
   a. Red discoloration (rose bengal)
   b. Green discoloration (lissamine green)
   c. Photosensitizer (rose bengal)

Probable
1. Inhibit polymerase chain reaction (PCR) detection of herpes simplex virus

Clinical Significance
Rose bengal, especially in concentrations above 1%, may cause significant ocular irritation after topical ocular instillation. It was thought that rose bengal was a vital dye, but it has now been shown to stain primarily epithelium not adequately covered by periocular tear film.[1] If the corneal or conjunctival epithelium is not intact, the topical application of rose bengal may cause long-term or rarely permanent stromal deposits of the dye. Lee et al reaffirmed that light augmentation

can enhance the toxic effects of rose bengal.[2] Manning et al showed that lissamine green had similar staining properties to rose bengal with much better patient acceptance with the duration of ocular discomfort significantly less.[3] Rose bengal and lissamine green may inhibit detection of herpes simplex virus by PCR.[4]

Generic Name:
Trypan blue.

Proprietary Name:
Visionblue.

Primary Use
This dye is used intraocularly to help visualize ocular structures. Trypan blue will stain dead tissue blue.

Ocular Side Effects
Local ophthalmic use or exposure – intracameral injection
Certain
1. Staining (Fig. 18.13)
   a. Endothelial cells
   b. Anterior and posterior capsule
   c. Internal limiting membrane
   d. Vitreous
   e. Retina
   f. Hydrogel intraocular lenses
   g. Amyloidosis
2. Lens capsule
   a. Reduction of elasticity
   b. Increased stiffness
3. Lens epithelial cell death

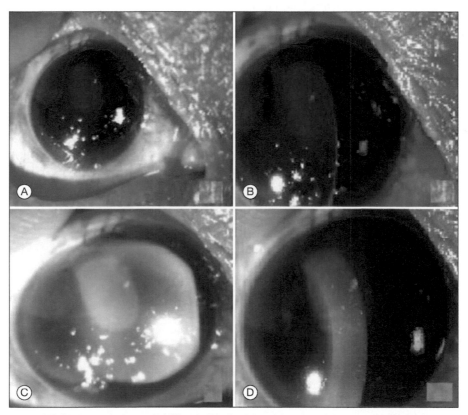

FIG. 18.13 **(A)** Slit-lamp photograph (diffuse) showing blue coloration of the cornea. **(B)** Slit-lamp photograph (slit) showing corneal edema and a mature senile cataract with a blue-stained anterior capsule. **(C)** Slit-lamp photograph (diffuse) at the end of 10 days showing clearing of the blue coloration. **(D)** Slit-lamp photograph (slit) showing decreasing corneal edema.[2]

Probable
1. Toxic anterior segment syndrome

Possible
1. Cystoid macular edema
2. Decreased elasticity of Descemet's membrane

Clinical Significance

Trypan blue has been reported to inadvertently stain the internal limiting membrane of the retina, corneal stroma, vitreous, fundus, and posterior lens capsule.[1-5] These stained structures usually lose the dye within 2 weeks. Trypan blue can cause significant retinal pigment abnormalities if dye is left in place allowing for prolonged exposure. This is primarily if the dye migrates to a subretinal space.[6] Dick et al showed that trypan blue causes a significant reduction in elasticity and increased stiffness of the lens capsule and Descemet's membrane.[7,8] Buzard et al reported 2 possible cases of toxic anterior segment syndrome after the injection of 0.1% trypan blue into the anterior chamber for capsulorhexis; Matsou et al reported 5 cases with 0.6% generic trypan blue.[9,10] Trypan blue can stain hydrogel intraocular lenses if used intraoperatively. Portes et al showed that trypan blue causes lens epithelial cell death, so it may decrease posterior capsular opacification after cataract surgery.[11] Trypan blue stains dead or damaged cells. A corneal endothelial leopard spot pattern occurred after the dye was used to visualize the lens capsule during cataract surgery.[11] The rubella virus was a possible reason for the damaged cells. The dye cleared after a number of weeks. This dye will stain corneal amyloid up to 7+ years without complications.[12]

CLASS: OPHTHALMIC IMPLANTS AND INJECTABLE GASES

Generic Names:

Organic pigments (metal salts), inorganic pigments (iron and zinc oxides).

Proprietary Name:

Eyelid tattoo (blepharopigmentation).

Primary Use

Used for cosmetic purposes anywhere on the dermis. The primary ocular use is to mimic eyeliner.

Ocular Side Effects

Eyelid tattoo
Probable
1. Eyelids

   a. Chronic irritation
   b. Deformity
   c. Meibomian gland loss
   d. Ulcerative blepharitis
   e. Granulomatous reactions
2. Eyelashes
   a. Loss
   b. Misdirection
3. Shortened tear film break-up time
4. Allergic reactions
   a. Acute
   b. Delayed
5. Uveitis

Possible
1. Lamellar keratitis

Skin tattoo (other than eyelids)
Probable
1. Uveitis

Clinical Significance

Tattoo dyes rarely cause ocular side effects; however, occasional significant reactions do occur. Kojima et al, Lee et al, and Bussell et al have shown that eyelid tattooing shortened tear film break-up time, increased fluorescein staining, and increased meibomian gland loss.[1-3] There are numerous reports of early and late granulomatous reactions to blepharopigmentation procedures.[3-6] Eyelid margin tattooing can lead to permanent scarring, lid deformity, eyelash loss, and lash misdirection.[7,8]

Probably of greatest clinical interest is the possibility of the causation of uveitis in rare instances, especially with specific dyes or in individuals with extensive areas of body tattooing.[9-11]

Recommendation

Be aware that extensive body tattooing has been associated with uveitis.

Generic Names:

1. Perfluorooctaine; 2. perfluoroperhydrophenanthrene.

Proprietary Names:

1. Perfluoron; 2. Vitreon.

Primary Use

Intracameral injections used in the management of complicated retinal detachments and proliferative vitreoretinopathy.

Ocular Side Effects
Local ophthalmic use or exposure – intracameral injections (retained liquid)
Certain
1. Decreased vision
2. Retina
   a. Local decrease in sensitivity
   b. Localized inflammation
   c. Precipitates
   d. Secondary membrane formation
   e. Pigment epithelium damage
3. Visual fields
   a. Absolute scotoma
   b. Relative scotoma
4. Cornea
   a. Edema
   b. Endothelial cell changes
   c. Precipitates
   d. Membrane formation

Possible
1. Orbit
   a. Proptosis
   b. Edema
2. Scleritis

Clinical Significance
These agents, retained in the eye and orbit, are fairly well tolerated. Only in rare cases involving large drug volumes, young eyes, large amounts of residual vitreous gel, or associated severe ocular injury are secondary side effects seen. As with epiretinal or retrocorneal membranes, some effects may be mechanical and not secondary to any toxic properties of the drug.

Elsing et al showed that retained perfluoro-n-octane (PFO) mechanically compressed residual vitreous, causing deposition of white proteinaceous deposits as early as 3–4 weeks postoperatively.[1] These precipitates were noncellular denatured proteins or compressed vitreous. Tewari et al reported reduced retinal sensitivity associated with retained subretinal PFO.[2] These changes may or may not be reversible.

These agents have found their way into the anterior chamber and settle inferiorly. Corneal endothelium changes are only seen in the area of contact, which speaks for mechanical rather than toxic effects.[3]

Orbital agents are found in extensive eye injuries to the eye, with the fluid leaking from the eye into the orbit.[4] Scleritis, proptosis, and orbital edema have been reported.

Generic Names:
1. Polydimethylsiloxane (PMDS); 2. silicone.

Proprietary Names:
1. Dimethicone (dimeticone); 2. Generic only.

Primary Use
Various silicone polymers of various viscosities or solids are used in ophthalmology as lubricants, implants, and volume expanders. PMDS belongs in the group of polymeric organosilicon compounds commonly referred to as *silicones*.

Ocular Side Effects
Local ophthalmic use or exposure – topical ocular application
Certain
1. Conjunctiva
   a. Irritation (minimal)
   b. Burning sensation (minimal)

Local ophthalmic use or exposure – intravitreal injection
Certain
1. Cornea
   a. Edema
   b. Opacity
   c. Vascularization
   d. Thinning
   e. Vacuoles
   f. Keratopathy – bullous and/or band
   g. Perforation (silicone in anterior chamber)
2. Chamber angle
   a. Glaucoma
   b. Vacuoles
3. Eyelid
   a. Vacuoles
   b. Ptosis
4. Iris – vacuoles
5. Retina
   a. Detachment
   b. Macula – vacuoles
   c. Microcystic
   d. Pseudohypopyon
6. Optic nerve – vacuoles
7. Glaucoma
   a. Pupillary block (Fig. 18.14)
   b. Ahmed valve (occlusion)
8. Migration of silicone into brain
   a. Visual field effects

Probable
1. Optic nerveatrophy
2. Cataract

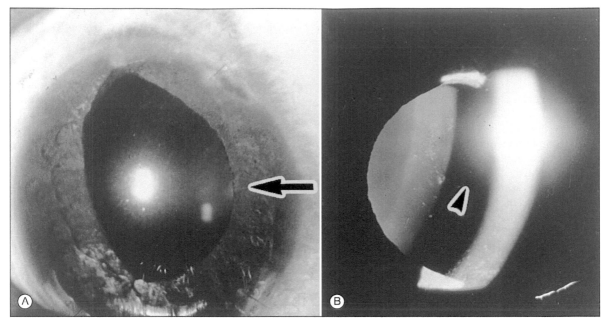

FIG. 18.14 (**A**) Anterior segment photo showing iridocorneal contact nasally (*arrow*) due to silicone oil between iris and lens. (**B**) Deep anterior chamber of same eye (*arrowhead*).[3]

3. Sympathetic ophthalmia
4. Vitreoretinopathy

***Local ophthalmic use or exposure – implants
(eyelid, lacrimal system, or ocular)***
Certain
1. Granulomatous reactions
2. Lens
   a. Intravitreal silicone may attach to silicone lenses
   b. Calcification – intraocular lenses (asteroid hyalosis)

Probable
1. Increase in infections

Clinical Significance
Silicone solutions or solids rarely cause adverse ocular reactions, but significant side effects may occur under certain circumstances. Silicone plugs are used frequently in the management of keratitis sicca. Like any foreign body buried within tissue, the implant, even if inert, may be encased by scar tissue or granulomatous tissue. Rapoza et al first reported pyogenic granulomas caused by these devices.[1] Most granulomas resolved after the plugs were removed. Granulomas may also form after retinal surgery

and when silicone is used in augmentation of the eyelids. Amemiya et al have shown that this latter procedure may also cause degeneration of the orbicularis muscle.[2]

As with silicone liquids placed in other areas of the body, the silicone liquid within the eye may migrate to new locations with time. Because the usual site of injection is intravitreal, occasionally the solution may come in contact with the lens or enter the anterior chamber, with the potential to affect the outflow channels, lens, cornea, or pupillary block glaucoma (see Fig. 18.14).[3,4] Apple et al reported 3 cases of intravitreal silicone oil injection migrating forward to come into contact with a silicone intraocular lens.[5] The silicone oil coated the intraocular lens as droplet formations. These adherences could not be removed with instrumentation or viscoelastics. They caused decreased vision and aberrations such as halos or rainbow patterns. Shalchi et al reported 4 cases of visual loss secondary to microcystic macular changes and focal severe loss of papillofoveal nerve-fiber layer after intravitreal silicone injections.[6] Nicholson et al are the first to report a central scotoma secondary to silicone oil tamponade years after multiple retinal surgeries.[7] Karth et al and Falavarjani et al reported cases of pseudohypopyon due to the migration of silicone emulsification subretinally secondary to heavy silicone oil.[8,9] Retinal detachments have been described after vitreous injections with the silicone entering through retinal breaks.[10] Shields et al have also shown that silicone liquids have the potential to migrate posteriorly to affect glaucomatous damaged optic nerves and enhance atrophy, probably on a mechanical basis.[11] Knecht et al reported that preexisting glaucomatous damage to the disc region and/or active transport mechanisms are involved in the development of silicone oil–associated optic neuropathy.[12] Multiple authors have reported on the potential for migration of silicone oil from the vitreous, through the optic nerve, and into the brain. Del Bufalo et al suspected that intravitreal silicone migrated into the lungs causing pulmonary symptoms.[13] Eckle et al have shown visual field defects in association with chiasmal migration of intraocular silicone oil, and Fangtian et al reported a case of migration of intraocular silicone oil into the cerebral ventricles.[14,15] There are also rare reports of eyelid swelling and blepharoptosis from migration into the eyelid from silicone oil instilled into the eye during vitreoretinal surgery. Corneal changes are probably not a toxic process, but rather, as pointed out by Norman et al, act as a nutritional barrier.[16] Silicone oils may increase permeability by dissolving substances such as cholesterol and other lipophilic substances out of membranes in the corneal endothelium and retina. Hutton et al have shown that silicone oil removal after anatomically successful retinal surgery significantly improved visual acuity with some slight increase of redetachment.[17] Stringham et al showed calcification of silicone lenses in eyes with asteroid hyalosis.[18] Nazemi et al showed migration of silicone oil into the subconjunctival space and orbit.[19]

Khoroshilova-Maslova et al reported 9 cases of enucleated eyes removed in part due to intravitreal injections of silicone.[20] Over a 2-year postsilicone injection period, inflammation surrounded the silicone, uveitis, and progressive loss of vision ensued. Various sequelae occurred, including traction detachments, proliferative vitreoretinopathy, formation of epiretinal and subretinal membranes, formation of bone in the internal choroidal surface, and retinal tissue atrophy with loss of neuronal structure and growth of glial tissue. These events happened over a 2- to 30-year period before enucleation.

CLASS: OPHTHALMIC PRESERVATIVES AND ANTISEPTICS

Generic Name:
Benzalkonium chloride (BAK).

Proprietary Names:
Benza, Zephiran.

Primary Use
This topical ocular quaternary ammonium agent is used as a preservative in ophthalmic solutions and as a germicidal cleaning solution for contact lenses.

Ocular Side Effects
Local ophthalmic use or exposure – topical ocular application
Certain
1. Irritation
   a. Lacrimation
   b. Hyperemia
   c. Photophobia
   d. Pain
   e. Burning sensation
2. Eyelids or conjunctiva
   a. Allergic reactions
   b. Hyperemia
   c. Erythema
   d. Blepharitis
   e. Conjunctivitis
   f. Edema
   g. Contact allergies
   h. Subconjunctival fibrosis
3. Cornea
   a. Punctate keratitis
   b. Edema
   c. Pseudomembrane formation
   d. Decreased epithelial microvilli
   e. Vascularization
   f. Scarring
   g. Delayed wound healing
   h. Increased transcorneal permeability
   i. Decreased stability of tear film
   j. Decreased goblet cells
   k. Increased inflammatory cells
   l. Disruption of cytoplasmic membrane and cell detachment
   m. Decreased tear-film break-up time
   n. Reduced aqueous tear production
   o. Endothelial cell damage
4. May aggravate or cause ocular sicca

Probable
1. Eyelids or conjunctiva – pemphigoid lesion with symblepharon (Fig. 18.15A)
2. Leukoplakia (Fig. 18.15B)

Possible
1. Cataracts
2. Cystoid macular edema

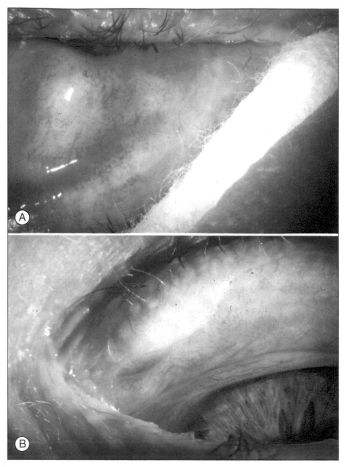

FIG. 18.15 **(A)** Cicatricial changes associated with topical ocular application of eye drops containing BAK. **(B)** Leukoplakia from topical ocular application of eye drops containing BAK.[16]

Clinical Significance

This bactericide is the most commonly used preservative because its antimicrobial effects cover a broad pH range of formulations and it allows medications to more easily penetrate the cornea. Adverse ocular reactions to BAK are not uncommon, even at exceedingly low concentrations, and may cause cell damage by emulsification of the lipids in the cell wall. De Saint Jean et al reported that this chemical can cause cell growth arrest and death at concentrations as low as 0.0001%.[1] Baudouin et al have a long history of studying BAK.[2-7] With short-term use in healthy corneas, most adverse effects are inconsequential after this agent is discontinued because the damage is fairly superficial. However, long-term use has caused extensive corneal

damage requiring corneal transplantation. BAK may destroy the corneal epithelial microvilli, and thereby possibly prevent adherence of the mucoid layer of the tear film to the cornea. Antiglaucoma medication containing BAK may cause further trabecular degeneration, thereby increasing resistance to outflow. Long-term topical ocular solutions containing BAK may allow this chemical to be deposited and retained in the trabecular meshwork. BAK can enhance the characteristics of the trabecular meshwork commonly seen in glaucoma, i.e. apoptosis, oxidative stress, and induction of inflammatory chemokines. Topical epithelial cell sensitization to BAK has been postulated to cause increased fibrosis and inflammation, decreasing the success of glaucoma filtration procedures.[2] Perez-Bartolome et al feel that these effects are more common with longer periods of treatment and older age.[8]

Means et al showed the toxicity of BAK from irrigating solutions on the endothelial cells of the cornea.[9] A case in the spontaneous reports showed irreversible corneal damage with vascularization when 1:1000 BAK was inadvertently placed in both eyes and irrigated out 20 minutes later. This agent, as pointed out by Lemp et al, is toxic to the corneal endothelium.[10] Even in the small amounts used in ophthalmic solutions, it may cause problems in diseased denuded corneas that receive multiple topical ocular applications daily.

An editorial by Brandt explored the possibility of cataracts.[11] Goto et al described the possible mechanism behind how this could occur.[12] It is "possible" that cataracts form after chronic therapy with BAK-containing products. Maculopathy has been postulated to occur by Miyake et al, and "pseudophakic preservative maculopathy" is poorly understood at this time; the authors feel it is only "possible."[13]

Stevens et al have shown that short-term BAK administration produced inflammation in the anterior segment of previously untreated patients whose blood–aqueous barrier was intact.[14] This was proven by the laser flare meter in BAK-treated patients versus controls.

BAK binds to soft contact lenses, and the use of preservatives has been said to concentrate in the contact lens, possibly causing increased epithelial breakdown.

Recommendations

1. Long-term use of topical ocular drugs containing BAK should be individualized based on potential side effects.
2. BAK-containing solutions should be avoided with mitochondrial deficiency, i.e. Leber hereditary optic neuropathy (LHON), LHON carriers, and possibly primary open-angle glaucoma patients.[15]

Generic Name:
Chlorhexidine gluconate.

Proprietary Names:
Betasept, Hibiclens, Oro Clense, Peridex, Periogard, PerioRx, Perisol.

Primary Use
Topical
This disinfectant is used as an antiseptic wound and general skin cleanser for preoperative preparation of the patient, as a surgical scrub, and as a hand wash for health care personnel.

Ophthalmic
A topical ocular antiseptic and surfactant commonly used in contact lens solutions and in the treatment of *Acanthamoeba* infection. Intravitreal injections used for antisepsis.

Ocular Side Effects
Inadvertent ocular exposure (4.0%)
Certain
1. Decreased vision, including blindness
2. Corneal
   a. Decreased endothelial counts
   b. Punctate keratitis
   c. Edema (including bullous)
   d. Opacification (all layers)
   e. Vascularization (all layers)
   f. Decreased sensation
   g. Stria
3. Conjunctiva
   a. Hyperemia
   b. Lacrimation
   c. Photophobia
   d. Pain
   e. Burning sensation
4. Iris
   a. Iritis
   b. Atrophy
5. Decreased intraocular pressure

Local ophthalmic use or exposure (0.02–0.04% for *Acanthamoeba*) – topical ocular application
Certain
1. Keratitis – transitory
2. Corneal edema – transitory
3. Cataracts – higher concentrations
4. Iris atrophy – higher concentrations
5. Loss of endothelial cells – higher concentrations
6. Conjunctiva
   a. Hyperemia
   b. Lacrimation
   c. Photophobia
   d. Pain
   e. Burning sensation

Local ophthalmic use or exposure (0.05–0.10% for antisepsis) – intravitreal injection
Certain
1. Pain
2. Allergic reaction

Clinical Significance
Serious and permanent eye injury may occur during inadvertent ocular exposure of 4.0% chlorhexidine,

mainly from preoperative scrub of the head with accidental ocular exposure. The head is usually turned, and gravity allows the chemical to be exposed to the dependent eye. The head drape covers this area; therefore a significant delay occurs before recognition of the problem and irrigation of the eye. Almost total destruction of the corneal endothelium can occur, with only variable success gained from conventional corneal grafting. In general, with immediate irrigation, only superficial punctate keratitis and mild corneal edema with conjunctivitis lasting 7–10-plus days occurs. The role of the detergent with this chemical is unclear, but it has been suggested that this enhances the penetration of chlorhexidine, allowing for stromal and anterior chamber concentration, with toxicity to the corneal endothelium.[1-5]

Chlorhexidine and propamidine in combination are commonly used for the treatment of *Acanthamoeba*. Propamidine may cause epithelial cysts, but chlorhexidine may cause conjunctival irritation and keratitis, especially at high dosage and prolonged therapy. Ehler et al suggested that, in rare instances with prolonged treatment and with already damaged corneas, chlorhexidine may more easily enter the anterior chamber.[6] This chemical can destroy the membrane of the *Acanthamoeba* cyst wall, keratocytes, and even fibrocytes, as well as the iris and lens membranes. There have been no other reports of iris, lens, or corneal endothelial damage from topical 0.02–0.04% chlorhexidine in the spontaneous reports.

Two series, Merani et al (40,535 patients) and Oakley et al (4322 patients), used intravitreal chlorhexidine 0.05–0.1% for antisepsis.[7,8] Safety profiles included only 1 allergic reaction in each series. One case had positive rechallenge.[7]

Concentrations of 0.002–0.005% chlorhexidine used as chemical disinfectants of soft contact lenses may rarely present problems of toxic anterior segment irritation. Transitory corneal edema and "chlorhexidine conjunctivitis" can occur. Okuda et al reported a case of anaphylactic shock secondary to an ophthalmic wash containing chlorhexidine.[9]

Generic Name:

Povidone-iodine (PVP-1) (iodopovidone).

Proprietary Names:

Betadine, Betadine Prep, GRx Dyne, GRx Dyne Scrub, Povidex, Povidex Peri.

Primary Use

Used in a 5% solution on periocular regions (eyelids, brows, and cheek) and irrigation of the ocular surface (cornea, conjunctiva, and palpebral fornices) to decrease bacterial counts at the operative site before surgery. A buffered PVP-1 solution of 2.5% can be used for the prevention of neonatal conjunctivitis.

Ocular Side Effects

Local ophthalmic use or exposure – using povidone-iodine preps repeatedly as with anti–vascular endothelial growth factor (VEGF) intravitreal injections
Certain
1. May aggravate or cause ocular sicca
2. Increased corneal staining
3. Increased tear film osmolarity

Local ophthalmic use or exposure – single ocular application
Certain
1. Decreased vision – transitory
2. Ocular sicca symptoms – transitory
3. Ocular irritation – transitory
4. Discharge – transitory
5. Lacrimation – transitory
6. Punctate keratitis

Conditional/unclassified
1. Thyroid complications (infants)

Clinical Significance

These products have been on the market for decades, yet this is the first time we have included this chemical. This is due to the new findings that repeated ocular preps with povidone-iodine statistically increased symptoms of ocular sicca.[1] Detrimental effects on the cornea and ocular tear film have also been documented.

Routine use as a prep in ocular surgery has stood the test of time that it is safe with few ocular side effects. Only in rare instances where irrigation is faulty, an overdose is given, or there are open wounds have complications occurred. It is probable that the inferior and superior cul-de-sac are areas where postinstillation irrigation is insufficient and where pathology is more likely to occur. Grzybowski et al and Ridder et al both gave recent overviews of ocular reactions to povidone-iodine.[2,3]

Hsu et al has shown no evidence that povidone-iodine 5% used repeatedly as with preps for anti-VEGF intravitreal injections promote bacterial resistance or a discernible change in conjunctiva flora.[4]

There is no evidence that this iodine compound interferes with adults with thyroid problems, although this is rarely a factor in infants.

True allergies to povidone-iodine do not exist; however, unsupported patient-reported allergies may confuse the issue.[5] Physicians may need more detailed histories to sort this out.

Generic Names:
1. Thiomersal (thimersal); 2. yellow mercuric oxide (hydrargyric oxide flavum).

Proprietary Names:
1. Aeroaid, Mersol; 2. Stye.

Primary Use
These topical ocular organomercurials are used as antiseptics, preservatives, and antibacterial or antifungal drugs.

Ocular Side Effects
Local ophthalmic use or exposure – topical ocular application
Certain
1. Irritation (thiomersal)
   a. Lacrimation
   b. Hyperemia
   c. Photophobia
   d. Pain
   e. Burning sensation
2. Eyelids or conjunctiva
   a. Allergic reactions
   b. Hyperemia
   c. Erythema
   d. Blepharitis
   e. Conjunctivitis – follicular
   f. Edema
   g. Urticaria
   h. Eczema
3. Bluish-gray mercury deposits (yellow mercuric oxide)
   a. Eyelids
   b. Conjunctiva
   c. Cornea
   d. Lens
4. Cornea (thiomersal)
   a. Punctate keratitis
   b. Opacities
   c. Edema
   d. Subepithelial infiltrates
   e. Vascularization
   f. Band keratopathy
   g. Hypersensitivity reactions
5. Decreased contact lens tolerance (thiomersal)

Clinical Significance
Adverse ocular side effects due to these organomercurials are rare and seldom of significance. The most striking side effect is mercurial deposits in various ocular and periocular tissues. This is an apparently harmless side effect because it is asymptomatic and no related visual impairments have been reported. These deposits are primarily seen with yellow mercuric oxide in 1–2% ointments.[1] Conjunctival mercurial deposits can be seen around blood vessels near the cornea. Corneal deposits are in the peripheral Descemet's membrane, and lens deposits are mainly in the visual axis. This usually takes many years of frequent application.[2-5] No deposits have been reported in any other ocular tissues with the topical ocular use of thiomersal.

Thiomersal is a preservative in some ophthalmic contact lens solutions. Mercurialentis has not been seen with thiomersal at concentrations of 0.005%, the concentration used as a preservative in some ophthalmic solutions. Hypersensitivity is not uncommon.[6-8] To evaluate this agent as a factor for ocular intolerance, thiomersal skin testing can be performed. Soft contact lenses cleaned and stored in thiomersal-containing solution may produce an ocular inflammatory process similar to superior limbic keratoconjunctivitis. The corneal changes are transient and range from faint epithelial opacities to a coarse, punctate epithelial keratopathy. The primary concern is a delayed hypersensitivity response. These patients develop conjunctival hyperemia, corneal infiltrates, and intolerance to soft contact lens solutions containing thiomersal. These clear with discontinuing thiomersal.[8]

CLASS: PROTEOLYTIC ENZYMES

Generic Name:
Ocriplasmin.

Proprietary Name:
Jetrea.

Primary Use
Intravitreal proteolytic enzyme used in the management of symptomatic vitreomacular adhesions.

Ocular Side Effects
Local ophthalmic use or exposure – intravitreal injection
Certain
1. Decreased vision – acute
2. Dyschromatopsia
3. Photopsia
4. Retina
   a. Edema
   b. Subretinal edema
   c. Macular edema
   d. Reflectivity
   e. Serous detachment

f. Abnormal electroretinogram (ERG)
5. Optical coherence tomography (OCT) abnormalities
6. Night blindness

Probable
1. Macular hole – enlargement
2. Postvitreous detachment
3. Afferent pupillary defect/sluggish pupil

Possible
1. Ocular inflammation
2. Visual field constriction – transitory
3. May aggravate or cause ocular sicca
4. Corneal edema

Conditional/unclassified
1. Lens
   a. Subluxated
   b. Phacodonesis
2. Retina
   a. Bleeds
   b. Rhegmatogenous detachment

Clinical Significance
The ocular side effects profile of this drug is incomplete, and until the ongoing phase IV data are available, much is controversial.[1,2] This drug is primarily used in the elderly population with significant ocular pathology, which may mask ocular side effects. Kaiser et al, in a placebo-controlled trial, reported that the drug is generally a safe and well-tolerated option to control a blinding ocular condition.[3] Others feel that the drug may have some problems and await future research and clinical data.

The most clinically significant ocular side effect is ocriplasmin retinopathy possibly occurring in some form in 40–50% of patients.[4] The data from Shah et al are closer to 17%.[2] This includes decreasing vision, which, in rare cases, decreases to hand motion or light perception. It may be associated with dyschromatopsia, bizarre photopsias, and night blindness. Even visual field constriction and afferent pupillary defects have been seen. These effects usually occur shortly after the intravitreal injection, and recovery occurs within hours to days with a median of 14 days. This appears to be a transitory effect with full recovery in most cases.[5,6] The cause is unknown, but theories include direct or indirect toxicity on the rods and cones.[3,5-7] These adverse retinal effects may be total.[7-9] Beebe pointed out that this enzyme affects many substrates, including laminin, which is found in the retina.[10] Support for panretinal problems comes from spectral domain OCT imaging and full-field ERGs.[11,12]

Subretinal fluid accumulation, which may include the fovea, has been estimated at around 10%.[2] Cases of chronic serous detachments have been reported.[13] Although incidence data vary, Shah et al, in a phase IV study, found progression of vitreomacular traction to macular hole in 8.7%, development of retinal detachment in 2.65%, and development of retinal tear in 1.8%.[2]

The drug may cause inflammation with severe sterile endophthalmitis.[14] There are cases of iritis in the spontaneous reports, which are supported by data in the *Physicians' Desk Reference* (PDR).[15]

Placebo-controlled studies show no increase over controls in intraocular pressure or intraocular bleeding. There are situations where the increased volume of the injection alone can cause a marked increase in pressure, which may require therapy.[16]

Cataracts are a common complication of vitreous procedures. Kaiser et al did not find an increase in cataract formation in their ocriplasmin-treated group.[3] Long-term follow-up is pending. Subluxation of the lens on the basis of enzymatic effects on the zonules has been reported by Keller et al.[17]

Kaiser et al also reported no increase in rhegmatogenous retinal detachments with ocriplasmin therapy compared with the placebo group.[17] This may be in part due to the drug lessening vitreoretinal tractions. There are a host of clinical case reports that feel there may be an association. Further studies are needed.

Intravitreal ocriplasmin has been implicated in causing transient corneal edema.[18] There are 5 cases of transient corneal edema in the spontaneous reports.

CLASS: SURGICAL ADJUNCTS

Generic Name:
Mitomycin.

Proprietary Names:
Mitosol, Mutamycin, Mytozytrex.

Primary Use
Mitomycin is used as an adjunct in the surgical treatment of pterygia and glaucoma. It may also be used in the management of carcinoma in situ and primary acquired melanosis.

Ocular Side Effects
Local ophthalmic use or exposure – intraocular injection or topical ocular application
Certain
1. Irritation
   a. Lacrimation

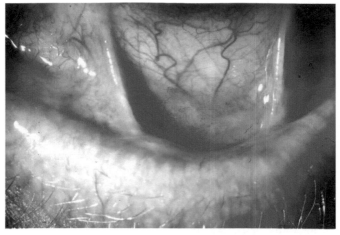

FIG. 18.16 Topical ocular mitomycin-induced symblepharon.[25]

  b. Hyperemia
  c. Photophobia
  d. Pain
  e. Epiphora
2. Eyelids or conjunctiva
  a. Allergic or irritative reactions
  b. Hyperemia
  c. Erythema
  d. Blepharitis
  e. Conjunctivitis
  f. Edema
  g. Granuloma
  h. Avascularity
  i. Symblepharon (Fig. 18.16)
3. Cornea
  a. Punctate keratitis
  b. Edema
  c. Delayed wound healing
  d. Erosion (epithelial and stromal)
  e. Perforation
  f. Crystalline epithelial deposits
  g. Recurrence of herpes simplex
  h. Astigmatism
  i. Ulceration
  j. Reorganization of cell density of anterior stromal cells
  k. Decrease in limbal stem cells
  l. Decrease in corneal endothelium
4. Sclera
  a. Erosion
  b. Delayed wound healing
  c. Perforation
  d. Avascularity
  e. Necrotizing scleritis
  f. Calcium deposits
  g. Yellowish plaques
  h. Scleritis (anterior and posterior)
5. Uvea
  a. Iridocyclitis
  b. Hypopigmentation of iris
6. Glaucoma
7. Punctal occlusion
8. Hypotony – occasionally persistent
9. Filtering blebs
  a. Thinned wall
  b. Excessive size
  c. Over filtration
  d. Spontaneous leaks
  e. Endothelial cell loss
10. Cataract
11. Choroidal effusions
12. May aggravate or cause ocular sicca

Clinical Significance

The topical ocular use of mitomycin has been in clinical use for over 2 decades. During this time much has been learned about how to limit local side effects and improve the risk–benefit ratio of this potent drug. Still, this antimetabolite is misused, and there are hundreds of published cases of ocular side effects to attest to this. The ocular complications that occur are due directly to the concentration, duration of application, and surface to which it is applied. Irritative signs and symptoms are usually short lived and seldom last more than a few weeks after discontinuing the drug. The most serious side effects are probably immune mediated. Although these may affect many areas, a long-term effect on limbal stem cells, keratocytes, and the sclera may be permanent.

In large part, the side effects due to topical and surgical adjunctive application is due to the condition being treated. For example, when mitomycin is used for glaucoma filtering surgery, there are reports of bleb problems, conjunctival and corneal pathology, cataracts, retinal effects, and ptosis.[1-10] When mitomycin is used in pterygium treatment, there are reports of corneal and scleral side effects, endothelial cell side effects, phorias, and tropias.[11-16] In eye-whitening procedures with mitomycin there are reports of persistent corneal defects, limbal stem-cell compromise, tendon scarring with diplopia, scleritis, necrotizing scleritis, increased intraocular pressure, and endophthalmitis.[17-19] In treating superficial premalignant or malignant lesions with mitomycin, there are reports of punctal stenosis and death of keratocytes and stem cells.[20-23] These can occur from any prolonged treatment of most any ocular condition. Abraham gave a complete overview of these side effects.[24]

CLASS: TOPICAL LOCAL ANESTHETICS

Generic Name:
Cocaine hydrochloride.

Proprietary Name:
Goprelto.

Street Names
Base, bernice, bernies, blow, C, coke, crack, flake, freebase, girl, gold dust, happy dust, heaven dust, pearl, rock, snow, toot.

Primary Use
Injection
Intravenous cocaine may be used by drug abusers.

Nasal or oral
Cocaine is a potent central nervous system stimulant that is commonly available on the illicit drug market.

Inhaled
Crack cocaine effect secondary to smoking.

Ophthalmic
This topical local anesthetic is used in diagnostic and surgical procedures.

Ocular Side Effects
Systemic administration – intravenous, nasal, or oral (solution)
Certain
1. Decreased vision
2. Visual hallucinations
3. Photosensitivity
4. Pupils
    a. Mydriasis
    b. Absence of reaction to light – toxic states
5. Decreased accommodation
6. Secondary optic nerve involvement (sinusitis)
    a. Optic neuritis
    b. Optic atrophy
    c. Inflammatory mass pressing on optic nerve
7. Retina (Fig. 18.17)
    a. Increased retinal artery branching angle
    b. Venular dilation
    c. Vasospasm
    d. Vascular occlusion

Possible
1. Exophthalmos
2. Madarosis
3. Iritis
4. Glaucoma
5. Maculopathy
6. Color vision defect – blue-yellow defect
7. Choroidal infarcts

Systemic administration – inhalation (crack cocaine)
Certain
1. Any and all of the earlier listed side effects
2. Significant ocular irritation
3. Madarosis

Local ophthalmic use or exposure – topical ocular application
Certain
1. Mydriasis – may precipitate angle-closure glaucoma
2. Corneal epithelium
    a. Punctate keratitis
    b. Gray, ground-glass appearance
    c. Edema
    d. Softening, erosions, and sloughing
    e. Filaments
    f. Ulceration
    g. Anesthesia
3. Corneal stroma
    a. Yellow-white opacities (Fig. 18.18)

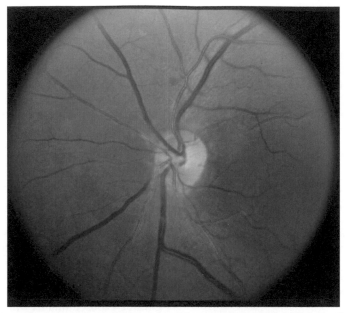

FIG. 18.17 A 30-degree fundus photograph image of the retina centered on the optic disc taken with a Zeiss fundus camera.[11]

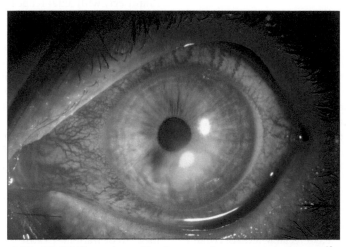

FIG. 18.18 Corneal opacities from cocaine exposure to the eye.[18]

    b. Vascularization
    c. Scarring
 4. Irritation
    a. Lacrimation
    b. Hyperemia
    c. Pain
    d. Burning sensation

 5. Eyelids or conjunctiva
    a. Allergic reactions
    b. Blepharoconjunctivitis
    c. Widening of palpebral aperture
 6. Decreased stability of corneal tear film
 7. Subconjunctival hemorrhages
 8. Decreased blink reflex

9. Hypopyon
10. Decreased vision
11. Conjunctival vasoconstriction
12. Decreased accommodation
13. Visual hallucinations – especially Lilliputian
14. Abnormal electroretinogram (ERG) (reduced blue-cone responses)
15. Delayed corneal wound healing

Possible
1. Iritis

Ocular teratogenic effects
1. Nystagmus
2. Strabismus
3. Optic nerve abnormalities
4. Retinal vascular abnormalities

Systemic Side Effects
Local ophthalmic use or exposure – topical ocular application
Certain
1. Nervousness
2. Tremors
3. Convulsion
4. Bradycardia
5. Asthma
6. Apnea

Clinical Significance
Most significant ocular side effects are due to abuse. Topical ocular cocaine can cause all the side effects that one sees from the topical abuse of local anesthetics. It differs, however, from other local anesthetics in that it causes conjunctival vasoconstriction. Mydriasis is always seen and, in some instances, may affect accommodation. Rarely does this precipitate angle-closure glaucoma, although there are many well-documented cases in the literature and spontaneous reports.[1–4] Visual hallucinations, especially Lilliputian, may occur. A potential problem is that a detectable level of cocaine may be present in the urine for 72 hours after the application of topical ocular cocaine by ophthalmologists. This has occasionally been a law enforcement problem, and the patient should be warned.[5,6] There has been a marked increase in the illicit use of cocaine with new and more potent drugs available. One of the most common methods of using this drug systemically is by applying it to the nasal mucosa. There have been a number of cases of optic neuropathies associated with chronic sinusitis and orbital inflammation secondary to chronic cocaine-induced nasal or optic nerve

pathology. These have included optic neuritis, optic atrophy, and blindness.[7–9] There are a few scattered reports of transitory blue-yellow color vision problems, especially in overdoses.[10] Ascaso et al reported a possible bilateral symmetrical maculopathy associated with chronic cocaine use.[10] Intracranial hemorrhages have occurred secondary to cocaine use, including bilateral and unilateral intranuclear ophthalmoplegia secondary to micro-infarcts in the medial longitudinal fasciculus. Cocaine has been shown to cause cerebral vasodilation, and Leung et al have shown this in the retina along with changes in arterial branching.[11] Vascular infarcts with secondary visual field changes and extraocular muscle dysfunction have been reported, including central artery occlusion.[12]

Ocular teratogenic effects secondary to cocaine administration probably occur. Dominguez et al reported that 9 infants had ophthalmic abnormalities, including strabismus, nystagmus, and hypoplastic optic discs.[13] Good et al reported 13 cocaine-exposed infants who had optic nerve abnormalities, delayed visual maturation, and prolonged eyelid edema.[14] Stafford et al, however, showed no significant effects of prenatal cocaine exposure on the infant eye, with axial lengths consistent with the statistical norm, along with other parameters that were normal for fetal growth.[15] Nucci et al reported a 24% incidence of congenital esotropia in infants who were cocaine-exposed newborns.[16] It is apparent, however, that many of the infants who have cocaine in their urine at birth may show increased congestion, engorgement, and bleeding of their retinal and iris vessels.

Another form of cocaine use is crack cocaine. This is the most addictive form of delivery with the most intense high. The fumes from the cocaine cause significant ocular irritation, dryness, and loss of eyebrows. It has become advisable to consider crack cocaine on the differential diagnosis if a young patient comes in with corneal ulcers or epithelial defects and no related medical or traumatic cause. Various bacterial and fungal organisms have been identified in these ulcers. Staphylomas have been seen probably secondary to severe vasoconstriction.[17] McHenry et al reported central retinal artery occlusions, unilateral mydriasis, cranial nerve palsies, and optic neuropathies with crack-cocaine use.[3]

Generic Names:
1. Oxybuprocaine (benoxinate); 2. proxymetacaine hydrochloride (proparacaine); 3. tetracaine (amethocaine).

Proprietary Names:

1. Novesin, Novesine; 2. Alcaine, Flucaine, Ophthetic, Paracaine; 3. Pontocaine.

Primary Use

These topical ocular local anesthetics are used in diagnostic and surgical procedures.

Ocular Side Effects

Local ophthalmic use or exposure – topical ocular application

Certain

1. Corneal epithelium
   a. Punctate keratitis
   b. Gray, ground-glass appearance
   c. Edema
   d. Softening, erosions, and sloughing
   e. Filaments
   f. Ulceration
2. Corneal stroma
   a. Yellow-white opacities
   b. Vascularization
   c. Scarring
   d. Ulceration
   e. Crystalline keratopathy
   f. Perforation
   g. Increased incidence of *Acanthamoeba* keratitis
   h. Increased incidence of *Candida* keratitis
   i. Melting (Fig. 18.19)
   j. Increased corneal thickness in females (oxybuprocaine)
3. Corneal endothelium
   a. Loss of cells
   b. Variation in cell size
4. Uveitis
   a. Fibrinous
   b. Hypopyon
5. Irritation
   a. Lacrimation
   b. Hyperemia
   c. Pain
   d. Burning sensation
6. Delayed wound healing
7. Eyelids or conjunctiva
   a. Allergic reactions
   b. Blepharoconjunctivitis
   c. Pruritus
   d. Erythema
   e. Contact dermatitis
8. Decreased stability of corneal tear film
9. Subconjunctival hemorrhages
10. Decreased blink reflex
11. Inhibits fluorescence of fluorescein
12. Decreased vision
13. Pupil
    a. Potentiate mydriatic topical ocular medications
    b. Atonic pupil
    c. Irregular pupil dilation

Systemic Side Effects

Local ophthalmic use or exposure – topical ocular application

Probable

1. Nervousness

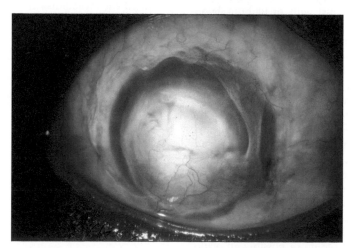

FIG. 18.19 Corneal melt and vascularization from topical proxymetacaine hydrochloride abuse.[14]

2. Tremors
3. Convulsion
4. Bradycardia
5. Asthma
6. Apnea

Clinical Significance

Few significant ocular side effects are seen with these drugs if they are given topically for short periods, but prolonged use will inevitably cause severe and possible permanent corneal damage, including visual loss.[1-3] Local anesthetics inhibit the rate of corneal epithelial cell migration by disruption of cytoplasmic action in filaments and destruction of superficial corneal epithelial microvilli. This allows for permanent epithelial defects and disruption of the corneal tear film with continued drug use. Chronic use of local anesthetics causes denuding of corneal epithelium, which may cause dense yellow-white rings in the corneal stroma. This may occur as early as the 6th or as late as the 60th day after initial use. The corneal ring resembles a Wessely ring and often resolves once the local anesthetic is discontinued. Moreira et al have shown a direct toxic effect of local anesthetics on stromal keratocytes.[4] Secondary infection is common, and an increase in the frequency of *Acanthamoeba* may be seen. Chern et al described 4 patients who, after local anesthetic abuse, developed *Candida* keratitis.[5] Infectious crystalline keratopathy has been reported due to topical local anesthetic abuse.[6] Risco et al have shown irreversible destruction of the endothelial cells secondary to topical ocular local anesthetic abuse.[7] With prolonged use, from one-third to two-thirds of endothelial loss may occur. Various degrees of uveitis have been reported, including fibrinous, with or without hypopyon. Rosenwasser et al reviewed this subject, including cases of ocular perforation requiring enucleation.[8] Topical ocular anesthetics potentiate the mydriatic effects of mydriatics.[1] Takkar et al have shown that proparacaine can be absorbed through bare sclera during surgery and can cause skewed dilation of the pupil.[9] Of the currently available anesthetics, proxymetacaine 0.5% was the least inhibitory on bacterial cultures.[10] Oxybuprocaine can cause a significant increase in corneal thickness in females, but not in males.[11]

Numerous systemic reactions from topical ocular applications of local anesthetics have been reported. Some are probably not drug induced if they occur immediately after the eye drop is administered, but may be emotionally mediated. They may occur, in part, from fear of the impending procedure or possibly an oculocardiac reflex. Side effects include syncope, convulsions, and anaphylactic shock. Liesegang et al described an

ophthalmologist with fingertip dermatitis secondary to exposure to proparacaine on a daily basis.[12] Taddio et al reported a preterm infant developing bradycardia and contact dermatitis on 4% tetracaine gel.[13]

CLASS: TOPICAL OCULAR NONSTEROIDAL ANTI-INFLAMMATORY DRUGS

Generic Names:

1. Bromfenac sodium; 2. diclofenac sodium; 3. ketorolac tromethamine; 4. nepafenac.

Proprietary Names:

1. Bromday, BromSite, Prolensa, Xibrom; 2. Voltaren, Voltaren XR; 3. Acular, Acular LS; 4. Ilevro, Nevanac.

Primary Use

These topical ocular nonsteroidal anti-inflammatory drugs (NSAIDs) are used in the management of inflammation associated with cataract surgery (diclofenac, bromfenac, nepafenac) and for relief of ocular itching due to seasonal allergies (ketorolac).

Ocular Side Effects
Local ophthalmic use or exposure – topical ocular application
Certain
1. Irritation
   a. Burning
   b. Stinging
   c. Lacrimation
2. Eyelids or conjunctiva
   a. Allergic reactions
   b. Edema
3. Cornea
   a. Superficial punctate keratitis
   b. Anesthesia
   c. Delayed epithelial healing
   d. Persistent epithelial defects
   e. Melting
   f. Perforation (Fig. 18.20)
4. Conjunctiva
   a. Conjunctivitis
   b. Erosions
   c. Hyperemia
5. Scleral
   a. Melting
   b. Perforation
6. Pupil
   a. Inhibits surgical-induced miosis
   b. Postsurgical atonic mydriasis

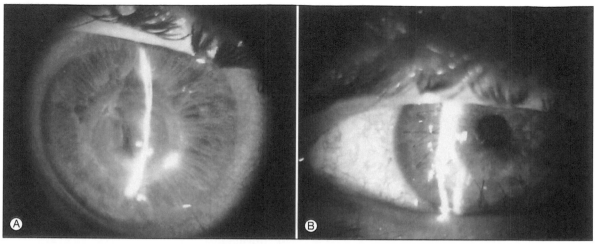

FIG. 18.20 **(A)** Central corneal perforation from topical ocular diclofenac. **(B)** Corneal transplant to repair (1-week after surgery).[6]

7. Potentiates ocular bleeding
8. Iritis
9. Visual hallucinations – usually Lilliputian

Probable
1. May aggravate or cause ocular sicca
2. Intraocular pressure increased

Systemic Side Effects
Local ophthalmic use or exposure – topical ocular application
Possible
1. Nausea and vomiting
2. Exacerbation of asthma
3. Abdominal pain
4. Asthenia
5. Chills
6. Dizziness
7. Facial edema
8. Headaches
9. Insomnia

Clinical Significance
The NSAIDs are probably the most common medications used in the United States.[1] Topical ocular NSAIDs seldom cause serious ocular side effects if used per the manufacturer's guidelines. These 4 NSAIDs are grouped together because they, in the main, have similar side effects. There are differences, but the differences are mainly regarding incidences rather than different ocular side effects. In the spontaneous reports, the number-one ocular side effect for diclofenac and ketorolac was

periorbital and eyelid edema; for bromfenac it was eye irritation and pain, and for nepafenac it was eye pain. The incidence of most ocular side effects (irritation, blurred vision, pain, pruritus, keratitis, and hyperemia) is from 1–10%.[2] All NSAIDs slow or delay wound healing and have the potential for cross-sensitivity, most NSAIDs increase bleeding (especially during surgery), and several NSAIDs may cause increased intraocular pressure if used for prolonger periods and may cause corneal anesthesia.[2] There are hundreds of literature reports and tens of thousands of cases in the spontaneous reports of ocular side effects confirming the earlier lists. Just a few are listed in Further Reading. Most preparations use benzalkonium chloride as a preservative, so the usual recommendations on soft contact lens use apply to these drugs.

Intravitreal diclofenac in chronic diabetic retinopathy may cause retinal toxicity in the form of inner retinal cystic spaces and splitting of the internal limiting membrane on the first follow-up day.[3] These resolve after the first month.

Systemic reactions, although rare and sometimes theoretical, can be serious. These include potentiation of vascular insufficiency in patients with depression, cerebral or coronary insufficiency, Raynaud phenomenon, orthostatic hypotension, or thromboangiitis obliterans. Many products contain sulfites, which may cause asthmatic or anaphylactic attacks.[1,4,5]

Generic Name:
Lifitegrast.

Proprietary Name:
Xiidra.

Primary Use
Topical ocular solution used in dry eye disease primarily acting as an anti-inflammatory. It is the first medication in the new class of drugs known as lymphocyte function-associated antigen (LFA-1) antagonists.

Ocular Side Effects
Local ophthalmic use or exposure – topical ocular application
Certain
1. Decreased vision – transitory
2. Eyelids or conjunctiva
   a. Discharge
   b. Hyperemia
   c. Pruritus

Systemic Side Effects
Local ophthalmic use or exposure – topical ocular application
Certain
1. Abnormal taste

Possible
1. Headaches
2. Sinusitis

Clinical Significance
This solution is well tolerated with no serious ocular side effects.[1] Transient decrease in vision occurred in up to 25% of patients.[2] The next most common ocular side effect reported was ocular irritation after instillation, which occurred in up to 18% of patients.[1] These symptoms of irritation usually abated within 3 minutes. Sheppard et al, Tauber et al, and Donnenfeld et al reported similar results as to Holland et al.[1,3–5]

The usual signs of ocular irritation – hyperemia, lacrimation, ocular discharge, or pruritus – occurred in 1–5% of patients.[2]

No serious ocular side effects have been seen in clinical trials. Spontaneous reports for serious adverse ocular effects, such as keratitis, corneal erosion, corneal ulcers, or acquired punctal occlusion, are few and may well be found in the usual population of ocular sicca patients.

Recommendations
Avoid use with contact lenses. Contact lenses should be removed before using the eye drops and not reinserted until 15 minutes after administration of the drug per the manufacturer's recommendations.

CLASS: TOPICAL OSMOTIC DRUGS

Generic Name:
Sodium chloride.

Proprietary Name:
Muro 128.

Primary Use
This topical ocular hypertonic salt solution is used to reduce corneal edema.

Ocular Side Effects
Local ophthalmic use or exposure – topical ocular application
Certain
1. Irritation
   a. Hyperemia
   b. Pain
   c. Burning sensation
2. Corneal dehydration
3. Subconjunctival hemorrhages
4. Nose bleeds
5. Decreased vision
6. Eyelid and orbit – edema

Probable
1. Lacrimation

Clinical Significance
Few significant adverse ocular reactions are seen with commercial topical sodium chloride solutions. The most frequent ocular side effects are irritation and discomfort, which are primarily related to the frequency of application. At suggested dosages, all ocular side effects are reversible and transient.[1] Kushner reported that nosebleeds may occur after use of topical ocular hypertonic salt solutions or ointment; cases in the spontaneous reports support this.[2] Subconjunctival hemorrhages are not uncommon if solutions or ointment are used excessively. It is felt that these occur purely on a strong osmotic effect.

CLASS: VISCOELASTICS

Generic Name:
Sodium hyaluronate.

Proprietary Names:
AMO Vitrax, Amvisc, Coease, Euflexxa, Gel-One, Healon, Hyalgan, Orthovisc, Provisc, Restylane, Shellgel, Supartz, Synvisc, Viscoat.

Primary Use

Primarily used as a viscoelastic material in ophthalmic surgery. It is also used as an ocular surface lubricant.

Ocular Side Effects

Local ophthalmic use of exposure – intraocular injection

Certain

1. Elevated intraocular pressure
2. Opacities (corneal injection)
3. Crystalline deposition on intraocular lenses (high molecular weight)
4. Myopia
5. Ciliary block glaucoma
6. Pupil
   a. Sluggish pupil
   b. Dilated
   c. Nonreactive

Possible

1. Uveitis – transient

Local ophthalmic use of exposure – topical ocular application

Certain – soft contact lens wear

1. Increased corneal aberration
2. Decreased vision

Clinical Significance

Improvements have been made in the manufacture of viscoelastics since the 1970s; many of the initial adverse events, such as uveitis or precipitation of calcium salts due to excessive phosphate in the buffer, have now been eliminated. Floren showed that because autoclaving degrades high-molecular-weight hyaluronic acid molecules, it may still be a problem to keep these products free of endotoxins.[1] This still occurs.[2] The sodium salt of hyaluronic acid is sodium hyaluronate, which is one of the more commonly used viscoelastics. All of the viscoelastics can cause transitory elevations in pressure, usually peaking between 6 and 12 hours and returning to normal within 24 hours. This pressure elevation seems to be more acute and lasting in patients with glaucoma. There is some evidence that lower-molecular-weight viscoelastics do not produce as great a pressure elevation as those with higher molecular weights. Tanaka et al have shown that viscosity is important as well.[3] It is recommended that washout times of at least 10 seconds are necessary to help prevent intraocular pressure elevations. Shammas, Holtz, and Reck et al described entrapment of a viscoelastic in the capsular bag.[4–6] This material is very slow to absorb and may require a surgical procedure, as it did in these 3 cases, to prevent myopia, shallow anterior chamber, and a distended capsular bag. Berger et al described a case of suspected ciliary block glaucoma caused by the viscoelastic agent being misdirected into the vitreous through an unsuspected small zonular dialysis.[7] This required a vitrectomy and peripheral iridectomy to resolve. Because postoperative uveitis is common, it is difficult to determine a true incidence of inflammation attributed directly to these agents. However, this was more of a problem initially than it is currently. Studies by Storr-Paulsen et al show little difference in the severity of iritis among the various viscoelastics.[8] In general, these products seldom cause a significant inflammatory response. Jensen et al described a series of patients with visually significant deposition of a high-molecular-weight sodium hyaluronate (Healon GV).[9] These deposits may remain up to 6 months and decrease vision to 20/40 or worse. Isolated cases have been reported of corneal opacities occurring after inadvertent corneal injection of viscoelastics, but they seem to absorb and resolve in a matter of months. Tan et al described partially reactive pupils after hyaluronate use in cataract surgery, and Eason et al showed fixed pupils could occur.[10,11] This is seldom a problem now because more attention is given to remove this material at surgery. Lee et al showed that 0.3% sodium hyaluronate caused primarily defocus aberrations in some soft contact lens wearers, which caused decreased vision.[12]

REFERENCES

Drugs: Aflibercept, bevacizumab, pegaptanib sodium, ranibizumab

1. Kitchens JW, Do DV, Boyer DS, et al. Comprehensive review of ocular and systemic safety events with intravitreal aflibercept injection in randomized controlled trials. *Ophthalmology.* 2016;123(7):1511–1520.
2. Yashkin AP, Hahn P, Sloan FA. Introducing anti-vascular endothelial growth factor therapies for AMD did not raise risk of myocardial infarction, stroke, and death. *Ophthalmology.* 2016;123(10):2225–2231.
3. Aflibercept: Package Insert. Tarrytown, NW: Regeneron Pharmaceuticals; 2018.
4. Bakri SJ, Thorne JE, Ho AC, et al. Safety and efficacy of anti-vascular endothelial growth factor therapies for neovascular age-related macular degeneration: a report by the American Academy of Ophthalmology. *Ophthalmology.* 2019;126(1):55–63.
5. Chang LK, Sarraf D. Tears of the retinal pigment epithelium: an old problem in a new era. *Retina.* 2007;27:523–524.
6. Hata M, Yamashiro K, Oishi A, et al. Retinal pigment epithelial atrophy after anti-vascular endothelial growth factor injections for retinal angiomatous proliferation. *Retina.* 2017;37(11):2069–2077.

7. Munk MR, Ceklic L, Ebneter A, et al. Macular atrophy in patients with long-term anti-VEGF treatment for neovascular age-related macular degeneration. *Acta Ophthalmol.* 2016;94(8):e757–e764.

8. Kabanarou SA, Kirou T, Mangouritsas G, et al. Full-thickness macular hole formation following anti-VEGF injections for neovascular age-related macular degeneration. *Clin Interv Aging.* 2017;12:911–915.

9. Kiss C, Michels S, Prager F, et al. Evaluation of anterior chamber inflammatory activity in eyes treated with intravitreal bevacizumab. *Retina.* 2006;26:877–881.

10. Ziemssen F, Warga M, Neuhann IM, et al. Does intravitreal injection of bevacizumab have an effect on the blood–aqueous barrier function? *Br J Ophthalmol.* 2006;90:922.

11. Spaide RF, Laud K, Fine HF, et al. Intravitreal bevacizumab treatment of choroidal neovascularization secondary to age-related macular degeneration. *Retina.* 2006;26:383–390.

12. Goldberg RA, Shah CP, Wiegand TW, et al. Noninfectious inflammation after intravitreal injection of aflibercept: clinical characteristics and visual outcomes. *Am J Ophthalmol.* 2014;158(4):733–737.

13. Fine HF, Roth DB, Shah SP, et al. Frequency and characteristics of intraocular inflammation after aflibercept injection. *Retina.* 2015;35(4):681–686.

14. VanderBeek BL, Bonaffini SG, Ma L. Association of compounded bevacizumab with postinjection endophthalmitis. *JAMA Ophthalmol.* 2015;133(10):1159–1164.

15. VEGF Inhibition Study in Ocular Neovascularization (VISION) Clinical Trial Group, Chakravarthy U, Adamis AP, et al. Year 2 efficacy results of 2 randomized controlled clinical trials of pegaptanib for neovascular age-related macular degeneration. *Ophthalmology.* 2006;113(9):1508. e1–e25.

16. Singer MA, Awh CC, Sadda SV, et al. HORIZON: an open-label extension trial of ranibizumab for choroidal neovascularization secondary to age-related macular degeneration. *Ophthalmology.* 2012;119:1175–1183.

17. Silva R, Axer-Siegel R, Eldem B, et al. The SECURE Study: Long-term safety of ranibizumab 0.5 mg in neovascular age-related macular degeneration. *Ophthalmology.* 2013;120:130–139.

18. Dedania VS, Bakri SJ. Sustained elevation of intraocular pressure after intravitreal anti-VEGF agents: what is the evidence? *Retina.* 2015;35(5):841–858.

19. Bakri SJ, Moshfeghi DM, Francom S, et al. Intraocular pressure in eyes receiving monthly ranibizumab in 2 pivotal age-related macular degeneration clinical trials. *Ophthalmology.* 2014;121(5):1102–1108.

20. Freund KB, Hoang QV, Saroj N, et al. Intraocular pressure in patients with neovascular age-related macular degeneration receiving intravitreal aflibercept or ranibizumab. *Ophthalmology.* 2015;122(9):1802–1810.

21. Atchison EA, Wood KM, Mattox CG, et al. The real-world effect of intravitreous anti-vascular endothelial growth factor drugs on intraocular pressure. *Ophthalmology.* 2018;125(5):676–682.

22. Bressler NM, Beaulieu WT, Glassman AR, et al. Persistent macular thickening following intravitreous aflibercept, bevacizumab, or ranibizumab for central-involved diabetic macular edema with vision impairment: a secondary analysis of a randomized clinical trial. *JAMA Ophthalmol.* 2018;136(3):257–269.

23. Lass JH, Benetz BA, Menegay HJ, et al. Effects of repeated intravitreal aflibercept injection on the corneal endothelium in patients with age-related macular degeneration: outcomes from the RE-VIEW study. *Cornea.* 2018;37(5):596–601.

24. Steffensmeier AC, Azar AE, Fuller JJ, et al. Vitreous injections of pegaptanib sodium triggering allergic reactions. *Am J Ophthalmol.* 2007;143:512–513.

25. Duan Y, Mo J, Klein R. AMD is associated with incident myocardial infarction among elderly Americans. *Ophthalmology.* 2007;114:732–737.

26. Polizzi S, Mahajan VB. Intravitreal anti-VEGF injections in pregnancy: case series and review of literature. *J Ocul Pharmacol Ther.* 2015;31(10):605–610.

27. Bakri SJ, Kitzmann AS. Retinal pigment epithelial tear after intravitreal ranibizumab. *Am J Ophthalmol.* 2007;143(3):505–507.

Drug: Verteporfin

1. Verteporfin. 2019. Retrieved from http://www.pdr.net.

2. Postelmans L, Pasteels B, Coquelet P, et al. Severe pigment epithelial alterations in the treatment area following photodynamic therapy for classic choroidal neovascularization in young females. *Am J Ophthalmol.* 2004;138:803–808.

3. Sugawara E, Machida S, Fujiwara T, et al. Development of retinal pigment epithelium alternation following single photodynamic therapy for age-related macular degeneration. *Retin Cases Brief Rep.* 2007;1(2):70–73.

4. Wachtlin J, Behme T, Heimann H, et al. Concentric retinal pigment epithelium atrophy after a single photodynamic therapy. *Graefes Arch Clin Exp Ophthalmol.* 2003;241:518–521.

5. Do DV, Bressler NM, Bressler SB. Large submacular hemorrhages after verteporfin therapy. *Am J Ophthalmol.* 2004;137(3):558–560.

6. Gelisken F, Inhoffen W, Partsch M, et al. Retinal pigment epithelial tear after photodynamic therapy for choroidal neovascularization. *Am J Ophthalmol.* 2001;131:518–520.

7. Gelisken F, Inhoffen W, Karim-Zoda K, et al. Subfoveal hemorrhage after verteporfin photodynamic therapy in treatment of choroidal neovascularization. *Graefes Arch Clin Exp Ophthalmol.* 2005;243:198–203.

8. Ojima Y, Tsujikawa A, Otani A, et al. Recurrent bleeding after photodynamic therapy in polypoidal choroidal vasculopathy. *Am J Ophthalmol.* 2006;141:958–960.

9. Theodossiadis GP, Panagiotidis D, Georgalas IG, et al. Retinal hemorrhage after photodynamic therapy in patients with subfoveal choroidal neovascularization caused by age-related macular degeneration. *Graefes Arch Clin Exp Ophthalmol.* 2003;241:13–18.

10. Theodossiadis GP, Grigoropoulos VG, Emfietzoglou I, et al. Evolution of retinal pigment epithelium detachment after photodynamic therapy for choroidal neovascularization in age-related macular degeneration. *Eur J Ophthalmol.* 2006;16:491–494.
11. Mennel S, Meyer CH, Eggarter F, et al. Transient serous retinal detachment in classic and occult choroidal neovascularization after photodynamic therapy. *Am J Ophthalmol.* 2005;140:758–760.
12. Hoz ER, Linare L, Meiler WF, et al. Exudative complications after photodynamic therapy. *Arch Ophthalmol.* 2003;121:1649–1652.
13. Ratanasukon M, Wongchaikunakorn N. Exudative retinal detachment after photodynamic therapy: a case report in an Asian patient. *Eye.* 2006;20:499–502.
14. Michels S, Aue A, Simader C, et al. Retinal pigment epithelium tears following verteporfin therapy with intravitreal triamcinolone. *Am J Ophthalmol.* 2006;141:396–398.
15. Pece A, Introini U, Bottoni F, et al. Acute retinal pigment epithelial tear after photodynamic therapy. *Retina.* 2001;21:661–665.
16. Srivastava S, Sternberg Jr P. Retinal pigment epithelial tear weeks following photodynamic therapy with verteporfin for choroidal neovascularization secondary to pathologic myopia. *Retina.* 2002;22:669–671.
17. Klais CM, Ober MD, Freund KB, et al. Choroidal infarction following photodynamic therapy with verteporfin. *Arch Ophthalmol.* 2005;123:1149–1153.
18. Koizumi H, Hatanaka H. Severe retinal vascular infarction after photodynamic therapy with verteporfin using the standard protocol. *Arch Ophthalmol.* 2010;128(2):259–262.
19. Van Dijk EHC, Dijkman G, Theelen T, et al. Short-term findings on optical coherence tomography and microperimetry in chronic central serous chorioretinopathy patients treated with half-dose photodynamic therapy. *Retin Cases Brief Rep.* 2018;12(4):266–271.
20. Mammo Z, Forooghian F. Incidence of acute exudative maculopathy after reduced-fluence photodynamic therapy. *Retin Cases Brief Rep.* 2017;11(3):217–220.
21. Tsai FY, Lau LI, Chen SJ, et al. Persistent exudative retinal detachment after photodynamic therapy and intravitreal bevacizumab injection for multiple retinal capillary hemangiomas in a patient with von Hippel-Lindau disease. *J Chin Med Assoc.* 2014;77(1):52–56.
22. Fujita K, Imamura Y, Shinoda K, et al. One-year outcomes with half-dose verteporfin photodynamic therapy for chronic central serous chorioretinopathy. *Ophthalmology.* 2015;122(3):555–561.
23. Leys AM, Silva R, Inhoffen W, et al. Neovascular growth following photodynamic therapy for choroidal hemangioma and neovascular regression after intravitreous injection of triamcinolone. *Retina.* 2006;26(6):693–697.
24. Colucciello M. Choroidal neovascularization complicating photodynamic therapy for central serous retinopathy. *Retina.* 2006;26:239–242.
25. Karacorlu M, Karacorlu S, Ozdemir H, et al. Nonarteritic anterior ischemic optic neuropathy after photodynamic therapy for choroidal neovascularization. *Jpn J Ophthalmol.* 2004;48:418–426.
26. Schnurrbusch UE, Jochmann C, Einbock W, et al. Complications after photodynamic therapy. *Arch Ophthalmol.* 2005;123(10):1347–1350.
27. Azab M, Benchaboune M, Blinder KJ, et al. Verteporfin therapy of subfoveal choroidal neovascularization in age-related macular degeneration: meta-analysis of 2-year safety results in three randomized clinical trials: treatment of age-related macular degeneration with photodynamic therapy and verteporfin in photodynamic therapy study report no. 4. *Retina.* 2004;24(1):1–12.
28. Fossarello M, Peiretti E. Acute respiratory distress due to verteporfin infusion for photodynamic therapy. *Arch Ophthalmol.* 2006;124:1508–1509.

Drug: Emedastine difumarate

1. Emedastine difumarate. 2019. Retrieved from http://www.pdr.net.
2. Vermeeren A, Ramaekers JG, O'Hanlon JF. Effects of emedastine and cetirizine, alone and with alcohol, on actual driving of males and females. *J Psychopharmocol.* 2002;16:57–64.

Drug: Loteprednol etabonate

1. Friedlander MH, Howes J. A double-masked, placebo-controlled evaluation of the efficacy and safety of loteprednol etabonate in the treatment of giant papillary conjunctivitis. *Am J Ophthalmol.* 1997;123(4):455–464.
2. Dell SJ, Shulman DG, Lowry GM, et al. A controlled evaluation of the efficacy and safety of loteprednol etabonate in the prophylactic treatment of seasonal allergic conjunctivitis. *Am J Ophthalmol.* 1997;123(6):791–797.
3. Loteprednol etabonate. 2018. Retrieved from http://www.pdr.net.
4. Lu E, Fujimoto LT, Vejabul PA, et al. Steroid-induced ocular hypertension with loteprednol etabonate 0.2%: a case report. *Optometry.* 2011;82(7):413–420.
5. Lin S, Gupta B, Rossiter J. Combined ab interno trabeculotomy and lens extraction: a novel management option for combined uveitic and chronic narrow angle raised intraocular pressure. *BMJ Case Rep.* 2016;2016 Feb 1.

Drugs: Olopatadine, hydrochloride

1. *Olopatadine Hydrochloride.* 2019. Retrieved from http://www.pdr.net.
2. McLaurin E, Narvekar A, Gomes P, et al. Phase 3 randomized double-masked study of efficacy and safety of once-daily 0.77% olopatadine hydrochloride ophthalmic solution in subjects with allergic conjunctivitis using the conjunctival allergen challenge model. *Cornea.* 2016;34(10):1245–1251.
3. Huang OS, Mehta JS, Htoon HM, et al. Incidence and risk factors of elevated intraocular pressure following deep anterior lamellar keratoplasty. *Am J Ophthalmol.* 2016;170:153–160.

4. Charters L. Olopatadine effect on TFBUT similar to tear substitute. *Ophthalmology Times.* 2006:28.

Drug: Apraclonidine hydrochloride

1. *Apraclonidine Hydrochloride.* 2019. Retrieved from http://www.pdr.net.
2. Araujo SV, Bond BB, Wilson RP, et al. Long-term effect of apraclonidine. *Br J Ophthalmol.* 1995;79:1098–1101.
3. Robin AL, Ritch R, Shin DH, et al. Short-term efficacy of apraclonidine hydrochloride added to maximum-tolerated medical therapy for glaucoma. Apraclonidine maximum-tolerated medical therapy study group. *Am J Ophthalmol.* 1995;120(4):423–432.
4. Cambron M, Maertens H, Crevits L. Apraclonidine and my pupil. *Clin Auton Res.* 2011;21(5):347–351.
5. Jampel HD. Hypotony following instillation of apraclonidine for increased intraocular pressure after trabeculoplasty. *Am J Ophthalmol.* 1989;108:191–192.
6. Stewart WC, Laibovitz R, Horwitz B, et al. A 90-day study of the efficacy and side effects of 0.25% and 0.5% apraclonidine vs 0.5% timolol. Apraclonidine Primary Therapy Study Group. *Arch Ophthalmol.* 1996;114:938–942.
7. Wright TM, Freedman SR. Exposure to topical apraclonidine in children with glaucoma. *J Glaucoma.* 2009;18(5):395–398.
8. Yarwood J, Bartholomew K. Systemic effects of topical ophthalmic agents. *Br J Anaesth.* 2010;105(2):238–239.
9. Fraunfelder FT. *Follicular Conjunctivitis Involving the Palpebral Conjunctiva of Lower Eyelid [Photograph].* Portland, OR: Casey Eye Institute, Oregon Health & Science University; ©1990:1 photograph: color.

Drugs: Betaxolol hydrochloride, levobunolol hydrochloride, timolol maleate

1. *Timolol Maleate.* 2019. Retrieved from http://www.pdr.net.
2. Feiler-Ofry V, Godel V, Lazar M. Nail pigmentation following timolol maleate therapy. *Ophthalmologica.* 1981;182(3):153–156.
3. Coppeto JR. Timolol associated myasthenia gravis. *Am J Ophthalmol.* 1984;98:244–245.
4. Fraunfelder FT, Meyer SM. Sexual dysfunction secondary to topical ophthalmic timolol. *JAMA.* 1985;253:3092–3093.
5. Schwab IR, Linberg JV, Gioia VM, et al. Foreshortening of the inferior conjunctival fornix associated with chronic glaucoma medications. *Ophthalmology.* 1992;99:197–202.
6. Zhang Y, Kam WR, Liu Y, et al. Influence of pilocarpine and timolol on human meibomian gland epithelial cells. *Cornea.* 2017;36(6):719–724.
7. Baffa Ldo P, Ricardo JR, Dias AC, et al. Tear film and ocular surface alterations in chronic users of antiglaucoma medications. *Arq Bras Oftalmol.* 2008;71(1):18–21.
8. Hong S, Lee CS, Seo KY, et al. Effects of topical antiglaucoma application on conjunctival impression cytology specimens. *Am J Ophthalmol.* 2006;142:185–186.

9. Servat JJ, Bernardino CR. Effects of common topical antiglaucoma medications on the ocular surface, eyelids and periorbital tissue. *Drugs Aging.* 2011;28(4):267–282.
10. Seider N, Miller B, Beiran I. Topical glaucoma therapy as a risk factor for nasolacrimal duct obstruction. *Am J Ophthalmol.* 2008;145(1):120–123.
11. Lee AJ, Wang JJ, Kifley A, et al. Open-angle glaucoma and cardiovascular mortality, the Blue Mountains Eye Study. *Ophthalmology.* 2006;113:1069–1076.
12. Lama PJ. Topical beta adrenergic blockers and glaucoma: a heart-stopping association? *Ophthalmology.* 2006;113:1067–1068.
13. Müskens RP, Wolfs RC, Witteman JC, et al. Topical β-blockers and mortality. *Ophthalmology.* 2008;115(11):2037–2043.
14. Frommelt P, Juern A, Siegel D, et al. Adverse events in young and preterm infants receiving topical timolol for infantile hemangioma. *Pediatr Dermatol.* 2016;33(4):405–414.
15. Bailey PL. Timolol and postoperative apnea in neonates and young infants. *Anesthesiology.* 1984;61(5):622.
16. Olson RJ, Bromberg BB, Zimmerman TJ. Apneic spells associated with timolol therapy in a neonate. *Am J Ophthalmol.* 1979;88(1):120–122.
17. Kiryazov K, Stefova M, Iotova V. Can ophthalmic drops cause central nervous systemic depression and cardiogenic shock in infants? *Pediatr Emerg Care.* 2013;29(11):1207–1209.
18. Bright RA, Everitt DE. Beta blockers and depression. *JAMA.* 1992;267:1783–1787.
19. Duch S, Duch C, Pasto L, et al. Changes in depressive status associated with topical beta blockers. *Int Ophthalmol.* 1992;16(4–5):L331–L335.
20. Orlando RG. Clinical depression associated with betaxolol. *Am J Ophthalmol.* 1986;102:275.
21. Kaiserman I, Kaiserman N, Elhayany A, et al. Topical beta blockers are not associated with an increased risk of treatment for depression. *Ophthalmology.* 2006;113:1077–1080.
22. Negi A, Thoung D, Dabbous F. Nightmares with topical beta-blocker. *Eye.* 2000;14(5):813–814.
23. Hackethal V. Visual hallucinations linked to timolol eye drops. *Psychiatric Times.* 2018;35(1).
24. Nanda T, Rasool N, Callahan AB, et al. Ophthalmic timolol hallucinations: a case series and review of the literature. *J Glaucoma.* 2017;26(9):e214–e216.
25. Shelley WB, Shelley ED. Chronic erythroderma induced by beta blocker (timolol maleate) eyedrops. *J Am Acad Derm.* 1997;37(5 Pt 1):799–800.
26. Muramatsu K, Nomura T, Shiiya C, et al. Alopecia induced by timolol eye-drops. *Acta Derm Venereol.* 2017;97(2):295–296.
27. Fraunfelder FT, Meyer SM, Menacker SJ. Alopecia possible secondary to topical ophthalmic beta-blockers. *JAMA.* 1990;263(11):1493–1494.
28. Swenson ER. Severe hyperkalemia as a complication of timolol, a topically applied beta-adrenergic antagonist. *Arch Inter Med.* 1986;146(6):1220–1221.

29. Madadi P, Koren G, Freeman DJ, et al. Timolol concentrations in breast milk of a woman treated for glaucoma. *J Glaucoma.* 2008;17(4):329–331.

30. Fraunfelder FT. *Hair Loss From Topical Ocular Timolol [Photograph].* Portland, OR: Casey Eye Institute, Oregon Health & Science University; ©1990:1 photograph: color.

Drugs: Bimatoprost, latanoprost, tafluprost, travoprost

1. Johnstone MA. Hypertrichosis and increased pigmentation of eyelashes and adjacent hair in the region of the ipsilateral eyelids of patients treated with unilateral topical latanoprost. *Am J Ophthalmol.* 1997;124:544–547.

2. Chiba T, Kashiwagi K, Ishijimia K, et al. A prospective study of iridal pigmentation and eyelash changes due to ophthalmic treatment with latanoprost. *Jpn J Ophthalmol.* 2004;48:141–147.

3. Uva MG, Avitabile T, Reibaldi M, et al. Long-term efficacy of latanoprost in primary congenital glaucoma. *Eye. (Lond).* 2014;28(1):53–57.

4. Huang P, Zhong Z, Wu L, et al. Increased iridial pigmentation in Chinese eyes after use of travoprost 0.004%. *J Glaucoma.* 2009;18(2):153–156.

5. Albert DM, Gangnon RE, Zimbric ML, et al. A study of iridectomy histopathologic features of latanoprost- and non-latanoprost-treated patients. *Arch Ophthalmol.* 2004;122:1680–1685.

6. Alm A, Grierson I, Shields MB. Side effects associated with prostaglandin analog therapy. *Surv Ophthalmol.* 2008;53(suppl 1):S93–S105.

7. Esteve E, Beau-Salinas F, Esteve L, et al. Melanoma during latanoprost therapy: three cases. *Ann Dermatol Venereol.* 2009;136(1):60–61.

8. Krohn J, Hove VK. Iris cyst associated with topical administration of latanoprost. *Am J Ophthalmol.* 1999;127:91–93.

9. Pruthi S, Kashani S, Ruben S. Bilateral iris cyst secondary to topical latanoprost. *Acta Ophthalmol.* 2008;86(2):233–234.

10. Miyake K, Ota I, Maekubo K, et al. Latanoprost accelerates disruption of the blood-aqueous barrier and the incidence of angiographic cystoid macular edema in early postoperative pseudophakias. *Arch Ophthalmol.* 1999;117:34–39.

11. Furuichi M, Chiba T, Abe K, et al. Cystoid macular edema associated with topical latanoprost in glaucomatous eyes with a normally functioning blood-ocular barrier. *J Glaucoma.* 2001;10:233–236.

12. Lin M, Schmutz M, Mosaed S. Latanoprost-induced skin depigmentation. *J Glaucoma.* 2017;26(11):e246–e248.

13. Doshi M, Edward DP, Osmanovic S. Clinical course of bimatoprost-induced periocular skin changes in Caucasians. *Ophthalmol.* 2006;113:1961–1967.

14. Calladine D, Harrison RJ. Severe darkening of a facial skin graft from latanoprost. *Arch Ophthalmol.* 2007;125(10):1427–1428.

15. Priluck JC, Fu S. Latisse-induced periocular skin hyperpigmentation. *Arch Ophthalmol.* 2010;128(6):792–793.

16. Shah M, Lee G, Lefebvre DR, et al. A cross-sectional survey of the association between bilateral topical prostaglandin analogue use and ocular adnexal features. *PLoS ONE.* 2013;8(5):e61638.

17. Peplinksi LS, Albiani Smith K. Deepening of the lid sulcus from topical bimatoprost therapy. *Optom Vis Sci.* 2004;81(8):574–577.

18. Yam JC, Yuen NS, Chan CW. Bilateral deepening of upper lid sulcus from topical bimatoprost therapy. *J Ocul Pharmacol Ther.* 2009;25(5):471–472.

19. Jayaprakasam A, Ghazi-Nouri S. Periorbital fat atrophy – an unfamiliar side effect of prostaglandin analogues. *Orbit.* 2010;29(6):357–359.

20. Ung T, Currie Z. Periocular changes following long-term administration of latanoprost 0.005%. *Ophthal Plast Reconstr Surg.* 2012;28(2):e42–e44.

21. Mocan MC, Uzunosmanoglu E, Kocabeyoglu S, et al. The association of chronic topical prostaglandin analog use with meibomian gland dysfunction. *J Glaucoma.* 2016;25(9):770–774.

22. Abedi F, Chappell A, Craig JE. Audible clicking on blinking: an adverse effect of topical prostaglandin analogue medication. *Clin Exp Ophthalmol.* 2017;45(3):304–306.

23. Kaufman HE, Varnell ED, Thompson HW. Latanoprost increases the severity and recurrence of herpetic keratitis in the rabbit. *Am J Ophthalmol.* 1999;127(5):531–536.

24. Kaufman HE, Varnell ED, Toshida H, et al. Effects of topical unoprostone and latanoprost on acute recurrent herpetic keratitis in the rabbit. *Am J Ophthalmol.* 2001;131(5):643–646.

25. Gordon YJ, Yates KA, Mah FS, et al. The effects of xalatan on the recovery of ocular herpes simplex virus type 1 (HSV-1) in the induced reactivation and spontaneous shedding rabbit models. *J Ocul Pharmacol Ther.* 2003;19(3):233–245.

26. Bean G, Reardon G, Zimmerman TJ. Association between ocular herpes simplex virus and topical ocular hypotensive therapy. *J Glaucoma.* 2004;13:361–364.

27. Gutierrez-Ortiz C, Teus MA. Alterations in anterior chamber depth in primary open-angle glaucoma patients during latanoprost therapy. *Acta Ophthalmol.* 2012;90(1):e76–e77.

28. Yalvac IS, Tamcelik N, Duman S. Acute angle-closure glaucoma associated with latanoprost. *Jpn J Ophthalmol.* 2003;47:530–531.

29. Latanoprost. 2018. Retrieved from http://www.pdr.net.

30. Goodwin D, Erickson DH. Accidental overdose of travoprost. *Optom Vis Sci.* 2014;91(12):e298–e300.

31. Fahim A, Morice AH. Heightened cough sensitivity secondary to latanoprost. *Chest.* 2009;136(5):1406–1407.

32. Tooley AA, Garrity JA. Antiglaucoma medications complicating the management of Graves' ophthalmopathy. *Ophthalmic Plast Reconstr Surg.* 2018;34(6):600–601.

33. Younus M, Schachar RA, Zhang M, et al. A long-term safety study of latanoprost in pediatric patients with glaucoma and ocular hypertension: a prospective cohort study. *Am J Ophthalmol.* 2018. 196–101–111.

Drug: Brimonidine tartrate

1. *Brimonidine Tartrate.* 2019. Retrieved from http://www.pdr.net.
2. Becker HI, Walton RC, Diamant JI, et al. Anterior uveitis and concurrent allergic conjunctivitis associated with long-term use of topical 0.2% brimonidine tartrate. *Arch Ophthalmol.* 2004;122:1063–1066.
3. Byles DB, Frith P, Salmon JF. Anterior uveitis as a side effect of topical brimonidine. *Am J Ophthalmol.* 2000;130:287–291.
4. Cates CA, Jeffrey MN. Granulomatous anterior uveitis associated with 0.2% topical brimonidine. *Eye.* 2003;17:670–671.
5. Goyal R, Ram AR. Brimonidine tartrate 0.2% (Alphagan) associated granulomatous anterior uveitis. *Eye.* 2000;14:908–910.
6. McKnight CM, Richards JC, Daniels D, et al. Brimonidine (Alphagan) associated anterior uveitis. *Br J Ophthalmol.* 2012;96(5):766–768.
7. Moorthy RS, Valluri S, Jampol LM. Drug-induced uveitis. *Surv Ophthalmol.* 1999;42:557–570.
8. Nguyen EV, Azar D, Papalkar D, et al. Brimonidine-induced anterior uveitis and conjunctivitis: clinical and histologic features. *J Glaucoma.* 2008;17(1):40–42.
9. Velasque L, Ducousso F, Pernod L, et al. Anterior uveitis and topical brimonidine: a case report. *J Fr Ophthalmol.* 2004;27:1150–1152.
10. Beltz J, Zamir E. Brimonidine induced anterior uveitis. *Ocul Immunol Inflamm.* 2016;24(2):128–133.
11. Maruyama Y, Ikeda Y, Yokoi N, et al. Severe corneal disorders developed after brimonidine tartrate ophthalmic solution use. *Cornea.* 2017;36(12):1567–1569.
12. Shah AA, Modi Y, Thomas B, et al. Brimonidine allergy presenting as vernal-like keratoconjunctivitis. *J Glaucoma.* 2015;24(1):89–91.
13. Besada E, Reed K, Najman P, et al. Pupillometry study of brimonidine tartrate 0.2% and apraclonidine 0.5%. *J Clin Pharmacol.* 2011;51(12):1690–1695.
14. Novitskaya ES, Dean SJ, Moore JE, et al. Effects of some ophthalmic medications on pupil size: a literature review. *Can J Ophthalmol.* 2009;44(2):193–197.
15. McDonald II JE, El-Moatassem Kotb AM, Decker BB. Effect of brimonidine tartrate ophthalmic solution 0.2% on pupil size in normal eyes under different luminance conditions. *J Cataract Refract Surg.* 2001;27:560–564.
16. Edwards JD, Burka JM, Bower KS, et al. Effect of brimonidine tartrate 0.15% on night-vision difficulty and contrast testing after refractive surgery. *J Cataract Refract Surg.* 2008;34:1538–1541.
17. Grueb M, Mielke J, Rohrbach JM, et al. Effect of brimonidine on corneal thickness. *J Ocul Pharmacol Ther.* 2011;27(5):503–509.
18. Walter KA, Gilbert DD. The adverse effect of perioperative brimonidine tartrate 0.2% on flap adherence and enhancement rates in laser in situ keratomileusis patients. *Ophthalmology.* 2001;108:1434–1438.
19. Hedge V, Robinson R, Dean F, et al. Drug-induced ectropion: what is the best practice? *Ophthalmology.* 2007;114(2):362–366.
20. Berlin RJ, Lee UT, Samples JR, et al. Ophthalmic drops causing coma in an infant. *J Pediatr.* 2001;138:441–443.
21. Carlsen JO, Zabriskie NA, Kwon YH, et al. Apparent central nervous system depression in infants after the use of topical brimonidine. *Am J Ophthalmol.* 1999;128(2):255–256.
22. Korsch E, Grote A, Seybold M, et al. Systemic adverse effects of topical treatment with brimonidine in an infant with secondary glaucoma (letter). *Eur J Peds.* 1999;158:685.
23. Mungan NK, Wilson TW, Nischal KK, et al. Hypotension and bradycardia in infants after the use of topical brimonidine and beta-blockers. *J Am Assoc Pediatr Ophthalmol Strabismus.* 2003;7:60–70.
24. Tomsak RL, Zaret CR, Weidenthal D. Charles Bonnet syndrome precipitated by brimonidine tartrate eye drops. *Br J Ophthalmol.* 2003;87:917–929.
25. Kim DD. A case of suspected Alphagan-induced psychosis. *Arch Ophthalmol.* 2000;118:1132–1133.
26. Rahman I, Fernando B, Harrison M. Charles Bonnet syndrome and brimonidine: comments. *Br J Ophthalmol.* 2004;88(5):724.
27. Garcia-Catalan MR, Arriola-Villalobos P, Santos-Bueso E, et al. Charles Bonnet syndrome precipitated by brimonidine. *Arch Soc Esp Oftalmol.* 2013;88(9):362–364.
28. Tooley AA, Garrity JA. Antiglaucoma medications complicating the management of Graves' ophthalmopathy. *Ophthal Plast Reconstr Surg.* 2018;34(6):600–601.
29. Fraunfelder FT. *Allergic Reaction to Topical Ocular Brimonidine in the Left Eye Only [Photograph]. Follicular Conjunctivitis From Topical Ocular Brimonidine [Photograph].* Portland, OR: Casey Eye Institute, Oregon Health & Science University; ©1990:2 photographs: color.

Drugs: Brinzolamide, dorzolamide hydrochloride

1. Konowal A, Morrison JC, Brown SVL, et al. Irreversible corneal decompensation in patients treated with topical dorzolamide. *Am J Ophthalmol.* 1999;127:403–406.
2. Carlsen J, Durcan J, Zabriskie N, et al. Nephrolithiasis with dorzolamide. *Arch Ophthalmol.* 1999;117:1087–1088.
3. Guedes GB, Karan A, Mayer HR, et al. Evaluation of adverse events in self-reported sulfa-allergic patients using topical carbonic anhydrase inhibitors. *J Ocul Pharmacol Ther.* 2013;29(5):456–461.
4. Tooley AA, Garrity JA. Antiglaucoma medications complicating the management of Graves' ophthalmopathy. *Ophthal Plast Reconstr Surg.* 2018;34(6):600–601.
5. *Brinzolamide.* 2019. Retrieved from http://www.pdr.net.
6. Tanimura H, Minamoto A, Narai A, et al. Corneal edema in glaucoma patients after the addition of brinzolamide 1% ophthalmic suspension. *Jpn J Ophthalmol.* 2005;49:332–333.

Drug: Carteolol hydrochloride

1. *Carteolol Hydrochloride.* 2019. Retrieved from http://www.pdr.net.
2. Baudouin C, de Lunardo C. Short-term comparative study of topical 2% carteolol with and without benzalkonium chloride in healthy volunteers. *Br J Ophthalmol.* 1998;82(1):39–42.
3. Brazier DJ, Smith SE. Ocular and cardiovascular response to topical carteolol 2% and timolol 0.5% in healthy volunteers. *Br J Ophthalmol.* 1988;72:101–103.
4. Kitazawa Y, Horie T, Shirato S. Efficacy and safety of carteolol hydrochloride: a new beta-blocking agent for the treatment of glaucoma. *Int Cong Ophthalmol.* 1983;1:683–685.
5. Stewart WC, Dubiner HB, Mundorf TK, et al. Effects of carteolol and timolol on plasma lipid profiles in older women with ocular hypertension or primary open-angle glaucoma. *Am J Ophthalmol.* 1999;127(2):142–147.

Drug: Metipranolol

1. Melles RB, Wong IG. Metipranolol-associated granulomatous iritis. *Am J Ophthalmol.* 1994;118:712–715.
2. Beck RW, Moke P, Blair RC, et al. Uveitis associated with topical beta blockers. *Arch Ophthalmol.* 1996;114(10):1181–1182.
3. Akingbehin T, Villada JR. Metipranolol-associated granulomatous anterior uveitis. *Br J Ophthalmol.* 1991;75:519–523.
4. Akingbehin T, Villada JR, Walley T. Metipranolol-induced adverse reactions: I. The rechallenge study. *Eye.* 1992;6:277–279.
5. Patel NP, Patel KH, Moster MR, et al. Metipranolol-associated nongranulomatous anterior uveitis. *Am J Ophthalmol.* 1997;123(6):843–846.
6. Watanabe TM, Hodes BL. Bilateral anterior uveitis associated with a brand of metipranolol. *Arch Ophthalmol.* 1997;115:421–422.
7. De Groot AC, Van Ginkel CJ, Bruynzeel DP, et al. Contact allergy to eye drops containing beta blockers. *Ned Tijdschr Geneeskd.* 1998;142(18):1034–1036.
8. Wolf S, Werner E, Schulte K, et al. Acute effect of metipranolol on the retinal circulation. *Br J Ophthalmol.* 1998;82:892–896.
9. *Metipranolol.* 2019. Retrieved from http://www.pdr.net.

Drug: Netarsudil

1. Serle JB, Katz LJ, McLaurin E, et al. Two phase 3 clinical trials comparing the safety and efficacy of netsarsudil to timolol in patients with elevated intraocular pressure: Rho kinase elevation IOP treatment trial 1 and 2 (ROCKET-1 and ROCKET-2). *Am J Ophthalmol.* 2018;186:116–127.
2. *Rhopressa [Package Insert].* Irvine, CA: Aerie Pharmaceuticals, Inc; 2017.
3. Wang S, Chang R. An emerging treatment option for glaucoma: Rho kinase inhibitors. *Clin Ophthalmol.* 2014;8:883–890.

4. Arnold JJ, Hansen MS, Gorman GS, et al. The effect of Rho-associated kinase inhibition on the ocular penetration of timolol maleate. *Invest Ophthalmol Vis Sci.* 2013;54(2):1118–1126.
5. Hahmann C, Schroeter T. Rho-kinase inhibitors as therapeutics: from pan inhibition to isoform selectivity. *Cell Mol Life Sci.* 2010;67(2):171–177.

Drug: Vancomycin

1. Intraocular injections of a compounded triamcinolone, moxifloxacin and vancomycin (TMV) formulation: not recommended for use during cataract surgery. *WHO Pharmaceuticals Newsletter.* 2017;6:12.
2. Nicholson LB, Kim BT, Jardon J, et al. Severe bilateral ischemic retinal vasculitis following cataract surgery. *Ophthalmic Surg Lasers Imaging Retina.* 2014;45(4):338–342.
3. Lenci LT, Chin EK, Carter C, et al. Ischemic retinal vasculitis associated with cataract surgery and intracameral vancomycin. *Case Rep Ophthalmol Med.* 2015;2015:683194.
4. Witkin AJ, Shah AR, Engstrom, et al. Postoperative hemorrhagic occlusive retinal vasculitis: expanding the clinical spectrum and possible association with vancomycin. *Ophthalmology.* 2015;122(7):1438–1451.
5. Balducci N, Savini G, Barboni P, et al. Hemorrhagic occlusive retinal vasculitis after first eye cataract surgery without subsequent second eye involvement. *Ophthalmic Surg Lasers Imaging Retina.* 2016;47(8):764–766.
6. Hsing YE, Park J. Haemorrhagic occlusive retinal vasculitis associated with intracameral vancomycin during cataract surgery. *Clin Exp Ophthalmol.* 2016;44(7):635–637.
7. Miller MA, Lenci LT, Reddy CV, et al. Postoperative hemorrhagic occlusive retinal vasculitis associated with intracameral vancomycin prophylaxis during cataract surgery. *J Cataract Refract Surg.* 2016;42(11):1676–1680.
8. Andreanos K, Petrou P, Kymionis G, et al. Early anti-VEGF treatment for hemorrhagic occlusive retinal vasculitis as a complication of cataract surgery. *BMC Ophthalmol.* 2017;17(1):238.
9. Ehmann DS. Hemorrhagic occlusive retinal vasculitis and nonhemorrhagic vasculitis after uncomplicated cataract surgery with intracameral vancomycin. *Retin Cases Brief Rep.* 2017;11(suppl 1):S155–S158.
10. Witkin AJ, Chang DF, Jumper JM, et al. Vancomycin-associated hemorrhagic occlusive retinal vasculitis: clinical characteristics of 36 eyes. *Ophthalmology.* 2017;124(5):583–595.
11. Todorich B, Faia LJ, Thanos A, et al. Vancomycin-associated hemorrhagic occlusive retinal vasculitis: a clinical-pathophysiological analysis. *Am J Ophthalmol.* 2018;188:131–140.

Drug: Acyclovir (aciclovir)

1. *Acyclovir.* 2019. Retrieved from http://www.pdr.net.
2. Chevret L, Debray D, Poulain C, et al. Neurological toxicity of acyclovir: report of a case in a six-month-old liver transplant recipient. *Pediatr Transplant.* 2006;10(5):632–634.

3. Colin J, Hoh HB, Easty DL, et al. Ganciclovir ophthalmic gel (Virgan; 0.15%) in the treatment of herpes simplex keratitis. *Cornea*. 1997;16(4):393–399.
4. Koliopoulos J. Acyclovir – a promising antiviral agent: a review of the preclinical and clinical data in ocular herpes simplex management. *Ann Ophthalmol*. 1984;16:19–24.
5. Ohashi Y. Treatment of herpetic keratitis with acyclovir: benefits and problems. *Ophthalmologica*. 1997;221(suppl 1):29–32.
6. Richards DM, Carmine AA, Brogden RN, et al. Acyclovir. A review of its pharmacodynamic properties and therapeutic efficacy. *Drugs*. 1983;26:378–438.
7. Wilhelmus KR, Keener MJ, Jones DB, et al. Corneal lipidosis in patients with the acquired immunodeficiency syndrome. *Am J Ophthalmol*. 1995;119:14–19.

Drug: Cidofovir

1. *Cidofovir*. 2019. Retrieved from http://www.pdr.net.
2. Taskintuna I, Rahhal FM, Rao NA, et al. Adverse events and autopsy findings after intravitreous cidofovir (HPMPC) therapy in patients with acquired immune deficiency syndrome (AIDS). *Ophthalmology*. 1997;104(11):1827–1836.
3. Taskintuna I, Rahhal FM, Arevalo JF, et al. Low-dose intravitreal cidofovir (HPMPC) therapy of cytomegalovirus retinitis in patients with acquired immune deficiency syndrome. *Ophthalmology*. 1997;104(6):1049–1057.
4. Chavez de la Paz E, Arevalo JF, Kirsch LS, et al. Anterior nongranulomatous uveitis after intravitreal HPMPC (cidofovir) for the treatment of cytomegalovirus retinitis. Analysis and prevention. *Ophthalmology*. 1997;104(3):539–544.
5. Kirsch LS, Arevalo JF, De Clercq E. Phase I/II study of intravitreal cidofovir for the treatment of cytomegalovirus retinitis in patients with the acquired immunodeficiency syndrome. *Am J Ophthalmol*. 1995;119(4):466–476.
6. Davis JL, Taskintuna I, Freeman WR, et al. Iritis and hypotony after treatment with intravenous cidofovir for cytomegalovirus retinitis. *Arch Ophthalmol*. 1997;115(6):733–736.
7. Akler ME, Johnson DW, Burman WJ, et al. Anterior uveitis and hypotony after intravenous cidofovir for the treatment of cytomegalovirus retinitis. *Ophthalmology*. 1998;105(4):651–657.
8. Friedberg DN. Hypotony and visual loss with intravenous cidofovir treatment of cytomegalovirus retinitis. *Arch Ophthalmol*. 1997;115:801–802.
9. Orssaud C, Wermert D, Roux A, et al. Urrets-Zavalia syndrome as a complication of ocular hypotonia due to intravenous cidofovir treatment. *Eye (Lond)*. 2014;28(6):776–777.
10. Accorinti M, Ciapparoni V, Pirraglia MP, et al. Treatment of severe ocular hypotony in AIDS patients with cytomegalovirus retinitis and cidofovir-associated uveitis. *Ocul Immunol Inflamm*. 2001;9(3):211–217.
11. Soltau JB. Treatment of severe ocular hypotony in AIDS patients with cytomegalovirus retinitis and cidofovir-associated uveitis. *Ocul Immunol Inflamm*. 2001;9(3):137–139.
12. Hillenkamp J, Reinhard T, Rudolf RS, et al. The effects of cidofovir 1% with and without cyclosporin A 1% as a topical treatment of acute adenoviral keratoconjunctivitis. A controlled clinical pilot study. *Ophthalmology*. 2002;109:845–850.

Drugs: Idoxuridine (IDU), trifluridine (F3T, trifluorothymidine), vidarabine (ara-A)

1. *Trifluridine*. 2019. Retrieved from http://www.pdr.net.
2. Falcon MG, Jones BR, Williams HP, et al. Adverse reactions in the eye from topical therapy with idoxuridine, adenine arabinoside and trifluorothymidine. In: Sundmacher R, ed. *Herpetische Augenerkrankungen*. Munich: JF Bergmann; 1981:263–268.
3. Shearer DR, Bourne WM. Severe ocular anterior segment ischemia after long-term trifluridine treatment for presumed herpetic keratitis. *Am J Ophthalmol*. 1990;109:346–347.
4. Jayamanne DGR, Vize C, Ellerton CR, et al. Severe reversible ocular anterior segment ischaemia following topical trifluorothymidine (F3T) treatment for herpes simplex keratouveitis (letter). *Eye*. 1997;11(Pt 5):757–759.
5. Spalton DJ, Hitchings RA, Hunter PA. *Atlas of Clinical Ophthalmology*. 3rd ed. London: Mosby Elsevier; 2005.

Drugs: Acetazolamide, methazolamide

1. Mancino R, Varesi C, Cerulli A, et al. Acute bilateral angle-closure glaucoma and choroidal effusion associated with acetazolamide administration after cataract surgery. *J Cat Refract Surg*. 2011;37(2):415–417.
2. Parthasarathi S, Myint K, Singh G, et al. Bilateral acetazolamide-induced choroidal effusion following cataract surgery. *Eye*. 2007;21(6):870–872.
3. Vela MA, Campbell DG. Hypotony and ciliochoroidal detachment following pharmacologic aqueous suppressant therapy in previously filtered patients. *Ophthalmology*. 1985;92:50–57.
4. De Rojas V, Gonzalez-Lopez F, Baviera J. Acetazolamide-induced bilateral choroidal effusion following insertion of a phakic implantable collamer lens. *J Refract Surg*. 2013;29(8):570–572.
5. Grigera JD, Grigera ED. Ultrasound biomicroscopy in acetazolamide-induced myopic shift with appositional angle closure. *Arq Bras Oftalmol*. 2017;80(5):327–329.
6. Hari-Kovacs A, Soos J, Gyetvai T, et al. Case report on choroidal effusion after oral acetazolamide administration: an unusual manifestation of a well-known idiosyncratic effect? *Orv Hetil*. 2017;158(50):1998–2002.
7. Szawarski P, Hall-Thompson B. Acetazolamide-induced myopia at altitude. *Wilderness Environ Med*. 2009;20(3):300–301.
8. Firth PG, Gray C, Novis CA. High-altitude corneal oedema associated with acetazolamide. *SAMJ*. 2011;101(7):462.
9. Apushkin MA, Fishman GA, Grover S, et al. Rebound of cystoids macular edema with continued use of acetazolamide in patients with retinitis pigmentosa. *Retina*. 2007;27:1112–1118.

10. *Acetazolamide*. 2019. Retrieved from http://www.pdr.net.
11. Shuster JN. Side effects of commonly used glaucoma medications. *Geriatr Ophthalmol.* 1986;2:30.
12. Barbey F, Nseir G, Ferrier C, et al. Carbonic anhydrase inhibitors and calcium phosphate stones. *Nephrologie.* 2004;25:169–172.
13. Au JN, Waslo CS, McGwin Jr G, et al. Acetazolamide-induced nephrolithiasis in idiopathic intracranial hypertension patients. *J Neuroophthalmol.* 2016;36(2):126–130.
14. Jachiet M, Bellon N, Assier H, et al. Cutaneous adverse drug reaction to oral acetazolamide and skin tests. *Dermatology.* 2013;226(4):347–352.
15. Flach AJ, Smith RE, Fraunfelder FT. Stevens-Johnson syndrome associated with methazolamide treatment reported in two Japanese-American women. *Ophthalmology.* 1995;102:1677–1680.
16. Tabbara KF, Al-Faisal Z, Al-Rashed W. Interaction between acetazolamide and cyclosporine. *Arch Ophthalmol.* 1998;116:832–833.
17. Keisu M, Wiholm BE, Ost A, et al. Acetazolamide-associated aplastic anemia. *J Int Med.* 1990;228:627–632.

Drugs: Naphazoline hydrochloride, tetryzoline hydrochloride (tetrahydrozoline)

1. Lasala GS, Vearrier D, Boroughf W, et al. Munchausen syndrome by proxy due to tetrahydrozoline poisoning. *Clin Toxicol.* 2014;52(7):746.
2. Al-Abri SA, Yang HS, Olson KR. Unintentional pediatric ophthalmic tetrahydrozoline ingestion: case files of the medical toxicology fellowship at the University of California, San Francisco. *J Med Toxicol.* 2014;10(4):388–391.
3. Nakatsuka AS, Beaver HA, Lee AG. Mydriasis due to Opcon-A: an indication to avoid pharmacologic testing for anisocoria. *Can J Ophthalmol.* 2018;53(1):e6–e7.
4. Cook Jr BE, Holtan SB. Mydriasis from inadvertent topical application of naphazoline hydrochloride *(Opcon-A, Bausch & Lomb)*. *CLAO J.* 1998;24(2):72.
5. Keklikoglu HD, Gilbert A, Torun N. Transient mydriasis due to Opcon-A. *Austin J Clin Ophthalmol.* 2015;2:1049.
6. Williams TL, Williams AJ, Enzenauer RW. Case report: unilateral mydriasis from topical Opcon-A and soft contact lens. *Aviat Space Environ Med.* 1997;68:1035–1037.
7. *Naphazoline Hydrochloride*. 2019. Retrieved from http://www.pdr.net.
8. Kisilevsky E, DeAngelis DD. Anterior and posterior segment vasculopathy associated with long-term use of tetrahydrozoline. *CMAJ.* 2018;190(40):e1208.
9. Soparkar CN, Wilhelmus KR, Koch DD, et al. Acute and chronic conjunctivitis due to over-the-counter ophthalmic decongestants. *Arch Ophthalmol.* 1997;115(1):34–38.
10. Mendonca TB, Lummertz AP, Bocaccio FJL, et al. Effect of low-concentration, nonmydriatic selective alpha-adrenergic agonist eyedrops on upper eyelid position. *Dermatol Surg.* 2017;43(2):270–274.
11. *Tetrahydrozoline*. 2019. Retrieved from https://toxnet.nlm.nih.gov.
12. Stillwell ME, Saady JJ. Use of tetrahydrozoline for chemical submission. *Forensic Sci Int.* 2012;221(1-3):e12–e16.

Drug: Acetylcholine chloride

1. *Product Information. Miochol* (acetylcholine chloride, intraocular). Duluth, GA: Ciba Vision Ophthalmics.
2. *Miochol-E Side Effects*. 2019. Retrieved from https://www.drugs.com.
3. Fraunfelder FT. Corneal edema after use of carbachol. *Arch Ophthalmol.* 1979;97:975.
4. Grimmett MR, Williams KK, Broocker G, et al. Corneal edema after miochol (letter). *Am J Ophthalmol.* 1993;116(2):236–238.
5. Lazar M, Rosen N, Nemet P. Miochol-induced transient cataract. *Ann Ophthalmol.* 1977;9:1142–1143.
6. Rosen N, Lazar M. The mechanism of the Miochol lens opacity. *Am J Ophthalmol.* 1978;86(4):570–571.
7. Hagan J. Severe bradycardia and hypotension following intraocular acetylcholine in patients who previously tolerated the medication. *Missouri Med.* 1990;87:231–233.
8. Gombos GM. Systemic reactions following intraocular acetylcholine instillation. *Ann Ophthalmol.* 1982;11:529–530.
9. Brinkley Jr JR, Henrick A. Vascular hypotension and bradycardia following intraocular injection of acetylcholine during cataract surgery. *Am J Ophthalmol.* 1984;97:40–42.

Drug: Echothiophate iodide (ecotiophate)

1. *Echothiophate Iodide*. 2019. Retrieved from http://www.pdr.net.
2. Eggers NM. Toxicity of drugs used in diagnosis and treatment of strabismus. In: Srinivasan D, ed. *Ocular Therapeutics*. New York: Masson; 1980:115–122.
3. Eshagian J. Human posterior subcapsular cataracts. *Trans Ophthalmol Soc UK.* 1982;102:364–368.
4. West RH, Cebon L, Gillies WE. Drop attack in glaucoma. The Melbourne experience with topical miotics, adrenergic and neuronal blocking drops. *Aust J Ophthalmol.* 1983;11:149–153.
5. Beasley H, Fraunfelder FT. Retinal detachments and topical ocular miotics. *Ophthalmology.* 1979;86(1):95–98.
6. Halperin LS, Goldman HB. Cystoid macular edema associated with topical ecothiophate iodide. *Ann Ophthalmol.* 1993;25(12):457–458.
7. Flore PM, Jacobs IH, Goldberg DB. Drug-induced pemphigoid. *Arch Ophthalmol.* 1987;105:1660–1663.
8. Pouliquen Y, Patey A, Foster CS, et al. Drug-induced cicatricial pemphigoid affecting the conjunctiva. *Ophthalmology.* 1986;93(6):775–783.
9. Schwab IR, Linberg JV, Gioia VM, et al. Foreshortening of the inferior conjunctival fornix associated with chronic glaucoma medications. *Ophthalmology.* 1992;99(2):197–202.
10. Adams SL, Mathews J, Grammer LC. Drugs that may exacerbate myasthenia gravis. *Ann Emerg Med.* 1984;13:532–538.
11. Mezer E, Krivoy N, Scharf J, et al. Ecothiophate iodide induced transient hyper- and hypothyroidism. *J Glaucoma.* 1996;5(3):191–192.

12. Adler AG, McElwain GE, Merli GJ, et al. Systemic effects of eye drops. *Arch Intern Med.* 1982;142:2293–2294.

Drug: Pilocarpine hydrochloride

1. Baudouin C, Pisella PJ, Fillacier K, et al. Ocular surface inflammatory changes induced by topical antiglaucoma drugs: Human and animal studies. *Ophthalmology.* 1999;106(3):556–563.
2. Naveh-Floman N, Stahl V, Korczyn AD. Effect of pilocarpine on intraocular pressure in ocular hypertensive subjects. *Ophthalmic Res.* 1986;18:34–37.
3. Nuzzi R, Finazzo C, Cerruti A. Adverse effects of topical antiglaucomatous medications on the conjunctiva and the lachrymal response. *Intern Ophthalmol.* 1998;22(1):31–35.
4. *Pilocarpine Hydrochloride.* 2019. Retrieved from http://www.pdr.net.
5. Abramson DH, MacKay C, Coleman J. Pilocarpine-induced retinal tear: an ultrasonic evaluation of lens movements. *Glaucoma.* 1981;3:9.
6. Beasley H, Fraunfelder FT. Retinal detachments and topical ocular miotics. *Ophthalmology.* 1979;86(1):95–98.
7. Benedict WL, Shami M. Impending macular hole associated with topical pilocarpine. *Am J Ophthalmol.* 1992;114(6):765–766.
8. Walker JD, Alvarez MM. Vitreofoveal traction associated with the use of pilocarpine to reverse mydriasis. *Eye.* 2007;21(11):1430–1431.
9. Schuman JS, Hersh P, Kylstra J. Vitreous hemorrhage associated with pilocarpine. *Am J Ophthalmol.* 1989;108(3):333–334.
10. Massry GG, Assil KK. Pilocarpine-associated allograft rejection in postkeratoplasty patients. *Cornea.* 1995;14(2):202–205.
11. Kobayashi H, Kobayashi K, Kiryu J, et al. Pilocarpine induces an increase in the anterior chamber angular width in eyes with narrow angles. *Br J Ophthalmol.* 1999;83:553–558.
12. Fraunfelder FT, Morgan R. The aggravation of dementia by pilocarpine. *JAMA.* 1994;271(22):1742–1743.
13. Reyes PF, Dwyer BA, Schwartzman RJ, et al. Mental status changes induced by eye drops in dementia of the Alzheimer type. *J Neurol Neurosurg Psychiatry.* 1987;50:113–115.
14. Fox C, Richardson K, Maidment ID, et al. Anticholinergic medication use and cognitive impairment in the older population: the medical research council cognitive function and ageing study. *J Am Geriatr Soc.* 2011;59(8):1477–1483.
15. Tsao J, Shah R, Leurgans S, et al. Impaired cognition in normal individuals using medications with anticholinergic activity occurs following several years. *60th Annual Meeting of the American Academy of Neurology.* 2008; abstr S51.001.
16. Crandall AS, Levy N, Dunbar Hoskins H, et al. Characterization of subtle corneal deposits. *J Toxicol Cut Ocular Toxicol.* 1984:263.

17. Sherwood MB, Grierson I, Millar L, et al. Long-term morphologic effects of antiglaucoma drugs on the conjunctiva and Tenon's capsule in glaucomatous patients. *Ophthalmology.* 1989;96(3):327–335.
18. Flore PM, Jacobs IH, Goldberg DB. Drug-induced pemphigoid. *Arch Ophthalmol.* 1987;105:1660–1663.
19. Pouliquen Y, Patey A, Foster CS, et al. Drug-induced cicatricial pemphigoid affecting the conjunctiva. *Ophthalmology.* 1986;93(6):775–783.
20. Schwab IR, Linberg JV, Gioia VM, et al. Foreshortening of the inferior conjunctival fornix associated with chronic glaucoma medications. *Ophthalmology.* 1992;99(2):197–202.
21. Samples JR, Meyer SM. Use of ophthalmic medications in pregnant and nursing women. *Am J Ophthalmol.* 1988;106(5):616–623.
22. Spalton DJ, Hitchings RA, Hunter PA. *Atlas of Clinical Ophthalmology.* 3rd ed. London: Mosby Elsevier; 2005.

Drugs: Cyclopentolate hydrochloride, tropicamide

1. Brooks AM, West RH, Gillies WE. The risks of precipitating acute angle-closure glaucoma with the clinical use of mydriatic agents. *Med J Aust.* 1986;145:34–36.
2. Mori M, Araie M, Sakurai M, et al. Effects of pilocarpine and tropicamide on blood–aqueous permeability in man. *Invest Ophthalmol Vis Sci.* 1992;33(2):416–423.
3. McCormack DL. Reduced mydriasis from repeated doses of tropicamide and cyclopentolate. *Ophthalmic Surg.* 1990;21(7):508–512.
4. Akkaya C, Zorlu Kocagoz S, Sarandol A, et al. Addiction to topically used cyclopentolate hydrochloride: a case report. *Prog Neuropsychopharmacol Biol Psychiatry.* 2008;32:1752–1753.
5. Buhrich N, Weller A, Kevans P. Misuse of anticholinergic drugs by people with serious mental illness. *Psychiatr Serv.* 2005;51:928–929.
6. Crouch BI, Caravati EM, Booth J. Trends in child and teen nonprescription drug abuse reported to a regional poison control center. *Am J Health Syst Pharm.* 2004;61:1252–1257.
7. Darcin AE, Dilbaz N, Yilmaz S, et al. Cyclopentolate hydrochloride eye drops addiction: a case report. *J Addict Med.* 2011;5(1):84–85.
8. Ostler HB. Cycloplegics and mydriatics. Tolerance, habituation, and addiction to topical administration. *Arch Ophthalmol.* 1975;93:423–513.
9. Pullen GP, Best NR, Maguire J. Anticholinergic drug abuse: a common problem? *Br Med J (Clin Res Ed).* 1984;289:612–613.
10. Sato EH, de Freitas D, Foster CS. Abuse of cyclopentolate hydrochloride (Cyclogyl) drops. *N Engl J Med.* 1992;326:1363–1364.
11. Kellner U, Esser J. Acute psychosis caused by cyclopentolate. *Klin Mbl Augenheilk.* 1989;194:458–461.
12. Shihab ZM. Psychotic reaction in an adult after topical cyclopentolate. *Ophthalmologica.* 1980;181:228–230.

13. Mirshahi A, Kohnen T. Acute psychotic reaction caused by topical cyclopentolate use for cycloplegic refraction before refractive surgery. *J Cataract Refract Surg.* 2003;29:1026–1030.
14. Marti J, Anton E, Ezcurra I. An unexpected cause of delirium in an old patient. *J Am Geriatr Soc.* 2005;52:545.
15. Hermansen MC, Sullivan LS. Feeding intolerance following ophthalmologic examination. *Am J Dis Child.* 1985;139:367–368.
16. Isenberg SJ, Abrams C, Hyman PE. Effects of cyclopentolate eyedrops on gastric secretory function in pre-term infants. *Ophthalmology.* 1985;92:698–700.
17. Sarici SU, Yurdakok M, Unal S. Acute gastric dilatation complicating the use of mydriatics in a preterm newborn. *Pediatr Radiol.* 2001;31:581–583.
18. Lim DL, Batilando M, Rajadurai VS. Transient paralytic ileus following the use of cyclopentolate-phenylephrine eye drops during screening for retinopathy of prematurity. *J Paediatr Child Health.* 2003;39:318–320.
19. Newman DK, Jordan K. Generalized urticaria induced by topical cyclopentolate. *Eye.* 1996;10(Pt 6):750–751.
20. Meyer D, Hamilton RC, Gimbel HV. Myasthenia gravis-like syndrome induced by topical ophthalmic preparations. a case report. *J Clin Neuro-Ophthalmol.* 1992;12(3):210–212.
21. Tayman C, Mete E, Catal F, et al. Anaphylactic reaction due to cyclopentolate in a 4-year-old child. *J Investig Allergol Clin Immunol.* 2010;20(4):347–348.

Drug: Hydroxyamphetamine hydrobromide (hydroxyamfetamine)

1. Rebecca Lurcott for Ophthalmology Management. *Unique Mydriatic Returns: the Combination Formula Fosters Patient Flow Efficiencies*; 2002.
2. Grant WM. *Toxicology of the Eye.* 2nd ed. Springfield, IL: Charles C Thomas; 1974:567–568.
3. Kronfeld PC, McGarry HI, Smith HE. The effect of mydriatics upon the intraocular pressure in so-called primary wide-angle glaucoma. *Am J Ophthalmol.* 1943;26:245.
4. Munden PM, Kardon RH, Denison CE, et al. Palpebral fissure responses to topical adrenergic drugs. *Am J Ophthalmol.* 1991;111:706–710.
5. Priest JH. Atropine response of the eyes in mongolism. *Am J Dis Child.* 1960;100:869–872.
6. Allergan Lamber J. letter advising of 3 serious adverse events following use of Paremyd. *January.* 1996;7.

Drugs: Botulinum toxin A (abobotulinumtoxinA, incobotulinumtoxinA, onabotulinumtoxinA), botulinum toxin B (rimabotulinumtoxinB)

1. Taylan Sekeroglu H, Kocabeyoglu S, Mocan MC, et al. Ocular surface changes following botulinum toxin injection for strabismus. *Cutan Ocul Toxicol.* 2015;34(3):185–188.
2. OnabotulinumtoxinA. 2019. Retrieved from http://www.pdr.net.
3. Kane MA, Brandt F, Rohrich RJ, et al. Evaluation of variable-dose treatment with a new US Botulinum Toxin Type A (Dysport) for correction of moderate to severe glabellar lines: results from a phase III, randomized, double-blind, placebo-controlled study. *Plast Reconstr Surg.* 2009;124:1619–1629.
4. Cavallini M, Cirillo P, Fundaro SP, et al. Safety of botulinum toxin A in aesthetic treatments: a systematic review of clinical studies. *Dermatol Surg.* 2014;40(5):525–536.
5. Chang YS, Chang CC, Shen JH, et al. Nonallergic eyelid edema after botulinum toxin type A injection: case report and review of literature. *Medicine (Baltimore).* 2015;94(38):e1610.
6. Wutthiphan S, Kowal L, O'Day J, et al. Diplopia following subcutaneous injections of botulinum A toxin for facial spasms. *J Pediatr Ophthalmol Strabismus.* 1997;34(4):229–234.
7. Pediatric Eye Disease Investigator Group, Christiansen SP, Chandler DL, et al. Tonic pupil after botulinum toxin-A injection for treatment of esotropia in children. *J AAPOS.* 2016;20(1):78–81.
8. Corridan P, Nightingale S, Mashoudi N, et al. Acute angle-closure glaucoma following botulinum toxin injection for blepharospasm. *Br J Ophthalmol.* 1990;74:309–310.
9. Keech RV, Morris RJ, Ruben JB, et al. Anterior segment ischemia following vertical muscle transposition and botulinum toxin injection. *Arch Ophthalmol.* 1990;108:176.
10. Sanders DB, Massey EW, Buckley EG. Botulinum toxin for blepharospasm. *Neurology.* 1986;36:545–547.
11. Roehm PC, Perry JD, Girkin CA, et al. Prevalence of periocular depigmentation after repeated botulinum toxin A injections in African American patients. *J Neuro-Ophthalmol.* 1999;19(1):7–9.
12. Friedland S, Burde RM. Porcelinizing discoloration of the periocular skin following botulinum A toxin injections. *J Neuroophthalmol.* 1996;16:70–71.
13. Nussgens Z, Roggenkamper P. Comparison of two botulinum-toxin preparations in the treatment of essential blepharospasm. *Graefes Arch Clin Exp Ophthalmol.* 1997;235(4):197–199.
14. Ramappa M, Jiya PY, Chaurasia S, et al. Reactivation of herpes simplex viral keratitis following botulinum toxin injection. *Indian J Ophthalmol.* 2018;66(2):306–308.
15. Gadient PM, Smith JH, Ryan SJ. Herpes zoster ophthalmicus following onabotulinumtoxinA administration for chronic migraine: a case report and literature review. *Cephalalgia.* 2015;35(5):443–448.
16. Vleming EN, Pérez-Rico C, Montes MA, et al. Persistent corneal defects treated with botulinum toxin-induced ptosis. *Arch Soc Esp Oftalmol.* 2007;82:547–550.

Drug: Fluorescein sodium

1. Kwiterovich KA, Maguire MG, Murphy RP, et al. Frequency of adverse systemic reactions after fluorescein angiography; results of a prospective study. *Surv Ophthalmol.* 1991;98(7):1139–1142.
2. Bregu M, Tesha PE, Wong DT, et al. Nausea and fluorescein injection speed. *Ophthalmology.* 2012;119(6). 1281–1281.
3. Bearelly S, Rao S, Fekrat S. Anaphylaxis following intravenous fluorescein angiography in a vitreoretinal clinic: report of 4 cases. *Can J Ophthalmol.* 2009;44(4):444–445.

4. Butrus SI, Negvesky GJ, Rivera-Velazques PM, et al. Serum tryptase: an indicator of anaphylaxis following fluorescein angiography. *Graefes Arch Clin Exp Ophthalmol.* 1999;237(5):433–434.

5. Hitosugi M, Omura K, Yokoyama T, et al. An autopsy case of fatal anaphylactic shock following fluorescein angiography: a case report. *Med Sci Law.* 2004;44:264–265.

6. Balbino M, Silva G, Correia GC. Anaphylaxis with convulsions following intravenous fluorescein angiography at an outpatient clinic. *Einstein (Sao Paulo).* 2012;10(3):374–376.

7. Danis RP, Stephens T. Phototoxic reactions caused by sodium fluorescein. *Am J Ophthalmol.* 1997;123(5):694–696.

8. Johnson RN, McDonald HR, Schatz H. Rash, fever, chills after intravenous fluorescein angiography. *Am J Ophthalmol.* 1998;126(6):837–838.

9. Hara T, Inami M, Hara T. Efficacy and safety of fluorescein angiography with orally administered sodium fluorescein. *Am J Ophthalmol.* 1998;126(4):560–564.

10. Kratz RP, Davidson B. A case report of skin necrosis following infiltration with IV fluorescein. *Ophthalmology.* 1980;12:654–656.

11. Brodsky ME, Bauerberg JM, Sterzovsky A. Case report: probably fluorescein-induced uveitis following radial keratotomy. *J Refract Surg.* 1987;3(1):29.

12. Valvano MN, Martin TP. Periorbital urticaria and topical fluorescein. *Am J Emerg Med.* 1998;16(5):525–526.

Drug: Indocyanine green (ICG)

1. Cheng S-N, Yang T-C, Ho J-D, et al. Ocular toxicity of intravitreal indocyanine green. *J Ocul Pharmacol Ther.* 2005;21:85–93.

2. Kanda S, Uemura A, Yamashita T, et al. Visual field defects after intravitreous administration of indocyanine green in macular hole surgery. *Arch Ophthalmol.* 2004;122:1447–1451.

3. Uemura A, Kanda S, Sakamoto Y, et al. Visual field defects after uneventful vitrectomy for epiretinal membrane with indocyanine green-assisted internal limiting membrane peeling. *Am J Ophthalmol.* 2003;136:252–257.

4. Thompson JT. Indocyanine green should be used to facilitate removal of the internal limiting membrane in macular hole surgery. *Surv Ophthalmol.* 2009;54(1):135–138.

5. Gale JS, Proulx AA, Gonder JR, et al. Comparison of the in vitro toxicity of indocyanine green to that of trypan blue in human retinal pigment epithelium cell cultures. *Am J Ophthalmol.* 2004;138:64–69.

6. Ho J-D, Tsai RJ, Chen S-N, et al. Toxic effect of indocyanine green on retinal pigment epithelium related to osmotic effects of the solvent. *Am J Ophthalmol.* 2003;135:258–259.

7. Ho J-D, Tsai RJ, Chen S-N, et al. Cytotoxicity of indocyanine green on retinal pigment epithelium. *Arch Ophthalmol.* 2003;121:1423–1429.

8. Gulkilik G, Balci O, Eliacik M, et al. Late phototoxicity after indocyanine green assisted internal limiting membrane peeling. *Ophthalmic Res.* 2016;56(suppl 1):23.

9. Hope-Ross M, Yannuzzi LA, Gragoudas ES, et al. Adverse reactions due to indocyanine green. *Ophthalmology.* 1994;101(3):529–533.

10. Bonte CA, Ceuppens J, Leys AM. Hypotensive shock as a complication of infracyanine green injection. *Retina.* 1998;18(5):476–477.

11. Nanikawa R, Hayashi T, Hayashi K, et al. A case of fatal shock induced by indocyanine green (ICG) test. *Jpn Leg Med.* 1978;32:209–214.

12. Olsen TW, Lim JI, Capone Jr A, et al. Anaphylactic shock following indocyanine green angiography (letter). *Arch Ophthalmol.* 1996;114(1):97.

13. Speich R, Saesseli B, Hoffmann U, et al. Anaphylactoid reactions after indocyanine green administration. *Ann Intern Med.* 1988;109:345–346.

Drugs: Lissamine green, rose bengal

1. Feensra RP, Tseng SC. What is actually stained by rose bengal? *Arch Ophthalmol.* 1992;110:984–993.

2. Lee YC, Park CK, Kim MS, et al. In vitro study for staining and toxicity of rose bengal on cultured bovine corneal endothelial cells. *Cornea.* 1996;15(4):376–385.

3. Manning FJ, Wehrly SR, Foulks GN. Patient tolerance and ocular surface staining characteristics of lissamine green versus rose bengal. *Ophthalmology.* 1995;102(12):1953–1957.

4. Seitzman GD, Cevallos V, Margoli TP. Rose bengal and lissamine green inhibit detection of herpes simplex virus by PCR. *Am J Ophthalmol.* 2006;141:756–758.

Drug: Trypan blue

1. Birchall W, Matthew R, Turner G. Inadvertent staining of the posterior lens capsule with trypan blue dye during phacoemulsification. *Arch Ophthalmol.* 2001;119:1082–1083.

2. Jhanji V, Agarwal T, Titiyal JS. Inadvertent corneal stromal staining by trypan blue during cataract surgery. *J Cataract Refract Surg.* 2008;34:161–162.

3. Kheirkhah A, Nazari R, Roohipour R. Inadvertent vitreous staining with trypan blue in pseudoexfoliation syndrome. *Arch Ophthalmol.* 2010;128(10):1372–1373.

4. Tsui I, Tsui IK, Auran JD, et al. Cerulean fundus: an unexpected complication of cataract surgery in an eye with aqueous misdirection. *Br J Ophthalmol.* 2010;94(8):1105–1106.

5. Pelit A. Unintentional staining of the posterior lens capsule with trypan blue dye during phacoemulsification: case report. *Intern Ophthalmol.* 2012;32(2):187–189.

6. Saeed MU, Heimann H. Atrophy of the retinal pigment epithelium following vitrectomy with trypan blue. *Intern Ophthalmol.* 2009;29(4):239–241.

7. Dick HB, Aliyeva SE, Hengerer F. Effect of trypan blue on the elasticity of the human anterior lens capsule. *J Cataract Refract Surg.* 2008;34(8):1367–1373.

8. John T, Patel A, Vasavada A, et al. Effect of trypan blue on Descemet membrane elasticity. *Cornea.* 2016;35(11):1401–1403.

9. Buzard K, Zhang JR, Thumann G, et al. Two cases of toxic anterior segment syndrome from generic trypan blue. *J Cataract Refract Surg.* 2010;36(12):e2195–e2199.

10. Matsou A, Tzamalis A, Chalvatzis N, et al. Generic trypan blue as possible cause of a cluster toxic anterior segment syndrome cases after uneventful cataract surgery. *J Cataract Refract Surg.* 2017;43(6):848–852.

11. Baldwin A, Risma J, Longmuir S. Transient leopard spot corneal endothelial staining with trypan blue during cataract surgery in a child with congenital rubella syndrome. *J AAPOS.* 2013;17(6):629–631.

12. Marcon A, Perillat N, Garcin T, et al. Transplantation blues: inadvertent staining of amyloid deposits with trypan blue. *Cornea.* 2018;37(7):824–828.

Drugs: Organic pigments (metal salts), inorganic pigments (iron and zinc oxides)

1. Kojima T, Dogru M, Matsumoto Y, et al. Tear film and ocular surface abnormalities after eyelid tattooing: a case report. *Ophthalmic Plast Reconstr Surg.* 2005;21(1):69–71.

2. Lee YB, Kim JJ, Hyon JY, et al. Eyelid tattooing induces Meibomian gland loss and tear film instability. *Cornea.* 2015;34(7):750–755.

3. Bussel II , Dhaliwal DK. Cosmetic eyeliner tattoo as risk factor for ocular surface disease. *Ophthalmology Times Jan.* 2018;1.

4. Tse DT, Folberg R, Moore K. Clinicopathologic correlate of a fresh eyelid pigment implantation. *Arch Ophthalmol.* 1985;103(10):1515–1517, 1985.

5. Bee CR, Steele EA, White KP, et al. Tattoo granuloma of the eyelid mimicking carcinoma. *Ophthalmic Plast Reconstr Surg.* 2014;30(1):e15–e17.

6. Schwarze HP, Giordano-Labadie F, Loche F, et al. Delayed-hypersensitivity granulomatous reaction induced by blepharopigmentation with aluminum-silicate. *J Am Acad Dermatol.* 2000;42(5 Pt 2):888–891.

7. Goldberg RA, Shorr N. Complications of blepharopigmentation. *Ophthalmic Surg.* 1989;20(6):420–423.

8. Vagefi MR, Dragan L, Hughes SM, et al. Adverse reactions to permanent eyeliner tattoo. *Ophthalmic Plast Reconstr Surg.* 2006;22(1):48–51.

9. Rorsman H, Brehmer-Andersson E, Dahlquist I, et al. Tattoo granuloma and uveitis. *Lancet.* 1969;2(7610):27–28.

10. Ostheimer TA, Burkholder BM, Leung TG, et al. Tattoo-associated uveitis. *Am J Ophthalmol.* 2014;158(3):637–643.

11. Pandya VB, Hooper CY, Essex RW, et al. Tattoo-associated uveitis. *Am J Ophthalmol.* 2014;158(6):1355–1356.

Drugs: Perfluorooctaine, perfluoroperhydrophenanthrene

1. Elsing SH, Fekrat S, Green R, et al. Clinicopathologic findings in eyes with retained perfluoro-n-octane liquid. *Ophthalmology.* 2001;108(1):45–48.

2. Tewari A, Eliott D, Singh CN, et al. Changes in retinal sensitivity from retained subretinal perfluorocarbon liquid. *Retina.* 2009;29(2):248–250.

3. Alharbi SS, Asiri MS. Reversible corneal toxicity of retained intracameral perfluoro-n-octane. *Middle East Afr J Ophthalmol.* 2016;23(3):277–279.

4. Nazarali S, Lapere S, Somani R, et al. A rare case of perfluoro-n-octane in the orbit following vitreoretinal surgery. *Can J Ophthalmol.* 2017;52(3):e113–e115.

Drugs: Polydimethylsiloxane (PMDS), silicone

1. Rapoza PA, Ruddat MS. Pyogenic granuloma as a complication of silicone punctal plugs. *Am J Ophthalmol.* 1992;113(4):454–455.

2. Amemiya T, Dake Y. Granuloma after augmentation of the eyelids with liquid silicone: an electron microscope study. *Ophthalmic Plast Reconstr Surg.* 1994;10(1):51–56.

3. Jackson TL, Thiagarajan M, Murthy R, et al. Pupil block glaucoma in phakic and pseudophakic patients after vitrectomy with silicone oil injection. *Am J Ophthalmol.* 2001;132:414–416.

4. Yusuf IH, Fung TH, Salmon JF, et al. Silicone oil pupil block glaucoma in a pseudophakic eye. *BMJ Case Reports Sept.* 2014;23.

5. Apple DJ, Federman JL, Krolicki TJ, et al. Irreversible silicone oil adhesion to silicone intraocular lenses. *Ophthalmology.* 1996;103(10):1555–1562.

6. Shalchi Z, Mahroo OA, Shunmugam M, et al. Spectral domain optic coherence tomography findings in long-term silicone oil-related visual loss. *Retina.* 2015;35(3):555–563.

7. Nicholson BP, Bakri SJ. Silicone oil emulsification at the fovea as a reversible cause of vision loss. *JAMA Ophthalmol.* 2015;133(4):484–486.

8. Karth PA, Moshfeghi DM. Spectral-domain optic coherence tomography of emulsified subretinal silicone oil presenting as a macular inverted pseudohypopyon. *Ophthalmic Surg Lasers Imaging Retina.* 2014;45(5):437–439.

9. Falavarjani GK, Modarres M. Double pseudohypopyon from emulsified heavy silicone oil. *Retin Cases Brief Rep.* 2017;11(2):126–127.

10. Gargallo Vaamonde A, Ibañez Muñoz D, Salceda Artola J, et al. Silicone oil migration along the optic nerve after intraocular tamponade. *Arch Soc Esp Oftalmol.* 2016;91(11):535–538.

11. Shields CL, et al. Silicone oil. Optic atrophy: case report. *Arch Ophthalmol.* 1989;107:683–686.

12. Knecht P, Groscurth P, Ziegler U, et al. Is silicone oil optic neuropathy caused by high intraocular pressure alone? A semi-biological model. *Br J Ophthalmol.* 2007;91:1293–1295.

13. Del Bufalo F, Mastronuzzi A, De Vito R, et al. Systemic granulomatosis after surgical injection of silicone oil for retinal detachment in a child affected by Fisher-Evans syndrome. *Eur Rev Med Pharmacol Sci.* 2015;19(3):375–380.

14. Eckle D, Kampik A, Hintschich C, et al. Visual field defect in association with chiasmal migration of intraocular silicone oil. *Br J Ophthalmol.* 2005;89:918–920.

15. Fangtian D, Rongping D, Lin Z, et al. Migration of intraocular silicone into the cerebral ventricles. *Am J Ophthalmol.* 2005;140:156–158.
16. Norman BC, Oliver J, Cheeks L, et al. Corneal endothelial permeability after anterior chamber silicone oil. *Ophthalmology.* 1990;97(12):1671–1677.
17. Hutton WL, Azen SP, Blumenkranz MS, et al. The effects of silicone oil removal. *Arch Ophthalmol.* 1994;112:778–785.
18. Stringham J, Werner L, Monson B, et al. Calcification of different designs of silicone intraocular lenses in eyes with asteroid hyalosis. *Ophthalmology.* 2010;117:1486–1492.
19. Nazemi PP, Chong LP, Varma R, et al. Migration of intraocular silicone oil into the subconjunctival space and orbit through the ahmed glaucoma valve. *Am J Ophthalmol.* 2001;132(6):929–931.
20. Khoroshilova-Maslova IP, Nabieva MK, Leparskaia NL. Morphogenesis of complications after long-term intraocular silicon oil filling (clinical histopathological study). *Vestn Oftalmol.* 2012;128(4):57–61.

Drug: Benzalkonium chloride (BAK)

1. De Saint Jean M, Brignole F, Bringuier AF, et al. Effects of benzalkonium chloride on growth and survival of change conjunctival cells. *Invest Ophthalmol Vis Sci.* 1999;40:619–630.
2. Baudouin C. Mechanisms of failure in glaucoma filtering surgery: a consequence of antiglaucoma drugs? *Int J Clin Pharm Res.* 1996;16(1):29–41.
3. Baudouin C, de Lunardo C. Short-term comparative study of topical 2% carteolol with and without benzalkonium chloride in healthy volunteers. *Br J Ophthalmol.* 1998;82(1):9–42.
4. Baudouin C, Denoyer A, Desbenoit N, et al. In vitro and in vivo experimental studies on trabecular meshwork degeneration induced by benzalkonium chloride (an American Ophthalmological Society thesis). *Trans Am Ophthalmol Soc.* 2012;110:40–63.
5. Baudouin C, Garcher C, Haouat N, et al. Expression of inflammatory membrane markers by conjunctival cells in chronically treated patients with glaucoma. *Ophthalmology.* 1994;101(3):454–460.
6. Baudouin C, Labbe A, Liang H, et al. Preservatives in eyedrops: the good, the bad and the ugly. *Prog Retin Eye Res.* 2010;29(4):312–334.
7. Baudouin C, Pisella PJ, Fillacier K, et al. Ocular surface inflammatory changes induced by topical antiglaucoma drugs: human and animal studies. *Ophthalmology.* 1999;106(3):556–563.
8. Perez-Bartolome F, Martinez-de-la-Casa JM, Arriola-Villalobos P, et al. Ocular surface disease in patients under topical treatment for glaucoma. *Eur J Ophthalmol.* 2017;27(6):694–704.
9. Means TL, Holley GP, Mehta KR, et al. Corneal edema from an intraocular irrigating solution containing benzalkonium chloride. *J Toxicol Cut Ocular Toxicol.* 1994;13(1):67–81.
10. Lemp MA, Zimmerman LE. Toxic endothelial degeneration in ocular surface disease treated with topical medications containing benzalkonium chloride. *Am J Ophthalmol.* 1988;105:670–673.
11. Brandt JD. Does benzalkonium chloride cause cataract? *Arch Ophthalmol.* 2003;121:892–893.
12. Goto Y, Ibaraki N, Miyake K. Human lens epithelial cell damage and stimulation of their secretion of chemical mediators by benzalkonium chloride rather than latanoprost and timolol. *Arch Ophthalmol.* 2003;121:835–839.
13. Miyake K, Ibaraki N, Goto Y, et al. ESCRS Binkhorts Lecture 2002: pseudophakic preservative maculopathy. *J Cataract Refract Surg.* 2003;29:1800–1810.
14. Stevens AM, Kestelyn PA, De Bacquer D, et al. Benzalkonium chloride induces anterior chamber inflammation in previously untreated patients with ocular hypertension as measured by flare meter: a randomized clinical trial. *Acta Ophthalmol.* 2012;90(3):e221–e224.
15. Datta S, Baudouin C, Brignole-Baudouin F, et al. The eye drop preservative benzalkonium chloride potently induces mitochondrial dysfunction and preferentially affects LHON mutant cells. *Invest Ophthalmol Vis Sci.* 2017;58:2406–2412.
16. Fraunfelder FT. *Cicatricial Changes Associated with Topical Ocular Application of Eye Drops Containing Bak [Photograph] and Leukoplakia From Topical Ocular Application of Eye Drops Containing Bak [Photograph].* Portland, OR: Casey Eye Institute, Oregon Health & Science University; ©1990:2 photographs: color.

Drug: Chlorhexidine gluconate

1. Apt L, Isenberg SJ. Hibiclens keratitis. *Am J Ophthalmol.* 1987;104:670–671.
2. Hamed LM, Ellis FD, Boudreault G, et al. Hibiclens keratitis. *Am J Ophthalmol.* 1987;104:50–56.
3. MacRae SM, Brown B, Edelhauser HF. The corneal toxicity of presurgical skin antiseptics. *Am J Ophthalmol.* 1984;97:221–232.
4. Nasser RE. The ocular danger of Hibiclens. *Plast Reconstr Surg.* 1992;89(1):164–165.
5. Shore JW. Hibiclens keratitis. *Am J Ophthalmol.* 1987;104:670–671.
6. Ehlers E, Hjortdal J. Are cataract and iris atrophy toxic complications of medical treatment of *Acanthamoeba keratitis*? *Acta Ophthalmol Scand.* 2004;82:228–231.
7. Merani R, McPherson ZE, Luckie AP, et al. Aqueous chlorhexidine for intravitreal injection antisepsis. *Ophthalmology.* 2016;123(12):2588–2594.
8. Oakley CL, Vote BJ. Aqueous chlorhexidine (0.1%) is an effective alternative to povidone – iodine for intravitreal injection prophylaxis. *Acta Ophthalmol.* 2016;94(8):e808–e809.
9. Okuda T, Funasaka M, Arimitsu M, et al. Anaphylactic shock by ophthalmic wash solution containing chlorhexidine. *Jpn J Anesthesiol.* 1994;43(9):1352–1355.

Drug: Povidone-iodine (PVP-1) (iodopovidone)

1. Saedon H, Nosek J, Phillips J, et al. Ocular surface effects of repeated application of povidone iodine in patients receiving frequent intravitreal injections. *Cutan Ocul Toxicol.* 2017;36(4):343–346.
2. Grzybowski A, Kanclerz P, Myers WG. The use of povidone-iodine in ophthalmology. *Curr Opin Ophthalmol.* 2018;29(1):19–32.
3. Ridder 3rd WH, Oquindo C, Dhamdhere K, et al. Effect of povidone iodine 5% on the cornea, vision, and subjective comfort. *Optom Vis Sci.* 2017;94(7):732–741.
4. Hsu J, Gerstenblith AT, Garg SJ, et al. Conjunctival flora antibiotic resistance patterns after serial intravitreal injections without postinjection topical antibiotics. *Am J Ophthalmol.* 2014;157(3):514–518.
5. Wykoff CC, Flynn HW, Han DP. Allergy to povidone-iodine and cephalosporins: the clinical dilemma in ophthalmic use. *Am J Ophthalmol.* 2011;151(1):4–6.

Drugs: Thiomersal (thimersal), yellow mercuric oxide (hydrargyric oxide flavum)

1. Ashkenazi I, Desatnik HR, Abraham FA. Yellow mercuric oxide: a treatment of choice from phthiriasis palpebrarum. *Br J Ophthalmol.* 1991;75(6):356–358.
2. Kern AB. Mercurial pigmentation. *Arch Dermatol.* 1969;99:129–130.
3. Lamar LM, Bliss BO. Localized pigmentation of the skin due to topical mercury. *Arch Dermatol.* 1966;93:450–453.
4. Long JC, Danielson RW. Mercurial discoloration of the eyelids. *Am J Ophthalmol.* 1951;34:753–756.
5. Wheeler M. Discoloration of the eyelids from prolonged use of ointment containing mercury. *Am J Ophthalmol.* 1948;31:441–444.
6. Wilson LA, McNatt J, Reitschel R. Delayed hypersensitivity to thimerosal in soft contact lens wearers. *Ophthalmology.* 1981;88:804–809.
7. Wilsonholt N, Dart JK. Thiomersal keratoconjunctivitis, frequency, clinical spectrum and diagnosis. *Eye.* 1989;3:581–587.
8. Mondino BJ, Salamon SM, Zaidman GW. Allergic and toxic reactions in soft contact lens wearers. *Surv Ophthalmol.* 1982;26:337–344.

Drug: Ocriplasmin

1. Hager A, Seibel I, Riechardt A, et al. Does ocriplasmin affect the RPE-photoreceptor adhesion in macular holes? *Br J Ophthalmol.* 2015;99(5):635–638.
2. Shah SP, Jeng-Miller KW, Fine HF, et al. Post-marketing survey of adverse events following Ocriplasmin. *Ophthalmic Surg Lasers Imaging Retina.* 2016;47(2):156–160.
3. Kaiser PK, Kampik A, Kuppermann BD, et al. Safety profile of ocriplasmin for the pharmacologic treatment of symptomatic vitreomacular adhesion/traction. *Retina.* 2015;35(6):1111–1127.
4. Johnson MW, Fahim AT, Rao RC, et al. Acute ocriplasmin retinopathy. *Retina.* 2015;35(6):1055–1058.
5. Freund KB, Shah SA, Shah VP. Correlation of transient vision loss with outer retinal disruption following intravitreal ocriplasmin. *Eye (Lond).* 2013;27(6):773–774.
6. Singh RP, Li A, Bedi R, et al. Anatomical and visual outcomes following ocriplasmin treatment for symptomatic vitreomacular traction syndrome. *Br J Ophthalmol.* 2014;98(3):356–360.
7. Fahim AT, Khan NW, Johnson MW. Acute panretinal structural and functional abnormalities after intravitreous ocriplasmin injection. *JAMA Ophthalmol.* 2014;132(4):484–486.
8. Tibbetts MD, Reichel E, Witkin AJ. Vision loss after intravitreal ocriplasmin: correlation of spectral-domain optic coherence tomography and electroretinography. *JAMA Ophthalmol.* 2014;132(4):487–490.
9. Barteselli G, Carini E, Invernizzi A, et al. Early panretinal abnormalities on fundus autofluorescence and spectral domain optical coherence tomography after intravitreal ocriplasmin. *Acta Ophthalmol.* 2016;94(2):e160–e162.
10. Beebe DC. Understanding the adverse effects of ocriplasmin. *JAMA Ophthalmol.* 2015;133(2):229.
11. Reiss B, Smithen L, Mansour S. Transient vision loss after ocriplasmin injection. *Retina.* 2015;35(6):1107–1110.
12. Birch DG, Benz MS, Miller DM, et al. Evaluation of full-field electroretinogram reductions after ocriplasmin treatment: results of the OASIS trial ERG substudy. *Retina.* 2018;38(2):364–378.
13. Luttrull JK. Chronic serous macular detachments and visual disturbance complicating consecutive cases of symptomatic vitreomacular adhesion with macular hole treated with ocriplasmin. *Ophthalmic Surg Lasers Imaging Retina.* 2015;46(9):976–978.
14. Han IC, Scott AW. Sterile endophthalmitis after intravitreal ocriplasmin injection: report of a single case. *Retin Cases Brief Rep.* 2015;9(3):242–244.
15. *Ocriplasmin.* 2018. Retrieved from http://www.pdr.net.
16. Novack RL, Staurenghi G, Girach A, et al. Safety of intravitreal ocriplasmin for focal vitreomacular adhesion in patients with exudative age-related macular degeneration. *Ophthalmology.* 2015;122(4):796–802.
17. Keller J, Haynes RJ. Zonular dehiscence at the time of combined vitrectomy and cataract surgery after intravitreal ocriplasmin injection. *JAMA Ophthalmol.* 2015;133(9):1091–1092.
18. Zhang TY, Vachon-Joannette E, Proulx S, et al. Delayed transient corneal edema after intravitreal injection of ocriplasmin. *Can J Ophthalmol.* 2018;53(2):e77–e79.

Drug: Mitomycin

1. DeBry PW, Perkins TW, Heatley G, et al. Incidence of late-onset bleb-related complications following trabeculectomy. *Arch Ophthalmol.* 2002;120:297–300.
2. Widder RA, Dietlein TS, Dinslage S, et al. The XEN45 gel stent as a minimally invasive procedure in glaucoma surgery: success rates, risk profile, and rates of re-surgery after 261 surgeries. *Graefes Arch Clin Exp Ophthalmol.* 2018;256(4):765–771.

3. Mietz H, Roters S, Krieglstein GK. Bullous keratopathy as a complication of trabeculectomy with mitomycin C. *Graefes Arch Clin Exp Ophthalmol.* 2005;243:1284–1287.

4. Shaheer M, Amjad A, Ahmed N. Comparison of mean corneal endothelial cell loss after trabeculectomy with and without mitomycin C. *J Coll Physicians Surg Pak.* 2018;28(4):301–303.

5. Daugelience L, Yamamoto T, Kitazawa Y. Cataract development after trabeculectomy with mitomycin C: a 1-year study. *Surv Ophthalmol.* 2000;45:165.

6. Fourman S. Scleritis after glaucoma filtering surgery with mitomycin C. *Ophthalmology.* 1995;102(10):1569–1571.

7. Danias J, Rosenbaum J, Podos SM. Diffuse retinal hemorrhages (ocular decompression syndrome) after trabeculectomy with mitomycin C for neovascular glaucoma. *Acta Ophthalmol Scand.* 2000;78:468–469.

8. Dev S, Herndon L, Shields MB. Retinal vein occlusion after trabeculectomy with mitomycin C. *Am J Ophthalmol.* 1996;122(4):574–575.

9. Figueiredo ARM, Sampaio IC, Meneres MJFDS, et al. Consecutive bilateral decompression retinopathy after mitomycin C trabeculectomy: a case report. *J Med Case Rep.* 2016;10:32.

10. Naruo-Tsuchisaka A, Maruyama K, Arimoto G, et al. Incidence of postoperative ptosis following trabeculectomy with mitomycin C. *J Glaucoma.* 2015;24(6):417–420.

11. Lu L, Xu S, Ge S, et al. Tailored treatment for the management of scleral necrosis following pterygium excision. *Exp Ther Med.* 2017;13(3):845–850.

12. Ji YW, Park SY, Jung JW, et al. Necrotizing scleritis after cosmetic conjunctivectomy with mitomycin C. *Am J Ophthalmol.* 2018;194:72–81.

13. Carrasco MA, Rapuano CJ, Cohen EJ, et al. Scleral ulceration after preoperative injection of mitomycin C in the pterygium head. *Arch Ophthalmol.* 2002;120:1585–1586.

14. Bahar I, Kaiserman I, Lange AP, et al. The effect of mitomycin C on corneal endothelium in pterygium surgery. *Am J Ophthalmol.* 2009;147:447–452.

15. McDermott ML, Wang J, Shin DH. Mitomycin and the human corneal endothelium. *Arch Ophthalmol.* 1994;112:533–537.

16. Dafgard-Kopp E, Seregard S. Epiphora as a side effect of topical mitomycin C. *Br J Ophthalmol.* 2004;88:1422–1424.

17. Leung TG, Dunn JP, Akepk EK, et al. Necrotizing scleritis as a complication of cosmetic eye whitening procedure. *J Ophthalmic Inflamm Infect.* 2013;3(1):39.

18. Vo RC, Stafeeva K, Aldave AJ, et al. Complications related to a cosmetic eye-whitening procedure. *Am J Ophthalmol.* 2014;158:967–973.

19. Lee S, Go J, Rhiu S, et al. Cosmetic regional conjunctivectomy with postoperative mitomycin C application with or without bevacizumab injection. *Am J Ophthalmol.* 2013;156:616–622.

20. Billing K, Karagiannis A, Selva D. Punctal-canalicular stenosis associated with mitomycin-C for corneal epithelial dysplasia. *Am J Ophthalmol.* 2003;136:746–747.

21. De Benito-Llopis L, Canadas P, Drake P, et al. Keratocyte density 3 months, 15 months, and 3 years after corneal surface ablation with mitomycin C. *Am J Ophthalmol.* 2012;153:17–23.

22. Dudney BW, Malecha M. Limbal stem cell deficiency following topical mitomycin C treatment of conjunctival-corneal intraepithelial neoplasia. *Am J Ophthalmol.* 2004;137:950–951.

23. Lichtinger A, Pe'er J, Frucht-Pery J, et al. Limbal stem cell deficiency after topical mitomycin C therapy for primary acquired melanosis with atypia. *Ophthalmology.* 2010;117(3):431–437.

24. Abraham LM, Selva D, Casson R, et al. Mitomycin: clinical application in ophthalmic practice. *Drugs.* 2006;66:321–340.

25. Fraunfelder FT. *Topical Ocular Mitomycin-Induced Symblepharon [Photograph].* Portland, OR: Casey Eye Institute, Oregon Health & Science University; ©1990:1 photograph: color.

Drug: Cocaine hydrochloride

1. Wilcsek GA, Vose MJ, Francis IC, et al. Acute angle closure glaucoma following the use of intranasal cocaine during dacryocystorhinostomy. *Br J Ophthalmol.* 2002;86:1312–1321.

2. French DD, Margo CE, Harman LE. Substance use disorder and the risk of open-angle glaucoma. *J Glaucoma.* 2011;20(7):452–457.

3. McHenry JG, Zeiter JH, Madion MP, et al. Ophthalmic complications of crack cocaine (letter). *Ophthalmology.* 1993;100(12):1747.

4. Mitchell JD, Schwartz AL. Acute angle-closure glaucoma associated with intranasal cocaine abuse. *Am J Ophthalmol.* 1996;122(3):425–426.

5. Jacobson DM, Berg R, Grinstead GF, et al. Duration of positive urine for cocaine metabolite after ophthalmic administration: implications for testing patients with suspected Horner syndrome using ophthalmic cocaine. *Am J Ophthalmol.* 2001;131:742–747.

6. Cruz OA, Patrinely JR, Reyna GS, et al. Urine drug screening for cocaine after lacrimal surgery. *Am J Ophthalmol.* 1991;111:703–705.

7. Goldberg RA, Weisman JS, McFarland JE, et al. Orbital inflammation and optic neuropathies associated with chronic sinusitis of intranasal cocaine abuse. *Arch Ophthalmol.* 1989;107:831–835.

8. Shen CC, Silver AL, O'Donnell TJ, et al. Optic neuropathy caused by naso-orbital mass in chronic intranasal cocaine abuse. *J Neuro-Ophthalmol.* 2009;29(1):50–53.

9. Siemerink MJ, Freling NJM, Saeed P. Chronic orbit inflammatory disease and optic neuropathy associated with long-term intranasal cocaine abuse: 2 cases. *Orbit.* 2017;36(5):350–355.

10. Ascaso FJ, Cruz N, Del Buey MA, et al. An unusual case of cocaine-induced maculopathy. *Eur J Ophthalmol.* 2009;19(5):880–882.

11. Leung IY, Lai S, Ren S, et al. Early retinal vascular abnormalities in African-American cocaine users. *Am J Ophthalmol.* 2008;146(4):612–619.

12. Gokoffski KK, Thinda S. Ophthalmic artery occlusion after cocaine use. *J Emerg Med.* 2015;49(1):61–62.

13. Dominguez R, Aguirre Vila-Coro A, Slopis JM, et al. Brain and ocular abnormalities in infants with in utero exposure to cocaine and other street drugs. *Am J Dis Child.* 1991;145:688–695.

14. Good WV, Ferriero DM, Golabi M, et al. Abnormalities of the visual system in infants exposed to cocaine. *Ophthalmology.* 1992;99(3):341–346.

15. Stafford Jr JR, Rosen TS, Zaider M, et al. Prenatal cocaine exposure and the development of the human eye. *Ophthalmology.* 1994;101(2):301–308.

16. Nucci P, Brancato R. Ocular effects of prenatal cocaine exposure (letter). *Ophthalmology.* 1994;101(8):1321–1324.

17. Vasconcelos SB, Guerra FM, Morato GM, et al. Acquired anterior staphyloma after corneal ulcer associated with the use of crack. *Arq Bras Oftalmol.* 2016;79(4):268–269.

18. Fraunfelder FT. *Corneal opacities from cocaine exposure to the eye [photograph].* Portland, OR: Casey Eye Institute, Oregon Health & Science University; ©1990. 1 photograph: color.

Drugs: Oxybuprocaine (benoxinate), proxymetacaine hydrochloride (proparacaine), tetracaine (amethocaine)

1. Burns RP, Gipson I. Toxic effects of local anesthetics. *JAMA.* 1978;240:347.

2. Fraunfelder FT, Sharp JD, Silver BE. Possible adverse effects from topical ocular anesthetics. *Doc Ophthalmol.* 1979;18:341.

3. Roche G, Brunette I, Le Francois M. Severe toxic keratopathy secondary to topical anesthetic abuse. *Can J Ophthalmol.* 1995;30(4):198–202.

4. Moreira LB, Kasetsuwan N, Sanchez D, et al. Toxicity of topical anesthetic agents to human keratocytes in vivo. *J Cataract Refract Surg.* 1999;25:975–980.

5. Chern KC, Meisler DM, Wilhelmus KR, et al. Corneal anesthetic abuse and *Candida* keratitis. *Ophthalmology.* 1996;103:37–40.

6. Kinter JC, Grossniklaus HE, Lass JH, et al. Infectious crystalline keratopathy associated with topical anesthetic abuse. *Cornea.* 1990;9(1):77–80.

7. Risco JM, Millar LC. Ultrastructural alterations in the endothelium in a patient with topical anesthetic abuse keratopathy. *Ophthalmology.* 1992;99(4):628–633.

8. Rosenwasser GO, Holland S, Pflugfelder SC, et al. Topical anesthetic abuse. *Ophthalmology.* 1990;97(8):967–972.

9. Takkar B, Sharma P, Gaur N, et al. Proparacaine-induced mydriasis during strabismus surgery. *Semin Ophthalmol.* 2018;33(3):367–370.

10. Pelosini L, Treffene S, Hollickk E. Antibacterial activity of preservative-free topical anesthetic drops in current use in ophthalmology departments. *Cornea.* 2009;28(1):58–61.

11. Fernandez-Garcia P, Cerviño A, Quiles-Guiñau L, et al. Corneal thickness differences between sexes after oxybuprocaine eye drops. *Optom Vis Sci.* 2015;92(1):89–94.

12. Lemagne JM, Michiels X, Van Causenbroeck S, et al. Purtscher-like retinopathy after retrobulbar anesthesia. *Ophthalmology.* 1990;97(7):859–861.

13. Taddio A, Lee CM, Parvez B, et al. Contact dermatitis and bradycardia in a preterm infant given tetracaine 4% gel. *Ther Drug Monit.* 2006;28:291–294.

14. Fraunfelder FT. *Corneal melt and vascularization from topical proxymetacaine hydrochloride abuse* [photograph]. Portland, OR: Casey Eye Institute, Oregon Health & Science University; ©1990. 1 photograph: color.

Drugs: Bromfenac sodium, diclofenac sodium, ketorolac tromethamine, nepafenac

1. Blumenthal KG, Lai KH, Huang M, et al. Adverse and hypersensitivity reactions to prescription nonsteroidal antiinflammatory agents in a large health care system. *J Allergy Clin Immunol Pract.* 2017;5(3):737–743.

2. *Bromfenac Sodium, Diclofenac Sodium, Ketorolac Tromethamine, Nepafenac.* 2019. Retrieved from http://www.pdr.net.

3. Chidambara L, Singhal R, Srinivasan P, et al. Unreported side effect of intravitreal diclofenac in chronic diabetic macular edema. *Retin Cases Brief Rep.* 2018;12(3):254–256.

4. Sitenga GL, Ing EB, Van Dellen RG, et al. Asthma caused by topical application of ketorolac. *Ophthalmology.* 1996;103:890–892.

5. Sharir M. Exacerbation of asthma by topical diclofenac. *Arch Ophthalmol.* 1997;115:294–295.

6. Gabison EE, Chastang P, Menashi S, et al. Late corneal perforation after photorefractive keratectomy associated with topical diclofenac. *Ophthalmology.* 2003;11:1626–1631.

Drug: Lifitegrast

1. Holland EJ, Luchs J, Karpecki PM, et al. Lifitegrast for the treatment of dry eye disease. *Ophthalmology.* 2017;124(1):53–60.

2. *Lifitegrast.* 2018. Retrieved from http://www.pdr.net.

3. Sheppard JD, Torkildsen GL, Lonsdale JD, et al. Lifitegrast ophthalmic solution 5.0% for treatment of dry eye disease: results of the OPUS-1 phase 3 study. *Ophthalmology.* 2014;121(2):475–483.

4. Tauber J, Karpecki P, Latkany R, et al. Lifitegrast ophthalmic solution 5.0% versus placebo for treatment of dry eye disease: results of the randomized phase III OPUS-2 study. *Ophthalmology.* 2015;122(12):2423–2431.

5. Donnenfeld ED, Karpecki PM, Majmudar PA, et al. Safety of lifitegrast ophthalmic solution 5.0% in patients with dry eye disease: a 1-year, multicenter.

Drug: Sodium chloride

1. *Sodium Chloride.* 2019. Retrieved from http://www.pdr.net.

2. Kushner FH. Sodium chloride eye drops as a cause of epistaxis. *Arch Ophthalmol.* 1987;105:1643.

Drug: Sodium hyaluronate

1. Floren I. Viscoelastic purity. *J Cataract Refract Surg.* 1998;24(2):145–146.
2. Althoumali TA. Viscoelastic substance in prefilled syringe as an etiology of toxic anterior segment syndrome. *Cutan Ocul Toxicol.* 2016;35(3):237–241.
3. Tanaka T, Inoue H, Kudo S, et al. Relationship between postoperative intraocular pressure elevation and residual sodium hyaluronate following phacoemulsification and aspiration. *J Cataract Refract Surg.* 1997;23(2):284–288.
4. Shammas HJ. Relaxing the fibrosis capsulorhexis rim to correct induced hyperopia after phacoemulsification. *J Cataract Refract Surg.* 1995;21:228–229.
5. Holtz SJ. Postoperative capsular bag distension. *J Cataract Refract Surg.* 1992;18:310–317.
6. Reck AC, Pathmanathan T, Butler RE. Post-operative myopic shift due to trapped intracapsular Healon (letter). *Eye.* 1998;12(Pt 5):900–901.
7. Berger RR, Kenyeres AM, Powell DA. Suspected ciliary block associated with Viscoat use. *J Cataract Refract Surg.* 1999;25(4):594–596.
8. Storr-Paulsen A, Larsen M. Long-term results of extracapsular cataract extraction with posterior chamber lens implantation. *Acta Ophthalmol.* 1991;69:766–769.
9. Jensen MK, Crandall AS, Mamalis N, et al. Crystallization on intraocular lens surfaces associated with the use of Healon GV. *Arch Ophthalmol.* 1994;112:1037–1042.
10. Tan AK, Humphry RC. The fixed dilated pupil after cataract surgery – is it related to intraocular use of hypromellose? *Br J Ophthalmol.* 1993;77:639–641.
11. Eason J, Seward HC. Pupil size and reactivity following hydroxypropyl methylcellulose and sodium hyaluronate. *Br J Ophthalmol.* 1995;79:541–543.
12. Lee JS, Park JM, Cho HK, et al. Influence of sodium hyaluronate concentration on corneal aberrations in soft contact lens wearers. *Korean J Ophthalmol.* 2018;32(2):89–94.

FURTHER READING
Aflibercept, bevacizumab, pegaptanib sodium, ranibizumab

Agrawal S, Joshi M, Christoforidis JB. Vitreous inflammation associated with intravitreal anti-VEGF pharmacotherapy. *Mediators Inflamm.* 2013;2013:943409.

Avery RL, Pearlman J, Pieramici DJ, et al. Intravitreal bevacizumab (Avastin) in the treatment of proliferative diabetic retinopathy. *Ophthalmology.* 2006;113:1695–1705.

Beaumont PE, Kang HK. Erratum. Ranibizumab and nonocular hemorrhage. *Ophthalmology.* 2010;117(8):1662–1663, author reply 1663–1664.

Brown DM. Erratum: Ranibizumab and nonocular hemorrhage (author reply). *Ophthalmology.* 2010;117(8):1663.

Carvounis PE, Kopel PE, Benz MS. Retinal pigment epithelium tears following ranibizumab for exudative age-related macular degeneration. *Am J Ophthalmol.* 2007;143(3):504–505.

Chandler RE, Aoki Y, Sandberg L. Aflibercept and deep vein thrombosis/pulmonary embolism. *WHO Pharmaceuticals Newsletter.* 2018;6:12.

Chen SN, Lin CJ, Li KH, et al. Choroidal infarction after photodynamic therapy combined with bevacizumab and triamcinolone reversed by tissue plasminogen activator: case report. *Retin Cases Brief Rep.* 2013;7(1):52–56.

Chun DW, Heier JS, Topping TM, et al. A pilot study of multiple intravitreal injections of ranibizumab in patients with center involving clinically significant diabetic macular edema. *Ophthalmology.* 2006;113:1706–1712.

Gillies MC. What we don't know about Avastin might hurt us. *Arch Ophthalmol.* 2006;123:1478–1479.

Hirata A, Hayashi K, Murata K, et al. Removal of choroidal neovascular membrane in a case of macular hole after anti-VEGF therapy for age-related macular degeneration. *Am J Ophthalmol Case Rep.* 2017;9:14–17.

Manzano RPA, Peyman GA, Khan P, et al. Testing intravitreal toxicity of bevacizumab (Avastin). *Retina.* 2006;26:257–261.

Nguyen QD, Shah SM, Khwaja A, et al. Two-year outcomes of the ranibizumab for edema of the macular in diabetes (READ-2) study. *Ophthalmology.* 2010;117:2146–2151.

Reis GM, Grigg J, Chua B, et al. Incidence of intraocular pressure elevation following intravitreal ranibizumab (Lucentis) for age-related macular degeneration. *J Curr Glaucoma Pract.* 2017;11(1):3–7.

Silva R, Axer-Siegel R, Eldem B, et al. The SECURE Study: Long-term safety of ranibizumab 0.5 mg in neovascular age-related macular degeneration. *Ophthalmology.* 2013;120:130–139.

Smith BT, Kraus CL, Apte RS. Retinal pigment epithelial tears in ranibizumab-treated eyes. *Retina.* 2009;29:335–339.

Van Der Reis MI, La Heij EC, De Jong-Hess Y, et al. A systematic review of the adverse events of intravitreal anti-vascular endothelial growth factor injections. *Retina.* 2011;31:1449–1469.

Wen JC, Chen CL, Rezaei KA, et al. Optic nerve head perfusion before and after intravitreal antivascular growth factor injections using optic coherence tomography-based microangiography. *J Glaucoma.* 2019;28(3):188–193.

Verteporfin

Beaumont P, Lim CS, Chang A, et al. Acute severe vision decrease immediately after photodynamic therapy. *Arch Ophthalmol.* 2004;122:1546–1547.

Hou Y, Le VNH, Clahsen T, et al. Photodynamic therapy leads to time-dependent regression of pathologic corneal (lymph) angiogenesis and promotes high-risk corneal allograft survival. *Invest Ophthalmol Vis Sci.* 2017;58(13):5862–5869.

Lai TY, Chan WM, Lam DS. Transient reduction in retinal function revealed by multifocal electroretinogram after photodynamic therapy. *Am J Ophthalmol.* 2004;137:826–833.

Mauget-Faysse M, Mimoun G, Ruiz-Moreno JM, et al. Verteporfin photodynamic therapy for choroidal neovascularization associated with toxoplasmic retinochoroiditis. *Retina.* 2003;26:396–403.

Mennel S, Meyer CH. Transient visual disturbance after photodynamic therapy. *Am J Ophthalmol.* 2005;139:748–749.

Noffke AS, Lee J, Weinberg DV, et al. A potentially life-threatening adverse reaction to verteporfin. *Arch Ophthalmol.* 2001;119:143.

Schnurrbusch UEK, Jochmann C, Einbock W, et al. Complications after photodynamic therapy. *Arch Ophthalmol.* 2005;123:1347–1350.

Scott LJ, Goa KL. Verteporfin. *Drugs Aging.* 2000;16:139–146.

TAP and VIP Study Groups. Acute severe visual acuity decrease after photodynamic therapy with verteporfin: case reports from randomized clinical trials. TAP and VIP report no 3. *Am J Ophthalmol.* 2004;137:683–696.

Tzekov R, Lin T, Zhang K-M, et al. Ocular changes after photodynamic therapy. *Invest Ophthalmol Vis Sci.* 2006;47:377–385.

Emedastine difumarate

AHSF Drug information. Emedastine difumarate. *Am Soc Health Syst Pharmacists.* 1998:1–15.

Horak F, Stubner P, Zieglmayer R, et al. Clinical study of the therapeutic efficacy and safety of emedastine difumarate versus cetirizine in the treatment of seasonal allergic rhinitis. *Arzneimittelforschung.* 2004;54:666–672.

Loteprednol etabonate

Noble S, Goa KL. Loteprednol etabonate: a review of its pharmacological properties and clinical potential in the management of giant papillary conjunctivitis and other ocular inflammation. *BioDrugs.* 1998;9(4):1–9.

Yu YJ, Yang HK, Hwang JM. Efficacy and safety of loteprednol 0.5% and fluorometholone 0.1% after strabismus surgery in children. *J Ocul Pharmacol Ther.* 2018;34(6):468–476.

Olopatadine hydrochloride

Anonymous. Olopatadine for allergic conjunctivitis. *Med Lett Drugs Ther.* 1997;39:108–109.

Ciprandi G, Buscaglia S, Cerqueti PM, et al. Drug treatment of allergic conjunctivitis: a review of the evidence. *Drugs.* 1995;45:1005–1008.

Galindez OA, Kaufman HE. Coping with itchy-burnies. the management of allergic conjunctivitis. *Ophthalmology.* 1996;103:1335–1336.

Apraclonidine hydrochloride

Butler P, Mannschreck M, Lin S, et al. Clinical experience with the long-term use of 1% apraclonidine. *Arch Ophthalmol.* 1995;113:293–296.

Coleman AL, Robin AL, Pollack IP. Cardiovascular and intraocular pressure effects and plasma concentrations of apraclonidine. *Arch Ophthalmol.* 1990;108:1264–1267.

Holdiness MR. Contact dermatitis to topical drugs for glaucoma. *Am J Contact Dermatitis.* 2001;12:217–219.

Jampel HD. Discussion: apraclonidine. *Ophthalmology.* 1993;100(9):1323.

Jampel HD, Robin AL, Quigley HA, et al. Apraclonidine. A one-week dose-response study. *Arch Ophthalmol.* 1988;106:1069–1073.

Juzych MS, Robin AL, Novack GD. Alpha-2 agonists in glaucoma therapy. *Ocular Pharmacology.* Philadelphia: Lippincott-Raven; 1997.

Lin SL, Liang SS. Evaluation of adverse reactions of apraclonidine hydrochloride ophthalmic solution. *J Ocul Pharmacol Ther.* 1995;11(3):267–278.

Morrison JC. Side effects of α-adrenergic agonists. *J Glaucoma.* 1995;4(suppl 1):S36–S38.

Munden PM, Kardon RH, Denison CE, et al. Palpebral fissure responses to topical adrenergic drugs. *Am J Ophthalmol.* 1991;111:706–710.

Nagasubramanian S, Hitchings RA, Demailly P, et al. Comparison of apraclonidine and timolol in chronic open-angle glaucoma. A three-month study. *Ophthalmology.* 1993;100(9):1318–1323.

Silvestre JF, Camero L, Ramon R, et al. Allergic contact dermatitis from apraclonidine in eyedrops. *Contact Dermatitis.* 2001;45:251.

Betaxolol hydrochloride, levobunolol hydrochloride, timolol maleate

Akingbehin T, Raj PS. Ophthalmic topical beta blockers: review of ocular and systemic adverse effects. *J Toxicol Cut Ocular Toxicol.* 1990;9:131–147.

Chun JG, Brodsky MA, Allen BJ. Syncope, bradycardia, and atrioventricular block associated with topical ophthalmic levobunolol. *Am Heart J.* 1994;127(3):689–690.

Coleman AL, Diehl DL, Jampel HD, et al. Topical timolol decreases plasma high-density lipoprotein cholesterol level. *Arch Ophthalmol.* 1990;106:1260–1263.

Doyle E, Liu C. A case of acquired iris depigmentation as a possible complication of levobunolol eye drops. *Br J Ophthalmol.* 1999;83:1403–1406.

Fraunfelder FT. Ocular beta blockers and systemic effects. *Arch Intern Med.* 1986;146:1073–1074.

Fraunfelder FT, Meyer SM. Systemic side effects from ophthalmic timolol and their prevention. *J Ocular Pharmacol.* 1987;3:177–184.

Geyer O, Neudorfer M, Lazar M. Recurrent choroidal detachment following timolol therapy in previously filtered eye. Choroidal detachment post filtering surgery. *Acta Ophthalmol.* 1992;70(5):702–703.

Gorlich W. Experience in clinical research with beta blockers in glaucoma. *Glaucoma.* 1987;9:21.

Hannaway PJ, Hopper GDK. Severe anaphylaxis and drug-induced beta-blockade. *N Engl J Med.* 1983;308:1536.

Harris LS, Greenstein SH, Bloom AF. Respiratory difficulties with betaxolol. *Am J Ophthalmol.* 1986;102:274–275.

Herreras JM, Pastor JC, Calonge M, et al. Ocular surface alteration after long-term treatment with an antiglaucomatous drug. *Ophthalmology.* 1992;99(7):1082–1088.

Jain S. Betaxolol-associated anterior uveitis. *Eye.* 1994;8(Pt 6):708–709.

Kaufman HS. Timolol-induced vasomotor rhinitis: a new iatrogenic syndrome. *Arch Ophthalmol.* 1986;104:967.

Mort JR. Nightmare cessation following alteration of ophthalmic administration of a cholinergic and a beta-blocking agent. *Ann Pharmacother.* 1992;26(7–8):914–916.

Nelson WL, Fraunfelder FT, Sills JM, et al. Adverse respiratory and cardiovascular events attributed to timolol ophthalmic solution. 1978–1985. *Am J Ophthalmol.* 1986;102:606–611.

Nuzzi R, Finazzo C, Cerruti A. Adverse effects of topical antiglaucomatous medications on the conjunctiva and the lachrymal (Brit. Engl) response. *Int Ophthalmol.* 1998;22(1):31–35.

Palmer EA. How safe are ocular drugs in pediatrics? *Ophthalmology.* 1986;93:1038–1040.

Sharir M, Nardin GF, Zimmerman TJ. Timolol maleate associated with phalangeal swelling. *Arch Ophthalmol.* 1991;109:1650.

Shore JH, Fraunfelder FT, Meyer SM. Psychiatric side effects from topical ocular timolol, a beta-adrenergic blocker. *J Clin Psychopharmacol.* 1987;7:264–267.

Verkijk A. Worsening of myasthenia gravis with timolol maleate eyedrops. *Ann Neurol.* 1985;17:211–212.

Vogel R. Surface toxicity of timolol (letter). *Ophthalmology.* 1993;100(3):293–294.

Vogel R. Topical timolol and serum lipoproteins (letter). *Arch Ophthalmol.* 1991;109:1341–1342.

Wilhelmus KR, McCulloch RR, Gross RL. Dendritic keratopathy associated with beta-blocker eyedrops. *Cornea.* 1990;9:335–337.

Bimatoprost, latanoprost, tafluprost, travuprost

Arranz-Marquez E, Teus MA, Saornil MA, et al. Analysis of irises with a latanoprost-induced change in iris color. *Am J Ophthalmol.* 2004;138:625–630.

Aslanides IM. Bilateral optic disk oedema associated with latanoprost. *Br J Ophthalmol.* 2000;84:673.

Avakian A, Renier SA, Butler PJ. Adverse effects of latanoprost on patients with medically resistant glaucoma. *Arch Ophthalmol.* 1998;116:679–680.

Ayyala RS, Cruz DA, Margo CE, et al. Cystoid macular edema associated with latanoprost in aphakic and pseudophakic eyes. *Am J Ophthalmol.* 1998;126:602–604.

Callanan D, Fellman RL, Savage JA. Latanoprost-associated cystoid macular edema. *Am J Ophthalmol.* 1998;126:134–135.

Eisenberg D. CME and anterior uveitis with latanoprost use. *Ophthalmology.* 1998;105:1978–1983.

Grierson I, Lee WR, Albert DM. The fine structure of an iridectomy specimen from a patient with latanoprost-induced eye color change. *Arch Ophthalmol.* 1999;117:394–396.

Heier JS. Cystoid macular edema associated with latanoprost use. *Arch Ophthalmol.* 1998;116:680–682.

Kroll DM, Schuman JS. Reactivation of herpes simplex virus keratitis after initiating bimatoprost treatment for glaucoma. *Am J Ophthalmol.* 2002;133(3):401–403.

Lai IC, Kuo MT, Teng IMC. Iris pigment epithelial cyst induced by topical administration of latanoprost. *Br J Ophthalmol.* 2003;87:366.

Lee H, Cho BJ. Long-term effect of latanoprost on central corneal thickness in normal-tension glaucoma: five-year follow-up results. *J Ocul Pharmacol Ther.* 2015;31(3):152–155.

Lee YC. Abdominal cramp as an adverse effect of travoprost. *Am J Ophthalmol.* 2005;139(1):202–203.

Morales J, Shihab ZM, Brown SM, et al. Herpes simplex virus dermatitis in patients using Latanoprost. *Am J Ophthalmol.* 2001;132(1):114–116.

Rowe JA, Hattenhauer MG, Herman DC. Adverse side effects associated with latanoprost. *Am J Ophthalmol.* 1997;124:683–685.

Stewart WC, Kolker AE, Stewart JA, et al. Conjunctival hyperemia in healthy subjects after short-term dosing with latanoprost, bimatoprost, and travoprost. *Am J Ophthalmol.* 2003;135:314–320.

Teus MA, Arranz-Marquez E, Lucea-Suescu P. Incidence of iris colour change in latanoprost treated eyes. *Br J Ophthalmol.* 2002;86:1085–1088.

Wand M. Latanoprost and hyperpigmentation of eyelashes. *Arch Ophthalmol.* 1997;115:1206–1208.

Wand M, Gilbert CM, Liesegang TJ. Latanoprost and herpes simplex keratitis. *Am J Ophthalmol.* 1999;127(5):602–604.

Wand M, Ritch R, Isbey Jr EK, et al. Latanoprost and periocular skin color changes. *Arch Ophthalmol.* 2001;119:614–615.

Warwar RE, Bullock JD, Ballal D. Cystoid macular edema and anterior uveitis associated with latanoprost use. *Ophthalmology.* 1998;105:263–268.

Yoo R, Choi YA, Cho BJ. Change in central corneal thickness after the discontinuation of latanoprost in normal tension glaucoma-change in central corneal thickness after stop of latanoprost. *J Ocul Pharmacol Ther.* 2017;33(1):57–61.

Brimonidine tartrate

Adkins JC, Balfour JA, Brimonidine. A review of its pharmacological properties and clinical potential in the management of open-angle glaucoma and ocular hypertension. *Drugs Aging.* 1998;12(3):225–241.

Derick RJ, Robin AL, Walters TR, et al. Brimonidine tartrate: a one-month dose response study. *Ophthalmology.* 1997;104:131–136.

Enyedi LB, Freedman SF. Safety and efficacy of brimonidine in children with glaucoma. *J Am Assoc Pediatr Ophthalmol Strabismus.* 2001;5:281–284.

LeBlanc RP, for Brimonidine Study Group. Twelve-month results of an ongoing randomized trial comparing brimonidine tartrate 0.2% and timolol 0.5% given twice daily in patients with glaucoma or ocular hypertension. *Ophthalmology.* 1998;105:1960–1967.

Manlapaz CA, Kharlamb AB, Williams LS, et al. IOP, pulmonary and cardiac effects of anti-glaucoma drugs brimonidine, timolol, and betaxolol. *Invest Ophthalmol Vis Sci.* 1997;38(suppl):S814.

Nordlund JR, Pasquale LR, Robin AL, et al. The cardiovascular, pulmonary, and ocular hypotensive effects of 0.2% brimonidine. *Arch Ophthalmol.* 1995;113:77–83.

Rosenthal AL, Walters T, Berg E, et al. A comparison of the safety and efficacy of brimonidine 0.2%, BID versus TID, in subjects with elevated intraocular pressure. *Invest Ophthalmol Vis Sci.* 1996;37(3):1102.

Schuman JS. Clinical experience with brimonidine 0.2% and timolol 0.5% in glaucoma and ocular hypertension. *Surv Ophthalmol.* 1996;41(suppl 1):27–37.

Schuman JS, Horwitz B, Choplin NT, et al. A 1-year study of brimonidine twice daily in glaucoma and ocular hypertension. *Arch Ophthalmol.* 1997;115:847–852.

Serle JB. A comparison of the safety and efficacy of twice daily brimonidine 0.2% versus betaxolol 0.25% in subjects with elevated intraocular pressure. *Surv Ophthalmol.* 1996;41(suppl 1):S39–S47.

Sodhi PK, Verma L, Ratan J. Dermatological side effects of brimonidine: a report of three cases. *J Dermatol.* 2003;30:697–700.

Tomsak RL, Zaret CR, Weidenthal D. Charles Bonnet syndrome precipitated by brimonidine tartrate eye drops. *Br J Ophthalmol.* 2003;87:917–929.

Waldock A, Snape J, Graham CM. Effects of glaucoma medications on the cardiorespiratory and intraocular pressure status of newly diagnosed glaucoma patients. *Br J Ophthalmol.* 2000;84:710–713.

Walters G, Taylor RH. Severe systemic toxicity caused by brimonidine drops in an infant with presumed juvenile xanthogranuloma (letter). *Eye.* 1999;13:797–798.

Whitson JT, Ochsner KI, Moster MR, et al. The safety and intraocular pressure-lowering efficacy of brimonidine tartrate 0.15% preserved with polyquaternium-1. *Ophthalmology.* 2006;113(8):1333–1339.

Brinzolamide, dorzolamide hydrochloride

Aalto-Korte K. Contact allergy to dorzolamide eyedrops. *Contact Dermatitis.* 1998;39:206.

Abelson MB, Howe AJ, Lane KJ, et al. An eye-opening look at morning eye. *Rev Ophthalmol.* 2009:86–88.

Anupama B, Puthran N, Hegde V. Choroidal detachment in an elderly patient who was treated post operatively with topical dorzolamide and timolol combination. *J Clin Diagn Res.* 2010;4(5):3230–3232.

Balfour JA, Wilde MI. Dorzolamide – a review of its pharmacology and therapeutic potential in the management of glaucoma and ocular hypertension. *Drugs Aging.* 1997;10:384–483.

Blondeau P, Rousseau JA. Allergic reactions to brimonidine in patients treated for glaucoma. *Can J Ophthalmol.* 2002;37:21–26.

Callahan C, Ayyala RS. Hypotony and choroidal effusion induced by topical timolol and dorzolamide in patients with previous glaucoma drainage device implantation. *Ophthalmic Surg Lasers Imaging.* 2003;34:467–469.

Clineschmidt CM, Williams RD, Snyder E, et al. A randomized trial in patients inadequately controlled with timolol alone comparing the dorzolamide-timolol combination to monotherapy with timolol or dorzolamide. *Ophthalmology.* 1998;105:1952–1958.

Epstein RJ, Brown SVL, Konowal A. Endothelial changes associated with topical dorzolamide do appear to be significant. *Arch Ophthalmol.* 2004;122:1089–1090.

Fineman MS, Katz LJ, Wilson RP. Topical dorzolamide-induced hypotony and ciliochoroidal detachment in patients with previous filtration surgery (letter). *Arch Ophthalmol.* 1996;114:1031–1032.

Florez A, Roson E, Conde A, et al. Toxic epidermal necrolysis secondary to timolol, dorzolamide, and latanoprost eyedrops. *J Am Acad Dermatol.* 2005;53:909–911.

Fraunfelder FT, Meyer S, Bagby GC. Hematologic reactions to carbonic anhydrase inhibitors. Reply. *Am J Ophthalmol.* 1985;100:746.

Fraunfelder FT, Meyer S, Bagby GC. Hematologic reactions to carbonic anhydrase inhibitors. Letter to the Ed. *Am J Ophthalmol.* 1986;101:129.

Goldberg S, Gallily R, Bishara S, et al. Dorzolamide-induced choroidal detachment in surgically untreated eye. *Am J Ophthalmol.* 2004;138:285–286.

Gupta R, Vernon SA. An unusual appearance of limbal conjunctival follicles in a patient on brimonidine and dorzolamide. *Eye.* 2004;19:353–356.

Harris A, Arend O, Martin B. Effects of topical dorzolamide on retinal and retrobulbar hemodynamics. *Acta Ophthalmol Scand.* 1996;74:569–572.

Hoffmanova I, Sanchez D. Metabolic acidosis and anaemia associated with dorzolamide in a patient with impaired renal function. *Br J Clin Pharmacol.* 2018;84(4):796–799.

Johnson T, Kass MS. Letter to the editor. *Am J Ophthalmol.* 1986;101:128–129.

Lee WW, Portaliou D, Sayed MS, et al. Diplopia and symblepharon following Meuller's muscle conjunctival resection in patients on long-term multiple antiglaucoma medications. *Ophthalmic Plast Reconstr Surg.* 2017;33(3S suppl 1):S79–S82.

Lichter PR. Carbonic anhydrase inhibitors, blood dyscrasias, and standard of care. *Ophthalmology.* 1988;95:711–712.

Menke B, Walters A, Payne JF. Paradoxical anatomic response to topical carbonic anhydrase inhibitor in X-linked retinoschisis. *Ophthalmic Surg Lasers Imaging Retina.* 2018;49(2):142–144.

Miller RD. Hematologic reactions to carbonic anhydrase inhibitors. *Am J Ophthalmol.* 1985;100:745–746.

Mogk LG, Cyrlin MN. Blood dyscrasias and carbonic anhydrase inhibitors. Letter to the editor. *Ophthalmology.* 1988;95:768–771.

Mohammadpour M, Jabbarvand M, Javadi MA. Focal corneal decompensation after filtering surgery with mitomycin C. *Cornea.* 2007;26(10):1285–1287.

Morris S, Geh V, Nischal KK, et al. Topical dorzolamide and metabolic acidosis in a neonate. *Br J Ophthalmol.* 2003;87:1052–1053.

Munshi V, Ahluwalia H. Erythema multiforme after use of topical dorzolamide. *J Ocul Pharmacol Ther.* 2008;24(1):91–93.

Pfeiffer N. Dorzolamide: development and clinical application of a topical carbonic anhydrase inhibitor. *Surv Ophthalmol.* 1997;42:137–151.

Schwartzenberg GWS, Trope G. Anorexia, depression and dementia induced by dorzolamide eyedrops (Trusopt). *Can J Ophthalmol.* 1999;34(2):93–94.

Sponsel WE, Harrison J, Elliott WR. Dorzolamide hydrochloride and visual function in normal eyes. *Am J Ophthalmol.* 1997;123:759–766.

Wirtitsch MG, Findl O, Kiss B, et al. Short-term effect of dorzolamide hydrochloride on central corneal thickness in humans with cornea guttata. *Arch Ophthalmol.* 2003;121:621–625.

Young JW, Clements JL, Morrison JC, et al. Brinzolamide-induced follicular conjunctivitis. *J Glaucoma.* 2018;27(11):e183–e184.

Zambarakji HJ, Spencer AF, Vernon SA. An unusual side effect of dorzolamide (letter). *Eye.* 1997;11:418–419.

Zhao JC, Chen T. Brinzolamide induced reversible corneal decompensation. *Br J Ophthalmol.* 2005;89:389–390.

Zimran A, Beutler E. Can the risk of acetazolamide-induced aplastic anemia be decreased by periodic monitoring of blood cell counts? *Am J Ophthalmol.* 1987;104:654–658.

Carteolol hydrochloride

Chrisp P, Sorkin EM. Ocular carteolol – A review of its pharmacological properties, and therapeutic use in glaucoma and ocular hypertension. *Drugs Aging.* 1992;2:58–77.

Freedman SF, Freedman NJ, Shields MB, et al. Effects of ocular carteolol and timolol on plasma high density lipoprotein cholesterol level. *Am J Ophthalmol.* 1993;116:600–611.

Grunwald JE, Delehanty J. Effect of topical carteolol on the normal human retinal circulation. *Inv Ophthalmol Vis Sci.* 1992;33:1853–1863.

Hoh H. Surface anesthetic effect and subjective compatibility of 2% carteolol and 0.6% metipranolol in eye-healthy people. *Lens Eye Toxicity Res.* 1990;7:347–352.

Scoville B, Mueller B, White BG, et al. Double-masked comparison of carteolol and timolol in ocular hypertension. *Am J Ophthalmol.* 1988;105:150–154.

Metipranolol

Akingbehin T, Villada JR. Metripranolol-associated granulomatous anterior uveitis. *Br J Ophthalmol.* 1991;75:519–523.

Cervantes R, Hernandez HH, Frati A. Pulmonary and heart rate changes associated with nonselective beta-blocker glaucoma therapy. *J Toxicol Cut Ocular Toxicol.* 1986;5:185–193.

Derous D, de Keizer RJ, de Wolff-Rouendaal D, et al. Conjunctival keratinization, an abnormal reaction to an ocular beta blocker. *Acta Ophthalmol.* 1989;67:333–338.

Flaxel C, Samples JR. Metipranolol. *J Toxicol Cut Ocular Toxicol.* 1991;10:171–174.

Hoh H. Surface anesthetic effect and subjective compatibility of 2% carteolol and 0.6% metipranolol in eye-healthy people. *Lens Eye Toxic Res.* 1990;7:347–352.

Kessler C, Christ T. Incidence of uveitis in glaucoma patients using metipranolol. *J Glaucoma.* 1993;2:166–170.

Schultz JS, Hoenig JA, Charles H. Possible bilateral anterior uveitis secondary to metipranolol (OptiPranolol) therapy. *Arch Ophthalmol.* 1993;111:1607.

Serle JB, Lustgarten JS, Podos SM. A clinical trial of metipranolol, a noncardioselective beta-adrenergic antagonist, in ocular hypertension. *Am J Ophthalmol.* 1991;112:302–307.

Stempel I. Different beta blockers and their short-time effect on break-up time. *Ophthalmologica.* 1986;192:11.

Netarsudil

Karmel M. Glaucoma pipeline drugs: targeting the trabecular meshwork. *EyeNet.* 2013:38–43.

Wheeler K. First in class drug for glaucoma: what pharmacists need to know: netarsudil ophthalmic solution (Rhopressa) for the treatment of elevated intraocular pressure. *Drug Topics.* 2018.

Vancomycin

Akova Budak B, Baykara M, Kivanc SA, et al. Comparing the ocular surface effects of topical vancomycin and linezolid for treating bacterial keratitis. *Cutan Ocul Toxicol.* 2016;35(2):126–130.

Arepalli S, Modi YS, Deasy R, et al. Mild bilateral hemorrhagic occlusive retinal vasculitis following intracameral vancomycin administration in cataract surgery. *Ophthalmic Surg Lasers Imaging Retina.* 2018;49(5):369–373.

Harrison L. Vancomycin in cataract procedures may cause blindness. *Internet Document.* 15 Aug 2016; Available from: http://www.medscape.com.

Lee JY, Lee EK, Lee HJ, et al. Postoperative hemorrhagic occlusive retinal vasculitis with intracameral vancomycin. *Korean J Ophthalmol.* 2018;32(5):430–431.

Tu EY, Jain S. Topical linezolid 0.2% for the treatment of vancomycin-resistant or vancomycin-intolerant gram-positive bacterial keratitis. *Am J Ophthalmol.* 2013;155(6):1095–1098.e1.

Acyclovir (aciclovir)

Auwerx J, Knockaert D, Hofkens P. Acyclovir and neurologic manifestations. *Ann Intern Med.* 1983;99:882–883.

Collum LM, Logan P, Ravenscroft T. Acyclovir (Zovirax) in herpetic disciform keratitis. *Br J Ophthalmol.* 1983;67:115–118.

de Koning EWJ, van Bijsterveld OP, Cantell K. Combination therapy for dendritic keratitis with acyclovir and α-interferon. *Arch Ophthalmol.* 1983;101:1866–1868.

Jones PG, Beier-Hanratty SA. Acyclovir: neurologic and renal toxicity. *Ann Intern Med.* 1986;104:892.

Cidofovir

Barrier JH, Bani-Sadr F, Gaillard F, et al. Recurrent iritis after intravenous administration of cidofovir. *CID.* 1997;25:337–338.

Fraunfelder FW, Rosenbaum T. Drug-induced uveitis – incidences, prevention and treatment. *Drug Safety.* 1997;17(3):197–207.

Jabs DA. Cidofovir. *Arch Ophthalmol.* 1997;115:785–786.

Kirsch LS, Arevalo JF, Chavez de la Paz E, et al. Intravitreal cidofovir (HPMPC) treatment of cytomegalovirus retinitis in patients with acquired immune deficiency syndrome. *Ophthalmology.* 1995;102(4):533–542.

Labetoulle M, Goujard C, Frau E, et al. Cidofovir ocular toxicity is related to previous ocular history. *AIDS.* 2000;14:622–623.

Lin AP, Holland GN, Engstrom Jr RE. Vitrectomy and silicone oil tamponade for cidofovir-associated hypotony with ciliary body detachment. *Retina*. 1999;19(1):75–76.

Scott RAH, Pavesio C. Ocular side-effects from systemic HPMPC (cidofovir) for a non-ocular cytomegalovirus infection. *Am J Ophthalmol*. 2000;130:126–127.

Idoxuridine (IDU), trifluridine (F3T, trifluorothymidine), vidarabine (ara-A)

Kaufman HE. Chemical blepharitis following drug treatment. *Am J Ophthalmol*. 1983;95:703.

Kremer I, Rozenbaum D, Aviel E. Immunofluorescence findings in pseudopemphigoid induced by short-term idoxuridine administration. *Am J Ophthalmol*. 1991;111(3):375–377.

Lass JH, Troft RA, Dohlman CH. Idoxuridine-induced conjunctival cicatrization. *Arch Ophthalmol*. 1983;101:747–750.

Maudgal PC, Van Damme B, Missotten L. Corneal epithelial dysplasia after trifluridine use. *Graefes Arch Clin Exp Ophthalmol*. 1983;220:6–12.

Patten JT, Cavanagh HD, Allansmith MR. Induced ocular pseudopemphigoid. *Am J Ophthalmol*. 1976;82:272–276.

Udell IJ. Trifluridine-associated conjunctival cicatrization. *Am J Ophthalmol*. 1985;99:363–364.

Acetazolamide, methazolamide

Aminlari A. Falling scalp hairs. *Glaucoma*. 1984;6:41–42.

Elinav E, Ackerman Z, Gotthehrer NP, et al. Recurrent life-threatening acidosis induced by acetazolamide in a patient with diabetic type IV renal tubular acidosis. *Ann Emerg Med*. 2002;40:259–260.

Epstein RJ, Allen RC, Lunde MW. Organic impotence associated with carbonic anhydrase inhibitor therapy for glaucoma. *Ann Ophthalmol*. 1987;19:48–50.

Falardeau J, Lobb BM, Golden S, et al. The use of acetazolamide during pregnancy in intracranial hypertension patients. *J Neuroophthalmol*. 2013;33(1):9–12.

Fraunfelder FT, Meyer SM, Bagby Jr GC, et al. Hematologic reactions to carbonic anhydrase inhibitors. *Am J Ophthalmol*. 1985;100:79–81.

Gallerani M, Manzoli N, Fellin R, et al. Anaphylactic shock and acute pulmonary edema after a single oral dose of acetazolamide. *Am J Emerg Med*. 2002;20:371–372.

Guven Yilmaz S, Palamar M, Gurgun C. Acute pulmonary oedema due to single dose acetazolamide after cataract surgery. *BMJ Case Rep*. 2016:2016.

Hu CY, Lee BJ, Cheng HF, et al. Acetazolamide-related life-threatening hypophosphatemia in a glaucoma patient. *J Glaucoma*. 2015;24(4):e31–e33.

Kodjikian L, Duran B, Burillon C, et al. Acetazolamide-induced thrombocytopenia. *Arch Ophthalmol*. 2004;122:1543–1544.

Lichter PR. Reducing side effects of carbonic anhydrase inhibitors. *Ophthalmology*. 1981;88:266–296.

Margo CE. Acetazolamide and advanced liver disease. *Am J Ophthalmol*. 1986;100:611–612.

Niven BI, Manoharan A. Acetazolamide-induced anaemia. *Med J Aust*. 1985;142:120.

Shirato S, Kagaya F, Suzuki Y, et al. Stevens-Johnson syndrome induced by methazolamide treatment. *Arch Ophthalmol*. 1997;115:550–553.

Söderman P, Hartvig P, Fagerlund C. Acetazolamide excretion into human breast milk. *Br J Clin Pharmacol*. 1984;17(5):599–600.

Vogt PH, Barr G, Maitland CG. Palinopsia: side effect of topiramate and acetazolamide. *J Neuroophthalmol*. 2016;36(3):347–348.

White GL, Pribble JP, Murdock RT. Acetazolamide and the sulfonamide sensitive patient. *Ophthalmol Times*. 1985;10:15.

Naphazoline hydrochloride, tetryzoline hydrochloride (tetrahydrozoline)

Abelson MB, Allansmith MR, Friedlaender MH. Effects of topically applied ocular decongestant and antihistamine. *Am J Ophthalmol*. 1980;90:254–257.

Abelson MB, Butrus SI, Weston JH, et al. Tolerance and absence of rebound vasodilation following topical ocular decongestant usage. *Ophthalmology*. 1984;91:1364–1367.

Abelson MB, Yamamoto GK, Allansmith MR. Effects of ocular decongestants. *Arch Ophthalmol*. 1980;98:856–858.

Cook Jr BE, Holtan SB. Mydriasis from inadvertent topical application of naphazoline hydrochloride. *Contact Lens Assoc Ophthalmol*. 1998;24(2):72.

Khan MAJ, Watt LL, Hugkulstone CE. Bilateral acute angle-closure glaucoma after use of Fenox nasal drops. *Eye*. 2002;16:662–663.

Rich LF. Toxic drug effects on the cornea. *J Toxicol Cut Ocular Toxicol*. 1982–1983;1:267.

Skilling Jr FC, Weaver TA, Kato KP, et al. Effects of two eye drop products on computer users with subjective ocular discomfort. *Optometry*. 2005;76:47–54.

Stamer UM, Buderus S, Wetegrove S, et al. Prolonged awakening and pulmonary edema after general anesthesia and naphazoline application in an infant. *Anesth Analg*. 2001;93:1162–1164.

Williams TL, Williams AJ, Enzenauer RW. Case report: unilateral mydriasis from topical Opcon-A and soft contact lens. *Aviat Space Environ Med*. 1997;68(11):1035–1037.

Acetylcholine chloride

Fraunfelder FT. Recent advances in ocular toxicology. In: Srinivasan BD, ed. *Ocular Therapeutics*. New York: Masson; 1980:123–126.

Hollands RH, Drance SM, Schulzer M. The effect of acetylcholine on early postoperative intraocular pressure. *Am J Ophthalmol*. 1987;103:749–753.

Leopold IH. The use and side effects of cholinergic agents in the management of intraocular pressure. In: Drance SM, Neufeld AH, eds. *Glaucoma: Applied Pharmacology in Medical Treatment*. New York: Grune & Stratton; 1984:357–393.

Rasch D, Holt J, Wilson M, et al. Bronchospasm following intraocular injection of acetylcholine in a patient taking metoprolol. *Anesthesiology*. 1983;59:583–585.

Echothiophate iodide (ecothiophate)

Hirst LW, Werblin T, Novak M, et al. Drug-induced cicatrizing conjunctivitis simulating ocular pemphigoid. *Cornea*. 1982;1:121.

Tseng SC, Maumenee AE, Stark WJ, et al. Topical retinoid treatment for various dry-eye disorders. *Ophthalmology*. 1985;92:717–727.

Wood JR, Anderson RL, Edwards JJ. Phospholine iodide toxicity and Jones' tubes. *Ophthalmology*. 1980;87:346–349.

Pilocarpine hydrochloride

Ancelin ML, Artero S, Portet F, et al. Non-degenerative mild cognitive impairment in elderly people and use of anticholinergic drugs: longitudinal cohort study. *BMJ*. 2006;332:455–459.

Kastl PR. Inadvertent systemic injection of pilocarpine. *Arch Ophthalmol*. 1987;105:28–29.

Koeppl C, Findl O, Menapace R. Pilocarpine-induced shift of an accommodating intraocular lens: AT-45 Crystalens. *J Cataract Refract Surg*. 2005;31:1290–1297.

Levine RZ. Uniocular miotic therapy. *Trans Am Acad Ophthalmol Otolaryngol*. 1975;79:376–380.

Littman L, Kempler P, Rohla M, et al. Severe symptomatic atrioventricular block induced by pilocarpine eye drops. *Arch Intern Med*. 1987;147:586–587.

Merritt JC. Malignant glaucoma induced by miotics postoperatively in open angle glaucoma. *Arch Ophthalmol*. 1977;95:1988–1989.

Mishra P, Calvey TN, Williams NE, et al. Intraoperative bradycardia and hypotension associated with timolol and pilocarpine eye drops. *Br J Anaesth*. 1983;55:897–899.

Mori M, Araie M, Sakurai M, et al. Effects of pilocarpine and tropicamide on blood-aqueous barrier permeability in man. *Invest Ophthalmol Vis Sci*. 1992;33(2):416–423.

Skaat A, Rosman MS, Chien JL, et al. Effect of pilocarpine hydrochloride on the Schlemm canal in healthy eyes and eyes with open-angle glaucoma. *JAMA Ophthalmol*. 2016;134(9):976–981.

Zhang Y, Kam WR, Liu Y, et al. Influence of pilocarpine and timolol on human meibomian gland epithelial cells. *Cornea*. 2017;36(6):719–724.

Cyclopentolate hydrochloride, tropicamide

Demayo AP, Reidenberg MM. Grand mal seizure in a child 30 minutes after Cyclogyl (cyclopentolate hydrochloride) and 10% Neo-Synephrine (phenylephrine hydrochloride) eye drops were instilled. *Pediatrics*. 2004;113:e499–e500.

Eggers MN. Toxicity of drugs used in diagnosis and treatment of strabismus. In: Srinivasan D, ed. *Ocular Therapeutics*. New York: Masson; 1980:115–122.

Fitzgerald DA, Hanson RM, West C, et al. Seizures associated with 1% cyclopentolate eyedrops. *J Paediatr Child Health*. 1990;26:106–107.

Jones LWJ, Hodes DT. Cyclopentolate. First report of hypersensitivity in children: 2 case reports. *Ophthalmic Physiol Opt*. 1991;11:16–20.

Rosales T, Isenberg S, Leake R, et al. Systemic effects of mydriatics in low weight infants. *Pediatr Ophthalmol*. 1981;18:42–44.

Rush R, Rush S, Nicolau J, et al. Systemic manifestations in response to mydriasis and physical examination during screening for retinopathy of prematurity. *Retina*. 2004;24:242–245.

Hydroxyamphetamine hydrobromide (hydroxyamfetamine)

Burde RM, Thompson HS. Hydroxyamphetamine. A good drug lost? *Am J Ophthalmol*. 1991;111(1):100–102.

Gartner S, Billet E. Mydriatic glaucoma. *Am J Ophthalmol*. 1957;43:975–976.

Botulinum toxin A (abobotulinumtoxinA, incobotulinumtoxinA, onabotulinumtoxinA), botulinum toxin B (rimabotulinumtoxinB)

Averbuch-Heller L, von Maydell RD, Poonyathalang A, et al. Inverse Argyll Robertson pupil in botulism: late central manifestation. *Ophthalmol Lit*. 1997;50(2):132.

Biglan AW, Gonnering R, Lockhart LB, et al. Absence of antibody production in patients treated with botulinum A toxin. *Am J Ophthalmol*. 1986;101:232–235.

Burns CL, Gammon A, Gemmill MC. Ptosis associated with botulinum toxin treatment of strabismus and blepharospasm. *Ophthalmology*. 1986;93(12):1621–1627.

Dutton JJ, Buckley EG. Long-term results and complications of botulinum A toxin in the treatment of blepharospasm. *Ophthalmology*. 1988;95(11):1529–1534.

Gunes A, Demirci S, Koyuncuoglu HR, et al. Corneal and tear film changes after botulinum toxin-A in blepharospasm or hemifacial spasm. *Cornea*. 2015;34(8):906–910.

Harris CP, Alderson K, Nebeker J, et al. Histologic features of human orbicularis oculi treated with botulinum A toxin. *Arch Ophthalmol*. 1991;109:393–395.

Ho MC, Hsu WC, Hsieh YT. Botulinum toxin type A injection for lateral canthal rhytids: effect on tear film stability and tear production. *JAMA Ophthalmol*. 2014;132(3):332–337.

Jia Z, Lu H, Yang X, et al. Adverse events of botulinum toxin type A in facial rejuvenation: a systematic review of meta-analysis. *Aesthetic Plast Surg*. 2016;40(5):769–777.

Kalra HK, Magoon EH. Side effects of the use of botulinum toxin for treatment of benign essential blepharospasm and hemifacial spasm. *Ophthalmic Surg*. 1990;21(5):335–338.

Kouris A, Agiasofitou E, Gregoriou S, et al. Generalized neurological symptoms following treatment of focal hyperhidrosis with botulinum toxin A. *Int J Dermatol*. 2014;53(11):e544–e547.

Mauriello JA, Coniaris H, Haupt EJ. Use of botulinum toxin in the treatment of one hundred patients with facial dyskinesias. *Ophthalmology*. 1987;94(8):976–979.

Repka MX, Savino PJ, Reinecke RD. Treatment of acquired nystagmus with botulinum neurotoxin A. *Arch Ophthalmol*. 1994;112:1320–1324.

Zheng L, Azar D. Angle-closure glaucoma following periorbital botulinum toxin injection. *Clin Exp Ophthalmol*. 2014;42(7):690–693.

Fluorescein sodium

Antoszyk AN, de Juan Jr E, Landers MB, et al. Subretinal hemorrhages during fluorescein angiography. *Am J Ophthalmol.* 1987;103:111–112.

Chishti MI. Adverse reactions to intravenous fluorescein. *Pak J Ophthalmol.* 1986;2:19.

Danis RP, Wolverton S, Steffens T. Phototoxicity from systemic sodium fluorescein. *Retina.* 2000;20:370–373.

Duffner LR, Pflugfelder SC, Mandelbaum S, et al. Potential bacterial contamination in fluorescein-anesthetic solutions. *Am J Ophthalmol.* 1990;110:199–202.

Foster RE, Kode R, Ross D, et al. Unusual reaction to fluorescein dye in patients with inflammatory eye disease. *Retina.* 2004;24:263–266.

Jacob AK, Dilger JA, Hebl JR. Status epilepticus and intrathecal fluorescein: anesthesia providers beware. *Anesth Analg.* 2008;107(1):229–231.

Karhunen U, Raitta C, Kala R. Adverse reactions to fluorescein angiography. *Acta Ophthalmol.* 1986;64:282–286.

Kurli M, Hollingworth K, Kumar V, et al. Fluorescein angiography and patchy skin discoloration: a case report. *Eye.* 2003;17:422–424.

Yannuzzi LA, Rohrer KT, Tindel LJ, et al. Fluorescein angiography complication survey. *Ophthalmology.* 1986;93:611–617.

Indocyanine green (ICG)

Aydin P, Tayanc E, Dursun D, et al. Anterior segment indocyanine green angiography in pterygium surgery with conjunctival autograft transplantation. *Am J Ophthalmol.* 2003;135:71–75.

Blem RI, Huynh PD, Thall EH. Altered uptake of infrared diode laser by retina after intravitreal Indocyanine green dye and internal limiting membrane peeling. *Am J Ophthalmol.* 2002;134:285–286.

Ciardella AP, Schiff W, Barile G, et al. Persistent indocyanine green fluorescence after vitrectomy for macular hole. *Am J Ophthalmol.* 2003;136:174–177.

Gaur A, Kayarkar VV. Inadvertent vitreous staining. *J Cataract Refract Surg.* 2005;31:649.

Guyer DR, Puliafito CA, Monés JM, et al. Digital indocyanine-green angiography in chorioretinal disorders. *Ophthalmology.* 1992;99:287–291.

Haritoglou C, Kampik A, Langhals H. Indocyanine green should not be used to facilitate removal of the internal limiting membrane in macular hole surgery. *Surv Ophthalmol.* 2009;54(1):138–141.

Iriyama A, Yanagi Y, Uchida S, et al. Retinal nerve fibre layer damage after indocyanine green assisted vitrectomy. *Br J Ophthalmol.* 2004;88:1606–1607.

Kampik A, Sternberg P. Indocyanine green in vitreomacular surgery – (why) it is a problem? *Am J Ophthalmol.* 2003;136:527–529.

Kogure K, David NJ, Yamanouchi U, et al. Infrared absorption angiography of the fundus circulation. *Arch Ophthalmol.* 1970;83:209–214.

Lee JE, Yoon TJ, Oum BS, et al. Toxicity of indocyanine green injected into the subretinal space. *Retina.* 2003;23:675–681.

Obana A, Miki T, Hayashi K, et al. Survey of complications of indocyanine green angiography in Japan. *Am J Ophthalmol.* 1994;118:749–753.

Rezai KA, Farrokh-Siar L, Ernest JT, et al. Indocyanine green induced apoptosis in human retinal pigment epithelial cells. *Am J Ophthalmol.* 2004;93:931–933.

Uemoto R, Yamamoto S, Takeuchi S. Changes in retinal pigment epithelium after indocyanine green–assisted internal limiting lamina peeling during macular hole surgery. *Am J Ophthalmol.* 2005;140:752–755.

Yannuzzi LA, Slakter JS, Sorenson JA, et al. Digital indocyanine green videoangiography and choroidal neovascularization. *Retina.* 1992;12:191–223.

Lissamine green, rose bengal

Chodosh J, Banks MC, Stroop WG. Rose bengal inhibits herpes simplex virus replication in vero and human corneal epithelial cells in vitro. *Invest Ophthalmol Vis Sci.* 1992;33(8):2520–2527.

Doughty MJ, Naase T, Donald C, et al. Visualization of "Marx's line" along the marginal eyelid conjunctiva of human subjects with lissamine green dye. *Ophthalmic Physiol Opt.* 2004;24:1–7.

Menon IA, Basu PK, Persad SD, et al. Reactive oxygen species in the photosensitization of retinal pigment epithelial cells by rose Bengal. *J Toxicol Cut Ocular Toxicol.* 1992;11(4):269–283.

Trypan blue

Ang GS, Ang AJ, Burton RL. Iatrogenic macula hole and consequent macular detachment caused by intravitreal trypan blue injection. *Eye.* 2004;18:759–760.

Balayre S, Boissonnot M, Paquereau J, et al. Evaluation of trypan blue toxicity in idiopathic epiretinal membrane surgery with macular function test using multifocal electroretinography: seven prospective case studies. *J Fr Ophtalmol.* 2005;28:169–176.

Bisol T, Rezende RA, Guedes J, et al. Effect of blue staining of expendable hydrophilic intraocular lenses on contrast sensitivity and glare vision. *J Cataract Refract Surg.* 2004;30:1732–1735.

Chowdhury PK, Raj SM, Vasavada AR. Inadvertent staining of the vitreous with trypan blue. *JCataract Refract Surg.* 2004;30:274–276.

Gaur A, Kayarkar VV. Inadvertent vitreous staining. *J Cataract Refract Surg.* 2005;31:649.

Gouws P, Merriman M, Goethals S, et al. Cystoid macular oedema with trypan blue use. *Br JOphthalmol.* 2004;88:1348–1349.

Portes AL, Almeida AC, Allodi S, et al. Trypan blue staining for capsulorhexis: ultrastructural effect on lens epithelial cells and capsules. *J Cataract Refract Surg.* 2010;36:582–587.

Rezai KA, Farrokh-Siar L, Gasyna EM, et al. Trypan blue induces apoptosis in human retinal pigment epithelial cells. *Am J Ophthalmol.* 2004;138:492–495.

Uno F, Malerbi F, Maia M, et al. Subretinal trypan blue migrapeeling. *Retina.* 2006;26:237–239.

van Dooren BT, DeWaard PW, Poort-van Nouhuys H, et al. Corneal endothelial cell density after trypan blue capsule staining in cataract surgery. *J Cataract Refract Surg.* 2002;28:574–575.

Werner L, Apple DJ, Crema AS, et al. Permanent blue discoloration of a hydrogel intraocular lens by intraoperative trypan blue. *J Cataract Refract Surg.* 2002;28:1279–1286.

Yuen HKL, Lam RF, Lam DSC, et al. Cystoid macular oedema with trypan blue use. *Br J Ophthalmol.* 2005;89:644–645.

Organic pigments (metal salts), inorganic pigments (iron and zinc oxides)
Lu CW, Liu XF, Zhou DD, et al. Bilateral diffuse lamellar keratitis triggered by permanent eyeliner tattoo treatment: a case report. *Exp Ther Med.* 2017;14(1):283–285.

1. Polydimethylsiloxane (PMDS); 2. silicone
Tanaka Y, Toyoda F, Shimmura-Tomita M, et al. Clinicopathological features of epiretinal membranes in eyes filled with silicone oil. *Clin Ophthalmol.* 2018;12:1949–1957.

Yu JH, Gallemore E, Kim JK, et al. Silicone oil droplets following intravitreal bevacizumab injections. *Am J Ophthalmol Case Rep.* 2017;10:142–144.

Benzalkonium chloride (BAK)
Bernal DL, Ubels JL. Quantitative evaluation of the corneal epithelial barrier: effect of artificial tears and preservatives. *Curr Eye Res.* 1991;10:645–656.

Bielory BP, Shariff A, Hussain RM, et al. Toxic anterior segment syndrome: inadvertent administration of intracameral lidocaine 1% and phenylephrine 2.5% preserved with 10% benzalkonium chloride during cataract surgery. *Cornea.* 2017;36(5):621–624.

Burstein NL. Corneal cytotoxicity of topically applied drugs, vehicles and preservatives. *Surv Ophthalmol.* 1980;25:15–30.

Chapman JM, Cheeks L, Green K. Interactions of benzalkonium chloride with soft and hard contact lenses. *Arch Ophthalmol.* 1990;108:244–246.

Gibran SK. Unilateral drug-induced ocular pseudopemphigoid. *Eye.* 2004;18:1270–1278.

Hughes EH, Pretorius M, Eleftheriadis H, et al. Long-term recovery of the human corneal endothelium after toxic injury by benzalkonium chloride. *Br J Ophthalmol.* 2007;91:1460–1463.

Ishibashi T, Yokoi N, Kinoshita S. Comparison of the short-term effects on the human corneal surface of topical timolol maleate with and without benzalkonium chloride. *J Glaucoma.* 2003;12:486–490.

Keller N, Moore D, Carper D, et al. Increased corneal permeability induced by the dual effects of transient tear film acidification and exposure to benzalkonium chloride. *Exp Eye Res.* 1980;30:203–210.

Lavine JB, Binder PS, Wickham MG. Antimicrobials and the corneal endothelium. *Ann Ophthalmol.* 1979;11:1517–1528.

Samples JR, Binder PS, Nayak S. The effect of epinephrine and benzalkonium chloride on cultured corneal endothelial and trabecular meshwork cells. *Exp Eye Res.* 1989;49:1–12.

Chlorhexidine gluconate
Khurana AK, Ahluwalie BK, Sood S. Savlon keratopathy, a clinical profile. *Acta Ophthalmol.* 1989;67:465–466.

Morgan JF. Complications associated with contact-lens solutions. *Ophthalmology.* 1979;86:1107–1119.

Murthy S, Hawksworth NR, Cree I. Progressive ulcerative keratitis related to the use of topical chlorhexidine gluconate (0.02%). *Cornea.* 2002;21(2):237–239.

Paugh JR, Caywood TG, Peterson SD. Toxic reactions associated with chemical disinfection of soft contact lenses. *Int Contact Lens Clin.* 1984;11:680.

Phinney RB, Mondino BJ, et al. Corneal edema related to accidental Hibiclens exposure. *Am J Ophthalmol.* 1988;106:210–215.

Sawyer WI, Burwick K, Jaworski J, et al. Corneal injury secondary to accidental Surgilube exposure. *Arch Ophthalmol.* 2011;129(9):1229–1230.

Scott WG. Antiseptic (Hibiclens) and eye injuries. *Med J Aust.* 1980;2:456.

Tabor E, Bostwick DC, Evans CC. Corneal damage due to eye contact with chlorhexidine gluconate. *JAMA.* 1989;261:557–558.

Povidone-iodine (PVP-1) (iodopovidone)
Caldwell DR, Kastl PR, Cook J, et al. Povidone-iodine: its efficacy as a preoperative conjunctival and periocular preparation. *Ann Ophthalmol.* 1984;16(6):577.

Thiomersal (thimersal), yellow mercuric oxide (hydrargyric oxide flavum)
Binder PS, Rasmussen DM, Gordon M. Keratoconjunctivitis and soft contact lens solutions. *Arch Ophthalmol.* 1981;99:87–90.

Brazier DJ, Hitchings RA. Atypical band keratopathy following long-term pilocarpine treatment. *Br J Ophthalmol.* 1989;73:294–296.

De la Cuadra J, Pujol C, Aliagia A. Clinical evidence of cross-sensitivity between thiosalicyclic acid, a contact allergen, and piroxicam, a photoallergen. *Cont Dermatol.* 1989;21:349–351.

Gero G. Superficial punctate keratitis with CSI contact lenses dispensed with the Allergan Hydrocare cold kit. *Int Contact Lens Clin.* 1984;11:674.

Rietschel RL, Wilson LA. Ocular inflammation in patients using soft contact lenses. *Arch Dermatol.* 1982;118:147–149.

Wright P, Mackie I. Preservative-related problems in soft contact lens wearers. *Trans Ophthalmol Soc UK.* 1982;102:3–6.

Mitomycin
Al-Hazmi A, Zwaan J, Awad A, et al. Effectiveness and complications of mitomycin C use during pediatric glaucoma surgery. *Ophthalmology.* 1998;105(10):1915–1919.

Bindish R, Condon GP, Schlosser JD, et al. Efficacy and safety of mitomycin-C in primary trabeculectomy. *Ophthalmology.* 2002;109:1336–1342.

Cartsburg O, Kallen C, Hillenkamp J, et al. Topical mitomycin C and radiation induce conjunctival DNA-polyploidy. *Anal Cell Pathol.* 2001;23:65–74.

Ditta LC, Shildkrot Y, Wilson MW. Outcomes in 15 patients with conjunctival melanoma treated with adjuvant topical mitomycin C: complications and recurrences. *Ophthalmology*. 2011;118:1754–1759.

Gupta S, Basti S. Corneoscleral, ciliary body, and vitreoretinal toxicity after excessive instillation of mitomycin C. *Am J Ophthalmol*. 1992;114:503–504.

Higginbotham EJ. Adjunctive use of mitomycin in filtration surgery: is it worth the risk? *Arch Ophthalmol*. 1997;115(8):969–974, 1068–1069.

Khong JJ, Muecke J. Complications of mitomycin C therapy in 100 eyes with ocular surface neoplasia. *Br J Ophthalmol*. 2006;90:819–822.

Kymionis GD, Tsiklis NS, Ginis H, et al. Dry eye after photorefractive keratectomy with adjuvant mitomycin C. *J Refract Surg*. 2006;22:511–513.

Mohammadpour M, Jabbarvand M, Javadi MA. Focal corneal decompensation after filtering surgery with mitomycin C. *Cornea*. 2007;26:1285–1287.

Nassiri N, Farahangiz S, Rahnavardi M, et al. Corneal endothelial cell injury induced by mitomycin-C in photorefractive keratectomy: nonrandomized controlled trial. *J Cataract Refract Surg*. 2008;34:902–908.

Oram O, Gross RL, Wilhelmus KR, et al. Necrotizing keratitis following trabeculectomy with mitomycin. *Arch Ophthalmol*. 1995;113:19–20.

Perez-Rico C, Benitez-Herreros J, Montes-Mollon MA, et al. Intraoperative mitomycin C and corneal endothelium after pterygium surgery. *Cornea*. 2009;28:1135–1138.

Pfister RR. Permanent corneal edema resulting from the treatment of PTK corneal haze with mitomycin. *Cornea*. 2004;23:744–747.

Price Jr FW. Corneal endothelial damage after trabeculectomy with mitomycin C in two patients with glaucoma with cornea guttata. *Cornea*. 2002;21:733.

Robin AL, Ramakrishnan R, Krishnadas R, et al. A long-term dose response study of mitomycin in glaucoma filtration surgery. *Arch Ophthalmol*. 1997;115:969–974.

Rubinfeld RS, Pfister RR, Stein RM, et al. Serious complications of topical mitomycin-C after pterygium surgery. *Ophthalmology*. 1992;99(11):1647–1654.

Sacu S, Ségur-Eltz N, Horvat R, et al. Intumescent cataract after topical mitomycin-C for conjunctival malignant melanoma. *Am J Ophthalmol*. 2003;136:375–377.

Sauder G, Jonas JB. Limbel stem cell deficiency after subconjunctival mitomycin C injection for trabeculectomy. *Am J Ophthalmol*. 2006;141:1129–1130.

Sihota R, Dada T, Gupta SD, et al. Conjunctival dysfunction and mitomycin C-induced hypotony. *J Glaucoma*. 2000;9:392–397.

Storr-Paulsen T, Norregaard JC, Ahmed S, et al. Corneal endothelial cell loss after mitomycin C-augmented trabeculectomy. *J Glaucoma*. 2008;17(8):654–657.

Suner IJ, Greenfield DS, Miller MP, et al. Hypotony maculopathy after filtering surgery with mitomycin C. *Ophthalmology*. 1997;104(2):207–215.

Vizel M, Oster MW. Ocular side effects of cancer chemotherapy. *Cancer*. 1982;49:1999–2002.

Wu SC. Central retinal vein occlusion after trabeculectomy with mitomycin C. *Can J Ophthalmol*. 2001;36:37–39.

You Y, Gu Y-S, Fang C-T, et al. Long-term effects of simultaneous subconjunctival and subscleral mitomycin C application in repeat trabeculectomy. *J Glaucoma*. 2002;11:110–118.

Young DC, Mitchell A, Kessler J, et al. Cortical blindness and seizures possibly related to cisplatin, vinblastine, and bleomycin treatment of ovarian dysgerminoma. *J Am Osteopath Assoc*. 1993;93:502–504.

Zarnowski T, Haszcz D, Rakowska E, et al. Corneal astigmatism after trabeculectomy. *Klin Oczna*. 1997;99(5):313–315.

Cocaine hydrochloride

Block SS, Moore BD, Scharre JE. Visual anomalies in young children exposed to cocaine. *Optom Vis Sci*. 1997;74(1):28–36.

Foster M, et al. Cocaine associated oculomotor nerve (CN III) palsy with pupil involvement. *North American Congress of Clinical Toxicology*. 2010; abstr 144.

Munden PM, Kardon RH, Denison CE, et al. Palpebral fissure responses to topical adrenergic drugs. *Am J Ophthalmol*. 1991;111:706–710.

Perinatal toxicity of cocaine. *Med Newslett*. 1988;30:59–60.

Reddy S, Goldman DR, Hubschman J-P, et al. Cocaine and choroidal infarction, revisiting the triangular sign of amalric. *Retin Cases Brief Rep*. 2011;5:91–93.

Sachs R, Zagelbaum BM, Hersh PS. Corneal complications associated with the use of crack cocaine. *Ophthalmology*. 1993;100(2):187–191.

Silva-Araujo AL, Tavares MA, Patacao MH, et al. Retinal hemorrhages associated with in utero exposure to cocaine. *Retina*. 1996;16:411–418.

Steinkamp PN, Watzke RC, Solomon JD, et al. An unusual case of solar retinopathy. *Arch Ophthalmol*. 2003;121:1798–1799.

Stominger MB, Sachs R, Hersh PS. Microbial keratitis with crack cocaine. *Arch Ophthalmol*. 1990;108:1672.

Tames SM, Goldenring JM. Madarosis from cocaine use. *N Engl J Med*. 1986;15:1324.

Zagelbaum BM, Tannenbaum MH, Hersh PS. Candida albicans corneal ulcer associated with crack cocaine. *Am J Ophthalmol*. 1991;111(2):248–249.

Zeiter JH, McHenry JG, McDermott ML. Unilateral pharmacologic mydriasis secondary to crack cocaine (letter). *Am J Emerg Med*. 1990;8:568–569.

Zeiter JH, Corder DM, Madion MP, et al. Sudden retinal manifestations of intranasal cocaine and methamphetamine abuse (letter). *Am J Ophthalmol*. 1992;114:780–781.

Oxybuprocaine (benoxinate), proxymetacaine hydrochloride (proparacaine), tetracaine (amethocaine)

Dannaker CJ, Maibach HI, Austin E. Allergic contact dermatitis to proparacaine with subsequent cross sensitization to tetracaine from ophthalmic preparations. *Am J Contact Dermatitis*. 2001;12:177–179.

Duffin RM, Olson RJ. Tetracaine toxicity. *Ann Ophthalmol*. 1984;16:836.

Gild WM, Posner KL, Caplan RA, et al. Eye injuries associated with anesthesia. *Anesthesiology.* 1992;76:204–208.

Haddad R. Fibrinous iritis due to oxybuprocaine. *Br J Ophthalmol.* 1989;73:76–77.

Hodkin MJ, Cartwright MJ, Kurumety UR. In vitro alteration of Schirmer's tear strip wetting by commonly instilled anesthetic agents. *Cornea.* 1994;13(2):141–147.

Liesegang TJ, Perniciaro C. Fingertip dermatitis in an ophthalmologist caused by proparacaine. *Am J Ophthalmol.* 1999;127(2):240–241.

Bromfenac sodium, diclofenac sodium, ketorolac tromethamine, nepafenac

Appiotti A, Gualdi L, Alberti M, et al. Comparative study of the analgesic efficacy of flurbiprofen and diclofenac in patients following excimer laser photorefractive keratectomy. *Clin Ther.* 1998;20:913–920.

Asai T, Nakagami T, Mochizuki M, et al. Three cases of corneal melting after instillation of new nonsteroidal anti-inflammatory drug. *Cornea.* 2006;25. 224–224.

Buckley MMT, Brogden RN. Ketorolac: a review of its pharmacodynamic and pharmacokinetic properties, and therapeutic potential. *Drugs.* 1990;39:86–109.

Eiferman RA, Hoffman RS, Sher NA. Topical diclofenac reduces pain following photorefractive keratectomy. *Arch Ophthalmol.* 1993;111:1022.

Evliyaoglu F, Akpolat C, Kurt MM, et al. Retinal vascular caliber changes after topical nepafenac treatment for diabetic macular edema. *Curr Eye Res.* 2018;43(3):357–361.

Flach AJ. Corneal melts associated with topically applied nonsteroidal anti-inflammatory drugs. *Trans Am Ophth Soc.* 2001;99:205–212.

Flach AJ. Cyclo-oxygenase inhibitors in ophthalmology. *Surv Ophthalmol.* 1992;36:259–285.

Flach AJ. Topically applied nonsteroidal anti-inflammatory drugs and corneal problems: an interim review and comment. *Ophthalmology.* 2000;107:1224–1226.

Flach AJ, Graham J, Kruger LP, et al. Quantitative assessment of postsurgical breakdown of the blood aqueous barrier following administration of 0.5% ketorolac tromethamine solution. *Arch Ophthalmol.* 1988;106:344–347.

Goes F, Richard C, Trinquand C. Comparative study of two nonsteroidal anti-inflammatory eyedrops, 0.1% indomethacin versus 0.1% diclofenac in pain control postphotorefractive keratectomy. *Bull Soc Belge Ophtalmol.* 1997;267:11–19.

Guidera AC, Luchs JI, Udell IJ. Keratitis, ulceration, and perforation associated with topical nonsteroidal anti-inflammatory drugs. *Ophthalmology.* 2001;108:936–944.

Hersh PS, Rice BA, Baer JC, et al. Topical nonsteroidal agents and corneal wound healing. *Arch Ophthalmol.* 1990;108:577–583.

Hettinger ME, Gill DJ, Robin JB, et al. Evaluation of diclofenac sodium 0.1% ophthalmic solution in the treatment of ocular symptoms after bilateral radial keratectomy. *Cornea.* 1997;16:406–413.

Jampol LM, Jain S, Pudzisz B, et al. Nonsteroidal anti-inflammatory drugs and cataract surgery. *Arch Ophthalmol.* 1994;112:891–893.

Koch DD. Corneal complications and NSAIDs. *Ophthalmology.* 2001;108:1519–1520.

Lin JC, Rapuano CJ, Laibson PR, et al. Corneal melting associated with use of topical nonsteroidal anti-inflammatory drugs after ocular surgery. *Arch Ophthalmol.* 2000;118:1129–1132.

Reid AL, Henderson R. Diclofenac and dry, irritable eyes. *Med J Aust.* 1994;160:308.

Seitz B, Sorken K, LaBree LD, et al. Corneal sensitivity and burning sensation. Comparing topical ketorolac and diclofenac. *Arch Ophthalmol.* 1996;114:921–924.

Singer DD, Kennedy J, Wittpenn JR. Topical NSAIDs effect on corneal sensitivity. *Cornea.* 2015;34(5):541–543.

Solomon KD, Turkalj JW, Whiteside SB, et al. Topical 0.5% ketorolac vs 0.03% flurbiprofen for inhibition of miosis during cataract surgery. *Arch Ophthalmol.* 1997;115:1119–1122.

Strelow SA, Sherwood MB, Broncata LJ, et al. The effect of diclofenac sodium ophthalmic solution on intraocular pressure following cataract extraction. *Ophthalmic Surg.* 1992;23:170–175.

Szerenyi K, Sorken K, Garbus JJ, et al. Decrease in normal human corneal sensitivity with topical diclofenac sodium. *Am J Ophthalmol.* 1994;118(3):312–315.

Yee RW, the Ketorolac Radial Keratotomy Study Group. Analgesic efficacy and safety of nonpreserved ketorolac tromethamine ophthalmic solution following radial keratotomy. *Am J Ophthalmol.* 1998;125:472–480.

Zaidman GW. Diclofenac and its effect on corneal sensation. *Arch Ophthalmol.* 1995;113:262.

Zanini M, Savini G, Barboni P. Corneal melting associated with topical diclofenac use after laser-assisted subepithelial keratectomy. *J Cataract Refract Surg.* 2006;32:1570–1572.

Sodium chloride

Barabino S, Rolando M, Camicione P, et al. Effects of a 0.9% sodium chloride ophthalmic solution on the ocular surface of symptomatic contact lens wearers. *Can J Ophthalmol.* 2005;40:45–50.

Ho Wang Yin G, Sampo M, Soare S, et al. Visual acuity, pachymetry and corneal density after 5% sodium chloride treatment in corneal edema after surgery. *J Fr Ophtalmol.* 2015;38(10):967–973.

Sodium hyaluronate

Alpar JJ. Comparison of healon and amvisc. *Ann Ophthalmol.* 1985;17:647–651.

Daily L. Caution on sodium hyaluronate (Healon) syringe. *Am J Ophthalmol.* 1982;94(4):59.

Glasser DB, Matsuda M, Edelhauser HF. A comparison of the efficacy and toxicity of an intraocular pressure response to viscous solutions in the anterior chamber. *Arch Ophthalmol.* 1986;104:1819–1824.

Goa KL, Benfield P. Hyaluronic acid: A review of its pharmacology and use as a surgical aid in ophthalmology, and its therapeutic potential in joint disease and wound healing. *Drugs.* 1994;47(3):563–566.

Hoover DL, Giangiacomo J, Benson RL. Descemet's membrane detachment by sodium hyaluronate. *Arch Ophthalmol.* 1985;103:805–808.

Kim EG, Eom TK, Kang SJ. Severe visual loss and cerebral infarction after injection of hyaluronic acid gel. *J Craniofac Surg.* 2014;25(2):684–686.

MacRae SM, Edelhauser HF, Hyndiuk RA, et al. The effects of sodium hyaluronate, chondroitin sulfate, and methylcellulose on the corneal endothelium and intraocular pressure. *Am J Ophthalmol.* 1983;95:332–341.

McDermott ML, Edelhauser HF. Drug binding of ophthalmic viscoelastic agents. *Arch Ophthalmol.* 1989;107:261–263.

Pape LG, Balazs EA. The use of sodium hyaluronate (Healon) in human anterior segment surgery. *Ophthalmology.* 1980;87(7):699–705.

Passo MS, Ernest JT, Goldstick TK. Hyaluronate increases intraocular pressure when used in cataract extraction. *Br J Ophthalmol.* 1985;69(8):572–575.

Sholohov G, Levartovsky S. Retained ophthalmic viscosurgical device material in the capsular bag 6 months after phacoemulsification. *J Cataract Refract Surg.* 2005;31:627–629.

Storr-Paulsen A. Analysis of the short-term effect of two viscoelastic agents on the intraocular pressure after extracapsular cataract extraction. *Acta Ophthalmol.* 1993;71:173–176.

CHAPTER 19

Herbal Medicine– and Dietary Supplement–Induced Ocular Side Effects

HERBAL OR SUPPLEMENT NAMES:

1. Aluminum nicotinate; 2. niacin (nicotinic acid); 3. niacinamide (nicotinamide); 4. nicotinyl alcohol.

Primary Use

Nicotinic acid and its derivatives are used as peripheral vasodilators, as vitamins, and as a first-line drug in the treatment of hyperlipidemia.

Ocular Side Effects
Systemic administration – oral
Certain
1. Decreased vision
2. Macula (Fig. 19.1)
   a. Edema
   b. Cystoid macular edema

Probable
1. Sicca sensation
2. Eyelids or conjunctiva
   a. Allergic reactions
   b. Hyperpigmentation
   c. Edema

Possible
1. Diplopia
2. Proptosis (minimal)
3. Decreased risk of cataracts
4. Eyelids or conjunctiva
   a. Urticaria
   b. Loss of eyelashes or eyebrows
   c. Edema

Clinical Significance

All of the signs and symptoms listed are dose related to niacin (nicotinic acid), although the other drugs may cause these symptoms as well. These drugs cause macular edema with resultant blurred vision. This may occur from even 1 dose and may last for 1–2 hours; however, with prolonged use, some can develop cystoid macular edema. If this goes unrecognized, permanent damage to the macula may occur. Spirn et al have shown that these cystoid spaces are in the inner nuclear and outer plexiform layers of the retina.[1] Macular edema occurs primarily in patients who are taking at least 3 g per day, although it has been seen in patients taking as little as 1.5 g per day. Macular edema is 10 times more common in men than in women, especially in the third to fifth decades of life. The edema usually disappears on discontinuation of the drug. This drug is also secreted in the tears and will aggravate patients who already have a sicca-type problem. There is also a group of patients who will develop lid or periorbital edema with or without minimal proptosis while taking niacin. Occasionally, a transitory, grayish discoloration of the eyelids occurs as well. There are a few cases in the spontaneous reports of superficial punctate keratitis and 2 cases of eyelash or eyebrow loss. A retrospective survey showed that 7% of patients had to discontinue niacin in dosages above 3 g per day secondary to adverse ocular effects.[2] All of these side effects seem to be dose related, and patients may consider titrating the drug. Freisberg et al demonstrated resolution of niacin-induced maculopathy with dosage decrease.[3] If decreased vision occurs, one needs to consider macular edema in the differential diagnosis. One of the hallmarks of niacin maculopathy is absence of leakage on fluorescein angiography even in the late phases. Although this drug decreases lipids, and lipid-lowering drugs have been linked to cataract formation, no relationship with niacin and cataracts has been established. In fact, a case-control study suggested that the antioxidant potential of niacin is inhibitory in the formation of cortical, nuclear, or mixed cataracts.[4] There is a single positive rechallenge case report of niacin-induced glaucoma that resolved with cessation of niacin therapy.[5] Niacin therapy has been used to treat central retinal vein occlusions.[6]

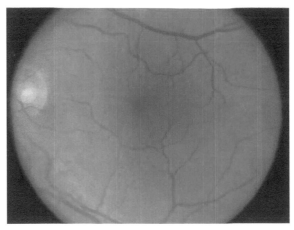

FIG. 19.1 Niacin maculopathy.[7]

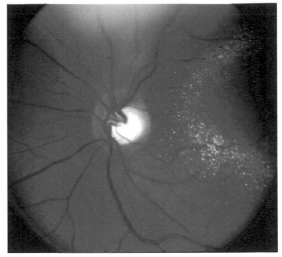

FIG. 19.2 Canthaxanthine crystalline retinopathy.[9]

HERBAL OR SUPPLEMENT NAME:

Canthaxanthine.

Primary Use

Used in cosmetics, as a food coloring, and to produce an artificial suntan when administered orally. It is naturally occurring and is found in crustaceans and chanterelle mushrooms.

Ocular Side Effects

Systemic administration – oral

Certain

1. Retina – extracellular yellow or gold-like particles (predisposed to macular area) (Fig. 19.2)
2. Decreased vision
3. Decreased dark adaptation
4. Electroretinogram (ERG)
   a. Hypernormal scotopic amplitudes (low doses)
   b. Increased scotopic latencies (higher doses)
   c. Depressed photopic activity

Clinical Significance

For over 2 decades canthaxanthine has been known to cause deposition of a crystalline in all layers of the retina, especially the superficial layers. These may cover retinal blood vessels. There is a predisposition for deposition in the macular area, areas of prior trauma, or areas of retinal pathology. The deposits are dose related and may be more common in the elderly and patients with preexisting ocular disease (i.e. glaucoma or pigmentary retinopathies). Chang et al described a case in which deposits significantly increased around a branch-vein occlusion.[1] The deposits will absorb with time if the supplement is discontinued, but this may take many years. In general, these crystals cause no visual problems, although in rare cases some visual complaints are seen. Static threshold perimetry, dark adaptation, and ERG can show abnormalities, which are reversible.[2-4] If 37 g of canthaxanthine are given over time to enhance skin tanning, 50% of individuals will have retinal deposition; at the 60-g level, 100% will show retinal deposits.[2] Cases in the literature and spontaneous reports suggest that in sensitive individuals, dietary intake may rarely show mild cases similar to those described here.[2,5] There have also been canthaxanthine retinopathy case reports without direct intake of canthaxanthine due to deposits from food coloring.[6] This naturally occurring carotenoid is a commonly used food coloring and can be found in crustaceans, chanterelle mushrooms, and some pink-colored fish. The most complete review of this subject is by Arden et al.[7] It is possible that canthaxanthine has a strong effect on lipid membranes and this somehow adversely affects the macular vascular system.[8]

HERBAL OR SUPPLEMENT NAME:
Chamomile (*Matricaria chamomilla*).

Primary Use
Chamomile is used to treat inflammation of the eye, as well as insomnia, indigestion, migraine headaches, bronchitis, fevers, colds, inflammation, and burns. The indications for the eye include eye irritation, styes, epiphora, and inflammation.

Ocular Side Effects
Local ophthalmic use or exposure – topical ocular application
Certain
1. Allergic conjunctivitis (severe)
2. Edema

Clinical Significance
Chamomile tea, which is a common drink worldwide, is made from the dried flower heads of the German or common chamomile plant. There is strong evidence that this tea, when applied topically in or around the eye, can cause a severe conjunctivitis. Subiza et al described 7 patients who rinsed their eyes with chamomile tea to treat styes and runny, irritated eyes.[1] All subjects developed severe conjunctivitis, with edema occurring in 2 patients. All 7 subjects had a history of seasonal allergic rhinitis. A possible mechanism for these patients' conjunctivitis could be sensitivity to the allergens present in *M. chamomilla* pollen. Cross-reactivity with other allergenic pollens to which the patient is already sensitive could lead to the severe conjunctivitis observed in Subiza's study. Because patients are using chamomile to treat their eyes, clinicians should recognize the possibility of *M. chamomilla* sensitivity in cases of what appears to be allergic conjunctivitis, especially in patients who already have an atopic history.

HERBAL OR SUPPLEMENT NAME:
Chrysanthemum (lice shampoo) (Fig. 19.3).

Primary Use
Pyrethrum (*Chrysanthemum cinerariifolium*) is used as an insecticide for scabies, head lice, crab lice, and their nits. Not Nice to Lice (NNTL) shampoo is used to kill head lice and their nits. The ingredients of the latter, according to the product label, include purified water, anionic/nonionic surfactant blend, glycerin, enzymes, and peppermint oil.

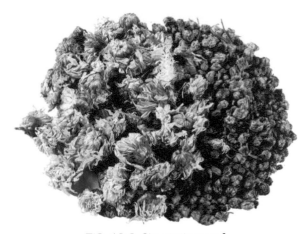

FIG. 19.3 Chrysanthemum.[3]

Ocular Side Effects
Inadvertent ocular exposure
Certain
1. Keratitis
2. Conjunctivitis
   a. Irritative
   b. Allergic (severe)
3. Corneal abrasions

Clinical Significance
From the spontaneous reports, there are 54 cases of keratitis and 19 cases of irritative conjunctivitis from topical use of pyrethrum, which presumably got into the eye of the patients inadvertently. In addition, there are 15 case reports of severe surface ocular reactions from NNTL, which got into the eyes of the user.[1,2] Seven of these cases were corneal abrasions. It may not be unusual for eye irritation to occur when a topical solution is used around the eyes (i.e. lice shampoo on the head), but it is unusual for the reaction to cause more than transient eye irritation or red eye. Specifically, reports of corneal abrasions are worrisome, as patients will need to seek emergency treatment due to severe ocular pain and the risk of a bacterial infection superimposed on the corneal epithelial defect. Corneal abrasions may be due to the proteolytic enzymes present in the shampoo preparation. From the available data, all adverse reactions were immediate and resolved after 1–2 days after discontinuation of the product. The dosage in all patients was per manufacturer instructions for use of NNTL; however, the concentration of pyrethrum is unknown in this and other products.

HERBAL OR SUPPLEMENT NAME:

Datura (angel's trumpet, Jimson weed, thorn apple).

Primary Use

The dried leaves of this flower are used to treat inflammation of the eye, as well as asthma, bronchitis, influenza, and coughs. The leaves contain alkaloids that are anticholinergic and parasympatholytic in extremely varying concentrations. Jimson weed (*Datura stramonium*) is the main member of this genus utilized for its potential therapeutic value.

Ocular Side Effects
Inadvertent ocular exposure
Certain
1. Mydriasis

Clinical Significance

Hayman reported *Datura wrightii* induced mydriasis in a 4-year-old girl as she was picking flowers in her garden.[1] Thin-layer chromatography showed large quantities of scopolamine, the highest concentration being in the seed pod. There were also trace amounts of hyoscyamine and atropine in all the samples. There are multiple case reports of dilated pupils reported in young adults who used this flower for its hallucinogenic properties in Europe.[2] There are also case reports of anisocoria associated with *Datura* in both humans and animals exposed to this herbal product.[3–6] Clinicians should remain aware of this ocular side effect from this wildflower, especially in the southwest United States, where it is most prevalent.

HERBAL OR SUPPLEMENT NAME:

Echinacea purpurea (Fig. 19.4).

Primary Use

This plant's roots, leaves, or the whole plant in various stages of development are used to treat the common cold, coughs, fevers, urinary tract infections, burns, and influenza.

Ocular Side Effects
Systemic administration – oral
Certain
1. Conjunctivitis
   a. Irritative
   b. Allergic

Clinical Significance

The evidence of efficacy for *Echinacea* has been studied through randomized placebo-controlled, double-blind

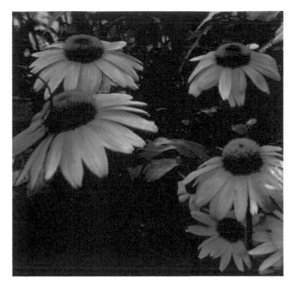

FIG. 19.4 Echinacea purpurea.[2]

studies, and the results are mixed, especially for upper respiratory infections. There are 7 cases in the spontaneous reports of eye irritation and conjunctivitis secondary to *Echinacea*. All reports were in adults, and in all cases the ocular symptoms resolved within at least a day after stopping *Echinacea*. The conjunctivitis may be due to an anaphylactic reaction. There is evidence that *Echinacea* may activate the autoimmune response, and therefore it has been suggested that it be avoided in patients with autoimmune diseases.[1]

HERBAL OR SUPPLEMENT NAME:

Ginkgo biloba.

Primary Use

The flower and seeds, when separated from their fleshy outer layer, provide medicinal effects similar to aspirin, in that they inhibit platelet aggregation. The therapeutic benefits have been studied for dementia, peripheral occlusive arterial disease, and equilibrium disorders. *G. biloba* is also used to treat tinnitus, asthma (inhibits bronchoconstriction), hypertonia, angina pectoris, and tonsillitis.

Ocular Side Effects
Systemic administration – oral
Certain
1. Spontaneous hyphema
2. Retinal hemorrhage

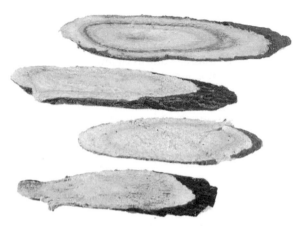

FIG. 19.5 Licorice.[4]

Clinical Significance

G. biloba is one of the best-selling and most popular herbal medicines in the world. Multiple manufacturers produce this product, either alone or in combination with other herbal medicines.

There are numerous case reports of bleeding tendencies in patients taking *G. biloba*. From 118 cases in the spontaneous reports, there are 16 cases of spontaneous hyphema and 4 reports of retinal hemorrhages in patients taking *G. biloba*. The literature reveals well-documented cases of spontaneous hyphema in a 70-year-old man and a retrobulbar hemorrhage in a 65-year-old woman after retrobulbar injection for cataract surgery.[1,2] The blood-thinning properties and propensity to bleed in patients taking *G. biloba* appear to be real; therefore it should be used with caution in patients who are also taking coumadin or aspirin, as the effects could be additive. There is no proof of a correlation between *G. biloba* use and glaucoma.

HERBAL OR SUPPLEMENT NAME:

Licorice (*Glycyrrhiza glabra*) (Fig. 19.5).

Primary Use

Used to treat patients with gastric ulcers, peptic ulcers, and hepatitis C. Indian medicine sometimes uses licorice for eye diseases, and it is frequently used by some patients to treat upper respiratory tract infections, ulcers of the gastrointestinal tract, appendicitis, constipation, and other conditions.

Ocular Side Effects
Systemic administration – oral
Certain

1. Transient visual loss similar to the visual symptoms associated with migraine headaches

Possible

1. Hypertensive retinopathy
2. Posterior reversible encephalopathy syndrome (PRES)

Clinical Significance

Licorice (*G. glabra*) root derives some of its medicinal properties from the isoflavonoid glabridin. Glabridin inhibits cyclooxygenase activity and has an anti-inflammatory and an antiplatelet effect. Dobbins et al reported 5 cases of transient visual loss after licorice ingestion.[1] The visual symptoms were similar to what one might see with an ocular migraine without headache. The authors postulate that vasospasm of the brain, retinal, and/or optic nerve blood vessels plays a role in the visual symptoms, as there is strong evidence that licorice, through its glucocorticoid and norepinephrine effects, can cause vasospasm throughout the body. Clinically, it appears subjects need to consume large amounts of licorice for the ocular side effects to occur. Licorice has been associated with PRES and with hypertensive retinopathy due to its vasoconstrictive effects and hypokalemic effects.[2,3] One should use caution if the patient has a history of migraine headaches due to vasospasm, as the effects could be additive.

HERBAL OR SUPPLEMENT NAME:

Retinol (vitamin A).

Proprietary Names

Aquasol A, A-25, Palmitate-A, Pedi-Vit-A, Retinol A.

Primary Use

Vitamin A is used as a dietary supplement, in the management of vitamin A–deficient states, and in the treatment of acne.

Ocular Side Effects
Systemic administration – oral or topical
Certain

1. Eyelids or conjunctiva
   a. Conjunctivitis – nonspecific
   b. Yellow or orange discoloration
   c. Loss of eyelashes or eyebrows

d. Irritation
2. Exophthalmos
3. Pseudotumor cerebri
   a. Paresis or paralysis of extraocular muscles
   b. Papilledema
   c. Visual fields
      i. Scotomas
      ii. Enlarged blind spot
   d. Diplopia
   e. Nystagmus
   f. 6th-nerve palsy
   g. Peripapillary hemorrhages
   h. Optic nerve atrophy
4. Color vision defect
   a. Objects have yellow tinge
   b. Improves red dyschromatopsia

Probable

1. Increased intraocular pressure – minimal
2. Subconjunctival or retinal hemorrhages

Possible

1. Eyelids or conjunctiva – exfoliative dermatitis

Clinical Significance

Vitamin A deficiency is a cause of blindness in the developing world. Severe xerophthalmia from vitamin A deficiency can lead to opacification of the cornea. Ocular manifestations from hypervitaminosis A are varied and dose related. Although some direct effects, such as loss of eyelashes, are evident, most are central effects due to increased intracranial pressure, such as diplopia and strabismus. Simultaneous use of vitamin A and tetracyclines, isotretinoin, or other drugs causing pseudotumor may increase the incidence of intracranial hypertension (ICH). To date, it is not known how excess vitamin A causes ICH. There is a case report of ICH from topical application of vitamin A containing compounds and also ICH from breast-feeding from a mother on vitamin A products systemically.[1,2] Ocular side effects due to hypervitaminosis A are much more frequent and extensive in infants and children than in adults. Nearly all ocular side effects are rapidly reversible if recognized early and if the vitamin therapy is discontinued. In some instances, it may be several months before these effects are completely resolved. This prolonged effect of vitamin A probably occurs because of the extensive storage of vitamin A in the liver. Papilledema, if untreated, may progress to permanent optic atrophy. Berson et al suggested that vitamin A may have beneficial effects on retinitis pigmentosa.[3] Other authors do not agree.[4,5] If exophthalmos is present, it may be secondary to thyroid changes because vitamin A has antithyroid activity. Hypercalcemia due to vitamin A is infrequent, and band keratopathy has not been reported in the literature or in the spontaneous reports. Dryness and irritation of the eyes have been reported in patients on high doses of vitamin A, probably because the vitamin has been found to be present in tears. Evans et al report an "hourglass" cornea and iris in an infant after the mother took excessive vitamin A products during pregnancy.[6]

HERBAL OR SUPPLEMENT NAME:

Saw palmetto.

Primary Use

Serenoa repens is the herbal extract of saw palmetto, and it is used in the treatment of benign prostatic hyperplasia (BPH), although the efficacy of treatment remains inconclusive.

Ocular Side Effects

Systemic administration – oral
Possible

1. Intraoperative floppy iris syndrome (IFIS)

Clinical Significance

IFIS is characterized by 3 main events during cataract surgery: (1) iris or uveal prolapse through the intraoperative wound, (2) progressive pupillary miosis during surgery, and (3) billowing and floppy iris that dilates poorly during surgery. Treatment for BPH with alpha-adrenergic antagonists has been associated with IFIS, and perhaps saw palmetto has some alpha-adrenergic blocking capacity. There are case reports that indicate saw palmetto is a potential contributor to IFIS syndrome when taken as an herbal supplement for BPH.[1-4]

HERBAL OR SUPPLEMENT NAME:

Vitamin D. The following preparations contain vitamin D as a single entity: calcifediol, calcitriol, cholecalciferol, dihydrotachysterol (DHT), doxercalciferol, ergocalciferol (calciferol), and paricalcitol.

Proprietary Names

Calciferol, Calcijex, Calderol, Delta-D, Delta D3, DHT, DHT Intensol, Drisdol, Hectorol, Hytakerol Rayaldee, Rocaltrol, Vitamin D, Zemplar.

Primary Use

Vitamin D is used as a dietary supplement and in the management of vitamin D–deficient states and hypoparathyroidism.

Ocular Side Effects

Systemic administration – intramuscular or oral

Certain

1. Calcium deposits or band keratopathy
   a. Conjunctiva
   b. Cornea
   c. Sclera
2. Papilledema
3. Optic atrophy
4. Narrowed optic foramina
5. Photophobia (late)

Probable

1. Decreased pupillary reaction to light
2. Small optic discs

Possible

1. Strabismus
2. Epicanthus
3. Nystagmus
4. Visual hallucinations
5. Amblyopia

Clinical Significance

Severe adverse ocular reactions due to vitamin D are caused by either a direct toxicity or an unusual sensitivity seen primarily in infants. Calcium deposits in or around the optic canal cause narrowing of the optic foramina, which may cause papilledema. If the vitamin intake is not discontinued, optic atrophy may result. Children with these toxic effects often have elf-like faces and prominent epicanthal folds. In adults, the toxic effects are few, and the main adverse reaction appears to be the calcium deposits in ocular tissue. Hypervitaminosis D can manifest a band keratopathy.[1] It is of interest that in addition to corneal calcification, white fleck–crystalline calcium deposits may also occur on the conjunctiva. One case of a presumed basilar artery insufficiency with hemianopsia due to vitamin D intake has been reported.[2]

REFERENCES

Herbals or Supplements: Aluminum nicotinate, niacin (nicotinic acid), niacinamide (nicotinamide), nicotinyl alcohol

1. Spirn MJ, Warren FA, Guyer DR, et al. Optical coherence tomography findings in nicotinic acid maculopathy. *Am J Ophthalmol*. 2003;135:913–914.
2. Fraunfelder FW, Fraunfelder FT, Illingworth DR. Adverse ocular effects associated with niacin therapy. *Br J Ophthalmol*. 1995;79:54–56.
3. Freisberg L, Rolle TJ, Ip MS. Diffuse macular edema in niacin-induced maculopathy may resolve with dosage decrease. *Retin Cases Brief Rep*. 2011;5:227–228.
4. Leske MC. The lens opacities case-control study. Risk factors for cataract. *Arch Ophthalmol*. 1991;109:244–251.
5. Tittler EH, De Barros DS, Navarro JB, et al. Oral niacin can increase intraocular pressure. *Ophthalmic Surg Lasers Imaging*. 2008;39(4):341–342.
6. Gaynon MW, Paulus YM, Rahimy E, et al. Effect of oral niacin on central retinal vein occlusion. *Graefes Arch Clin Exp Ophthalmol*. 2017;255(6):1085–1092.
7. Fraunfelder FT. *Niacin Maculopathy [photograph]*. Portland: Casey Eye Institute, Oregon Health & Science University; 1988. 1 photograph: color.

Herbal or Supplement: Canthaxanthine

1. Chang TS, Aylward W, Clarkson JG, et al. Asymmetric canthaxanthin retinopathy. *Am J Ophthalmol*. 1995;119(6):801–802.
2. Harnois C, Cortin P, Samson J, et al. Static perimetry in canthaxanthin maculopathy. *Arch Ophthalmol*. 1988;106:58–60.
3. Philipp W. Carotinoid deposits in the retina. *Klin Mbl Augenheilk*. 1985;187:439–440.
4. Weber U, Kern W, Novotny GE, et al. Experimental carotenoid retinopathy. I. Functional and morphological alterations of the rabbit retina after 11 months dietary carotenoid application. *Graefes Arch Clin Exp Ophthalmol*. 1987;225:198–205.
5. Sharkey JA. Idiopathic canthaxanthine retinopathy. *Eur J Ophthalmol*. 1993;3(4):226–228.
6. Oosterhuis JA, Remky H, Nijman NM, et al. Canthaxanthin retinopathy without intake of canthaxanthin. *Klin Monatsbl Augenheilkd*. 1989;194:110–116.
7. Arden GB, Barker FM. Canthaxanthin and the eye: A critical ocular toxicologic assessment. *J Toxicol Cut Ocul Toxicol*. 1991;10(1&2):115–155.
8. Sujak A. Interactions between canthaxanthin and lipid membranes – possible mechanisms of canthaxanthin toxicity. *Cell Mol Biol Lett*. 2009;14(3):395–410.
9. Chan A, Ko TH, Duker JS. Ultrahigh-resolution optical coherence tomography of canthaxanthine retinal crystals. *Ophthalmic Surg Lasers Imaging*. 2006;37:138–139.

Herbal or Supplement: Chamomile *(Matricaria chamomilla)*

1. Subiza J, Subiza JL, Alonso M, et al. Allergic conjunctivitis to chamomile tea. *Ann Allergy.* 1990;65:127–132.

Herbal or Supplement: Chrysanthemum (lice shampoo)

1. Fraunfelder FW. Adverse ocular effects from lice shampoo. *Arch Ophthalmol.* 2004;122(10):1575.
2. Fraunfelder FW, Fraunfelder FT, Goetsch RA. Adverse ocular effects from over-the-counter lice shampoo. *Arch Ophthalmol.* 2003;121:1790–1791.
3. Ayurvedic Medicine. *The Principles of Traditional Practice.* London: Elsevier; 2006.

Herbal or Supplement: *Datura* (angel's trumpet, Jimson weed, thorn apple)

1. Hayman J. Datura poisoning – the angel's trumpet. *Pathology.* 1985;17:465–466.
2. Reader AL. Mydriasis from *Datura wrightii. Am J Ophthalmol.* 1977;82:263–264.
3. El Ouazzani Chahdi K, Benharbit M, Mansouri I, et al. Acute toxic anisocoria. *J Fr Ophthalmol.* 2012;35(4):288. e1–e3.
4. Hansen P, Clerc B. Anisocoria in the dog provoked by a toxic contact with an ornamental plant: *Datura stramonium. Vet Ophthalmol.* 2002;5(4):277–279.
5. Firestone D, Sloane C. Not your everyday anisocoria: angel's trumpet ocular toxicity. *J Emerg Med.* 2007;33(1):21–24.
6. Macchiaiolo M, Vignati E, Gonfiantini MV, et al. An unusual case of anisocoria by vegetal intoxication: a case report. *Ital J Pediatr.* 2010;36:50.

Herbal or Supplement: *Echinacea purpurea*

1. Blumenthal M, ed. *The Complete German Commission E Monographs: Therapeutic Guide to Herbal Medicines.* American Botanical Council; 1998:121–123. 327–328, 391–5393.
2. Ayurvedic Medicine. *The Principles of Traditional Practice.* London: Elsevier; 2006.

Herbal or Supplement: *Ginkgo biloba*

1. Rosenblatt M. Spontaneous hyphema associated with ingestion of ginkgo biloba extract. *N Engl J Med.* 1997;336:1108.
2. Fong KC, Kinnear PE. Retrobulbar haemorrhage associated with chronic gingko biloba ingestion. *Postgrad Med J.* 2003;79:532–533.

Herbal or Supplement: Licorice *(Glycyrrhiza glabra)*

1. Dobbins KR, Saul RF. Transient visual loss after licorice ingestion. *J Neuroophthalmol.* 2000;20:38–41.
2. O'Connell K, Kinsella J, McMahon C, et al. Posterior reversible encephalopathy syndrome (PRES) associated with liquorice consumption. *Ir J Med Sci.* 2016;185(4):945–947.
3. Schröder T, Hubold C, Muck P, et al. A hypertensive emergency with acute visual impairment due to excessive liquorice consumption. *Neth J Med.* 2015;73(2):82–85.

4. Ayurvedic Medicine. The Principles of Traditional Practice. London: Elsevier; 2006.

Herbal or Supplement: Retinol (vitamin A)

1. Mohammad YM, Raslan IR, Al-Hussain FA. Idiopathic intracranial hypertension induced by topical application of vitamin A. *J Neuroophthalmol.* 2016;36(4):412–413.
2. Ramkumar HL, Verma R, Crow J, et al. A baby with a lot of nerve. *Surv Ophthalmol.* 2016;61(4):506–511.
3. Berson EL, Rosner B, Sandberg MA, et al. Vitamin A supplementation for retinitis pigmentosa (letter). *Arch Ophthalmol.* 1993;111(11):1456–1459.
4. Clowes DD. A randomized trial of vitamin A and vitamin E supplementation for retinitis pigmentosa (letter). *Arch Ophthalmol.* 1993;111(6):761–772.
5. Massof RW, Finkelstein D. Supplemental vitamin A retards loss of ERG amplitude in retinitis pigmentosa. *Arch Ophthalmol.* 1993;111(6):751–754.
6. Evans K, Hickey-Dwyer MU. Cleft anterior segment with maternal hypervitaminosis A. *Br J Ophthalmol.* 1991;75(11):691–692.

Herbal or Supplement: Saw palmetto

1. Bell CM, Hatch WV, Fischer HD, et al. Association between tamsulosin and serious ophthalmic adverse events in older men following cataract surgery. *JAMA.* 2009;301(19):1991–1996.
2. Chang DF, Campbell JR. Intraoperative floppy iris syndrome associated with tamsulosin. *J Cataract Refract Surg.* 2005;31:664–673.
3. Neff KD, Sandoval HP, Fernandez de Castro LE, et al. Factors associated with intraoperative floppy iris syndrome. *Ophthalmology.* 2009;116(4):658–663.
4. Yeu E, Grostern R. Saw palmetto and intraoperative floppy-iris syndrome. *J Cataract Refract Surg.* 2007;33:927–928.

Herbal or Supplement: Vitamin D

1. Ziaie H, Razmjou S, Jomhouri R, et al. Vitamin D toxicity; stored and released from adipose tissue? *Arch Iran Med.* 2016;19(8):597–600.
2. Streeto JM. Acute hypercalcemia simulating basilar-artery insufficiency. *N Engl J Med.* 1969;280(8):427–429.

FURTHER READING

Aluminum nicotinate, niacin (nicotinic acid), niacinamide (nicotinamide), nicotinyl alcohol

Callanan D, Blodi BA, Martin DF. Macular edema associated with nicotinic acid. *JAMA.* 1998;279(21):1702.

Chazin BJ. Effect of nicotinic acid on blood cholesterol. *Geriatrics.* 1960;15:423–429.

Choice of cholesterol-lowering drugs. *Med Lett Drugs Ther.* 1991;33(835):2.

Courtney RJ, Singh RP. Spectral domain optical coherence tomography features in niacin maculopathy. *Eye (Lond).* 2014;28(5):629–632.

Gass JD. Nicotinic acid maculopathy. *Am J Ophthalmol.* 1973;76:500–510.

Harris JL. Toxic amblyopia associated with administration of nicotinic acid. *Am J Ophthalmol.* 1963;55:133–144.

Jampol LM. Niacin maculopathy. Author reply, Millay RH. *Ophthalmology.* 1988;95(12):1704–1705.

Metelitsina TI, Grunwald JE, DuPont JC, et al. Effect of niacin on the choroidal circulation of patients with age related macular degeneration. *Br J Ophthalmol.* 2004;88:1568–1572.

Millay RH, Klein ML, Illingworth DR. Niacin maculopathy. *Ophthalmology.* 1988;95(7):930–936.

Parsons Jr WB, Flinn JH. Reduction in elevated blood cholesterol levels by large doses of nicotinic acid. *JAMA.* 1957;165:234–238.

Peczon JD, Grant WM, Lambert BW. Systemic vasodilator, intraocular pressure and chamber depth in glaucoma. *Am J Ophthalmol.* 1971;72:74–78.

Rahman W, Errera MH, Egan C. A rare case of cystoid maculopathy. *J Fr Ophtalmol.* 2013;36(2):e33–e36.

Zahn K. The effect of vasoactive drugs on the retinal circulation. *Trans Ophth Soc UK.* 1966;86:529–536.

Canthaxanthine

Arden GB, Oluwole JO, Polkinghorne P, et al. Monitoring of patients taking canthaxanthin and carotene: An electroretinographic and ophthalmological survey. *Hum Toxicol.* 1989;8:439–450.

Barker FM. Canthaxanthin retinopathy. *J Toxicol Cut Ocul Toxicol.* 1988;7:223–236.

Bluhm R, Branch R, Johnston P, et al. Aplastic anemia associated with canthaxanthin ingested for "tanning" purposes. *JAMA.* 1990;264:1141–1142.

Cortin P, Corriveau LA, Rousseau AP, et al. Gold sequin maculopathy. *Can J Ophthalmol.* 1982;17:103–106.

Espaillat A, Aiello LP, Arrigg PG, et al. Canthaxanthine retinopathy. *Arch Ophthalmol.* 1999;113:412–413.

Harnois C. Canthaxanthine retinopathy. Anatomic and functional reversibility. *Arch Ophthalmol.* 1989;107:538–540.

Leyon H, Ros AM, Nyberg S, et al. Reversibility of canthaxanthin within the retina. *Acta Ophthalmol.* 1990;68:607–611.

Lonn LI. Canthaxanthin retinopathy. *Arch Ophthalmol.* 1987;105:1590.

Weber U, Goerz G. Carotinoid-Retinopathie III. Reversibilitat. *Klin Mbl Augnheilk.* 1986;188:20–22.

Datura (angel's trumpet, Jimson weed, thorn apple)

Andreola B, Piovan A, Da Dalt L, et al. Unilateral mydriasis due to Angel's Trumpet. *Clin Toxicol.* 2008;46(4):329–331.

Havelius U, Asman P. Accidental mydriasis from exposure to Angel's trumpet (Datura suaveolens). *Acta Ophthalmol Scand.* 2002;80(3):332–335.

Levecq L. Didatic case: gardener's eye. *Bull Soc Belge Ophthalmol.* 2011;37:69.

Raman SV, Jacob J. Mydriasis due to Datura inoxia. *Emerg Med J.* 2005;22:310–311.

Roemer HC, Both HV, Foellmann W, et al. Angel's trumpet and the eye. *J R Soc Med.* 2000;93(6):319.

Echinacea purpurea

Grimm W, Müller H. A randomized controlled trial of the effect of fluid extract of *Echinacea purpurea* on the incidence and severity of colds and respiratory infection. *Am J Med.* 1999;106:138–143.

Mullins RJ. Echinacea-associated anaphylaxis. *Med J Aust.* 1998;168:170–171.

Ginkgo biloba

Benjamin JT, Muir T, Briggs K. A case of cerebral haemorrhage: can ginkgo biloba be implicated? *Postgrad Med J.* 2001;77:112–113.

Jia L-Y, Sun L, Fan DS, et al. Effect of topical gingko biloba extract on steroid-induced changes in the trabecular meshwork and intraocular pressure. *Arch Ophthalmol.* 2008;126(12):1700–1706.

Licorice *(Glycyrrhiza glabra)*

Chatterjee N, Domoto-Reilly K, Fecci PE, et al. Licorice-associated reversible cerebral vasoconstriction with PRES. *Neurology.* 2010;75(21):1939–1941.

Van Beers EJ, Stam J, van den Bergh WM. Licorice consumption as a cause of posterior reversible encephalopathy syndrome: a case report. *Crit Care.* 2011;15(1):R64.

Retinol (vitamin A)

Baadsgaard O, Thomsen NH. Chronic vitamin A intoxication. *Danish Med Bull.* 1983;30:51–52.

Baxi SC, Dailey GE. Hypervitaminosis. A cause of hypercalcemia. *West J Med.* 1982;137:429–431.

Clowes DD. A randomized trial of vitamin A and vitamin E supplementation for retinitis pigmentosa. *Arch Ophthalmol.* 1993;111(11):1461–1462.

LaMantia RS, Andrews CE. Acute vitamin A intoxication. *South Med J.* 1981;74:1012–1014.

Marcus DF, Turgeon P, Aaberg TM, et al. Optic disk findings in hypervitaminosis A. *Ann Ophthalmol.* 1985;17:397–402.

Morrice G, Havener WH, Kapetansky F. Vitamin A intoxication as a cause of pseudotumor cerebri. *JAMA.* 1960;173:1802–1805.

Ng EW, Congdon NG, Sommer A. Acute sixth nerve palsy in vitamin A treatment of xerophthalmia. *Br J Ophthalmol.* 2000;84:931–932.

Oliver TK, Havener WH. Eye manifestations of chronic vitamin A intoxication. *Arch Ophthalmol.* 1958;60:19–22.

Pasquariello Jr PS. Benign increased intracranial hypertension due to chronic vitamin A overdosage in a 26-month-old child. *Clin Pediatr.* 1977;16:379–382.

Pearson MG, Littlewood SM, Bowden AN. Tetracycline and benign intracranial hypertension. *BMJ.* 1981;1:292.

Stirling HF, Laing SC, Barr DGD. Hypercarotenaemia and vitamin A overdose from proprietary baby food. *Lancet.* 1986;1:1089.

Ubels JL, MacRae SM. Vitamin A is present as retinol in the tears of humans and rabbits. *Curr Eye Res.* 1984;3:815–822.

Van Dyk HJL, Swan KC. Drug-induced pseudotumor cerebri. In: Leopold IH, ed. *Symposium on Ocular Therapy.* 4th ed. St Louis: Mosby; 1969:71–77.

Wason S, Lovejoy Jr FH. Vitamin A toxicity. *Am J Dis Child.* 1982;136:174.

White JM. Vitamin-A-induced anaemia. *Lancet.* 1984;2:573.

Vitamin D

Baxi SC, Dailey GE. Hypervitaminosis. A cause of hypercalcemia. *West J Med.* 1982;137:429.

Burton JM, Costello FE. Vitamin D in multiple sclerosis and central nervous system demyelinating disease: a review. *J Neuroophthalmol.* 2015;35(2):194–200.

Cogan DC, Albright F, Bartter FC. Hypercalcemia and band keratopathy. *Arch Ophthalmol.* 1948;40:624.

Cohen HN, Fogelman I, Boyle IT, et al. Deafness due to hypervitaminosis D. *Lancet.* 1978;1:973.

Gartner S, Rubner K. Calcified scleral nodules in hypervitaminosis D. *Am J Ophthalmol.* 1955;39:658.

Harley RD, DiGeorge AM, Mabry CC, et al. Idiopathic hypercalcemia of infancy: optic atrophy and other ocular changes. *Trans Am Acad Ophthalmol Otolaryngol.* 1965;69:977–992.

Wagener HP. The ocular manifestations of hypercalcemia. *Am J Med Sci.* 1956;231:218–230.

Index of Side Effects

Note: Page numbers followed by "f" indicate figures and "t" indicate tables.

Choroiditis

Probable

atezolizumab, 300
ipilimumab, 300
nivolumab, 300
pembrolizumab, 300
ritonavir, 409

Possible

bacillus Calmette-Guérin vaccine, 381

Color perception heightened

Certain

binimetinib, 301
cobimetinib, 301
oxygen, 183
oxygen-ozone, 183
trametinib, 301

Color vision abnormal

Certain

acetaminophen, 155
acetohexamide, 279
adrenal cortex injection, 242
alcohol, 116
amfetamine, 91
amobarbital, 122
amyl/butyl nitrite, 203
aspirin, 156
atropine, 192
azithromycin, 24
beclomethasone dipropionate, 242
betamethasone dipropionate, 242
broxyquinoline, 19
budesonide, 242
butabarbital sodium, 122
butalbital, 122
carbachol, 195
carbamazepine, 102
carbon dioxide, 182
chloramphenicol, 29
chloroquine phosphate, 52
chlorothiazide, 220
chlorpromazine hydrochloride, 109
chlorpropamide, 279
cisplatin, 312
clarithromycin, 24
clindamycin, 24
cocaine hydrochloride, 464
cortisone acetate, 242
deferoxamine mesylate, 364
dexamethasone, 242
dicyclomine hydrochloride, 194
digoxin, 209
diiodohydroxyquinoline, 19
dimethyl sulfoxide, 378
disulfiram, 361
dronabinol, 119
epinephrine, 224
erythromycin, 24
estrogen and progestogen
    combination products, 251
ethambutol hydrochloride, 62
fludrocortisone acetate, 242
fluorometholone, 242
fluphenazine hydrochloride, 109

Color vision abnormal *(Continued)*

fluticasone propionate, 242
furosemide, 222
gabapentin, 87
glimepiride, 279
glipizide, 279
glyburide, 279
glycopyrrolate, 194
hashish, 119
homatropine, 192
hydrochlorothiazide, 220
hydrocortisone, 242
hydroxychloroquine sulfate, 52
indapamide, 220
indomethacin, 152
isoniazid, 65
lidocaine, 181
linezolid, 40
lysergic acid diethylamide (LSD), 121
lysergide, 121
marihuana, 119
medroxyprogesterone acetate, 251
mepacrine hydrochloride, 21
mepenzolate bromide, 194
mescaline, 121
methanol, 118
methazolamide, 439
methohexital sodium, 122
methyclothiazide, 220
methylene blue, 267
methylphenobarbital, 122
methylprednisolone, 242
metolazone, 220
metronidazole, 60
morphine sulfate, 162
nalidixic acid, 42
nicotine, 143
nitrofurantoin, 43
norepinephrine bitartrate, 224
ocriplasmin, 461
opium, 162
oxcarbazepine, 102
pentobarbital sodium, 122
perphenazine, 109
phenobarbital, 122
phenytoin, 96
prednisolone, 242
prednisone, 242
primidone, 122
prochlorperazine, 109
promethazine hydrochloride, 109
propantheline bromide, 194
psilocybin, 121
quinine sulfate, 59
retinol, 506
rifampin, 67
rimexolone, 242
secobarbital sodium, 122
sildenafil citrate, 249
sulfacetamide sodium, 45
sulfadiazine, 45
sulfafurazole, 45
sulfamethizole, 45

Color vision abnormal *(Continued)*

sulfamethoxazole, 45
sulfanilamide, 45
sulfasalazine, 45
sulfathiazole, 45
tadalafil, 249
tamoxifen citrate, 337
thiethylperazine, 109
thioridazine hydrochloride, 109
tolazamide, 279
tolbutamide, 279
tolterodine tartrate, 194
tranexamic acid, 271
triamcinolone acetonide, 242
vardenafil hydrochloride, 249
vigabatrin, 89
voriconazole, 50

Probable

acitretin, 375
alendronate sodium, 362
docetaxel, 319
ergometrine maleate, 201
ergotamine tartrate, 201
etidronate disodium, 362
hydroxyamphetamine
    hydrobromide, 448
ibandronate sodium, 362
ibuprofen, 151
iodide and iodine solutions and
    compounds, 248
isotretinoin, 375
lorazepam, 93
methylergometrine, 201
nitroglycerin, 206
oxazepam, 93
pamidronate disodium, 362
pioglitazone, 282
piperazine, 21
radioactive iodine, 248
reserpine, 218
risedronate sodium, 362
rosiglitazone maleate, 282
thiabendazole, 22
zoledronic acid, 362

Possible

carboplatin, 307
cimetidine, 189
estradiol, 253
ethionamide, 64
influenza virus vaccine, 386
isocarboxazid, 104
metoclopramide, 190
naproxen sodium, 154
oxaliplatin, 333
penicillamine, 367
phenelzine sulfate, 104
pilocarpine hydrochloride, 445
quinidine gluconate or sulfate, 212
ranitidine hydrochloride, 189
tranylcypromine sulfate, 104
vincristine sulfate, 341
warfarin sodium, 272
zidovudine, 407

Decreased contact lens tolerance *(Continued)*

> nortriptyline hydrochloride, 101
> orphenadrine citrate, 294
> oxybutynin chloride, 119
> procyclidine hydrochloride, 291
> trihexyphenidyl hydrochloride, 291
> trimipramine maleate, 100

Possible

> estradiol, 253
> pralidoxime chloride, 293

Decreased dark adaptation

Certain

> acitretin, 375
> alcohol, 116
> canthaxanthine, 502
> carbon dioxide, 182
> chloroquine phosphate, 52
> deferoxamine mesylate, 364
> dronabinol, 120
> hashish, 120
> hydroxychloroquine sulfate, 52
> isotretinoin, 375
> lysergic acid diethylamide (LSD), 121
> lysergide, 121
> marihuana, 120
> mescaline, 121
> nilutamide, 331
> oxygen, 183
> oxygen-ozone, 183
> pilocarpine hydrochloride, 445
> psilocybin, 121

Probable

> ergometrine maleate, 201
> ergotamine tartrate, 201
> methylergometrine, 201
> pioglitazone, 282
> rosiglitazone maleate, 282

Possible

> lithium carbonate, 113
> vincristine sulfate, 341

Delayed corneal wound healing

Certain

> adrenal cortex injection, 242
> amphotericin B, 48
> bacitracin, 25
> beclomethasone dipropionate, 242
> benzalkonium chloride, 457
> betamethasone dipropionate, 242
> betaxolol hydrochloride, 422
> bromfenac sodium, 468
> budesonide, 242
> cetuximab, 310
> cocaine hydrochloride, 466
> colchicine, 146
> cortisone acetate, 242
> dexamethasone, 242
> diclofenac sodium, 468
> erlotinib, 310
> fludrocortisone acetate, 242
> fluorometholone, 242
> fluorouracil, 322
> flurbiprofen, 150

Delayed corneal wound healing *(Continued)*

> fluticasone propionate, 242
> gefitinib, 310
> gentamicin sulfate, 38
> hydrocortisone, 242
> idoxuridine, 437
> iodide and iodine solutions and compounds, 248
> ketorolac tromethamine, 468
> levobunolol hydrochloride, 422
> methylprednisolone, 242
> mitomycin, 463
> nepafenac, 468
> osimertinib, 310
> oxybuprocaine, 467
> panitumumab, 310
> prednisolone, 242
> prednisone, 242
> proxymetacaine hydrochloride, 467
> radioactive iodine, 248
> rimexolone, 242
> sulfacetamide sodium, 45
> sulfadiazine, 45
> sulfafurazole, 45
> sulfamethizole, 45
> sulfamethoxazole, 45
> sulfanilamide, 45
> sulfasalazine, 45
> sulfathiazole, 45
> tetracaine, 467
> thiotepa, 340
> timolol maleate, 422
> triamcinolone acetonide, 242
> trifluridine, 437
> vidarabine, 437

Probable

> azathioprine, 370

Dermatochalasis

Certain

> bimatoprost, 425
> latanoprost, 425
> tafluprost, 425
> travoprost, 425

Descemet's membrane wrinkling, folds, or stria

Certain

> bupivacaine hydrochloride, 181
> chloroprocaine hydrochloride, 181
> cytarabine, 315
> lidocaine, 181
> melphalan, 328
> mepivacaine hydrochloride, 181
> prilocaine, 181
> procaine hydrochloride, 181

Diplopia

Certain

> adrenal cortex injection, 242
> alcohol, 116
> aspirin, 156
> beclomethasone dipropionate, 242
> benzathine benzylpenicillin, 26
> betamethasone dipropionate, 242

Diplopia *(Continued)*

> betaxolol hydrochloride, 421
> botulinum toxin A, 449
> botulinum toxin B, 449
> broxyquinoline, 19
> budesonide, 242
> bupivacaine hydrochloride, 180
> carbon dioxide, 182
> chloroprocaine hydrochloride, 180
> codeine, 158
> cortisone acetate, 242
> crizotinib, 314
> cytarabine, 315
> dexamethasone, 242
> dextropropoxyphene, 158
> dicyclomine hydrochloride, 194
> diiodohydroxyquinoline, 19
> divalproex sodium, 94
> dronabinol, 120
> flecainide acetate, 205
> fludrocortisone acetate, 242
> fluorometholone, 242
> fluticasone propionate, 242
> gabapentin, 87
> gentamicin sulfate, 39
> glycopyrrolate, 194
> hashish, 120
> hydrocortisone, 242
> insulin, 280
> iomeprol, 369
> iopamidol, 369
> iopromide, 369
> ketamine hydrochloride, 177
> lamotrigine, 87
> levobunolol hydrochloride, 421
> levodopa, 291
> lidocaine, 180
> marihuana, 120
> mepenzolate bromide, 194
> mepivacaine hydrochloride, 180
> methylprednisolone, 242
> metoclopramide, 190
> metronidazole, 60
> morphine sulfate, 162
> opium, 162
> oxcarbazepine, 102
> penicillamine, 367
> phencyclidine, 121
> phenytoin, 96
> pralidoxime chloride, 293
> prednisolone, 242
> prednisone, 242
> pregabalin, 88
> prilocaine, 180
> procaine hydrochloride, 180
> propantheline bromide, 194
> propofol, 179
> retinol, 506
> rimexolone, 242
> succinylcholine chloride, 175
> timolol maleate, 421
> tolterodine tartrate, 194
> triamcinolone acetonide, 242

Diplopia *(Continued)*
valproate sodium, 94
valproic acid, 94
vincristine sulfate, 341
zonisamide, 99
Probable
abacavir, 407
amoxicillin, 23
ampicillin, 23
atezolizumab, 299
atorvastatin calcium, 191
azithromycin, 24
carisoprodol, 94
chloroquine phosphate, 52
chlorpromazine hydrochloride, 109
ciprofloxacin, 31
clarithromycin, 24
clomifene citrate, 255
danazol, 246
demeclocycline hydrochloride, 33
didanosine, 407
digoxin, 209
doxycycline, 33
emtricitabine, 407
erythromycin, 24
ethotoin, 96
fluphenazine hydrochloride, 109
fluvastatin sodium, 191
hydromorphone hydrochloride, 160
hydroxychloroquine sulfate, 52
ibuprofen, 151
interferon, 325
ipilimumab, 299
kanamycin sulfate, 40
lamivudine, 407
lithium carbonate, 113
lovastatin, 191
mefloquine hydrochloride, 58
meprobamate, 94
minocycline hydrochloride, 33
nafcillin sodium, 23
neomycin sulfate, 42
nitrofurantoin, 43
nivolumab, 299
oxaliplatin, 333
oxprenolol hydrochloride, 211
oxymorphone hydrochloride, 160
oxytetracycline, 33
pembrolizumab, 299
pentazocine, 163
perphenazine, 109
piperacillin, 23
pitavastatin, 191
polymyxin B sulfate, 44
pravastatin sodium, 191
prochlorperazine, 109
promethazine hydrochloride, 109
propranolol hydrochloride, 211
quetiapine fumarate, 114
quinine sulfate, 59
rosuvastatin calcium, 191
simvastatin, 191
sparfloxacin, 31

Diplopia *(Continued)*
stavudine, 407
telithromycin, 46
tetracycline hydrochloride, 33
thiethylperazine, 109
thioridazine hydrochloride, 109
ticarcillin monosodium, 23
tobramycin, 46
topiramate, 98
tosufloxacin, 31
trihexyphenidyl hydrochloride, 291
zidovudine, 407
Possible
acebutolol, 213
alprazolam, 93
aluminum nicotinate, 501
amitriptyline hydrochloride, 100
aripiprazole, 108
atenolol, 213
auranofin, 148
benzfetamine hydrochloride, 92
bortezomib, 304
brompheniramine maleate, 286
carbamazepine, 102
carbinoxamine maleate, 286
carvedilol, 213
cetirizine hydrochloride, 287
chlordiazepoxide, 93
chlorphenamine maleate, 286
cisplatin, 312
citalopram hydrobromide, 103
clemastine fumarate, 286
clindamycin, 25
clomipramine hydrochloride, 100
clonazepam, 93
clorazepate dipotassium, 93
cyproheptadine hydrochloride, 288
dantrolene sodium, 293
desloratadine, 287
dexchlorphenamine maleate, 286
diazepam, 93
diethylpropionate hydrochloride, 92
diphenhydramine hydrochloride, 286
doxepin hydrochloride, 100
doxylamine succinate, 286
edrophonium chloride, 285
escitalopram oxalate, 103
ethionamide, 64
ethosuximide, 96
fenoprofen calcium, 149
fentanyl, 160
fexofenadine hydrochloride, 287
fluorouracil, 322
fluoxetine hydrochloride, 103
flurazepam hydrochloride, 93
flurbiprofen, 150
fluvoxamine maleate, 103
gatifloxacin, 36
hepatitis A vaccine, 383
hepatitis B vaccine, 383
iotalamic acid, 370
isocarboxazid, 104
labetalol hydrochloride, 213

Diplopia *(Continued)*
levofloxacin, 36
levonorgestrel, 254
levothyroxine sodium, 257
liothyronine sodium, 257
loratadine, 287
lorazepam, 93
meperidine hydrochloride, 161
methadone hydrochloride, 161
methsuximide, 96
methylene blue, 267
metoprolol tartrate, 213
midazolam hydrochloride, 93
moxifloxacin hydrochloride, 36
nadolol, 213
niacin, 501
niacinamide, 501
nicotinyl alcohol, 501
nilutamide, 331
norfloxacin, 36
ofloxacin, 36
orphenadrine citrate, 294
oxazepam, 93
paroxetine hydrochloride, 103
phendimetrazine tartrate, 92
phenelzine sulfate, 104
phentermine hydrochloride, 92
pindolol, 213
procainamide hydrochloride, 205
quinidine gluconate or sulfate, 212
rabies immune globulin, 388
rabies vaccine, 388
selegiline hydrochloride, 292
sertraline hydrochloride, 103
sulfacetamide sodium, 45
sulfadiazine, 45
sulfafurazole, 45
sulfamethizole, 45
sulfamethoxazole, 45
sulfanilamide, 45
sulfasalazine, 45
sulfathiazole, 45
temazepam, 93
thyroid, 257
tranylcypromine sulfate, 104
trazodone hydrochloride, 107
triazolam, 93
trimipramine maleate, 100
tripelennamine, 287
triprolidine hydrochloride, 286
verteporfin, 415
vinblastine sulfate, 341
Discharge
Certain
aflibercept, 413
apraclonidine hydrochloride, 420
bevacizumab, 413
brimonidine tartrate, 427
cyclosporine, 371
gentamicin sulfate, 38
influenza virus vaccine, 386
lifitegrast, 470
pazopanib, 333

Erythema *(Continued)*
cefazolin sodium, 28
cefditoren pivoxil, 28
cefoperazone sodium, 28
cefotaxime, 28
cefotetan disodium, 28
cefoxitin sodium, 28
cefradine, 28
ceftazidime, 28
ceftizoxime sodium, 28
ceftriaxone sodium, 28
cefuroxime, 28
cefuroxime axetil, 28
cetirizine hydrochloride, 287
chlordiazepoxide, 92
chlorphenamine maleate, 286
clemastine fumarate, 286
clonazepam, 92
clorazepate dipotassium, 92
cyproheptadine hydrochloride, 287
desloratadine, 287
dexchlorphenamine maleate, 286
dextran, 273
diazepam, 92
diltiazem hydrochloride, 202
diphenhydramine hydrochloride, 286
disulfiram, 361
doxylamine succinate, 286
fexofenadine hydrochloride, 287
flurazepam hydrochloride, 92
ibuprofen, 151
labetalol hydrochloride, 213
loratadine, 287
lorazepam, 92
meperidine hydrochloride, 161
metoprolol tartrate, 213
midazolam hydrochloride, 92
nadolol, 213
naltrexone hydrochloride, 158
nifedipine, 202
oxazepam, 92
pentazocine, 163
pindolol, 213
temazepam, 92
triazolam, 92
tripelennamine, 287
triprolidine hydrochloride, 286
verapamil hydrochloride, 202
Possible
acyclovir, 435
botulinum toxin A, 449
botulinum toxin B, 449
diazoxide, 216
ethionamide, 64
flurbiprofen, 150
influenza virus vaccine, 386
measles virus vaccine live, 387
measles, mumps and rubella virus
vaccine live, 387
measles, mumps, rubella, and
varicella virus vaccine live, 387
mumps virus vaccine live, 387
pimozide, 114

Erythema *(Continued)*
rubella and mumps virus vaccine
live, 387
rubella virus vaccine live, 387
tetanus immune globulin, 390
tetanus toxoid, 390
trazodone hydrochloride, 107
Erythema multiforme
Probable
isoniazid, 65
Possible
acetazolamide, 439
amlodipine besylate, 202
amoxicillin, 24
ampicillin, 24
atorvastatin calcium, 191
bacillus Calmette-Guérin vaccine, 381
botulinum toxin A, 449
botulinum toxin B, 449
carbamazepine, 102
carisoprodol, 94
cefaclor, 28
cefadroxil, 28
cefalexin, 28
cefazolin sodium, 28
cefditoren pivoxil, 28
cefoperazone sodium, 28
cefotaxime, 28
cefotetan disodium, 28
cefoxitin sodium, 28
cefradine, 28
ceftazidime, 28
ceftizoxime sodium, 28
ceftriaxone sodium, 28
cefuroxime, 28
cefuroxime axetil, 28
ciprofloxacin, 31
dapsone, 51
demeclocycline hydrochloride, 33
diltiazem hydrochloride, 202
diphtheria vaccine, 382
diphtheria and tetanus vaccine, 382
diphtheria, tetanus, and pertussis
vaccine, 382
doxycycline, 33
estrogen and progestogen
combination products, 251
ethosuximide, 96
ethotoin, 96
fluvastatin sodium, 191
gabapentin, 87
gatifloxacin, 36
griseofulvin, 49
levofloxacin, 36
lovastatin, 191
medroxyprogesterone acetate, 251
mefloquine hydrochloride, 58
meprobamate, 94
methazolamide, 439
methotrexate, 329
methsuximide, 96
minocycline hydrochloride, 33
moxifloxacin hydrochloride, 36

Erythema multiforme *(Continued)*
nafcillin sodium, 24
nifedipine, 202
nitrofurantoin, 43
norfloxacin, 36
ofloxacin, 36
oxcarbazepine, 102
oxprenolol hydrochloride, 211
oxytetracycline, 33
phenytoin, 97
piperacillin, 24
pitavastatin, 191
pravastatin sodium, 191
propranolol hydrochloride, 211
quinine sulfate, 59
rosuvastatin calcium, 191
simvastatin, 191
sparfloxacin, 31
sulfacetamide sodium, 45
sulfadiazine, 45
sulfafurazole, 45
sulfamethizole, 45
sulfamethoxazole, 45
sulfanilamide, 45
sulfasalazine, 45
sulfathiazole, 45
tetracycline hydrochloride, 33
thiabendazole, 22
thioacetazone, 68
ticarcillin monosodium, 24
tosufloxacin, 31
verapamil hydrochloride, 202
voriconazole, 50
Erythema nodosum
Possible
ciprofloxacin, 31
gatifloxacin, 36
levofloxacin, 36
moxifloxacin hydrochloride, 36
norfloxacin, 36
ofloxacin, 36
sparfloxacin, 31
tosufloxacin, 31
Exfoliative dermatitis
Probable
isoniazid, 65
Possible
amoxicillin, 24
ampicillin, 24
azithromycin, 24
bupivacaine hydrochloride, 181
carbamazepine, 103
carisoprodol, 94
cefaclor, 28
cefadroxil, 28
cefalexin, 28
cefditoren pivoxil, 28
cefoperazone sodium, 28
cefotaxime, 28
cefotetan disodium, 28
cefoxitin sodium, 28
cefradine, 28
ceftazidime, 28

Eyelid and/or conjunctival deposits

Eyelid and/or conjunctival discoloration

Eyelid and/or conjunctival edema

Eyelid and/or conjunctival edema *(Continued)*

Eyelid and/or conjunctival edema *(Continued)*

Hyperemia *(Continued)*
clindamycin, 24
cocaine hydrochloride, 465
colchicine, 146
cyclopentolate hydrochloride, 447
cyclophosphamide, 314
cyclosporine, 371
cytarabine, 315
diclofenac sodium, 468
diethylcarbamazine citrate, 20
dimethyl sulfoxide, 378
dronabinol, 119
dupilumab, 288
echothiophate iodide, 443
emedastine difumarate, 418
emetine hydrochloride, 19
ephedrine sulfate, 224
erythromycin, 24
ether, 176
etidronate disodium, 362
ferrous fumarate, 266
ferrous gluconate, 266
ferrous sulfate, 266
flurbiprofen, 150
gatifloxacin, 36
gentamicin sulfate, 38
glycerol, 222
guanethidine monosulfate, 217
hashish, 119
homatropine, 192
hydralazine hydrochloride, 217
hyoscine butylbromide, 174
hyoscine hydrobromide, 174
hyoscine methobromide, 174
ibandronate sodium, 362
idoxuridine, 437
iron dextran, 266
iron sucrose, 266
ketorolac tromethamine, 468
latanoprost, 424
levobunolol hydrochloride, 422
levofloxacin, 36
loteprednol etabonate, 418
marihuana, 119
methotrexate, 329
methoxsalen, 366
methyl ethyl ketone peroxide, 379
metipranolol, 433
mitomycin, 463
moxifloxacin hydrochloride, 36
nafcillin sodium, 24
naphazoline hydrochloride, 442
neomycin sulfate, 42
nepafenac, 468
netarsudil, 433
norfloxacin, 36
ofloxacin, 36
olopatadine hydrochloride, 419
oprelvekin, 332
oxprenolol hydrochloride, 211
oxybuprocaine, 467
pamidronate disodium, 362

Hyperemia *(Continued)*
phenoxybenzamine
hydrochloride, 223
phenylephrine, 227
piperacillin, 24
piroxicam, 154
polysaccharide iron complex, 266
pralidoxime chloride, 293
propranolol hydrochloride, 211
proxymetacaine hydrochloride, 466
reserpine, 218
rifabutin, 66
risedronate sodium, 362
sildenafil citrate, 249
sodium chloride, 470
sparfloxacin, 31
tadalafil, 249
tafluprost, 424
tetracaine, 467
tetryzoline hydrochloride, 442
thiomersal, 461
ticarcillin monosodium, 24
timolol maleate, 421
topiramate, 97
tosufloxacin, 31
travoprost, 424
trifluridine, 437
trimethoprim, 48
tropicamide, 447
vardenafil hydrochloride, 249
vidarabine, 437
zoledronic acid, 362
Probable
epoetin alfa, 265
epoetin beta, 265
ketoprofen, 153
vinblastine sulfate, 341
Possible
acetylcholine chloride, 443
edrophonium chloride, 285
filgrastim, 35
penicillamine, 367
Hypertrichosis
Certain
thioacetazone, 68
Possible
methoxsalen, 366
zidovudine, 407
Hyphema
Certain
alteplase, 268
amphotericin B, 48
Ginkgo biloba, 504
reteplase, 268
streptokinase, 271
tenecteplase, 268
warfarin sodium, 272
Possible
echothiophate iodide, 443
Hypopyon
Certain
cocaine hydrochloride, 466

Hypopyon *(Continued)*
oxybuprocaine, 466
proxymetacaine hydrochloride, 466
rifabutin, 66
tetracaine, 467
Hypotony
Certain
bupivacaine hydrochloride, 181
chloroprocaine hydrochloride, 181
cidofovir, 436
lidocaine, 181
mepivacaine hydrochloride, 181
mitomycin, 463
prilocaine, 181
procaine hydrochloride, 181
Probable
brinzolamide, 430
dorzolamide hydrochloride, 430

I

Inability to cry
Possible
citalopram hydrobromide, 103
escitalopram oxalate, 103
fluoxetine hydrochloride, 103
fluvoxamine maleate, 103
paroxetine hydrochloride, 103
sertraline hydrochloride, 103
Intraocular pressure decreased
Certain
acebutolol, 213
aflibercept, 413
alcohol, 117
amyl/butyl nitrite, 203
aspirin, 156
atenolol, 213
bevacizumab, 413
bupivacaine hydrochloride, 180
carbachol, 195
carteolol hydrochloride, 432
carvedilol, 213
chlorhexidine gluconate, 459
chloroprocaine hydrochloride, 180
cidofovir, 436
clonidine hydrochloride, 216
dronabinol, 119
echothiophate iodide, 443
ephedrine sulfate, 224
epinephrine, 224
ether, 176
glycerol, 222
hashish, 119
labetalol hydrochloride, 213
lidocaine, 180
mannitol, 223
marihuana, 120
mepivacaine hydrochloride, 180
methacholine chloride, 211
metipranolol, 433
metoprolol tartrate, 213
morphine sulfate, 162
nadolol, 213

Miosis *(Continued)*
    codeine, 158
    dextropropoxyphene, 158
    diacetylmorphine, 159
    dronabinol, 120
    echothiophate iodide, 443
    edrophonium chloride, 285
    ergotamine tartrate, 201
    ether, 176
    fluphenazine hydrochloride, 109
    gatifloxacin, 37
    guanethidine monosulfate, 217
    hashish, 120
    hydromorphone hydrochloride, 160
    levodopa, 291
    levofloxacin, 37
    lidocaine, 180
    marihuana, 120
    mepivacaine hydrochloride, 180
    methacholine chloride, 211
    methadone hydrochloride, 161
    methohexital sodium, 122
    methylphenobarbital, 122
    morphine sulfate, 162
    moxifloxacin hydrochloride, 37
    naltrexone hydrochloride, 158
    nitrous oxide, 178
    norfloxacin, 37
    ofloxacin, 37
    opium, 162
    oxprenolol hydrochloride, 211
    oxymor phone hydrochloride, 160
    pentazocine, 163
    pentobarbital sodium, 122
    perphenazine, 109
    phencyclidine, 121
    phenobarbital, 122
    phenoxybenzamine
       hydrochloride, 223
    phenylephrine, 227
    pilocarpine hydrochloride, 444
    prilocaine, 180
    primidone, 122
    procaine hydrochloride, 180
    prochlorperazine, 109
    promethazine hydrochloride, 109
    propranolol hydrochloride, 211
    pyridostigmine bromide, 285
    secobarbital sodium, 122
    thiethylperazine, 109
    thioridazine hydrochloride, 109
  Probable
    droperidol, 112
    fentanyl, 159
    haloperidol, 112
    meperidine hydrochloride, 160
    piperazine, 22
  Possible
    midazolam hydrochloride, 93
    reserpine, 218
Multiple evanescent white dot
syndrome
Possible
    hepatitis A vaccine, 383

Multiple evanescent white dot
syndrome *(Continued)*
    influenza virus vaccine, 386
    rabies immune globulin, 388
    rabies vaccine, 388
    yellow fever vaccine, 390
Myasthenia gravis, aggravated
Certain
    betaxolol hydrochloride, 421
    echothiophate iodide, 443
    levobunolol hydrochloride, 421
    penicillamine, 367
    timolol maleate, 421
Probable
    amoxicillin, 23
    ampicillin, 23
    atezolizumab, 299
    azithromycin, 24
    bacitracin, 25
    chloroquine phosphate, 52
    ciprofloxacin, 31
    clarithromycin, 24
    demeclocycline hydrochloride, 33
    doxycycline, 33
    erythromycin, 24
    gabapentin, 87
    gentamicin sulfate, 38
    hydroxychloroquine sulfate, 52
    interferon, 325
    ipilimumab, 299
    kanamycin sulfate, 40
    lithium carbonate, 113
    minocycline hydrochloride, 33
    nafcillin sodium, 23
    neomycin sulfate, 42
    nitrofurantoin, 43
    nivolumab, 299
    oxprenolol hydrochloride, 211
    oxytetracycline, 33
    pembrolizumab, 299
    phenytoin, 97
    piperacillin, 23
    polymyxin B sulfate, 44
    procainamide hydrochloride, 205
    propranolol hydrochloride, 211
    quetiapine fumarate, 114
    quinine sulfate, 59
    sparfloxacin, 31
    telithromycin, 46
    tetracycline hydrochloride, 33
    ticarcillin monosodium, 23
    tobramycin, 46
    tosufloxacin, 31
    trihexyphenidyl hydrochloride, 291
Possible
    acebutolol, 213
    apixaban, 269
    atenolol, 213
    atorvastatin calcium, 191
    auranofin, 148
    botulinum toxin A, 449
    botulinum toxin B, 449
    carvedilol, 213
    cisplatin, 312

Myasthenia gravis, aggravated
(Continued)
    dabigatran etexilate mesylate, 269
    ethosuximide, 96
    fluvastatin sodium, 191
    iotalamic acid, 370
    isocarboxazid, 104
    ketoprofen, 153
    labetalol hydrochloride, 213
    levonorgestrel, 254
    levothyroxine sodium, 257
    liothyronine sodium, 257
    lovastatin, 191
    methsuximide, 96
    metoprolol tartrate, 213
    nadolol, 213
    phenelzine sulfate, 104
    pindolol, 213
    pitavastatin, 191
    pravastatin sodium, 191
    quinidine gluconate or sulfate, 212
    rivaroxaban, 269
    rosuvastatin calcium, 191
    simvastatin, 191
    sulfacetamide sodium, 45
    sulfadiazine, 45
    sulfafurazole, 45
    sulfamethizole, 45
    sulfamethoxazole, 45
    sulfanilamide, 45
    sulfasalazine, 45
    sulfathiazole, 45
    tacrolimus, 373
    thyroid, 257
    tranylcypromine sulfate, 104
    verapamil hydrochloride, 202
Myasthenia gravis, unmask
Possible
    azithromycin, 24
    clarithromycin, 24
    clindamycin, 24
    erythromycin, 24
Mydriasis
Certain
    acetaminophen, 155
    acetylcholine chloride, 443
    adrenal cortex injection, 242
    albuterol, 219
    alcohol, 116
    amfetamine, 91
    amobarbital, 122
    amyl/butyl nitrite, 203
    apraclonidine hydrochloride, 420
    aspirin, 156
    atomoxetine, 101
    atropine, 192
    beclomethasone dipropionate, 242
    benzathine benzylpenicillin, 26
    benztropine mesylate, 291
    betamethasone dipropionate, 242
    biperiden, 291
    bromfenac sodium, 468
    brompheniramine maleate, 285
    budesonide, 242

Retinal vascular spasms
Certain
oxygen, 183
oxygen-ozone, 183
Probable
ergometrine maleate, 201
ergotamine tartrate, 201
methylergometrine, 201
Possible
estradiol, 254
Retinal vasculitis
Certain
cefaclor, 28
cefadroxil, 28
cefalexin, 28
cefazolin sodium, 28
cefditoren pivoxil, 28
cefoperazone sodium, 28
cefotaxime, 28
cefotetan disodium, 28
cefoxitin sodium, 28
cefradine, 28
ceftazidime, 28
ceftizoxime sodium, 28
ceftriaxone sodium, 28
cefuroxime, 28
cefuroxime axetil, 28
rifabutin, 66
vancomycin, 434
Probable
amfetamine, 91
dextroamfetamine sulfate, 91
methamfetamine hydrochloride, 91
Possible
influenza virus vaccine, 386
Retinopathy
Certain
melphalan, 328
vigabatrin, 89
Possible
bacillus Calmette-Guérin vaccine, 381
deferasirox, 363
insulin, 280
licorice, 505
Retinopathy, crystalline
Possible
amfetamine, 91
dextroamfetamine sulfate, 91
methamfetamine hydrochloride, 91
nitrofurantoin, 43
Retinopathy of prematurity
Certain
adrenal cortex injection, 242
beclomethasone dipropionate, 242
betamethasone dipropionate, 242
budesonide, 242
cortisone acetate, 242
dexamethasone, 242
fludrocortisone acetate, 242
fluorometholone, 242
fluticasone propionate, 242
hydrocortisone, 242

Retinopathy of prematurity (Continued)
methylprednisolone, 242
prednisolone, 242
prednisone, 242
rimexolone, 242
triamcinolone acetonide, 242
Possible
epoetin alfa, 265
epoetin beta, 265
Retrobulbar optic neuritis
Certain
chloramphenicol, 29
disulfiram, 361
ethambutol hydrochloride, 62
isoniazid, 65
metronidazole, 60
Probable
cisplatin, 312
vincristine sulfate, 341
Possible
adalimumab, 146
amobarbital, 122
butabarbital sodium, 122
butalbital, 122
etanercept, 146
hepatitis a vaccine, 383
ibuprofen, 151
infliximab, 146
methohexital sodium, 122
methylphenobarbital, 122
naproxen sodium, 154
penicillamine, 367
pentobarbital sodium, 122
phenobarbital, 122
primidone, 122
rabies immune globulin, 388
rabies vaccine, 388
secobarbital sodium, 122
Retrolental fibroplasia
Certain
oxygen, 183
oxygen-ozone, 183

S

Sarcoidosis or ocular sarcoid
Probable
interferon, 326
Possible
adalimumab, 147
etanercept, 147
infliximab, 147
Scleral deposits
Certain
ferrous fumarate, 266
ferrous gluconate, 266
ferrous sulfate, 266
iron dextran, 266
iron sucrose, 266
mitomycin, 463
polysaccharide iron complex, 266
vitamin D, 507

Scleral discoloration
Certain
adrenal cortex injection, 242
beclomethasone dipropionate, 242
betamethasone dipropionate, 242
budesonide, 242
cortisone acetate, 242
dexamethasone, 242
ferrous fumarate, 266
ferrous gluconate, 266
ferrous sulfate, 266
fludrocortisone acetate, 242
fluorometholone, 242
fluticasone propionate, 242
hydrocortisone, 242
iron dextran, 266
iron sucrose, 266
methylprednisolone, 242
polysaccharide iron complex, 266
prednisolone, 242
prednisone, 242
rimexolone, 242
triamcinolone acetonide, 242
Scleral perforation
Certain
bromfenac sodium, 468
diclofenac sodium, 468
ketorolac tromethamine, 468
mitomycin, 463
nepafenac, 468
Scleral pigmentation
Certain
demeclocycline hydrochloride, 33
doxycycline, 33
etoposide, 320
minocycline hydrochloride, 33
mitoxantrone hydrochloride, 331
oxytetracycline, 33
tetracycline hydrochloride, 33
Scleral rigidity decreased
Certain
echothiophate iodide, 443
pilocarpine hydrochloride, 445
Scleritis
Certain
alendronate sodium, 362
etidronate disodium, 362
ibandronate sodium, 362
melphalan, 328
mitomycin, 463
pamidronate disodium, 362
risedronate sodium, 362
zoledronic acid, 362
Probable
atropine, 192
homatropine, 192
Possible
adrenal cortex injection, 242
amfetamine, 91
beclomethasone dipropionate, 242
betamethasone dipropionate, 242
budesonide, 242

Visual hallucinations *(Continued)*
  ephedrine sulfate, 224
  ergometrine maleate, 201
  ergotamine tartrate, 201
  ethosuximide, 96
  fentanyl, 159
  gentamicin sulfate, 38
  hydromorphone hydrochloride, 160
  ibuprofen, 151
  imipramine hydrochloride, 101
  iodide and iodine solutions and
    compounds, 248
  ketoprofen, 153
  lamotrigine, 87
  leuprolide acetate, 247
  maprotiline hydrochloride, 105
  meperidine hydrochloride, 161
  methsuximide, 96
  methylergometrine, 201
  methylphenidate hydrochloride, 105
  metronidazole, 60
  nalidixic acid, 42
  nifedipine, 202
  nortriptyline hydrochloride, 101
  oxymorphone hydrochloride, 160
  phenytoin, 97
  piperazine, 22
  quetiapine fumarate, 114
  radioactive iodine, 248
  sparfloxacin, 31
  thiabendazole, 22
  tosufloxacin, 31
  triprolidine hydrochloride, 286
  verapamil hydrochloride, 202
  verteporfin, 415
  zonisamide, 99
Possible
  atomoxetine, 101
  clozapine, 111
  codeine, 158
  cyproheptadine hydrochloride,
    288
  dextropropoxyphene, 158
  duloxetine, 101
  epoetin alfa, 265
  epoetin beta, 265
  ethionamide, 64
  levodopa, 292
  loxapine, 111
  olanzapine, 111
  orphenadrine citrate, 294
  phenylephrine, 227
  prazosin hydrochloride, 218
  procainamide hydrochloride, 205
  quinidine gluconate or sulfate, 212
  selegiline hydrochloride, 292
  venlafaxine hydrochloride, 101
  vitamin D, 507

Visual loss, transient
Certain
  amyl/butyl nitrite, 203
  licorice, 505
Possible
  Iomeprol, 369
  Iopamidol, 369
  Iopromide, 369
Visual sensations, abnormal
Certain
  amiodarone hydrochloride, 206
  binimetinib, 301
  ciprofloxacin, 31
  clomifene citrate, 255
  cobimetinib, 301
  digoxin, 209
  flecainide acetate, 205
  ketamine hydrochloride, 177
  nalidixic acid, 42
  phenytoin, 96
  quinine sulfate, 59
  sildenafil citrate, 249
  sparfloxacin, 31
  tadalafil, 249
  tosufloxacin, 31
  trametinib, 301
  trazodone hydrochloride, 106
  tryparsamide, 61
  vardenafil hydrochloride, 249
  voriconazole, 50
Probable
  ibuprofen, 151
  norfloxacin, 36
  paroxetine hydrochloride, 103
  piperazine, 22
  thiabendazole, 22
Possible
  hydralazine hydrochloride, 217
Vitreous detachment
Certain
  aflibercept, 413
  bevacizumab, 413
  pegaptanib sodium, 413
  ranibizumab, 413
Probable
  ocriplasmin, 462
Vitreous floaters
Certain
  aflibercept, 413
  bevacizumab, 413
  crizotinib, 314
  pegaptanib sodium, 413
  ranibizumab, 413
Possible
  ciprofloxacin, 31
  digoxin, 210
  sparfloxacin, 31
  tosufloxacin, 31

Vitreous opacities
Certain
  aflibercept, 413
  bevacizumab, 413
  carmustine, 309
  gentamicin sulfate, 39
  pegaptanib sodium, 413
  ranibizumab, 413
  rifabutin, 66
Vitritis
Certain
  cidofovir, 437
  rifabutin, 66
Probable
  abacavir, 407
  didanosine, 407
  emtricitabine, 407
  lamivudine, 407
  ritonavir, 409
  stavudine, 407
  zidovudine, 407
Possible
  bacillus Calmette-Guérin vaccine, 381
Vogt-Koyangi-Harada disease
Possible
  atezolizumab, 300
  ipilimumab, 300
  nivolumab, 300
  pembrolizumab, 300
Vortex keratopathy
Certain
  amiodarone hydrochloride, 206
  clofazimine, 50
  ibuprofen, 151
  netarsudil, 433
  suramin sodium, 61

X
Xanthelasma decreased
Possible
  atorvastatin calcium, 191
  fluvastatin sodium, 191
  lovastatin, 191
  pitavastatin, 191
  pravastatin sodium, 191
  rosuvastatin calcium, 191
  simvastatin, 191

Z
Zoster keratitis, exacerbation
Possible
  herpes zoster vaccine, 384
  measles, mumps, rubella, and
    varicella virus vaccine live, 384
  varicella vaccine, 384

Subject Index

Note: Page number followed by *f* indicates figure, by *t* table, and by *b* box.